Design of
Enzyme Inhibitors as Drugs
Volume 2

Design of
Enzyme Inhibitors
as Drugs
Volume 2

Edited by

Merton Sandler

Professor of Chemical Pathology,
University of London

and

H. John Smith

Senior Lecturer in Medicinal Chemistry,
University of Wales

OXFORD NEW YORK TOKYO
OXFORD UNIVERSITY PRESS
1994

Oxford University Press, Walton Street, Oxford OX2 6DP

Oxford   New York   Toronto
Delhi   Bombay   Calcutta   Madras   Karachi
Kuala Lumpur   Singapore   Hong Kong   Tokyo
Nairobi   Dar es Salaam   Cape Town
Melbourne   Auckland   Madrid
and associated companies in
Berlin   Ibadan

Oxford is a trade mark of Oxford University Press

Published in the United States
by Oxford University Press Inc., New York

A catalogue record for this book is available from the British Library

Library of Congress Cataloging in Publication Data
Design of enzyme inhibitors as drugs.
Includes bibliographies and index.
1. Enzyme inhibitors—Therapeutic use—Testing.
2. Enzyme inhibitors—Structure-activity relationships.
3. Chemistry, Pharmaceutical.   4. Enzyme Inhibitors.
I. Sandler, Merton.   II. Smith, H. J., 1930–
RM666.E548D47   1989   615'.7   88–1432
ISBN 0–19–261537–8 (v. 1)
ISBN 0–19–262134–3 (v. 2)

Typeset by Apex Products, Singapore
Printed in Great Britain by
Bookcraft (Bath) Ltd, Midsomer Norton

Preface

In Volume I of this series, we set the scene and identified a range of enzymes which had, at that time, become established as targets for drug development. We tried to show how their inhibition might provide new therapeutic opportunities and demonstrated how basic knowledge of the characteristics of different types of inhibitors might be helpful in the quest for potent analogues.

This volume updates some of that earlier information but its main task is to introduce new enzyme targets which have clearly emerged as a result of academic and industrial research in the intervening period. In addition, we have added a chapter which serves to introduce some of the concepts we had rather taken for granted in the earlier volume.

We wish to thank the many expert contributors to this text who have helped to bring our work to fruition and excited us with their visions.

London   M. S.
Cardiff   H. J. S.
February 1993

Preface to Volume I

At first sight, it may seem strange and paradoxical that a drug can exert a beneficial effect by impairing a particular body function. And yet, when enzyme inhibitors are used as drugs, that is precisely what we design them to do! Increasingly, in recent years, drugs have been developed which work by inhibiting a selected target enzyme in a metabolic chain—for a variety of reasons, which will become clear when the chapters which follow are consulted.

Although specialized aspects of this topic have been reviewed earlier in more limited compilations, comprehensive coverage in one volume has not previously been attempted. Such a book seemed badly overdue in this rapidly advancing field of drug design. Accordingly, we decided to provide a wide overview of the main target enzymes and their known inhibitors and, within this framework of knowledge, to demonstrate how the drug designer uses all available information to develop a specific therapeutic agent. Paramount in our minds was the need to tackle the subject in interdisciplinary fashion so as to appeal to the widest range of biological interests. Thus, chemical and biochemical data concerning inhibitor structures and the way these compounds inhibit are presented, together with pharmacological and clinical material on their toxicity, bioavailability, and pharmacokinetics. Another prominent aspect of the text relates to modern computerized techniques of drug design such as QSAR and molecular graphics. This topic has been dealt with in a general introductory manner and built on in particular chapters where appropriate. The authors of each of the chapters which follow are acknowledged world experts and it is a pleasure to express our gratitude to them for their willing cooperation.

London   M. S.
Cardiff   H. J. S.
July 1987

Contents

Contributors

A. Aitken, Laboratory of Protein Structure, National Institute for Medical Research, The Ridgeway, Mill Hill, London NW7 1AA, UK.

B. Anderson, Experimental Retrovirology Section, National Cancer Institute, National Institutes of Health, Bethesda, MD 20892, USA.

M. J. Ashton, Rhône-Poulenc Ltd, Dagenham Research Centre, Rainham Road South, Dagenham, Essex RM10 7XS, UK.

D. Berg, Institute of Biotechnology, Agrochemicals Division, Bayer AG, D-5090 Leverkusen-Bayerwerk, Germany.

K. M. K. Bottomley, Research Centre, Roche Products Ltd, PO Box 8, Welwyn Garden City, Herts AL7 3AY, UK.

J. Bralet, UER de Pharmacie, 7 Boulevard Jeanne d'Arc, 21033 Dijon Cédex, France.

M. J. Broadhurst, Research Centre, Roche Products Ltd, PO Box 8, Welwyn Garden City, Herts AL7 3AY, UK.

A. Brodie, Department of Pharmacology and Experimental Therapeutics, School of Medicine, University of Maryland at Baltimore, 655 West Baltimore Street, Baltimore, MD 21201, USA.

J. R. Brooks, Merck Sharp & Dohme Research Laboratories, PO Box 2000, Rahway, NJ 07065, USA.

P. A. Brown, Research Centre, Roche Products Ltd, PO Box 8, Welwyn Garden City, Herts AL7 3AY, UK.

D. D. Buechter, Department of Biology, Massachusetts Institute of Technology, Cambridge, MA 02139, USA.

Y.-C. Cheng, Yale University School of Medicine, Department of Pharmacology, New Haven, CT 06520, USA.

E. De Clercq, Rega Institute for Medical Research, Katholieke Universiteit Leuven, B-3000, Leuven, Belgium.

Z. Debyser, Rega Institute for Medical Research, Katholieke Universiteit Leuven, B-3000, Leuven, Belgium.

L. Duhamel, Laboratoire de Chimie Organique, UA 464 CNRS, Faculte des Sciences et des Techniques, 76130 Mònt Saint Aignon, France.

P. Duhamel, Laboratoire de Chimie Organique, UA 464 CNRS, Faculte des Sciences et des Techniques, 76130 Mont Saint Aignon, France.

D. Dvornik, 174 Moore Street, Princeton, NJ 08540, USA.

A. M. Edelman, Department of Pharmacology and Therapeutics, State University of New York at Buffalo, Buffalo, NY 14214, USA.

G. Fenton, Rhône-Poulenc Ltd, Dagenham Research Centre, Rainham Road South, Dagenham, Essex RM10 7XS, UK.

J. F. Fisher, Upjohn Laboratories, Medicinal Chemistry Research, The Upjohn Company, Kalamazoo, MI 49001, USA.

J. Fostel, Anti-infective Research Division, Abbott Laboratories, Abbott Park, IL 60064, USA.

S. A. Foster, Yale University School of Medicine, Department of Pharmacology, New Haven, CT 06520, USA.

C. Gros, Unite de Neurobiologie et Pharmacologie, U109 de l'INSERM, Centre Paul Broca, 2 ter rue d'Alesia, 75014 Paris, France.

G. S. Harris, Merck Sharp & Dohme Research Laboratories, PO Box 2000, Rahway, NJ 07065, USA.

N. Higuchi, Suntory Ltd, Pharmaceutical Division, The Garden Court, 4–1 Kioicho, Chiyoda-ku, Tokyo 102, Japan.

C. H. Hill, Research Centre, Roche Products Ltd, PO Box 8, Welwyn Garden City, Herts AL7 3AY, UK.

W. H. Johnson, Research Centre, Roche Products Ltd, PO Box 8, Welwyn Garden City, Herts AL7 3AY, UK.

S. Kaakkola, Department of Neurology, University of Helsinki, Haartmaninkatu 4, SF-00290, Helsinki, Finland.

D. Keeling, Astra Hässle AB, Preclinical Research and Development, S-431 83 Mölndal, Sweden.

P. J. Kennelly, Department of Biochemistry and Nutrition, Virginia Polytechnic Institute and State University, Blacksburg, VA 24061, USA.

G. L. Kenyon, Department of Pharmaceutical Chemistry, University of California, San Francisco, CA 94143, USA.

J. M. Lecomte, Laboratoire Bioprojet, 30 rue des Francs Bourgeois, 75003 Paris, France.

R. Lindahl, Department of Biochemistry and Molecular Biology, University of South Dakota School of Medicine, Vermillion, SD 57069, USA.

P. Lindberg, Astra Hassle AB, Preclinical Research and Development, S-431 83 Mölndal, Sweden.

D. K. Luscombe, Welsh School of Pharmacy, UWCC, PO Box 13, Cardiff, UK.

P. T. Männistö, Department of Pharmacology and Toxicology, P. O. Box 8 (Siltavuorenpenger 10, Helsinki) SF-00014 University of Helsinki, Finland.

H. Mitsuya, Experimental Retrovirology Section, National Cancer Institute, National Institutes of Health, Bethesda, MD 20892, USA.

D. Mobilio, Wyeth-Ayerst Research, Princeton, NJ 08543–8000, USA.

H. Moereels, Janssen Research Foundation, B-2340 Beerse, Belgium.

P. J. Nicholls, Welsh School of Pharmacy, UWCC, PO Box 13, Cardiff, UK.

J. S. Nixon, Research Centre, Roche Products Ltd, PO Box 8, Welwyn Garden City, Herts AL7 3AY, UK.

P. Nussbaumer, Sandoz Forschungsinstitut, Brunnerstrasse 59, A-1235 Vienna, Austria.

B. K. Park, Department of Pharmacology and Therapeutics, The University of Liverpool, P. O. Box 147, Liverpool, U.K.

E. Peles, Department of Chemical Immunology, Weizmann Institute of Science, Rehovot 76100, Israel.

T. M. Penning, Department of Pharmacology, School of Medicine, University of Pennsylvania, 36th Street and Hamilton Walk, Philadelphia, PA 19104–6084, USA.

C. J. Pepper, Welsh School of Pharmacy, UWCC, PO Box 13, Cardiff, UK.

M. Pirmohamed, Department of Pharmacology and Therapeutics, The University of Liverpool, P. O. Box 147, Liverpool, U.K.

M. Plempel, Institute of Chemotherapy, Pharmaceuticals Division, Bayer AG, D-5090 Leverkusen-Bayerwerk, Germany.

J. C. Powers, School of Chemistry, Georgia Institute of Technology, Atlanta, GA 30332-0400, USA.

A. Purohit, Unit of Metabolic Medicine, St Mary's Hospital Medical School, Imperial College of Science, Technology and Medicine, London W2 1PG, UK.

T. Rademacher, Glycobiology Unit, Department of Biochemistry, University of Oxford, South Parks Road, Oxford OX1 3QU, UK.

G. H. Rasmusson, Merck Sharp & Dohme Research Laboratories, PO Box 2000, Rahway, NJ 07065, USA.

M. J. Reed, Unit of Metabolic Medicine, St Mary's Hospital Medical School, Imperial College of Science, Technology and Medicine, London W2 1PG, UK.

N. S. Ryder, Sandoz Forschungsinstitut, Brunnerstrasse 59, A-1235 Vienna, Austria.

M. Sandler, Department of Chemical Pathology, Queen Charlotte's and Chelsea Hospital, Goldhawk Road, London W6 OXG, UK.

G. A. Schiehser, Wyeth-Ayerst Research, Princeton, NJ 08543–8000, USA.

D. Schols, Rega Institut for Medical Research, Kathiolieke Universiteit Leuven, B-3000 Leuven, Belgium.

J. C. Schwartz, Unite de Neurobiologie et Pharmacologie, U109 de l'INSERM, Centre Paul Broca, 2 ter rue d'Alésia, 75014 Paris, France.

C. P. Selitrennikoff, Department of Cellular and Structural Biology, University of Colorado Health Sciences Centre, Denver, CO 80262, USA.

L. L. Shen, Anti-infective Research Division, Abbott Laboratories, Abbott Park, IL 60064, USA.

R.-S. Shen, Department of Human Biological Chemistry and Genetics, University of Texas Medical Branch, Galveston, TX 77550, USA.

A. M. Slater, Zeneca Pharmaceuticals, Alderley Park, Macclesfield, Cheshire, SK10 4TG, UK.

H. J. Smith, Welsh School of Pharmacy, UWCC, PO Box 13, Cardiff, UK.

A. Stuetz, Sandoz Forschungsinstitut, Brunnerstrasse 59, A-1235, Vienna, Austria.

W. G. Tarpley, Upjohn Laboratories, Cancer and Infectious Diseases Research, The Upjohn Company, Kalamazoo, MI 49001, USA.

J. Taskinken, Orion Pharmaceutical Research Centre, Orionintie 1, SF-02101 Espoo, Finland.

S. Thaisrivongs, Upjohn Laboratories, Medicinal Chemistry Research, The Upjohn Company, Kalamazoo, MI 49001, USA.

D. Timms, Zeneca Pharmaceuticals, Alderley Park, Macclesfield, Cheshire SK10 4TG, UK.

M. Tucker, Zeneca Pharmaceuticals, Alderley Park, Macclesfield, Cheshire SK10 4TJ, UK.

I. Ulmanen, Orion Corporation, Laboratory of Molecular Genetics, Valimotie 7, SF-00380, Helsinki, Finland.

A.-M. Vandamme, Rega Institute for Medical Research, Katholieke Universiteit Leuven, B-3000 Leuven, Belgium.

H. Vanden Bossche, Janssen Research Foundation, B-2340, Beerse, Belgium.

B. Wallmark, Astra Hässle AB, Preclinical Research and Development, S-431 83 Mölndal, Sweden.

A. J. Wilkinson, Zeneca Pharmaceuticals, Alderley Park, Macclesfield, Cheshire SK10 4TG, UK.

Y. Yarden, Department of Chemical Immunology, Weizmann Institute of Science, Rehovot 76100, Israel.

Abbreviations

ACE	angiotensin-converting enzyme
ACG	acyclovir
ACTH	corticotropin
ADH	alcohol dehydrogenase
AdV	adenoviruses
AG	aminoglutethimide
AGP	α_1-acid glycoprotein
AIDS	acquired immunodeficiency syndrome
AK	adenylate kinase (EC 2.7.4.3)
ALDHs	mammalian aldehyde dehydrogenases (EC 1.2.1.3)
AMPAL	4-amino-4-methyl-2-pentyne-1-al
ANF	atrial natriuretic factor
ANF-ir	ANF immuno-reactivity
ANP	atrial natriuretic peptide
AP-1	transcription factor
$Ap_3 dT$	P'-(adenosine-5')-P^3-(2'-deoxythimidine-5')-triphosphate
Ap_3 glucose	P'-(adenosine-5')-P^3-glucose-6-triphosphate
AR	aldose reductase (L-alditol, $NADP^+$ 1-oxidoreductase, EC 1.1.1.21)
AraA	1-(β-D-arabinofuranosyl) adenine (vidarabine)
ARC	AIDS-related complex
ARDS	adult respiratory distress syndrome
AUC	area under the plasma concentration curve
AZA	3'-azido-2',3'-dideoxyadenosine
AZddU	3'-azido-2',3'-dideoxyuridine
AZG	3'-azido-2',3'-dideoxyguanosine
AZT	3'-azido-2',3'-dideoxythymidine (zidovudine)
BH_4	L-*erythro*-5,6,7,8-tetrahydrobiopterin
BHAPs	bis(heteroaryl)piperazines
BMN	benzylidene malonitrile
BNP	brain natriuretic peptide
BPB	p-bromophenacyl bromide
BPH	benign prostatic hypertrophy
BSA	bovine serum albumin
BuDNJ	*N*-butyldeoxy nojirimycin
BUN	blood urea nitrogen
BVDU	(*E*)-5-(2-bromovinyl)-2'-deoxyuridine
CA	capsid protein
cAMP	cyclic adenosine monophosphate
CCDPK	Ca^{2+}-calmodulin-dependent protein kinase

CHD	coronary heart disease
CMPA	chiral mobile phase additive
CMV	human cytomegalovirus
CNS	central nervous system
COMFA	comparative molecular field analysis
COMT	catechol-O-methyltransferase (EC 2.1.1.6)
COPP	cyclophosphamide, vincristine, prednisone, and procarbazine
CP	cyclophosphamide
CSCC	cholesterol side-chain cleavage enzyme
CSF-1	colony-stimulating factor
CSP	chiral stationary phase
CYS	cystein-rich domains
DAG	diacylglycerol
ddA	2',3'-dideoxyadenosine
ddC	2',3'-dideoxycytidine (zalcitabine)
ddG	2',3'-dideoxyguanosine
ddI	2',3'-dideoxyinosine (didanosine)
DEAB	4-(diethylamino) benzaldehyde
DHA-S	dehydroepiandrosterone sulphate
DHEA	dehydroepiandrosterone
DHFR	dihydrofolate reductase (EC 1.5.1.3)
DHPG	ganciclovir
DHPR	dihydropteridine reductase (DADH: 6,7-dihydropteridine oxidoreductase, EC 1.6.99.7)
DHT	dihydrotestosterone
DMAPP	dimethyl-allyl-pyrophosphate
DMARDs	disease-modifying anti-rheumatic drugs
DNJ	1-deoxynojirimycin
dNTP	deoxyribonucleoside triphosphates
DOC	11-deoxycorticosterone
DOPAC	3,4-dihydroxyphenyl acetic acid
DOPP	12-deoxyphorbol-13-phenylacetate
DOPPA	deoxyphorbol
DPM	dipyridamole
DSC	differential scanning calorimetry
d4T	2',3'-didehydro-2',3'-dideoxythymidine (2',3'-dideoxythymidinene)
dTMP	deoxythymidine monophosphate
DTMT	dithiobis (1-methyltetrazole)
dTTP	deoxythymidine triphosphate
E1	oestrone
E2	oestradiol
EBV	Epstein−Barr virus
ECDGF	embryonal carcinoma-derived growth factor

ECL	enterochromaffin-like
EGF	epidermal growth factor
ElS	oestrone sulphate
EtDNJ	N-ethyldeoxynojirimycin
ETYA	5,8,11,14-eicosatetraynoic acid
6-FD	6-fluoro-L-dopa
FEP	free energy perturbation
FGFs	fibroblast growth factors
FPP	farnesyl pyrophosphate
FSH	follicle-stimulating hormone
GABA	γ-aminobutyric acid
GFR	glomerular filtration rate
GMCSF	granulocyte macrophage colony-stimulating factor
GPI	glycosylphosphatidylinositol
GPP	geranyl-pyrophosphate
hCG	human chorionic gonadotrophin
HEPT	1-((2-hydroxyethoxy) methyl)-6-(phenylthio)-thymine
HFC	human fibroblast
HIV	human immunodeficiency virus
HMG	3-hydroxy-3-methylglutaric acid
HMG CoA	3-hydroxy-3-methylglutaryl-coenzyme A
HMPA	[(S)-9-(3-hydroxy-2-phosphonylmethoxypropyl)] adenine
HMW	high molecular weight
HMWK	high molecular mass kininogen
HNC	human neutrophil procollagenase
HPMPC	[(S)-9(3-hydroxy-2-phosphorylmethoxypropyl)] cytosine
H_2RAs	histamine H_2-receptor antagonists
17β-HSD	17β-hydroxysteroid dehydrogenase
HSV	herpes simplex virus
HUM	human polymerase α
HVA	homovanillic acid
IDU	5-iodo-2'-deoxyuridine (idoxuridine)
IFNα	interferon α
Ig	immunoglobulin
IGF-1	insulin-like growth factor
IL-(1 or 2)	interleukin-(1 or 2)
IN	integrase
IP$_3$	inositol-1,4,5-triphosphate
IPP	isopentenylpyrophosphate
KCIP-1	kinase C inhibitor protein
KL	kit ligand
LAB	1,4-dideoxy-1,4-imino-L-arabinitol
LDH	lactate dehydrogenase
LDL	low density lipoprotein

LH	luteinizing hormone
LH-RH	luteinizing-hormone-releasing hormone
LMW	low molecular weight
5-LO	5-lipoxygenase
LTRs	long terminal repeats
lyso-PAF	lyso-platelet-activating factor
lysoPC	lysophosphatidylcholine
MA	matrix protein
4-MA	N,N-diethyl-4-methyl-3-oxo-4-aza-5α-androstan-17β-carboxamide (DMAA)
MAO	monoamine oxidase
MAP	microtubule associated protein
α-MAPI	pepstatins
MB-COMT	membrane bound catechol O-methyltransferase (EC 2.1.1.6)
MCD	multiple copy dynamics
MDR	multiple drug resistance
MeDNJ	N-methyldeoxynojirimycin
mEH	microsomal epoxide hydrolase
MEL	mouse erythroleukaemic
MEP	membrane metalloendopeptidase (atriopeptidase, enkephalinase, neutral endopeptidase, EC 3.4.24.11)
MGF	mast cell growth factor
MHC	major histocompatibility complex
MMP	matrix metalloproteinase
MRSA	methicillin-resistance *staphylococcus aureus*
MTT	methyltetrazolethiol
MTX	methotrexate
NC	nucleocapsid proteins
NGF	nerve growth factor
N-PLA$_2$	*Naja naja naja* phospholipase A$_2$
NSAIDs	non-steroidal anti-inflammatory drugs
4-OHA	4-hydroxyandrostenedione
3-OMD	3-O-methyldopa
3-OMFD	3-O-methyl-6-fluoro-L-dopa
OSBP	cytosolic oxysterol binding protein
P450 17	17α-hydroxylase: C-17,20-lyase
P450 arom	aromatase (oestrogen synthetase)
P450 C21	21-hydroxylase
P450 cam	camphor hydroxylase of *Pseudomonas putida*
P450 scc	cholesterol side chain cleavage enzyme
PA	phosphatidic acid
PAA	phosphonoacetic acid
PAF	platelet-activating factor
PAP	prostatic acid phosphatase

PAPs	3′-phosphoadenosine-5′-phosphosulphate
PBs	primer binding site
PCA	principal components analysis
PCA	prostatic carcinoma
PCR	polymerase chain reaction
PCZ	procarbazine
PDBu	phorbol dibutyrate
PDGF	platelet-derived growth factor
PEP	phosphoenol pyruvate
PFA	phosphonoformate
PGE	prostaglandin
PHA	phytohaemagglutinin
PI-K	phosphatidylinositol kinase
PIP$_2$	phosphatidylinositol-4,5-biphosphate
PK-A	cAMP-dependent protein kinase
PKC	protein kinase C (Ca^{2+}-phospholipid-dependent protein kinase)
PKCI	protein kinase C inhibitor proteins
PKI	protein kinase inhibitor
PKM	protein kinase M
PLA$_2$	phospholipase A$_2$
PLC	phospholipase C
PLD	phospholipase D
PLP	pyridoxal-5′-phosphate
PLS	principal least squares
PMEA	9-(2-phosphonylmethoxyethyl) adenine
PMNs	polymorphonuclear leucocytes
PR	protease (HIV)
PS	phosphatidyl serine
PSA	prostatic specific antigen
PTKs	protein tyrosine kinases
PUVA	psoralens and ultraviolet light
RACKs	receptor for activated C kinase
RFLP	fragment length polymorphism
RMSD	root mean squared deviation
RNase	ribonuclease
RRE	*rev* responsive element
RT	reverse transcriptase
RTK	receptor tyrosine kinases
SAM	*S*-adenosylmethionine
SAP A	sapintoxin
SAR	structure–activity relationship
SBIs	sterol biosynthesis inhibitors
SCF	stem cell factor

S-COMT	soluble catechol *O*-methyltransferase (EC 2.1.1.6)
SDS	sodium dodecyl sulphate
SH	Src homology
SIBLINKS	suicide inhibitory bifunctionally linked substrates
SIV	simian immunodeficiency virus
TAR	*trans*-activation regions
3TC	2′,3′-dideoxy-3′-thiacytidine
TCR	T-cell receptor
TFT	trifluorothymidine (trifluridine)
TGF-(α or β)	transforming growth factor (α or β)
TIBO	tetrahydro-imidazo (4,5,1-jk)(1,4)-benzo-diazepin-2(IH)-one and thione
TIMP	tissue inhibitors of metalloproteinases
TMP	trimethoprim
TNF	tumour necrosis factor
TPA	12-*O*-tetradecanoylphorbol 13-acetate
TPFA	thiophosphonoformate
TRE	phorbol ester-responsive element
TRH	thyrotropin-releasing hormone
tRNA$_{lys}$	lysine tRNA-3
TURP	transurethral prostatic resection
UDP-GA	uridine diphosphoglucuronic acid
UDPGT	UDP-glucuronyl transferases
VV	vaccinia virus
VZV	varicella-zoster virus

1

Enzyme inhibitors as drugs: from design to the clinic

D.K. Luscombe, M. Tucker, C.J. Pepper, P.J. Nicholls,

M. Sandler, and H.J. Smith

1.1   Introduction

Characterization of the biochemical pathways involved in many of the physiological activities which take place within the cell, and their relevance to disease processes, has resulted in the development of a number of clinically useful drugs which owe their effectiveness to the ability to inhibit a specific enzyme. This particular approach to the development of new therapeutic agents has gathered momentum over the past decade, not least because it offers a means of increasing the selectivity of a substance for a particular target site. It should be stressed that, once an enzyme system involved in disease has been identified, the design of a suitable inhibitor is a lengthy procedure. It is likely to be at least 10 years before a substance identified as a potentially useful enzyme inhibitor in the laboratory will reach the clinic and establish itself as a useful therapeutic agent. During this period, steps are taken to ensure that a drug is designed which will not only elicit the desired clinical response, but will be relatively free of side-effects and lack toxicity. The aim of this chapter is to provide the reader with an overview of many of the factors that have to be considered when developing a drug for clinical use. Attention is focused on factors influencing drug absorption, distribution, and elimination, the problems associated with drug stereoisomerism, and finally a brief outline of the toxicity tests that are required to demonstrate drug safety.

If an enzyme inhibitor is to prove useful as a medicine, it must be capable of presenting itself in an appropriate concentration at its pharmacological site of action in the body. Whilst clearly a function of the amount of substance administered, the concentration of drug reached at the site of action will also depend on the extent and rate of its absorption, distribution, metabolism, and excretion. The interrelationship between these factors is known as 'pharmacokinetics'. Since the absorption, distribution, metabolism, and excretion of any substance will involve its passage across cell membranes, such characteristics as molecular size and shape, solubility at the site of absorption, degree of ionization, and relative lipid solubility of the ionized and non-ionized forms will all play an essential part in determining the pharmacodynamic activity of the drug. Thus a basic knowledge of the physical and chemical principles that govern the active and passive transfer and distribution of drugs across biological membranes is required when deciding whether an enzyme inhibitor is likely to be a potential therapeutic agent. Information is also required on how the drug is metabolized and subsequently eliminated from the body, since these factors will dictate the pharmacodynamic activity of any administered drug. Furthermore, if any drug is to be therapeutically useful, it is vitally important that, in addition to possessing pharmacodynamic activity, it is free from intolerable side-effects and is relatively safe.

In addition to the references quoted in this chapter, the reader is referred to the following publications for further relevant information: Smith and Rawlins 1976; Benet *et al*. 1984; Laurence *et al*. 1984; Smith 1985; Poole and Leslie 1989; Davies 1991; Gibaldi 1992; Laurence and Bennett 1992.

1.2 Absorption

Drugs are seldom applied directly to their sites of action but are administered at points of entry, such as the gastrointestinal tract, from which they are absorbed into the bloodstream. When administering any therapeutic agent, a route of administration, as well as a suitable dose and dosage form (e.g. tablet or capsule), must be selected to ensure that the drug will reach its site of action in a pharmacologically effective concentration and be maintained at this concentration for an adequate period of time for a pharmacodynamic response to take place. Although most medicines are taken by mouth and swallowed, they may also be administered sublingually, rectally, by application to epithelial surfaces (e.g. skin, cornea, vagina, or nasal mucosa), by inhalation, and by injection (e.g. intravenous, intramuscular, or subcutaneous). With the exception of the intravenous route, in which the drug is administered directly into the bloodstream, a drug must initially be absorbed from its site of administration before it passes into the plasma. Consequently the process of absorption is of fundamental importance in determining the pharmacodynamic and hence therapeutic activity of a medicine. Delays or losses of drug during the absorption phase may contribute to variability in drug response and may even result in failure of drug therapy. For the process of absorption to take place, a drug must cross one or more cell membranes. The ease with which this occurs will reflect the concentration of drug achieved in body fluids and tissues.

1.2.1 Transfer of drugs across cell membranes

Passive diffusion is the commonest and most important mechanism by which drugs are transferred across biological membranes (Pratt 1990). Water-soluble substances are able to diffuse through the aqueous channels or 'pores' in biological membranes, provided that their molecular weights are no larger than 100–200 Da. However, transfer is usually along a concentration gradient, by virtue of the solubility of the drug in the lipid bilayer of the cell membrane. Thus lipid–water partition is important; the greater the partition coefficient, the higher is the concentration of drug in the membrane and the faster its rate of diffusion. Many drugs are weak acids or weak bases which, in aqueous solution, exist as an equilibrium mixture of non-ionized and ionized species. The non-ionized form is more lipid soluble than the ionized molecule and diffuses more readily across cell membranes; the ionized form is usually unable to penetrate the lipid membrane owing to low lipid solubility. Thus the transfer of a weak electrolyte can be influenced by its pK_a value and the pH gradient across the membrane. The relationship between pK_a and pH and the extent of ionization is given by the Henderson–Hasselbalch equation. Most basic drugs are so highly ionized in the acid fluids of the stomach that absorption is negligible. In contrast, many weakly acidic drugs are absorbed to some extent in the stomach since they exist largely in the non-ionized state at acidic pH values. However, restrictions imposed by the relatively small surface area of the gastric mucosa and its covering blanket of mucus renders the stomach a less than ideal site for the absorption of orally administered dose formulations. In the upper segments of the small intestine, the presence of finger-like villi and microvilli results in a markedly expanded surface area. This allows for efficient absorption not only of weak bases (which tend to be less ionized in the near-neutral fluids in this part of the intestine) but also of weak acids that may have escaped absorption higher in the alimentary canal.

Active transport is an alternative mechanism for the transmembrane movement of substances. Whilst specific for iodide and amino acids, it is relatively unusual for drugs to be transported this way, although the enzyme inhibitors methotrexate and 5-fluorouracil are exceptions. The renal tubular secretion of weak acids and weak bases employs a similar mechanism of transfer, and this can be an important process for some drugs and their acidic metabolites. In active transport the substrate is carried through the membrane against a concentration gradient, with expenditure of metabolic energy. Such processes can effect rapid transfer of solutes across membranes. However, the carrier mechanism has a finite capacity and the system can be readily saturated in the presence of a high concentration of the molecules being transported. Where two compounds are transferred by the same system, competition may occur, resulting in the inhibition of transport of one agent by the other. Facilitated diffusion is a similar carrier-mediated transport process in which no energy is required, so that movement of a substance against an electrochemical gradient cannot take place. This latter mechanism is not important for drugs, although it may be highly selective for specific conformational structures of some substances.

Pinocytosis is a term which describes the active uptake of substances by a process similar to phagocytosis. Microscopic invaginations of a cell membrane engulf drops of extracellular fluid such that solute molecules are carried through the membrane in the resulting vacuoles. Although important for the absorption of large molecules such as proteins and nucleic acids, this process is of little importance in the transport of drug molecules across cell membranes, with the exception, perhaps, of oral vaccines. However, efforts are currently being directed towards incorporating drugs into liposomes as a means of directing them to their required sites of action. These may then be taken up selectively by cells that are capable of pinocytosis.

1.2.2   Oral dosing

Oral administration is convenient, relatively safe, and economical, and is the dosage route preferred by patients, subject to the drug's being presented in a palatable and suitable form (Wagner 1975). However, this route has a number of disadvantages. For example, the drug may cause irritation of the gastrointestinal mucosa, resulting in nausea and vomiting. This is often the case with anti-inflammatory drugs. The drug may become mixed with food, it may be destroyed by digestive enzymes or gastric acid, it may pass too rapidly along the gastrointestinal tract for absorption to take place, or it may interact with other drugs being taken concurrently. The most important site for the absorption of drugs administered orally is the small bowel. This is largely due to its structure (see §1.2.1), which offers a far greater epithelial surface area for drug absorption to take place than is provided by the stomach. Thus any factor that promotes gastric emptying will tend to result in an increased rate of absorption of most drugs. Prompt gastric emptying is particularly important for drugs that are unstable in stomach fluids. It may be increased by fasting or hunger, alkaline buffer solutions, anxiety, diseases such as hyperthyroidism, and some drugs such as the anti-emetic metoclopramide. Liquids generally pass through the stomach at a much faster rate than solid food or solid dosage forms such as tablets and capsules. This is one reason for recommending that solid dosage forms should always be taken orally with at least half a tumblerful of water.

1.2.2.1   *Drug stability in gastric acid*
When administered orally, many drugs such as penicillins (inhibitors of bacterial transpeptidases) are absorbed to differing degrees, depending largely on their stability in gastric acid. Benzylpenicillin, the only naturally occurring penicillin in clinical use, is destroyed by gastric acid. It is also adsorbed on food and so, for efficient use, needs to be administered by injection. Phenoxymethylpenicillin is closely related to benzylpenicillin, having a similar, although less potent, spectrum of antimicrobial activity, but it is acid stable and consequently can be administered by mouth. However, the absorption of phenoxymethylpenicillin tends to be variable and unpredictable. The more recent development of the β-lactam-resistant

penicillins (cloxacillin, flucloxacillin, dicloxacillin, and nafcillin) has resulted in penicillins which are sufficiently acid stable to be given orally, as they are rapidly absorbed from the gastrointestinal tract although the process is incomplete. Methicillin is acid labile, and hence this useful penicillin has to be administered to patients by injection.

One of the most widely used antibiotics is ampicillin which possesses a broader spectrum of antibacterial activity than benzylpenicillin. Since it is acid resistant, it is administered orally although absorption is variable and incomplete. In an attempt to improve absorption, lipophilic esters have been prepared with some success. Whilst simple aliphatic esters of penicillins are inactive *in vivo*, once absorbed they are hydrolysed to release the active penicillin. As a result, a number of these so-called 'prodrugs' have been developed. Pivampicillin, bacampicillin, and talampicillin are all readily absorbed as inactive prodrugs when administered orally. Once absorbed, they are all converted to active ampicillin by enzymic hydrolysis.

The prodrug approach to overcoming poor gastrointestinal absorption has also been used with angiotensin-converting enzyme (ACE) inhibitors which are used to inhibit the conversion of angiotensin I to angiotensin II. They are widely used in the treatment of hypertension and as adjuncts in congestive heart failure. Modification of captopril, the first ACE inhibitor, by increasing its resemblance to a peptide led to the discovery of the potent second-generation inhibitor enalaprilat. This was poorly absorbed after oral dosing but conversion to the ethyl ester enalapril, which is hydrolysed to the active enalaprilat *in vivo*, resulted in good intestinal absorption of the prodrug. Likewise, the orally inactive prodrug cilazapril, which is the ethyl ester prodrug of cilazaprilat, is converted to the active dicarboxylic acid *in vivo* and, as a result, is therapeutically effective. Interestingly, lisinopril, the lysine analogue of enalaprilat, is itself active on oral dosing although it is only slowly and relatively incompletely (30 per cent) absorbed.

1.2.2.2 *Presence of food in the intestines*

In general, drug absorption following oral dosing is favoured when the stomach is empty. Food not only has the effect of reducing the concentration of drug in the gastrointestinal tract but will limit the rate of drug absorption, although not the total amount of drug absorbed, and delay gastric emptying (Melander 1983). Thus drugs such as antibiotics are recommended to be taken on an empty stomach because a rapid onset of action is required. Only when a drug is irritating to the gastric mucosa is it reasonable to administer the dosage form either with or after a meal (i.e. anti-inflammatory agents). This may result in a significant decrease in the rate of drug absorption, although the total amount absorbed would be expected to be unchanged. In some instances, the absorption of a drug is promoted when taken after food. Interestingly, the absorption of oral griseofulvin appears to be doubled following postprandial administration.

Whilst the ACE inhibitor captopril is rapidly absorbed when administered orally, only about 65 per cent of the ingested dose is absorbed into the bloodstream and this is significantly reduced in the presence of food. For this reason, the drug should generally be administered approximately an hour before meals. In contrast, the second-generation ACE inhibitor enalapril is rapidly and more completely absorbed, and in consequence the total amount of drug absorbed is little affected by food. Similarly, oral doses of the older penicillins, such as ampicillin, are less than half absorbed, and this factor is further decreased if the drugs are administered orally with food. In contrast, absorption of the newer ampicillin esters pivampicillin and talampicillin is little affected by the presence of food. Consequently, they may be given at any time relative to meals, although compliance is probably improved if they are administered at meal times.

In the case of orally administered irreversible monoamine oxidase (MAO) inhibitors such as phenelzine, isocarboxazid, and tranylcypromine, which are sometimes used in the treatment of depression, particular care has to be taken to avoid eating certain foods which could prove dangerous if consumed during the period of enzyme inhibition. This is because drugs of this kind potentiate the pressor effect of the indirectly acting sympathomimetic substance tyramine, which may be present in foods such as cheese, pickled herrings, and yeast products. This effect stems from inhibition of its metabolism by gastrointestinal and hepatic MAO.

1.2.2.3 *Bioavailability*

The term 'bioavailability' is used to indicate the overall proportion of administered drug that passes unchanged into the systemic blood circulation. Thus, it takes into account absorption and any local metabolic degradation that takes place in the stomach and small bowel following oral dosing. It is also influenced by the so-called 'first-pass' or pre-systemic effect. Once absorbed in the gastrointestinal tract, an orally administered drug will enter the portal circulation and pass immediately to the liver before reaching the systemic circulation where it is transported around the body to its site(s) of action, enabling expression of its pharmacodynamic action to occur. On passing through the liver, a fraction of the drug may be metabolized (in many cases resulting in activation) by hepatic microsomal enzymes or excreted in the bile. The result is that less unchanged (active) drug is available to exert its action than was absorbed following oral dosing. For drugs which undergo extensive first-pass metabolism, bioavailability will be relatively low. Bioavailability is also influenced by gastrointestinal motility, gastric pH, drug solubility, the presence or absence of food, and the formulation of the dosage form administered. This latter factor may be particularly important when dosing with a drug prepared by different manufacturers. Because of variations in the manufacturing process, perhaps resulting in variable particle sizes for example, one dosage form may have a markedly different bioavailability from another preparation. Single doses of different formulations of digoxin (an inhibitor of sodium and potassium ATPase) have been reported to give rise to up to a sevenfold variation in peak plasma levels (Lindenbaum et al. 1971). Clinically, the result is that different blood drug concentrations will occur, despite the fact that the drug content of the tablets or capsules is identical. This may lead to toxicity or inactivity of one of the dosage forms owing to variability in bioavailability. A change in the tablet formulation (replacement of calcium sulphate with lactose as excipient) of phenytoin was responsible for an outbreak of toxicity by increasing the bioavailability of this anti-epileptic drug (Tyrer et al. 1970).

1.2.3   Sublingual dosing

A drug may be absorbed through the mucosa of the buccal cavity (Anon 1987) when it is given in a dosage form which can be placed under the tongue and allowed to dissolve. Once absorbed, the drug enters the blood circulation directly, avoiding first-pass metabolism. Since it does not have to enter the stomach or small bowel to exert its effect, absorption is generally more rapid than after swallowing and the drug is likely to be effective at a lower dose. In addition, the drug effect may be terminated once therapeutic relief has been achieved simply by removal of the medicine. Unfortunately, high molecular weight substances are not well absorbed by this route, and clearly it cannot be used for drugs with an unpleasant taste. Indeed, few drugs are administered in this way although it is useful for dosing with glyceryl trinitrate at the first sign of an acute attack of angina pectoris.

1.2.4   Parenteral dosing

The term parenteral (*par*—beyond, *enteral*—intestinal) implies that a drug is given by a route which takes it directly into body fluids, thus avoiding the need for gastrointestinal absorption. The most common method of introducing a drug directly into the systemic circulation is to inject it into a vein. This route is useful when a rapid therapeutic response is required, such as in status asthmaticus, cardiac arrhythmias, epileptic seizures, and the induction of anaesthesia. When administered intravenously, the drug is rapidly removed from the injection site, being carried first to the heart and then to other tissues. Since the total circulation time in man is of the order of 15 s, the onset of drug action is almost immediate. Drugs administered intravenously may be given as a single rapid injection lasting 1–2 min known as a 'bolus' injection, or as a slow infusion over a period of several hours or even longer. This latter choice is preferred when a sustained level of drug in the bloodstream is required over a relatively long period of time (e.g. antibiotics for life-threatening infections).

A prerequisite of an intravenous injection is that the drug is water soluble, and furthermore the dosage form must be sterile. Thus intravenous injections are expensive to manufacture and require administration by trained personnel. However, for some enzyme inhibitors such as benzylpenicillin, the intravenous route is the only means of administering this still useful antibiotic since, as previously stated, it is inactivated by gastric acid if given orally. Because of stability problems, the sodium salt (unbuffered) of benzylpenicillin is reconstituted in water for injection immediately before clinical use. Cloxacillin, flucloxacillin, temocillin, amoxycillin, ampicillin, piperacillin, and carbenicillin may all be administered by the intravenous route when rapid action for life-threatening infections is indicated. Each is supplied as a dry sterile powder (i.e. sodium salt) to be reconstituted with water for injection before use.

Intramuscular and subcutaneous injection may be used for the localized delivery of an exact quantity of drug, although the rate of drug absorption may be variable. Factors influencing absorption include vascularity of the injection site, degree of ionization and lipid solubility of the drug, volume of injection, and osmolarity. The intramuscular route is often used in patients who are unable to receive oral medication, for drugs which are poorly absorbed from the gastrointestinal tract, or for drugs which undergo extensive first-pass metabolism. For example, 4-hydroxyandrostenedione is a potent mechanism-based enzyme inactivator of aromatase used to lower oestrogen levels in post-menopausal women with breast cancer. This has to be administered as an intramuscular injection to avoid extensive first-pass metabolism to the glucuronidated conjugate which takes place following oral dosing.

In general, drugs administered by intramuscular injection are absorbed and exert their pharmacological effect more rapidly than after oral dosing. However, intramuscular injections tend to be painful and do not generally find favour with patients. They are also expensive to manufacture. Nevertheless, a number of penicillins are administered by this route. For example, in early syphilis, procaine penicillin is injected intramuscularly for 10 days. Cloxacillin, flucloxacillin, methicillin, and ampicillin may also be given intramuscularly as an alternative to oral dosing. Subcutaneous injection is suitable only for small dose volumes, and few drugs are currently administered by this route, a notable exception being insulin. In general, a subcutaneous injection results in faster absorption than a corresponding intramuscular injection, although the difference is not marked and is of little clinical significance.

Absorption from intramuscular or subcutaneous sites of dosing can be delayed by administering the drug in a relatively insoluble 'slow-release' dosage form. It might be converted into a poorly soluble salt, ester, or complex, which is injected either as an aqueous suspension or an oily solution. Procaine penicillin is a salt of penicillin which is only slightly water soluble. When injected as an aqueous suspension, it is only slowly absorbed, thus exerting a prolonged therapeutic effect.

1.2.5   Topical application

Drug application to the skin or to mucous membranes, such as conjunctiva, nasopharynx, or vagina, is used primarily for local effects, although novel transdermal dosage forms (i.e. skin patches or dressings) have now been successfully developed to permit a drug to pass across the skin into the systemic circulation to produce a generalized effect.

Few drugs readily penetrate the intact healthy skin, and absorption of those that do is proportional to their lipid solubility. This is because the epidermis acts as a lipid barrier. In contrast, the dermis is freely permeable to many solutes and therefore systemic absorption occurs more readily through broken skin. Absorption through the skin is increased by occlusive dressings which retain moisture and 'macerate' the epidermis. Recently introduced dosage forms of glyceryl trinitrate depend upon percutaneous absorption for therapeutic activity. Applied to the skin as a self-adhesive patch or dressing, glyceryl trinitrate is slowly and continuously released, providing prophylactic treatment of angina pectoris for a 24 h period. The transdermal preparation is replaced every 24 h, siting the replacement dressing on a different area of the body.

1.3   Distribution

Once circulating in the bloodstream, most drugs are distributed throughout body fluids and tissues with relative ease. In contrast with the process of elimination, distribution represents a reversible transfer of drug between tissue sites and plasma. The pattern of distribution depends on the drug's permeability, lipid solubility, and capacity to bind to macromolecules.

For those drugs of molecular weight up to about 600 Da, which are free in solution in plasma water, penetration into interstitial fluid is rapid. The reason appears to be that the capillary wall generally behaves like a leaky sieve. The lining endothelial cells of the capillary have junctions with each other that are discontinuous (loose), and these allow free passage of small molecules of up to 600 Da. This is an important route for polar compounds. However, both this route and diffusion through the actual capillary wall are available pathways for lipid-soluble compounds.

The apparent volume of distribution, V_D is a useful term for describing the pattern of a drug's distribution in the body. It represents the volume in which the drug appears to be dissolved and is a proportionality constant relating plasma drug concentration to the total amount of drug in the body. An apparent volume of distribution of 0.04 1 kg^{-1} would be compatible with the restriction of a drug to the plasma compartment (e.g. heparin,

0.05 1 kg^{-1}). Values in excess of total body water (about 0.6 1 kg^{-1}) indicate that a drug is being accumulated or stored in extravascular sites (e.g. nortriptyline, 22–27 1 kg^{-1}). In general, weak bases have a large volume of distribution, owing to their lipid solubility, and therefore will be present in low concentrations in plasma. The reverse situation tends to apply to weak acids.

1.3.1 Binding

Distribution depends partly on whether a drug is bound to macromolecules such as albumin and other plasma proteins. This binding is usually a reversible process and will influence the concentration of drug that is freely available in the plasma for diffusion and distribution (Craig and Welling 1983). This is because a drug–protein binding complex has such a high molecular weight that it will not cross cell membranes. Drugs also bind intracellularly, and the binding gradient is important in affecting the distribution equilibrium. Cerebrospinal fluid possesses a very low level of protein compared with plasma, thus limiting the possibility for binding within this particular biological fluid.

The extent to which drugs are bound to plasma proteins is variable. The sulphonamides, which owe their bacteriostatic action to dihydropteroate synthetase inhibition, are bound in varying degrees to plasma proteins, particularly albumin. Sulphadimidine is 60–80 per cent bound, while sulphadiazine is 25–55 per cent bound and sulphafurazole only 25 per cent bound. The dihydrofolate reductase inhibitor methotrexate, which is widely used in antineoplastic chemotherapy, is readily absorbed from the gastrointestinal tract at low dosage, although larger amounts have to be administered orally because of incomplete intestinal absorption at higher doses. Between 35 and 50 per cent of methotrexate is bound to plasma protein, with the drug being distributed throughout the body fluids including exudates and effusions. Since it is a weak organic acid with low lipid solubility, it diffuses only slowly across physiological membranes such as the blood–brain barrier. Thus neoplastic cells in the brain and spinal cord are unlikely to be killed at standard dosage regimens, since the concentration of methotrexate in the central nervous system (CNS) will only be about 3 per cent of the plasma concentration. This is in contrast with the anticancer drug 5-fluorouracil which inhibits thymidilate synthetase. After oral or intravenous dosing, this drug is rapidly distributed throughout body water ($V_D = 0.25 \pm 0.12$ 1 kg^{-1}) and readily crosses the blood–brain barrier. Binding is almost negligible, with only 8–12 per cent of the drug being bound to plasma proteins.

1.3.2 Blood–brain barrier

The passage of a drug from the bloodstream into the brain and cerebrospinal fluid is restricted by the nature of the absorption surface presented

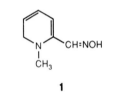

1

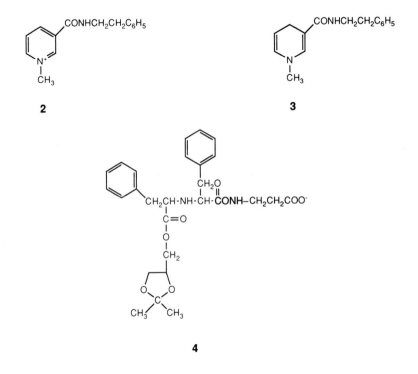

2   **3**

4

(Lorenzo and Spector 1976). The endothelial cells of the brain capillaries have tight junctions. In addition, layers of glial cells closely surround the capillaries. Thus a profoundly lipid barrier, the so-called blood–brain barrier, must be crossed if a drug is to gain access to central neurones. Whilst highly lipid-soluble compounds reach the brain rapidly following dosing, more polar compounds penetrate at a much slower rate. As the rate of penetration of a drug depends on its degree of ionization in plasma and its lipid solubility, these variables can be exploited to influence its distribution into the brain. An established success story in this respect is the development of the dopa-decarboxylase inhibitors carbidopa and benserazide (see below).

Highly polar drugs do not cross the blood—brain barrier (Nicholls 1980). However, penetration of the nerve gas antagonist pralidoxime into the CNS has been achieved by using a non-polar inactive prodrug **1** which readily crosses the blood—brain barrier. Once within the brain, the prodrug is rapidly oxidized to the active substance pyridine-2-aldoxime (pralidoxime). Conversion of the methiodide to its 1,4-dihydro base facilitates passage into the CNS and has been developed as a means of delivering other drugs into the brain which either do not readily cross the blood—brain barrier or else are rapidly metabolized. Phenylethylamine has been condensed with nicotinic acid and then quaternized to give **2** followed by reduction to the 1,4-dihydro derivative **3**. The prodrug **3** crosses into rat brain, where it is oxidized and trapped as the quaternary ammonium salt **2**. This is slowly cleaved by enzymatic action in the brain, with sustained release of the biologically active substance phenylethylamine and the facile elimination of the carrier molecule. Interestingly, elimination of the drug from the general circulation was accelerated, and was in the form of **2** or **3** or as cleavage products. This contrasts with most drugs where plasma levels must be maintained to produce the required central effect, frequently leading to systemic side-effects.

Thiorphan is a potent inhibitor of enkephalinase *in vitro* (Roques *et al.* 1980) and possesses anti-nociceptive activity when administered into the cerebral ventricles of animals. It is inactive when given parenterally. However, acetorphan is a prodrug of thiorphan in which the ionizable COOH group of thiorphan has been converted to the benzyl ester and the thiol group is acetylated. The prodrug is parenterally active because it is able to cross the blood—brain barrier. Once within the brain, it is hydrolysed by esterases to the parent drug (Lecomte *et al.* 1986). Likewise, the potent enkephalinase inhibitor SCH-34826 **4** exhibits anti-nociceptive action when administered orally owing to facilitated passage across the blood—brain barrier as the half glycerol acetal ester. The prodrug is subsequently hydrolysed by brain esterases to the potent dicarboxylic acid (Chipkin *et al.* 1988).

1.3.3   Placental barrier

Fetal blood is separated from maternal blood by a cellular barrier composed of trophoblastic layer, mesenchymal tissue, and fetal capillary endothelium (Maxwell 1984). The thickness of this composite barrier is greater in early pregnancy (25 μm) than in late pregnancy (2 μm). Although specific transport systems for endogenous materials are present in the placenta and may provide a method for transporting some drugs (e.g. α-methyl dopa, 5-fluorouracil), it appears that most drugs cross the placenta by passive diffusion. Therefore penetration is rapid with lipid-soluble un-ionized drugs and slow with very polar compounds. However, some degree of fetal exposure is likely to occur with virtually all drugs and, in view of the uncertain effects of such drugs on the fetus, caution is required with drug administration during pregnancy. Sulphonamides readily pass across the placenta and enter the fetal blood circulation. The clinical significance is that the sulphonamides reach concentrations sufficient to be antibacterial in the fetus and toxicity may supervene.

1.3.4   Partition into fat

Lipid-soluble drugs may achieve high concentrations in adipose tissue, being stored by physical solution in the neutral fat. Since fat is normally 15 per cent of body weight (in grossly obese subjects it can be as high as 50 per cent), it can serve as an important reservoir for such drugs. It also has a role in terminating the effects of highly lipid-soluble compounds by acting as an acceptor of the drug during a redistribution phase. Thus, after intravenous injection, thiopentone enters the brain rapidly, but also leaves it rapidly because of falling plasma levels and this terminates the action. It then slowly redistributes into fatty tissues where as much as 70 per cent of the drug may be found 3 h after administration (Brodie *et al.* 1952).

1.4   Metabolism

Many drugs have to undergo biotransformation (metabolism) in order to be removed from the body. While the liver is the major organ for this process, drugs may also be metabolized at other sites, e.g. lung, gut wall, kidney, and skin. Two general kinds of biochemical reaction may take place, known as phase I reactions (asynthetic changes) and phase II reactions (conjugations). As the original compound is chemically altered by these means, metabolism can be considered as a means of inactivating a drug although the problem of excreting the metabolites remains. In most instances the metabolites have a markedly different partition character from the parent compound, usually being more polar. Such products tend to be more easily excreted and not so readily reabsorbed from the renal tubular fluid. Therefore metabolism usually results in reduced pharmacodynamic activity of the parent substance, although occasionally a drug may be transformed into a metabolite possessing a pharmacological effect of comparable intensity. This is true for nortriptyline and desipramine which are as active as their respective parent compounds, amitriptyline and imipramine. Some drugs and other chemicals may be metabolized to products that induce or initiate toxic reactions (e.g. paracetamol, paraquat, phenytoin, polycyclic hydrocarbons) (see Timbrel 1982, 1989). For a small number of prodrugs which are biologically inactive *per se*, metabolic activation is a prerequisite for therapeutic utility. Thus the antiscabies drug malathion is metabolized by the mite *Sarcoptes scabiei*, which invades the epidermis, to the anticholinesterase malaoxon which is lethal to the mite.

1.4.1   Phase I metabolism

Phase I reactions consist of oxidation, reduction, and hydrolysis, with the products sometimes being more reactive, and some occasionally more toxic, than the parent drug. Many of the oxidation reactions, such as aliphatic and aromatic hydroxylation, epoxidation, dealkylation, deamination, *N*-oxidation, and *S*-oxidation are catalysed by a complex enzyme system known as the mixed-function oxidase system which resides on the smooth endoplasmic reticulum. At least four separate groups of enzymes are involved, the most important being the cytochrome P450 family. This enzyme is coupled to the flavoprotein enzyme, cytochrome P450 reductase, and linked to NADPH as a source of electrons. Under the influence of cytochrome P450, an oxygen atom from molecular oxygen is transferred to a drug molecule (DH→DOH). The remaining oxygen atom combines with two protons to yield a molecule of water. However, not all drug oxidation reactions depend on the mixed-function oxygenase system. Ethanol is metabolized by the soluble cytoplasmic enzyme alcohol dehydrogenase. The non-microsomal enzyme xanthine oxidase is responsible for inactivation of 6-mercaptopurine, an anticancer agent which acts as an inhibitor of riboxyl amidotransferase. Another enzyme which occurs in many tissues other than the liver is MAO which inactivates a broad range of biologically active monoamines such as noradrenaline, tyramine, and 5-hydroxytryptamine.

Reductive reactions are much less common than oxidative reactions. However, some drugs are metabolized by reductases which are located at both microsomal and non-microsomal sites. Some reductases are also found in the micro-organisms of the large bowel.

Hydrolytic reactions occur in many tissues. Drugs containing an ester group may be hydrolysed by esterases which have both microsomal and non-microsomal locations, the former tending to be concentrated in the liver. Such an enzyme is responsible for the hydrolysis of the analgesic pethidine. Procaine, a local anaesthetic, is rapidly inactivated by plasma cholinesterase. The esterases also hydrolyse amides, such as procainamide, although at a much slower rate than the corresponding esters.

1.4.2   Phase II metabolism

Phase II metabolism involves the coupling of a drug or its metabolites with various endogenous components. The reaction, which is carried out by a transferase enzyme, produces a conjugate which is usually pharmacodynamically inactive. It is less lipid soluble than its precursor and accordingly may be excreted in the urine or bile.

Glucuronide formation is probably the most common conjugation pathway. The combination with glucuronic acid occurs with compounds possessing a functional group with a reactive proton, usually attached to a heteroatom (e.g. hydroxyl, carboxyl, amino, or sulphydryl). These functional groups may already be present in the drug molecule (e.g. paracetamol) or may be acquired by phase I metabolism (e.g. phenytoin hydroxylation). Depending on the grouping through which conjugation takes place, these metabolites can be described as O-glucuronides (ether type combination through a hydroxyl group, e.g. hydroxyl metabolites of barbiturates; ester type combination through a carboxyl group, e.g. salicylic acid), N-glucuronides (via amino groups, e.g. meprobamate), or S-glucuronides (via sulphydryl groups, e.g. 2-mercaptobenzothiazole). Glucuronic acid is derived enzymatically from glucose and its active form, uridine diphosphoglucuronic acid (UDP-GA), is utilized by UDP-glucuronyltransferase to effect the conjugation.

Glucuronides are very polar and relatively strong acids ($pK_a \approx 3$). Thus they are extensively ionized at the pH of blood and urine, which makes them good candidates for excretion.

Sulphate conjugation is mediated by non-microsomal sulphotransferases. Sulphate esters are formed by the soluble fraction (i.e. 100 S supernatant), with the high energy sulphate being 3′-phosphoadenosine-5′-phosphosulphate (PAPS) and the other component substrate being either a phenol (e.g. paracetamol, salicylamide) or an aliphatic and steroid alcohol (e.g. ethanol, androsterone). Sulphamates may also be formed in a similar manner from aromatic amines. The capacity to form sulphate conjugates is rather limited, and this appears to be related to the poor availability of sulphate.

Methylation is an important physiological process for the conversion of noradrenaline into adrenaline (N-methylation). Both these catecholamines are also metabolized by O-methylation under the influence of catechol-O-methyltransferase (COMT). The methyl group is derived from methionine, the active methyl donor form of which is S-adenosylmethionine. Drugs or their metabolites containing primary aliphatic amine, phenolic, or sulphydryl groups may be N-, O- or S-methylated respectively by methyltransferases.

Acylation involves the reaction between an amine and a carboxylic acid to yield an amide; the high energy molecule required is a coenzyme A derivative of the carboxylic acid. The drug, or its metabolite, can be either of the conjugating molecules. Thus aromatic primary amines (e.g. sulphonamides, aminoglutethimide) and hydrazine derivatives (e.g. isoniazid) are acetylated utilizing acetyl coenzyme A. It should be noted that acetylation has little influence on the polarity of a drug.

Glutathione conjugation is an important process for a number of drugs. The tripeptide glutathione (cysteine-glycine-glutamate) may be coupled via its sulphydryl group to various compounds possessing an electrophilic centre. In the case of paracetamol, such a site is introduced as a result of oxidative metabolism. This conjugation reaction is an important mechanism for the effective disposal of electrophiles (e.g. reactive epoxides) before they are able to react with nucleophilic centres of nucleic acids and enzymes to initiate toxic responses. Myleran (busulphan), azathioprine, and urethane are examples of drugs conjugated by this pathway. Glutathione conjugates are polar and of high molecular weight (above 300 Da), and are eliminated as such in the bile. However, the glutathione portion of the conjugate may be further metabolized (via the peptide bonds) to mercapturic acids which are the normal urinary products of this conjugation pathway.

1.4.3   Induction of microsomal enzymes

Many drugs, when repeatedly administered, are able to produce an increase (induction) in the synthesis of hepatic microsomal mixed-function oxidases and certain other enzymes (Park and Breckenridge 1983). In each case, the rate of metabolism of the inducing agent is increased, as is the metabolism of any other drug being administered concurrently and also metabolized by these enzymes. An example of a powerful enzyme inducer is pheno-barbitone which increases the level of cytochrome P450 and its associated reductase. Aminoglutethimide, the aromatase inhibitor used in the treatment of oestrogen-mediated breast cancer, is also an enzyme inducer. Thus patients receiving concomitant therapy with warfarin or other coumarin anticoagulants, or with oral hypoglycaemic drugs, may require increased dosages owing to their increased hepatic metabolism. Enzyme induction is maximal after 2–3 weeks of repeated administration, returning to normal within 3–4 weeks once dosing has been discontinued. For drugs such as paracetamol, whose hepatotoxicity is mainly due to phase I metabolites, the presence of an enzyme inducer may enhance toxicity.

1.4.4   Inhibition of metabolism

Drugs which inhibit metabolism fall into two groups, those which act as non-specific inhibitors of metabolic processes and those acting on specific metabolic pathways (Park and Breckenridge 1983). Disulfiram inhibits the metabolism of acetaldehyde which accumulates in the body causing unpleasant symptoms such as abdominal colic, flushing, dizziness, tachycardia, and vomiting. Since alcohol is metabolized to acetaldehyde, which in turn is normally broken down to carbon dioxide and water, disulfiram has been used for its enzyme inhibitor properties in attempts to stop alcoholics drinking. Allopurinol is an example of a drug which reversibly inhibits a specific enzyme—xanthine oxidase. Therefore, during its use in the treatment of gout, allopurinol will reduce the metabolism of concurrently administered drugs such as 6-mercaptopurine and azathioprine (of which 6-mercapto-purine is a metabolite) which are themselves metabolized by xanthine oxidase. A reduced dosage would thus be required.

Carbidopa and benserazide are both inhibitors of dopa-decarboxylase. This is made use of therapeutically in the treatment of Parkinson's disease in which striatal levels of the neurotransmitter dopamine are reduced. When L-dopa is administered orally, it is decarboxylated to dopamine throughout the body, with only a limited amount of the amino acid itself gaining access to the brain to exert its antiparkinsonian effect. Drugs such as carbidopa and benserazide decrease peripheral metabolism but, as they are unable to cross the blood−brain barrier, leave dopamine formation in the brain unaffected. The net result is that more L-dopa is available for entry into the brain, with a subsequent build-up of dopamine. At the same time, the dose of administered L-dopa can be reduced. A series of new COMT inhibitors, which have a similar L-dopa-sparing effect, have recently come into experimental use (see Chapter 12).

1.5   Removal of drugs from the body

The main routes for drug excretion from the body are the kidneys, biliary system, and lungs (Pratt 1990). Drugs may also be eliminated in secretions such as milk, saliva, or sweat, but these are quantitatively unimportant compared with excretion by the kidneys, the major route by which most drugs leave the body. Some drugs are excreted into the bile (e.g. ampicillin), but in most instances reabsorption occurs in the small bowel (enterohepatic recycling). Excretion in expired air occurs only with highly volatile or gaseous agents.

Three basic processes are involved in drug elimination by the kidneys: glomerular filtration, active tubular secretion, and passive diffusion across the renal tubule.

1.5.1   Glomerular filtration

The glomerular capillaries trap compounds with a molecular weight of 66 000 Da or above, including plasma proteins and drugs bound to these proteins. With the exception of a few macromolecular substances (heparin, dextrans), all non-protein-bound drugs pass freely across the glomerulus so that the concentration of drug in the glomerular filtrate is the same as that of free drug in the plasma.

1.5.2   Active tubular secretion

Active transport from the peritubular capillaries (which bring blood to the kidneys) to the lumen of the proximal tubules is the major mechanism of removal of acidic drugs and glucuronide metabolites. It is unlikely that the secretion of unmetabolized basic compounds contributes substantially to their removal from the body, although a transport system exists to handle basic substances. This system, together with an independent non-selective carrier system for acidic drugs, can transport drug molecules against an electrochemical gradient and is potentially the most rapid mechanism for renal elimination. In contrast to glomerular filtration, carrier-mediated transport in the proximal tubules can achieve maximal drug clearance even when most of the drug is bound to plasma proteins.

Drugs which are actively secreted by the proximal tubules include the penicillins and probenecid. Penicillin elimination from the body is mainly renal and occurs rapidly, usually on one passage through the kidney. Whilst penicillin is 80 per cent protein bound and therefore cleared only slowly by glomerular filtration, proximal tubular secretion is rapid and complete, and is responsible for the relatively short elimination half-life of 30–60 min. Hence it is necessary to dose frequently if penicillin is to be clinically effective. In an effort to prolong the action of the early penicillins, the drug probenecid was co-administered. Probenecid acts competitively for the same transport system as the penicillins in the proximal tubules. The result is reduced elimination of penicillins, increasing plasma concentrations and prolonged antibacterial action. With the development of newer longer-acting penicillins, the concurrent administration of probenecid and penicillin is no longer necessary.

For a drug such as the anticancer agent methotrexate, renal excretion involves both glomerular filtration and tubular secretion. Approximately 90 per cent of a large dose and nearly half of a small dose of methotrexate is eliminated unchanged in the urine, mostly within 12 h of dosing.

1.5.3   Passive diffusion across the renal tubule

Following glomerular filtration, water is progressively reabsorbed from the filtrate so that only about 1 per cent of the original filtered volume is voided as urine. The renal tubule acts like a lipid barrier, particularly at its distal part. The result is that lipid-soluble drugs in the glomerular filtrate are reabsorbed back into the bloodstream until the concentrations in plasma water and in urine in the distal tubule are similar. Therefore drugs with high lipid solubility are only slowly eliminated from the plasma into urine until they have been metabolized to more polar substances, primarily by the liver. If the drug is highly polar and therefore of low tubular permeability, the filtered drug will not be reabsorbed and urinary elimination will be rapid. Reabsorption of weak acids or weak bases is highly pH dependent, and since urinary pH can vary over a considerable range, urinary excretion rates may exhibit corresponding degrees of variability. A basic drug will be more rapidly excreted in an acid urine since the low pH within the tubule will favour ionization, thus inhibiting reabsorption. Likewise, an acidic drug will be most rapidly eliminated if the urine is made alkaline.

The development of a series of compounds may give rise to drugs for the treatment of a variety of clinical conditions. Thus sulphonamides are particularly useful for treating both urinary tract infections and intestinal infections. For the former complaint, sulphonamides have been developed for their high aqueous solubility so that rapid elimination takes place with little tubular reabsorption. The result is that high concentrations of the sulphonamide are obtained in the urine where it is required for its anti-bacterial activity. For example, sulphafurazole and sulphamethizole are relatively strong acids, with pK_a values of 4.9 and 5.5 respectively. Thus they are almost completely ionized at physiological pH. The additional high solubility of their acetyl metabolites avoids unwanted crystallization in the renal tubules, which was a problem with earlier sulphonamides. In contrast, N^4-succinyl and phthalyl sulphathiazoles have low water solu-bilities but are highly ionized in the alkaline pH of the intestinal fluid. Therefore they are only poorly absorbed after oral dosing, and most of the administered drug is retained within the intestinal tract. The carboxy-amide group becomes hydrolysed by digestive and bacterial proteinases, releasing the parent sulphonamide which is then available to treat intestinal infections such as bacillary dysentery.

1.5.4   Biliary elimination

Following biotransformation in the liver, many drug metabolites are actively transported into bile by carrier systems similar to those which carry sub-stances across renal tubules (Smith 1973). On entering the small bowel, lipid-soluble metabolites are reabsorbed and become involved in the process of enterohepatic cycling. In contrast, highly water-soluble metabolites will remain in the intestinal tract and be excreted with the faeces. Formation of a glucuronide or other conjugate in the liver results in a metabolite which is polar and therefore is not reabsorbed in the small bowel. However, in some instances deconjugation may take place in the intestine, with the liberated parent drug being free for reabsorption.

Anions, cations, and un-ionized molecules containing both polar and lipophilic groups may be candidates for biliary excretion in man, provided that their molecular weights exceed about 400–500 Da. Substances of lower molecular weight may undergo reabsorption during their passage through the small canaliculi of the liver and thus will not be available to pass into the bile. Examples of drugs which have a significant biliary component to their excretion pattern include the penicillins. In particular, ampicillin is well excreted in the bile and, since appreciable quantities of ampicillin are excreted in the faeces, this may induce diarrhoea in the patient after several days of treatment with the antibiotic. The reason for this is that the ampicillin, on entering the large bowel, will kill many of the commensal organisms living in it, resulting in an overgrowth of antibiotic-resistant bacteria which initiates diarrhoea.

1.6   Adverse effects and toxicity

Enzyme inhibitors, in common with all other therapeutic agents, may be potentially harmful, causing drug-induced adverse effects and toxicity. Many of these unwanted effects are simply due to an extension of the drug's pharmacological properties and are dose related. The following statement attributed to Paracelsus (1493−1541) remains true today: 'All substances are poisons; there is none which is not a poison. The right dose differentiates a poison from a remedy.' While many drugs are not themselves toxic, they may be activated to toxic metabolites by enzymatic biotransformation. Since the liver is the main organ for the detoxification of foreign substances administered to the body, this organ is often the target of toxicity although any other organ or tissue may be affected.

1.6.1   Adverse effects

Drugs of the same therapeutic class often exhibit similar adverse effect profiles (Rawlins and Thompson 1991). The non-steroidal anti-inflammatory drugs (NSAIDs), such as aspirin, paracetamol, and ibuprofen, owe their therapeutic effectiveness to a large extent to their ability to inhibit prostaglandin synthetase. Unfortunately, these weak organic acids, which are non-ionized in the stomach, are absorbed and inhibit prostaglandin synthesis in the gastric mucosa. This frequently results in gastrointestinal damage, dyspepsia, nausea, and gastritis, requiring the patient to stop medication. More serious adverse drug reactions to NSAIDs include gastrointestinal bleeding and perforation. Since inhibition of prostaglandin formation leads to these effects, misoprostol, a synthetic analogue of prostaglandin E_1 (alprostadil), may be administered to prevent the gastrointestinal toxicity induced by NSAIDs.

Following the first dose of an ACE inhibitor (Todd and Heel 1986), a rapid fall in blood pressure frequently occurs in patients with severe hypertension who have been on multiple drug therapy including a diuretic. This is associated with sodium depletion resulting from diuretic treatment. Less serious side-effects induced by ACE inhibitors include a persistent dry cough (Gibson 1989), loss of taste, sore mouth, abdominal pain, and skin rash. Rare but serious adverse effects include angioneurotic oedema, proteinuria, and neutropenia. ACE inhibitors occasionally cause impairment of renal function, particularly in patients with pre-existing renal disease or impairment and in the elderly.

1.6.2   Hypersensitivity reactions

Although the penicillins have a very low toxicity, in a few patients they produce a hypersensitivity reaction causing skin rashes and, rarely, an anaphylactic reaction which is fatal in approximately 10 per cent of cases. Patients who are hypersensitive or allergic to one penicillin will be hypersensitive to all, since the antigen appears to be the penicilloyl moiety formed when the β-lactam ring is opened. Hypersensitivity reactions may also occur with salicylate type analgesics and are more likely to be observed in asthmatics or patients suffering from other allergic disorders.

1.7   Drug stereoisomerism

Macroscopic life shows a high degree of symmetry, but at the molecular level asymmetry predominates. Consequently, biological macromolecules such as enzymes or receptors are frequently capable of distinguishing between the asymmetric forms of drugs. This ability has far-reaching consequences, since it may determine which form (stereoisomer) of a drug will be accepted by the appropriate registration authorities as suitable for marketing. Here, a brief account is given of the different pharmacological effects that may arise due to stereoisomerism in a drug, the problems associated with obtaining pure stereoisomeric forms and assessment of their purity, and the views of the regulatory bodies on the marketing of stereoisomers.

1.7.1   Chirality

The principle of *chirality* was most elegantly studied by Pasteur in the nineteenth century (Geison and Secord 1988). This followed the observations of Biot, another French scientist, that salts of tartaric acid, which were apparently identical by chemical analysis, were different in one respect, namely in their effects on plane-polarized light. Pasteur solved this paradox by demonstrating that the optically inactive salt of paratartaric acid (racemic acid, hence the term racemic) could be separated into two *optical isomers* (*enantiomers*)—the 'natural' form, which rotated plane-polarized light to the right (*dextrorotatory* (*d* or +)), and a previously unknown form, which rotated the light in an equal but opposite direction (*laevorotatory* (*l*, or −)). A racemate, i.e. 1:1 ratio of a pair of enantiomers, does not rotate the plane of polarized light at all. The molecular basis for asymmetry was described by van't Hoff, who recognized that when four different groups are attached to a tetravalent carbon (the most common form of molecular asymmetry), a pair of molecules which are mirror-image related are possible. It follows from this that if one enantiomer aligns three of its groups to interact with three complementary sites in a receptor, its mirror image will only be able to align two of these groups with the same receptor at any one time. Synthetic chemical routes not involving other stereochemicals generally result in a 1:1 mixture of enantiomers (racemate) when one chiral centre is in the final molecule.

The nomenclature for describing enantiomers and their effect on plane-polarized light can be quite confusing: $(+)/(-)$ or d/l used as a prefix for a compound indicates the direction of rotation of plane-polarized light caused by an isomer in solution; however, it gives no indication of absolute geometry. The absolute configuration was once assigned by relating the structure to one of two reference compounds, serine, the natural enanti-omer of which was designated L, or glyceraldehyde, with a natural con-figuration designated D. While this system was used to describe amino acids and sugars, it was of limited applicability, and absolute configuration is now usually related to the relative orientation in space of the atoms attached to a chiral centre using the Cahn–Ingold–Prelog convention otherwise described as the R/S system. The system assigns *a priori*ty based on the atomic number of each of the substituent groups attached to the chiral atom. Once the absolute configuration of a compound has been determined, the R/S assignments for an enantiomeric pair can be cor-related with the $(+)/(-)$ or d/l information for the enantiomers. When two or more different chiral centres occur in a molecule then, there are 2^n optically active forms in total, where n is the number of chiral centres. When $n = 2$, this gives rise to two pairs of enantiomers (RS,SR, and RR,SS); any one form of one pair is a diastereoisomer of any one form of the other pair. Diastereoisomers have different physical properties and can be separated by fractional crystallization using a suitable solvent system.

1.7.2 Pharmacological consequences of the use of racemic drugs

Stereoisomers may differ in their pharmacological activities for the follow-ing reasons: (a) one isomer is metabolized in a different manner or at a different rate from its related isomer; (b) one isomer is preferentially bound to plasma proteins causing a difference in circulating free drug and hence differences in concentrations at active sites, and there may also be a stereo-selective process of elimination; (c) there are differences in the interaction of isomers at active sites by which pharmacological action is mediated. Therefore a range of possibilities exists for the relative actions of the stereoisomers *in vivo*

1. All the pharmacological action may reside in one of the isomers, or the isomers may have similar activity but to different degrees, or the activities may be similar in character and degree. However, these features can be further complicated by differences in rates of metabolism and distribution of the isomers.

2. The isomers may have distinctly different pharmacological actions because of selective binding at different receptor sites.

3. The isomers may exhibit different toxic actions because of the difference in binding at receptor sites through which toxic actions are mediated.

4. One isomer may react at an active site to synergize or antagonize the action of the other isomer.

The stereoselective action of drugs may be important from a pharmacological or therapeutic point of view, particularly when enantiomers differ considerably in pharmacological properties. For example, the biotransformation of the isomer responsible for the pharmacological effect may be influenced by the metabolizing enzyme interaction or pharmacokinetic effects, such as are observed in the metabolism of amphetamine (Jackman et al. 1981) or propranolol (Nies et al. 1973). β-Adrenergic blocking agents such as propranolol and timolol (5) (*shows chiral centre) are enantioselectively taken up into extravascular tissue (Aula et al. 1988), and this is thought to reflect the enantioselective binding of (−)-enantiomers to β-receptors. Interestingly, the binding of S-timolol to melanin in the iris is not affected by S-propranolol or by R-propranolol, suggesting that timolol is not bound to β_1-receptors in this tissue. Kupfer et al. (1981) have shown, in human studies on the anticonvulsant mephenytoin (6), that the proportion of S- and R-enantiomers in the urine is different. The 4-hydroxy derivative of the S-enantiomer is by far the most prominent metabolite; the R-enantiomer undergoes N-demethylation. This enantioselectivity for product formation is likely to be the result of different modes of binding of the substrate molecule, resulting in different target groups being in close proximity to the catalytic site of the metabolizing enzymes.

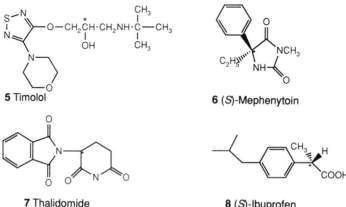

5 Timolol

6 (S)-Mephenytoin

7 Thalidomide

8 (S)-Ibuprofen

Perhaps the most infamous chiral drug is thalidomide (7). It has been shown by Blaschke *et al.* (1979) that $S(-)$thalidomide, but not $R(+)$-thalidomide, is transformed *in vivo* into *l*-*N*-phthaloylglutamine and *l*-*N*-phthaloylglutamic acid, products that are both embryotoxic and teratogenic in SWS mice and Natal rats. $R(+)$thalidomide is transformed into *d*-*N*-phthaloylglutamine and *d*-*N*-phthaloylglutamic acid which are neither embryotoxic nor teratogenic in these species. According to work done by Fabro *et al.* (1967), the enantiomers are equi-active in terms of hypnotic potency. Subject to further *in vivo* testing, to ascertain whether the metabolites of $R(+)$ thalidomide are enzymatically racemized or inverted, it would seem that $R(+)$ thalidomide might have been a useful hypnotic drug.

A relatively rare, but highly significant, stereoselective metabolic reaction is inversion of the chirality of one enantiomer to that of its optical antipode. This reaction is illustrated by the 2-arylpropionic acids (the profens) (8) which are used as non-steroidal anti-inflammatory drugs. These compounds contain a chiral centre in the propionate side-chain and undergo a metabolic inversion of the *R*-enantiomer to the biologically active *S*-enantiomer. The reaction is believed to proceed via formation of an acyl coA ester with the $R(-)$-acid which inverts and is hydrolysed to give the $S(+)$-acid; the initial ester formation is apparently unavailable to the $S(+)$-acid, thus giving enantioselectivity. Here, the racemate is equi-active with the $S(+)$-enantiomer (Kaye 1991).

There are many examples of elimination of enantiomers at very different rates; one such is the hypnotic drug hexobarbital. In man, the elimination half-life of the more active $(+)$-isomer is about three times longer than that of the less active $(-)$-isomer (Breimer and Van Rossum 1973). This is due to a difference in hepatic clearance and not to differences in volumes of distribution or plasma protein binding between the enantiomers. A particularly marked difference in clearance of enantiomers is found in the case of the anticoagulant acenocoumarol. In man, the $R(+)$-enantiomer is cleared approximately 15 times more rapidly than the $S(-)$-enantiomer, essentially due to differences in intrinsic hepatic clearance (Thijssen *et al.* 1986).

The binding of drug molecules at the active site of drug-metabolizing enzymes often leads to enantioselective discrimination in the substrate and/or products. These stereochemical aspects of drug disposition are often complex, with differences being observed between species and, in human populations, in individual variability in rates of metabolism which may be under genetic control. Chiral metabolism is only one of the many factors to consider, along with relative biological potency and economic feasibility for example in the decision to take a particular drug or one of its isomers into the development process. If an enantiomer rather than a racemate is preferred, and this will not always be the case, the added financial costs of development and production will have to be weighed against potential clinical benefit.

In the light of the evidence surrounding stereoselectivity in biological systems, there has been increasing pressure to prepare or separate enantiomers by commercially acceptable routes. Fractional crystallization (Anson *et al*. 1954) and seeding methods (Kleeman and Martens 1982) have been used, but neither has general applicability and they are time-consuming. They frequently require optically pure reagents and so often fail to achieve total separation of enantiomers. Acceptable routes involve either stereoselective synthesis of enantiomers or large-scale chromatographic separation of racemates. In view of this, chiral separation technology plays a vital role in determining acceptable levels of chiral purity. Chiral separation is also a precondition for *in vivo* studies of enantiomers in terms of metabolism, pharmacokinetics, and pharmacodynamics.

Stereochemistry of enzyme inhibitors with a chiral centre(s) is usually important in determining their potency towards a specific enzyme. Whereas the literature abounds with examples of activity residing mainly in one enantiomer following *in vitro* studies, very few of these compounds have, as yet, reached the clinic or been subjected to registration requirements and *in vivo* information is not available from animal studies.

Aminoglutethimide (AG) **(9)**, a long-established aromatase inhibitor, is used clinically as the racemate in the treatment of breast cancer in postmenopausal women (after surgery) to decrease their oestrogen levels. The $(+)(R)$-form is about 38 times more potent as an inhibitor than the $(-)$-(S)-form (Graves and Salhanick 1979). AG is also an inhibitor of the side-chain cleavage enzyme (CSCC) which converts cholesterol to pregnenolone in the adrenal steroidogenic pathway. Depletion of corticosteroids in this manner requires adjuvant hydrocortisone administration with the drug. Here the $(+)(R)$-form is about 2.5 times more potent than the $(-)(S)$-form (Salhanick 1982).

For pyridoglutethimide (Rogletimide) **(10)**, an analogue of AG without the undesirable depressant effect and now in clinical trials as the racemate, the inhibitory potency resides mainly in the $(+)(R)$-form (20 times that of the $(-)(S)$-form) (McCague *et al*. 1989). 1-Alkylation improves potency *in vitro* but the activity for the most potent inhibitor in the series, the 1-octyl, resides in the $(-)(S)$-form (Laughton *et al*. 1990) owing to a change in the mode of binding of inhibitor to enzyme.

A more selective inhibitor of aromatase than AG is the triazole R76713 **(11)** which is about 1000-fold more potent as an inhibitor. The aromatase inhibitory activity mainly resides in the $(+)$-form (32 times that of the $(-)$-form) (Van den Bossche *et al*. 1990), but the very small inhibitory activity of the racemate towards other steroidogenic pathway enzymes, 11β-hydroxylase and 17,20-lyase, originates in the $(-)$- and $(+)$-forms respectively.

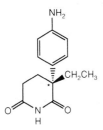

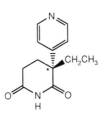

9 (*R*)-Aminoglutethimide   **10** (*R*)-Pyridoglutethimide

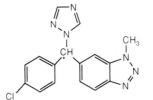

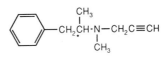

11 R76713   **12** Deprenyl

3-Cyclohexylaminoglutethimide, which is in clinical trials as the racemate, is a selective inhibitor of aromatase not requiring adjuvant hydrocortisone in treatment and lacking the undesirable CNS effects of AG. The (+)(*S*)-enantiomer, with the same configuration as (*R*)-AG, possesses the inhibitory activity of the drug (30 times that of the (−)(*R*)-form) (Hartmann *et al.* 1990).

MAO occurs in two forms, MAO-A and MAO-B (McDonald *et al.* 1989). The use of MAO inhibitors as antidepressants is complicated by a dangerous hypertensive reaction with tyramine-containing foods (the 'cheese-effect') which is due to inhibition of MAO-A located in the gastro-intestinal tract which would otherwise remove the tyramine. L-deprenyl (selegiline) (**12**), a selective inhibitor of MAO-B (16-fold), is widely employed to limit dopamine breakdown in Parkinson's disease in selective inhibitory dosage; however, its usefulness as an antidepressant is extremely limited (Johnson and Sandler 1992). The (−)-isomer is much more potent than the (+)-isomer and, since the products of metabolism are (−)-metamphetamine and (+)-metamphetamine respectively, the more potent (+)-metamphetamine side-effects are removed from the racemate by use of L-deprenyl (Reynolds *et al.* 1978).

γ-Aminobutyric acid (GABA) transaminase inhibitors allow a build-up of the inhibitory neurotransmitter GABA and are potential drugs in the treatment of epilepsy. The inhibitory action of γ-vinyl GABA (vigabatrin), a drug used clinically in the treatment of refractory forms of this disease, resides mainly in the (S)-enantiomer (Jung and Danzin 1989).

1.7.3 Separation of stereoisomers

Enantiomers cannot be resolved by conventional separation techniques because they have identical physicochemical properties. There are three methods for resolution of enantiomers by liquid chromatography: two of them exploit conventional column technology, either by formation of diastereoisomeric derivatives or by the use of chiral mobile phase additives; the third involves the use of a chiral stationary phase (CSP). The formation of diastereoisomers is achieved by reacting a pair of enantiomers with an optically pure chiral agent. Unlike enantiomers, these diastereoisomers have different physical properties and therefore can be separated by conventional methods. This approach is limited by the purity of the chiral derivatizing agent. There may also be a difference in the rate of reaction between the chiral derivatizing agent and the enantiomers, leading to inaccurate values for the enantiomeric ratio. However, this method has been used successfully in chiral drug development (Allenmark 1988).

A chiral complexing additive in the mobile phase can promote stereo-selective retention by one or more of the following mechanisms:

(1) stereoselective complexation in the mobile phase;

(2) formation of diastereoisomeric complexes with different distribution properties between the mobile and stationary phases.

One such chiral mobile phase additive (CMPA) which has been used to great effect is cyclodextrin. Cyclodextrins are toroidal cyclic oligosaccharides, which resemble open truncated cones in shape. The wider rim consists of secondary hydroxyl groups, while the inner surface is primarily hydrophobic. The recognition model is considered to rely on inclusion of a bulky hydrophobic group into the cyclodextrin cavity, while other groups on or close to the chiral centre are postulated to interact with the secondary hydroxyl groups on the outer rim (Armstrong et al. 1986). As with any chiral separation, a three-point interaction between the analyte and the chiral discriminator is required. This three-point interaction model was originally proposed by Dalgliesh (1952) and later emphasized by Pirkle et al. (1981). At least three simultaneous interactions (hydrogen bonding, π-π interactions, dipole stacking, steric repulsion, and van der Waals forces) between the enantiomeric solute and the chiral mobile phase are necessary to discriminate and separate the enantiomers. Two interactions only are not sufficient to produce enough difference in the binding strength between the R- or S-enantiomer and the chiral complexing agent to allow separation.

CSPs have been classified by Wainer and Drayer (1988) into five categories, based on their proposed method of chiral recognition. The first of these are the Pirkle phases (Pirkle *et al.* 1981). These are based on dinitrobenzoyl derivatives of amino acids bonded to silica. They function by facilitating the formation of transient diastereomeric analyte–CSP complexes. Although these phases are the most widely characterized in the literature, derivatization of the analyte is often required to provide the necessary three interaction sites with the CSP. In addition, biological samples require extraction into organic solvent before analysis, since the Pirkle phases need an aprotic environment to function.

The next two types of stationary phase are both based on derivatives of cellulose. The recognition mechanism of these phases is believed to be due largely to the formation of attractive interactions between the solute and the CSP, with part of the molecule entering a cavity within the structure of the stationary phase. Microcrystalline triacetyl cellulose has a high degree of cross-linking in the cellulose and this offers the possibility of inclusion complexing. The most common of the commercially available inclusion-type phases are the cyclodextrins developed by Armstrong *et al.* (1986). These columns operate in a reversed-phase mode and are bonded to silica via a hydrocarbon linkage. The method of separation is believed to be similar to that described earlier for cyclodextrins in the mobile phase.

The fourth category is based on chiral ligand exchange chromatography, developed by Davankov in the early 1970s (Davankov *et al.* 1973). Separation involves the use of an achiral column (e.g. ODS-silica) with a chiral mobile phase containing a transition metal ion, such as Cu^{2+} together with a single enantiomer of an amino acid, e.g. L-proline (Takeuchi *et al.* 1984). The resolution occurs due to the formation of a diastereoisomeric mixed-chelate complex with the drug.

The final category of CSP is based on protein as a chiral selector bonded to a silica support. There are three types of protein column commercially available: one based on bovine serum albumin (BSA) (Allenmark *et al.* 1984), another based on a_1-acid glycoprotein (AGP) (Hermansson 1984), and a third based on ovomucoid isolated from chicken egg white (Miwa *et al.* 1987). The separation mechanism of protein columns is based on the principles of bioaffinity, which include hydrophobic interactions (similar to true reversed phase) of polar groups and steric effects. These columns have shown the widest range for chiral recognition of any CSPs developed so far (Dappen *et al.* 1986).

CSPs have been used very effectively in the analysis of chiral compounds. However, some doubt remains concerning their use on a preparative scale. Although there are some semipreparative and preparative CSPs available, it seems impracticable for the protein columns to be used in this way. As the internal width of the column is increased, the flow dynamics change and separation is undoubtedly altered.

1.7.4   Analysis of chiral compounds

Enantiomeric purity is an entirely different concept from the chemical purity of organic compounds as commonly determined. The methods used for establishing enantiomeric purity may or may not lead to separation of the two forms. Polarimetry, NMR, isotopic dilution, differential scanning calorimetry (DSC), and enzymatic reactions do not separate enantiomers but are used for determination of enantiomeric composition. All these methods except NMR require information about the pure enantiomer for comparison (Martens and Bhushan 1990). Polarimetry, though widely used, requires knowledge of the specific rotation of the compound in optically pure form. The specific rotation is strongly dependent on solvent, solute concentration, and temperature.

Determination of enantiomeric purity, using NMR, requires the conversion of enantiomers into diastereomers by interaction with a suitable chiral agent, e.g. cyclodextrins (see earlier). Alternatively, a chiral solvent such as 2,2,2-trifluoro-1-phenylethanol is used, which induces a chemical shift difference between the enantiomers. The solvent-induced chemical shift is a consequence of the preferential interaction of one of the enantiomers with the chiral solvent. However, the enantioselective interaction is often too small to be of practical use. The isotopic dilution method requires mixing the unknown sample with an isotopically labelled racemate of the same compound. This mixture is then recrystallized and the optical rotation measured (polarimetry). Since the isotopic content of this sample is known, the optical purity of the original sample can be calculated. Both DSC and enzymatic reactions are of limited use in the routine situation.

1.7.5   Drug registration requirements

The principles for assessment of a medicine are a demonstration of appropriate safety, of an ability to manufacture the medicine consistently to an acceptable specification, and of efficacy in the intended indications for use of the product. The data must be scientifically rigorous and the conclusions must be justified. Justification and validation are therefore the keywords. Until recently, no data were required by the Drug Registration Authorities for the separate enantiomers or diastereoisomers of a proposed drug; however, the climate is changing. In 1987, the Japanese adopted rational requirements for racemic products; both pharmacological and toxicological data are now required for the enantiomers and the racemate. In the case of the racemate, it seems likely that only pharmacokinetics based on chiral assays would be accepted. The EC, in *Rules governing medicinal products in the European Community*, Vol. II, 1989, extended the section on stereoisomerism, and requires that when a submission for a new active substance (NAS) containing one or more chiral centres is made, it must specify whether specific isomers or a mixture of stereoisomers was used in the animal and human studies, and the form of the active ingredient in the final marketed product. At present, it is not a mandatory requirement for isomers to be separated and single enantiomers marketed. However, it is a requirement for the possible problems in relation to stereoisomerism to be discussed. The US authorities (FDA) have assumed a comparable approach to that of the Japanese and the EC, which took effect in 1992. At the moment, it is still possible to make a successful marketing application for a racemic mixture, as long as information on the activity of the separate enantiomers is available and enantioselective methods of chemical and biological analysis are used in both animal and human studies.

The importance of molecular asymmetry impinges on many areas of drug design and synthesis, and on all aspects of pharmacology. Indeed, pharmacological enantioselectivities question the rationale for the continued use of racemic drug preparations, although the decision as to which racemic drugs already being used might most effectively be resolved is a matter of much debate. It is unquestionable that the use of single enantiomeric drugs would simplify the interpretation of pharmacodynamic and phar-macokinetic data. Indeed, Ariens (1984) believes that it is the only way to avoid the production of 'sophisticated nonsense in clinical pharmacology'. This view is not shared by every scientist, but one thing is acknowledged, and that is that a chiral approach is required if an intrinsically chiral discipline is to be understood.

1.8   Toxicity testing

Enzyme inhibitors are frequently highly potent chemicals which, when administered at the high (non-therapeutic) doses required in standard toxi-city tests, disrupt the homeostasis of many physiological functions. They produce pathological and toxicological changes which may have little or no relevance to their therapeutic use in man. Of course, this applies to many different classes of drugs and not just to enzyme inhibitors. None the less, marketing any compound designed for long-term use in man requires a package of toxicology studies designed to demonstrate the safety of the compound to the satisfaction of regulatory authorities.

It is not proposed to discuss the regulatory requirements or the design of studies in detail. There are no published regulations on the design of toxicology studies, only guidelines. Because of this lack of defined regu-lations, there is some variation in the design and performance of regulatory toxicity studies from one laboratory to another, but the major studies required to satisfy the authorities in the United Kingdom, the United States, and Japan are well defined (Table 1.1). The type of investigations normally undertaken during the course of a toxicity study are shown in Table 1.2. Standard toxicity tests have many design features in common; in the same

Table 1.1 Major toxicity studies required for product license

Toxicity study	Species	Dose groups (no. of animals)	Duration (months)
Preliminary	Rat	4 (10/sex/group)	
	Dog or primate	4 (4/sex/group)	1
Preclinical	Rat	4 (25/sex/group)	
	Dog or primate	4 (5/sex/group)	6
Oncogenicity	Rat	4 (50/sex/group)	
	Mouse or other	4 (50/sex/group)	24
Teratogenicity	Rat	4 (30/sex/group)	
	Rabbit	4 (10/sex/group)	Organogenesis
Additional tests for US FDA	Rat	4 (25/sex/group)	
	Dog or primate	4 (5/sex/group)	12
Fertility test	Rat	4 (25/sex/group)	5

Table 1.2 Routine examinations in a standard toxicity test

In-life examinations	Blood and urine samples	Necropsy
Body weights	Haematology	Major organs weighed
Food intake	Chemical pathology	
Daily examination	Pharmacokinetics	
Ophthalmology	Urinanalysis	40 tissues sampled
Cardiovascular physiology	Urine cytology	

species, dose levels may be the same and the clinical parameters measured are likely to be identical from one test to another. The chief difference is duration of dosing and route of administration. It is common practice for studies of shorter duration to be dosed by gavage, while administration in the diet is more common in oncogenicity tests. Dose selection is one of the most difficult facets of the design of toxicity studies; the doses must take account of the pharmacokinetics of the drug so that levels achieved in animals can be related to the human therapeutic blood level. The highest dose must satisfy the regulatory criterion of a maximum tolerated level without producing so severe an effect that mortality compromises the study. The lowest dose is usually a multiple of the therapeutic dose which, it is hoped, will not produce any toxic effects so that a no-effect level can be defined, while the middle dose is usually at a median point between the two. A variety of small range-finding studies will usually be necessary to define suitable doses for all the species to be used in the pivotal studies, listed in Table 1.1, to begin. A withdrawal group is often included in the studies to determine the reversibility of any changes observed. The whole package of studies required to obtain a product licence is likely to take a minimum of 6 years; if problems which require further investigation are encountered, additional studies may add considerably to the package time.

Toxic effects can be divided into two broad categories; those which are known, or might be expected because of the pharmacology of the compound, and those which are 'unexpected'. The first company to develop a compound with a novel pharmacological action frequently encounters unique toxic effects. As similar drugs are developed and toxicological findings published, it becomes possible to identify 'class' toxicology, but owing to the time taken to develop drugs, this can be a lengthy process. To illustrate some of these problems, examples of three different classes of drugs have been selected to demonstrate how they may affect the design and interpretation of toxicology tests.

1.8.1   Angiotensin-converting enzyme inhibitors

Angiotensin II is the most potent vasoconstrictor known; thus, in hypertensive conditions where the renin–angiotensin–aldosterone system is involved, reducing the availability of angiotensin II to its receptors will lower blood pressure. In the last decade, a range of ACE inhibitors have been shown to be useful agents in the treatment of hypertension. In toxicity tests with the inhibitor captopril, changes were observed in the kidney, including swelling and hyperplasia of the juxtaglomerular apparatus, in both rats and dogs (Hashimoto et al. 1981; Imai et al. 1981). Such a change would be of concern to the toxicologist if the nature of this change and its functional significance in the kidney were not known. Further investigations (Zaki et al. 1982) showed that enlargement of the cells was due to an increase in granules in the renin-secreting cells of the juxtaglomerular apparatus; this was caused by lack of feedback inhibition by angiotensin II. Subsequently, this effect has been observed with several other ACE inhibitors (La Rocca et al. 1986; Donabauer and Mayer 1988; Dominick et al. 1989), and is now recognized as a pharmacological effect which is dose dependent and reversible. Other renal effects with ACE inhibitors are species dependent. Blood urea nitrogen (BUN) levels are elevated in rats dosed with captopril (Keim 1980) and with enalapril and Sch 31846 (Bagdon *et al.* 1985a). The elevation is slight but rapid and is not accompanied by any pathological changes which would account for it. Neither captopril nor Sch 31846 have any effect on BUN in dogs, but enalapril, in the dog, causes marked BUN elevation, renal tubular degeneration, and death at doses greater than 30 mg kg^{-1} (Bagdon *et al.* 1985b). This effect can be ameliorated by supplementation with physiological saline (Macdonald 1984), suggesting that alterations in fluid balance may be involved. A decrease in haemoglobin and haematocrit values in rats has been observed with some ACE inhibitors, but not with all. The mechanisms for this effect have not been defined; it could relate to a haemolytic action or to alteration in the release of renal erythropoietic factor.

1.8.2   Thymidylate synthetase inhibitors

Thymidylate synthetase catalyses the conversion of de-deoxyuridylate to thymidine and therefore is a key enzyme in the synthesis of DNA. Inhibitors of this enzyme are of interest only in the treatment of neoplastic diseases so that the toxicology programme for this type of drug would be reduced, and oncogenicity and teratogenicity studies would not usually be required. Fluorouracil (Heidelberger *et al.* 1957) is an example of this type of drug; it is a potent agent used clinically in the treatment of breast and colon cancer. The toxicology of fluorouracil exemplifies the problems facing the toxicologist with this type of drug which is highly cytotoxic. This could be described as the 'pharmacological' effect of this type of inhibitor. In animals, cytotoxic agents destroy cells in those organs where there is a rapid turnover, i.e. the intestinal tract, the lymphoreticular system, the bone marrow, and the testis. The degree to which these organs are affected varies with the compound, the dose, and the species. This means that toxicity tests with thymidylate synthetase inhibitors are likely to be extensively modified from the standard format. It would be impossible to dose a compound which produces widespread destruction of the intestinal tract for a long period of time; the animals would not survive. The therapeutic aim of this type of compound is to maintain the cytotoxic effect in the neoplastic tissue while keeping the generalized cytotoxic effects to a minimum. Depending on potency, dose levels are likely to be much closer to the human therapeutic level and the duration of dosing short, possibly less than a week. The rapidity of recovery from the cytotoxic effects is important and can be studied in animals withdrawn from the study at specific intervals after the dosing period. As a consequence of the cytotoxicity, many of the variables usually measured in toxicity studies may be profoundly deranged; haematological values could be greatly reduced because of bone marrow effects, and body and organ weights may be reduced because of intestinal changes. As with all drugs, unexpected toxic effects remain a possibility.

1.8.3   Aromatase and 5α-reductase inhibitors

These two classes of drug have quite different actions but represent another type of inhibitor, one which affects hormone synthesis. The complexity of the interrelationships between endocrine organs is such that it is not possible to affect the activity of one hormone without introducing effects in other organs. These types of inhibitor present the toxicologist with other problems of design and interpretation. When intended only for the treatment of neoplastic diseases, the toxicology programme, as with thymidylate synthetase inhibitors, would be modified to exclude some of the studies. If non-neoplastic diseases are either the main or an additional target for treatment, then the whole package will be necessary. There are a number of toxicological problems associated with these types of drugs; it is well recognized that a constant increase in any hormone which has a trophic effect in a target tissue will, after long treatment, produce hyperplasia and neoplasia in the target organ. Inhibitors which affect the synthesis of a hormone interfere with regulatory feedback mechanisms to other organs. In addition, there are both major and subtle differences between the endocrinology of man and experimental animals; for example, in women, oestrogen is the important hormone in the control of breast function, in the dog it is growth hormone, and in the rat prolactin.

Aromatase is the enzyme involved in the final stages of oestrogen biosynthesis. Inhibition of this enzyme results in an oestrogen deficiency, and deprivation of oestrogen is well established as an effective therapy in the treatment of oestrogen-dependent breast cancer. Aminoglutethimide, a non-selective inhibitor, has been shown to be effective in this condition (Brodie and Santen 1986) and has spurred the development of a new generation of more potent specific inhibitors (see Chapter 9). Although a drug may be targeted at a condition only occurring in males or females, it is very unlikely that the toxicological studies would be confined to a single sex; to repeat the studies in the other sex at a later date, to support trials under other conditions, would be untenable in terms of cost and time.

An understanding of the normal endocrinology of the experimental animal and the way it is modified by the inhibitor is essential to the design and interpretation of toxicological studies; measurement of appropriate hormone levels is critical in understanding the effects so that a reasoned explanation, not mere speculation, can be proposed for any observed effects. Many of the 'toxic' effects can be predicted; in female animals changes will occur in those organs (ovary and uterus) which are oestrogen dependent, but the severity of the effects will depend on potency and specificity. There would be different effects in rats and dogs because the negative feedback mechanisms are different in the two species; in the male rat the feedback loop from testis to hypothalamus is androgen dominated, while in the dog aromatization of androgen to oestrogen also occurs in the hypothalamus and oestrogen influences the release of luteinizing hormone (LH) from the pituitary. Therefore hyperplasia of testicular interstitial cells should occur in the dog but not in the rat. After long-term treatment, it is possible that a new homeostasis can be established but high doses of a very potent inhibitor could overwhelm the feedback controls and produce effects which are not easy to explain.

The membrane-bound enzyme 5α-reductase is responsible for the conversion of testosterone to dihydrotestosterone (DHT), the hormone-controlling prostate function. Inhibitors of this enzyme, such as finasteride (Stoner 1990), are designed for use in the treatment of benign prostatic hypertrophy (BPH) and hormone-dependent prostate cancer (see Chapter 9). In toxicological studies, one would expect to see changes associated with an excess of testosterone or a decrease of DHT. Both hormones inhibit LH production but DHT is much more potent in this action (Bookstaff *et al.* 1990); an increase in LH would result in hyperplasia of testicular Leydig cells and, on prolonged treatment, Leydig cell tumours.

The examples of enzyme inhibitors as drugs which have been described here illustrate the problems which such compounds present to the toxicologist in the design and interpretation of studies. This is likely to be a continuing process, as more inhibitors with new activity and greater potency are developed.

1.9   Summary

To be effective *in vivo*, and therefore to be of potential clinical value, any biologically active agent must be capable of reaching its site of action in an adequate concentration which must be maintained there for an appropriate time. The processes of absorption, distribution, metabolism, and excretion are thus important determinants that must be taken into account in the drug design strategy. In addition, the medicinal chemist must also consider the biological implication of chirality, particularly inasmuch as it may influence the pharmacological/biochemical activity profile and processes of disposition such as metabolism and excretion. Finally, a promising new compound must satisfy regulatory authorities as to its 'safety' by appropriate toxicological examination in animal species before it can be studied in man. It is then that 'The best laid schemes o' mice an' men gang aft a-gley' (Robert Burns, *To a mouse*)!

References

Allenmark, S. (1988). *Chromatographic enantioseparations*. Wiley, Chichester.
Allenmark, S., Bomgren, B., Boren, H., and Lagerstrom, P.-O. (1984). Direct optical resolution of a series of pharmacologically active racemic sulphoxides by high-performance liquid chromatography. *Analytical Biochemistry*, **136**, 293–97.

Anon. (1987). Administration of drugs by the buccal route (Editorial). *Lancet*, **i**, 666–7.

Anson, M. L., Bailey, K., and Edsall, J. T. (eds.) (1954). *Advances in protein chemistry*. Academic Press, New York.

Ariens, E. J. (1984). Stereochemistry, a basis for sophisticated nonsense in pharmacokinetics and clinical pharmacology. *European Journal of Clinical Pharmacology*, **26**, 663–8.

Armstrong, D. W., Ward, T. J., Armstrong, R. D., and Beesley, T. E. (1986). Separation of drug stereoisomers by the formation of b-cyclodextrin inclusion complexes. *Science*, **232**, 1132–5.

Aula, P., Kaila, T., Huupponen, R., and Salminen, L. (1988). Timolol binding to bovine ocular melanin *in vitro*. *Journal of Ocular Pharmacology*, **4**, 29–36.

Bagdon, W. J., Bokelman, D. L., and Stone, C. A. (1985a). Subacute, chronic toxicity studies, saline supplementation, saline depletion studies in the rat. *Japanese Journal of Pharmacology and Therapeutics*, **13**, 425–66.

Bagdon, W. J., Bokelman, D. L., and Stone, C. A. (1985b). Subacute and one year studies in beagle dogs. *Japanese Journal of Pharmacology and Therapeutics*, **13**, 467–518.

Benet, L. Z., Massoud, N., and Gambertoglio, J. G. (1984). *Pharmacokinetic basis for drug treatment*. Raven Press, New York.

Blaschke, G., Kraft, H. P., Fickentscher, K., and Kohler, F. (1979). Chromatographische Racemattrennung von Thalidomide und teratogene Wirkung der Enantiomer. *Arzneimittel-Forschung*, **29**, 1640–2.

Bookstaff, R. C., Moore, R. W., and Peterson, R. E. (1990). Androgen deficiency in male rats treated with perfluorodecanoic acid. *Toxicology and Applied Pharmacology*, **104**, 212–24.

Breimer, D. D. and Van Rossum, J. M. (1973). Pharmacokinetics of (+)- and (−)-hexobarbitone in man after oral administration. *Journal of Pharmacy and Pharmacology*, **25**, 762–3.

Brodie, A. M. M. and Santen, R. J. (1986). Aromatase in breast cancer and the role of aminoglutethamide and other aromatase inhibitors. *CRC Critical Review in Oncology and Hematology*, **5**, 361–96.

Brodie, B. B., Bernstein, E., and Mark, L. C. (1952). The role of body fat in limiting the duration of action of thiopental. *Journal of Pharmacology and Experimental Therapeutics*, **105**, 421–6.

Chipkin, R. E., Berger, J. C., Billard, W., Iovio, L. C., Chapman, R., and Barnett, A. (1988). Pharmacology of SCH 34826, an orally active enkeplialinase inhibitor analpsic. *Journal of Pharmacology and Experimental Therapeutics*, **245**, 829–38.

Craig, W. A. and Welling, P. G. (1983). Protein binding of antimicrobials: clinical pharmacokinetic and therapeutic implications. In *Handbook of clinical pharmacokinetics* (ed. M. Gibaldi and L. Prescott), pp. 55–74. ADIS, Press, Balgowlah, Australia.

Dalgliesh, C. E. (1952). The optical resolution of aromatic amino acids on paper chromatograms. *Journal of the Chemical Society*, **3**, 3940–5.

Dappen, R., Arm, H., and Meyer, V. R. (1986). Applications and limitations of commercially available chiral stationary phases for high-performance liquid chromatography. *Journal of Chromatography*, **373**, 1–20.

Davankov, V. A., Kurganov, A. A., and Bochkov, A. S. (1973). Resolution of racemates by high performance liquid chromatography. In *Advances in chromatography* (ed. J. C. Giddings, E. Gruchka, J. Cazes, and P. R. Brown) Vol. 22, pp. 432–6, Marcel Dekker, New York.

Davies, D. M. (1991). *Textbook of adverse drug reactions*, 4th edn. Oxford University Press.

Dominick, M. A., Susick, R. L., and Macdonald, J. R. (1989). Effects of the angiotensin converting enzyme inhibitor quinapril on renal structure and function. *Toxicologist*, **9**, 175–6.

Donabauer, H. H. and Mayer, D. (1988). Acute, sub chronic and chronic toxicity of the new angiotensin converting enzyme inhibitor rampipril. *Arzneimittel-Forschung*, **38**, 14–20.

Fabro, S., Smith, R. L., and Williams, R. T. (1967). Toxicity and teratogenicity of optical isomers of thalidomide. *Nature, London*, **215**, 296.

Geison, G. L. and Secord, J. A. (1988). Pasteur and the process of discovery. The case for optical isomerism. *Isis*, **79**, 6–36.

Gibaldi, M. (1992). *Biopharmaceutics and clinical pharmacokinetics*, 4th edn. Lea & Febiger, Philadelphia, PA.

Gibson, G. R. (1989). Enalapril-induced cough. *Archives of Internal Medicine*, **149**, 2701–3.

Graves, P. E. and Salhanick, H. A. (1979). Stereoselective inhibition of aromatase by enantiomers of aminoglutethimide. *Endocrinology*, **105**, 52–7.

Hartmann, R. W., Batzl, Mannschreck, A., and Pongratz, T. (1990). Stereoselective aromatase inhibition by the enantiomers of 3-cyclohexyl-3(4-aminophenyl)-2,6-piperidinedione. In *Chirality and biological action* (ed. B. Holmstedt, H. Frank, and B. Testa), pp. 185–90. Alan R. Liss, New York.

Hashimoto, K., Yoshimura, S., Ohtki, T., and Imai, K. (1981). Toxicological studies of captopril, an inhibitor of angiotensin converting enzyme. Three twelve-month studies—the chronic toxicity of captopril in beagle dogs. *Journal of Toxicological Science*, **6** (Suppl 2), 215–46.

Heidelberger, C., Chaudhuri, N. K., Dannenberg, P., Mooren, D., Griesbach, L., Duschinsky, R., *et al.* (1957). Fluorinated pyrimidines, a new class of tumour inhibiting compounds. *Nature, London*, **179**, 663–6.

Hermansson, J. (1984). Liquid chromatographic resolution of racemic drugs using a chiral α_1-glycoprotein column. *Journal of Chromatography*, **298**, 67–8.

Imai, K., Yoshimura, S., Ohtaki, T., and Hashimoto, K. (1981). Toxicological studies of captopril, an inhibitor of angiotensin converting enzyme. Two one-month studies in the subacute toxicity of captopril in rats. *Journal of Toxicological Science*, **6** (Suppl. 2), 189–214.

Jackman, G. P., McLean, A. J., Jennings, G. L., and Bobik, A. (1981). No stereoselective first-pass hepatic extraction of propranolol. *Clinical Pharmacology and Therapeutics*, **30**, 291–6.

Johnson, F. N. and Sandler, M. (1992). The pharmacology of selegiline. *Reviews in contemporary pharmacotherapy*, **3**, 51–65.

Jung, M. J. and Danzin, C. (1989). New developments in enzyme-activated irreversible inhibitors of pyridoxal phosphate-dependent enzymes of therapeutic interest. In *Design of enzyme inhibitors as drugs* (ed. M. Sandler and H. J. Smith), pp. 257–93. Oxford University Press.

Kaye, B. (1991). Chiral drug metabolism: a perspective. *Biochemical Society Transactions*, **19**, 456–9.

Keim, G. R. (1980). Toxicology and drug metabolic studies of SQ 14,225 in animals. In *Captopril and hypertension* (ed. D. B. Case, E. H. Sonnenblick, and J. H. Laragh), pp. 137–47. Plenum Press, New York.

Kleeman, A. and Martens, J. (1982). Optical resolution of racemic *S*-(carboxymethyl) cysteine. *Annalen der Chemie*, **7**, 1995–8.

Kupfer, A., Roberts, R. K., Schenker, S., and Branch, R. A. (1981). Stereoselective metabolism of mephenytoin in man. *Journal of Pharmacology and Experimental Therapeutics*, **218** (1), 193–9.

La Rocca, P. T., Squibb, R. E., Powell, M. L., Szot, R. J., Black, H. E., and Schwartz, E. (1986). Acute and sub chronic toxicity of a non-sulphydril angiotensin converting enzyme inhibitor. *Toxicology and Applied Pharmacology*, **82**, 104–11.

Laughton, C. A., McKenna, R., Neidle, S., Jarman, M., McCague, R., and Rowlands, M. G. (1990). Crystallographic and molecular modelling studies on 3-ethyl-3-(4-pyridyl) piperidine-2, 6-dione and its butyl analogue, inhibitors of mammalian aromatase. Comparison with natural substrates: prediction of enantioselectivity for *N*-alkyl derivatives. *Journal of Medicinal Chemistry*, **33**, 2673–9.

Laurence, D. R. and Bennett, P. N. (1992). *Clinical pharmacology*. Churchill Livingstone, New York.

Laurence, D. R., McLean, A. E. M., and Weatherall, M. (1984). *Safety testing of new drugs*. Academic Press, London.

Lecomte, J.-M., Costentin, J., Valaiculesci, H., Chaillet, P., Llorens-Cortes, C., Leboyer, M., and Schwartz, J.-C. (1986). *Journal of Pharmacology and Experimental Therapeutics*, **237**, 937–44.

Lindenbaum, J., Mellow, M. H., Blackstone, M. O., and Butler, V. (1971). Variation in biologic availability of digoxin from four preparations. *New England Journal of Medicine*, **285**, 1344–7.

Lorenzo, A. V. and Spector, R. (1976). The distribution of drugs in the central nervous system. In *Transport phenomena in the central nervous system* (ed. G. Levi, L. Battistin, and A. Lajtha), pp. 447–61. Plenum Press, New York.

Macdonald, J. (1984). *FDA Committee review of enalopril*. US Government Printing Office, Washington, DC.

McCague, R., Jarman, M., Rowlands, M. G., Mann, J., Thickitt, C. P., Clissold, D. W., *et al*. (1989). Synthesis of the aromatase inhibitor 3-ethyl-3-(4-pyridyl) piperidine-2, 6-dione and its enantiomers. *Journal of the Chemical Society Perkin Transactions I*, 196–8.

McDonald, I. A., Bey, P., and Palfreyman, M. G. (1989). Monoamine oxidase inhibitors. In *Design of enzyme inhibitors as drugs* (ed. M. Sandler and H. J. Smith), pp. 227–44. Oxford University Press.

Martens, J. and Bhushan, R. (1990). Importance of enantiomeric purity and its control by thin-layer chromatography. *Journal of Pharmaceutical and Biomedical Analysis*, **8**, 259–69.

Maxwell, G. M. (1984). *Principles of paediatric pharmacology*. Croom-Helm, London.

Melander, A. (1983). Influence of food on the bioavailability of drugs. In *Handbook of clinical pharmacokinetics* (ed. M. Gibaldi and L. Prescott), pp. 39–54. ADIS Press, Balgowlah, Australia.

Miwa, T., Miyakawa, T., and Kayano, M. (1987). Application of an ovomucoid-conjugated column for the optical resolution of some pharmaceutically important drugs. *Journal of Chromatography*, **218**, 193–9.

Nicholls, P. J. (1980). Neurotoxicity of penicillin. *Journal of Antimicrobial Chemotherapy*, **6**, 161–72.

Nies, A. S., Evans, G. H., and Shand, D. G. (1973). The hemodynamic effects of beta adrenergic blockade on the flow-dependent hepatic clearance of propranolol. *Journal of Pharmacology and Experimental Therapeutics*, **184**, 716–20.

Park, B. K. and Breckenridge, A. M. (1983). Clinical implications of enzyme induction and enzyme inhibition. In *Handbook of clinical pharmacokinetics* (ed. M. Gibaldi and L. Prescott), pp. 243–66. ADIS Press, Balgowlah, Australia.

Pirkle, W. H., Finn, J. M., Schreiner, J. L., and Hamper, B. C. (1981). A widely useful chiral stationary phase for the high-performance liquid chromatography separation of enantiomers. *Journal of the American Chemical Society*, **103**, 3964–6.

Poole, A. and Leslie, G. B. (1989). *A practical approach to toxicological investigations*. Cambridge University Press.

Pratt, W. B. (1990). The entry, distribution and elimination of drugs. In *Principles of drug action* (ed. W. B. Pratt and P. Taylor), 3rd edn., pp. 201–96. Churchill Livingstone, New York.

Rawlins, M. D. and Thompson, J. W. (1991). Mechanisms of adverse drug reactions. In *Textbook of adverse drug reactions* (ed. D. M. Davies), 4th edn., pp. 18–45. Oxford University Press.

Reynolds, G. P., Elsworth, J. D., Blau, K., Sandler, M., Lees, A. J., and Stern, G. M. (1978). Deprenyl is metabolised to methamphetamine and amphetamine in man. *British Journal of Clinical Pharmacology*, **6**, 542–4.

Roques, B. P., Fournie-Zaluski, M. C., Soraca, E., Lecomte, J.-M., Malfray, B., Llorens, C., and Schwartz, J.-C. (1980). The encephalinase inhibitor, thiorphan, shows antinociceptive activity in mice. *Nature, London*, **288**, 286–8.

Salhanick, H. A. (1982). Basic studies on aminoglutethimide. *Cancer Research*, **42**, 3315S–21S.

Smith, R. B. (1985). *The development of a medicine*. Macmillan, London.

Smith, R. L. (1973). *The excretory function of bile*. Chapman & Hall, London.

Smith, S. E. and Rawlins, M. D. (1976). *Variability in human drug response*. Butterworths, London.

Stoner, E. (1990). The clinical development of a 5-alpha reductase inhibitor, finasteride. *Journal of Steroid Biochemistry and Molecular Biology*, **37**, 375–8.

Takeuchi, T., Horikava, R, and Tanimura, T. (1984). Enantioselective solvent extraction of neutral D,L-amino acids in two-phase system containing *N*-n-alkyl-L-proline and copper ions. *Analytical Chemistry*, **56**, 1152–4.

Thijssen, H. H. W., Janssen, G. M. J., and Baars, L. G. M. (1986). Lack of effect of cimetidine on pharmacodynamics and kinetics of single oral doses of *R*- and *S*- acenocoumarol. *European Journal of Clinical Pharmacology*, **30**, 619–23.

Timbrel, J. A. (1982). *Principles of biochemical toxicology*. Taylor & Francis, London.

Timbrel, J. A. (1989). *Introduction to toxicology*. Taylor & Francis, London.

Todd, P. A. and Heel, R. C. (1986). Enalapril. A review of its pharmacodynamic and pharmacokinetic properties, and therapeutic use in hypertension and congestive heart failure. *Drugs*, **31**, 198–248.

Tyrer, J. H., Eadie, M. J., Sutherland, J. M., and Hooper, W. D. (1970). *British Medical Journal*, **4**, 271.

Van den Bossche, Willemsens, G., Roels, I., Bellens, D., Moereels, H., Coene, M.-C., Le Jeune, L., Lauwers, W., and Janssen, P. A. J. (1990). R76713 and enantiomers: selective non-steroidal inhibitors of the cytochrome P450-dependent oestrogen synthesis. *Biochemical Pharmacology*, **40**, 1707–18.

Wagner, J. G. (1975). *Fundamentals of clinical pharmacokinetics*. Drug Intelligence Publications, Hamilton, IL.

Wainer, I. W. and Drayer, D. E. (eds.) (1988). *Drug stereochemistry—analytical methods and pharmacology*. Marcel Dekker, New York.

Zaki, F. G., Keim, G. R., Taku, Y., and Ingomai, T. (1982). Hyperplasia of the juxtaglomerular cells and renin localisation in the kidneys of normotensive animals given captopril. *Annals of Clinical Laboratory Science*, **12**, 200–15.

2

Computer-aided molecular design of enzyme inhibitors

A.M. Slater, D. Timms, and A.J. Wilkinson

2.1   Introduction

Historically, inhibitors of enzymes have been discovered by random screening or designed by analogy with elements of the enzyme's catalytic pathway. Thus inhibitors based on substrates, transition states, and products have been produced by a procedure that relies on an understanding of the enzyme mechanism, together with some innovative chemical thinking. Molecular modelling techniques can significantly enhance this process, and in addition they provide the opportunity to aid the discovery of completely novel inhibitors.

In most instances, the chemist starts with a lead compound discovered via the more conventional methodology referred to above. If the inhibitor is required to function as a drug, there will usually be a need to modify this compound to achieve a desired profile of some form. This may involve attempts to find a compound of higher intrinsic inhibitory potency or increased selectivity. Additionally, physical and chemical properties may need modification to attain compounds that are, for example, orally active or which have better *in vivo* activity or reduced toxic side-effects. Modelling may be directed at optimizing activity within a defined chemical series or at generating completely novel compounds. The particular objective for inhibitor design will influence the techniques and approaches used.

Molecular graphics and molecular modelling techniques have developed significantly over the last 10–15 years. The development of the molecular modelling workstation has made realistic the concept of every scientist having access to substantial computing power and high resolution graphics. A number of powerful high quality molecular modelling software packages are now available to complement these developments in hardware. Molecular modelling techniques themselves have also undergone substantial development. Thus both *ab initio* and semi-empirical quantum-mechanical techniques have developed significantly, and software for both is commonly available (Clark 1985). Molecular mechanics force-field methodology continues to evolve, although there is still a need for a high quality general force field (Dinur and Hagler 1991). Molecular dynamics techniques (van Gunsteren and Berendsen 1985) have become more widely applied, enabling a more realistic view of enzyme–inhibitor interactions to develop in which the flexibility of the solutes and the nature of the solvent environment are explicitly included.

One area which has significantly increased our understanding of enzyme structure and function has been the determination of protein structure by protein X-ray crystallography and NMR spectroscopy. Since the first determination of the structure of an enzyme, lysozyme (Phillips 1966), several hundred enzyme structures have been solved. If the structure of the enzyme of interest is known, molecular modelling techniques can provide a powerful impetus to inhibitor design studies, and a number of approaches will be described later. Often the structure of the enzyme of interest is not known, and a number of computational techniques have evolved to aid inhibitor design in these circumstances. These approaches are reviewed briefly in the next section. The general strategy for applying computational techniques is shown schematically in Fig. 2.1.

2.2 No model of the enzyme structure exists

Without knowing the structure of the target enzyme, the chemist must rely on knowledge of the enzyme mechanism and the known structure activity within defined chemical series. It is possible to use the known or calculated physical, chemical, electronic, and conformational properties of a series of molecules to rationalize their enzyme inhibitory capability and to derive pharmacophore models. These pharmacophores postulate the relative positions of key chemical groups found in the bioactive conformation of inhibitors of a given enzyme. The bioactive conformation is the conformation that an inhibitor must adopt in order to bind to the enzyme.

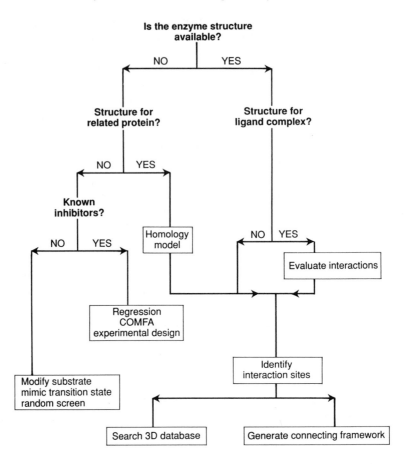

Fig. 2.1 Schematic diagram of the ligand design process.

One approach is to define the pharmacophore by superposing molecules in a way that emphasizes the similarity between active molecules. This has been achieved by overlaying key functional groups, overlaying electrostatic potential minima, matching common volumes, or by a number of other criteria (McLachlan 1982; Danziger and Dean 1985; Sheridan *et al*. 1986; Papadopoulos and Dean 1991). These techniques work well with fairly rigid molecules, but with flexible molecules they are dependent on the correct identification of the bioactive conformation which may differ significantly from its favoured conformation when free in solution.

A technique that attempts to identify such bioactive conformations is the active analogue approach (Marshall *et al*. 1979). The conformational space available to a range of inhibitors is examined and attempts are made to define the common space available to active analogues and to distinguish this from the conformational space available to inactive or less active analogues. Using this approach, Marshall and colleagues were able to derive a pharmacophore for angiotensin-converting enzyme (ACE) inhibitors (Mayer *et al*. 1987).

More recently, chemometric methods have been used to correlate a wide range of physicochemical properties with biological activity. These techniques involve calculating or determining a large number of atomic and molecular properties associated with a series of molecules (Franke 1984). Thus the number of such properties far outweighs the number of observables (e.g. inhibition constants) and this precludes the use of simple regression techniques. Therefore the first stage in any chemometric analysis is to reduce the number of variables in some way. One example of this is the use of principal components analysis (PCA) in an approach known as PC regression. With this technique, the original variables are replaced by a reduced set of new variables, called principal components, which are linear combinations of the original variables. The principal components are orthogonal to one another and this has the effect of removing any correlations inherent in the original set of properties. The result is that a much smaller number of variables can represent virtually all the variance in the data. It is quite common to be able to replace 30 or 40 physical properties with fewer than 10 principal components. The simplest way to use these components is to identify those which show any significant correlation with biological activity and then to carry out a standard multilinear regression. By definition, this methodology can only be predictive within the bounds of a training set from which the model has been derived. Extrapolating beyond this is unlikely to yield useful results. This approach is more suited to ranking lists of molecules according to predicted inhibitory potency than to the design of new molecules, as the principal components can be difficult to interpret directly.

A variation on this approach is called comparative molecular field analysis (COMFA) (Cramer *et al*. 1988). The interaction energy of a probe is calculated at a number of points around a molecule. These energies are equivalent to the physical properties described above, and a more sophisticated form of PC regression called principal least squares (PLS) is used to define a model for activity. The power of this technique is that the results can easily be interpreted visually. Areas around a molecule in which substitutions of different kinds affect activity can be contoured. New molecules can be designed, and a quantitative prediction of the effects of substitutions is provided. The approach is critically dependent on the correct identification of the bioactive conformation, and thus may be less suited to series of flexible molecules. However, it has been successfully applied to a number of enzyme systems including ACE (Marshall and Cramer 1988) and DNA gyrase (Dolmella *et al*. 1989).

As demonstrated by the approaches described above, without knowledge of the enzyme structure the chemist requires a large amount of structure activity data before a rationalization of inhibitory activity and the design of inhibitors can be attempted. However, if a degree of understanding of the enzyme mechanism is available, it is possible to use this, in combination with computational techniques, to aid inhibitor design. The best example of this is probably the discovery of potent ACE inhibitors. Working from the knowledge that ACE is a metalloprotease and knowing its specificity from substrate studies, Ondetti *et al.* (1977) were able to work by analogy with the structure and mechanism of carboxypeptidase A to design inhibitors containing a strong zinc ligand but with the desired specificity for ACE.

2.3   Model of the enzyme structure exists

2.3.1   Structure generation

If a model of the enzyme structure exists, then opportunities for the use of molecular modelling techniques to aid the rational design of enzyme inhibitors increase. Ideally, the model should be derived directly from experimental data using X-ray crystallography or NMR spectroscopy, but models built using homology modelling techniques have also proved useful. However, techniques such as secondary structure prediction are unlikely to be of value in this context. Below, we briefly consider the different routes to the structure of an enzyme and the confidence that we can have in the resulting model.

2.3.1.1   *X-ray crystallography*

X-ray crystallography involves directing a beam of X-rays at a single crystal of the protein and measuring the intensity of the diffracted X-rays (Blundell and Johnson 1976). Combination of these intensities with phase information derived via isomorphous substitution, for example, allows transformation to a three-dimensional structural model of the protein. Protein crystal structures vary considerably in quality and accuracy. To obtain structures revealing atomic detail, data with resolution to better than 3.0 Å are required. A high resolution structure is normally judged as one where the data have been collected with resolution to better than 2.0 Å. One indicator as to the quality of a structure is the R factor which reflects how well the structural model fits the experimental data. A well refined model would normally have an R factor below 20.0 per cent. In considering an X-ray structure, the temperature factors that have been reported should be carefully examined. High temperature factors (>50 Å^2) associated with a group of atoms suggest that this region of the structure is particularly uncertain. In addition, stereochemical and other criteria have been developed (Morris *et al.* 1992) for the assessment of structural quality.

Several hundred protein structures are now available within the Brookhaven Protein Database (Abola *et al.* 1987), and a large proportion of these are enzymes. This information, together with kinetic, mechanistic, and protein engineering studies, have provided a detailed characterization of the structure and mechanism of several enzyme families.

2.3.1.2   *NMR spectroscopy*

The use of NMR spectroscopy to determine protein structure has developed in recent years (Clore and Gronenborn 1991). Well over a hundred protein structures have already been determined by NMR. There are significant limitations to the range of application of this technique. In particular, it is currently only applicable to proteins with $M_r < 20\ 000$ at a concentration of 0.5–10.0 mM. Nevertheless, the structures of several enzymes have been solved by NMR, including phospholipase A2, lysozyme, and dihydrofolate reductase. Indeed, NMR experiments have the advantage of being carried out in solution and can provide insight into the dynamics of protein structure.

Several NMR techniques have been developed which allow the conformation of bound ligand to be studied in the absence of detailed knowledge of the protein structure. Knowledge of the bioactive conformation of an inhibitor provides a powerful stimulus to inhibitor design. An excellent review of these techniques is given by Fesik (1991).

NMR studies usually generate less precisely defined structures than crystallography, and atomic positions are often known only to within 1 Å. Usually, a number of structures that fit the NMR data are calculated. The root mean squared deviation (RMSD) between these structures is one indicator of the confidence that can be had in the precise structure of particular regions of the protein. Current methods under development involving relaxation matrix refinement (Bonvin *et al.* 1991) enable an *R* factor to be calculated in the same way as for X-ray crystallography.

2.3.1.3   *Homology modelling*

If the structure of a related enzyme and the sequence of the target enzyme are known, it is possible to build a model of the enzyme of interest by a technique known as homology modelling (Stewart *et al.* 1987; Sali *et al.* 1990). The target enzyme should normally exhibit at least 30 per cent sequence identity to the enzyme of known structure. The greater the sequence identity and similarity, the more accurate the resulting model is likely to be. In the most favourable cases, this can result in a model of the enzyme structure which is comparable with a low to medium resolution X-ray structure. If a number of structures are known for related proteins, these can be used cooperatively to produce a single 'best' model for the target enzyme. Alternatively, a number of homology models can be generated which, as for the NMR structures, can be used to evaluate the uncertainties in the models. The regions of greatest uncertainty will generally reflect insertions or deletions with respect to the known structures.

2.3.2 Utilization of structural model

The use of enzyme structural information in design can be considered in stages. The first step begins with familiarization with the enzyme structure and, if possible, structures of enzyme–inhibitor complexes. Attempts can be made to 'dock' other inhibitors, either by analogy or using the approaches to be described below.

A major aim at this stage is the identification of key binding sites and the nature and magnitude of potential interactions. As we shall show this information can be used as the basis for the design of inhibitors with completely novel chemistry which bear little or no obvious relationship to known inhibitors, i.e. *de novo* design. Regarding bound ligands as part of the protein structure enables the same design techniques to be used to improve the affinity and specificity of known inhibitors.

We now examine, in more detail, the ways in which inhibitor binding modes and key interaction sites can be identified, and the exploitation of this information in the design of inhibitors.

2.3.2.1 *Identification of the binding mode of inhibitors*

Normally, in attempting to discover novel enzyme inhibitors, one starts from an existing, possibly weak, inhibitor. This may have been discovered by mimicking the structure of known elements of the enzyme's catalytic pathway (e.g. substrate, transition state, or product) or by random screening. Alternatively, it may be a naturally occurring inhibitor of the enzyme's activity.

To maximize the chances of success in using computational approaches to aid inhibitor design, the binding mode of this inhibitor, or a related structure, needs to have been determined experimentally by X-ray crystallography or NMR spectroscopy. The best example of this to date is that of the Agouron group (Appelt *et al*. 1991), who have determined the structures of a number of thymidylate synthase inhibitors bound to the enzyme. They have embarked on an iterative design cycle, designing modifications to their existing lead inhibitor, synthesizing this new molecule, and then determining its structure when bound to the enzyme. Thus they have been continually checking the success of their design philosophy.

If experimental information on the binding mode is not available, a variety of predictive approaches can be used. However, enzymes often change their active site conformation on binding ligands and so, unless the structure of the complex is known experimentally, it can be difficult to predict from the isolated enzyme. Indeed, knowledge of the nature of any major conformation change on binding could generate opportunities for the design of allosteric non-competitive inhibitors.

Nevertheless, some progress in the development of techniques that 'dock' a ligand into a protein active site has been made over the last few years. Recent techniques which look promising include constrained simulated annealing (Goodsell and Olson 1990) and methods which allow 'soft docking' (Jiang and Kim 1991). The latter approach involves representing the molecular surfaces of protein and ligand as three-dimensional or two-dimensional patterns and searching for a complementary pattern match. The 'softness' of such representations may allow for conformational adaptation by the partners in complex formation.

2.3.2.2   *Identification of key binding sites*

An important element in inhibitor design is the identification of the key binding sites within an enzyme. The nature of such interaction sites can be considered in terms of the various forces which contribute to binding including steric, electrostatic, hydrogen bonding, and desolvation. Most substrate−enzyme interactions occur within cavities in the protein surface, and algorithms have been developed (Ho and Marshall 1990) which identify and define the extent of candidate binding regions within protein structures. In order to visualize these pockets and grooves more clearly, the molecular surface of the enzyme can be calculated (Connolly 1983).

If the electrostatic potential around the active site is calculated and displayed on the molecular surface, this should provide an insight into the electrostatic nature of the site. The steric accessibility for ligand atoms at the surface of the protein is used in the program DOCK (DesJarlais *et al.* 1988) to construct spheres which represent the locations of candidate ligand atoms. The positions of potential hydrogen-bonding ligand atoms can be constructed based on the known geometry of such interactions. This approach forms the basis of the program HSITE (Danziger and Dean 1989a,b) and has been used more recently in the LUDI suite of programs (Bohm 1992).

Useful though these approaches are, they each treat only a single element of the interaction energy. Additional tools for identifying key binding sites have been developed. The program GRID (Goodford 1985) calculates the spatial distribution of the interaction energy between probe atoms and a protein. This can then be contoured by energy value if required, thus providing a more comprehensive view of the binding preferences of a particular protein. However, the use of a single-atom probe ignores the fact that binding is a multi-atom phenomenon. We have developed a program GROPE (Timms and Wilkinson 1990) which defines the optimum binding orientations around a protein for small to medium functional groups. An imaginary grid is placed around the enzyme active site. In separate calculations, functional group probes (e.g. phenyl, naphthyl, amide, acetate, etc.) are placed at each grid point in turn. They are then allowed to move, without bond rotation, to find the orientation with the most favourable interaction energy in the locality. With standard minimization routines, movements of greater than 0.5 Å would be unlikely and so grid separations of 0.5 Å or smaller would be required to ensure that all low energy binding orientations are identified. In GROPE, we use the conformational search technique SNIFR (Donnelly and Rogers 1988), which allows movements of 4.0 Å or greater, and thus relatively coarse grids can be used and the problem becomes computationally tractable. We have tested GROPE against a number of protein—inhibitor systems, including trypsin—benzamidine, DNA gyrase—ATP and dihydrofolate reductase (DHFR)—methotrexate with a fair degree of success. This work is summarized in Table 2.1. Experimental binding positions are well reproduced apart from the ribose in the gyrase—ATP complex where there are few specific interactions with the enzyme. It is interesting to note that one of the carboxylate positions in methotrexate was only identified after inclusion in the calculation of a bound water molecule observed in the X-ray structure.

One problem with this approach is that it treats both the ligand and the protein as rigid. While it might be feasible to incorporate a small number of variable torsions into GROPE, it is not practical to allow for any

Table 2.1 Results of test calculations carried out using GROPE on known enzyme—inhibitor complexes

	RMSD[a] (Å)	Ranking[b]	Grid size (Å)
Trypsin—benzamidine			
Benzamidine	0.3	1/3	4.0
DHFR—MTX			
Pteridinium	0.8	1/3	3.0
	0.4	2/3	3.0
Carboxylate (1)	1.2	1/12	3.0
	0.5	4/12	3.0
Carboxylate (2)	0.8[c]	12/12	3.0
Gyrase—ATP			
Adenine	1.5	2/2	4.0
Ribose	2.5	5/6	4.0
Triphosphate	0.2	1/1	4.0

[a] RMS deviation from the experimentally defined complex found in the protein database.

[b] The second number refers to the number of ligand binding sites identified. The first indicates the ranking of the specific site within the total identified.

[c] This carboxylate site was only found if a single key water molecule from the X-ray structure was included as part of the protein.

substantial flexibility in the protein. A recent method (Miranker and Karplus 1991) which has the potential to overcome these problems is multiple copy dynamics (MCD), where the dynamics of a protein active site together with a large number of ligands are simulated. The ligands do not 'see' one another, and the total interaction of all the ligands with the protein is normalized. While the published applications of this method are fairly limited so far, it has considerable potential.

2.3.2.3 *Exploiting bound water*
One type of ligand that is often overlooked is bound solvent. The positions and thermal *B* factors of such solvent molecules are often available from X-ray diffraction studies. As for bound ligands in general, these water molecules can be regarded as part of the protein structure that forms the basis for *de novo* design. In this way they can allow water-bridged inter-actions between the protein and candidate functional groups.

Water molecules that interact strongly with the protein exhibit low thermal factors and can be regarded as docked hydrogen-bonding groups; hence they can be replaced by appropriate ligand atoms. There is an addi-tional benefit in replacing such 'immobilized' water molecules which stems from the gain in entropy on releasing them to bulk solvent.

In the absence of experimentally determined solvent positions, a number of techniques exist to generate them. A geometric approach has been used by Pitt and Goodfellow (1991); alternatively, the protein can be immersed in a pre-equilibrated box of water molecules and the system allowed to relax using energy optimization or molecular dynamics techniques. Mole-cular dynamics can also be used to gauge the persistence of bound water molecules and hence their value in the design process (Hermann and Dow 1991). In addition, simulations can identify structured water in the vicinity of apolar groups (Brooks and Karplus 1989). Careful analysis of the behaviour of water in such simulations can thus identify binding positions for both polar and apolar groups.

2.3.2.4 *Structure generation of putative inhibitors*
Given that a number of key binding sites and associated functional groups have been identified, what chemical framework can we use to link these sites to each other or to an existing inhibitor lead? Until recently, this has depended on a chemist interacting directly with the modelling system and trying out various linking groups one by one. We and others were able to use this approach with some success in the design of renin inhibitors (Bradbury *et al.* 1990), but it can be a difficult and tedious exercise. For this reason a number of automated techniques have been developed that can aid the process.

One of the most powerful is the use of three-dimensional database searching. Given a database of three-dimensional structures, it is possible

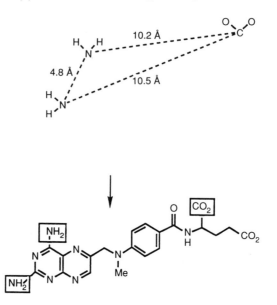

Fig. 2.2 Three-dimensional database searching illustrated with a demonstration of how methotrexate could be found from the DHFR active site. Binding sites for the three functional groups (two amino and one carboxylate) would be found using an approach such as GROPE or multiple copy dynamics. A database is searched for groups with a similar spatial disposition.

to search for those which match a defined pharmacophoric pattern. This approach requires an ability to generate a database of three-dimensional structures from simple chemical descriptions of molecules and some means of searching it. Programs such as CONCORD (Rusinko *et al.* 1988) and WIZARD (Dolata *et al.* 1987) address the former requirement, and there are now several packages, in various stages of development, which allow the databases to be searched (van Drie *et al.* 1989). Despite the limitations in current systems (most do not allow for conformational flexibility), we and others have used this technique with considerable success. The concept of three-dimensional database searching is depicted schematically in Fig. 2.2.

A limitation of the three-dimensional database approach is that molecules of interest must exist in the database. Generally, such databases have been derived from collections of compounds synthesized by chemical and pharmaceutical companies or from structural sources such as the Cambridge Crystallographic Database (Allen *et al.* 1979). To enlarge the range of chemistry available to this approach, 'virtual' databases have been introduced (Nilakantan *et al.* 1991). In these, candidate structures are assembled from randomly chosen fragments and assessed against the

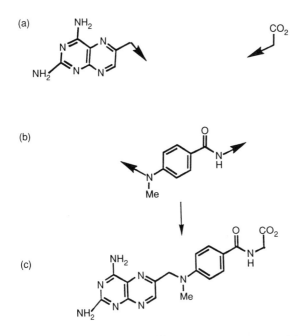

Fig. 2.3 The concept of the spacer skeleton demonstrated with fragments of methotrexate. (a) Binding site for pteridine and carboxylate fragments have been identified by applying a technique such as GROPE to the DHFR active site. Their substituent bond vectors are represented by arrows. A database of spacer skeletons is then searched for equivalent bond vectors in the correct orientation to link the two groups. The relative spatial orientation of the bond vectors is described by one distance, two angles, and a dihedral angle. (b) If *p*-anilino benzamide were in the spacer skeleton database, it would fit the required spatial distribution of bond vectors in this case and (c) would lead to the design of a fragment of methotrexate.

current search criteria. If the search problem is formulated in terms of the required directions of bonds connecting protein-bound functional groups to a framework fragment, then a database of spacer skeletons, represented as substituent vectors, can be searched (Bartlett *et al.* 1989). Bohm has incorporated this approach into a suite of programs (LUDI) which are directed at the whole process of automated ligand design (Bohm 1992). The spacer skeleton concept is demonstrated schematically in Figure 2.3 using fragments of methotrexate.

A number of workers have attempted to develop non-database or *ab initio* approaches to structure generation. Some of these use a standard lattice (e.g. tetrahedral or hexagonal) to link functional groups of interest (Lewis and Dean 1989a,b). Difficulties can occur when attempting to mix and match lattices of different types. To avoid this problem, we have developed

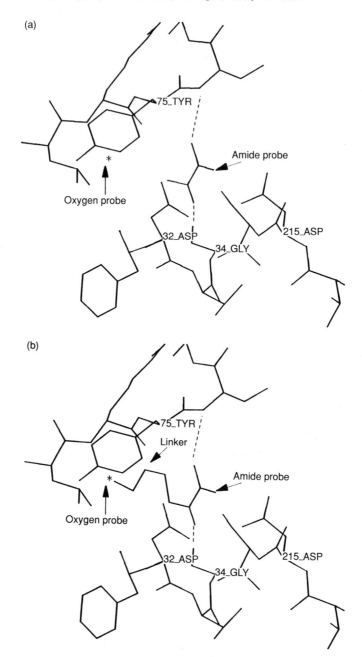

Fig. 2.4 (a) GROPE results for two probes and a model of renin. Hydrogen bonds are represented by broken lines. (b) One example of a connecting path derived by CLINK. A phenyl ring is implied by linker torsion angles.

a program CLINK which 'grows' a chain of generic atoms from some point on an existing ligand to the desired functional group, saving all feasible routes. Examination of combinations of routes can highlight potential ring systems which can act as rigid linker groups. Thus we are attempting to combine the creative talent of a molecular modeller or medicinal chemist with an automated computational approach. This is exemplified in Fig. 2.4 with its application to a model of the aspartyl protease renin. A similar philosophy has been incorporated into the program BUILDER (Lewis 1991), which is derived from the lattice approach.

2.3.2.5 *Single-step design: the future*

A method of growing peptides in protein binding sites has been developed (Moon and Howe 1991) which iteratively adds amino acid fragments in a variety of feasible conformations and evaluates the energy of interaction with the static protein structure. This is a limited attempt at what might be termed single-step design in which the characterization of the binding site and the generation of molecular structures is carried out in a single step.

The intriguing promise of the MCD approach to locating key binding sites is that this step could be combined with the computer generation of candidate inhibitor molecules to provide a more general approach to single-step design (Miranker and Karplus 1991). A collection of functional groups or probe atoms could be introduced into the binding site, along with framework fragments. By allowing probes to coalesce in the course of a dynamics simulation, inhibitor molecules may emerge which optimally make use of the available structural and dynamic information. Although there are clear technical problems to be overcome, it is our understanding that this approach is currently being investigated by Karplus and his group at Harvard.

2.3.2.6 *Prediction of binding energy*

Having identified novel ligands with the desired properties, ideally we would like to be able to estimate their probable binding affinities. This would allow candidates for synthesis to be chosen on the basis of feasibility and probable affinity.

Potential energies of interaction are inadequate for this purpose because of an inability to allow for the changes in solvation of the protein and ligand on complexation and difficulties associated with estimating the contributions from conformational, orientational, and librational entropy. The development of molecular dynamics and, in particular, free energy perturbation (FEP) calculations (Beveridge 1989) has meant that useful estimates of relative binding affinity within a chemical series are now feasible. These calculations are extremely computer intensive. A more pragmatic and rapid approach is to estimate the solvation energetics empirically, frequently using the concept of solvent-accessible surface or volume (Vila *et al.* 1991).

The entropic contributions to binding can also be estimated (Novotny 1991, Williams *et al.* 1991) from simple thermodynamic relations. Such estimates are system dependent, but freezing a single bond on binding costs $2-8$ kJ mol^{-1} and the loss of orientational entropy contributes $36-60$ kJ mol^{-1}. In conjunction with potential energy calculations, these approximate methods have been useful in ranking the affinities of related inhibitors and in interpreting the contributions to binding.

2.4   Lessons from experimental and theoretical studies

The number of experimentally determined structures of protein–ligand complexes and associated theoretical investigations is steadily increasing. Although the information database is still rather limited, some interesting and to some extent surprising insights from the point of view of inhibitor design are now available.

2.4.1   The importance of electrostatic effects

When the inhibitor methotrexate (MTX) binds to DHFR, the pK_a for protonation of the N(1) atom increases from 5.3 to more than 10.0 (Cocco *et al.* 1983). Similar shifts are seen for other inhibitors and this reflects the environment of the binding site, in particular the presence of a carboxyl group whose apparent pK_a is raised to 6.5 (Fierke *et al.* 1987).

Thus these environmental effects on the protonation states of ligand and protein groups need to be taken into account in the design process. Electrostatic potential surfaces can be useful in visualizing the possible effects of such perturbations, and methods are available for the semiquantitative estimation of shifts in pK_a arising from the electrostatic environment (Matthew and Gurd 1986).

Recently, Bajorath *et al.* (1991) have calculated the electron distribution of ligands in the free state and bound to DHFR. Their results indicate that the enzyme polarizes the ligands such that the atom-centred charges normally used in calculating interaction energies are different in the two states. Similarly, such polarization effects can occur with respect to protein atoms. In particular, hydrogen-bonded relays and peptide groups are polarized by buried charged groups. A dramatic example is provided by the crystal structure for the complex between sulphate and its periplasmic binding protein (Quiocho *et al.* 1987). The sulphate dianion is not directly juxtaposed to a complementary positively charged group but is hydrogen bonded to NH groups at the N termini of three helices and via peptide groups to an arginine and a histidine residue.

The design of carboxy-containing analogues of the DHFR inhibitor trimethoprim (TMP) (Kuyper 1989) is representative of attempts to exploit electrostatic interactions. Three candidate positively charged residues were considered. Of these, Arg 57 was the most successful target. In the native structure, this residue is the most buried and sterically restricted of the three candidates. These findings may illustrate the value of targeting interactions in which part of the entropic and desolvation cost of binding has already been paid in the structure of the unbound enzyme.

In summary, the assignment of the probable protonation states for ligand and enzyme and the adequate treatment of electrostatic interactions represent significant challenges for inhibitor design.

2.4.2   The binding modes of chemical analogues

The pteridine ring of dihydrofolate, the substrate for DHFR, is also found in the inhibitor MTX but with a 4-amino substituent in place of the 4-oxo group of folate. Despite this chemical analogy, the pteridine ring of MTX binds in an inverse orientation to that of folate (Oefner *et al.* 1988), reflecting the different hydrogen-bonding capabilities of the 4-substituents.

A similar inversion of binding orientation is found for antiviral analogues binding to the coat protein of rhinovirus (Badger *et al.* 1988). The introduction of a single methyl substituent in the ligand results in rotation of the ligand binding mode by approximately 180 °.

Peptide substrates and inhibitors of serine proteases are located in the binding site by main-chain hydrogen bonds to and from the enzyme, forming a β-sheet structure. Thus there are two possible orientations for peptide inhibitors, depending on whether a parallel or antiparallel β-sheet is formed. In general, an antiparallel orientation is favoured, however, CF_3CO-Lys-Ala-NH-C_6H_4-p-CF_3 binds in a parallel fashion to elastase (Bode *et al.* 1989).

A major assumption, often adopted when modelling chemical analogues, is that equivalent atoms should be superposed. In particular, this assumption has governed the modelling of binding conformations and the generation of pharmacophore models. In the cases cited above, such assumptions have prove invalid. This may arise because of the existence of elements of imperfect symmetry in the ligand, the protein binding site, or indeed both partners in complex formation. Thus there is a need to supersede atom-by-atom superposition in considering the relationships between analogues. In this respect, electrostatic surfaces for ligands and also for enzyme binding sites can prove useful.

2.4.3   The importance of simple substituents to affinity

The important contribution of simple substituents to affinity is exemplified by the effect of incorporating hydroxyl substituents in a variety of enzyme ligands (Wolfenden and Kati 1991). The potentially predictive concept that such substitutions can be characterized by an intrinsic or perhaps a differential binding contribution is belied by the variation in the observed effects. Each substitution and each system provides a unique balance of contributions from direct binding, desolvation, entropic, and environmental effects. These considerations are illustrated in the two systems considered below.

In the case of adenosine deaminase, the $-OH$ group of 6R-hydroxy-1,6-dihydro purine ribonucleoside contributes almost 40 kJ mol^{-1} to binding in comparison with the $-H$ group of 1,6-dihydro purine ribonucleoside. The interaction is highly stereospecific, and recent structural studies (Wilson *et al.* 1991) indicate that hydrogen bonding, zinc complexation, and possibly, ionization may all play a part in imitating an intermediate on the normal reaction pathway.

The $>NH$ group of phosphonamidate inhibitors of thermolysin forms a hydrogen bond to the carbonyl group of Ala 113 of the enzyme. Replacement of this $>NH$ group by $-O$ (i.e. phosphonates) does not change the binding orientation but results in a loss of binding energy of the order of 16 kJ mol^{-1} (Bartlett and Marlowe 1987). However, if the $>NH$ group is replaced by $>CH_2$ (i.e. phosphinates), then binding energy is retained (Morgan *et al.* 1991). Although a hydrogen bond is lost in both cases, this is counterbalanced by desolvation effects for the phosphinates, whereas desolvation effects are additionally deleterious for the phosphonates.

2.4.4   The pursuit of selectivity

If enzyme inhibitors are required in a pharmaceutical context, selectivity of action is often an important prerequisite. This selectivity may be required between a target human enzyme and similar human enzymes, or to discriminate between, for example, a bacterial target and corresponding human enzyme.

In the former situation, the restricted specificity of thrombin, the target enzyme for fibrinogen, has been used to generate selective inhibitors. These hirulog inhibitors exploit a unique *exo* site involved in binding fibrinogen and hirudin, the natural inhibitor from leeches (Skrzypczak-Jankun *et al.* 1991).

The DHFR inhibitor TMP, which is 35 000 times more selective for bacterial than mammalian enzymes, provides an example of discrimination between species. The basis for this selectivity has been the subject of considerable study. The conformation adopted by TMP when bound to the *Escherichia coli* enzyme differs from that found with the chicken liver enzyme. This results in a significantly different position for the trimethoxy-phenyl group within the two active sites. In addition, there are differences of hydrogen bonding from the heterocyclic ring and in the environment of the NADPH cofactor, as well as the adoption of different side-chain conformations in the proteins (Matthews *et al.* 1985).

A recent structure determination for the co-crystallized ternary complex of TMP, NADPH, and mouse DHFR (Groom *et al.* 1991) suggests that the structure of the chicken liver complex may be artefactual. The structure determination involved soaking the inhibitor into crystals of the binary NADPH−enzyme complex. A discrepancy may have arisen because the crystal lattice of the binary complex prevented appropriate access and adoption of the bioactive conformation during soaking. If further studies confirm this interpretation, co-crystallization would seem to be the method of choice in such experiments.

None the less, the main reason for the enhanced selectivity of TMP for bacterial enzymes does not appear to derive from a difference in conformation or from a significant reduction in direct interactions with the enzyme. It is possible that the deletion of residues at the rim of the binding pocket of bacterial enzymes allows greater exposure to solvent for the methoxy groups of the inhibitor, and that it is this differential solvation that accounts for the selectivity of inhibition (Kuyper 1990).

2.5 Conclusions

In cases where the structure of the enzyme is unknown, a number of statistically sophisticated techniques for inhibitor design have been developed. These can prove valuable if sufficient structure activity data are available. However, assumptions such as the atom-by-atom superposition of analogues may need to be superseded by more flexible approaches and considerations.

Where enzyme structure is available, the exciting prospect of an iterative cycle of design and structural evaluation is now a reality. The ability to create and search three-dimensional structural databases has provided a powerful stimulus to inhibitor design. More recent developments suggest that the methodology is evolving towards a single-step process in which factors such as the role of solvent and structural accommodation can be taken into account, although many technical problems remain. In addition, the incorporation of an element of synthetic feasibility into automated design programs has not yet been addressed. As the structural database of ligand−protein complexes enlarges, we can anticipate further insights which will improve our ability to design and evaluate potential inhibitors.

References

Abola, E. E., Bernstein, F. C., Bryant, S. H., Koetzle, T. F., and Weng, J. (1987). Protein data bank. In *Crystallographic databases—information content, software systems, scientific applications* (ed. F. H. Allen, G. Bergerhoff, and R. Sievers), pp. 107−32. Data Commission of the International Union of Crystallography, Bonn.

Allen, F. H., Bellard, S., Brice, M. D., Cartwright, B. A., Doubleday, A., Higgs, H., *et al.* (1979). The Cambridge Crystallographic Data Centre: computer-based search, retrieval, analysis and display of information. *Acta Crystallographica, Section B*, **35**, 2331–9.

Appelt, K., Bacquet, R. J., Bartlett, C. A., Booth, C. L. J., Freer, S. T., Fuhry, M. A. M., *et al.* (1991). Design of enzyme inhibitors using iterative protein crystallographic analysis. *Journal of Medicinal Chemistry*, **34**, 1925–34.

Badger, J., Minor, I., Kremer, M. J., Oliveira, M. A., Smith, T. J., Griffith, J. P., *et al.* (1988). Structural analysis of a series of antiviral agents complexed with human rhinovirus 14. *Proceedings of the National Academy of Sciences*, **85**, 3304–8.

Bajorath, J., Li, Z., Fitzgerald, G., Kitson, D. H., Farnum, M., Fine, R. M., *et al.* (1991). Changes in the electron density of the cofactor NADPH on binding to *E. coli* dihydrofolate reductase. *Proteins: Structure, Function and Genetics*, **11**, 263–70.

Bartlett, P. A. and Marlowe, C. K. (1987). Evaluation of intrinsic binding energy from a hydrogen bonding group in an enzyme inhibitor. *Science*, **235**, 568–71.

Bartlett, P. A., Shea, G. T., Telfer, S. J., and Waterman, S. (1989). CAVEAT: a program to facilitate the structure-derived design in biologically active molecules. *Special Publication of the Royal Society of Chemistry*, **78**, 182–96.

Beveridge, D. L. (1989). Free energy via molecular simulation: a primer. In *Computer simulation of biomolecular systems* (ed. W. F. Van Gunsteren and P. K. Weiner), pp. 1–26. Escom, Leiden.

Blundell, T. L. and Johnson, L. N. (1976). *Protein crystallography*. Academic Press, London.

Bode, W., Meyer, E., Jr., and Powers, J. C. (1989). Human leukocyte and porcine pancreatic elastase: X-ray crystal structures, mechanism, substrate specificity, and mechanism-based inhibitors. *Biochemistry*, **28**, 1951–63.

Bohm, H.-J. (1992). The computer program LUDI: a new method for the *de-novo* design of enzyme inhibitors. *Journal of Computer Aided Molecular Design*, **6**, 61–78.

Bonvin, A. M. J. J., Boelens, R., and Kaptein, R. (1991). Direct NOE refinement of biomolecular structures using 2D NMR data. *Journal of Biomolecular NMR*, **1**, 305–9.

Bradbury, R. H., Major, J. S., Oldham, A. A., Rivett, J. E., Roberts, D. A., Slater, A. M., *et al.* (1990). 1,2,4-Triazolo[4,3-a]pyrazine derivatives with human renin inhibitory activity. 2. Synthesis, biological properties and molecular modelling of hydroxyethylene isostere derivatives. *Journal of Medicinal Chemistry*, **33**, 2335–42.

Brooks, C. L., III and Karplus, M. (1989). Solvent effects on protein motion and protein effects on solvent motion. Dynamics of the active site region of lysozyme. *Journal of Molecular Biology*, **208**, 159–81.

Clark, T. (1985). *A handbook of computational chemistry: a practical guide to chemical structure and energy calculations*. Interscience, New York.

Clore, G. M. and Gronenborn, A. M. (1991). Structures of larger proteins in solution: three- and four-dimensional heteronuclear NMR spectroscopy. *Science*, **252**, 1390–9.

Cocco, L., Roth, B., Temple, C., Jr., Montgomery, J. A., London R. E., and Blakley, R. L. (1983). Protonated state of methotrexate, trimethoprim, and pyrimethamine bound to dihydrofolate reductase. *Archives of Biochemistry and Biophysics*, **226**, 567–77.

Connolly, M. L. (1983). Solvent accessible surface of proteins and nucleic acids. *Science*, **221**, 709–13.

Cramer, R. D., Patterson, D. E., and Bunce, J. D. (1988). Comparative molecular field analysis (CoMFA). 1. Effect of shape on binding of steroids to carrier proteins. *Journal of the American Chemical Society*, **110**, 5959–67.

Danziger, D. J. and Dean, P. M. (1985). The search for functional correspondences in molecular structure between two dissimilar molecules. *Journal of Theoretical Biology*, **116**, 215–24.

Danziger, D. J. and Dean, P. M. (1989a). Automated site-directed drug design: a general algorithm for knowledge acquisition about hydrogen-bonding regions at protein surfaces. *Proceedings of the Royal Society of London, Series B*, **236**, 101–13.

Danziger, D. J. and Dean, P. M. (1989b). Automated site-directed drug design: the prediction and observation of ligand point positions at hydrogen-bonding regions on protein surfaces. *Proceedings of the Royal Society of London, Series B*, **236**, 115–24.

Desjarlais, R. L., Sheridan, R. P., Seibel, G. L., Dixon, J. S., Kuntz, I. D., and Venkataraghavan, R. (1988). Using shape complementarity as an initial screen in designing ligands for a receptor binding site of known three-dimensional structure. *Journal of Medicinal Chemistry*, **31**, 722–9.

Dinur, U. and Hagler, A. T. (1991). New approaches to empirical force fields. *Reviews in Computational Chemistry*, **2**, 99–164.

Dolata, D. P., Leach A. R., and Prout K. (1987). WIZARD: AI in conformational analysis. *Journal of Computer Aided Molecular Design*, **1**, 73–85.

Dolmella, A., Leahy, D. E., and Wilkinson, A. J. (1989). Comparative molecular field analysis of quinolone acid DNA gyrase inhibitors. *Zeneca Pharmaceuticals Library Report, PH32961*.

Donnelly, R. A. and Rogers, J. W. (1988). A discrete search technique for global optimisation. *International Journal of Quantum Chemistry*, **S22**, 507–13.

Fesik, S. W. (1991). NMR studies of molecular complexes as a tool in drug design. *Journal of Medicinal Chemistry*, **34**, 2937–45.

Fierke, C. A., Johnson, K. A., and Benkovic, S. J. (1987). Construction and evaluation of the kinetic scheme associated with dihydrofolate reductase from *Escherichia coli*. *Biochemistry*, **26**, 4085–92.

Franke, R. (1984). *Theoretical drug design methods*. Elsevier, Amsterdam.

Goodford, P. J. (1985). A computational procedure for determining energetically favourable binding sites on biologically important macromolecules. *Journal of Medicinal Chemistry*, **28**, 849–57.

Goodsell, D. S. and Olson, A. J. (1990). Automated docking of substrates to proteins by simulated annealing. *Protein: Structure, Function and Genetics*, **8**, 195–202.

Groom C. R., Thillet J., North A. C. T., Pictet, R., and Geddes, A. J. (1991). Trimethoprim binds in a bacterial mode to the wild-type and E30D mutant of mouse dihydrofolate reductase. *Journal of Biological Chemistry*, **266**, 19890–3.

Hermann, R. B. and Dow, E. (1991). Construction of a human synovial phospholipase A$_2$ model. *Cray Channels*, **13**(3), 2–5.

Ho, C. M. W. and Marshall, G. R. (1990). Cavity search: an algorithm for the isolation and display of cavity-like binding regions. *Journal of Computer Aided Molecular Design*, **4**, 337–54.

Jiang, F. and Kim, S. (1991). 'Soft docking': matching of molecular surface cubes. *Journal of Molecular Biology*, **219**, 79–102.

Kuyper, L. F. (1989). Inhibitors of dihydrofolate reductase. In *Computer-aided drug design. Methods and applications* (ed. T. J. Perun and C. L. Propst), pp. 327–69. Marcel Dekker, New York.

Kuyper, L. F. (1990). The potential role of solvation in the dihydrofolate reductase species selectivity of trimethoprim. In *Crystallographic and molecular modelling methods in molecular design* (ed. C. E. Bugg and S. E. Ealick), pp. 56–79. Springer-Verlag, Berlin.

Lewis, R. A. (1991). Rational methods for site-directed drug design: novel approaches for the discovery of potential ligands. *Biochemical Society Transactions*, **19**, 883–7.

Lewis, R. A. and Dean, P. M. (1989a). Automated site-directed drug design: the concept of spacer skeletons for primary structure generation. *Proceedings of the Royal Society of London, Series B*, **236**, 125–40.

Lewis, R. A. and Dean, P. M. (1989b). Automated site-directed drug design: the formation of molecular templates in primary structure generation. *Proceedings of the Royal Society of London, Series B*, **236**, 141–62.

McLachlan, A. D. (1982). Rapid comparison of protein structures. *Acta Crystallographica, Section A*, **38**, 871–3.

Marshall, G. R. and Cramer, R. D. (1988). Three dimensional structure–activity relationships. *Trends in Pharmacological Sciences*, **9**, 285–9.

Marshall, G. R., Barry, C. D., Bosshard, H. E., Dammkoehler, R. A., and Dunn, D. A. (1979). The conformational parameter in drug design: the active analog approach. *Computer-Assisted Drug Design*, **112**, 205–26.

Matthew, J. B. and Gurd, F. R. N. (1986). Calculation of electrostatic effects in proteins. *Methods in Enzymology*, **130**, 413–36.

Matthews, D. A., Bolin, J. T., Burridge, J. M., Filman, D. J., Volz, K. W., and Kraut, J. (1985). Dihydrofolate reductase. The stereochemistry of inhibitor selectivity. *Journal of Biological Chemistry*, **260**, 392–9.

Mayer, D., Naylor, C. B., Motoc, I., and Marshall, G. R. (1987). A unique geometry of active site of angiotensin converting enzyme consistent with structure–activity studies. *Journal of Computer Aided Molecular Design*, **1**, 3–16.

Miranker, A. and Karplus, M. (1991). Functionality maps of binding sites: a multiple copy simultaneous search method. *Proteins: Structure, Function and Genetics*, **11**, 29–34.

Moon, J. B. and Howe, W. J. (1991). Computer design of bioactive macromolecules: a method for receptor-based *de-novo* ligand design. *Proteins: Structure, Function and Genetics*, **11**, 314–28.

Morgan, B. P., Scholtz, J. M., Ballinger, M. D., Zipkin, I. D., and Bartlett, P. A. (1991). Differential binding energy: a detailed evaluation of the influence of hydrogen-bonding and hydrophobic groups on the inhibition of thermolysin by phosphorus-containing inhibitors. *Journal of the American Chemical Society*, **113**, 297–307.

Morris, A. L., MacArthur, M. W., Hutchinson, E. G., and Thornton, J. M. (1992). Stereochemical quality of protein coordinates. *Proteins: Structure, Function and Genetics*, **12**, 345–64.

Nilakantan, R., Bauman, N., and Venkataraghavan, R. (1991). A method for automatic generation of novel chemical structures and its potential applications to drug discovery. *Journal of Chemical Information and Computer Science*, **31**, 527–30.

Novotny, J. (1991). Protein antigenicity: a thermodynamic approach. *Molecular Immunology*, **28**, 201–7.

Oefner, C., D'Arcy, A., and Winkler, F. K. (1988). Crystal structure of human dihydrofolate reductase complexed with folate. *European Journal of Biochemistry*, **174**, 377–85.

Ondetti, M. A., Rubin, B., and Cushman, D. W. (1977). Design of specific inhibitors of angiotensin converting enzyme: new class of orally active antihypertensive agents. *Science*, **196**, 441–4.

Papadopoulos, M. C. and Dean, P. M. (1991). Molecular structure matching by simulated annealing: IV Classification of atom correspondences in sets of dissimilar molecules. *Journal of Computer Aided Molecular Design*, **5**, 119–33.

Phillips, D. C. (1966). The three dimensional structure of an enzyme. *Scientific American*, **215**, 78–90.

Pitt, W. R. and Goodfellow, J. M. (1991). Modelling of solvent positions around polar groups in proteins. *Protein Engineering*, **4**, 531–7.

Quiocho, F. A., Sack, J. S., and Vyas, N. K. (1987). Stabilization of charges on isolated ionic groups sequestered in proteins by peptide units. *Nature, London*, **329**, 561–4.

Rusinko, A., Shell, J. K., Balducci, R., McGarity, C. M., and Pearlman, R. S. (1988). *CONCORD, A program for the rapid generation of high quality approximate 3-dimensional molecular structures*. University of Texas at Austin, distributed by Tripos Associates.

Sali, A., Overington, J. P., Johnson, M. S., and Blundell, T. L. (1990). From comparisons of protein sequences and structures to protein modelling and design. *Trends in Biochemical Sciences*, **15**, 235–40.

Sheridan, R. P., Nilakantan, R., Dixon, J. S., and Venkataraghavan, R. (1986). The ensemble approach to distance geometry: application to the nicotinic pharmacophore. *Journal of Medicinal Chemistry*, **29**, 899–906.

Skrzypczak-Jankun, E., Carperos, V. E., Ravichandran, K. G., Tulinsky, A., Westbrook, M., and Marganore, J. M. (1991). Structure of the hirugen and hirulog 1 complexes of alpha-thrombin. *Journal of Molecular Biology*, **221**, 1379–93.

Stewart, D. E., Weiner, P. K., and Wampler, J. E. (1987). Prediction of the structure of proteins using related structures, energy minimisation and computer graphics. *Journal of Molecular Graphics*, **5**, 133–40.

Timms, D. and Wilkinson, A. J. (1990) *De-novo* ligand design at ICI Pharmaceuticals. *Chemical Design Automation News*, **5**, 20–3.

van Drie, J. H., Weininger, D., and Martin, Y. C. (1989). ALADDIN: An integrated tool for computer-assisted molecular design and pharmacophore recognition from geometric, steric and substructure searching of three dimensional molecular structures. *Journal of Computer Aided Molecular Design*, **3**, 225–51.

van Gunsteren, W. F. and Berendsen, H. (1985). Molecular dynamics simulations: techniques and applications to proteins. In *Molecular dynamics and protein structure* (ed. J. Hermans), pp. 5–15. Polycrystal Book Service, Dayton, Ohio.

Vila, J., Williams, R. L., Vasquez, M., and Scheraga, H. A. (1991). Empirical solvation models can be used to differentiate native from near-native conformations of bovine pancreatic trypsin inhibitor. *Proteins: Structure, Function and Genetics*, **10**, 199–218.

Williams, D. H., Cox, J. P. L., Doig, A. J., Gardner, M., Gerhard, U., Kaye, P. T., *et al*. (1991). Toward the semiquantitative estimation of binding constants. Guides for peptide-peptide binding in aqueous solution. *Journal of the American Chemical Society*, **113**, 7020–30.

Wilson, D. K., Rudolph, F. B., and Quiocho, F. A. (1991). Atomic structure of adenosine deaminase complexed with a transition-state analog: understanding catalysis and immunodeficiency mutations. *Science*, **252**, 1278–84.

Wolfenden, R. and Kati, W. M. (1991). Testing the limits of protein–ligand binding discrimination with transition-state analogue inhibitors. *Accounts of Chemical Research*, **24**, 209–15.

Protein serine–threonine kinases

Section 3A

General introduction to protein serine–threonine kinases

Peter J. Kennelly and Arthur M. Edelman

3A.1   Protein phosphorylation: a ubiquitous regulatory mechanism

In nature, a broad range of proteins become modified via the covalent bonding of phosphate to nucleophilic functional groups located on the side-chains of their constituent amino acids. Although numerous amino acids can be modified in this way, by far the most widespread and quantitatively significant phosphorylation events take place on the hydroxyl groups of serine and threonine (Hunter 1991). Protein phosphorylation is a truly ubiquitous phenomenon, both in terms of the range of proteins modified—a murine fibroblast contains several hundred phosphoproteins (Levenson and Blackshear 1989) and a *Escherichia coli* contains over a hundred (Cortay *et al.* 1991)—as well as the diversity of organisms in which it has been observed. Virtually all living cells, regardless of function, habitat, or phylogeny, are sites of protein phosphorylation.

Although the addition or subtraction of a phosphoryl group represents a relatively minute change in terms of the mass or charge of a protein comprised of hundreds of amino acids, phosphorylation often dramatically alters its functional properties. Phosphorylation is essential for the catalytic activation of many enzymes, while for others it attenuates their catalytic efficiency. Affinities for substrates or other ligands, including subunits that target enzymes to particular intracellular locations, may be increased or decreased manyfold. Although other post-translational modification events such as methylation or glycosylation can also affect the functions of the proteins that they target, phosphorylation stands out by virtue of its widespread utilization and readily reversible nature. The ability to alter the functions of proteins rapidly, dramatically, and reversibly via phosphorylation provides cells with a powerful and versatile means of meeting the challenges of existence in a dynamic external environment. Some of the processes that are regulated, in whole or in part, by the phosphorylation of proteins on serine and threonine residues are listed below:

- glycogen metabolism (Cohen 1988);
- fatty acid biosynthesis (Hardie 1989; Hardie *et al.* 1989);
- cholesterol biosynthesis (Hardie *et al.* 1989; Kennelly 1991);
- progression through the cell division cycle (Cyert and Thorner 1989);
- muscle contraction (Sellers and Adelstein 1987);
- hormonal signal transduction (Cohen 1988);
- protein translation rates (Hershey 1989; Erikson 1991);
- neuronal signal transduction (Walaas and Greengard 1991).

The intimate involvement of protein phosphorylation events in the co-ordination and regulation of this broad spectrum of cell functions has rendered the process a prominent and attractive target for pharmacological intervention.

3A.2   Protein kinases: nomenclature and classification

The class of enzymes that catalyse the covalent phosphorylation of proteins is referred to as the protein kinases. In the overwhelming majority of cases, the source of the modifying phosphoryl moiety is the γ phosphate of an ATP molecule that is complexed to a divalent metal ion, usually Mg^{2+}. Although most protein kinases show a very high selectivity for ATP as the phosphoryl donor some, such as casein kinase 2, can utilize other nucleotide triphosphates such as GTP (Pinna 1990).

To date, the existence of over a hundred protein serine–threonine kinases has been documented with a rate of discovery that is increasing in logarithmic fashion (Hunter 1987). For further information concerning their individual identities, as well as descriptions of their physical and functional characteristics, the reader is referred to a number of extensive reviews and the references contained therein (Edelman *et al*. 1987; Hunter and Sefton 1991a,b). The explosive growth in membership of the protein kinase family has given rise to a complex and unsystematic nomenclature. The earliest means of designating individual protein kinases, first employed for phosphorylase kinase (Krebs *et al*. 1958), was to name them after a substrate protein. While this is often one of the enzyme's physiological targets, as is the case for myosin light-chain kinase or the β-adrenergic receptor kinase, in some instances it may be an exogenous substrate protein of questionable physiological relevance but which played a pivotal role in the identification of the enzyme, as was the case for casein kinases 1 and 2. The second means employed historically was to name them after the cellular second messengers that modulate their activity. This became necessary as it was realized, initially for phosphorylase kinase kinase and later for other protein kinases, that these enzymes were capable of phosphorylating multiple protein substrates. As a consequence, phosphorylase kinase kinase was renamed the cAMP-dependent protein kinase (Walsh *et al*. 1968). More recently, the breakthroughs made possible by molecular genetic techniques have led to the designation of new protein kinases using the acronyms for the genes that encode them, i.e. *raf* kinase or c-*mos* kinase. Occasionally, shortened trivial names have come into common use because of their simplicity and convenience, as with protein kinase C, the Ca^{2+}- and phospholipid-dependent protein kinase.

As more and more protein kinases continue to be discovered, the drawbacks of this eclectic unsystematic approach to their nomenclature have become increasingly apparent. This is particularly true with regard to substrate-based nomenclature, as it has been found that phosphorylation of a common substrate protein is not generally indicative of a close genetic relationship. Hanks and coworkers, in a set of classic papers (Hanks *et al*. 1988; Hanks and Quinn 1991), have provided the first truly systematic classification scheme for protein kinases, which is based upon their primary structure. It remains to be seen whether this will give rise, in turn, to a more systematic nomenclature for these enzymes.

3A.3   Protein serine–threonine kinase structure

Amino acid sequences—many derived from DNA clones—from the catalytic domains of nearly a hundred protein serine–threonine kinases have been accumulated to date. Comparison of these sequences reveals that the protein serine–threonine kinases belong to a single genetic superfamily that includes, as one of its branches, the protein tyrosine kinases (Hanks *et al*. 1988; Hanks and Quinn 1991). These enzymes share a common catalytic core spanning about 280 amino acids that is marked by several conserved sequence motifs such as the Gly-Xaa-Gly-Xaa-Xaa-Gly-Xaa$_{14-23}$-Lys sequence from the ATP binding site. The components of this nucleotide-binding fold dominate the N-terminal portion of the common catalytic core, leaving the function of binding protein substrates to the C-terminal region.

Recently, the first X-ray crystal structure of a protein kinase, that of the catalytic subunit of the cAMP-dependent protein kinase, was solved by Knighton and colleagues (1991a,b). The catalytic subunit is globular in nature and is composed of two distinct lobes that correspond to the N-terminal nucleotide-binding and C-terminal protein-binding domains suggested from sequence comparisons. Peptide and protein substrates bind in a distinct furrow on the surface of the C-terminal region that continues along the interface of the two lobes (Knighton *et al.* 1991b). The phospho-acceptor threonine or serine is positioned near the interface of the two lobes with the phosphoryl binding portion of the nucleotide-binding domain positioned directly above. Immediately adjacent is Asp_{166}, whose carboxylate group, located on a very short loop joining two helical segments of the C-terminal lobe, is believed to act as a base during catalysis.

Although sequence comparisons and X-ray crystallographic data indicate that the C-terminal portion of the catalytic core participates in substrate protein binding, it is not clear whether this function resides exclusively in this domain for every protein serine–threonine kinase. Studies of skeletal muscle myosin light-chain kinase have implicated the involvement of regions N-terminal to the common catalytic core in the recognition of protein and peptide substrates. Early work indicated that partial proteolysis of the N-terminal region with trypsin, which left the catalytic core and regulatory domains intact, nevertheless significantly attenuated the catalytic efficiency of the enzyme (Edelman *et al.* 1985). Monoclonal antibodies whose binding maps to areas N-terminal to the core competitively inhibited the binding of peptide substrates (Nunnally *et al.* 1987), and mutagenesis of certain amino acids in this region increased the enzyme's K_m for substrate peptides about tenfold (Herring *et al.* 1990). Thus, areas outside the common catalytic core may contribute to substrate protein binding and recognition for myosin light-chain kinase and, by implication, for other protein kinases as well.

3A.4 Recognition of protein and peptide substrates by protein serine–threonine kinases

Despite its prolific nature, protein phosphorylation is a precisely targeted process. For example, while most phosphorylated proteins contain many serine and threonine residues, a given protein serine–threonine kinase will generally modify only one or two discrete members of this set. Yet many of these same protein kinases phosphorylate a number of proteins that differ widely in their size, shape, amino acid composition, and function.

The explanation for this paradoxically broad yet narrow substrate specificity is that protein serine–threonine kinases appear to recognize discrete sites on proteins rather than the protein as a whole.

The most widely accepted paradigm for the structure of these recognition sites is the consensus sequence model (Pinna 1988; Kemp and Pearson 1991; Kennelly and Krebs 1991). This model defines the basic substrate recognition unit as the amino acid sequence of the polypeptide chain immediately surrounding the phosphoacceptor threonine or serine. The presence of particular amino acids within this unit and their positioning relative to the phosphoacceptor amino acid forms a code, known as a consensus sequence, that is characteristic of each particular kinase. Such consensus sequences generally range in size from four to eight amino acids, although at least one contains nearly 20.

Not all of the amino acids surrounding the site of phosphorylation form essential parts of a consensus sequence. Some positions appear to be recognition-neutral. Charge factors appear to play an important role since most consensus sequences prominently feature amino acids with ionizable side-chains such as lysine, arginine, glutamate, aspartate, and even the modified amino acids phosphoserine and phosphothreonine. One notable exception is the proline-directed protein kinases, whose dominant recognition feature is a proline residue immediately C-terminal to the phosphoacceptor group (Vulliet *et al.* 1989). Examples of consensus sequences are Arg-Xaa-Xaa-Ser*/Thr* for the calmodulin-dependent protein kinase type II (where the asterisk denotes the amino acid that becomes phosphorylated) (Payne *et al.* 1983; Pearson *et al.* 1985) and Ser*/Thr*-Xaa-Xaa-Xaa-Phosphoserine for glycogen synthase kinase 3 (Fiol *et al.* 1990). Unfortunately not all consensus sequences can be defined with such precision. Protein kinase C, for example, avidly phosphorylates serine and threonine residues bracketed by basic amino acids. However, the enzyme will also efficiently phosphorylate substrates whose phosphorylation sites contain basic amino acids on *either* the C- or N-terminal sides of the phosphoacceptor group.

Although the consensus sequence model has been successfully applied to understanding the behaviour of several protein kinases, it is unlikely that phosphorylation site sequence alone will prove to be the sole factor in determining substrate recognition. Some protein kinases, such as phosphorylase kinase, display substrate specificities that cannot be fully explained on the basis of local primary sequence factors (Graves 1983). Moreover, not all sites on proteins that conform to a particular consensus sequence are actually phosphorylated. Presumably, factors such as the geometry of the phosphorylation site or the features of distant portions of the polypeptide chain, which nevertheless may be closely proximate in space, play important and sometimes dominant roles in substrate recognition by protein serine–threonine kinases.

3A.5   Regulation of protein serine–threonine kinases

As key intermediaries in cellular regulatory and signal transduction networks, the activities of many protein serine–threonine kinases are themselves stringently regulated (Edelman *et al*. 1987). In some cases this is accomplished via the binding of second messengers, such as cAMP, Ca^{2+}, or diacylglycerol, or a cellular metabolite such as AMP. Often the activity of a particular protein kinase is itself regulated by either autophosphorylation or phosphorylation by another protein kinase. Since protein kinases function catalytically, this latter event (often referred to as a protein kinase cascade) provides an important means for the intracellular amplification of extracellular signals (Krebs 1989). Another, less frequently employed, mechanism is substrate level regulation. Glycogen synthase kinase 3 phosphorylates glycogen synthase, for example, but only after the latter has been phosphorylated by a second protein kinase, casein kinase 2 (Roach 1991), while the β-adrenergic receptor kinase only phosphorylates β-adrenergic receptors that are in the agonist-bound state (Benovic *et al*. 1986). Intracellular localization may also play a role in protein kinase regulation, as seen in the agonist and phorbol-ester-induced translocation of protein kinase C to membranes (Nishikuza 1989; Nelsestuen and Bazzi 1991). To date, few intracellular inhibitors of protein kinases with potential physiological significance have been discovered. One exception is the protein kinase inhibitor PKI, which potently blocks the activity of the cAMP-dependent protein kinase (Walsh *et al*. 1971). However, its precise role in the control of cAMP-dependent protein kinase remains a mystery (Scott 1991; Walsh and Glass 1991).

3A.6   Protein serine–threonine kinases as drug targets: some general considerations

The involvement of protein serine–threonine kinases in controlling and coordinating aspects of virtually every process in the life of a mammalian cell renders them natural targets for the design of inhibitors for scientific study as well as for pharmacological intervention in disease states (see Section 3C). There are essentially three sites on a typical protein serine–threonine kinase that might be targeted by such inhibitors: the ATP substrate binding site, the protein substrate binding site, and the binding site for regulatory molecules. Since many vitally important enzymes bind ATP and most cellular second messengers also possess multiple target sites, the design of specific high affinity inhibitors acting through either of these sites represents a daunting task. Nevertheless, there have been some notable successes in this area, such as H-89 and (Rp)cAMPs, which specifically inhibit cAMP-dependent protein kinase through its ATP- and cAMP-binding sites respectively (Van Haastert *et al*. 1984; Chijiwa *et al*. 1990). In general, however, it would appear that the most promising site to consider for producing highly specific inhibitors of protein serine–threonine kinases is the protein substrate binding site, as compounds directed thereto would be the least likely to have secondary sites of action elsewhere in the cell.

Early attempts to design a potent protein kinase inhibitor focused on substituting a non-phosphorylatable alanine for the phosphoacceptor serine in a high affinity substrate peptide for the cAMP-dependent protein kinase. However, this produced a disappointingly poor inhibitor (Kemp et al. 1977; Feramisco and Krebs 1978). Since then, progress in the design of peptide-based inhibitors of protein kinases has been greatly facilitated by the confirmation of a hypothesis, first proposed by Corbin, that many protein kinases contain 'autoinhibitory' domains within their structures (Soderling 1990). Under basal conditions, these domains block substrate accessibility to the active site by virtue of the ability of the autoinhibitor to mimic a substrate (hence the term pseudosubstrate). Inhibition is then subject to relief by the binding of allosteric activators such as cAMP or Ca_4^{2+}–calmodulin. Initial studies demonstrated that both smooth and skeletal muscle myosin light-chain kinases could be inhibited by peptides modelled after their autoinhibitor domains (Kemp et al. 1987; Kennelly et al. 1987), and subsequent work has seen the development of potent pseudosubstrate inhibitor peptides for a number of protein kinases (Kemp et al. 1991). With the advent of the first three-dimensional structure of a protein kinase catalytic domain (Knighton et al. 1991a,b), even more refined approaches to inhibitor design should now prove possible.

Although recent discoveries presage the design of more specific and more potent protein serine–threonine kinase inhibitors, the successful utilization of these compounds still represents a formidable task. Once it was thought that protein kinases functioned simply as catalytic amplification units in linear signal transduction cascades. However, it has become increasingly clear that these enzymes actually form an interlocking network in which the various signalling cascades engage in active 'cross-talk' with one another. This is perhaps most clearly demonstrated by the phenomenon of hierarchical phosphorylation, where phosphorylation by one protein kinase may be an essential prerequisite for phosphorylation by a second or, in other instances, acts as a block to phosphorylation by the second (Roach 1991). Understanding the complex interrelationships in this interlocking cellular control and coordination network will be a vital factor in the successful application of protein serine–threonine kinase inhibitors to the study and manipulation of living cells.

References

Benovic, J. L., Strasser, R. H., Caron, M. G., and Leftkowitz, R. J. (1986). β-Adrenergic receptor kinase: identification of a novel protein kinase that phosphorylates the agonist-occupied form of the receptor. *Proceedings of the National Academy of Sciences of the United States of America*, **83**, 2797–801.

Chijiwa, T., Mishima, A., Hagiwara, M., Sano, M., Hayashi, K., Inoue, T., *et al.* (1990). Inhibition of forskolin-induced neurite outgrowth and protein phosphorylation by a newly-synthesized selective inhibitor of cyclic AMP-dependent protein kinase, *N*-[2-(p-bromocinnamylamino)ethyl]-5-isoquinolinesulfonamide (H-89), of PC12D pheochromocytoma cells. *Journal of Biological Chemistry*, **265**, 5267–72.

Cohen, P. (1988). Protein phosphorylation and hormone action. *Proceedings of the Royal Society of London, Series B*, **234**, 115–44.

Cortay, J.-C., Negré, D., and Cozzone, A.-J. (1991). Analyzing protein phosphorylation in prokaryotes. *Methods in Enzymology*, **200A**, 214-27.

Cyert, M. S. and Thorner, J. (1989). Putting it on and taking it off: phosphoprotein phosphatase involvement in cell cycle regulation. *Cell*, **57**, 891–3.

Edelman, A. M., Takio, K., Blumenthal, D. K., Hansen, R. S., Walsh, K. A., Titani, K., and Krebs, E. G. (1985). Characterization of the calmodulin-binding and catalytic domains in skeletal muscle myosin light chain kinase. *Journal of Biological Chemistry*, **260**, 11275–85.

Edelman, A. M., Blumenthal, D. K., and Krebs, E. G. (1987). Protein serine/ threonine kinases. *Annual Review of Biochemistry*, **56**, 567–613.

Erikson, R. L. (1991). Structure, expression, and regulation of protein kinases involved the phosphorylation of ribosomal protein S6. *Journal of Biological Chemistry*, **266**, 6007–10.

Feramisco, J. R. and Krebs, E. G. (1978). Inhibition of cyclic AMP-dependent protein kinase by analogues of a synthetic peptide substrate. *Journal of Biological Chemistry*, **253**, 8968–71.

Fiol, C. J., Wang, Y., Roeske, R. W., and Roach, P. J. (1990). Ordered multisite protein phosphorylation. Analysis of glycogen synthase kinase 3 action using model peptide substrates. *Journal of Biological Chemistry*, **265**, 6061–5.

Graves, D. J. (1983). Use of peptide inhibitors to study the specificity of phosphorylase kinase phosphorylation. *Methods in Enzymology*, **99**, 268–78.

Hanks, S. K. and Quinn, A. M. (1991). Protein kinase catalytic domain sequence database: identification of conserved features of primary structure and classification of family members. *Methods in Enzymology*, **200A**, 38–62.

Hanks, S. K., Quinn, A. M., and Hunter, T. (1988). The protein kinase family: conserved features and deduced phylogeny of the catalytic domains. *Science*, **241**, 42–52.

Hardie, D. G. (1989). Regulation of fatty acid synthesis via phosphorylation of acetyl-CoA carboxylase. *Progress in Lipid Research*, **28**, 117–46.

Hardie, D. G., Carling, D., and Sim, A. T. R. (1989). The AMP-activated protein kinase: a multisubstrate regulator of lipid metabolism. *Trends in Biochemical Sciences*, **14**, 20–3.

Herring, B. P., Fitzsimons, D. P., Stull, J. T., and Gallagher, P. J. (1990). Acidic residues comprise part of the myosin light chain-binding site on skeletal muscle myosin light chain kinase. *Journal of Biological Chemistry*, **265**, 16588–91.

Hershey, J. W. B. (1989). Protein phosphorylation controls translation rates. *Journal of Biological Chemistry*, **264**, 20823–6.

Hunter, T. (1987). A thousand and one protein kinases. *Cell*, **50**, 823–9.

Hunter, T. (1991). Protein kinase classification. *Methods in Enzymology*, **200A**, 3–37.

Hunter, T. and Sefton, B. M. (ed.) (1991a). Protein phosphorylation, part A. Protein kinases: assays, purification, antibodies, functional analysis, cloning, and expression. *Methods in Enzymology*, **200A**.

Hunter, T. and Sefton, B. M. (ed.) (1991b). Protein phosphorylation, part B. Analysis of protein phosphorylation, protein kinase inhibitors, and protein phosphatases. *Methods in Enzymology*, **201B**.

Kemp, B. E. and Pearson, R. B. (1990). Protein kinase recognition sequence motifs. *Trends in Biochemical Sciences*, **15**, 342–6.

Kemp, B. E., Graves, D. J., Benjamini, E., and Krebs, E. G. (1977). Role of multiple basic residues in determining the substrate specificity of cyclic AMP-dependent protein kinase. *Journal of Biological Chemistry*, **252**, 4888–94.

Kemp, B. E., Pearson, R. B., Guerriero, V., Jr., Bagchi, I., and Means, A. R. (1987). The calmodulin binding domain of chicken smooth muscle myosin light chain kinase contains a pseudosubstrate sequence. *Journal of Biological Chemistry*, **262**, 2542–8.

Kemp, B. E., Pearson, R. B., and House, C. B. (1991). Pseudosubstrate-based peptide inhibitors. *Methods in Enzymology*, **201B**, 287–304.

Kennelly, P. J. (1991). New perspectives on the role of protein phosphorylation in the regulation of 3-hydroxy-3-methylglutaryl coenzyme A reductase. *Advances in Lipids Research*, **1**, 19–26.

Kennelly, P. J. and Krebs, E. G. (1991). Consensus sequences as substrate specificity determinants for protein kinases and protein phosphatases. *Journal of Biological Chemistry*, **266**, 15555–8.

Kennelly, P. J., Edelman, A. M., Blumenthal, D. K., and Krebs, E. G. (1987). Rabbit skeletal muscle myosin light chain kinase: The calmodulin-binding domain as a potential active site-directed inhibitory domain. *Journal of Biological Chemistry*, **262**, 11958–3.

Knighton, D. R., Zheng, J., Ten Eyck, L. F., Ashford, V. A., Xuong, N.-H., Taylor, S. S., and Sowadski, J. M. (1991a) Crystal structure of the catalytic subunit of cyclic adenosine monophosphate-dependent protein kinase. *Science*, **253**, 407–14.

Knighton, D. R., Zheng, J., Ten Eyck, L. F., Xuong, N.-H., Taylor, S. S., and Sowadski, J. M. (1991b). Structure of a peptide inhibitor bound to the catalytic subunit of cyclic adenosine monophospnate-dependent protein kinase. *Science*, **253**, 414–20.

Krebs, E. G. (1989). Role of the cyclic AMP-dependent protein kinase in signal transduction. *Journal of the American Medical Association*, **262**, 1815–18.

Krebs, E. G., Kent, A. B., and Fischer, E. H. (1958). The muscle phosphorylase b kinase reaction. *Journal of Biological Chemistry*, **231**, 78–83.

Levenson, R. M. and Blackshear, P. J. (1989). Insulin-stimulated protein tyrosine phosphorylation in intact cells evaluated by giant two-dimensional gel electrophoresis. *Journal of Biological Chemistry*, **264**, 19984–93.

Nelsestuen, G. L. and Bazzi, M. D. (1991). Activation and regulation of protein kinase C enzymes. *Journal of Bioenergetics and Biomembranes*, **23**, 43–61.

Nishizuka, Y. (1989). The family of protein kinase C for signal transduction. *Journal of the American Medical Association*, **262**, 1826–33.

Nunnally, M. H., Hsu, L.-C., Mumby, M. C., and Stull, J. T. (1987). Structural studies of rabbit skeletal muscle myosin light chain kinase with monoclonal antibodies. *Journal of Biological Chemistry*, **262**, 3833–8.

Payne, M. E., Schworer, C. M., and Soderling, T. R. (1983). Purification and characterization of rabbit liver calmodulin-dependent glycogen synthase kinase. *Journal of Biological Chemistry*, **258**, 2376–82.

Pearson, R. B., Woodgett, J. R., Cohen, P., and Kemp, B. E. (1985). Substrate specificity of a multifunctional calmodulin-dependent protein kinase. *Journal of Biological Chemistry*, **260**, 14471–6.

Pinna, L. A. (1988). Structural basis for the specificity of protein phosphorylation and dephosphorylation processes. *Advances in Experimental Medicine and Biology*, **231**, 433–3.

Pinna, L. A. (1990). Casein kinase 2: an 'eminence grise' in cellular regulation? *Biochimica et Biophysica Acta*, **1054**, 267–84.

Roach, P. J. (1991). Multisite and hierarchical protein phosphorylation. *Journal of Biological Chemistry*, **266**, 14139–142.

Scott, J. D. (1991). Cyclic nucleotide-dependent protein kinases. *Pharmacology and Therapeutics*, **50**, 123–45.

Sellers, J. R. and Adelstein, R. S. (1987). Regulation of contractile activity. *Enzymes*, **18**, 381–418.

Soderling, T. R. (1990). Protein kinases. Regulation by autoinhibitory domains. *Journal of Biological Chemistry*, **265**, 1823–6.

Van Haastert, P. J. M., Van Driel, R., Jastorff, B., Baraniak, J., Stec, W. J., and De Wit, R. J. W. (1984). Competitive cAMP antagonists for cAMP-receptor proteins. *Journal of Biological Chemistry*, **259**, 10020–4.

Vulliet, P. R., Hall, F. L., Mitchell, J. P., and Hardie, D. G. (1989). Identification of a novel proline-directed serine/threonine protein kinase in rat pheochromocytoma. *Journal of Biological Chemistry*, **264**, 16292–8.

Walaas, S. I. and Greengard, P. (1991). Protein phosphorylation and neuronal function. *Pharmacological Reviews* **43**, 299–349.

Walsh, D. A. and Glass, D. B. (1991). Utilization of the inhibitor of adenosine cyclic monophosphate-dependent protein kinase, and peptides derived from it, as tools to study adenosine cyclic monophosphate-mediated cellular processes. *Methods in Enzymology*, **201B**, 304–16.

Walsh, D. A., Perkins, J. P., and Krebs, E. G. (1968). An adenosine 3′,5′-monophosphate-dependent protein kinase from rabbit skeletal muscle. *Journal of Biological Chemistry*, **243**, 3763–5.

Walsh, D. A., Ashby, C. D., Gonzalez, C., Calkins, D., Fischer, E. H., and Krebs, E. G. (1971). Purification and characterization of a protein inhibitor of adenosine 3′,5′-monophosphate-dependent protein kinase. *Journal of Biological Chemistry*, **246**, 1977–85.

Section 3B

Protein kinase C: its properties and role in signal transduction

Alastair Aitken

3B.1 Introduction

Protein kinase C (PKC) is a widespread enzyme involved in a broad range of biological processes. It has a key role in mediating second-messenger signals inside the cell and consists of a large number of isoforms that are (mostly) distinct gene products. These isoforms may have distinct properties, such as tissue distribution and intracellular localization, distinct mechanisms of activation (e.g. regulation by proteolysis and Ca^{2+} dependency of some isoforms), and distinct substrate specificity. Therefore there is flexibility in the function of PKC isoforms that may permit them to be possible targets for different drugs. Activation (or inhibition) of specific isoforms by distinct phorbol esters indicates that they are potential targets of structurally manipulated phorbol esters in the design of novel drugs.

3B.2   Purification, enzymatic properties, and distribution of PKC

PKC was first discovered by Nishizuka and coworkers (Inoue et al. 1977) who described it as a proteolytically activated enzyme which was present in many tissues. It was later shown to be a Ca^{2+}-activated phospholipid-dependent enzyme. The role of the kinase in signal transduction was later established by the demonstration that diacylglycerol (DAG) is essential for the activation of this kinase. DAG is a second messenger, a product of the hydrolysis of phosphatidylinositol-4,5-bisphosphate (PIP_2) which is stimulated by a wide range of hormones and neurotransmitters (Michel 1983; Berridge 1984).

3B.2.1   Phosphatidylinositol turnover

The role of DAG in activating kinase C is illustrated in Fig. 3B.1. On activation by either DAG or phorbol esters, PKC, which is mainly associated with the cytoplasm, becomes attached to the inside of the plasma membrane (Kraft and Anderson 1983). It has been suggested that the increase in intracellular calcium directs PKC association with the membrane while DAG enhances this association, leading to activation of at least some isoforms of the enzyme. Although it is now membrane associated, PKC is still capable of phosphorylating specific intracellular proteins.

Different PKC signal pathway responses may apply when cells are presented with different agonists. For example, PKC has been shown to be partially activated by phorbol esters without association with phospholipid, indicating that at least some isoforms may function without binding to membrane phospholipid (Da Silva et al. 1990). PKC stimulation by platelet-activating factor is independent of translocation. Therefore, this phospholipid mediator may directly modulate activity of pre-existing membrane-associated PKC by a novel mechanism, rather than eliciting its recruitment from the cytosol (Pelech et al. 1990). There may be selective translocation of PKC isoforms in cells stimulated with phorbol esters (Fournier et al. 1989). Association of thyrotropin-releasing hormone (TRH) and phorbol dibutyrate-activated PKC a isoform with detergent-solublilized material suggests that activated a-PKC may be associated through its pseudosubstrate region (see §3B.3) with membrane and cytoskeletal components (Kiley and Jaken 1990). Other authors studying the site(s) of interaction of PKC with the plasma membrane have produced evidence for association with a 'receptor for activated C kinase' protein(s) ('RACKs') (Mochly-Rosen et al. 1991).

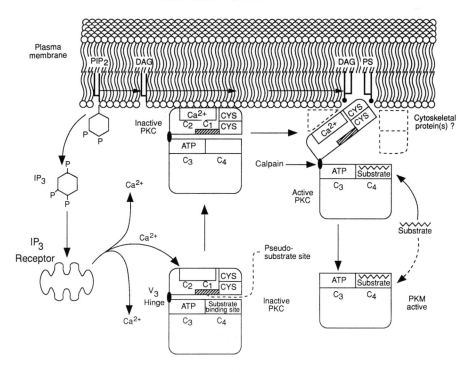

Fig. 3B.1 Phosphatidylinositol hydrolysis and activation of PKC. On binding to its receptor on the cell surface, the agonist stimulates hydrolysis of PIP_2, catalysed by a phospholipase C, to produce the two second messengers inositol-1,4, 5-trisphosphate (IP_3) and DAG. The former is responsible for triggering release of Ca^{2+} ions from internal stores in the endoplasmic recticulum. The increased level of Ca^{2+} then activates Ca^{2+}-dependent protein kinases and regulates many other intracellular events. In the other branch of the response to the agonist, DAG activates the Ca^{2+}- and phospholipid-dependent PKC. The phospholipid, normally phosphatidylserine, is indicated as PS. The figure is described for the α, β, and γ (group A) isoforms of PKC. The other forms may be calcium independent, since they lack the putative Ca^{2+}-binding region in the regulatory domain (Fig. 3B.3). The potential role of cytoskeletal proteins in the association of PKC with the plasma membrane is also illustrated. In addition to this active (intact) membrane-associated PKC, proteolysis by calpain may occur to form the constitutively active (second-messenger-independent) catalytic fragment protein kinase M (PKM). The positions in the linear amino acid sequence of the constant (C_x) and variable (V_y) regions, as well as the cysteine-rich domains (CYS) in PKC isoforms, are shown in Fig. 3B.3.

As well as functioning as a second messenger in the stimulation of PKC activity, DAG may also be a precursor for the release of arachidonic acid which is required for the synthesis of prostaglandins, leukotrienes, and thromboxane. Preferential hydrolysis of phosphoinositides with arachidonic acid (the most common fatty acid) in the 2-position may occur (Mahadevappa and Holub 1983).

In addition to PIP_2 hydrolysis, DAG may be derived from phosphoinositides or phosphatidylcholine (PC). Sequential action of a specific phospholipase D (Mattila 1991) and a phosphatase may produce DAG. Lacal *et al*. (1987) have attributed this to the actions of vasopressin, platelet-derived growth factor (PDGF), bombesin, and interleukin-1.

Phorbol-ester-mediated activation of PKC may also enhance production of DAG through hydrolysis of PC and synthesis of this phospholipid (Daniel *et al*. 1986; Kolesnick 1987). Phosphatidic acid (PA) generated from the hydrolysis of PC by phospholipase D (PLD) may also be regulated by PKC and G_o protein (Bocckino *et al*. 1987). The PC–PLD–PA pathway regulated by the muscarinic-acetylcholine receptor may be a novel mechanism for activation of PKC resulting from production of DAG from PC (Qian and Drewes 1990). Activation of PKC by DAG generated from either PIP_2 or PC could perpetuate further production of DAG from PC (a larger pool of membrane phospholipid). This could stimulate membrane bound PKC without causing a persistent rise in calcium and may also cause a sustained response. Potentially, this could be a mechanism for the specific activation of 'group B' isoforms of PKC that are not Ca^{2+}-dependent.

A third main source of DAG may be from the inositol-containing glycolipid glycosylphosphatidylinositol, which is the membrane anchor of many proteins attached to the outside of the plasma membrane (Ferguson and Williams 1988). The action of a distinct phospholipase C would produce a structurally distinct DAG, perhaps mediated by the action of insulin (Salteil and Cuatrecasas 1988 (see Fig. 3B.2).

Some of the novel forms of PKC that have been described recently have been shown to be preferentially activated by other phospholipids, for example PKC δ (Mizuno *et al*. 1991) which is most potently activated by phosphatidylinositol (PI).

Normally, after induction of phosphatidylinositol breakdown by agonists, degradative pathways would remove these two second messengers (DAG and IP_3) rapidly when the external signal, the agonist, is removed. DAG is converted either to phosphatidic acid (by a diacylglycerol kinase) or to a monoacylglycerol. This is an important point to consider when seeking a basis for the tumour-promoting and other effects of phorbol esters (see §3B.4). Their biological effects may be due to the fact that the activation of PKC by phorbol esters is of longer duration than would be seen on activation by DAG. Evidence that the relative importance of each branch of the phosphatidylinositol hydrolysis pathway may vary with time has been obtained in a comparative study of the effects of 12-*O*-tetradecanoyl-phorbol-13-acetate (TPA) on platelet myosin phosphorylation (§3B.4.5.6). Calcium may be involved in the initiation of some of the effects, while

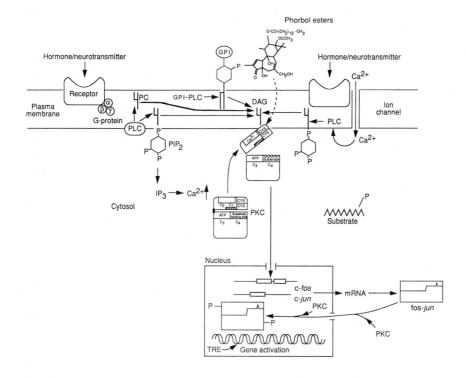

Fig. 3B.2 Activation of PKC by alternative pathways. As well as through PIP_2 hydrolysis, illustrated in Fig. 3B.1, PKC can be activated by hydrolysis of PC by a specific phospholipase C (PLC), also linked to a G-protein-coupled receptor (left-hand side of figure). The classes of receptor coupled to phosphatidylinositol hydrolysis (see Fig. 3B.2) include the a_1-adrenergic, H_1-histaminergic, muscarinic-cholinergic, V_1-vasopressin, and cytokine receptors (including interleukins). PLC may also be activated directly via binding of a hormone or neurotransmitter to a receptor (e.g. glutamate, NMDA receptor), which causes a calcium channel to open (right-hand side of figure). The influx of calcium may then activate the PLC resulting in hydrolysis of PIP_2. Growth hormone may activate PLC-γ on binding to their receptors (see Section 3B.4.5.1). PKC may also be activated by DAG released from the protein anchor glycosylphosphatidylinositol (GPI) by the action of a particular phospholipase C (GPI-PLC, centre of figure). Some of these pathways may be more important for the activation of the Ca^{2+}-independent forms of PKC. The direct activation of PKC by phorbol esters is also illustrated. The effects of PKC on gene transcription are shown in the lower portion of the figure. An early event that occurs when PKC is translocated to the nucleus in response to phorbol ester treatment is induction of 'TPA inducible sequences', including the proto-oncogenes c-*fos* and c-*jun*. These proteins form a heterodimer (AP-1 complex) and, after phosphorylation by PKC (inside or outside the nucleus), bind to a specific DNA sequence, the 'TPA response element' (TRE). This results in activation of specific genes in a long-term response (Rozengurt and Sinnett-Smith 1987).

diacylglycerol may be more important in the maintenance of the response to agonists. This type of synergistic effect has been observed where a combination of growth hormone (insulin or epidermal growth factor) and PIP_2 agonist has led to much greater activation of cell proliferation than one type of agonist alone. PDGF and epidermal growth factor (EGF) have been shown to possess the ability both to stimulate tyrosine kinase activity and to enhance PIP_2 breakdown (Berridge 1984) by stimulation of a γ-PLC.

In most systems so far studied, the stimulation of phosphatidylinositol metabolism is independent of an increase in the intracellular level of calcium. However, in a few cases, such as neutrophils (Cockroft 1981), stimulation of phosphatidylinositol turnover does appear to be dependent on calcium. There is evidence that, besides the formation of inositol-1, 4,5-trisphosphate (IP_3) which releases Ca^{2+} from internal stores, phosphatidylinositol metabolism may also be responsible for increasing the permeability of the plasma membrane to calcium.

The affinity of PKC for calcium is greatly increased in the presence of DAG such that some forms of the enzyme may be activated in a physiological system without an increase in intracellular calcium (Takai *et al.* 1979; Kishimoto *et al.* 1980). Some recently discovered members of the family have been shown to be calcium independent and are discussed in §3B.3.

3B.2.2   Purification and properties of PKC

The enzyme was first purified from rat brain by Nishizuka and coworkers (Kikkawa *et al.* 1982). PKC has also been purified to homogeneity from bovine brain by Parker *et al.* (1984) using a combination of ion-exchange, gel exclusion, and hydrophobic interaction chromatography.

The purified brain enzyme (a mixture of a, β, and γ forms) is dependent on Ca^{2+} (with a K_a in the micromolar range) and phospholipid (particularly phosphatidylserine). Five other phospholipids (phosphatidylinositol, phosphatidylethanolamine, phosphatidylcholine, phosphatidic acid, and sphingomyelin) were shown to be ineffective in stimulating brain PKC. Indeed, phosphatidylcholine and sphingomyelin inhibited the enzyme (Kaibuchi *et al.* 1981) The latter class of molecule (sphingosine and lysosphingolipids) binds at the DAG–phorbol dibutyrate site (Hannun and Bell 1987), and sphingosine may act as a natural regulator of PKC owing to its high concentration in cells (Hannun *et al.* 1986; Bell and Burns 1991).

The purified enzyme from bovine brain exhibits two apparent K_a values for phosphatidylserine of approximately 0.6–2.0 and 35–80 μg ml^{-1}. Single K_a values of 6–20 μg ml^{-1} were reported for the enzyme from other tissues. In the presence of 1,2-diacylglycerol (diolein), the K_a for Ca^{2+} is reduced from 10 to 1 μm (Kaibuchi *et al.* 1981).

The naturally occuring 1,2-*sn*-DAG (but not 1,3-*sn*-DAG) activates PKC (Boni and Rando 1985). The structural requirements are strict (Ganong *et al.* 1986): both carboxyl moieties of the oxygen esters are required, and any replacement of the 3-hydroxyl group or addition of a single carbon atom in the glycerol backbone results in loss of biological activity (Huang 1989).

PKC may also be directly activated by other metabolites resulting from the receptor-mediated phospholipase A_2 hydrolysis of phospholipids. These include lysophosphatidylcholine (lysoPC) (Oishi *et al.* 1988), lipoxin A (Hannson *et al.* 1986), and free arachidonate (McPhail *et al.* 1984). The δ isoform of PKC shows a different sensitivity to arachidonate (Ono *et al.* 1988). LysoPC can stimulate PKC at low concentration but inhibit it at high concentrations in the *in vitro* assay (Oishi *et al.* 1988). LysoPC-mediated activation of PKC is synergistic with activation by DAG. The membrane concentration of PC is much higher than that of PI; therefore the potential for cells to generate free fatty acid and lysoPC is greater than that for DAG. Recent studies (Shinomura *et al.* 1991) have shown synergistic effects of DAG with a wide range of unsaturated fatty acids on individual isoforms of PKC.

The enzyme from bovine and rat brain has been shown to bind close to 1 mol ^{3}H-phorbol dibutyrate, furnishing proof that PKC is the phorbol ester receptor. The bovine and rat brain preparations bound this phorbol ester with K_a values of 15 nM and 8 nM respectively. The binding is competitively inhibited by DAG (Sharkey *et al.* 1984). The presence of DAG or phorbol dibutyrate lowered the K_a values for phosphatidylserine in bovine brain PKC by a factor of 2–3.

3B.2.3 Assay for PKC

There are two methods for the assay of PKC activity *in vitro* which provide the opportunity of observing different effects of activators and inhibitors.

Assay methods employing phospholipid vesicles produced by sonication of phosphatidylserine have been widely accepted (Castagna *et al.* 1982; Parker *et al.* 1984), while, more recently, the use of mixed micelles has allowed independent variation of phospholipid and other cofactors (Hannun *et al.* 1985). The latter method has facilitated the demonstration of a higher degree of phospholipid specificity owing to lower artefact effects of calcium-dependent activation by the anionic surface of the phospholipid vesicles. Activation by DAG or phorbol esters may be greater in Triton X-100 mixed micelles.

3B.2.4 PKC isoforms

3B.2.4.1 *Separation of individual PKC isoforms*

The major isoforms of PKC expressed in mammalian brain can be separated on a hydroxylapatite column. The enzymes are eluted with a gradient of phosphate (Jaken and Kiley 1987; Marais and Parker 1989). This method has been used to study the biochemical properties of individual isoforms. The isoforms are separated into three peaks of activity, eluting at 80, 100, and 145 mM phosphate. These were designated types I, II, and III, which correspond to PKC γ, β, and α respectively. The β_I and β_{II} isoforms do not separate under these conditions, and in other tissues or cell types (e.g. platelets), the δ isoform coelutes with the β isoform(s) (Mischak *et al*. 1991).

Type I PKC (γ) was reported to be less calcium dependent than types II and III (Jaken and Kiley 1987; Kosaka *et al*. 1988). Type I was shown to be less sensitive to DAG but more responsive to arachidonic acid (Naor *et al*. 1988), while type III was most responsive to DAG.

Additional evidence for the differential regulation of isoforms of PKC has been obtained from the work of El Touny *et al*. (1990). Oleic acid preferentially activated non-membrane-bound forms of PKC that were relatively resistant to inhibition by sphingosine, although neither this soluble form nor the membrane-bound (particulate) form was assigned to a particular isoform(s).

The individual PKC isoforms have been expressed in a variety of cell types, for example PKC ε in baculovirus vector (Schaap and Parker 1990) and PKC δ, η, ζ in COS-7 cells (Ono *et al*. 1988; Olivier and Parker 1991). For a detailed study of potential inhibitors of specific isoforms, purification from these sources may be preferable to ensure that each form is free from contamination with another isoform. References to the primary publications will be found in the discussion of the particular isoforms.

3B.2.4.2 *Distribution of PKC isoforms*

Kinase C is widely distributed among phyla, ranging from yeast (Farago and Nishizuka 1990) through insects (*Drosophila*) to mammals. It has been purified from many of these sources and has also been reported to be present in the bacterium *Escherichia coli* (Norris *et al*. 1991).

PKC has been identified in many cellular subcompartments (e.g. Dunphy *et al*. 1981) and immunocytochemical studies have been carried out (Capitani *et al*. 1987). Tissue distribution of isoforms of PKC varies widely (Nishizuka 1988). α PKC appears to be expressed in all tissues and cell types examined to date, although its localization in brain tissue shows that it is heavily involved in control of specific functions of some neurones (Ito *et al*. 1990).

PKC β_I and β_{II} are expressed in different ratios in the brain and other tissues. In the brain, immunocytochemical analysis has shown that β_I is located mainly in the granular layer of the cerebellar cortex while β_{II} is found mainly in the presynaptic nerve endings (Nishizuka 1988). PKC γ is expressed only in neural tissue such as brain and spinal cord (Farago and Nishizuka 1990). In the rat, it is expressed postnatally and reaches a maximum 3 weeks after birth. In the mammalian brain, particularly high levels of PKC γ are found in the hippocampus, the amygdaloid complex, and the cerebellar cortex (Nishizuka 1988). Isoforms have been shown to be specifically expressed in certain types of central nervous system tumour (Shimosawa *et al.* 1990).

Of the more recently described isoforms, PKC ε is expressed mainly in brain tissue (Ono *et al.* 1988). An isoform that may be related to PKC ζ has been isolated from the nuclei of nerve cells (Hagiwara *et al.* 1990).

3B.2.4.3 *Nuclear PKC*

PKC has been shown to bind DNA (Testori *et al.* 1988); however, the physiological relevance is unknown, since it is a basic protein. PKC isoforms have been identified in the nucleus (Masmoudi *et al.* 1989), and translocation of PKC to the nucleus has been reported in cells treated with tumour-promoting phorbol esters (Vilgrain *et al.* 1984; Costa-Casnellie *et al.* 1985; Kiss *et al.* 1988; Leach *et al.* 1989). An early event that occurs on translocation of PKC to the nucleus is induction of 'TPA inducible sequences' including the proto-oncogenes c-*fos* and c-*jun* (Sheng and Greenberg 1990). The effects of PKC on gene transcription are illustrated in Fig. 3B.2.

Irvine and coworkers have recently reported evidence for a polyphosphoinositide cycle in the nucleus of Swiss 3T3 cells (Divecha *et al.* 1991). This leads to an increase in the nuclear concentration of DAG and induces translocalization of PKC to the nucleus. This response was due to an insulin-like growth factor (IGF-1) receptor in the plasma membrane, in contrast with the effects of bombesin which did not stimulate translocation of PKC to the nucleus.

3B.3 Sequence and domain structure of PKC

3B.3.1 Sequences of PKC isoforms

Cloning and DNA sequencing have confirmed the existence of a large number of isoforms in the PKC 'family'. cDNA clones that encode the α, β_I, β_{II}, and γ isoforms were initially isolated from brain cDNA libraries from a range of mammalian species (Coussens *et al.* 1986; Knopf *et al.* 1986; Ono *et al.* 1986; Parker *et al.* 1986; Kikkawa *et al.* 1987a,b). Genomic analysis revealed that the β_I and β_{II} subspecies are derived from a single mRNA transcript by alternative splicing. They differ from each other only in a short stretch of 50 amino acids at the carboxy terminal end (Kubo *et al.* 1987; Ono *et al.* 1987a). An additional group of cDNA clones encoding the δ, ε and ζ isoforms have been isolated from a rat cDNA library (Ono *et al.* 1988; Parker *et al.* 1989).

Purified PKC is a single polypeptide chain of 77–85 kDa and consists of two domains, regulatory and catalytic. The holoenzyme can be cleaved by the calcium-dependent proteinase calpain into two fragments of 51 kDa and 26 kDa (Kikkawa *et al.* 1982; Kishimoto *et al.* 1983). The larger (catalytic) domain is active in the *absence* of the cofactors and is hydrophilic. The smaller fragment is hydrophobic, contains the regulatory binding sites, and is membrane associated (Lee and Bell 1986). This may be a physiological mechanism for conversion of the enzyme to a cytosolic cofactor-independent, i.e. 'constitutively active', kinase (Pontremoli *et al.* 1988, 1990).

3B.3.2   Down-regulation (or down-modulation)

The process of proteolysis of PKC may also be a mechanism for initiating the degradation of the enzyme. Activation of PKC causes translocation from the cytosol to the plasma membrane (see §3B.2). This is true, at least, for the δ, β, γ, ('group A') isoforms. The Ca^{2+}-independent forms (e.g. ζ) show no translocation or down-regulation. This is followed by depletion of enzyme activity (Blackshear *et al.* 1985; Stabel *et al.* 1987; Borner *et al.* 1988).

Evidence that independent regulation of the levels of isoforms of PKC may occur at the post-transcriptional, i.e. protein, level has been obtained by chronic treatment of a human leukaemic T-cell line with phorbol ester. This resulted in loss, of CD2 and CD3 receptors, accompanied by reduction in α PKC. Levels of mRNA for α, β, and γ were all unaffected (Isakov *et al.* 1990).

The regulatory fragment which contains the zinc-finger-like motif consensus sequence, similar to a DNA-binding motif, may also have a distinct biological role (Ono *et al.* 1989b). Down-regulation by endogenous calcium-dependent proteinases (calpains) may be specific for different isoforms. Calpain treatment of the β isoform(s) results in a cofactor-independent form of protein kinase C (PKM) that is only 50 per cent active while α PKM retains full activity (Pontremoli *et al.* 1990).

3B.3.3   Domain structure of the kinase C isoforms

There are four conserved regions labelled C_1-C_4 (Fig. 3B.3) and five variable regions (V_1-V_5). The pseudosubstrate sequence (§3B.3.6) is located in C_1. This may be responsible for maintaining an inactive form in the absence of cofactors. The phorbol ester–diacylglycerol binding domain is also located in this conserved region where the tandem repeat of the cysteine-rich zinc-finger-like sequence is located (Kaibuchi *et al.* 1989; Ono *et al.* 1989b). The ζ isoform has only one Cys-rich repeat and is not activated by DAG or phorbol ester (Ono *et al.* 1989a).

The C_2 domain may be responsible for Ca^{2+} dependence and in the α isoform contains a potential calcium-binding motif [the F helix of the EF hand motif of the calmodulin class of calcium-binding proteins (Huang

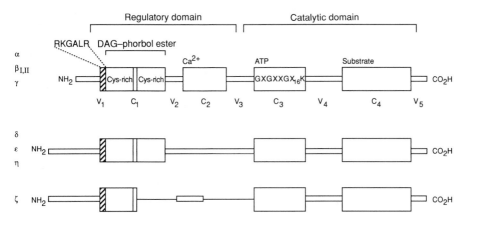

Fig. 3B.3 Domain structure and the linear amino acid sequence of PKC isoforms. There are four conserved regions (C_1–C_4) and five variable regions, (V_1–V_5). The pseudosubstrate sequence for the α, β, and γ isoforms (-RKGALR- in single-letter code for amino acids) is located in C_1. This is shown as a hatched bar. The phorbol ester–diacylglycerol-binding domain is also located in this conserved region where the tandem repeat of the cysteine-rich zinc-finger-like sequence is located. The ζ isoform has only one Cys-rich repeat and has a shorter stretch of primary structure between C_1 and C_3. The variable region V_4 is shorter in the γ isoform. The C_2 domain may be responsible for Ca^{2+} dependence and is absent from the δ, ε, η, and ζ isoforms. The C_3 and C_4 regions have the features of a typical protein kinase catalytic domain with the ATP binding site motif GXGXXG..K (single-letter code for amino acids where X is any residue) in the C_3 region and the substrate binding site located in C_4. The exact nomenclature for the alternately spliced β isoforms may differ between authors. The terms β_I and β_{II} have been used throughout this text.

1989)]. The C_3 and C_4 regions contain the features of a typical protein kinase catalytic domain. The ATP binding site motif is located in the C_3 region.

Now that the X-ray crystal structure of the catalytic subunit of cAMP-dependent protein kinase has been determined (Knighton *et al.* 1991), computer graphic modelling can be carried out on a range of other kinases, since all protein kinases, including protein tyrosine kinases, have homo-logies or conserved features in the catalytic domain (Hanks *et al.* 1988). This should facilitate design of suitable inhibitor compounds specific for a particular class of kinase. However, it will probably be necessary to wait for the three-dimensional structure determination on an isoform of PKC itself before compounds that interact with specific regions of the regulatory domain can be modelled.

The V_3 region contains the site of calpain (and trypsin) cleavage of the group A forms (Kishimoto *et al.* 1983; Huang 1989), i.e. it is the 'hinge' that separates the catalytic and regulatory domains (Coussens *et al.* 1986). Therefore the regions C_3 to V_5 are the catalytic domain fragment that express the constitutively active fragment that is independent of the cofactor effectors Ca^{2+}, phospholipid, and DAG.

Additional evidence for the roles of the different regions has come from mutagenesis, including alteration of the pseudosubstrate site from Ala to Glu (Pears *et al.* 1990) and deletion of the cysteine-rich regions which removed the DAG–phorbol ester binding (Kaibuchi *et al.* 1989; Ono *et al.* 1989b). It has been suggested that, with two cysteine-rich regions in α, β, and γ types, there may be two phorbol ester binding sites (Bell and Burns 1991).

3B.3.4   Differences in distinct isoforms

All isoforms of PKC are phospholipid and DAG dependent. However, forms of PKC that are Ca^{2+} independent, including δ and ε (Schaap and Parker 1990; Mizuno *et al.* 1991) have been characterized. These are members of the so-called 'group B' (Fig. 3B.3). For example, PKC ε distribution between soluble and particulate fractions is independent of Ca^{2+}. The association of the α and β forms with the membrane requires the presence of excess free calcium (Kiley and Jaken 1990).

It has been suggested (Maraganore 1987) that there may be some similarity between phospholipase A_2 and the cysteine repeat region of PKC which is essential for phorbol ester and, by inference, diacylglycerol binding (see above). This could suggest a possible evolutionary origin of this phospholipid- and calcium-requiring protein kinase and the calcium-dependent phospholipase with respect to phospholipid binding site.

3B.3.5   PKC substrate consensus sequences

There are a large number of basic amino acids surrounding the site of phosphorylation (a threonine residue) in the EGF receptor (Hunter *et al.* 1984). Other sites of phosphorylation in the basic proteins histone H1, H2B, and myelin basic protein (all phosphoserine residues) are preceded by basic amino acid residues. The primary structure requirements of PKC would therefore appear to be similar to that of many other protein kinases, particularly cAMP- and cGMP-dependent protein kinases which also have a requirement for basic residues, generally at the N-terminus of the phosphorylatable serine or threonine (Aitken 1990). In fact, there is a clear distinction in substrate site preference and optimal positions of the basic residues are different for each class of kinase, although there are examples of the phosphorylation of identical sites on one substrate protein by three of the kinases (Campbell *et al.* 1986, Hardie *et al.* 1986).

The consensus sequence of substrates for this kinase is based on known *in vivo* sites of phosphorylation. The C-terminal basic residue may be a more important determinant than those at the N-terminus (Woodgett *et al.* 1986; Ferrari *et al.* 1987), in contrast with AMP kinase where a hydrophobic residue on the C-terminal side of the phosphoamino acid is a positive determinant. Additional basic amino acids at the N- and C-terminals enhance the rate of phosphorylation of substrates for PKC (House *et al.* 1987).

Different isoforms have been shown to prefer distinct substrates. This has been demonstrated using different histone preparations (Parker *et al.* 1989). Histones may not be good substrates for 'group B' PKC isoforms (Parker *et al.* 1989). PKC γ has a marked preference (compared with α and β) for synthetic peptides with a basic residue C-terminal to the site of phosphorylation (Marais and Parker 1989). Synthetic peptides from glycogen synthase are phosphorylated best by an isoform that prefers C-terminal basic residues. Other examples include the neuronal specific protein GAP 43 which is a preferred substrate for the β_{II} isoform (Sheu *et al.* 1990) (see §3B.4.5)

The PKC consensus is

$$\text{-Baa}_{1-5}\text{-Ser/Thr-Xaa-Baa-}$$
$$\overset{\text{P}}{\underset{\mid}{\mid}}$$

where Xaa is an uncharged residue and Baa is one to five basic (lysine or arginine) residues N-terminal to the phosphorylatable serine or threonine. This knowledge of the consensus sequence proves useful in the study of the regulation of the activity of many kinases, including PKC, where replacement of the phosphorylatable residue (often by an alanine) converts a peptide substrate into an inhibitor that may be specific for that particular protein kinase and could be a basis for modelling studies for peptide analogues with high affinity. These 'pseudosubstrate' sites are discussed in the next section.

3B.3.6 Pseudosubstrate sequences

For many kinases that have a requirement for basic residues around the phosphorylatable serine or threonine, there is a sequence in the regulatory domain that is homologous with the consensus sequence, where the basic residues and the other elements necessary for a recognition site are in the correct positions but the phosphorylatable serine or threonine is replaced by another residue (particularly alanine). This hypothesis has been proposed to account for the inhibitory sequences in the regulatory domains of a wide range of second-messenger-dependent protein kinases (Hardie 1988; Soderling 1990). Competitive inhibition by this domain is relieved by the conformational change induced by second-messenger binding.

Synthetic peptides containing these so-called 'pseudosubstrate' sequences (Hardie 1988; Pearson *et al.* 1988) may be competitive inhibitors of the kinase (Eicholtz *et al.* 1990), while mutagenesis of the pseudosubstrate site can lead to activation of the enzyme (Pearson *et al.* 1988). Antibodies raised against the pseudosubstrate site have been reported to activate PKC in the absence of cofactors (Farago and Nishizuka 1990).

3B.3.7   Protein inhibitors of PKC

There are now a number of well-characterized proteins that have potent inhibitory activity specific for PKC. We recently described the isolation and characterization of a PKC inhibitor protein from sheep brain named kinase C inhibitor protein 1 (KCIP-1) (Toker *et al.* 1990). This inhibitory activity (IC$_{50}$ 0.85 μM for a dimer of ca. 60 kDa) consisted of several proteins of 29–33 kDa.

The amino acid sequence of KCIP-1 has no similarity to the 17 kDa or 12 kDa PKC inhibitor proteins (termed PKCI-1 and PKCI-2 respectively) isolated by Walsh and co-workers (McDonald *et al.* 1987; Pearson *et al.* 1990). The 17 kDa PKCI-1 has been shown to be a zinc-binding protein. Like PKCI-1, the inhibitory mechanism of KCIP-1 does not appear to involve competition with PKC, its substrates, ATP, or cofactors (calcium or diacylglycerol). There was also no effect on [^{3}H]-phorbol dibutyrate binding. They are members of the same family as 14–3–3 protein, which Yamauchi *et al.* (1981) showed was an activator of tyrosine and tryptophan hydroxylases, the rate-limiting enzymes involved in catecholamine and serotonin biosynthesis respectively, vital for the synthesis of dopamine and other neurotransmitters.

Although tyrosine hydroxylase is phosphorylated and activated by kinase C and cAMP-dependent protein kinase, the protein 14–3–3 was necessary for the activation after phosphorylation by Ca^{2+}-calmodulin-dependent kinase II. All three kinases phosphorylate an identical site on tyrosine hydroxylase, but kinase II phosphorylates an additional unique site. The proposed mechanism involves binding of the acidic C-terminus of 14–3–3 to the regulatory domain of the phospho form of the hydroxylase to induce an active conformation. This is a distinct second step that is not directly linked to phosphorylation of the enzyme.

One region of KCIP–14–3–3 shows close similarity with the conserved carboxy terminus of the family of calcium-, lipid-, and membrane-binding proteins, variously called annexins, lipocortins, etc. This could be the binding site for the regulatory domain of PKC (KCIP-1 does not inhibit PKM (Aitken *et al.* 1990)). This part of the regulatory domain of PKC could be the site of interaction with the plasma membrane or associated cytoskeletal proteins, since synthetic peptides based on this sequence similarity between KCIP and annexins inhibit the interaction of PKC with RACKs (Mochly-

Rosen *et al.* 1991) (see §3B.2.1). The primary structure of KCIP–14–3–3 has a sequence reminiscent of the 'pseudosubstrate' domain of PKC. The mechanism of inhibition could therefore involve association to PKC at the above binding site (in the regulatory domain of PKC) which then localizes this 'pseudosubstrate' site at the active site of PKC.

3B.4 Effects of phorbol esters and other compounds on the activities of PKC

3B.4.1 Phorbol esters

The role of PKC in regulating cellular function has been extensively studied using the specific activators phorbol esters, a group of toxic diterpenes isolated from the plant families Euphorbiaceae and Thymelaceae (Hecker 1968; Evans and Edwards 1987). There are a number of structural types, and these diterpenes, of the tigliane, daphnane, and ingenane classes, have been shown to elicit a wide range of biological responses in different tissues such as tumour promotion, cell proliferation, and lymphocyte mitogenesis (Blumberg 1980), inflammation and erythema of the skin (Evans and Edwards 1987), and prostaglandin production, stimulation of neutrophil degranulation, and platelet activation (Cockroft 1981). TPA administration induces terminal differentiation into macrophages in normal bone marrow promyelocytes and in myeloid leukaemic cells (Feuerstein and Cooper 1983).

All the biologically active phorbol esters are able to activate PKC *in vitro*. However, the structural requirements for phorbol-ester-stimulated platelet aggregation and tumour promotion do not correlate directly with inflammation, lymphocyte mitogenesis, or PKC activation *in vitro*. This is due to an additional requirement of a primary hydroxyl group at C20 of the hydrocarbon nucleus for the aggregatory response which is also essential for tumour-promoting activity (Evans 1986). These results suggest that some derivatives may act through distinct biochemical pathways, possibly through interaction with different receptors.

Further anomalies have been identified since neither of the aggregatory C20 primary hydroxyl derivatives, 12-deoxyphorhol-13-phenylacetate (DOPP) or sapintoxin A (SAP A), have been shown to be first- or second-stage tumour-promoting compounds (Brooks *et al.* 1987a), although the latter was shown to promote the formation of tumours when applied to mouse skin in the presence of a non-promoting dose of Ca^{2+} ionophore. These results could indicate that the less Ca^{2+}-dependent PKC isozymes are important in phorbol-ester-induced tumour promotion.

Phorbol itself belongs to the tigliane group, and its esters have been found in the genera *Croton*, *Sapium*, and *Euphorbia* (Evans 1986). One of these, 12-*O*-tetradecanoylphorbol-13-acetate (TPA), is particularly potent and has been used in many studies of biological activity.

3B.4.2   The stimulation of PKC by structurally diverse phorbol esters

Compounds that are are biologically active (including a wide range of tigliane and ingenane diterpenoids) stimulate PKC with K_a values of 20–50 nmol. In contrast, biologically inactive compounds, including α-sapinine and phorbol-12,13,20-triacetate (Ellis *et al*. 1987a), the daphnane derivative mezerein (Miyake *et al*. 1984), and phorbol 12-retinoate-13-acetate, 4-*O*-methylphorbol-12-myristate-13-acetate, and 12-deoxyphorbol-13-isobutyrate (Leach and Blumbery 1985) activate PKC only at high concentrations (approximately 3 μM required for maximal stimulation compared with 100 nM for TPA).

Compounds that do not activate PKC, or do so only at very high concentrations (such as α-sapinine (Ellis *et al*. 1987a)), still bind competitively with active daphnane and tigliane esters and may effectively act as inhibitors of PKC.

A study of the effects of many of these phorbol esters on individual isoforms of PKC has recently been undertaken (Ryves *et al*. 1991).

3B.4.2.1   In vivo *phosphorylation in response to phorbol esters of distinct biological activity*

Studies of *in vivo* phosphorylation by PKC, using phorbol esters that have different activities *in vitro*, have shown that activation of different isoforms of PKC may underlie the diverse biological effects of phorbol esters. This has been carried out, for example, using platelets as a model system, as well as other cell lines where PKC appears to play an important role.

Administration of a range of tigliane and ingenane diterpenoids, with a different spectrum of biological activity, leads to stimulation of phosphorylation of distinct substrate proteins in GH3 cells, a human pituitary cell line (Brooks *et al*. 1987b). In this cell line, the effects of thyrotropin-releasing hormone are mediated via phosphatidylinositol hydrolysis. Compounds used included 12-deoxyphorbol-13-phenylacetate-20-acetate (DOPPA) which has pro-inflammatory properties but is essentially non-tumour-promoting and non-platelet-aggregatory. A wide range of phorbol esters has also been shown to have distinct effects on differentiation in HL60 promyelocytes (Evans *et al*. 1989).

An acidic protein(s) of apparent M_r 80–87 kDa (called MARCKS Stumpo *et al*. 1989) is phosphorylated in response to treatment of intact cells with a variety of agonists which stimulate phosphatidylinositol turnover. It is also phosphorylated in response to phorbol esters and membrane-permeable diacylglycerols. Phosphorylation of this protein provides a useful marker for the activation state of PKC *in vivo*. The widespread tissue distribution and rapid high level of phosphorylation of this protein make it a likely mediator of a major function(s) of PKC. A role in macrophage activation, neurosecretion, and growth-factor-dependent mitogenesis has been suggested (Seykora *et al.* 1991). Phosphorylation displaces the protein from the membrane which may be part of a regulatory mechanism for actin—membrane interaction.

In fibroblasts, the state of phosphorylation of this protein is increased in response to phorbol esters and the growth factors PDGF and EGF, and by stimulation with the polypeptide mitogen embryonal carcinoma-derived growth factor (ECDGF) (Mahadevan *et al.* 1987). There was a distinction in the preferred site of phosphorylation on the MARCKS protein when PKC was stimulated by the tumour-promoting phorbol ester TPA, or by the non-tumour-promoting esters SAP A and DOPPA (Amess *et al.* 1992). Results from many different studies suggest that those phorbol esters may act *in vivo* by stimulating protein kinases with distinct substrate specificities. This would explain the ability of certain derivatives to evoke a limited range of biological responses. Whether these 'receptors' for phorbol esters are different forms of PKC or distinct protein kinases is the subject of continuing investigation.

It should be noted that a number of proteins of distinct function have been shown to contain regions similar in sequence to the cysteine-rich repeats of PKC. These include the brain-specific *n*-chimaerin (Ahmed *et al.* 1990) and diacylglycerol kinase (Schaap *et al.* 1990). The former has been shown to bind phorbol esters.

3B.4.3   Non-phorbol activators and inhibitors

Other naturally occurring and synthetic inhibitors of PKC include trifluoroperazine, which is a calmodulin antagonist of the phenothiazine type (although PKC is not a Ca^{2+}-dependent enzyme), and dibucaine and adriamycin which interfere with the binding of diacylglycerol to the regulatory domain of PKC (Geseher and Dale 1989). Cremophor EL (Zhao *et al.* 1989) and calphostin C (Bruns *et al.* 1991) also prevent DAG binding to PKC. H-7 and K-252 inhibit the enzyme by competing with ATP (Hidaka *et al.* 1984). The use of these compounds is limited in studies of regulatory mechanisms by their lack of specificity towards PKC. One of the most potent PKC inhibitors recently described is the microbial alkaloid staurosporine (see Section 3C), which interacts with the catalytic site and inhibits the kinase with a K_i of 2.7 nM (Tamaoki *et al.* 1986).

Many inhibitors of PKC have been shown to have a distinct effect on different isoforms; for example H7 has an effect (Pelosin *et al.* 1990) but staurosporin does not (Schaap and Parker 1990).

The bryostatins, isolated from marine bryozoans (Petit *et al.* 1970) also activate PKC. Their effect is variable in different cell types, and instead of activating PKC they may, in fact, antagonize the effect of phorbol esters. This may be explained by different modulation of the activity of PKC (Kraft *et al.* 1986; Wender *et al.* 1988; Fields *et al.* 1989).

A calcium-independent PKC isolated from neutrophils has been shown to be inhibited by fatty acyl-CoA (Majumdar *et al.* 1991).

3B.4.4 Activation by bacterial lipolysaccharide and its precursors

Brain PKC has been shown to be activated by lipopolysaccharide, a component of the outer surface of Gram-negative bacteria (Rosoff and Cantley 1985; Seykora *et al.* 1991). Precursors of the lipid A part of this complex were also shown to activate PKC *in vitro*. This does not compete with the phorbol ester–DAG binding site but appears to substitute for PS in the activation of PKC (Wightman and Raetz 1984; Ellis *et al.* 1987b).

3B.4.5 PKC substrate specificity, physiological role, and involvement in signal transduction pathways

Activation of PKC results in the phosphorylation of a wide range of proteins, leading to the regulation of many physiological processes such as neurotransmitter release, smooth muscle contraction, regulation of ion channels, growth control, and gene transcription (Nishizuka 1986; Kilimann 1991). In this section we cannot cover extensively the physiological role of PKC but we shall attempt to give an overview with references to more extensive recent reviews on particular topics and concentrate on aspects where targeting PKC function may be a useful guide for drug design.

PKC, in common with many other classes of protein kinase, has the ability to autophosphorylate. In this case, there is no known physiological significance of the reaction. The PKC family of kinases phosphorylates many substrates *in vitro* but appears to be more specific *in vivo*, which may be a reflection of the location of at least some of the isoforms in the active state at the inner surface of the plasma membrane (Nishizuka 1986; Woodgett *et al.* 1987)

3B.4.5.1 *Involvement with growth hormone receptors*

PKC has been shown to phosphorylate growth hormone receptors. The best studied example is the EGF receptor, which is phosphorylated by PKC on a threonine residue, nine amino acids from the cytoplasmic end of a proposed transmembrane domain (Hunter *et al.* 1984). Of the brain enzymes, the EGF receptor is most rapidly phosphorylated by the α isoform and most slowly by the γ isoform (Ido *et al.* 1987). The *in vivo* phosphorylation of the EGF receptor by PKC has been shown in A431 cells to lead to a reduction in the ability of EGF to bind to its receptor and to reduce the tyrosine protein kinase activity. Both TPA and the indole alkaloid tumour promoter teleocidin stimulated this phosphorylation. EGF has been shown to increase the hydrolysis of PIP_2. The role of this phosphorylation may therefore be a feedback mechanism to modulate the response of the ECF receptor.

Recently, the mechanism through which growth hormone receptors activate PKC has become clearer. Platelet derived growth factor and EGF undergo autophosphorylation on a group of specific tyrosine residues to which a specific phopholipase C (PLC-γ) binds and is activated (reviewed in Berridge 1993). The region on PLC-γ that binds to the tyrosine phosphorylated receptor subunit has a so-called SH2 (or src-homology) region. SH2 domains are named after the similarity to a region of sequence in the oncogene product, src. The PLC-γ, which is normally cytosolic, becomes associated with the receptor at the membrane. The PLC is activated and, in addition, is brought into contact with its substrate, PIP_2.

3B.4.5.2 *Gene transcription*
The role of PKC in regulating gene transcription through phosphorylation of the transcription factors c-*fos* and c-*jun* has been the subject of detailed study (Sheng and Greenberg 1990) (see Fig. 3B.2).

In addition, TPA can stimulate phosphorylation of ribosomal protein S6 in hepatoma cells (Trevillyan *et al.* 1984). This H35 rat hepatoma cell line has been shown to have increased ornithine decarboxylase activity and thus polyamine synthesizing ability in response to tumour-promoting phorbol esters. The growth hormones insulin and insulin-like growth factor have also been shown to enhance phosphorylation in protein S6. A function for ribosomal protein S6 phosphorylation has been suggested in transition into the G1 phase of the cell cycle and in altering the affinity of the ribosome for certain classes of mRNA.

Phosphorylation of topoisomerase by PKC results in activation of the enzyme (Alsner *et al.* 1991). Topoisomerases are involved in supercoiling/relaxation and catenation of DNA and have a role in the regulation of DNA replication, transcription of specific genes, and chromatid segregation.

3B.4.5.3 *Insulin and glycogen metabolism*
PKC phosphorylates both rat liver and skeletal muscle glycogen synthase *in vitro* (Ahmad *et al.* 1984). According to other authors, this phosphorylation may not be accompanied by a decrease in the activity of glycogen synthase (Imazu *et al.* 1984). In rat hepatocytes, the state of phosphorylation in sites on glycogen synthase associated with PKC is increased in response to phorbol esters, while those associated with other Ca^{2+}-dependent protein kinases were unaffected (Roach and Goldman 1983). This provided additional evidence that one part of the phosphatidylinositol hydrolysis pathway, namely activation of PKC, is involved, while the other branch, stimulation of release of Ca^{2+} from internal stores, is unaffected.

Administration of insulin has been shown to lead to the stimulation of the phosphorylation of a protein with $M_r = 47\,000$ in rat hippocampus

(Akers and Routtenberg 1984). This substrate, protein F1, is probably identical with the central nervous system B50 protein, also known as neuromodulin or GAP43a. It has been shown to be a preferential substrate for the β isoform of PKC (Sheu *et al.* 1990). This is in agreement with the results of Tanaka *et al.* (1991) who showed that β_{II} is the major form associated with membrane cytoskeleton elements in synaptosomes with which neuromodulin colocalizes (presynaptic region and growth cones).

The effects of PKC on fatty acid metabolism include phosphorylation of acetyl CoA carboxylase (on a different site to that phosphorylated by cAMP-dependent protein kinase (Hardie *et al.* 1986)). The phosphorylation does not result in activation of the enzyme. In ATP–citrate lyase, however, the same serine residue is phosphorylated by both kinases and the state of phosphorylation is increased by insulin (Kelleher *et al.* 1984).

3B.4.5.4 *Membrane proteins, ion channels, and neurotransmitters*

Increase in the intracellular level of Ca^{2+} and activation of an Na^+/H^+ exchange carrier are the main ionic events responsible for the onset of cell proliferation (Moolenaar *et al.* 1983). PKC phosphorylates and activates this neutral Na^+/H^+ exchanger (Rosoff *et al.* 1984). Induction of differentiation in a murine prelymphocyte cell line is accomplished by activation of this Na^+-uptake system. In 3T3 cells, administration of phorbol esters has been shown to increase internal pH (Burns and Rozengurt 1983).

The Ca^{2+}-ATPase (responsible for maintaining the intracellular Ca^{2+} concentration) is phosphorylated by PKC, in particular the γ isoform (Wang *et al.* 1991) in human erythrocytes. Phosphorylation was in the calmodulin-binding domain and decreased calmodulin activation of the enzyme. The effect of phosphorylation on the protein depended on the isoform of PKC and on the lipid associated with the Ca^{2+}-ATPase.

PKC phosphorylates a number of cardiac sarcolemma proteins including phospholamban (Allen and Katz 1991). This protein, which is also phosphorylated by a Ca^{2+}–calmodulin-dependent protein kinase, regulates the sarcoplasmic reticulum Ca^{2+}–ATPase and provides evidence for the involvement of PKC in the regulation of cardiac contraction. The β-adrenergic and nicotinic-acetylcholine (ligand-gated ion channel) receptors have been shown to be phosphorylated by PKC (Kilimann 1991). Tyrosine and tryptophan hydroxylases are the rate-limiting enzymes in the synthesis of the neurotransmitters dopamine and serotonin respectively, and are major substrates for PKC. The potential role of the family of PKC inhibitor proteins related to an activator protein of the hydroxylases is discussed in §3B.3.7.

Other membrane receptors phosphorylated by PKC include those for transferrin and IgE receptors, as well as for a number of other growth factors including insulin, IGF-1 and somatomedin C (Nishizuka 1988).

3B.4.5.5 *Cytoskeletal proteins: the role of PKC in morphology*

Phorbol esters cause morphological changes in many cells, a consequence of the effects of PKC on cytoskeletal organization.

Phosphorylation of the cytoskeletal protein vinculin in fibroblasts and Swiss 3T3 cell cultures is increased in response to TPA and phorbol dibutyrate (Werth and Pastar 1984). Vinculin is also a substrate for the transforming protein of Rous sarcoma virus when it is phosphorylated on a tyrosine residue. Vinculin has a role in the morphological changes seen in Rous sarcoma virus transformation, which suggests a link with the morphological changes induced by phorbol esters.

Other cytoskeletal proteins that are substrates for PKC include talin, filamin, profilin, and desmin, as well as the nuclear membrane protein lamin B. The microtubule associated protein MAP2 has a reduced ability to interact with actin when phosphorylated by PKC. The colocalization of PKC a has suggested a role for this isoform in mediating the effects of phosphorylation on cytoskeleton organization (Jaken *et al*. 1989).

In the study of the mechanism of enteropathogenic *E. coli*, the strong stimulation of phosphorylation of a number of epithelial cell proteins has been observed (Baldwin *et al*. 1990). One of these has been identified as myosin light chain, and the increase in phosphorylation mediated by activators of PKC affects its cytoskeletal association (Manjarrez-Hernandez *et al*. 1991).

3B.4.5.6 *Platelet aggregation*

In platelets, substrates for PKC include myosin light chains (20 kDa), a substrate for Ca^{2+}–calmodulin-dependent myosin light-chain kinase (Naka *et al*. 1983), and a 47 kDa protein (p47, a specific substrate for PKC now called 'pleckstrin'). p47 is rapidly phosphorylated in response to a variety of agonists including phorbol esters (Castagna *et al*. 1982; Connolly *et al*. 1986). The state of phosphorylation of this protein is also increased by thrombin on an identical site. A role for pleckstrin phosphorylation in serotonin release has been suggested.

When phorbol esters with different biological activities were tested for their ability to induce the phosphorylation of human platelet proteins, only the potent platelet aggregatory phorbol esters were able to stimulate phosphorylation. The less potent aggregatory esters show a greater calcium dependence for PKC activation. This correlated with their ability to cause platelet aggregation. When a non-platelet aggregatory deoxyphorbol (DOPPA) was combined with a subthreshold dose of the Ca^{2+} ionophore A23187, a large increase in phosphorylation of p47 and a fourfold decrease in K_a was observed. This contrasted with a barely detectable stimulation of phosphorylation at micromolar levels of this phorbol ester in the absence of the ionophore. This synergism was not evident for the potent platelet aggregatory derivatives. In the presence of calcium, DOPPA was shown to stimulate preferentially one of the isoforms of PKC (Brooks *et al.* 1990).

Type II PKC in platelets (Tsukuda *et al.* 1988; Watanabe *et al.* 1988) is not identical to β_I and β_{II} from brain, although the elution position on hydroxylapatite is similar. It is probably the δ isoform (see §3B.3).

The effect of thrombin on PIP_2 hydrolysis to form inositol trisphosphate (which leads to activation of Ca^{2+}–calmodulin-dependent myosin light-chain kinase and phosphorylation of platelet myosin light chain) was much faster than the effect of TPA on PKC (Naka *et al.* 1983). The sites of phosphorylation identified in the study also suggested a possible effect of PKC on PIP_2 hydrolysis which would subsequently raise Ca^{2+} levels to activate the Ca^{2+}–calmodulin-dependent protein kinase.

Many studies have also shown that the effects of the two second messengers can be mimicked in cells other than platelets (lymphocytes, insulin-secreting pancreatic cells, release of acetylcholine from ileum, etc.) by the addition of Ca^{2+} ionophores acting synergistically with activators of PKC (e.g. 1-oleoyl-2-acetylglycerol and TPA) which results in a full secretory response (Michell 1983; Berridge 1984; Wolf *et al.* 1985; Nishizuka 1988).

3B.5   Conclusions

This chapter has given a necessarily brief overview of the properties and biological roles of PKC—a large family of enzymes with distinct tissue distribution and a wide involvement in distinct biological events. The literature is now quite extensive. Different isoforms are regulated, to a different extent, by calcium and lipids, by translocation to the plasma membrane, or by translocation to the nucleus. Isoforms of PKC can be classified in different subgroupings of regulatory domain structure, and distinct isoforms can be activated or inhibited, to different extents, by a wide range of natural and synthetic compounds. This makes the PKC family of protein kinases a good potential target for the design of specific drugs which would be selective for isoforms of the enzyme and specifically influence the regulation of distinct biological and physiological processes.

References

Ahmad, Z., Lee, F. T., DePaoli-Roach, A., and Roach, P. J. (1984). Phosphorylation of glycogen synthase by the Ca^{2+}- and the phospholipid-activated protein kinase (protein kinase C). *Journal of Biological Chemistry*, **259**, 8743–7.

Ahmed, S., Kozma, R., Monfries, C., Hall, C., Lim, H. H., Smith, P., and Lim, L. (1990). Human brain n-chimaerin cDNA encodes a novel phorbol ester receptor. *Biochemical Journal*,, **272**, 767–73.

Aitken, A. (1990). *Identification of protein consensus sequences*, pp. 1–167. Ellis Horwood, Chichester.

Aitken, A., Ellis, C. A., Harris, A., Sellers, L. A., and Toker, A. (1990). Kinase and neurotransmitters. *Nature, London*, **344**, 594.

Akers, R. F. and Routtenberg, A. (1984). Brain protein phosphorylation *in vitro*: selective substrate action of insulin. *Life Science*, **35**, 809–13.

Allen, B. G. and Katz, S. (1991). Cardiac protein kinase C isozymes: phosphorylation of phospholamban in longitudinal and junctional sarcoplasmic reticulum. *NATO ASI Series*, **H56**, 239–43.

Alsner, J., Kjeldsen, E., Svejstrup, J. Q., Christiansen, K., and Westergaard, O. (1991). Stimulation of human DNA topoisomerase I by protein kinase C. *NATO ASI Series*, **H56**, 430–3.

Amess, R. H., Manjarrez-Hernandez, H. A., Howell, S. A., Learmonth, M. P., and Aitken, A. (1992). Multisite phosphorylation of the 80 kDa (MARCKS) protein kinase C substrate in C3H/10T1/2 fibroblasts. *Federation of European Biochemical Societies Letters*, **297**, 285–91.

Baldwin, T. J., Brooks, S. F., Knutton, S., Manjarrez-Hernandez, H. A., Aitken, A., and Williams, P. H. (1990). Protein phosphorylation by protein kinase C in HEp-2 cells, infected with enteropathogenic *Escherichia coli*. *Infection and Immunity*, **58**, 761–5.

Bell, R. M. and Burns, D. J. (1991). Lipid activation of protein kinase C. *Journal of Biological Chemistry*, **266**, 4661–4.

Berridge, M. J. (1984). Inositol trisphosphate and diacylglycerol as second messengers. *Biochemical Journal*, **220**, 345–60.

Berridge, M. J. (1993). Inositol trisphosphate and calcium signalling. *Nature, London*, **361**, 315–25.

Blackshear, P. J., Witters, L. A., Girard, P. R., Kuo, J. F., and Quamo, S. N. (1985). Growth factor stimulated protein phosphorylation in 3T3-L1 cells. *Journal of Biological Chemistry*, **260**, 13304–15.

Blumberg, P. (1980). *In vitro* studies on the mode of action of the phorbol esters. Potent tumour promoters. *CRC Critical Reviews in Toxicology*, **8**, 153–232.

Bocckino, S. B., Blackmor, P. F., Wilson, P. B., and Exton, J. H. (1987). Phosphotidate accumulation in hormone-treated hepatocytes via a phospholipase D mechanism. *Journal of Biological Chemistry* **262**, 15309–15.

Boni, L. T. and Rando, R. R. (1985). The nature of protein kinase C activation by physically defined phospholipid vesicles and diacylglycerols. *Journal of Biological Chemistry*, **260**, 10819–25.

Borner, C., Eppenberger, U., Wyss, R., and Fabbro, D. (1988). Continuous synthesis of two protein kinase C-related proteins after down regulation by phorbol esters. *Proceedings of the National Academy of Sciences of the United States of America*, **85**, 2110–14.

Brooks, G., Evans, A. T., Aitken, A., and Evans, F. J. (1987a). Sapintoxin A, a fluorescent phorbol ester that is a potent activator of protein kinase C but is not a tumour promoter. *Cancer Letters*, **38**, 165–70.

Brooks, S. F., Evans, F. J., and Aitken, A. (1987b). The stimulation of phosphorylation of intracellular proteins in GH$_3$ rat pituitary tumour cells by phorbol esters of distinct biological activity. *Federation of European Biochemical Societies Letters*, **224**, 109–16.

Brooks, S. F., Gordge, P. C., Toker, A., Evans, A. T., Evans, F. J., and Aitken, A.

(1990). Platelet protein phosphorylation and protein kinase C activation by phorbol esters with different biological activity and a novel synergistic response with Ca^{2+} ionophore *European Journal of Biochemistry*, **188**, 431–7.

Bruns, R. F., Miller, F. D., Merriman, R. L., Howbert, J. J., Heath, W. F., Kobayashi, E., *et al.* (1991). Inhibition of protein kinase C by calphostin C is light dependent. *Biochemical and Biophysical Research Communications*, **176**, 288–93.

Burns, C. P. and Rozengurt, E. (1983). Serum, platelet-derived growth factor, vasopressin, and phorbol esters increase intracellular pH in Swiss 3T3 cells. *Biochemical and Biophysical Research Communications*, **116**, 931–8.

Campbell, D. G., Hardie, D. G., and Vulliet, P. R. (1986). Identification of four phosphorylation sites in the N-terminal region of tyrosine hydroxylase. *Journal of Biological Chemistry*, **261**, 10489–92.

Capitani, S., Girard, P. R., Mazzei, G. J., Kuo, J. F., Berezney, R., and Manzoli, F. A. (1987). Immunochemical characterization of protein kinase C in rat liver nuclei and subnuclear fractions. *Biochemical and Biophysical Research Communications*, **142**, 367–75.

Castagna, M., Takai, Y., Kaibuchi, Y., Sano, K., Kikkawa, U., and Nishizuka, Y. (1982). Direct activation of calcium-activated, phospholipid-dependent protein kinase by tumor-promoting phorbol esters. *Journal of Biological Chemistry*, **257**, 7847–51.

Cockroft, S. (1981). Does phosphatidylinositol breakdown control the Ca^{2+} gating mechanism? *Trends in Pharmacological Sciences*, **2**, 340–3.

Connolly, T. M., Lawing, W. J., Jr, and Majerus, P. W. (1986). Protein kinase C phosphorylates human platelet inositol trisphosphate 5′-phosphomonoesterase, increasing the phosphatase activity. *Cell*, **46**, 951–8.

Costa-Casnellie, M. R., Segel, G. B., and Litchman, M. A. (1985). Concanavalin A and phorbol ester cause opposite subcellular redistribution of protein kinase C. *Biochemical and Biophysical Research Communications*, **133**, 1139–44.

Coussens, L., Parker, P. J., Rhee, L., Yang-Feng, T. L., Chen, E., Waterfield, M. D., *et al.* (1986). Multiple, distinct forms of bovine and human protein kinase C suggest diversity in cellular signaling pathways. *Science*, **233**, 859–66.

Daniel, L. W., Waite, M., and Wykle, R. L. (1986). A novel mechanism of diglyceride formation. *Journal of Biological Chemistry*, **261**, 9128–32.

Da Silva, C., Fan, X., Martelly, I., and Castagna, M. (1990). Phorbol esters mediate phospholipid-free activation of rat brain protein kinase C. *Cancer Research*, **50**, 2081–7.

Divecha, N., Banfic, H., and Irvine, R. F. (1991). Translocation of protein kinase C to the nucleus. *EMBO Journal*, **10**, 3207–14.

Dunphy, W. G., Kochenberger, R. J., Castagna, M., and Blumberg, P. M. (1981). Kinetics and subcellular localization of specific [^{3}H] phorbol 12, 13-dibutyrate binding by mouse brain. *Cancer Research*, **41**, 2640–7.

Eichholtz, T., Alblas, J., Van Overveld, M., Moolenaar, W., and Ploegh, H. (1990). A pseudosubstrate peptide inhibits protein kinase C-mediated phosphorylation in permeabilized Rat-1 cells. *Federation of European Biochemical Societies Letters*, **261**, 147–50.

Ellis, C. A., Aitken, A., Takayama, K., and Qureshi, N. (1987a). Substitution of phosphatidylserine by lipid A in the activation of purified rabbit brain protein kinase C. *Federation of European Biochemical Societies Letters*, **218**, 238–42.

Ellis, C. A., Brooks, S. F., Brooks, G., Evans, A. T., Morrice, N., Evans, F. J., and Aitken, A. (1987b). The effects of phorbol esters with different biological activities on protein kinase C. *Phytotherapy Research*, **1**, 187–90.

El Touny, S., Khan, W., and Hannun, Y. (1990). Regulation of platelet protein kinase C by oleic acid. *Journal of Biological Chemistry*, **265**, 16437–43.

Evans, F. J. (1986). Phorbol: its esters and derivatives. In *Naturally occurring phorbol esters* (ed. F. J. Evans), pp. 171–216. CRC Press, Boca Raton, FL.

Evans, F. J. and Edwards, M. C. (1987). Activity correlations in the phorbol ester series. *Botanical Journal of the Linnean Society*, **94**, 231–46.

Evans, A. T., MacPhee, C. H., Beg, F., Evans, F. J., and Aitken, A. (1989). The ability of diterpene esters with selective biological effects to activate protein kinase C and induce HL60 cell differentiation. *Biochemical Pharmacology*, **38**, 2925–7.

Farago, A. and Nishizuka, Y. (1990). Protein kinase C in transmembrane signalling. *Federation of European Biochemical Societies Letters*, **268**, 350–4.

Ferguson, M. A. J. and Williams, A. F. (1988). Cell-surface anchoring of proteins via glycosyl-phosphatidylinositol structures. *Annual Review of Biochemistry*, **57**, 285–320.

Ferrari, S., Marchiori, F., Marin, O., and Pinna, L. A. (1987). Ca^{2+} phospholipid-dependent and independent phosphorylation of synthetic peptide substrates by protein kinase C. *European Journal of Biochemistry*, **163**, 481–7.

Feuerstein, N. and Cooper, H. L. (1983). Rapid phosphorylation—dephosphorylation of specific proteins induced by phorbol ester in HL-60 cells, further characterization of the phosphorylation of 17-kilodalton and 27-kilodalton proteins in myeloid leukaemic cells and human monocytes. *Journal of Biological Chemistry*, **259**, 2782–8.

Fields, A. P., Picus, S. M., Kraft, A. S., and May, W. S. (1989). Interleukin-3 and Bryostatin 1 mediate rapid nuclear envelope protein phosphorylation in growth factor dependent FDC-P1 hematoporetic cells: a possible role for nuclear protein kinase C. *Journal of Biological Chemistry*, **264**, 21896–901.

Fournier, A., Hardy, S. L., Clark, K. J., and Murray, A. W. (1989). Phorbol ester induces differential membrane-association of protein kinase C subspecies in human platelets. *Biochemical and Biophysical Research Communications*, **161**, 556–61.

Ganong, B. R., Loomis, C. R., Hannun, Y. A., and Bell, R. M. (1986). Specificity and mechanism of protein kinase C activation by sn-1, 2-diacylglycerols. *Proceedings of the National Academy of Sciences of the United States of America*, **83**, 1184–8.

Gescher, A., Dale, I. L. (1989). Protein kinase C—a novel target for rational anti-cancer drug design? *Anti-Cancer Drug Design*, **4**, 93–105.

Hagiwara, M., Uchida, C., Usuda, N., Nagata, T., and Hidaka, H. (1990). ζ-related protein kinase C in nuclei of nerve cells. *Biochemical and Biophysical Research Communications*, **168**, 161–8.

Hanks, S. K., Quinn, A. M., and Hunter, T. (1988). The protein kinase family: conserved features and deduced phylogeny of the catalytic domains. *Science*, **241**, 42–52.

Hannun, Y. and Bell, R. M. (1987). Lysosphingolipids inhibit protein kinase C. Implications for the sphingolipidoses. *Science*, **235**, 670–4.

Hannun, Y., Loomis, C., and Bell, R. M. (1985). Activation of protein kinase C by Triton X-100 mixed micelles containing diacylglycerol and phosphatidylserine. *Journal of Biological Chemistry*, **260**, 10039–43.

Hannun, Y., Loomis, C., and Bell, R. M. (1986). Protein kinase C activation in mixed micelles. *Journal of Biological Chemistry*, **261**, 7184–90.

Hansson, A., Serhan, C. N., Haeggstrom, J., Ingelman-Sundberg, M., and Samuelsson, B. (1986). Activation of protein kinase C by lipoxin A and other eicosanoids. Intracellular action of oxygenation products of arachidonic acid. *Biochemical and Biophysical Research Communications*, **134**, 1215–22.

Hardie, D. G. (1988). Pseudosubstrates turn off protein kinases. *Nature, London*, **335**, 592–3.

Hardie, D. G., Carling, D., Ferrari, S., Guy, P. S., and Aitken, A. (1986). Characterisation of the phosphorylation of rat mammary ATP-citrate lyase and acetyl-CoA carboxylase by Ca^{2+} and calmodulin-dependent multiprotein kinase and Ca^{2+} and phospholipid-dependent protein kinase. *European Journal of Biochemistry*, **157**, 553–61.

Hecker, E. (1968). Cocarcinogenic principles from the seed oil of *Croton tiglium* and from other Euphorbiaceae. *Cancer Research*, **31**, 2338–49.

Hidaka, H., Inagaki, M., Kawamoto, S., and Sasaki, Y. (1984). Isoquinolinesulphonamides; novel and potent inhibitors of cyclic nucleotide dependent protein kinase and protein kinase C. *Biochemistry*, **23**, 5036–41.

House, C., Wettenhall, R. E. H., and Kemp, B. E. (1987). The influence of basic residues on the substrate specificity of protein kinase C. *Journal of Biological Chemistry*, **262**, 772–7.

Huang, K-P. (1989). The mechanism of protein kinase C activation. *Trends in Neurosciences*, **12**, 425–31.

Hunter, T., Ling, N., and Cooper, J. A. (1984). Protein kinase C phosphorylation of the EGF receptor at a threonine residue close to the cytoplasmic face of the plasma membrane. *Nature, London*, **311**, 480–3.

Ido, M., Sekiguchi, K., Kikkawa, U., and Nishizuka, Y. (1987). Phosphorylation of the EGF receptor from A431 epidermoid carcinoma cells by three distinct types of protein kinase C. *Federation of European Biochemical Societies Letters*, **219**, 215–18.

Imazu, M., Strickland, W. G., Chrisman, T. D., and Exton, J. H. (1984). Phosphorylation and inactivation of liver glycogen synthase by liver protein kinases. *Journal of Biological Chemistry*, **259**, 1813–26.

Inoue, M., Kishimoto, A., Takai, Y., and Nishizuka, Y. (1977). Studies on a cyclic nucleotide independent protein kinase and its proenzyme in mammalian tissues. *Journal of Biological Chemistry*, **252**, 7610–16.

Isakov, N., McMahon, P., and Altman, A. (1990). Selective post-transcriptional down-regulation of protein kinase C isoenzymes in leukemic T cells chronically treated with phorbol ester. *Journal of Biological Chemistry*, **265**, 2091–7.

Ito, A., Saito, N., Hirata, M., Kose, A., Tsujino, T., Yoshihara, C., *et al.* (1990). Immunocytochemical localisation of the α subspecies of protein kinase C in rat brain. *Proceedings of the National Academy of Sciences of the United States of America*, **87**, 3195–9.

Jaken, S. and Kiley, S. C. (1987). Purification and characterisation of three types of protein kinase C from rabbit brain cytosol. *Proceedings of the National Academy of Sciences of the United States of America*, **85**, 4418–22.

Jaken, S., Leach, K., and Klauck, T. (1989). Association of type 3 protein kinase C with focal contacts in rat embryo fibroblasts. *Journal of Cell Biology*, **109**, 697–704.

Kaibuchi, K., Takai, Y., and Nishizuka, Y. (1981). Cooperative role of various membrane phospholipids in the activation of calcium-activated phospholipid dependent protein kinase. *Journal of Biological Chemistry*, **256**, 7146–9.

Kaibuchi, K., Fukumoto, Y., Oku, N., Takai, Y., Arai, K-I., and Muramatsu, M-A. (1989). Molecular genetic analysis of the regulatory and catalytic domain of protein kinase C. *Journal of Biological Chemistry*, **264**, 13489–96.

Kelleher, D. J., Pessin, I. E., Ruoho, A. E., and Johnson, G. L. (1984). Phorbol ester induces desensitisation of adenylate cyclase and phosphorylation of the β-adrenergic receptor in turkey erthrocytes. *Proceedings of the National Academy of Sciences of the United States of America*, **81**, 4316–20.

Kikkawa, U., Takai, Y., Minakuchi, R., Inohara, S., and Nishizuka, Y. (1982). Calcium-activated, phospholipid-dependent protein kinase from rat brain. *Journal of Biological Chemistry*, **257**, 13341–8.

Kikkawa, U., Ono, Y., Ogita, T., Fujii, T., Asaoka, Y., Sekiguchi, K., *et al.* (1987a). Identification of the structures of multiple sub-species of protein kinase C expressed in rat brain. *Federation of European Biochemical Societies Letters*, **217**, 227–31.

Kikkawa, U., Ogita, K., Ono, Y., Asaoka, Y., Shearman, M. S., Fujii, T., *et al.* (1987b). The common structure and activities of four subspecies of rat brain protein kinase C family. *Federation of European Biochemical Societies Letters*, **223**, 212–16.

Kiley, S. C. and Jaken, S. (1990). Activation of a-protein kinase C leads to association with detergent-insoluble components of GH_4C_1 cells. *Molecular Endocrinology*, **4**, 59–68.

Kilimann, M. W. (1991). Protein phosphorylation in the nervous system. *NATO ASI Series*, **H56**, 389–396.

Kishimoto, A., Takai, Y., Mori, T., Kikkawa, U., and Nishizuka, Y. (1980). Activation of calcium and phospholipid-dependent protein kinase by diacylglycerol. *Journal of Biological Chemistry*, **255**, 2273–6.

Kishimoto, A., Kajikawa, N., Shiota, M., and Nishizuka, Y. (1983). Proteolytic activation of calcium activated phospholipid dependent protein kinase by a calcium dependent neutral protease. *Journal of Biological Chemistry*, **258**, 1156–64.

Kiss, Z., Deli, E., and Kuo, J. F. (1988). Temporal changes in intracellular distribution of protein kinase C during differentiation of human leukemia HL60 cells induced by phorbol ester. *Federation of European Biochemical Societies Letters*, **231**, 41–6.

Knighton, D. R., Zheng, J., Ten Eyck, L. F., Ashford, V. A., Xuong, N. H., Taylor, S. S., and Sowadski, J. M. (1991). Crystal structure of the catalytic subunit of cyclic adenosine monophosphate-dependent protein kinase. *Science*, **253**, 407–14.

Knopf, J. L., Lee, M. H., Sultzman, L. A., Kriz, R. W., Loomis, C. R., Hewick, R. M., and Bell, R. M. (1986). Cloning and expression of multiple protein kinase C cDNAs. *Cell*, **46**, 491–502.

Kolesnick, R. N. (1987). Thyrotropin-releasing hormone and phorbol esters induce phosphatidylcholine synthesis in GH_3 pituitary cells. Evidence for stimulation via protein kinase C. *Journal of Biological Chemistry*, **262**, 14525–30.

Kosaka, Y., Ogita, K., Ase, K., Nomura, H., Kikkawa, U., and Nishizuka, Y. (1988). The heterogeneity of protein kinase C in various rat tissues. *Biochemical and Biophysical Research Communications*, **151**, 973–81.

Kraft, A. S. and Anderson, W. B. (1983). Phorbol esters increase the amount of Ca^{2+}, phospholipid dependent protein kinase associated with plasma membrane. *Nature, London*, **301**, 621–3.

Kraft, A. S., Smith, J. B., and Berkow, R. L. (1986). Bryostatin, an activator of the calcium phospholipid-dependent protein kinase, blocks phorbol ester-induced differentiation of human promyelocytic leukemia cells HL-60. *Proceedings of the National Academy of Sciences of the United States of America*, **83**, 1334–8.

Kubo, K., Ohno, S., and Suzuki, K. (1987). Primary structures of human protein kinase C βI and βII differ only in their C-terminal sequences. *Federation of European Biochemical Societies Letters*, **223**, 138–42.

Lacal, J. C., Moscat, J., and Aaronson, S. A. (1987). Novel source of 1,2-diacylglycerol elevated in cells transformed by Ha-ras oncogene. *Nature, London*, **330**, 269–72.

Leach, K. L. and Blumberg, P. M. (1985). Modulation of protein kinase C activity and [^{3}H]phorbol-12,13-dibutyrate binding by various tumour promoters in mouse brain cytosol. *Cancer Research*, **45**, 1958–3.

Leach, K., Powers, E. A., Ruff, V. A., Jaken, S., and Kaufman, S. (1989). Type 3 protein kinase C localisation to the nuclear envelope of phorbol ester-treated NIH 3T3 cells. *Journal of Cell Biology*, **109**, 685–95.

Lee, M-H. and Bell, R. M. (1986). The lipid binding, regulatory domain of protein kinase C. *Journal of Biological Chemistry*, **261**, 14867–70.

McDonald, J. R., Gröschel-Stewart, U., and Walsh, M. P. (1987). Properties and distribution of the protein inhibitor (M_r 17000) of protein kinase C. *Journal of Biochemistry*, **242**, 695–705.

McPhail, L. C., Clayton, C. C., and Snyderman, R. (1984). A potential second messenger for unsaturated fatty acids: activation of Ca^{2+}-dependent protein kinase. *Science*, **224**, 622–5.

Mahadevan, L. C., Aitken, A., Heath, J., and Foulkes, J. G. (1987). Embryonal carcinoma derived growth factor activates protein kinase C *in vivo* and *in vitro*. *EMBO Journal*, **6**, 921–6.

Mahadevappa, V. G. and Holub, B. J. (1983). Degradation of different molecular species of phosphatidylinositol in thrombin-stimulated human platelets. Evidence for preferential degradation of 1-acyl-2-arachidonyl species. *Journal of Biological Chemistry*, **258**, 5337–9.

Majumdar, S., Rossi, M. W., Fujiki, T., Phillips, W. A., Disa, S., Queen, C. F., *et al*. (1991). Protein kinase C isotypes and signaling in neutrophils. *Journal of Biological Chemistry*, **266**, 9285–94.

Manjarrez-Hernandez, H. A., Amess, B., Sellers, L., Baldwin, T. J., Knutton, S., Williams, P. H., and Aitken, A. (1991). Purification of a 20 kDa phosphoprotein from epithelial cells and identification as a myosin light chain. *Federation of European Biochemical Societies Letters*, **292**, 121–7.

Maraganore, J. M. (1987). Structural elements for protein-phospholipid interactions may be shared in protein kinase C and phospholipases A_2. *Trends in Biochemical Sciences*, **12**, 176–7.

Marais, R. M. and Parker, P. J. (1989). Purification and characterisation of bovine brain protein kinase C isotypes α, β and γ. *European Journal of Biochemistry*, **182**, 129–37.

Masmoudi, A., Labourdette, G., Mersel, M., Huang, F. L., Huang, K-P., Vicendon,

G., and Malviya, A. N. (1989). Protein kinase C located in rat liver nuclei. *Journal of Biological Chemistry*, **264**, 1172–9.

Mattila, P. (1991). Protein kinase C subtypes in endothelial cells. *Federation of European Biochemical Societies Letters*, **289**, 86–90.

Michell, R. H. (1983). Ca^{2+} and protein kinase C: two synergistic cellular signals. *Trends in Biochemical Sciences*, **8**, 263–5.

Mischak, H., Bodenteich, A., Kolch, W., Goodnight, J., Hofer, F., and Mushinski, F. (1991). Mouse protein kinase C-δ, the major isoform expressed in mouse hemopoietic cells: sequence of the cDNA, expression patterns and characterization of the protein. *Biochemistry*, **30**, 7925–31.

Miyake, R., Tanaka, Y., Tsuda, T., Kaibuchi, K., Kikkawa, U., and Nishizuka, Y. (1984). Activation of protein kinase C by non-phorbol tumor promoter, mezerein. *Biochemical and Biophysical Research Communications*, **121**, 649–56.

Mizuno, K., Kubo, K., Saido, T. C., Akita, Y., Osada, S. I., Kuroki, T., *et al.* (1991). Structure and properties of a ubiquitously expressed protein kinase C, nPKCδ. *European Journal of Biochemistry*, **202**, 931–40.

Mochly-Rosen, D., Khaner, H., Lopez, J., and Smith, B. L. (1991). Intracellular receptors for activated protein kinase C. *Journal of Biological Chemistry*, **266**, 14866–8.

Moolenaar, W. H., Tsien, R. Y., van der Saag, P. T., and de Laat, S. W. (1983). Na^+/H^+ exchange and cytoplasmic pH in the action of growth factors in human fibroblasts. *Nature, London*, **304**, 645–8.

Naka, M., Nishikawa, M., Adelstein, R. S., and Hidaka, H. (1983). Phorbol ester-induced activation of human platelets is associated with protein kinase C phosphorylation of myosin light chains. *Nature, London*, **306**, 490–2.

Naor, Z., Shearman, M. S., Kishimoto, A., and Nishizuka, Y. (1988). Calcium-independent activation of hypothalamic type I protein kinase C by unsaturated fatty acids. *Molecular Endocrinology*, **2**, 1043–8.

Nishizuka, Y. (1986). Studies and perspective of protein kinase C. *Science*, **233**, 305–12.

Nishizuka, Y. (1988). The molecular heterogeneity of protein kinase C and its implications for cellular regulation. *Nature, London*, **334**, 661–5.

Norris, V., Baldwin, T. J., Sweeney, S. T., Williams, P. H., and Leach, K. L. (1991). A protein kinase C-like activity in *Escherichia coli*. *Molecular Microbiology*, **5**, 2977–81.

Oishi, K., Raynor, R. L., Charp, P. A., and Kuo, J. F. (1988). Regulation of protein kinase C by lysophospholipids. *Journal of Biological Chemistry*, **263**, 6865–71.

Olivier, A. R. and Parker, P. J. (1991). Expression and characterization of protein kinase C-δ. *European Journal of Biochemistry*, **200**, 805–10.

Ono, Y., Fujii, T., Ogita, K., Kikkawa, U., Igarashi, K., and Nishizuka, Y. (1987a). Identification of three additional members of rat protein kinase C family: δ-, ε-, and ζ- subspecies. *Federation of European Biochemical Societies Letters*, **226**, 125–8.

Ono, Y., Kurokawa, T., Fujii, T., Kawahara, K., Igarashi, K., Kikkawa, U., *et al.* (1986). Two types of cDNAs of rat brain protein kinase C. *Federation of European Biochemical Societies Letters*, **206**, 347–52.

Ono, Y., Kikkawa, U., Ogita, Y., Fujii, T., Kurokawa, T., Asaoka, Y., *et al.* (1987b). Expression and properties of two types of protein kinase C. Alternative splicing from a single gene. *Science*, **236**, 1116–20.

Ono, Y., Fujii, T., Ogita, K., Kikkawa, U., Igarashi, K., and Nishizuka, Y. (1988). The structure, expression, and properties of additional members of the protein kinase C family. *Journal of Biological Chemistry*, **263**, 6927−32.

Ono, Y., Fujii, T., Ogita, K., Kikkawa, U., Igarashi, K., and Nishizuka, Y. (1989a). Protein kinase C-ζ subspecies from rat brain: its structure, expression and properties. *Proceedings of the National Academy of Sciences of the United States of America*, **86**, 3099−103.

Ono, Y., Fujii, T., Igarashi, K., Kuno, T., Tanaka, C., Kikkawa, U., and Nishizuka, Y. (1989b). Phorbol ester binding protein kinase C requires a cysteine-rich zinc-finger-like sequence. *Proceedings of the National Academy of Sciences of the United States of America*, **86**, 4868−71.

Parker, P. J., Stabel, S., and Waterfield, M. D. (1984). Purification to homogeneity of protein kinase C from bovine brain—identity with the phorbol ester receptor. *EMBO Journal*, **3**, 953−9.

Parker, P. J., Coussens, L., Totty, N., Rhee, L., Young, S., Chen, E., *et al.* (1986). The complete primary structure of protein kinase C—the major phorbol ester receptor. *Science*, **233**, 853−9.

Parker, P. J., Kour, G., Marais, R. M., Mitchell. F., Pears, C., Schaap, D., *et al.* (1989). Protein kinase C—a family affair. *Molecular and Cellular Endocrinology*, **65**, 1−11.

Pears, C. J., Kour, G., House, C., Kemp, B. E., and Parker, P. J. (1990). Mutagenesis of the pseudosubstrate site of protein kinase C leads to activation. *European Journal of Biochemistry*, **194**, 89−94.

Pearson, R. B., Wettenhall, R. E. H., Means, A. R., Hartshorne, D. J., and Kemp, B. E. (1988). Autoregulation of enzymes by pseudosubstrate prototopes: Myosin light chain kinase. *Science*, **241**, 970−72.

Pearson, J. D., DeWald, D. B., Mathews, W. R., Mozier, N. M., Zurcher-Neely, H. A., Heinrikson, R. L., *et al.* (1990). Amino acid sequence and characterisation of a protein inhibitor of protein kinase C. *Journal of Biological Chemistry*, **265**, 4583−91.

Pelech, S. L., Charest, D. L., Howard, S. L., Paddon, H. B., and Salari, H. (1990). Protein kinase C activation by platelet activating factor is independent of enzyme translocation. *Biochimica et Biophysica Acta*, **1051**, 100−7.

Pelosin, J. M., Keramidas, M., Souvignet, C., and Chambaz, E. M. (1990). Differential inhibition of protein kinase C subtypes. *Biochemical and Biophysical Research Communications*, **169**, 1040−8.

Pettit, G. R., Day, J. F., Hartwell, J. L., and Wood, H. B. (1970). Antineoplastic components of marine animals. *Nature, London*, **227**, 962−3.

Pontremoli, S., Melloni, E., Damiani, G., Salamino, F., Sparatore, B., Michetti, M., and Horecker, B. L. (1988). Isozymes of protein kinase C in human neutrophils and their modification by two endogenous proteinases. *Journal of Biological Chemistry*, **263**, 1915−19.

Pontremoli, S., Melloni, E., Sparatore, B., Michetti, M., Salamino, F., and Horecker, B. L. (1990). *Journal of Biological Chemistry*, **265**, 706−12.

Qian, Z. and Drewes, L. R. (1990). A novel mechanism for acetylcholine to generate diacylglyerol in brain. *Journal of Biological Chemistry*, **265**, 3607−10.

Roach, P. J. and Goldman, M. (1983). Modification of glycogen synthase activity in isolated rat hepatocytes by tumour-promoting phorbol esters: evidence for differential regulation of glycogen synthase and phosphorylase. *Proceedings* of the National Academy of Sciences of the United States of America, **80**, 7170–2.

Rosoff, P. M. and Cantley, L. C. (1985). Lipopolysaccharide and phorbol esters induce-differentiation but have opposite effects on phosphatidylinositol turn-over and Ca^{2+} mobilization in 70Z/3 pre-B lymphocytes. *Journal of Biological Chemistry*, **260**, 9209–15.

Rosoff, P. M., Stein, L. F., and Cantley, L. C. (1984). Phorbol esters induce differentiation in a pre-B lymphocyte cell line by enhancing Na$^+$/H$^+$ exchange. *Journal of Biological Chemistry*, **259**, 7056–60.

Rozengurt, E. and Sinnett-Smith, J. W. (1987). Bombesin induction of c-*fos* and c-*myc* protooncogenes in Swiss 3T3 cells: significance for the mitogenic response. *Journal of Cellular Physiology*, **131**, 218–35.

Ryves, W. J., Evans, A. T., Olivier, A. R., Parker, P. J., and Evans, F. J. (1991). Activation of the PKC-isotopes a, β, γ, and ε by phorbol esters of different bio-logical activities. *Federation of European Biochemical Societies Letters*, **288**, 5–9.

Saltiel, A. R. and Cuatrecasas, P. (1988). Insulin-stimulated hydrolysis of a novel glycolipid generates modulators of cAMP phosphodiesterase. *American Journal of Physiology*, **225**, 1–11.

Schaap, D. and Parker, P. J. (1990). Expression purification and characterization of protein kinase C-ε. *Journal of Biological Chemistry*, **265**, 7301–7.

Schaap, D., Parker, P. J., Bristol, A., Kriz, R., and Knopf, J. (1989). Unique substrate specificity and regulatory properties of PKC-ε: a rationale for diversity. *Federation of European Biochemical Societies Letters*, **243**, 351–7.

Schaap, D., de Widt, J., van der Wal, J., Vandekerckhove, J., van Damme, J., Gussow, D., *et al.* (1990). Purification, cDNA-cloning and expression of human diacylglycerol kinase. *Federation of European Biochemical Societies Letters*, **275**, 151–8.

Seykora, J. T., Ravetch, J. V. J., and Aderem, A. (1991). Cloning and molecular characterization of the murine macrophage "68-kDa" protein kinase C substrate and its regulation by bacterial lipopolysaccharide. *Proceedings of the National Academy of Sciences of the United States of America*, **88**, 2205–9.

Sharkey, N. A., Leach, K. L., and Blumberg, P. M. (1984). Competitive inhibition by diacylglycerol of specific phorbol ester binding. *Proceedings of the National Academy of Sciences of the United States of America*, **81**, 607–10.

Sheng, M. and Greenberg, M. E. (1990). The regulation and function of c-*fos* and other early genes in the nervous system. *Neuron*, **4**, 477–85.

Sheu, F. S., Marais, R. M., Parker, P. J., Bazan, N. G., and Routtenberg, A. (1990). Neuron-specific protein F1/GAP-43 shows substrate specificity for the beta subunit of protein kinase C. *Biochemical and Biophysical Research Communications*, **171**, 1236–43.

Shimosawa, S., Hachiya, T., Hagiwara, M., Usuda, N., Sugita, K., and Hidaka, H. (1990). Type-specific expression of protein kinase C isozymes in CNS tumor cells. *Neuroscience Letters*, **108**, 11–16.

Shinomura, T., Asaoka, Y., Oka, M., Yoshida, K., and Nishizuka, Y. (1991), Synergistic action of diacylglycerol and unsaturated fatty acid for protein kinase C activation: its possible implications. *Proceedings of the National Academy of Sciences of the United States of America*, **88**, 5149–53.

Soderling, T. R. (1990). Protein kinases. Regulation by autoinhibitory domains. *Journal of Biological Chemistry*, **265**, 1823–6.

Stabel, S., Rodriguez-Pena, A., Young, S., Rozengurt, E., and Parker, P. J. (1987). Quantitation of protein kinase C by immunoblot—expression in different cell lines and response to phorbol esters. *Journal of Cellular Physiology*, **130**, 111–17.

Stumpo, D. J., Graff, J. M., Albert, K. A., Greengard, P., and Blackshear, P. J. (1989). Molecular cloning, characterization, and expression of a cDNA encoding the "80- to 87-kDa" myristoylated alanine-rich C kinase substrate: A major cellular substrate for protein kinase C. *Proceedings of the National Academy of Sciences of the United States of America*, **86**, 4012–16.

Takai, Y., Kishimoto, A., Kikkawa, U., Mori, T., and Nishizuka, Y. (1979). Unsaturated diacylglycerol as a possible messenger for the activation of calcium-activated, phospholipid-dependent protein kinase system. *Biochemical and Biophysical Research Communications*, **91**, 1218–24.

Tamaoki, T., Nomoto, H., Takahashi, I., Kato, Y., Morimoto, M., and Tomita, F. (1986). Staurosporine, a potent inhibitor of phospholipid/Ca^{++} dependent protein kinase. *Biochemical and Biophysical Research Communications*, **135**, 397–402.

Tanaka, S. I., Tominaga, M., Yasuda, I., Kishimoto, A., Nishizuka, Y. (1991). Protein kinase C in rat brain synaptosomes. βII-Subspecies as a major isoform associated with membrane-skeleton elements. *Federation of European Biochemical Societies Letters*, **294**, 267–70.

Testori, A., Hii, C. S. T., Fournier, A., Burgoyne, L. A., and Murray, A. W. (1988). DNA-binding proteins in protein kinase C preparations. *Biochemical and Biophysical Research Communications*, **156**, 222–7.

Toker, A., Ellis, C. A., Sellers, L. A., and Aitken, A. (1990). Protein kinase C inhibitor proteins: purification from sheep brain and sequence similarity to lipocortins and 14–3-3 protein. *European Journal of Biochemistry*, **191**, 421–9.

Trevillyan, J. M., Kulkarni, R. K., and Byus, C. V. (1984). Tumour-promoting phorbol esters stimulate the phosphorylation of ribosomal protein S6 in quiescent Reuber H35 hepatomacells. *Journal of Biological Chemistry*, **259**, 897–902.

Tsukuda, M., Asaoka, Y., Sekiguchi, K., Kikkawa, U., and Nishizuka, Y. (1988). Properties of protein kinase C subspecies in human platelets. *Biochemical and Biophysical Research Communications*, **155**, 1387–95.

Vilgrain, I., Cochet, C., and Chambaz, E. M. (1984). Hormonal regulation of a calcium-activated, phospholipid-dependent protein kinase in bovine adrenal cortex. *Journal of Biological Chemistry*, **259**, 3404–6.

Wang, K. K. W., Wright, L. C., Machan, C. L., Allen, B. G., Conigrave, A. D., and Roufogalis, B. D. (1991). Protein kinase C phosphorylates the carboxyl terminus of the plasma membrane Ca^{2+}-ATPase from human erythrocytes. *Journal of Biological Chemistry*, **266**, 9078–85.

Watanabe, M., Hagiwara, M., Onoda, K., and Hidaka, H. (1988). Monoclonal antibody recognition of two subtype forms of protein kinase C in human platelets. *Biochemical and Biophysical Research Communications*, **152**, 642–8.

Wender, P. A., Cribbs, C. M., Koehler, K. F., Sharkey, N. A., Herald, C. L., Kamano, Y., *et al.* (1988). Modelling of the bryostatins to the phorbol ester pharmacophore on protein kinase C. *Proceedings of the National Academy of Sciences of the United States of America*, **85**, 7197–201.

Werth, D. K. and Pastan, I. (1984). Vinculin phorphorylation in response to calcium and phorbol esters in intact cells. *Journal of Biological Chemistry*, **259**, 5264–70.

Wightman, P. D. and Raetz, C. R. H. (1984). The activation of protein kinase C by biologically active lipid moieties of lipopolysaccharide. *Journal of Biological Chemistry*, **259**, 10048–52.

Wolf, M., LeVine III, H., May, W. S., Jr, Cuatrecasas, P., and Sahyoun, N. (1985). A model for intracellular translocation of protein kinase C involving synergism between Ca^{2+} and phorbol esters. *Nature, London*, **317**, 546–49.

Woodgett, J. R., Gould, K. L., and Hunter, T. (1986). Substrate specificity of protein-kinase C. *European Journal of Biochemistry*, **161**, 177–84.

Woodgett, J. R., Hunter, T., and Gould, K. L. (1987). In *Cell Membranes— Methods and Reviews* (ed. Elson, E. L., Frazier, W. A., and Glaser, L.), Vol. 3, pp. 215–340. Plenum Press, New York.

Yamauchi, T., Nakata, H., and Fujisawa, H. (1981). A new activator protein that activates tryptophan 5-monooxygenase and tyrosine 3-monooxygenase in the presence of Ca^{2+}-, calmodulin-dependent protein kinase. *Journal of Biological Chemistry*, **256**, 5404–9.

Zhao, F-K., Chuang, L. F., Israel, M., and Chuang, R. Y. (1989). Cremophor EL, a widely used parenteral vehicle, is a potent inhibitor of protein kinase C. *Biochemical and Biophysical Research Communications*, **159**, 1359–67.

Section 3C

Protein kinase C inhibitors

Christopher H. Hill

3C.1 Introduction

A general role for protein kinases in cellular regulation was first recognized by Walsh *et al.* (1968) with the discovery of cAMP-dependent protein kinase (PKA). Subsequently, other serine–threonine-specific protein kinases, such as the Ca^{2+}–phospholipid-dependent protein kinase (protein kinase C (PKC)), and the Ca^{2+}–calmodulin-dependent protein kinase (CCDPK), have been identified.

Traditional biochemical techniques were initially employed to isolate and characterize these novel enzymes, but the advent of gene cloning and sequencing led to the discovery of well over a hundred distinct genes for protein kinases (Hanks *et al.* 1988). Although molecular biology has allowed the rapid identification of new members of the protein kinase family, the role of these enzymes in cellular systems has remained unclear. Progress has been impeded by the lack of potent selective inhibitors of protein kinases which could be used as biochemical tools to determine whether a particular kinase elicits a specific cellular response.

3C.2   Protein kinase C

The rapidly expanding PKC isoenzyme family currently comprises at least eight members (S. Osada *et al.* 1990). Each isoenzyme consists of a 30 kDa amino-terminal diacylglycerol (DAG)–phospholipid-binding regulatory domain and a 50 kDa protein–ATP binding catalytic domain. Proteolytic cleavage releases into the cytosol the free catalytic fragment (PKM), which is fully functional in the absence of cofactors but has no known physiological role (Kishimoto *et al.* 1983; Melloni *et al.* 1985).

The transduction of signals from a number of mediators across the cell membrane relies upon the pivotal role played by PKC (Farago and Nishizuka 1990). Receptor occupation by a variety of cytokines, hormone, and neurotransmitters promotes the phospholipase-C-mediated hydrolysis of phosphotidylinositolbisphosphate (PIP_2), via a G-protein or tyrosine kinase mechanism, to give the two second messengers DAG and inositol-1, 4,5-trisphosphate (IP_3), (Berridge 1987). DAG can also be formed from phosphatidylcholine (Rosoff *et al.* 1988; Augert *et al.* 1989) and is required for the activation of PKC, whilst IP_3 promotes the release of calcium from internal stores. On activation, PKC propagates the signal by transfer of the γ-phosphate of ATP to protein serine or threonine residues, resulting in phosphorylated proteins exhibiting modified properties. Therefore PKC is able to regulate gene expression, cell proliferation, and secretion. Consequently, an examination of the patent literature reveals PKC inhibitors claimed for the treatment of an extensive range of disease states. Indeed, selective inhibitors of PKC might well provide therapy for diseases ranging from asthma, cancer, dermatological disorders, and rheumatoid arthritis to viral diseases such as AIDS.

Investigations into the role of PKC in cellular processes have centred primarily on the use of phorbol esters (DAG mimics) as 'specific activators' of the enzyme or on the use of non-selective and/or weakly active inhibitors.

The problems associated with the latter are evident, but results of experiments with phorbols must also be carefully interpreted owing to the downregulation of PKC observed on prolonged exposure with these agents. Clearly, there is a need for potent and selective PKC inhibitors to allow the complex signal transduction pathways to be unravelled.

3C.3   Phospholipid–DAG competitive inhibitors

The regulatory domain of PKC was believed to be the only physiological receptor for phorbol esters, and it has been argued that inhibitors which are competitive with phorbol esters should be highly selective for this enzyme (Ruegg and Burgess 1989). However, other phorbol ester receptors have recently been reported (Ahmed *et al*. 1990).

Sphingosine (Fig. 3C.1) is a potent reversible inhibitor of PKC and of phorbol ester binding in mixed micellular assays (Hannun *et al*. 1986). The essential structural requirements for inhibition of PKC have been identified as the overall hydrophobic nature of the molecule and the presence of a primary amine. The 1-hydroxyl group is not required for activity, and substitution via a glycosidic linkage has resulted in a series of potent lysosphingolipid inhibitors. It has been proposed that these lysosphingolipids represent the missing functional link between the accumulation of sphingolipids and the pathogenesis of sphingolipidoses (Hannun and Bell 1987). The same authors also suggest that lysosphingolipids might exist as normal cellular constituents and function to regulate PKC activity.

Calphostin C has also been shown to be competitive with [^{3}H]phorbol dibutyrate (PDBu) and to possess potent cytotoxic and antitumour activity. This perylenequinone is three orders of magnitude more potent against PKC ($IC_{50} = 50$ nM) than any other protein kinase tested (Kobayashi *et al*. 1989a,b). The calphostin family represented a promising lead for the design of more potent inhibitors, however, it has recently become apparent that exposure to light is a prerequisite for the observed inhibitory activity. Indeed, this photoactivation of calphostin C generates a short-lived species that reacts with PKC, resulting in permanent inactivation of phorbol dibutyrate (PDBu) binding (Bruns *et al*. 1991).

Modification of phospholipid analogues has led to the synthesis of the alkyllysophospholipid, ilmofosine (BM 41440 (Fig. 3C.1)), in which the O—alkyl bond is replaced by a thioether linkage and the β-hydroxyl group is substituted by a methoxymethyl ether (Herrmann and Bicker 1988). Ilmofosine exhibits lipid competitive inhibition ($K_i = 0.56$ μM) of PKC and shows anti-neoplastic activity *in vitro* as well as *in vivo* antitumour activity. Although other mechanisms cannot be excluded, it has been shown that ilmofosine inhibits PKC in intact cells at therapeutic concentrations (Hofmann *et al*. 1989).

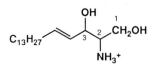

Sphingosine

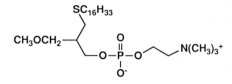

Ilmofosine

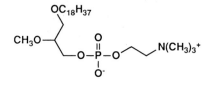

Et-18-OMe

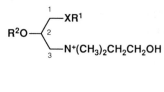

Quaternary ammonium
salts

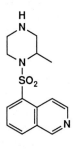

H7

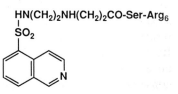

Bisubstrate inhibitor

Fig. 3C.1

Alkylated analogues of phosphatidylcholine such as rac-1-*O*-octadecyl-2-*O*-methylglycerophosphocholine (Et-18-OMe; (Fig. 3C.1)) have been shown to inhibit PKC selectively and to block the growth and metastasis of a variety of cancer cell lines (Helfman *et al.* 1983; Parker *et al.* 1987). Alkyl phospholipids also possess antineoplastic activity against human tumour cell lines (Morris-Natschke *et al.* 1986), one of which (racemic 1-octadecyl-2-methylglycero-3-phosphocholine) is undergoing phase I clinical trials (Berdel *et al.* 1981).

More recently, a series of novel quaternary ammonium derivatives of alkylglycerols (Fig. 3C.1) has been described (Marasco *et al.* 1990). These structures contain an 'inverse choline' moiety which apparently retains the hydrophilic nature of the phosphocholine moiety but is not susceptible to degradation by phospholipase C (PLC) or phospholipase D (PLD). However, the compounds in this series do require a free hydroxyl group and the dialkylether moiety to retain activity. They are competitive with phosphatidylserine and it was found to be essential to retain a long-chain alkyl ether (X = O or S) at position 1. Small alkyl ethers were tolerated at position 2 ($R^2 = CH_3$, CH_2CH_3). The antineoplastic activity of these compounds is currently under investigation.

Other inhibitors which have been reported to bind to the regulatory domain include adriamycin-iron(III) (Hannun *et al.* 1989), aminoacridines (Hannun and Bell 1988), dequalinium (Rotenberg *et al.* 1990), AMG-C16 (Kramer *et al.* 1989), *N*-Myr-KRTLR (O'Brian *et al.* 1990), and tamoxifen (Su *et al.* 1985).

3C.4 Protein competitive inhibitors

The regulatory domain of PKC contains a conserved basic-residue-rich amino acid sequence analogous to a substrate phosphorylation site. Small synthetic peptides corresponding to this sequence have been synthesized and shown to be potent and relatively selective inhibitors of PKC (House and Kemp 1987; Smith *et al.* 1990). The synthetic peptide corresponding to residues 19–36 in PKC inhibits both autophosphorylation and protein substrate phosphorylation. The shortest peptide sequence retaining inhibitory activity corresponds to residues 19–31 in PKC (IC_{50} = 92 nM). Replacement of Ala by Ser transforms this pseudosubstrate peptide into an excellent substrate (K_m = 0.2 μM), and it has been proposed that this conserved region of the regulatory domain may be responsible for maintaining the enzyme in the inactive form in the absence of activators.

More recently, the benzophenanthridine alkaloid chelerythrine has been described as a potent and 'specific' inhibitor of PKC, with a reported IC_{50} of 0.66 μM (Herbert *et al.* 1990). Surprisingly, this compound was found to be competitive with a range of phosphate acceptors. It is the only potent non-peptidic inhibitor reported to act at this site to date.

3C.5 ATP competitive inhibitors

3C.5.1 Isoquinoline sulphonamides

Extensive use of this class of compound has been made in an effort to evaluate the role of PKC in cellular systems. The most commonly used example of this series is 1-[5-isoquinolinesulphonyl]-2-methyl-piperazine dihydrochloride (H7) (Fig. 3C.1), which inhibits rat brain PKC with a K_i of 6 μM, but also inhibits PKA and cGMP-dependent protein kinase (PKG) at similar concentrations (Hidaka *et al.* 1984).

The concentration of ATP used in a typical isolated enzyme assay is in the 5–10 μM range (Nixon *et al.* 1991), whereas the concentration of ATP commonly found to be in intact cells is in the millimolar region. Therefore it is not surprising that the ATP-competitive H7 does not inhibit TPA-induced 47 kDa protein phosphorylation in intact platelets or PDBu-induced down-regulation of CD3 and CD4 in T-cells at concentrations up to 100 μM (Nixon *et al.* 1991). In contrast with the effects seen with H7 in phorbol-ester-driven systems, the IC_{50} obtained for H7 in many other cellular experiments is similar to that observed in the isolated enzyme assays (1–20 μM). Nixon *et al.* (1991) argue that these effects of H7 are unlikely to result from PKC inhibition since low micromolar concentrations of H7 do not inhibit cellular responses directly mediated by PKC activation.

Clearly, H7 is not an ideal choice as a probe for PKC involvement in cellular processes. It is neither selective nor potent enough to attribute its cellular effects to inhibition of PKC.

3C.5.2   Indolocarbazoles

The microbial metabolite staurosporine (Table 3C.1) has been widely used to investigate the role of PKC in signal transduction processes following the initial report describing it as a potent inhibitor of this kinase (Tamaoki *et al.* 1986). However, it rapidly became apparent that this indolocarbazole was also a potent inhibitor of a variety of other kinases (Ruegg and Burgess 1989; Elliott *et al.* 1990).

Many of the observed cellular effects of staurosporine, including its marked cytostatic effects, have been attributed to inhibition of PKC. In view of the poor selectivity profile of this compound (Table 3C.1), the conclusions drawn from such experiments must remain questionable. Nevertheless, staurosporine represents an attractive lead for inhibitor design, and the search for more selective analogues has concentrated on synthesizing derivatives of the amine group in the sugar moiety and modification of the lactam (Table 3C.1). The hydroxylactam UCN-01 retains the activity of staurosporine against PKC, but also exhibits some tenfold selectivity over PKA. The epimeric compound (UCN-02) displays less selectivity and is less potent. Clearly, the configuration at C-7 is important, but the methyl ethers of the hydroxylactams both exhibit improved activity and selectivity. The corresponding imide is also as active as staurosporine against PKC.

The methylamino substituent on the pyranose ring apparently contributes significantly to the potent activity of staurosporine, since the 4′-desmethylamino-4′-hydroxy analogue (RK-286C) is 500-fold less active (Osada *et al.* 1990). However, the bioactive conformation of the pyranose ring system is not known, since the protonated amine in staurosporine

Table 3C.1 Selectivity profile for staurosporine analogues

	R¹	X	Y	R²	IC₅₀(µM)			Reference
					PKC	PKA	PhK	
Staurosporine	H	H	H	NHCH₃	0.006	0.015	0.003	Meyer et al. 1989
CGP 41251	H	H	H	NCH₃COPh	0.050	2.4	0.048	Meyer et al. 1989
CGP 42700	PhCH₂	H	H	NCH₃COPh	>100	>100	>100	Meyer et al. 1989
RK286C	H	H	H	OH	3	ND	ND	H. Osada et al. 1990
UCN-01	H	H	OH	NHCH₃	0.004	0.042	ND	Takahashi et al. 1990
UCN-02	H	OH	H	NHCH₃	0.062	0.250	ND	Takahashi et al. 1990
UCN-01-Me	H	H	OCH₃	NHCH₃	0.001	0.240	ND	Takahashi et al. 1990
UCN-02-Me	H	OCH₃	H	NHCH₃	0.028	0.380	ND	Takahashi et al. 1990
UCN-01,02-Et	H	H, OCH₂CH₃	OCH₂CH₃, H	NHCH₃	0.140	0.780	ND	Takahashi et al. 1990
	H	O	O	NHCH₃	0.004	0.027	ND	Murakata et al. 1989

ND, not determined.

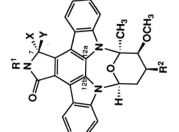

prefers the boat form in solution and the free base adopts a chair conformation. In view of the low pK_a of the amine (5.3), the possibility of free-base binding cannot be discounted and therefore both pyranose conformations should be considered when designing analogues (Davis *et al.* 1991).

Benzoylation of the amine in staurosporine gives a compound (CGP 41251) which demonstrates a significant selectivity improvement for PKC over PKA. However, this is achieved at the expense of some loss in potency and this analogue is still a potent inhibitor of phosphorylase kinase (PhK). Alkylation of the lactam nitrogen results in total abrogation of kinase inhibitory activity and indicates that the lactam NH is an important H-bond donor.

Other indolocarbazole systems bearing a common aglycone to staurosporine but which are attached to a furanose ring, such as K252a (Table 3C.2), have also been isolated. Such compounds have shown very little selectivity for any protein kinases; however, it has recently been reported that K252a is a potent and selective inhibitor of phosphorylase kinase (Elliott *et al.* 1990). The physiological implications of this are not clear, but this compound is known to possess *in vivo* anti-inflammatory activity (Ohmori *et al.* 1988). Within this series of compounds (Table 3C.2), the reported structure–activity relationships parallel those seen with staurosporine. *N*-alkylation of the lactam abolishes activity, and introduction of a second carbonyl to give the corresponding imide appears to be well tolerated, producing surprisingly selective inhibitors. Introduction of an amino substituent into the furanose ring has also resulted in more potent inhibitors of PKC in this series (Hachisu *et al.* 1989). It is likely that these structure–activity relationships indicate that these compounds share a common mode of binding with staurosporine and analogues, and that the amino substituent is able to access a common putative cationic binding site.

In view of the intense synthetic interest shown in the common aglycone unit (Sarstedt and Winterfeldt 1983; Magnus and Sear 1984; Bergman and Pelcman 1989; Hughes *et al.* 1990; Moody and Rahimtoola 1990), structure–activity studies are surprisingly sparse. However, it is apparent that alkylation of the indolocarbazole nitrogen atoms may be beneficial to activity (Table 3C.3). In addition, we have seen that alkylation of the lactam abrogates activity in parallel with results seen by others on staurosporine and K252a. The corresponding imide also appears to be tolerated, although an accurate IC_{50} was not obtained owing to the inherent insolubility of the compound. However, the hydroxylactam lost activity.

In conclusion, it has been possible to generate potent indolocarbazole inhibitors of PKC which display some degree of selectivity. This is both encouraging and surprising, bearing in mind the close homology between the ATP-binding sites of protein kinases (Hanks *et al.* 1988). However, it

Table 3C.2 Selectivity profile for K252 analogues

	R^1	R^2	R^3	R^4	X	Y	IC$_{50}$ (or K$_i$) (μM)			Reference
							PKC	PKA	PhK	
–	H	H	H	H	O	O	0.028	5.5	ND	Kleinschroth *et al.* 1991
–	PhCH$_2$	H	H	H	O	O	>10	ND	ND	Kleinschroth *et al.* 1991
K252a	H	OH	CO$_2$CH$_3$	CH$_3$	H	H	**0.025**	**0.018**	**0.0016**	Kase *et al.* 1987
K252b	H	OH	CO$_2$H	CH$_3$	H	H	**0.020**	**0.090**	ND	Kase *et al.* 1987
KT5720	H	OH	CO$_2$(CH$_2$)$_5$CH$_3$	CH$_3$	H	H	**> 2**	**0.060**	ND	Kase *et al.* 1987
KT5822	H	OCH$_3$	CO$_2$CH$_3$	CH$_3$	H	H	**0.079**	**0.037**	ND	Kase *et al.* 1987
NAO344	H	OH	CH$_2$N(CH$_3$)$_2$	CH$_3$	H	H	0.114	ND	ND	Hachisu *et al.* 1989
NAO345	H	OH	CH$_2$NHCH$_3$	CH$_3$	H	H	0.068	ND	ND	Hachisu *et al.* 1989
NAO346	H	OH	CH$_2$NH$_2$	CH$_3$	H	H	0.062	ND	ND	Hachisu *et al.* 1989

ND, not determined.

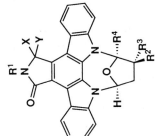

Table 3C.3 Aglycone analogues

R^1	R^2	R^3	R^4	R^5	X	Y	IC_{50} (μM) PKC	Reference
H	H	H	H	H	H	H	0.214	Kase et al. 1986
CH_2CH_3	CH_2CH_3	H	H	H	H	H	0.066	Hartenstein et al. 1989
H	CH_2CH_3	Cl,H	H,Cl	H	H	H	0.310	Kleinschroth et al. 1990
H	H	H	H	$PhCH_2$	H	H	>10	Wilkinson, personal communication
H	H	H	H	H	OH	H	4.6	Wilkinson personal communication
H	H	H	H	H	O	O	1	Wilkinson personal communication

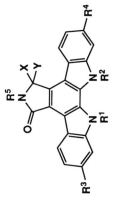

should be noted that none of these compounds have yet been demonstrated to display any selectivity for PKC over PhK.

3C.5.3   Bisindolylmaleimides

A series of compounds has been synthesized in which the 12a — 12b bond in the staurosporine aglycone has been formally removed in order to investigate the requirement for a planar indolocarbazole (Davis *et al.* 1989). An extra carbonyl was also introduced into the lactam ring, since it was reasoned that no low energy conformation could then have an indole group coplanar with the five-membered ring due to steric inter-actions. These bisindolylmaleimides inhibit PKC and are fully competitive with ATP (e.g. isothiourea (Table 3C.4), $K_i = 3$ nM). The most sur-prising result, however, was the observation that these compounds are much more selective than the staurosporine-like analogues. Modification of the imide moiety gave structure–activity relationships which resemble those of the aglycone. Two carbonyls are required for optimal activity since the lactam was somewhat less active than the imide, but *N*-alkylation of either gave essentially inactive compounds (Table 3C.4). Alkylation of the indole nitrogens gave some small increase in activity.

Structure–activity relationships have shown that one indole can be re-placed by other aryl rings only at the expense of potency. Bicyclic aromatics such as benzothiophene and naphthalene were the best replacements, but none was as good as indole. Substitution around the indole ring was also detrimental to activity in general. However, small lipophilic substituents were tolerated at the 2,4,5- and 7-positions. In contrast, substitution on the indole nitrogen was allowed without any significant loss of activity (Davis *et al.* 1992a).

Based on the results obtained on imide modification, a common mode of binding for the bisindolylmaleimides and staurosporine has been postulated. A molecular graphics approach was adopted whereby the imide moiety of the bisindolylmaleimides is matched onto the lactam of staurosporine. The indoles were allowed to approach the plane of the indolocarbazole as far as possible without energy penalty and a cationic-substituent-con-taining side-chain was attached to an indole nitrogen, the only position in the molecule known to tolerate any significant substitution. The graphics model predicted that a variety of chain lengths (2–5 methylenes) should all be able to access the putative amine-binding site for staurosporine. Indeed, such compounds were all significantly more active than the parent bisindolylmaleimide (Davis *et al.* 1992b).

Other cationic analogues have also been prepared, and, since isothioureas such as Ro 31–8220 proved to be even more potent inhibitors of PKC, it is likely that such a bifurcated cationic species is interacting with a carboxylate in the enzyme active site.

Table 3C.4 Selectivity profile for arylindolylmaleimides

X	Y	R^1	R^2	Ar	IC$_{50}$ (μM)		Reference
					PKC	PKA	
O	O	H	H	3-indolyl	0.55	11.8	Davis *et al.* 1992a
O	O	CH$_3$	H	3-indolyl	>100	>100	Davis *et al.* 1992a
H	OH	H	H	3-indolyl	45	ND	Davis *et al.* 1992a
H	H	H	H	3-indolyl	10	ND	Davis *et al.* 1992a
O	O	H	CH$_3$	1-methyl-3-indolyl	0.30	16	Davis *et al.* 1992a
O	O	H	CH$_3$	Ph	7.7	>100	Davis *et al.* 1989
O	O	H	CH$_3$	3-benzothienyl	0.90	>100	Davis *et al.* 1992a
O	O	H	CH$_3$	1-naphthyl	0.81	>100	Davis *et al.* 1992a
O	O	H	CH$_3$	1-methyl-2-indolyl	>100	>100	Davis *et al.* 1992a
O	O	H	CH$_3$	1-indolyl	3.0	ND	Davis *et al.* 1992a
O	O	H	(CH$_2$)$_2$NH$_2$	1-methyl-3-indolyl	0.06	8.9	Davis *et al.* 1992b
O	O	H	(CH$_2$)$_3$NH$_2$	1-methyl-3-indolyl	0.08	5.1	Davis *et al.* 1989
O	O	H	(CH$_2$)$_4$NH$_2$	1-methyl-3-indolyl	0.06	9.4	Davis *et al.* 1992b
O	O	H	(CH$_2$)$_3$SC(=NH)NH$_2$	1-methyl-3-indolyl	0.01	1.5	Davis *et al.* 1989

ND, not determined.

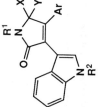

Table 3C.5 Selectivity profile of bisindolylmaleimides bearing a conformationally restricted side-chain

	R	IC$_{50}$ (μM)				Reference
		PKC	PKA	CCDPK	PhK	
Ro 31–8425	H	0.008	2.8	19	15	Muid et al. 1991
Ro 31–8830	CH$_3$	0.040	8.5	ND	11.4	Mulqueen et al. 1992

ND, not determined.

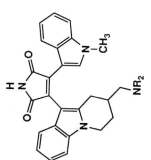

More potent inhibitors in this series have also been prepared by conformationally restricting the amine side-chain (Bit *et al*. 1991). This has culminated in the synthesis of Ro 31–8425, which has been shown to be as potent as staurosporine against PKC but displays a significantly improved selectivity profile (Table 3C.5). Not only is Ro 31–8425 highly selective for PKC over PKA and CCDPK but, unlike the indolocarbazoles, it is significantly selective for PKC over PhK (Muid *et al*. 1991).

These inhibitors have been shown to block PKC in intact cells and inhibit a mixed lymphocyte reaction (Muid *et al*. 1991; Davis *et al*. 1992b). The plasma levels of primary amines in this series are significantly lower than those of the corresponding tertiary amine, following oral administration to rats and mice. The tertiary amine Ro 31–8830 (Table 3C.5) is also active in *in vivo* models of inflammation. It antagonizes a phorbol-ester-induced paw oedema in mice with an MED of 20 mg kg^{-1} (Mulqueen *et al*. 1992) and is also active in the secondary phase of the developing adjuvant arthritis model in the rat with an MED < 25 mg kg^{-1}. These compounds represent exciting new agents for the potential therapy of autoimmune diseases such as rheumatoid arthritis.

3C.5.4   Other inhibitors

The antitumour nucleoside sangivamycin selectivity inhibits PKC (apparent $K_i = 11$ μM) compared with PKA ($IC_{50} = 50$ μM), but the inhibition of PKA was not strictly competitive with ATP (Loomis and Bell 1988).

Many plant flavonoids such as quercetin also inhibit PKC. Although these flavonoids are not very potent inhibitors, a model of the minimum essential features required for PKC inhibition has been postulated involving a coplanar flavone structure with free hydroxyl groups at the 3′-, 4′-, and 7-positions (Ferriola *et al*. 1989).

Erbstatin is a peptidic-substrate-competitive inhibitor of EGF receptor tyrosine kinase ($K_i = 5.6$ μM) and is non-competitive with respect to ATP (Imoto *et al*. 1987). More recently it has been shown to inhibit PKC ($K_i = 11$ μM) competitively with ATP (Bishop *et al*. 1990).

A series of oxazolones has been patented for use in the treatment of HIV infection, hypertension, and asthma (Cheng *et al*. 1991; Sunkara and Jones 1991a,b). One of these compounds, MDL 27032, is certainly a novel vasodilator but displays no selectivity for PKC inhibition over PKA (Robinson *et al*. 1990).

3C.6   A bisubstrate approach

It has been estimated that the binding of two substrates in their ground states could lead to rate enhancements of the order of 10^8 (Page and Jencks 1971). Similarly, the combination of two substrates required by an enzyme to form a single molecule could enhance its binding affinity through a significant entropic contribution by a factor as large as 10^8 compared with the product of the association constants of the individual molecules. This bisubstrate approach has been adopted by Ricouart *et al.* (1991) in an attempt to obtain potent inhibitors of PKC. Mimics of both the ATP and protein substrates separated by an appropriate length linker were designed (Fig. 3C.1). For the protein substrate, the primary sequence recognition motif is not clearly defined for PKC but it is known to be important to have basic residues close to the phosphorylation site. Therefore a cluster of arginine residues (Arg_4 or Arg_6) was chosen to interact with the peptidic recognition site. Naphthalene- and isoquinoline-sulphonyl groups were chosen as the ATP mimics, since the corresponding sulphonamides are known to be ATP-competitive inhibitors. Since no X-ray crystal structure had been reported for a protein kinase, it was assumed that the crystal data obtained with phosphoglycerate kinase (Bryant *et al.* 1974) could be extended to protein kinases. The distance between the carbon-bearing phosphorylated hydroxyl and N-9 of the adenine was thus found to be 16.3 Å. A flexible linker consisting of two β-alanine residues in an extended conformation was predicted by molecular modelling to allow the desired spacing between the two moieties.

Interestingly, all the active inhibitors reported demonstrated a selectivity for PKA and not PKC. The most potent inhibitor has an IC_{50} of 3 nM against PKA and 300 nM against PKC and was found to be competitive with ATP for both enzymes. However, it was not competitive with the peptidic substrates, and the authors concluded that this indicates an ordered mechanism of inhibition in which interaction with the ATP-binding site is required before interaction of the peptidic moiety.

3C.7   The future

At least eight different isoforms of PKC have been reported. Since the isoenzyme ratio in a particular target cell line and tissue type varies considerably, it might well be important in terms of obtaining a drug to design isoenzyme-selective inhibitors of PKC. To date there have been no reports of such compounds, but it can only be a matter of time before isoenzyme-selective inhibitors come to light. Recent years have seen an explosion of interest in the way in which cellular processes are controlled by phosphorylation state, and in the decades to come it is possible that inhibitors of a whole array of kinases and phosphatases will be synthesized. These will allow the elucidation of many signal transduction pathways and ultimately, it is hoped, to the creation of whole new classes of drugs.

References

Ahmed, S., Kozma, R., Monfries, C., Hall, C., Lim, H. H., Smith, P., and Lim, L. (1990). Human brain *n*-chimaerin cDNA encodes a novel phorbol ester receptor. *Biochemical Journal*, **272**, 767–73.

Augert, G., Bocckino, S. B., Blackmore, P. F., and Exton, J. H. (1989). Hormonal stimulation of diacylglycerol formation in hepatocytes. *Journal of Biological Chemistry*, **264**, 21689–98.

Berdel, W. E., Bausert, W. R., Fink, U., Rastetter, J., and Munder, P. G. (1981). Antitumor action of alkyl-lysophospholipids. *Anticancer Research*, **1**, 345–51.

Bergman, J. and Pelcman, B. (1989). Synthesis of indolo[2,3-a]pyrrolo[3,4-c]-carbazoles by double Fischer indolizations. *Journal of Organic Chemistry*, **54**, 824–8.

Berridge, M. J. (1987). Inositol trisphosphate and diacylglycerol: two interacting second messengers. *Annual Review of Biochemistry*, **56**, 159–93.

Bishop, W. R., Petrin, J., Wang, L., Ramesh, U., and Dol, R. J. (1990). Inhibition of protein kinase C by the tyrosine kinase inhibitor erbstatin. *Biochemical Pharmacology*, **40**, 2129–35.

Bit, R. A., Davis, P. D., Hill, C. H., Keech, E., and Vesey, D. (1991). A Dieckmann/ring expansion approach to tetrahydropyrido- and tetrahydroazepino-[1,2-a]indoles. *Tetrahedron*, **47**, 4645–64.

Bruns, R. F., Miller, F. D., Merriman, R. L., Howbert, J. J., Heath, W. F., Kobayashi, E., *et al.* (1991). Inhibition of protein kinase C by calphostin C is light-dependent. *Biochemical and Biophysical Research Communications*, **176**, 288–93.

Bryant, T. N., Watson, H. C., and Wendell, P. C. (1974). Structure of yeast phosphoroglycerate kinase. *Nature, London*, **247**, 14–17.

Cheng, H. C., Dage, R. C., Jones, W. D., and Robinson, P. J. (1991). Novel pyridyloxazole-2-ones useful as protein kinase C inhibitors. European Patent Application EP 428106, 1–10.

Davis, P. D., Hill, C. H., Keech, E., Lawton, G., Nixon, J. S., Sedgwick, A. D., *et al.* (1989). Potent selective inhibitors of protein kinase C. *Federation of European Biochemical Societies Letters*, **259**, 61–3.

Davis, P. D., Hill, C. H., Thomas, W. A., and Whitcombe I. W. A. (1991). The design of inhibitors of protein kinase C; the solution conformation of staurosporine. *Journal of the Chemical Society Chemical Communications*, 182–3.

Davis, P. D., Hill, C. H., Lawton, G., Nixon, J. S., Wilkinson, S. E., Hurst, S. A., *et al.* (1992a). Inhibitors of protein kinase C (1): 2,3-bisarylmaleimides. *Journal of Medicinal Chemistry*, **35**, 177–84.

Davis, P. D., Elliott, L. H., Harris, W., Hill, C. H., Hurst, S. A., Keech, E., *et al.* (1992b). Inhibitors of protein kinase C (2): substituted bisindolylmaleimides with improved potency and selectivity. *Journal of Medicinal Chemistry*, **35**, 994–1001.

Elliott, L. H., Wilkinson, S. E., Sedgwick, A. D., Hill, C. H., Lawton, G., Davis, P. D., and Nixon, J. S. (1990). K252a is a potent and selective inhibitor of phosphorylase kinase. *Biochemical and Biophysical Research Communications*, **171**, 148–54.

Farago, A. and Nishizuka, Y. (1990). Protein kinase C in transmembrane signalling. *Federation of European Biochemical Societies Letters*, **268**, 350–4.

Ferriola, P. C., Cody, V., and Middleton, E., Jr, (1989). Protein kinase C inhibition by plant flavonoids. *Biochemical Pharmacology*, **38**, 1617–24.

Hachisu, M., Hiranuma, T., Koyama, M., and Sezaki, M. (1989). Antihypertensive compounds with potent protein kinases inhibitory activity. *Life Sciences*, **44**, 1351–62.

Hanks, S. K., Quinn, A. M., and Hunter, T. (1988). The protein kinase family: conserved features and deduced phylogeny of the catalytic domains. *Science*, **241**, 42–52.

Hannun, Y. A. and Bell, R. M. (1987). Lysosphingolipids inhibit protein kinase C: implications for the sphingolipidoses. *Science*, **235**, 670–4.

Hannun, Y. A. and Bell, R. M. (1988). Aminoacridines, potent inhibitors of protein kinase C. *Journal of Biological Chemistry*, **263**, 9960–6.

Hannun, Y. A., Loomis, C. R., Merrill, A. H., and Bell, R. J. (1986). Sphingosine inhibition of protein kinase C activity and of phorbol dibutyrate binding *in vitro* and in human platelets. *Journal of Biological Chemistry*, **261**, 12604–9.

Hannun, Y. A., Foglesong, R. J., and Bell, R. J. (1989). The adriamycin-iron(III) complex is a potent inhibitor of protein kinase C. *Journal of Biological Chemistry*, **264**, 9960–6.

Hartenstein, J., Barth, H., Schachtele, C., Rudolf, C., and Weinheimer, G. (1989). Indolocarbazole Derivate, Verfahren zu deren Herstellung und diese enthaltende Arzneimittel. European Patent Application EP 328000, 1–14.

Helfman, D. M., Barnes, K. C., Kinkade, J. M., Vogler, W. R., Shoji, W. M., and Kuo, J. F. (1983). Phospholipid-sensitive Ca^{2+}-dependent protein phosphorylation system in various types of leukemic cells from human patients and in human leukemic cell lines HL60 and K562, and its inhibition by alkyl-lysophospholipid. *Cancer Research*, **43**, 2955–61.

Herbert, J. M., Augereau, J. M., Gleye, J., and Maffrand, J. P. (1990). Chelerythrine is a potent and specific inhibitor of protein kinase C. *Biochemical and Biophysical Research Communications*, **172**, 993–9.

Herrmann, D. B. J. and Bicker, U. (1988). Ilmofosine (BM41440), a new cytotoxic ether phospholipid. *Drugs of the Future*, **13**, 543–54.

Hidaka, H., Inaguki, M., Kawamoto, S., and Susaki, Y. (1984). Isoquinoline sulfonamides, novel and potent inhibitors of cyclic nucleotide dependent protein kinase and protein kinase C. *Biochemistry*, **23**, 5036–41.

Hofmann, J., Ueberall, F., Posch, L., Maly, K., Herrmann, D. B. J., and Grunicke, H. (1989). Synergistic enhancement of the antiproliferative activity of *cis*-diamminedichloroplatinum(II) by the ether lipid analogue BM41440, an inhibitor of protein kinase C. *Lipids*, **24**, 312–17.

House, C. and Kemp, B. E. (1987). Protein kinase C contains a pseudosubstrate prototype in its regulatory domain. *Science*, **238**, 1726–8.

Hughes, I., Nolan, W. P., and Raphael, R. A. (1990). Synthesis of the indolo-[2,3-a]carbazole natural products staurosporine and arcyriaflavin B. *Journal of the Chemical Society, Perkin Transactions I*, 2475–80.

Imoto, M., Umezawa, K., Isshika, K., Kunimoto, S., Sawa, T., Takeuchi, T., and Umezawa, H. (1987). Kinetic studies of tyrosine kinase inhibition by erbstatin. *Journal of Antibiotics*, **40**, 1471–3.

Kase, H., Iwahashi, K., and Matsuda, Y. (1986). K252b, c, and d, potent inhibitors of protein kinase C from microbial origin. *Journal of Antibiotics*, **39**, 1066–71.

Kase, H., Iwahashi, K., Nakanishi, S., Matsuda, Y., Yamada, K., Takahishi, M., et al. (1987). K252 compounds, novel and potent inhibitors of protein kinase C and cyclic nucleotide-dependent protein kinases. *Biochemical and Biophysical Research Communications*, **142**, 436–40.

Kishimoto, A., Kojikawa, N., Shiota, M., and Nishizuka, Y. (1983). Proteolytic activation of calcium-activated, phospholipid-dependent protein kinase by calcium-dependent natural protease. *Journal of Biological Chemistry*, **258**, 1156–64.

Kleinschroth, J., Barth, H., Hartenstein, J., Schachtele, C., Rudolf, C., and Osswald, H. (1990). Indolocarbazole Derivate, Verfahren zu deren Herstellung und deren Verwendung als Arzneimittel. German Patent Application DE 3835842, 1–12.

Kleinschroth, J., Schachtele, C., Hartenstein, J., and Rudolf, C. (1991). Indolo-carbazol und dessen Verwendung. European Patent Application EP 410389, 1–5.

Kobayashi, E., Ando, K., Nakano, H., and Tamaoki, T. (1989a). UCN-1028A, a novel and specific inhibitor of protein kinase C, from *Cladosporium*. *Journal of Antibiotics*, **42**, 153–5.

Kobayashi, E., Nakano, H., Morimoto, M., and Tamaoki, T. (1989b). Calphostin C (UCN-1028A), a novel microbial compound, is a highly potent and specific inhibitor of protein kinase C. *Biochemical and Biophysical Research Communications*, **159**, 548–53.

Kramer, I. M., van der Bend, R. C., Tool, A. T. J., van Blitterswijk, W. J., Roas, D., and Verhoeven, A. J. (1989). 1-*O*-Hexadecyl-2-*O*-methylglycerol, a novel inhibitor of protein kinase C, inhibits the respiratory burst in human neutrophils. *Journal of Biological Chemistry*, **264**, 5876–84.

Loomis, C. R. and Bell, R. M. (1988). Sangivamycin, a nucleoside analogue, is a potent inhibitor of protein kinase C. *Journal of Biological Chemistry*, **263**, 1682–92.

Magnus, P. D. and Sear, N. L. (1984). Indole-2,3-quinodimethanes. *Tetrahedron*, **40**, 2795–7.

Marasco, C. J., Jr, Piantadosi, C., Meyer, K. L., Morris-Natschke, S., Ishaq, K. S., Small, G. W., and Daniel, L. W. (1990). Synthesis and biological activity of novel quaternary ammonium derivatives of alkylglycerols as potent inhibitors of protein kinase C. *Journal of Medicinal Chemistry*, **33**, 985–92.

Melloni, E., Pontremolli, S., Michetti, M., Sacco, O., Sparatore, B., Salamino, F., and Horecker, B. L. (1985). Binding of protein kinase C to neutrophil membranes in the presence of calcium and its activation by a calcium-requiring proteinase. *Proceedings of the National Academy of Sciences of the United States of America*, **82**, 6435–9.

Meyer, T., Regenass, U., Fabbro, D., Alteri, E., Rosel, J., Muller, M., et al. (1989). A derivative of staurosporine (CGP 41251) shows selectivity for protein kinase C and *in vitro* antiproliferative as well as *in vivo* anti-tumor activity. *International Journal of Cancer*, **43**, 851–6.

Moody, C. J. and Rahimtoola, K. F. (1990). Synthesis of the staurosporine aglycone. *Journal of the Chemical Society Chemical Communications*, 1667–8.

Morris-Natschke, S., Surles, J. R., Daniel, L. W., Berens, M., Modest, E. J., and Piantados, C. (1986). Synthesis of sulphur analogues of alkyl lysophospholipid and neoplastic cell growth inhibitory properties. *Journal of Medicinal Chemistry*, **29**, 2114–17.

Muid, R. E., Dale, M. M., Davis, P. D., Elliott, L. H., Hill, C. H., Kumar, H., *et al.* (1991). A novel conformationally restricted protein kinase inhibitor, Ro 31–8425, inhibits human neutrophil superoxide generation by soluble, particulate and post-receptor stimuli. *Federation of European Biochemical Societies Letters*, **293**, 169–72.

Mulqueen, M. J., Bradshaw, D., Davis, P. D., Elliott, L. H., Griffiths, T. A., Hill, C. H., *et al.* (1992). Oral, antiinflammatory activity of a potent, selective protein kinase C inhibitor. *Agents and Actions*, **37**, 85–9.

Murakata, C., Sato, M., Kasai, M., Morimoto, M., and Akinaga, S. (1989). World Patent Application WO 89/07105.

Nixon, J. S., Wilkinson, S. E., Davis, P. D., Sedgwick, A. D., Wadsworth, J., and Westmacott, D. (1991). Modulation of cellular processes by H7, a non-selective inhibitor of protein kinases. *Agents and Actions*, **32**, 188–93.

O'Brian, C. A., Ward, N. A., Liskamp, R. M., de Bont, D. B., and van Boom, G. H. (1990). *N*-Myristyl-Lys-Arg-Thr-Leu-Arg: a novel protein kinase C inhibitor. *Biochemical Pharmacology*, **39**, 49–57.

Ohmori, K., Ishii, H., Manabe, H., Satoh, H., Tamura, T., and Kase, H. (1988). Antiinflammatory and antiallergic effects of a novel metabolite of Nocardiopsis sp. as a potent protein kinase C inhibitor of microbial origin. *Arzneimittelforschung*, **38**, 809–14.

Osada, H., Takahashi, H., Tsunoda, K., Kusabe, H., and Isono, K. (1990). A new inhibitor of protein kinase C, RK-286C (4′-Demethylamino-4′-hydroxy-staurosporine). *Journal of Antibiotics*, **43**, 163–7.

Osada, H., Mizuno, K., Saido, T. C., Akita, Y., Suzuki, K., Kuroki, T., and Ohno, S. (1990). A phorbol ester receptor/protein kinase, nPKC eta, a new member of the protein kinase C family predominantly expressed in lung and skin. *Journal of Biological Chemistry*, **265**, 22434–40.

Page, M. I. and Jencks, W. P. (1971). Entropic contributions to rate accelerations in enzymic and intramolecular reactions and the chelate effect. *Proceedings of the National Academy of Sciences of the United States of America*, **68**, 1678–83.

Parker, J., Daniel, L. W., and Waite, M. (1987). Evidence of protein kinase C in phorbol diester-stimulated arachidonic acid release and prostaglandin synthesis. *Journal of Biological Chemistry*, **262**, 5385–93.

Ricouart, A., Gesquiere, J. C., Tartar, A., and Sergheraert, C. (1991). Design of protein kinase inhibitors using the bisubstrate approach. *Journal of Medicinal Chemistry*, **34**, 73–8.

Robinson, P. J., Cheng, H. C., Black, C. K., Schmidt, C. J., Karita, T., Jones, D. W., and Dage, R. C. (1990). MDL 27032 [4-propyl-5-(4-pyridinyl)-2(3H)-oxazolone], an active site-directed inhibitor of protein kinase C and cyclic AMP-dependent protein kinase that relaxes vascular smooth muscle. *Journal of Pharmacology and Experimental Therapeutics*, **255**, 1392–8.

Rosoff, P. M., Savage, N., and Dinarello, C. A. (1988). Interleukin-1 stimulates diacylglycerol production in T lymphocytes by a novel mechanism. *Cell*, **54**, 73–81.

Rotenberg, S. A., Smiley, S., Ueffiney, M., Krauss, R. S., Chen, L. B., and Weinstein, B. (1990). Inhibition of rodent protein kinase C by the anticarcinoma agent dequalinium. *Cancer Research*, **50**, 677–85.

Ruegg, U. T. and Burgess, G. M. (1989). Staurosporine, K252 and UCN-01: potent but nonspecific inhibitors of protein kinases. *Trends in Pharmacological Sciences*, **10**, 218–20.

Sarstedt, B. and Winterfeldt, E. (1983). A simple synthesis of the staurosporine aglycon. *Heterocycles*, **20**, 469–76.

Smith, M. K., Colbran, R. J., and Soderling, T. R. (1990). Specificities of autoinhibitory domain peptides for four protein kinases. *Journal of Biological Chemistry*, **265**, 1837–40.

Su, H., Mazzei, G. J., Vogler, W. R., and Kuo, J. F. (1985). Effect of tamoxifen, a non-steroidal antiestrogen, on phospholipid/calcium-dependent protein kinase and phosphorylation of its endogenous substrate proteins from the rat brain and ovary. *Biochemical Pharmacology*, **34**, 3649–53.

Sunkara, S. P. and Jones, W. D. (1991a). Prevention of glycoprotein enveloped virus infectivity by pyridyloxazole-2-ones. European Patent Application EP 428103, 1–11.

Sunkara, S. P. and Jones, W. D. (1991b). Prevention of glycoprotein enveloped virus infectivity by quinolyl- and isoquinolyloxazole-2-ones. European Patent Application EP 428105, 1–16.

Takahashi, I., Kobayashi, E., Nakano, H., Murakata, C., Saitoh, H., Suzuki, K., and Tamaoki, T. (1990). Potent selective inhibition of 7-O-Methyl UCN-01 against protein kinase C. *Journal of Pharmacology and Experimental Therapeutics*, **255**, 1218–21.

Tamaoki, T., Nomoto, H., Takahashi, I., Kato, Y., Morimoto, M., and Tomita, F. (1986). *Biochemical and Biophysical Research Communications*, **135**, 397–402.

Walsh, D. A., Perkins, J. P., and Krebs, E. G. (1968). An adenosine 3′,5′-monophosphate-dependent protein kinase from rabbit skeletal muscle. *Journal of Biological Chemistry*, **243**, 3763–5.

4

Inhibitors of protein tyrosine kinases

Yosef Yarden and Elior Peles

4.1 Overview

Phosphorylation of tyrosine residues of proteins is an extremely rare post-translational covalent modification, accounting for less than 0.1 per cent of overall cellular phosphoproteins. Nevertheless, this modification appears to be uniquely involved in the regulation of cell growth and differentiation by extracellular signals. Close to 50 protein tyrosine kinases (PTKs) are already known, falling into two groups: the receptor tyrosine kinases (RTKs) are transmembrane glycoproteins that bind polypeptide growth factors, whereas the soluble PTKs reside in the cytoplasm. The catalytic function of both groups is activated, either directly or indirectly, by exoplasm-facing proteins and leads to self-phosphorylation of the stimulated kinase as well as modification of a set of cytoplasmic proteins. Loss of regulation of this catalytic function usually results in rapid cell proliferation and neoplastic transformation.

The rarity of tyrosine phosphorylation and its critical role in cell regulation made it an excellent pharmacological target. Natural or synthetic compounds were identified as potent inhibitors of the catalytic function. These agents compete for either the nucleotide binding site of the kinase, or displace the peptide substrate from the enzyme. The latter inhibitors are more specific to PTKs over other kinases and are usually more potent on a molar basis. Moreover, it appears that subtle substitutions of such synthetic inhibitory molecules can confer selectivity toward certain PTKs. However, the mechanism of action and degree of specificity of many other inhibitors is not yet known. Despite uncertainty as to their cellular targets, PTK inhibitors have been extensively used as research tools, primarily to obtain indications for the existence of a tyrosine phosphorylation step in complex biological processes such as signal transduction and differentiation, and for elucidation of the mechanistic role of such steps.

Although the biological effects of PTK inhibitors have been tested mostly on cultured mammalian cells *in vitro*, their specific growth inhibitory effects, and even differentiation induction by certain compounds, hold promise for clinical application, including treatment of diseases associated with non-malignant hyperproliferative states (e.g. psoriasis, atherosclerosis, and hypertension) and attempts to arrest the growth of cancers of rapidly dividing cells (e.g. leukaemias and adenocarcinomas).

4.2 Introduction

Covalent phosphorylation of proteins, because of its rapid reversibility and profound effects on protein conformation, is considered to be the most important post-translational mode of protein modification in animal cells. Whereas phosphorylation of serine and threonine residues constitutes over 99.9 per cent of phosphoproteins, tyrosine modification is rare and appears to be limited to certain proteins. Phosphotyrosine was first detected in immunoprecipitates of oncogenic viral proteins that were allowed to undergo phosphorylation *in vitro* by incubation with a nucleotide triphosphate (Eckhart *et al.* 1979; Hunter and Sefton 1980; Witte *et al.* 1980). The viral oncoproteins, as well as their cellular counterparts, were later found to possess an intrinsic protein tyrosine kinase activity, which is shared by almost 50 known cellular proteins. All these PTKs share extensive structural homology of their catalytic sequences, not only among themselves but also with a larger family of protein kinases (Hanks *et al.* 1988). The catalytic function of many PTKs appears to be under negative regulation under physiological conditions. This is achieved by a complex allosteric type of regulation that is released through inter- or intramolecular interactions (Soderling 1990). Some of the allosteric activators are humoral polypeptides, mostly growth factors which, upon binding to the regulatory exoplasmic domain of a receptor tyrosine kinase (RTK), initiate an array of cellular responses collectively termed the pleiotropic response (Yarden and Ullrich 1988a). PTKs that do not span the plasma membrane are also coupled to a similar pleiotropic response (Hunter 1989; Klausner and Samelson 1991). Therefore it is apparent that activation of tyrosine phosphorylation is the point at which the biochemical signal diverges to multiple cellular targets. Indeed, the tyrosine kinase activity of both soluble and transmembrane PTKs is strictly essential for all their biological activities (Yarden and Ullrich 1988b; Ullrich and Schlessinger 1990). Therefore it is predictable that successful inhibition of this initial step of tyrosine phosphorylation will block all biological effects of a given tyrosine kinase.

Several strategies have been employed to achieve inhibition of PTK activity. Bioflavonoids (Hagiwara *et al.* 1988) and other compounds were used as competitors of the phosphate donor group (usually ATP), whereas other agents, like erbstatin (Umezawa *et al.* 1986), were used to bind to the peptide substrate site. Levitzki and his collaborators went a step further by introducing a systematic synthetic approach based on the structure of natural compounds (Levitzki 1990). Yet another possibility is offered by the existence of physiological protein inhibitors of PTKs (Auberger *et al.* 1989). In this chapter we shall describe the pharmacology of the main inhibitory compounds that have been used to inhibit PTKs, their biological effects, and their potential value as research tools and pharmacological agents. Our main aim is to guide researchers in the selection of an appropriate drug and, at the same time, to draw their attention to possible caveats. We have also aimed at familiarizing the reader with the structural and functional background of the target tyrosine kinases, and the multiple potential sites for blocking their action. An extensive description of the family of PTKs and their involvement in signalling processes is beyond the scope of this chapters. The reader is referred to other reviews on these aspects (Hunter and Cooper 1985; Yarden and Ullrich 1988a; Hunter 1989; Ullrich and Schlessinger 1990; Cantley *et al.* 1991).

4.3 Protein tyrosine kinases: structural aspects

Tyrosine-specific protein kinases are mosaic proteins that share a well-conserved catalytic sequence 250 amino acids long which is fused to a

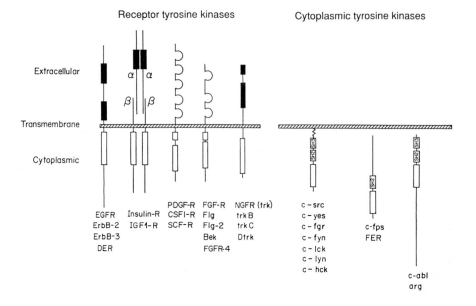

Fig. 4.1 Schematic illustration of the structures of known PTKs. The structure of each group of PTKs is schematically represented by drawing the amino acid backbones. Members of each group are listed below the scheme. The hatched horizontal box represents the plasma membrane. Closed boxes symbolize cysteine-rich regions and open boxes represent tyrosine kinase domains. Immunoglobulin-like domains are shown as open loops. Src homology (SH) domains are indicated.

variety of non-catalytic regulatory domains. The architecture of the latter regions not only modulates enzymatic activity by internal molecular constraints, but also determines the type of interaction between the enzyme and other molecules such as growth factors, cytoplasmic proteins, or membrane lipids. Therefore it is appropriate to relate to PTKs as to allosteric enzymes. On the basis mostly of structural landmarks of the regulatory sequences, the known PTKs are divided into two groups (Fig. 4.1): receptor tyrosine kinases (RTKs), whose non-catalytic amino termini traverse the plasma membrane once, and soluble PTKs which reside mostly in the cytoplasm.

4.3.1 Catalytic sequences

Usually located at the carboxy terminal half of PTK molecules, the enzymatic portion can easily be defined through analysis of conserved sequences (Hunter and Cooper 1985). Although the catalytic portions of serine- and threonine-specific protein kinases display remarkable homology to tyrosine kinases, a few blocks of sequences unequivocally distinguish each subfamily of protein kinases (for detailed comparison of amino acid sequences see Hanks *et al.* 1988). However, within the PTK subfamily relatively minor sequence variations characterize RTKs compared with soluble PTKs. This observation was utilized for isolation of new transmembrane PTKs (Raz *et al.* 1991).

Eleven short stretches of conserved amino acids can be recognized within the catalytic core of PTKs (Hanks *et al.* 1988). The functional roles of these protein motifs are only partially known. This is based on protein chemistry and mutagenesis studies, and on an analogy with other protein kinases such as cAMP-dependent protein kinase (PK-A) (Taylor *et al.* 1990). Affinity labelling experiments localized the nucleotide binding site of protein kinases to the amino terminal part of the catalytic region (Zoller *et al.* 1981) and, more specifically, to a lysine residue, analogous to lysine-72 of PK-A. Amino terminally to this subdomain lies a glycine-rich loop which, based on the crystal structures of nucleotide binding proteins, constitutes the site of interaction with the phosphate moieties of the nucleotide (Rossman *et al.* 1974). Other stretches of conserved amino acids located carboxy terminally to the nucleotide binding site are also involved in nucleotide binding. In contrast with the nucleotide site, certain subdomains display heterogeneity that depends on the amino acid specificity of the kinase. These subdomains probably play a role in recognition of the substrate hydroxyamino acid, as is also implied by studies with a peptide analogue (Bramson *et al.* 1982).

A structural feature that characterizes some RTKs over soluble PTKs is the existence of a variable-length non-catalytic domain within the catalytic core. This kinase insert is usually hydrophilic and exhibits sequence heterogeneity among various receptors (Yarden *et al.* 1987). It has been shown that the corresponding sequences of the receptors for the platelet-derived growth factor (PDGF) (Kazlauskas and Cooper 1989) and the colony-stimulating factor 1 (CSF-1) (Tapley *et al.* 1990; Van der Geer and Hunter 1990) serve as autophosphorylation sites.

4.3.2 Non-catalytic sequences

Amino acid stretches flanking both sides of the catalytic core function as regulatory domains, cellular localization signals, and sites of interactions with cytoplasmic or extracellular proteins. The presence of a hydrophobic stretch that functions as a transmembrane domain distinguishes RTKs from soluble PTKs (Fig. 4.1).

4.3.3 Receptor tyrosine kinases

At least six groups of receptors with intrinsic tyrosine kinase activity are known today. Each receptor has a single hydrophobic stretch of amino acids located 40–130 amino acids amino terminally to the catalytic sequence. This domain functions as a transmembrane region separating the receptor into two large domains, the exoplasmic ligand binding domain and the cytoplasmic catalytic sequence flanked by the non-catalytic juxtamembrane and the carboxy terminal stretches. Several structural landmarks characterize each group of receptors (Yarden and Ullrich 1988a; Ullrich and Schlessinger 1990). The receptor for the epidermal growth factor (EGF) and the putative receptors Neu/ErbB-2 and ErbB-3 contain two cysteine-rich domains at their exoplasmic portion. The heterotetrameric receptors for insulin and insulin-like growth factor 1 (IGF-1) are each composed of two α and two β subunits. The extracellular α subunit carries one cysteine-rich region whereas the β subunit traverses the plasma membrane and contains the catalytic core. The third group of RTKs includes the receptors for CSF-1, the stem cell factor (SCF), which is also called the kit ligand (KL) or the mast cell growth factor (MGF), and two receptors for the PDGFs. Their landmarks are five immunoglobulin (Ig) loops in the ectodomain and a split tyrosine kinase. The fourth group of RTKs appears to be the most divergent. Members of this group are characterized by three Ig loops at the ligand binding portion which all bind heparin-binding peptides belonging to the family of fibroblast growth factors (FGFs). The recent discovery that the nerve growth factor (NGF) and the biologically related neuronal factors NT-3 and BDNF bind to proteins encoded by the *trk* group of genes established the last group of receptors, which are characterized by a short carboxy terminal tail and a large and complex exoplasmic domain that includes cysteine-rich regions (Hempsted *et al.* 1991; Kaplan *et al.* 1991a,b; Klein *et al.* 1991a,b). Perhaps the first member of the sixth group of RTKs is the *met* gene product, which functions as a receptor for the hepatocyte growth factor (HGF) (Bottaro *et al.* 1991). It is important to note that many more receptor-like tyrosine kinases (e.g. *eph*, *eck*, *elk*, *flt*, *ros*, *sea*, *ret*, and others) have been discovered, but the identity of their ligands is currently unknown.

The cytoplasmic non-catalytic regions of RTKs also display extensive structural heterogeneity, even within each group of related receptors, implying receptor-specific functions. One proven function is the acceptor site for autophosphorylation: the EGF receptor undergoes autophosphorylation on multiple sites at the carboxy terminal tail (Downward *et al.* 1984), whereas the sub-type III receptors are self-phosphorylated at the interkinase region (Kazlauskas and Cooper 1989). However, autophosphorylation within the tyrosine kinase sequences occurs in the case of the insulin receptor (Herrera and Rosen 1986) and the PDGF receptor (Kazlauskas and Cooper 1989).

4.3.4   Non-receptor PTKs

The known soluble tyrosine kinases fall into three families. The largest is the *src* family which includes the protein products of the following genes:

src, *yes*, *fgr*, *fyn*, *lck*, *lyn*, and *hck*. The *fps* family includes the *fes/fps* and the *fer/flk* proteins, whereas the *abl* family has two mammalian members: *abl* and *arg*. By analogy with some genes that encode RTKs (e.g. *erb*-B, *fms*, and *kit*), genetically altered variants of soluble PTKs are encoded by retroviral oncogenes. Thus chicken sarcoma viruses encode *src*, *yes*, and *fps* (and also *erb*-B), feline retroviruses carry the viral forms of *fgr* and *fes* (and also *kit* and *fms*), and a mouse lymphoma virus encodes the viral *abl* gene. As well as the catalytic core, the non-receptor PTKs contain two types of conserved non-catalytic sequence, denoted *src* homology domains (SH2 and SH3). These motifs were originally defined in the $pp60^{src}$ protein (Sadowski *et al.* 1986), but later extended to other soluble PTKs and even proteins that are not kinases (Koch *et al.* 1991). In the src protein, the catalytic domain is located at the carboxy terminal half, whereas the amino terminal half that comprises the regulatory part includes one SH2 domain of about 100 amino acids adjacent to an SH3 domain 45 amino acids long. A myristylation site that is required for membrane association lies at the amino terminus. The regulatory role of the SH2 and SH3 domains was initially inferred from corresponding mutants which displayed alterations in kinase activity and interactions with substrates. The identification of SH2 domains in several substrates of PTKs, and particularly in the v-*crk* oncogene, made it apparent that the SH2 region regulates protein–protein associations that involve a phosphorylated tyrosine residue (Matsuda *et al.* 1990). The function of the SH3 domain is less understood, but there are indications that it functions in subcellular localization.

In addition to the proto-oncogenic forms of viral PTKs, normal tissues, particularly spleen and brain, contain high levels of PTK activity. The activity is defined primarily in catalytic terms like K_m values, dependence on cations, pH optima, and apparent molecular weight (Srivastava 1990). Although in most cases these activities are not defined in molecular terms, it appears that many more soluble PTKs exist in healthy cells.

4.4   Functional aspects of PTKs

4.4.1   Catalytic function

Consistent with a common evolutionary source, all PTKs display similar catalytic properties that are partially distinct from other protein kinases. The most important characteristic is specificity to tyrosine residues. However, not every tyrosine will be phosphorylated, but only those residues located close to one or more acidic amino acids (Hunter 1982). Finer requirements in terms of substrate selectivity appear to distinguish PTKs from RTKs (Srivastava and Chiasson 1989), and perhaps also individual PTKs, as was shown with synthetic substrates (Braun *et al.* 1983). Most PTKs show an apparent preference for Mn^{2+} over Mg^{2+} and for ATP over GTP. In the case of the EGF receptor, the enzymatic reaction displays a Bi Bi mechanism that implies no phosphoenzyme intermediate and substrate binding that precedes nucleotide binding (Erneux *et al.* 1983). In addition, PTKs are relatively heat sensitive and also undergo inactivation by alkylation. The catalytic property of PTKs that is experimentally most valuable is their ability to undergo autophosphorylation *in vitro*. This property is also retained in living cells, although here, the phosphorylation is mediated, at least in part, by intermolecular interactions (Weinmaster *et al.* 1984; Honegger *et al.* 1989).

4.4.2   Mechanism of activation

The critical role of PTKs in cellular function and the absolute requirement of the tyrosine kinase activity demand very stringent regulation mechanisms. Perhaps the best demonstration for a failure of these mechanisms is provided by the oncogenic capability of many PTKs activated virally and otherwise. Apparently, under normal conditions, the catalytic activity is under repression, i.e. mediated by 'autoinhibitory' domains (Soderling 1990). Removal of the repressive effects is achieved via the interactions of allosteric activators. Polypeptide growth factors that bind to the extracellular domains of RTKs exert kinase activation that is preceded by receptor dimerization (Yarden and Schlessinger 1987a,b) and involves conformational changes (Williams 1989). The latent state of the protein kinase of $pp60^{src}$ is maintained by phosphorylation of a single tyrosine residue (tyr_{527}) located at the carboxy terminus (Cooper *et al.* 1986). Folding the C-tail over the catalytic core appears to inactivate the enzyme. It follows that dephosphorylation of tyr_{527} or prevention of the folding-over would abolish the inhibitory effect. Whereas there is no direct evidence for the first mechanism, the latter is accomplished by several proteins, including the v-crk, the polyomavirus middle T protein, and probably also the PDGF receptor and the T-cell receptor (Cantley *et al.* 1991; Klausner and Samelson 1991). In contrast with tyr_{527}, which is phosphorylated by a distinct soluble tyrosine kinase, the tyr_{416} residue lying within the catalytic core of Src undergoes autophosphorylation which positively regulates the enzyme (Kmiecik and Shalloway 1987; Piwinica-Worms *et al.* 1987). Similarly, autophosphorylation of the insulin receptor within the catalytic core up-regulates the tyrosine kinase activity (Ellis *et al.* 1986). Autophosphorylation of other RTKs, on sites located outside the catalytic sequences, are less effective in terms of kinase activation.

4.4.3   Cellular function of PTKs

The mechanism by which activation of tyrosine kinase activity is translated into stimulation of metabolic pathways is currently the subject of intensive research. The emerging picture for RTKs attributes a pivotal role to auto-phosphorylated tyrosine residues on the receptors. According to the current model, these sites function as anchors for proteins with SH2 domains, and probably other structural motifs that are yet to be defined. SH2-containing proteins may either carry their own enzymatic function (e.g. phosphatidylinositol-specific phospholipase in the case of PLC$_y$, or GTPase activation in the case of ras-GAP), or be adaptor proteins that multimerize signalling proteins (e.g. *crk* and p85) (Koch *et al*. 1991). Potentially, the known spectrum of SH2-containing proteins may enable simultaneous association to occur with DNA binding proteins (e.g. *vav*), protein phos-phatases, and serine–threonine protein kinases. Simultaneous association of an activated RTK may thus create a signalling complex which, in the case of the PDGF receptor, includes PLC$_y$, *ras*-GAP, phosphatidylinositol 3' kinase (PI3K) and perhaps also the *Rafl* protein kinase (Kaplan *et al*. 1990; Ullrich and Schlessinger 1990). Catalytic activation of the substrate proteins is probably achieved by their phosphorylation on tyrosine residues (Morrison *et al*. 1989; Nishibe *et al*. 1990) or by cellular redistribution. Apparently, the complex dissociates in order simultaneously to generate second-messenger molecules which, in turn, stimulate serine–threonine protein kinases such as protein kinase C or the MAP kinase. The latter is the first example of stimulation of a protein kinase cascade, as MAP kinase phosphorylates S6 kinase which, by itself, phosphorylates the ribo-somal S6 protein. The end result is probably enhanced rate of protein synthesis (Ballou *et al*. 1988). Tyrosine-specific protein phosphatases and cellular routing are believed to terminate the signals arising from the tyrosine-phosphorylated RTK.

Signal transduction by the cytoplasmic PTKs is less well understood. However, once the non-receptor PTK protein is tyrosine phosphory-lated, it may potentially interact, in a fashion similar to RTKs, with signal-generating molecules. This is demonstrated well by the interaction between the T-cell surface protein CD4 and the *lck* tyrosine kinase. This is followed by activation of phospholipase C and its downstream dual pathway (Klausner and Samelson 1991).

4.4.4 Biological function of PTKs

As implied by their oncogenic counterparts, PTKs are certainly involved in the regulation of cell proliferation. However, in the past few years it has become apparent that tyrosine phosphorylation plays a central role in a variety of other and previously unexpected cellular functions. Thus platelet activation by thrombin (Ferrell and Martin 1989), T-cell activation by mitogen (Mustelin *et al*. 1990), cellular responses to lymphokines (Nakajima and Wall 1991), and the differentiation induced by NGF and other neuronal factors (Klein *et al*. 1991a,b) are all mediated by the

Table 4.1 Pharmacological and biochemical parameters of PTK inhibitors

Inhibitor	Site of inhibition	Source	Enzyme speciticity[a]	
			PTK autophosphorylation	Substrate
Genistein	Nucleotide site	Natural (*Pseudomonas sp.*)	EGF-R (2.6) v-fes (22) v-src v-abl (30) lck	H2B (22) Casein (24) *src* peptide (40)
Lavendustin A	Nucleotide site	Natural (*Streptomyces grisolavendus*)	EGF-R (0.01)	
Erbstatin	Peptide site	Natural (*Streptomyces*)	EGF-R(14) c-src erbB-2	
Tyrphostins RG 50864	Peptide site	Synthetic	EGF-R (40, living cells) PDGF-R (2.3) p120-bcr-abl I-R	PolyGAT (2.4) PolyGT (640)
RG 50872			PDGF-R EGF-R	polyGAT (460)
Cinnamamides (ST638,4HC)	Peptide site	Synthetic	EGF-R(0.85-1.1) v-fgr (4.2) c-src (18) v-fps (70) v-src (87)	
Hydroxy-2 naphtalenylmethyl phosphonic acid	Peptide site	Synthetic (also prodrug derivatives)	Insulin-R (200)	AII (100)
Herbimycin A	Undefined (interaction with reactive SH groups)	Natural (*Streptomyces*)	v-src (12) fyn lck	

Other enzymes	Biological effects[b]	Reference
PK-C(>360) PK-A(>360) Topoisomerase (5)	Inhibition of EGF(121)-, PDGF(40)-, and insulin(19)-induced mitogenicity, EGF-dependent inositolphosphate generation, and keratinocyte differentiation; induction of differentiation of erythroleukemia cells	Akiyama et al. 1987 Linassier et al. 1990
PK-A(>220) PK-C(>220) PI-K(14.5)		Onoda et al. 1989
Topoisomerases PK-A(550) PK-C(970) PI-K(140)	Inhibition of EGF-induced cell proliferation and PLC activation; PAF-induced protein tyrosine phosphorylation, and phosphoinositide hydrolysis in platelets TGF-precursor expression in human gastric carcinoma cells,	Umezawa et al. 1986 Imoto et al. 1987a Imoto et al. 1990 Onoda et al. 1989
	Inhibition of EGF-induced proliferation (40), DNA synthesis(10), keratinocyte proliferation (15), PLC phosphorylation, phosphoinositide breakdown (19.5) and Ca^{2+} increase in B cells	Levitzki and Gilon 1991 Yaish et al. 1988 Gazit et al. 1989 Lyall et al. 1989
	Inhibition of PDGF(0.01)- and EGF(0.22)-induced DNA synthesis in vascular smooth muscle cells	Bilder et al. 1991
PK-A(>100) PK-C(>100) Casein kinase I(>100) Na^+/K^+ ATPase (>100)	Inhibition of GM-CSF-induced tyrosine phosphorylation and superoxide production in human neutrophils Induction of differentiation of erythroleukemia cells, in synergy with mitomycin C	Shiraishi et al. 1989 Shiraishi et al. 1990
EGF-R(250)	Inhibition of glucose oxidation in isolated rat (10)	Saperstein et al. 1989
	Inhibition of TCR-mediated PLC activation Inhibition of leukaemic cell differentiation, morphological reversion of the transforming phenotype induced by v-Src, v-Fps, v-ErbB, v-Abl, and v-Ros	June et al. 1990 Uehara et al. 1989

Table 4.1 (*continued*)

Inhibitor	Site of inhibition	Source	Enzyme speciticity[a]	
			PTK autophosphorylation	Substrate
Staurosporine	Undefined	Natural (*Streptomyces*)	v-src (0.006) EGF-R I-R v-abl PDGF-R	AII (0.025) *src* peptide (0.06)
Thiazolidinediones (compound 2)	Undefined	Synthetic	EGF-R (5) c-src v-abl	AII (1) PolyGT (3) AII (100)

Numbers in parentheses indicate IC_{50} values in μM.

Abbreviations: EGF-R, I-R and PDGF-R, EGF, insulin, and PDGF receptors respectively; TCR T-cell receptor; AII, angiotensin II; H2B, histone H2B; polyGAT, synthetic copolymer of glutamic acid-alanine-tyrosine; polyGT, synthetic copolymer of glutamic acid-tyrosine; PK-A, refer to protein kinase A (cAMP dependent); PK-C, protein kinase C; PI-K, phosphatidylinositol kinase.

[a] Assays performed *in vitro* with isolated enzymes.

[b] Studies performed with living cultivated cells.

phosphorylation of tyrosine residues. Importantly, the membrane receptors involved are not necessarily tyrosine kinases, but nevertheless soluble PTKs are stimulated.

4.5   Pharmacological strategies for inhibition of PTKs

Chemotherapy based on inhibition of tyrosine kinase activity is a relatively new branch of the pharmacology of signal transduction processes. Unlike inhibition of specific enzymes involved in signalling, cytoskeletal organization, and synthesis of macromolecules, tyrosine kinase inhibitors are aimed at apparently the earliest cytoplasmic event common to diverse metabolic pathways. The extremely low abundance of tyrosine phosphorylation in normal cells, its defined specificity and the involvement of tyrosine phosphorylation in clinically relevant phenomena make it an appropriate target. It is conceivable, although yet unproved, that tyrosine kinase inhibitors will selectively act on the diseased tissue and will leave the adjacent normal cells relatively unaffected. Motivated by these considerations, over the last decade researchers have tested an impressive list of chemicals (Table 4.1) for their potential to act as tyrosine kinase inhibitors. These chemicals were natural products, synthetic compounds, or even endogeneous proteins. Two main approaches have been used: design of inhibitors to the nucleotide binding site or to the peptide substrate site. The latter offer the advantage

Other enzymes	Biological effects[b]	Reference
S6 kinase(0.005) PK-C(0.006) PK-A(0.05)	Inhibition of proliferation of various cell lines (0.029–0.13) Induction of increased high affinity EGF binding	Meyer *et al.* 1989 Herbert *et al.* 1990 Nakano *et al.* 1987 Meyer *et al.* 1989 Uehara *et al.* 1989
PK-C(>500) PK-A(>500)	Inhibition of EG(1)- and IL-3-dependent cell proliferation	Geissler *et al.* 1990

of being specific to PTKs, and sometimes even to a single PTK. Nevertheless, the ATP-like compounds, although potentially acting on any nucleotide-binding protein, display some selectivity towards PTKs over serine–threonine kinases. A large group of inhibitors show a mixed type of inhibition, which may also indicate non-specific interactions with tyrosine kinases. Before we discuss each group of inhibitors, it is worthwhile reviewing the common experimental tests and the pharmacological parameters commonly used to characterize a new tyrosine kinase inhibitor.

Most inhibition assays have been performed *in vitro* with isolated tyrosine kinases, using either peptide substrates (e.g. polymers of glutamine, alanine, and tyrosine in different ratios (Braun *et al.* 1984)) or a protein substrate (e.g. histone, angiotensin II, or casein). Autophosphorylation of the tested PTK has been used frequently. A superior assay is an *in vivo* test in which the inhibitor is added to living cultured cells, where tyrosine phosphorylation of the receptor (Geissler *et al.* 1990), or preferably an endogeneous substrate protein is being examined (Margolis *et al.* 1989; Bilder *et al.* 1991). The last variant is probably the most relevant, as it reflects inhibition of signal transduction and depends on the efficiency of penetration of the drug across the plasma membrane. Nevertheless, new problems, e.g. drug decomposition in serum, may arise when inhibitory drugs are eventually tested in living animals. Despite a lack of *in vivo* tests, the biological effects of many inhibitors have been tested on living cells. The cytotoxic effects of the compound have to be determined first, after which its cytostatic effect can be conveniently determined. It is essential that the specificity of the cytostatic or other effects are analysed. For example, the inhibition of EGF-dependent cell growth, compared with the response to whole serum (Dvir *et al.* 1991), may indicate specificity of an inhibitor for the EGF receptor. The results of the enzymatic and biological assays are

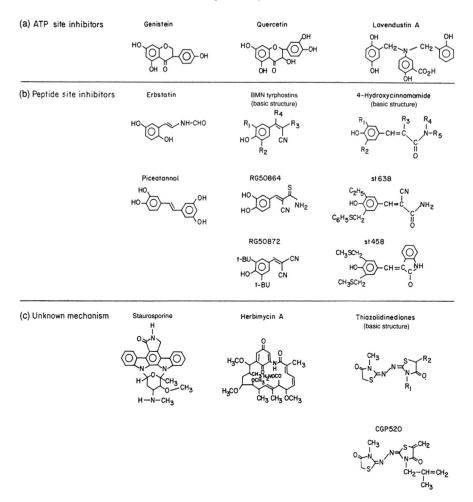

Fig. 4.2 Chemical structures of the most commonly used inhibitors of tyrosine kinases. The inhibitors are classified according to their type of enzymatic inhibition. In some cases, where more than one inhibitor exists, the basic structure and the major variant(s) are indicated.

best described by the concentration of inhibitor needed for 50 per cent maximal effect (IC_{50}). It is also useful to compare the relative efficiency of the inhibitor on kinases that are specific to serine or threonine, and even on related tyrosine kinases. The greater this difference, the higher is the chance for selective action. We now give a description of the more commonly used PTK inhibitors with respect to their structure, inhibition mechanism, and biochemical characterization. The basic chemical structures are presented in Fig. 4.2, and the main pharmacological and biochemical parameters of the compounds described are given in Table 4.1.

4.5.1 Nucleotide site inhibitors

4.5.1.1 *Bioflavonoids (genistein, quercetin and myricetin)*

The flavone quercetin has been reported to inhibit the tyrosine kinase activity of $pp60^{src}$ (Graziani *et al.* 1983), as well as the activities of several serine–threonine protein kinases (Graziani *et al.* 1981; Gschwendt *et al.* 1984) and ATPases (Lang and Racker 1974; Shoshan and MacLennan 1981). These results led to a search for a more specific flavone compound. The inhibitor found in fermentation broth of *Pseudomonas sp.*, genistein (4′,5,7-trihydroxyisoflavone), was indeed specific for tyrosine kinases (*src*, *fes*, and EGF receptor) and had only minor effects on serine- and threonine-specific kinases (Akiyama *et al.* 1987). The inhibition of the EGF-receptor tyrosine kinase was competitive with ATP, as predicted by similar studies done with quercetin. The selectivity of genistein to PTKs argues against the attribution of the inhibitory action to similarity in charge distribution in the pyranone ring of the flavone and the pyrimidine ring of ATP (Ferrell *et al.* 1979). More recent structure–activity studies indicated that selectivity towards tyrosine kinases increases with the number of hydroxyl groups on the flavone ring (Hagiwara *et al.* 1988). Similar to the isoflavone, genistein, synthetic flavonoid analogues, and particularly compound 17C, were found to be more selective to PTKs than to serine–threonine kinases (Cushman *et al.* 1991). Genistein is the most widely used tyrosine kinase inhibitor among those that affect the nucleotide site. Therefore it is important to examine its specificity for PTKs critically. Several *in vitro* studies have clearly indicated specificity towards tyrosine kinases over serine–threonine kinases. This observation was extended to living cells; genistein inhibited both EGF- and PDGF-induced mitogenesis and second-messenger generation in living fibroblasts with IC_{50} values of 10 μM and 40 μM respectively (Dean *et al.* 1989; Hill *et al.* 1990). In contrast, the biological effects of agents that are not involved in PTK activation, namely angiotensin II and ATP, were not inhibited by genistein. However, the drug blocked the mitogenic effect of thrombin at a concentration comparable with that required for blocking of insulin and EGF action on mouse fibroblasts (Linassier *et al.* 1990). Moreover, although the induction of c-*myc* mRNA by EGF is strictly dependent on the tyrosine kinase function of the EGF receptor, genistein did not block it (Linassier *et al.* 1990). This observation raises the possibility that genistein may have other cellular targets, in addition to PTKs. This was also implied by the cytotoxic effect of genistein at a concentration that is only two- or threefold higher than the cytostatic IC_{50}. In addition to its action on protein kinases and other nucleotide-binding proteins, genistein was found to interfere with the function of topoisomerase II both *in vitro* and in living cells (Markovits *et al.* 1989). Thus the apparent selectivity of genistein to PTKs is probably due to their relatively low K_m values for ATP. Other ATP-binding proteins may also be affected by genistein, particularly at relatively high concentrations (> 50 μM). With this reservation in mind, we should consider the numerous studies that have employed genistein as a pharmacological tool. In T-cells, genistein inhibited cell proliferation, IL-2 and IL-2 receptor expression in response to activation by antibodies to CD3 or CD28 surface antigens, and tyrosine phosphorylation of p56^{lck} and the ζ chain of the T-cell receptor (Mustelin *et al.* 1990; Trevillyan *et al.* 1990; Atluro and Atluro 1991). In platelets, stimulation by an endoperoxide analogue of genistein exerted an inhibitory effect on the formation of phosphatidylinositol-derived second messengers (Gaudette and Holub 1990). Similarly, genistein inhibited the mitogenic effects and various signalling events of EGF and PDGF on fibroblasts and smooth muscle cells (Clegg and Sambhi 1989; Dean *et al.* 1989; Zwiller *et al.* 1991). In contrast, genistein was shown to induce *in vitro* differentiation of mouse erythroleukaemia cells (Watanabe *et al.* 1989, 1991) but it inhibited the development of one-cell mouse pre-implantation embryos (Besterman and Schultz 1990).

4.5.1.2   *Lavendustin A*

This novel compound, containing substituted phenyl and benzyl groups, was isolated by Umezawa and his collaborators from *Streptomyces grisolavendus* (Onoda *et al.* 1989). When tested on the tyrosine kinase activity of the EGF-receptor an extremely low IC$_{50}$ value of 10 nM was obtained. Lavendustin did not affect protein kinases A or C, but was, nevertheless, competitive with ATP. The basis for this unexpected selectivity of lavendustin A is unknown, but it may reflect structural differences between the nucleotide sites of PTKs and other kinases. It remains to be seen how useful this compound will be, as its very high potency may compensate for the non-selective nature of its target site.

4.5.1.3   *Other compounds*

Inhibitors that affect the ATP site at relatively high IC$_{50}$ values (> 50 μM) have low potential to be useful as therapeutic or research tools. The compounds, amiloride and cibacron blue (Davis and Czech, 1985), are examples of such agents.

4.5.2   Inhibitors of the substrate site

Both natural and synthetic inhibitors that function at the peptide substrate site of PTKs have been described. Their low IC$_{50}$ values and the observation that they may be selective to specific PTKs promise the superiority of this type of inhibitor over ATP-site drugs. The principle behind this approach is to design compounds that will mimic the substrate and thereby block the accessibility of endogeneous substrates or prevent autophosphorylation of PTKs. As has been discussed already, natural autoregulatory sequences of protein kinases may act as pseudosubstrates to regulate kinase activity (Hardie 1988; Grandori 1989). Synthetic tyrosine-containing polymers of amino acids were, indeed, shown to have an inhibitory action on several PTKs and had different potencies depending on the identity of the kinase (Braun *et al.* 1983). Synthetic peptides corresponding to autophosphorylation sites of RTKs (Stadtmaver and Rosen 1983; Downward *et al.* 1984; Bertics and Gill 1985; Walker *et al.* 1987; Shoelson *et al.* 1989), or viral tyrosine kinases (Hunter 1982) were found to behave as substrates and weak inhibitors of the corresponding tyrosine kinases. Non-phosphorylatable analogues of such a peptide derived from the insulin receptor, in which tyrosine residues were replaced by either 4-methoxyphenylalanine or phenylalanine, had differential inhibitory potentials on autophosphorylation of the insulin-receptor, EGF receptor and pp60^{Src} (Shoelson *et al.* 1989). Similarly, gastrin, an analogue of the PTK substrate in which the tyrosine residue is replaced by a tetrafluorinated tyrosine, displayed inhibition of the catalytic function of the insulin receptor with an inhibitory constant of 100 μM (Yuan *et al.* 1990). In contrast with tyrosyl-containing peptides that correspond to autophosphorylation sites, a fully denatured derivative of lysozyme was found to be a very potent inhibitor of the insulin-receptor kinase (K_i = 0.6 μM) (Kohanski and Lane 1986). Importantly, native lysozyme was completely inactive, and derivatives that failed to inhibit autophosphorylation of the receptor were still able to function as substrates of the insulin receptor (Meyerovitch *et al.* 1990). An apparently different mechanism of inhibition of the insulin receptor kinase was displayed by two peptides derived from the major histocompatibility complex class I antigens (Hansen *et al.* 1989). These peptides are not competitive substrates, yet they completely inhibited the kinase *in vitro* at 10 μM concentration. In addition to peptidergic inhibitors, low molecular weight synthetic and other compounds, aimed at the substrate site, were also examined as described below.

4.5.2.1 *Erbstatin*

This analogue of tyrosine was originally isolated from an *Actinomycetes* broth, and was found to be a potent inhibitor of the tyrosine kinase activity of pp60^{src} and the EGF receptor (IC$_{50}$ $\approx$ 14 μM *in vitro*) (Umezawa *et al.* 1986). As inferred from its hydroxylated phenyl ring, the inhibition by erbstatin is competitive with a peptide substrate but not with ATP. When tested on cultured cells, erbstatin inhibited autophosphorylation and internalization of the EGF receptor (Imoto *et al.* 1987a). It also inhibited EGF-induced growth of six different human carcinoma cell lines

(Takekura *et al.* 1991). This effect appears to be due to a delay in the induction of DNA synthesis (Umezawa *et al.* 1990). Erbstatin was further reported to inhibit, in A431 cells, the activation of phospholipase C by EGF (Imoto *et al.* 1990). Oncogene-induced morphological changes of cells infected with temperature-sensitive retroviruses were also inhibited by erbstatin (Unezawa *et al.* 1991). The action of erbstatin *in vivo* appears to be limited by efficient inactivation of the drug by animal serum (Imoto *et al.* 1987b). This problem can be bypassed by using methyl 2,5-di-hydroxycinnamate as a stable analogue of erbstatin (Umezawa *et al.* 1990), or by giving erbstatin together with an iron-chelating agent (Imoto *et al.* 1987b). Such intraperitoneal administration of erbstatin and the iron chelator foroxymithine inhibited the growth of MCF-7 human breast carcinoma cells in nude mice (Toi *et al.* 1990). Erbstatin also retarded the growth of four oesophageal tumours, suggesting an anti-neoplastic potential due to inhibition of tyrosine kinase activity. However, this interpretation is challenged by the lack of effect on the Br-10 human breast carcinoma cell line (Toi *et al.* 1990). Moreover, the *in vitro* cytostatic effect of erbstatin is not limited to EGF-induced mitogenesis but extends to serum stimulation (Takekura *et al.* 1991). Although it can be argued that erbstatin is a non-specific tyrosine kinase inhibitor, as implied by inhibition of pp60^{src} and a soluble tyrosine kinase from HL-60 cells (Ernould *et al.* 1990), a recent study indicated inhibition of protein kinase C (Bishop *et al.* 1990). The inhibition (IC$_{50}$ = 20 μM) was competitive with ATP and limited to the trihydroxy derivative of erbstatin. Therefore it is possible that erbstatin also affects cellular targets that are not related to tyrosine kinases. This possibility is reinforced by the observations that erbstatin decreases membrane association of the transforming growth factor a (TGF-a) precursor (Takekura *et al.* 1991) and chemotaxis of neutrophils (Naccache *et al.* 1990). Direct involvement of tyrosine phosphorylation was not reported in either process.

4.5.2.2   *Tyrphostins*
Levitzki, Gilon, and collaborators synthesized a systematic series of compounds based on the structure of erbstatin that showed progressive capacity to inhibit the tyrosine kinase activity of the EGF receptor (Gazit *et al.* 1989). These molecules, termed 'tyrphostins', are derivatives of benzylidene malonitrile (BMN) and generally compete with the peptide substrate, rather than with ATP (Levitzki 1990; Levitzki and Gilon 1991). Impressively, the IC$_{50}$ values of various tyrphostins for inhibition of the EGF receptor kinase *in vitro* differed by three orders of magnitude. Nevertheless, the same tyrphostins were much less efficient as inhibitors of related tyrosine kinases, such as the insulin and the PDGF receptor (Gazit *et al.* 1989), probably reflecting differences in substrate selectivity of these kinases. Despite overall similarity to erbstatin, structure–activity analysis of

tyrphostins indicated differential effects of chemical substitutions in the structures, the most significant being the positions of the cyano group (in tyrphostins) and the formamide group (in erbstatin) and the number of hydroxyl groups on the phenolic ring (Gazit *et al*. 1989). The most studied class of tyrphostins is the one directed to the EGF receptor, and particularly the compound RG50864. Tyrphostins reversibly inhibit both EGF receptor autophosphorylation in living cells and also tyrosine phosphorylation of endogenous substrates in intact cells (Lyall *et al*. 1989). At similar concentrations, they also inhibit EGF-dependent proliferation of A431 cells that have been adapted to depend on EGF (Yaish *et al*. 1988; Gazit *et al*. 1989). Importantly, tyrphostins also inhibit PDGF- or serum-induced mitogenesis of cultured A431 cells or human keratinocytes, but higher concentrations are required (Lyall *et al*. 1989; Dvir *et al*. 1991). Thus the antiproliferative effect is partially selective for the EGF receptor. It has also been shown that tyrphostins inhibit EGF-induced breakdown of phosphoinositides (Posner *et al*. 1989), probably by preventing tyrosine phosphorylation of the phosphatidylinositol-specific PLC_γ (Margolis *et al*. 1989). Once again, tyrphostins inhibit the EGF-induced effect more efficiently than the response obtained with a calcium ionophore (Posner *et al*. 1989). The antiproliferative action of tyrphostins generally correlated with their relative kinase inhibitory potential (Dvir *et al*. 1991), but 10-fold higher concentrations were required for the anti-proliferative effect. Similarly, relatively high concentrations of tyrphostins ($> 40\ \mu M$) and prolonged incubation periods (16–17 h) were required for the effect on DNA synthesis and PLC_γ modification. This discrepancy could be due to instability or slow rate of cellular uptake of tyrphostins. However, a recent study which addressed this possibility raised an alternative interpretation, namely that tyrphostin does not directly interact with tyrosine phosphorylation. This was based on the use of electrochemical detection of the drug which indicated rapid (ca. 1 h) uptake of tyrphostin with no concomitant effect on tyrosine phosphorylation of the EGF receptor (Faaland *et al*. 1991).

In addition to inhibitors of the EGF receptor tyrosine kinase, structurally different tyrphostins have been used for blocking the biological effects of the receptors for PDGF and insulin. Compounds with a phenyl-malonitrile nucleus effectively inhibited the PDGF receptor kinase *in vitro* with IC_{50} values as low as 10 nM (Bilder *et al*. 1991). Slightly higher concentrations were required for 50 per cent inhibition of PDGF-induced DNA synthesis of vascular smooth muscle cells. The selectivity of the inhibitory action was implied by comparison with the effect on the EGF receptor kinase and the DNA synthesis induced by whole serum. Another series of compounds was found to inhibit insulin receptor kinase. Of these molecules, tBoc Tyr-aminomalonate was the most effective kinase inhibitor ($K_i = 2.4$ mM), and also blocked insulin-dependent lipogenesis and the insulin-dependent anti-lipolytic effect of rat adipocytes (Shechter *et al.* 1989).

4.5.2.3   *Cinnamamides*

Of seven synthetic 4-hydroxycinnamamide derivatives, the compound ST-638 was the most efficient tyrosine kinase inhibitor (Shiraishi *et al.* 1989). The IC_{50} values for different kinases were in the range 1–90 μM, with the EGF receptor being the most sensitive target. The inhibition of phosphorylation exhibited a substrate competition pattern, which is probably due to structural similarity to tyrosine. When tested on A431 cells, ST-638 (at 25 μM) inhibited the EGF-induced phosphorylation of whole-cell proteins, including lipocortin I, but had only a negligible effect on receptor autophosphorylation or serine–threonine phosphorylation (Shiraishi *et al.* 1990). In human neutrophils, ST-638 inhibited tyrosine phosphorylation of several cellular proteins (p92, p78, p54, and p40) in response to cellular activation by the granulocyte macrophage colony-stimulating factor (GMCSF) (Shiraishi and Shaafi 1989).

4.5.2.4   *(Hydroxy-2-naphthalenylmethyl)phosphonic acid*

This drug and its (acyloxy)methyl pro-drug derivatives have been shown to inhibit the insulin receptor kinase *in vitro* (IC_{50} = 200 μM for autophosphorylation). When added to cells that over express the insulin receptor, the pro-drug inhibited insulin-stimulated autophosphorylation of the receptor (Saperstein *et al.* 1989). Insulin-stimulated glucose oxidation in rat adipocytes was also blocked by the pro-drug (IC_{50} = 10 μM).

4.5.2.5   *Aeroplysinin-1*

This tyrosine metabolite from a marine sponge was found to inhibit *in vitro* tyrosine phosphorylation of lipocortin-like proteins by the EGF receptor. In addition, it inhibited the EGF-dependent growth of human breast cancer cells (Kreuter *et al.* 1990). It was further found to be cytotoxic to tumour cells at a concentration of 0.25–0.5 μM, but did not affect the growth of normal fibroblasts even at higher concentrations.

4.5.3   **Drugs with an undefined mode of inhibition**

This heterogeneous class of inhibitors of tyrosine kinases includes compounds that have a mixed type of competition (ATP and peptide sites) and also drugs that indirectly lead to reduction in tyrosine phosphorylation. The latter include the tumour-promoting phorbol ester TPA which functions as a ligand for protein kinase C (Nishizuka 1984). Phosphorylation of the EGF receptor by the activated protein kinase C enzyme (Cochet *et al.* 1984) results in the disappearance of high affinity EGF binding sites and an almost complete inactivation of the EGF-induced tyrosine phosphorylation of the receptor (Friedman *et al.* 1984). The mechanism of this inhibition is as yet unknown, but it probably involves covalent modification of the cytoplasmic portion of the EGF receptor kinase. The combination of psoralens and ultraviolet light (PUVA chemotherapy) which is widely used for clinical treatment of certain skin diseases may inhibit tyrosine phosphorylation of the EGF receptor by an analogous mechanism (Mermelstein *et al.* 1989). This is supported by increased serine phosphorylation of the EGF receptor in PUVA-treated A431 cells. Natural proteinaceous inhibitors of tyrosine kinases also appear to utilize indirect mechanisms. A phosphoprotein of relative molecular mass 63 kDa was isolated from the rat hepatocytes medium and found to inhibit insulin receptor tyrosine kinase and receptor autophosphorylation (Auberger *et al.* 1989). Only the phosphorylated form of the glycoprotein was active in kinase inhibition and blocking the growth-promoting action of insulin. A hint as to the mechanism of kinase inhibition is provided by the primary structure of the inhibitor, which shows homology with members of the transforming growth factor β (TGF-β) family (Auberger *et al.* 1989) and the cystatin superfamily of serum proteins (Haasemann *et al.* 1991). TGF-β interfers with the function of the EGF receptor tyrosine kinase through an as yet unknown mechanism (Massague 1990). A heat-stable protein that selectively inhibits PTK activity has been partially purified from lymphoid cells but its mechanism of action was not analysed (Hall et al. 1989).

4.5.3.1   *Herbimycin A*

This benzquinonoid antibiotic was originally found to reverse transformation by the Rous sarcoma virus. The inhibition is due to irreversible inactivation of the tyrosine kinase function of pp60^{src} (Uehara *et al.* 1988, 1989). Importantly, all the biological effects of herbimycin are abolished by sulphydryl compounds, indicating the presence of essential thiol groups in the viral *src* protein. Indeed, the sulphydryl alkylating agent *N*-ethylmaleimide also inactivated the pp60^{v-src} kinase (Uehara *et al.* 1989). Therefore it is possible that herbimycin A leads to alkylation that irreversibly inactivates the PTK. As well as reversion of the transformed morphology of *src*-transformed cells, herbimycin A was found to induce phenotypic differentiation of cultured K562 human leukaemic cells (Honma *et al.* 1989). When incubated with T-cells, herbimycin A inhibited substrate tyrosine phosphorylation, inositol phospholipid turnover, and calcium elevation (June *et al.* 1990). Similarly, the drug abrogated surface immunoglobulin-mediated signal transduction in B-cells, but it did not affect signalling in response to aluminium fluoride (Lane *et al.* 1991).

4.5.3.2   *Staurosporine*

Analysis of the binding of staurosporine to various protein kinases indicated that it bound both protein kinase A and TPKs with similar affinities

($K_d \approx 2$–3 nM), and also bound protein kinase C ($K_d \approx 10$ nM). This analysis confirmed the non-selective interaction of staurosporine with protein kinases (Meyer *et al.* 1989; Herbert *et al.* 1990). Nevertheless, staurosporine was a more efficient inhibitor of the PDGF receptor than of the EGF receptor, and at relatively low concentration ($IC_{50} = 70$ nM) it specifically prevented tyrosine phosphorylation of the asialoglycoprotein receptor (Fallon 1990). In contrast, the H7 protein kinase C inhibitor was ineffective. The effect of staurosporine on the EGF receptor is perhaps more complicated, as it involves enhancement of high affinity EGF binding and a decrease in overall phosphorylation of the receptor (Friedman *et al.* 1990).

4.5.3.3   *Other inhibitors*

A few other compounds have been found to inhibit PTKs with low selectivity and by an unknown mechanism. For example, doxorubicin inhibits the *abl* tyrosine kinase and spleen PTK ($IC_{50} = 20$ μM), whereas the sulphonylbenzoyl-nitrostyroles are more specific to the EGF receptor. Adriamycin, the lipid-interacting anticancer agent, has also been found to inhibit spleen PTK (Donella-Deanna *et al.* 1989). The mechanism involves the nucleotide site of the PTK, but other sites also appear to be affected. Other kinases are minimally affected by adriamycin. Finally, derivatives of thiazolidinediones (see basic structure and the formula of compound CGP520 in Fig. 4.2) have been identified as specific inhibitors of the EGF receptor and the *src* protein, but not the *abl* kinase or serine–threonine kinases (Geissler *et al.* 1990). When tested on intact murine and human cells, these compounds inhibited autophosphorylation of the EGF receptor and EGF-induced cell growth.

4.6   Tyrosine kinase inhibitors as research tools

The central role that PTKs play in signal transduction and the relative rarity of tyrosine phosphorylation call for specific inhibitors as molecular tools. Indeed, PTK inhibitors have been used as indicators for the existence of a tyrosine phosphorylation step in complex biological processes such as T- and B-cell activation, signalling by growth factors and lymphokines, and chemotaxis. In addition, PTK inhibitors have been used to dissect some of these processes into tyrosine-kinase-dependent and tyrosine-kinase-independent steps. Finally, the role of PTKs in the induction of cellular differentiation and malignant transformation has been investigated with blockers of tyrosine phosphorylation. The use of metabolic inhibitors, like PTK blockers, as an experimental strategy is based on the assumption that they have only a single cellular target. This assumption is not completely proven for the reported PTK inhibitors and has been repeatedly challenged in the cases of genistein (Markovits *et al.* 1989; Linassier *et al.*

1990), erbstatin (Takekura *et al.* 1991) and a tyrphostin (Faaland *et al.* 1991). The existence of non-PTK targets for the inhibitors is also implied by the requirement of prolonged incubation time, and concentrations that are much higher than the kinase inhibition constants (K_i). If these implications are correct, the action of PTK inhibitors via alternative targets may complicate their use as molecular tools. Consequently, this experimental approach should be critically considered, and conclusions preferably supported by independent evidence.

4.6.1   Dispensability of the tyrosine kinase function

To study the requirement of the PTK function in signalling pathways, the ultimate approach is to use a kinase-negative mutant of the PTK of interest. Inhibitors offer an alternative approach and can provide more useful information; some tyrphostins directed against the insulin receptor kinase blocked lipogenesis but failed to inhibit the antilipolytic effect of insulin (Shechter *et al.* 1989). This observation raised the possibility that insulin actions may be mediated by two separate pathways, in which the one leading to an antilipolytic signal is independent of tyrosine phosphorylation of protein substrates. A similar study, in which the EGF receptor kinase was blocked with genistein, showed that activation of c-*myc* mRNA synthesis and phosphorylation of an 80 kDa substrate were not affected by genistein, despite its cytostatic effect. Even so, stimulation of the S6 kinase was prevented (Linassier *et al.*) 1990). Perhaps the induction of *myc* by EGF is independent of tyrosine phosphorylation. However, this conclusion contradicts results obtained with a kinase-defective EGF receptor (Honegger *et al.* 1987). The role of tyrosine phosphorylation in endocytosis of the EGF receptor was also addressed by using tyrphostins (Yaish *et al.* 1988; Lyall *et al.* 1989). The latter completely inhibited tyrosine phosphorylation of endogenous protein substrates but only partially blocked receptor auto-phosphorylation. Nevertheless, internalization of EGF and its receptor were not affected by tyrphostins. In contrast, erbstatin, another PTK inhibitor, inhibited internalization of the EGF receptor (Imoto *et al.* 1987a). The reason for this discrepancy is not known, but it may reflect differential specificities of erbstatin and tyrphostin. Another aspect of the EGF receptor that was studied with a PTK inhibitor is the formation of high affinity EGF binding sites; staurosporine, an effective PTK inhibitor, enhanced the appearance of high affinity receptors and antagonized the inhibition of high affinity EGF binding by phorbol esters (Friedman *et al.* 1990).

4.6.2   Involvement of tyrosine phosphorylation in biological processes

Inhibition of biological effects by PTK blockers has been inferred as an indication of the involvement of a tyrosine phosphorylation step. Examples include inhibition by erbstatin or ST-638 of neutrophil chemotaxis and superoxide production that were induced by the formylated Met-Leu-Phe chemotactic factor (Shiraishi *et al.* 1989; Naccache *et al.* 1990). Similarly, genistein inhibited IL-1-stimulated prostaglandin production and the induction of prostaglandin endoperoxide synthase in cultured glomerular mesangial cells (Coyne and Morrison 1990). Tyrphostin was employed, together with direct analysis of tyrosine phosphorylation, to establish the existence of a tyrosine phosphorylation step in the activation of B-cells with IL-6 (Nakajima and Wall 1991). A similar approach using ST-638 has been used to show that neutrophil activation by GM-CSF involves tyrosine phosphorylation of two cellular proteins (Shiraishi and Sha'afi 1989). Evidence for the participation of tyrosine phosphorylation in early embryonic development was obtained by treating single-cell embryos with genistein (Besterman and Shultz 1990). Reversible and apparently specific inhibition of cell cleavage was observed.

4.6.3   Stimulation of mesenchymal cells by growth factors

The signal transduction pathways employed by EGF and PDGF were studied in fibroblasts by using PTK inhibitors. Tyrphostins inhibited EGF-induced Ca^{2+} mobilization (Margolis *et al.* 1989) and breakdown of phosphatidylinositol bisphosphate (Posner *et al.* 1989). These effects were probably due to inhibition of tyrosine phosphorylation and physical association of PLC_y with the activated EGF receptor (Margolis *et al.* 1989). The cytostatic effects of tyrphostins are correlated with their ability to inhibit the generation of intracellular second messengers (Posner *et al.* 1989; Levitzki and Gilon 1991), and the cytostatic effect of genistein correlates well with inhibition of S6 kinase activation but not with enhanced *myc* transcription in response to EGF (Linassier *et al.* 1990). By analogy with the EGF receptor system, genistein was used to inhibit PDGF-induced mitogenesis of mouse fibroblasts. Treatment with genistein exerted a cytostatic effect on PDGF-challenged cells (Dean *et al.* 1989; Hill *et al.* 1990). However, removal of PDGF and genistein 4 h after their application resulted in progression of the cells through the G1 phase of the cell cycle. This was accompanied by elevated transcription of *fos*, *jun*, and *jun* B (Zwiller *et al.* 1991), but no activation of PLC took place (Hill *et al.* 1990). Therefore it was concluded that activation of PLC by PDGF is not required for the induction of DNA synthesis.

4.6.4   T-cell activation

The multicomponent T-cell receptor (TCR) undergoes stimulation by antigen, monoclonal antibody to CD3, or lectin mitogens. Several signal transduction pathways are activated by the TCR, including enhanced metabolism of phosphatidylinositol lipids which is mediated by PLC. TCR activation involves tyrosine phosphorylation of the ζ subunit of the receptor. The exact relationships among these events have been extensively studied using PTK inhibitors. Activation of PLC was inhibited by genistein, suggesting that tyrosine phosphorylation is essential for the production of inositol phosphates and diacylglycerol (Mustelin et al. 1989). The T-cell PTK p56[lck] was inhibited by genistein with an IC_{50} of 40 μM (Trevillyan et al. 1990). Similarly, inhibition of PTK activity with herbimycin A led to inhibition of substrate tyrosine phosphorylation, TCR-mediated inositol phospholipid hydrolysis, and calcium elevation (June et al. 1990). The production of the T-cell growth factor IL-2 was also inhibited by genistein, herbimycin, and tyrphostin (Stanley et al. 1990), suggesting that activation of PTK also precedes the secretion of IL-2. The unresponsiveness (anergy) that follows antigenic stimulation was not inhibited by genistein (Norton et al. 1991), indicating a PTK-independent regulation of this process.

4.6.5   B-cell activation

Cross-linking of surface immunoglobulins of B lymphocytes causes activation of protein tyrosine phosphorylation (Campbell and Sefton 1990; Gold et al. 1990) and stimulation of phospholipase C with subsequent increase in production of inositol phosphates and diacylglycerol (Bijsterbosch et al. 1985). Using specific PTK inhibitors it was possible to demonstrate that PTK activation acts as an intermediary between the B-cell antigen receptor and phospholipase C. Herbimycin and genistein inhibited new tyrosine phosphorylation after receptor-linked activation of B-cells, and this was associated with inhibition of inositol phospholipid turnover and abrogation of the increase in intracellular calcium (Lane et al. 1991). Similarly, preincubation of B-lymphocytes with two different tyrphostins (AG126 and AG30) blocked anti-IgM-induced proliferation, fos expression, tyrosine phosphorylation, increase in intracellular Ca^{2+} and production of inositol phosphates (Padeh et al. 1991). In contrast with surface-Ig-mediated activation, the PTK inhibitors did not affect B-cell proliferation induced by phorbol esters and cation ionophores, or by aluminum fluoride, indicating specificity to PTK activity.

4.6.6   Induction of differentiation

Haemin induces erythroid differentiation of K562 human chronic myelogenic leukaemic cell line, and this process involves reduction in tyrosine phosphorylation. Similarly, PTK inhibitors also induce differentiation in vitro, implicating tyrosine phosphorylation in the process of differentiation. Herbimycin A rapidly induced reduction of tyrosine phosphorylation and subsequent differentiation of K562 cells (Honma et al. 1989).

Genistein and ST-638, when incubated with mouse erythroleukaemic (MEL) cells, also induced terminal erythroid differentiation (Watanabe *et al.* 1989). Simultaneous incubation with agents that block DNA synthesis (e.g. mitomycin C) enhanced the effect of PTK blockers on MEL differentiation, whereas known differentiation inducers of K562 cells (e.g. adriamycin) enhanced the effect of herbimycin A on K562 differentiation. Nevertheless, different phenotypes were induced by conventional inducing agents of MEL cells (e.g. dimethyl sulphoxide) and PTK inhibitor (genistein). The latter treatment induced earlier appearance of differentiated cells, and their phenotype was insensitive to dexamethasone (Watanabe *et al.* 1991). In contrast with erythroid differentiation, PTK inhibitors blocked differentiation of primary keratinocytes in culture (Filvaroff *et al.* 1990); incubation of these epithelial cells with calcium or phorbol ester caused early induction of PTK activity. This event appears to be critical for the appearance of the differentiated state as its inhibition blocked the whole process.

4.7   Clinical potential of PTK inhibitors

The realization that PTKs function as transducers of extracellular and intercellular signals for cell proliferation and differentiation identified this family of enzymes as a potential pharmacological target. This relatively young field of research (systematic search for PTK inhibitors started in 1985) has already brought drugs to phase I clinical trial and is promising for both malignant and benign diseases. Clinical applications of PTK inhibitors are expected to be most useful where activated forms of membrane-associated PTKs exist. Nevertheless, recent reports demonstrating activation of PTKs by various extracellular stimuli, including thrombin, interleukins, antigens and gap-junction-mediated cell–cell communication, suggest even broader chemotherapeutic application of PTK inhibitors.

Mutated or overexpressed PTKs are usually associated with elevated intrinsic tyrosine phosphorylation activity (Yarden and Ullrich 1988b; Cantley *et al.* 1991). Overexpression of the neu/erbB-2 gene in mammary and ovarian carcinomas (Slamon *et al.* 1989) and the EGF receptor in squamous carcinomas (Hendler *et al.* 1984) are believed to contribute to transformation by elevated basal activity of the overexpressed tyrosine kinase. Alternatively, autocrine or paracrine loops may result in increased tyrosine phosphorylation. This mechanism is relevant to the proliferation of smooth muscle cells that is mediated, in part, by secreted PDGF (Ross 1989). Diseases that may be affected by this mechanism are atherosclerosis and hypertension. The latter case may also involve activation of the EGF receptor (Clegg and Sambhi 1989). Accumulation of the growth factor is an alternative mechanism which is exemplified in psoriatic keratinocytes (Elder *et al.* 1989). Increased synthesis of the transforming growth factor

a, which binds to the EGF receptor, is believed to support hyperproliferation of keratinocytes in the psoriatic epidermis. Both keratinocyte proliferation (Dvir *et al.* 1991) and PDGF-mediated smooth muscle cell proliferation (Bilder *et al.* 1991) are susceptible to inhibition *in vitro* by tyrphostins. Proliferation of haematopoietic cells is also affected by PTKs. Altered forms of the *abl*-encoded tyrosine kinase are present in chronic myelogenic leukaemia cells, and PTKs function as relay systems for activation of T- and B-lymphocytes (Klausner and Samelson 1991). The observations that PTK inhibitors lead to erythroid differentiation of erythroleukaemic cells (Honma *et al.* 1989; Watanabe *et al.* 1989) promise that chemotherapy directed at PTKs may be clinically relevant.

Medical application of PTK inhibitors is expected to face problems that are not well represented by the current *in vitro* model systems. The existence of non-PTK targets may result in side-effects in the treated tissue or in remote organs. The drug may be rapidly cleared from serum by degradation or by binding to serum proteins, as is the case with erbstatin (Imoto *et al.* 1987b). Rapid clearance may require repeated administration of relatively high doses of the drug or development of more long-lived compounds. Certainly, prior to therapeutic application, improved drugs require to be synthesized and their effects tested in model animal systems such as athymic mice. In addition, the potential of combination therapy should be investigated; suboptimal doses of PTK inhibitors may exert synergistic effects with conventional drugs directed at inhibition of DNA synthesis, serine–threonine kinases, inositol lipid metabolism, and induction of differentiation (Tritton and Hickman 1990; Powis 1991).

4.8   Perspective and the future

The development of inhibitors of PTKs is dependent on an in-depth understanding of the physiological role of tyrosine kinases. The great progress that has been made in the past decade in elucidating the role of PTKs in signal transduction, mitogenesis, cell cycle control, and differentiation opened up a wide field for pharmacological experimentation. The realization that surface receptors are functionally linked to a cytoplasmic network of soluble PTKs and serine–threonine kinases is expected to extend further into the nucleus. This will probably result in a comprehensive picture that will explain the mechanism by which extracellular stimuli are coupled to regulation of gene expression and DNA replication. Once established, this model will provide a solid basis for reliable tests of the specificity of PTK inhibitors.

The design of new PTK inhibitors is probably entering a new phase where synthetic, rather than natural, compounds will be continuously improved by rigorous structure–function analysis. Although inhibitors aimed at the substrate site appear to be more promising, molecules that compete for the nucleotide binding site of PTKs are surprisingly selective and efficient. As is often the case with pharmacological reagents, conclusive proof that PTKs are the exclusive target of a given inhibitor remains the major obstacle. Several recent studies have indicated that this is not the case for some of the currently used PTK inhibitors. This will continue to limit the usefulness of tyrosine kinase inhibitors as research tools. However, the clinical potential of this pharmacological approach is less severely affected. We shall probably witness more and more PTK inhibitors reaching clinical trial after successful testing in animal model systems. At present, the latter are rarely used although this is the only method for early evaluation of side-effects of PTK inhibitors. The performance of *in vivo* tests is particularly important, as species-dependent variation of the biological effects of tyrosine kinase inhibitors is not expected. Chemotherapy employing inhibitors of tyrosine kinases may thus develop into a routine clinical treatment; malignancies involving secretory epithelia (e.g. breast, colon, and ovary) or haematopoietic cells (e.g. leukaemias) are predictable target diseases. In addition, benign states associated with hyperproliferation of poorly differentiated cells (e.g. early adenomas) or specific tissues (e.g. endothelial and smooth muscle cells of the atherosclerotic plaque) may also serve as clinical targets for PTK inhibitors.

Acknowledgements

We thank Zvika Kelman and Alexander Levitzki for useful comments. Our laboratory is supported by grants from the National Institutes of Health and the Wolfson Foundation administered by the Israel Academy of Sciences and Humanities. YY is an incumbent of the Armour Family Chair for Cancer Research.

References

Akiyama, T., Ishida, J., Nakagawa, S., Ogawara, H., Watanabe, S., Itoh, N., Shibuya, M., and Fukami, Y. (1987). Genistein, a specific inhibitor of tyrosine-specific protein kinases. *Journal of Biological Chemistry*, **262**, 5592–5.

Atluro, S. and Atluro D. (1991). Evidence that genistein, a protein tyrosine inhibitor, inhibits CD28 monoclonal antibody stimulated human T cell proliferation. *Transplantation*, **51**, 448–50.

Auberger, P., Falquerho, L., Contreres, J. O., Pages, G., LeCam, G., Rossi, B., and LeCam, A. (1989). Characterization of a natural inhibitor of the insulin receptor kinase: cDNA cloning, purification and anti-mitogenic activity. *Cell*, **58**, 631–40.

Ballou, I. M., Jeano, P., and Thomas, G. (1988). Control of S6 phosphorylation during the mitogenic response. *Advances in Experimental Medicine and Biology*, **231**, 445–52.

Bertics, P. J. and Gill, G. N. (1985). Self-phosphorylation enhances the protein-tyrosine kinase activity of the epidermal growth factor receptor. *Journal of Biological Chemistry*, **260**, 14642–7.

Besterman, B. and Schultz, R. M. (1990). Regulation of mouse preimplantation development: inhibitory effect of genistein, an inhibitor of tyrosine protein phosphorylation on cleavage of one cell embryos. *Journal of Experimental Zoology*, **256**, 44–53.

Bijsterbosch, M. K., Meade, C. J., Turner, G. A., and Klans, G. G. B. (1985). B lymphocyte receptors and polyphosphoinositide degradation. *Cell*, **41**, 999–1006.

Bilder, G. E., Krawiec, J. A., McVety, K. J., Gazit, A., Gilon, C., Lyall, R., *et al.* (1991). Tyrphostins inhibit PDGF-induced DNA synthesis and associated early events in smooth muscle cells. *American Journal of Physiology*, **260**, 721–30.

Bishop, W. R., Petrin, J., Wang, L., Ramesh, U., and Doll, R. J. (1990). Inhibition of protein kinase C by the tyrosine kinase inhibitor erbstatin. *Biochemical Pharmacology*, **40**, 2129–35.

Bottaro, D. P., Rubin, J. S., Faletto, D. L., Chan, A. M.-L., Kemieck, T. E., Van de Woude, G. F., and Aaronson, S. T. (1991). Identification of the hepatocyte growth factor receptor as the c-*met* proto-oncogene product. *Science*, **251**, 802–4.

Bramson, H. N., Thomas, N., Matsuda, R., Nelson, N. C., and Taylor, S. S. (1982). Modification of the catalytic subunit of bovine heart cAMP-dependent protein kinase with affinity labels related to peptide substrates. *Journal of Biological Chemistry*, **257**, 10575–81.

Braun, S., Abdel Ghany, M., and Racker, E. (1983). A rapid assay for protein kinases phosphorylating small polypeptides and other substrates. *Analytical Biochemistry*, **135**, 369–78.

Braun, S., Raymond, W. E., and Racker, E. (1984). Synthetic tyrosine polymers as substrates and inhibitors of tyrosine-specific protein kinases. *Journal of Biological Chemistry*, **259**, 2051–4.

Campbell, M. A. and Sefton, B. M. (1990). Protein tyrosine phosphorylation is induced in murine B lymphocytes in response to stimulation with anti-immunoglobulin. *EMBO Journal*, **9**, 2125–31.

Cantley, L. C., Auger, K. R., Carpenter, C., Duckworth, B., Graziani, A., Kapeller, R., and Soltoff, S. (1991). Oncogenes and signal transduction. *Cell*, **64**, 281–302.

Clegg, K. B. and Sambhi, M. P. (1989). Inhibition of epidermal growth factor-mediated DNA synthesis by a specific tyrosine kinase inhibitor in vascular smooth muscle cells of the spontaneously hypertensive rat. *Journal of Hypertension* (*Suppl.*) **7**, 144–5.

Cochet, C., Gill, G. N., Meisenheider, J., Cooper, J. A., and Hunter, T. (1984). C-kinase phosphorylates the epidermal growth factor-receptor and reduces its epidermal growth factor stimulated tyrosine protein kinase activity. *Journal of Biological Chemistry*, **259**, 2553–8.

Cooper, J. A., Gould, K. L., Cartwright, C. A., and Hunter, T. (1986). Tyr[527] is phosphorylated in pp60[src]. Implications for regulation. *Science*, **231**, 1431–4.

Coyne, D. U. and Morrison, A. R. (1990). Effect of tyrosine kinase inhibitor genistein on interleukin-1 stimulated PGE_2 production in mesangial cells. *Biochemical and Biophysical Research Communications*, **173**, 718–24.

Cushman, M., Nagarathnam, D., Burg, D. L., and Geahlen, R. L. (1991). Synthesis and protein tyrosine kinase inhibitory activity of flavonoid analogues. *Journal of Medicinal Chemistry*, **34**, 798–806.

Dean, N. M., Kanemitsu, M., and Boynton, A. L. (1989). Effects of the tyrosine kinase inhibitor genistein on DNA synthesis and phospholipid derived second messenger generation in mouse 10T 1/2 fibroblasts and rat liver T51B cells. *Biochemical and Biophysical Research Communications*, **165**, 795–801.

Donella-Deanna, A., Monti, E., and Pinna, L. A. (1989). Inhibition of tyrosine protein kinases by the antineoplasic agent adriamycin. *Biochemical and Biophysical Research Communications*, **160**, 1309–15.

Downward, J., Parker, P., and Waterfield, M. D. (1984). Autophosphorylation and protein kinase phosphorylation of the epidermal growth factor receptor. *Journal of Biological Chemistry*, **260**, 14538–46.

Dvir, A., Milner, Y., Chomsky, O., Gilon, C., Gazit, A., and Levitzki, A. (1991). The inhibition of EGF-dependent proliferation of keratinocytes by tyrphostin tyrosine kinase blockers. *Journal of Cell Biology*, **113**, 857–65.

Eckhart, W., Hutchinson, M. A., and Hunter, T. (1979). An activity phosphorylating tyrosine in polyoma T antigen immunoprecipitates. *Cell*, **18**, 925–33.

Elder, J. T., Fisher, G. J., Lindquist, P. B., Bennet, G. L., Pittelkow, M. R., Coffey, R. J., *et al.* (1989). Overexpression of transforming growth factor *a* in psoriatic epidermis. *Science*, **243**, 811–14.

Ellis, L., Clamsey, E., Morgan, D. O., Edery, M., Roth, R. A., and Rutter, W. J. (1986). Replacement of insulin receptor tyrosine kinase residues 1162 and 1163 compromises insulin-stimulated kinase activity and uptake of 2-deoxyglucose. *Cell*, **45**, 721–32.

Erneux, C., Cohen, S., and Garbers, D. L. (1983). The kinetics of tyrosine phosphorylation by the purified epidermal growth factor receptor kinase of A431 cells. *Journal of Cell Biology*, **258**, 4137–42.

Ernould, A. P., Ferry, G., Genton, A., Cudennee, C. A., and Boutin, J. A. (1990). Use of main tyrosine protein kinase activity purified from HL60 in the search for a new class of anticancer compounds. *Anticancer Research*, **10**, 197–201.

Faaland, C. A., Mermelstein, F. H., Hagashi, J., and Laskin, J. D. (1991). Rapid uptake of tyrphostin into A431 human epidermoid cells is followed by delayed inhibition of epidermal growth factor (EGF)-stimulated EGF receptor tyrosine kinase activity. *Molecular and Cell Biology*, **11**, 2697–703.

Fallon, R. J. (1990). Staurosporine inhibits a tyrosine protein kinase in human hepatoma cell membranes. *Biochemical and Biophysical Research Communications*, **170**, 1191–6.

Ferrell, J. E., Jr. and Martin, G. S. (1989). Platelet tyrosine-specific protein phosphorylation is regulated by thrombin. *Molecular and Cell Biology*, **8**, 3603–8.

Ferrell, J. E., Chang Sing, P. D. G., Loew, G., King, R., Mansour, J. M., and Mansour, T. E. (1979). Structure/activity studies of flavonoids as inhibitors of cAMP, phosphodiesterase and relationship to quantum chemical indices. *Molecular Pharmacology*, **16**, 556–68.

Filvaroff, E., Stern, D. F., and Dotto, G. P. (1990). Tyrosine phosphorylation is an early and specific event involved in primary keratinocyte differentiation. *Molecular and Cell Biology*, **10**, 1164–73.

Friedman, B. A., Frackelton, A. R., Jr, Ross, A. H., Connors, J. M., Fujiki, H., Sugimura, T., and Rosner, M. R. (1984). Tumor promoter blocks tyrosine-specific phosphorylation of the epidermal growth factor receptor. *Proceedings of the National Academy of Sciences of the United States of America*, **81**, 3034–8.

Friedman, B. A., Fujiki, H., and Rosner, M. R. (1990). Regulation of the epidermal growth factor receptor by growth-modulating agent: effect of staurosporine, a protein kinase inhibitor. *Cancer Research*, **50**, 533–8.

Gaudette, D. C. and Holub, B. J. (1990). Effect of genistein, a tyrosine kinase inhibitor on U46619-induced phosphoinositide phosphorylation in human platelets. *Biochemical and Biophysical Research Communications*, **170**, 238–42.

Gazit, A., Yaish, P., Gilon, C., and Levitzki, A. (1989). Tyrphostins I: synthesis and biological activity of protein tyrosine kinase inhibitors. *Journal of Medicinal Chemistry*, **32**, 2344–52.

Geissler, J. F., Traxler, P., Regenass, U., Murray, B. J., Roesel, J. L., Meyer, T., *et al.* (1990). Thiazolidine-diones: biochemical and biological activity of a novel class of tyrosine protein kinase inhibitors. *Journal of Biological Chemistry*, **265**, 22255–61.

Gold, M. R., Law, D. A., and DeFranco, A. L. (1990). Stimulation of protein tyrosine phosphorylation by the B lymphocyte antigen receptor. *Nature, London*, **345**, 810–813.

Grandori, C. (1989). Regulation of kinase activity. *Nature, London*, **338**, 467.

Graziani, Y., Chayoth, R., Karny, N., Feldman, B., and Levy, J. (1981). Regulation of protein kinase activity by quercetin in Ehrlich ascites tumor cells. *Biochimica et Biophysica Acta*, **714**, 415–21.

Graziani, Y., Erikson, E., and Erikson, R. L. (1983). The effect of quercetin on the phosphorylation activity of Rous sarcoma virus transforming gene product *in vitro* and *in vivo*. *European Journal of Biochemistry*, **135**, 583–9.

Gschwendt, M., Horn, F., Kittstein, W., Furstenberger, G., Besemfelder, E., and Marks, F. (1984). Calcium and phospholipid-dependent protein kinase activity in mouse epidermis cytosol; stimulation by complete and incomplete tumor promoter and inhibition by various compounds. *Biochemical and Biophysical Research Communications*, **124**, 63–8.

Haasemann, M., Nawratil, P., and Muller-Esterl, W. (1991). Rat tyrosine kinase inhibitors show sequence similarity to human alpha H3 glycoprotein and bovine fetuin. *Biochemical Journal*, **274**, 899–902.

Hagiwara, M., Inoue, S., Tanaka, T., Nunoki, K., Ito, M., and Hidaka, H. (1988). Differential effects of flavonoids as inhibitors of tyrosine protein kinases and serine/threonine kinases. *Biochemical Pharmacology*, **37**, 2987–92.

Hall, B. S., Hoffbrand, A. V., and Wickramasinghe, R. G. (1989). An endogenous inhibitor of tyrosine kinase activity of normal and malignant human lymphoid cells. *Oncogene*, **4**, 1225–31.

Hanks, S. K., Quinn, A. M., and Hunter, T. (1988). The protein kinase family: conserved features and deduced phylogeny of the catalytic domains. *Science*, **241**, 42–52.

Hansen, T., Stagsted, J., Pedersen, L., Roth, R. A., Goldstein, A., and Olsson, L. (1989). Inhibition of insulin receptor phosphorylation by peptides derived from major histocompatibility complex class I antigens. *Proceedings of the National Academy of Sciences of the United States of America*, **86**, 3123–6.

Hardie, G. (1988). Pseudosubstrates turn off protein kinases. *Nature, London* **335**, 592–3.

Hempsted, B. L., Martin-Zanca, D., Kaplan, D. R., Parada, L. F., and Chao, M. V.

(1991). High affinity NGF binding requires coexpression of the *trk* proto-oncogene and low-affinity NGF receptor. *Nature, London*, **350**, 678–83.

Hendler, F., Shum, A., Richards, C., Cassels, D., Guasterson, B., and Ozanne, B. (1984). Evidence for increased epidermal growth factor receptors in epidermal malignancies. *Cancer Cells*, **1**, 41–50.

Herbert, J. M., Seban, E., and Maffrand, P. (1990). Characterization of a specific binding site for [³H]-staurosporine and various protein kinases. *Biochemical and Biophysical Research Communications*, **171**, 189–95.

Herrera, R. and Rosen, O. M. (1986). Autophosphorylation of the insulin receptor *in vitro*. *Journal of Biological Chemistry*, **261**, 11980–5.

Hill, T. D., Dean, N. M., Mordan, L. J., Lau, A. F., Kanemitsu, M. Y., and Boynton, A. L. (1990). PDGF-induced activation of phospholipase C is not required for induction of DNA synthesis. *Science*, **248**, 1660–3.

Honegger, A. M., Szapary, D., Schmidt, A., Lyall, R., Van Obberghen, E., Dull, T., *et al.* (1987). A mutant epidermal growth factor receptor with defective protein tyrosine kinase is unable to stimulate proto-oncogene expression and DMA synthesis. *Molecular and Cell Biology*, **7**, 4568–71.

Honegger, A. M., Kris, R. M., Ullrich, A., and Schlessinger, J. (1989). Evidence that autophosphorylation of solubilized receptors for epidermal growth factor is mediated by intermolecular cross-phosphorylation. *Proceedings of the National Academy of Sciences of the United States of America*, **86**, 925–9.

Honma, Y., Okabe-Kado, J., Hozumi, M., Uehara, Y., and Mizuno, S. (1989). Induction of erythroid differentiation of K562 human leukemic cells by herbimycin A, an inhibitor of tyrosine kinase activity. *Cancer Research*. **49**, 331–4.

Hunter, T. (1982). Synthetic peptide substrates for a tyrosine protein kinase. *Journal of Biological Chemistry*, **257**, 4843–8.

Hunter, T. (1989). Protein modification: phosphorylation on tyrosine residues. *Current Opinion in Cell Biology*, **1**, 1168–81.

Hunter, T. and Cooper, J. A. (1985). Protein-tyrosine kinases. *Annual Review of Biochemistry*, **54**, 897–930.

Hunter, T. and Sefton, B. M. (1980). Transforming gene product of Rous sarcoma virus phosphorylates tyrosine. *Proceedings of the National Academy of Sciences of the United States of America*, **77**, 1311–15.

Imoto, M., Umezawa, K., Sawa, T., Takeuchi, T., and Umezawa, H. (1987a). *In situ* inhibition of tyrosine protein kinase by erbstatin. *Biochemistry International*, **15**, 989–95.

Imoto, M., Umezawa, K., Kamuro, K., Sawa, T., Takeuchi, T., and Umezawa, H. (1987b). Antitumor activity of erbstatin, a tyrosine protein kinase inhibitor. *Japanese Journal of Cancer Research* (*Gann*), **78**, 329–32.

Imoto, M., Shimura, N., Ui, H., and Umezawa, K. (1990). Inhibition of EGF-induced phospholipase C activation in A431 cells by erbstatin, a tyrosine kinase inhibitor. *Biochemical and Biophysical Research Communications*, **173**, 208–211.

June, C. H., Fletcher, M. C., Ledbetter, J. A., Schieven, G. L., Siegel, J. N., Phillips, A. F., and Samelson, L. E. (1990). Inhibition of tyrosine phosphorylation prevents T cell receptor-mediated signal transduction. *Proceedings of the National Academy of Sciences of the United States of America*, **87**, 7722–6.

Kaplan, D. R., Hempsted, B. L., Martin-Zanca, D., Chao, M. V., and Parada, L. F. (1991a). The *trk* proto-oncogene product: a signal transducing receptor for nerve growth factor. *Science*, **252**, 554–8.

Kaplan, D. R., Martin Zanca, D., and Parada, L. F. (1991b). Tyrosine phosphorylation and tyrosine kinase activity of *trk* protooncogene product induced by NGF. *Nature, London*, **350**, 158–60.

Kaplan, D. R., Morrison, D. K., Wong, G., McCormick, F., and Williams, L. T. (1990). PDGF β-receptor stimulates tyrosine phosphorylation of GAP and association of GAP with a signalling complex. *Cell*, **61**, 125–33.

Kazlauskas, A. and Cooper, A. J. (1989). Autophosphorylation of the PDGF receptor in the kinase insert region regulates interactions with cell proteins. *Cell*, **58**, 1121–33.

Klausner, R. D. and Samelson, L. E. (1991). T cell antigen receptor activation pathways: the tyrosine kinase connection. *Cell*, **64**, 875–8.

Klein, R., Jing, S., Nanduri, V., O'Rourke, E., and Barbacid, M. (1991a). The *trk* protooncogene encodes a receptor for nerve growth factor. *Cell*, **65**, 189–97.

Klein, R., Nanduri, V., Jing, S., Lamballe, F., Tapley, P., Bryant, S., *et al.* (1991b). The TrkB tyrosine protein kinase is a receptor for brain-derived neurotrophic factor and neurotrophin-3. *Cell*, **66**, 395–403.

Kmiecik, T. E. and Shalloway, D. (1987). Activation and suppression of pp60[c-src] transforming activity by mutation of its primary sites of tyrosine phosphorylation. *Cell*, **49**, 65–73.

Koch, C. A., Anderson, D., Moran, M. F., Ellis, C., and Pawson, T. (1991). SH2 and SH3 domains: elements that control interactions of cytoplasmic signalling proteins. *Science*, **252**, 668–74.

Kohanski, R. A. and Lane, D. M. (1986). Kinetic evidence for activating and non-activating components of autophosphorylation of the insulin receptor protein kinase. *Biochemical and Biophysical Research Communications*, **134**, 1312–18.

Kreuter, M. H., Leake, R. E., Rinaldi, F., Muller-Klieser, W., Maindof, A., Muller, W. E., and Schroder, H. C. (1990). Inhibition of intrinsic protein tyrosine kinase activity of EGF-receptor kinase ccmplex from human breast cancer cells by the marine sponge metabolite (+)-aeroplysinin-1. *Comparative Biochemistry and Physiology*, **97**, 151–8.

Lane, P. J., Ledbetter, J. A., McConnell, F. M., Draves, K., Deans, J., Shieven, G. L., and Clark, E. A. (1991). The role of tyrosine phosphorylation in signal transduction through surface Ig in human B cells: Inhibition of tyrosine phosphorylation prevents intracellular calcium release. *Journal of Immunology*, **146**, 715–22.

Lang, D. R. and Racker, E. (1974). Effect of quercetin and F1 inhibition on mitochondrial ATPase and energy-linked reactions in submitochondrial particles. *Biochimica et Biophysica Acta*, **333**, 180–6.

Levitzki, A. (1990). Tyrphostins—potential antiproliferative agents and novel molecular tools. *Biochemical Pharmacology*, **40**, 913–18.

Levitzki, A. and Gilon, C. (1991). Tyrphostins as molecular tools and potential antiproliferative drugs. *Trends in Pharmacological Sciences*, **12**, 171–4.

Linassier, C., Pierre, M., LePecq, J. B., and Pierre, J. (1990). Mechanism of action in NIH-3T3 cells of genistein: an inhibitor of EGF receptor tyrosine kinase activity. *Biochemical Pharmacology*, **39**, 187–93.

Lyall, R. M., Zilberstein, A., Gazit, A., Gilon, C., Levitzki, A., and Schlessinger, J. (1989). Tyrphostins inhibit epidermal growth factor (EGF)-receptor tyrosine kinase activity living cells and EGF-stimulated cell proliferation. *Journal of Biological Chemistry*, **264**, 14503–9.

Margolis, B., Rhee, S. G., Felder, S., Mervic, M., Lyall, R., Levitzki, A., *et al.* (1989). EGF induces tyrosine phosphorylation of phospholipase C-II: a potential mechanism for EGF receptor signalling. *Cell*, **57**, 1101–7.

Markovits, J., Linassier, C., Fosse, P., Couprie, J., Pierre, J., Jacquemin-Sablon, A., *et al.* (1989). Inhibitory effect of the tyrosine kinase inhibitor genistein on mammalian DNA topoisomerase II. *Cancer Research*, **49**, 5111–7.

Massague, J. (1990). The transforming growth factor-β family. *Annual Review of Cell Biology*, **6**, 597–641.

Matsuda, M., Mayer, B. J., Fukami, Y., and Hanafura, H. (1990). Binding of transforming protein p45$^{gag-crk}$ to a broad range of phosphotyrosine containing proteins. **Science**, **248**, 1537–9.

Mermelstein, F. H., Abidi, T. F., and Laskin, J. D. (1989). Inhibition of epidermal growth factor tyrosine kinase activity in A431 human epidermoid cells following psoralen/ultraviolet light treatment. *Molecular Pharmacology*, **36**, 848–55.

Meyer, T., Regenass, U., Fabbro, D., Alteri, E., Rosel, J., Muller, M., *et al.* (1989). A derivative of staurosporine (CGP 41 251) shows selectivity for protein kinase C inhibition and *in vitro* anti-proliferative as well as *in vivo* anti tumor activity. *International Journal of Cancer*, **43**, 851–6.

Meyerovitch, J., Kahn, C. R., and Shechter, Y. (1990). A family of substrates and inhibitors of insulin receptor kinase. *Biochemistry*, **29**, 3654–60.

Morrison, D. K., Kaplan, D. R., Escobedo, J. A., Rapp, U. R., Roberts, T. M., and Williams, L. T. (1989). Direct activation of the serine/threonine kinase activity of raf through tyrosine phosphorylation by the PDGF β-receptor. *Cell*, **58**, 649–57.

Mustelin, T., Coggeshall, K. M., Isakov, N., and Altman, A. (1990). T cell antigen receptor-mediated activation of phospholipase C requires tyrosine phosphorylation. *Science*, **247**, 1584–7.

Naccache, P. H., Gilbert, C., Caon, A. C., Gaudry, M., Huang, C. K., Bonak, V. A., *et al.* (1990). Selective inhibition of human neutrophil functional responsiveness by erbstatin an inhibitor of tyrosine protein kinase. *Blood*, **76**, 2098–104.

Nakajima, N. and Wall, R. (1991). Interleukln-6 signals activating junB and TIS11 gene transcription in a B-cell hybridoma. *Molecular Cell Biology*, **11**, 1409–18.

Nakano, H., Kobagashi, E., Takahashi, I., Tamaoki, T., Kuzuu, Y. J., and Iba, H. (1987). Staurosporine inhibits tyrosine-specific protein kinase activity of Rous sarcoma virus transforming protein p60. *Journal of Antibiotics, Tokyo*, **40**, 706–8.

Nishibe, S., Wahl, M. I., Hernandez-Stomayor, T., Tonks, N. K., Rhee, S. G., and Carpenter, G. (1990). Increase of the catalytic activity of phospholipase C-γ1 by tyrosine phosphorylation. *Science*, **250**, 1253–6.

Nishizuka, Y. (1984). The role of protein kinase C in cell surface signal transduction and tumour promotion. *Nature, London*, **308**, 693–8.

Norton, S. D., Hrinen, D., and Jenkins, M. K. (1991). IL-2 secretion and T cell clonal anergy are induced by distinct biochemical pathways. *Journal of Immunology*, **146**, 1125–9.

Onoda, T., Iinuma, H., Sasaki, Y., Hamada, M., Issihiki, K., Naganawa, H., *et al.* (1989). Isolation of a novel tyrosine kinase inhibitor, lavendustin A, from *Streptomyces grisolavendus*. *Journal of Natural Products*, **52**, 1252–7.

Padeh, S., Levitzki, A., Gasit, A., Mills, G. B., and Roifman, C. M. (1991).

Activation of phospholipase C in human B cell is dependent on tyrosine phosphorylation. *Journal of Clinical Investigation*, **87**, 1114–18.

Piwinica-Worms, H., Saunders, K. B., Roberts, T. M., Smith, A. E., and Cheng, S. H. (1987). Tyrosine phosphorylation regulates the biochemical and biological properties of pp60[c-src]. *Cell*, **49**, 75–82.

Posner, I., Gazit, A., Gilon, C., and Levitzki, A. (1989). Tyrphostins inhibit the epidermal growth factor receptor-mediated breakdown of phosphoinositide. *Federation of European Biochemical Societies Letters*, **257**, 287–91.

Powis, G. (1991). Signalling targets for anticancer drug development. *Trends in Pharmacological Sciences*, **12**, 188–94.

Raz, V., Kelman, Z., Avivi, A., Neufeld, G., Givol, D., and Yarden, Y. (1991). PCR-based identification of new receptors: molecular cloning of a receptor for fibroblast growth factors. *Oncogene*, **6**, 753–60.

Ross, R. (1989). Platelet derived growth factor. *Lancet*, **1**, 1179–82.

Rossman, M. G., Moras, D., and Olsen, K. (1974). Chemical and biological evolution of nucleotide binding proteins. *Nature, London*, **250**, 194–9.

Sadowski, I., Stone, J. C., and Pawson, T. (1986). A non-catalytic domain conserved among cytoplasmic protein tyrosine kinases modifies the kinase function and transforming activity of Fujinami sarcoma virus p130[gag-fps]. *Molecular Cell Biology*, **6**, 4396–408.

Saperstein, R., Vicario, P. P., Strout, H. V., Brady, E., Slater, E. E., Greenlee, W. J., *et al.* (1989). Design of a selective insulin receptor tyrosine kinase inhibitor and its effect on glucose uptake and metabolism in intact cells. *Biochemistry*, **28**, 5694–701.

Shechter, Y., Yaish, P., Chorev, M., Gilon, C., Braun, S., and Levitzki, A. (1989). Inhibition of insulin-dependent lipogenesis and anti-lipolysis by protein tyrosine kinase inhibitors. *EMBO Journal*, **8**, 1671–6.

Shiraishi, T. and Sha'afi, R. I. (1989). Tyrosine phpsphorylation in human neutrophil. *Biochemical and Biophysical Research Communications*, **162**, 1478–85.

Shiraishi, T., Owada, M. K., Tatsuka, M., Yamashita, T., Watanabe, K., and Kakunaga, T. (1989). Specific inhibitors of tyrosine-specific protein kinases: properties of *N*-hydroxycinnamamide derivatives *in vitro*. *Cancer Research*, **49**, 2374–8.

Shiraishi, T., Owada, M. K., Tatsuka, M., Fuse, Y., Watanabe, K., and Kakunaga, T. (1990). A tyrosine-specific protein kinase inhibitor, alpha-cyano-3-ethoxy-4-hydroxy-5-phenylthiomethylcinnamamide blocks the phosphorylation of tyrosine kinase substrate in intact cells. *Japanese Journal of Cancer Research*, **81**, 645–52.

Shoelson, S. E., White, M. F., and Kahn, C. R. (1989). Non-phosphorylatable substrate analogs selectively block autophosphorylation and activation of the insulin receptor epidermal growth factor receptor and pp60[v-scr] kinases. *Journal of Biological Chemistry*, **264**, 7831–6.

Shoshan, V. and MacLennan, D. H. (1981). Quercetin interaction with the $(Ca^{2+} + Mg^{2+})$-ATPase of sarcoplasmic reticulum. *Journal of Biological Chemistry*, **256**, 887–92.

Slamon, D. J., Godolphin, W., Jones, L. A., Holt, J. A., Wong, S. G., Keith, D. E., *et al.* (1989). Studies of the HER-2/neu protooncogene in human breast and ovarian cancer. *Science*, **244**, 707–12.

Soderling, T. R. (1990). Protein kinase regulation by autoinhibitory domains. *Journal of Biological Chemistry*, **265**, 1823–6.

Srivastava, A. K. (1990). Non-receptor protein tyrosine kinases of normal tissues. *International Journal of Biochemistry*, **22**, 1229–34.

Srivastava, A. K. and Chiasson, J. L. (1989). Comparative characterization of receptor and non-receptor associated protein kinases. *Biochimica et Biophysica Acta*, **996**, 13–18.

Stadtmaver, L. A. and Rosen, O. M. (1983). Phosphorylation of exogenous substrates by the insulin receptor-associated protein kinases. *Journal of Biological Chemistry*, **258**, 6682–5.

Stanley, J. B., Gorczynski, R., Hung, C. K., Love, J., and Mills, G. B. (1990). Tyrosine phosphorylation is an obligatory event in IL-2 secretion. *Journal of Immunology*, **145**, 2189–98.

Takekura, N., Yasui, W., Kgo, E., Yoshida, K., Kenada, T., Kitadai, Y., *et al*. (1991). Effect of tyrosine kinase inhibitor, erbstatin, a cell growth and growth factor receptor gene expression in human gastric carcinoma cells. *International Journal of Cancer*, **47**, 936–42.

Tapley, P., Kazlauskas, A., Cooper, J. A., and Rohrschneider, L. R. (1990). Macrophage colony-stimulating factor-induced tyrosine phosphorylation of c-*fms* proteins expressed in FDC-P1 and Balb/C 3T3 cells. *Molecular Cell Biology*, **10**, 2528–38.

Taylor, S. S., Buechler, J. A., and Yonemoto, W. (1990). cAMP-dependent protein kinase: framework for a diverse family of regulatory enzymes. *Annual Review of Biochemistry*, **59**, 971–1005.

Toi, M., Mukaida, H., Wada, T., Hirabyashi, N., Toge, T., Hori, T., and Umezawa, K. (1990). Antineoplastic effect of erbstatin on human mammary and esophageal tumors in athymic nude mice. *European Journal of Cancer*, **26**, 722–4.

Trevillyan, J. M., Lu, Y. L., Atluro, D., Phillips, C. A., and Bjorndahl, J. M. (1990). Differential inhibition of T cell receptor signal transduction and early activation events by a selective inhibitor of protein tyrosine kinase. *Journal of Immunology*, **145**, 3223–30.

Tritton, T. R. and Hickman, J. A. (1990). How to kill cancer cells: membranes and cell signalling as targets in cancer chemotherapy. *Cancer Cells*, **2**, 95–105.

Uehara, Y., Murakami, Y., Mizuho, S., and Kawai, S. (1988). Inhibition of transforming activity of tyrosine kinase oncogenes by herbimycin A. *Virology*, **164**, 294–8.

Uehara, Y., Fukazawa, H., Murakami, Y., and Mizuno, S. (1989). Irreversible inhibition of v-src tyrosine kinase activity by herbimycin A and its abrogation by sulfhydryl compounds. *Biochemical and Biophysical Research Communications*, **103**, 803–9.

Ullrich, A. and Schlessinger, J. (1990). Signal transduction by receptors with tyrosine kinase activity. *Cell*, **61**, 203–12.

Umezawa, H., Imoto, M., Sawar, T., Issihiki, K., Matsuda, N., Uchida, T., *et al*. (1986). Studies on a new epidermal growth factor kinase inhibitor, erbstatin, produced by MH435-hF3. *Journal of Antibiotics*, **39**, 170–3.

Umezawa, K., Hori, T., Tajima, H., Imoto, M., Issihiki, K., and Takeuchi, T. (1990). Inhibition of epidermal growth factor-induced DNA synthesis by tyrosine kinase inhibitors. *Federation of European Biochemical Societies Letters*, **260**, 198–200.

Umezawa, K., Tanaka, K., Hori, T., Abe, S., Sekizawa, K., and Imoto, M. (1991). Induction of morphological changes by tyrosine kinase inhibitors in Rous sarcoma virus-transformed rat kidney cells. *Federation of European Biochemical Societies Letters*, **279**, 132–6.

Van der Geer, P. and Hunter, T. (1990). Identification of tyrosine 706 in the kinase insert as the major colony-stimulating factor 1 (CSF-1)-stimulated autophosphorylation site in the CSF-1 receptor in a murine macrophage cell line. *Molecular Cell Biology*, **10**, 2991–3002.

Walker, D. H., Kupuswamy, D., Visvanathan, A., and Pike, L. J. (1987). Substrate specificity and kinetic mechanism of human placental insulin receptor/kinase. *Biochemistry*, **26**, 1428–33.

Watanabe, T., Shiraishi, T., Sasaki, H., and Oishi, M. (1989). Inhibitors for protein tyrosine kinases, ST698 and genistein, induce differentiation of mouse erythroleukemia cells in a synergistic manner. *Experimental Cell Research*, **183**, 335–42.

Watanabe, T., Kondo, K., and Oishi, M. (1991). Induction of *in vitro* differentiation of mouse erythroleukemia cells by genistein, an inhibitor of tyrosine protein kinases. *Cancer Research*, **51**, 764–8.

Weinmaster, G., Zoller, M. J., Smith, M., Hinze, E., and Pawson, T. (1984). Mutagenesis of Fujinami sarcoma virus: evidence that tyrosine phosphorylation of p130$^{gag-fps}$ modulates its biological activity. *Cell*, **37**, 559–68.

Williams, L. T. (1989). Signal transduction by the platelet-derived growth factor receptor. *Science*, **243**, 1564–70.

Witte, O. N., Dasgupta, A., and Baltimore, D. (1980). Abelson murine leukemia virus proteins phosphorylated *in vitro* to form phosphotyrosine. *Nature, London*, **283**, 826–31.

Yaish, P., Gazit, A., Gilon, C., and Levitzki, A. (1988). Blocking of EGF-dependent cell proliferation by EGF receptor kinase inhibitors. *Science*, **242**, 933–5.

Yarden, Y. and Schlessinger, J. (1987a). Self-phosphorylation of epidermal growth factor receptor: evidence for a model of intermolecular allosteric activation. *Biochemistry*, **26**, 1434–42.

Yarden, Y. and Schlessinger, J. (1987b). EGF induces rapid, reversible aggregation of the purified epidermal growth factor receptor. *Biochemistry*, **26**, 1443–51.

Yarden, Y. and Ullrich, A. (1988a). Growth factor receptor tyrosine kinases. *Review of Biochemistry*, **57**, 443–8.

Yarden, Y. and Ullrich, A. (1988b). Molecular analysis of signal transduction by growth factors. *Biochemistry*, **27**, 3113–9.

Yarden, Y., Kuang, W.-J., Yang-Feng, T., Coussens, L., Munemitsu, S., Dull, T. J., *et al.* (1987). Human proto-oncogene c-*kit*: a new cell surface receptor tyrosine kinase for an unidentified ligand. *EMBO Journal*, **6**, 3341–51.

Yuan, C.-Y., Jakes, S., Elliott, S., and Graves, D. J. (1990). A rationale for the design of an inhibitor of tyrosyl kinase. *Journal of Biological Chemistry*, **265**, 16205–9.

Zoller, M. N., Nelson, N. C., and Taylor, S. S. (1981). Affinity labelling of cAMP-dependent kinase with *p*-fluorosulfonylbenzoyl adenosine. *Journal of Biological Chemistry*, **256**, 10837–42.

Zwiller, J., Sassone-Corsi, P., Kakazu, K., and Boynton, A. L. (1991). Inhibition of PDGF-induced c-*jun* and c-*fos* expression by a tyrosine protein kinase inhibitor. *Oncogene*, **6**, 219–21.

5

Inhibitors of non-protein kinases

Douglas D. Buechter and George L. Kenyon

5.1   Introduction

Small molecule (non-protein) kinases are ubiquitous enzymes that catalyse the transfer of a phosphoryl group, usually from a nucleoside triphosphate donor (e.g. ATP), to a non-protein acceptor molecule. A few kinases are able to utilize pyrophosphate as the phosphoryl donor (e.g. pyrophosphate-dependent phosphofructokinase (Reeves *et al.* 1974)). Non-protein kinases are key enzymes in numerous critical cellular processes. These include the generation of 'high-energy phosphate' compounds in glycolysis, cellular storage of such compounds, salvage, and *de novo* synthesis of nucleotides/ nucleosides for nucleic acid synthesis and phospholipid biosynthesis. Inhibitors of non-protein kinases are of importance in mechanistic and enzymological investigations and in the elucidation of their physiological roles. Because these enzymes catalyse critical biochemical reactions, cellular growth and metabolism are often highly dependent upon their activity. As a result, many of these enzymes are attractive targets for anticancer and antiviral agents. Of particular importance is the design of inhibitors that are selective either for certain isozymes of one organism (e.g. fetal versus adult isozymes) or for enzymes from different organisms (e.g. viral versus host enzymes). The design of such inhibitors is facilitated by an understanding of the mechanism and structure of the enzyme at the molecular level. Thus investigations of the three-dimensional structure, kinetics, chemical mechanism, and active site residues of kinases are of considerable importance in modern drug design.

Some of the progress that has been made in recent years in the design of inhibitors of non-protein kinases is discussed in this chapter. Because of the large number of kinases and inhibitors that are of potential importance, an exhaustive survey is not possible and only those that are of the greatest interest are reviewed. Much of the recent literature up to 1985 has been reviewed previously (Kenyon and Reddick 1984; Kenyon and Garcia 1987).

5.2   Deoxythymidine kinase

Deoxythymidine kinase (EC 2.7.1.21) catalyses the phosphorylation of deoxythymidine to deoxythymidine monophosphate (dTMP) utilizing MgATP as the phosphoryl group donor. Deoxythymidine kinase is a key enzyme in the pyrimidine salvage pathway which is one of the two pathways responsible for deoxythymidine triphosphate (dTTP); the other is *de novo* synthesis of dTMP via the methylation of deoxyuridine 5′-monophosphate catalysed by thymidylate synthetase. Cytosolic and mitochondrial de-oxythymidine isozymes are present in humans. Deoxythymidine kinase is of interest from the drug design point of view for several reasons. First, it is important as a target for anticancer agents. There is a direct cor-relation between deoxythymidine kinase activity in rat tumour tissue and tumour growth rate (McDonald *et al.* 1975), and deoxythymidine kinase shows increased activity in neoplastic tissue (Kit 1976; Lai and Weber 1983). In this regard, inhibitors of both the salvage and *de novo* pathways for deoxythymidine synthesis are of potential importance in combination therapy (Hampton *et al.* 1982a, Weber *et al.* 1990). Second, the enzyme has received attention as a target for anti-viral agents, particularly those directed against herpes simplex virus (HSV) types 1 and 2. Upon infection of cells by HSV, a virus-specific deoxythymidine kinase is expressed. Studies have shown that this viral-encoded deoxythymidine kinase activity is important in HSV replication, in neurovirulence, and in the reactivation of latent virus from neural tissue (Field and Darby 1980; Darby *et al.* 1981; Coen *et al.* 1989; Tenser *et al.* 1989). The viral enzymes have different substrate tolerances from those of the mammalian enzymes, particularly with respect to substituents at the 5-position of the pyrimidine ring (Cheng 1977, 1978; Sim *et al.* 1988). These findings have stimulated interest in the design of inhibitors that show selectivity for the viral enzyme (Martin *et al.* 1989). Third, deoxythymidine kinases are responsible for converting a large number of antiviral and anticancer nucleoside analogues to their active phosphorylated derivatives (for examples, see Washtien and Santi 1982; Balzarini *et al.* 1985; Elwell *et al.* 1987). Therefore the design of effective antiviral and anticancer agents must take into consideration whether such compounds are appropriate substrates or inhibitors of both mam-malian and viral deoxythymidine kinases. Finally, inhibitors of mammalian

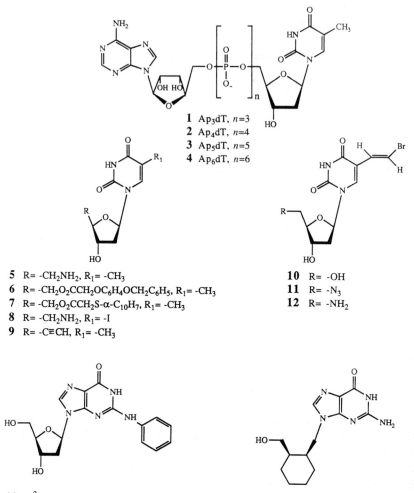

1   Ap₃dT, *n*=3
2   Ap₄dT, *n*=4
3   Ap₅dT, *n*=5
4   Ap₆dT, *n*=6

5   R= -CH₂NH₂, R₁= -CH₃
6   R= -CH₂O₂CCH₂OC₆H₄OCH₂C₆H₅, R₁= -CH₃
7   R= -CH₂O₂CCH₂S-α-C₁₀H₇, R₁= -CH₃
8   R= -CH₂NH₂, R₁= -I
9   R= -C≡CH, R₁= -CH₃

10   R= -OH
11   R= -N₃
12   R= -NH₂

13   N²-Phenyl-2'-deoxyguanosine   14   (±)-9-[[(Z)-2-(Hydroxymethyl)cyclohexyl]methyl]guanine

Fig. 5.1   Inhibitors of deoxythymidine kinase.

deoxythymidine kinases have the potential to decrease the toxicity associated with the phosphorylation of antiviral nucleoside analogues to antimetabolites that may occur in host tissues (Hampton *et al.* 1982a; Fischer
et al. 1983; Martin *et al.* 1989).

Dinucleotide analogues have been tested extensively as inhibitors of deoxythymidine kinase (Fig. 5.1). P^1-(Adenosine-5′)-P^3-(2′-deoxythymidine-
5′)-triphosphate (Ap₃dT (1)) is a potent and selective inhibitor of rat

cytoplasmic deoxythymidine kinase with a K_i versus ATP of 5 μM (Hampton *et al.* 1982b). However, it is considerably less potent as an inhibitor of the mitochondrial enzyme ($K_i = 260$ μM). Ap$_3$dT appears to bind to both nucleotide sites of the enzyme and to behave as a true substrate inhibitor. Ap$_4$dT (2), Ap$_5$dT (3), and Ap$_6$dT (4) have also been synthesized and tested as inhibitors (Bone *et al.* 1986b; Davies *et al.* 1988; Orr *et al.* 1988). These compounds are also inhibitors of mammalian cytosolic deoxythymidine kinase with Ap$_5$dT being the most potent ($K_i = 0.32$ μM versus ATP (Bone *et al.* 1986b)). They exhibit little selective inhibition of the cytosolic compared with the mitochondrial enzyme. Interestingly, these dinucleotide analogues also appear to bind to a second site of the enzyme that stabilizes the enzyme to thermal inactivation (Bone *et al.* 1986b). These compounds are also inhibitors of the enzyme thymidylate kinase (Davies *et al.* 1988; Orr *et al.* 1988).

A series of deoxythymidine analogues substituted either in the pyrimidine or the deoxyribose ring have been synthesized and tested for their ability to inhibit rat cytoplasmic or mitochondrial deoxythymidine kinase selectively (Hampton *et al.* 1982a). 5'-Amino-2',5'-dideoxythymidine (5) is a 400-fold better inhibitor of the cytosolic enzyme than the mitochondrial enzyme. This compound also decreases the ability of 5-trifluoromethyl-2'-deoxyuridine (a clinically useful antiherpes agent that requires phosphorylation for activation) to kill HeLa cells without antagonizing its ability to inhibit replication of HSV-2 in these same cells (Fischer *et al.* 1983). 5'-Amino-2',5'-dideoxythymidine has a K_i value of 2.2 μM for the deoxythymidine kinase purified from HeLa cells but of only 36 μM for the HSV-2 enzyme.

Several deoxythymidine derivatives with bulky substituents at the 5'-position have been reported to be effective inhibitors of the deoxythymidine kinase from cancer tissue (Baker and Neenan 1972; Neenan and Rohde 1973). In particular, 5'-[[4-(benzyloxy)phenoxy]acetoxy]-2',5'-dideoxythymidine (6) and 5'-[α-(naphthylthio)acetoxy]-2',5'-dideoxythymidine (7) showed good activity as inhibitors. Barrie *et al.* (1984) have re-examined these compounds and, by replacing the possibly labile ester linkages with either amide or ether linkages, have demonstrated that they are not particularly potent inhibitors of deoxythymidine kinase. The previous results are likely to be due to hydrolysis of the parent compounds to deoxythymidine which effectively dilutes the radiolabelled deoxythymidine used in the enzyme assay (Barrie *et al.* 1984). In related work, a number of derivatives of 5'-amino-2',5'-dideoxy-5-iodouridine (8) and 5'-amino-2',5'-dideoxythymidine (5) containing additional substituents at the 5'-position were tested as inhibitors of the deoxythymidine kinases from HSV types 1 and 2 (Sim *et al.* 1988). In general, those derivatives that retained the iodine at the 5-position of the pyrimidine ring were more effective inhibitors and also showed greater selectivity for the type 2 compared with the type 1 enzyme. Increasing the lipophilicity of the substituent at the 5'-position also tended to increase the inhibition. Other 5'-substituted nucleoside derivatives also have inhibitory activity. These include 5'-ethynl-2',5'-dideoxythymidine (9) which has K_i values of 0.09 μM and 0.38 μM against HSV-1 and HSV-2 deoxythymidine kinase respectively (Nutter et al. 1987). This same compound has no effect on human cytosolic deoxythymidine kinase at a concentration of 150 μM. Unfortunately, it also has no appreciable antiviral activity, although its ability to inhibit deoxythymidine kinase in vivo can be demonstrated by its antagonism of the antiviral activity of agents that require phosphorylation for activation.

Several analogues of the known antiviral agent (E)-5-(2-bromovinyl)-2'-deoxyuridine (BVDU, 10) (De Clercq et al. 1979), have been investigated as substrates/inhibitors of mammalian, HSV-1, and HSV-2 deoxythymidine kinases (Busson et al. 1981; Zou et al. 1984). The 5'-azido (11) and 5'-amino (12) derivatives of BVDU have considerably greater affinity for the HSV-1 enzyme and thus may be useful as tools to distinguish this enzyme from the HSV-2 enzyme (Zou et al. 1984). Most of the compounds tested did not possess anti-viral activity but did have K_i values for the viral deoxythymidine kinases in the 0.5–10 μM range. A series of derivatives of 5-ethyl-2'-deoxyuridine have also been synthesized and tested as inhibitors of the viral enzymes (Martin et al. 1989). The most potent of these compounds was the $5'-[2,4-Cl_2C_6H_3OCH(CH_3)CO]$ derivative of 5'-amino-5-ethyl-2'-deoxyuridine. This compound had an IC_{50} value (at 0.33 μM deoxythymidine) of 0.03 μM and was ca. 50 000-fold more selective for the viral enzyme compared with the mammalian enzyme. It does not have antiviral activity in the assay used in this study but does antagonize the antiviral activity of acyclovir.

The other class of nucleoside analogues that has been investigated for potential inhibition of the HSV deoxythymidine kinases is the N^2-substituted deoxyguanines. N^2-phenyl-2'-deoxyguanosine (13) has an IC_{50} value of 0.3 μM versus HSV-1 deoxythymidine kinase at a deoxythymidine concentration of 1 μM (Focher et al. 1988). The inhibition is competitive with respect to deoxythymidine, and the inhibitor is not a substrate for the viral enzyme. N^2-phenyl-2'-deoxyguanosine has no effect on the deoxythymidine kinase from HeLa cells at concentrations up to 1 mM, and interferes with the incorporation of [^{3}H]deoxythymidine into cellular DNA only in a deoxythymidine-kinase-deficient HeLa cell line that had been transformed with the HSV deoxythymidine kinase gene. Following this work, a number of N^2-phenylguanines have been investigated as inhibitors of the HSV enzymes (Hildebrand et al. 1990). Because these compounds are derivatives of the nucleic acid bases rather than the nucleosides, they have the potential advantage of not being substrates for either the viral or mammalian enzymes. Derivatives of N^2-phenylguanine with electron-attracting groups in the *meta* position of the phenyl ring tended to be the most potent inhibitors of the viral enzymes, with the *m*-trifluoromethyl derivative exhibiting an IC_{50} value of ca. 0.1 μM against both the HSV-1 and HSV-2 enzymes at a deoxythymidine concentration of 1 μM. Several of the derivatives tested were slightly more potent as inhibitors of the type 2 enzyme, and none significantly inhibited the enzyme from HeLa cells. Both N^2-phenyl-2′-deoxyguanosine and N^2-(*m*-trifluoromethylphenyl)guanine decrease the frequency of virus reactivation from latently infected murine trigeminal ganglia (Leib *et al.* 1990).

Finally, ($\pm$)-9-[[(Z)-2-(hydroxymethyl)cyclohexyl]methyl]guanine (14) was found to be a potent inhibitor of HSV-1 deoxythymidine kinase with an IC_{50} value of 0.07 μM (Ashton *et al.* 1989). This compound is not a substrate for the viral enzyme and does not inhibit the HeLa enzyme at concentrations up to 800 μM. It fails to inhibit HSV-1 replication in MRC-5 cells but delays and decreases the reactivation of virus from explants of mouse trigeminal ganglia. The difficulties associated with the development of clinically useful inhibitors of viral deoxythymidine kinases are highlighted by the finding that oral treatment of HSV-1-infected mice with ($\pm$)-9-[[(Z)-2-(hydroxymethyl)cyclohexyl]methyl]guanine actually led to the development of more severe lesions than those seen in control animals.

5.3   Adenylate kinase

Adenylate kinase (EC 2.7.4.3) catalyses the transfer of a phosphoryl group from ATP to AMP resulting in the generation of two molecules of ADP. Adenylate kinase is found in the cytosol of mammalian muscle (AK1), the mitochondrial intermembrane space (AK2), and the mitochondrial matrix (AK3). The enzymes from different sources range in relative molecular mass from 20 to 25 kDa. Inhibitors of adenylate kinase (Fig. 5.2) have been used to study the role of this enzyme in cellular ATP utilization (Humphrey *et al.* 1986), and it has been proposed that specific inhibition of isozymes that predominate in neoplastic tissue may be a viable approach to chemotherapy (Kappler *et al.* 1982). X-ray structures of the porcine (Schulz *et al.* 1974), yeast (Egner *et al.* 1987), and *Escherichia coli* (Miwa *et al.* 1984) enzymes are known. Extensive NMR studies have also been performed on the enzyme (Fry *et al.* 1985; McDonald *et al.* 1975). Despite these efforts, the locations of the substrate binding sites and the roles played by individual amino acid residues in catalysis remain controversial. The relative merits of the so-called X-ray and NMR models have recently been discussed (Tsai and Yan 1991) and will not be covered in detail here.

Potassium ferrate (K_2FeO_4) is a structural analogue of orthophosphate that irreversibly inactivates porcine adenylate kinase (Crivellone *et al.* 1985). The loss of activity is primarily associated with oxidation of Tyr-95 although Cys-25 is also modified. The bisubstrate analogue Ap_5A protects against inactivation, suggesting that modification has occurred at the active

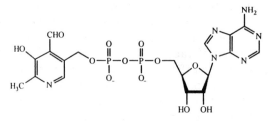

15   Adenosine diphosphopyridoxal

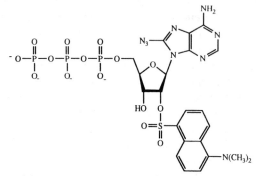

16   8-Azido-2'-*O*-dansyl-ATP

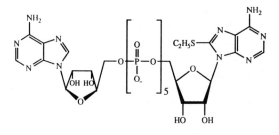

17   8-SEt-Ap₅A

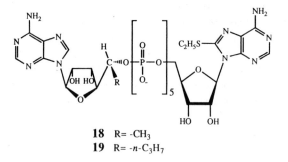

18   R= -CH₃
19   R= -*n*-C₃H₇

Fig. 5.2   Inhibitors of adenylate kinase.

site. Site-directed mutagenesis studies (Tian *et al.* 1988) and the X-ray structure (Dreusicke *et al.* 1988) of the enzyme indicate that both these residues are either in or near the active site. Adenosine diphosphopyridoxal (**15**) covalently modifies Lys-21 of rabbit muscle adenylate kinase after sodium borohydride reduction of the affinity label–enzyme complex (Tagaya *et al.* 1987; Yagami *et al.* 1988). In the X-ray model of the enzyme (Pai *et al.* 1977), this residue is interacting with the γ-phosphate of ATP. However, mutagenesis studies (Tian *et al.* 1990; Tsai and Yan 1991) are inconclusive as to whether Lys-21 plays a role in the chemical steps of catalysis or plays solely a structural role. 8-Azido-2′-*O*-dansyl-ATP (**16**) is a photoreactive analogue of ATP that labels Leu-115, Cys-25, and His-36 of rabbit muscle adenylate kinase (Chuan *et al.* 1989). His-36 is located near the phosphate region of ATP in the X-ray model (Dreusicke *et al.* 1988) and near the adenine ring of ATP in the NMR model (Smith and Mildvan 1982). Interestingly, recent mutagenesis studies suggest that His-36 plays a structural rather than a functional role in catalysis (Tian *et al.* 1988; Tsai and Yan 1991).

Hampton *et al.* (1982c) prepared a series of 6- and 8-substituted ATP analogues and tested their ability to inhibit specifically the muscle and liver isozymes of rat adenylate kinase. The 6-substituted derivatives were more effective inhibitors of the muscle isozyme than the liver isozymes. However, P^1-[8-(ethylthio)adenosine-5′]-P^5-(adenosine-5′)pentaphosphate (8-SEt-Ap$_5$A, **17**) and 8-SEt-ATP were considerably better inhibitors of the rat isozymes II and III compared with the rat muscle isozyme. 8-SEt-Ap$_5$A acted as a bisubstrate inhibitor of these enzymes and exhibited ca. 1000-fold better inhibition compared with 8-SEt-ATP.

In related work, a number of derivatives of AMP, substituted at several positions in both the purine and sugar rings, were prepared and tested for specific inhibition of the rat isozymes (Hai *et al.* 1982b). Several of these compounds, including 2-NHMe-AMP, 2′-*O*-Me-AMP, and 5′(*S*)-Et-AMP, were more effective inhibitors of the muscle isozyme. Placing substituents at the N1, N6, or C8 positions of AMP abolished inhibition. Three additional derivatives of 8-SEt-Ap$_5$A have been synthesized and tested (Kappler *et al.* 1982). P^1-[8-(ethylthio)adenosine-5′]-P^5-[5′(*R*)-*C*-methyl-adenosine-5′] pentaphosphate (**18**), its 5′(*R*)-*C*-*n*-Pr analogue (**19**), and di(8-SEt)-Ap$_5$A were all found to act as bisubstrate inhibitors of adenylate kinase with K_i values less than the K_m values for ATP and AMP. The 5′(*R*)-*C*-*n*-propyl derivative was a more potent inhibitor of the rat muscle enzyme, while the 5′(*R*)-*C*-methyl derivative exhibited greater selectivity for the rat adenylate kinase II isozyme.

5.4 Adenosine kinase

Adenosine kinase (EC 2.7.1.20) catalyses the phosphorylation of adenosine to AMP using ATP as the phosphoryl donor. Specific inhibitors of

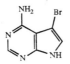

20 4-Amino-5-bromopyrrolo[2,3]pyrimidine

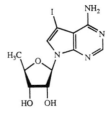

21 5'-Deoxy-5-iodotubercidin

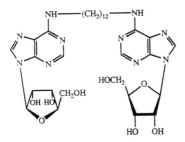

22 1,12-Di(adenosin-N^6-yl)dodecane

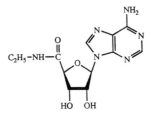

23 5'-N-Ethylcarboxamidoadenosine

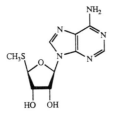

24 5'-Methylthioadenosine

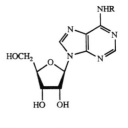

25 R= -C$_6$H$_{11}$
26 R= -CH(CH$_3$)CH$_2$C$_6$H$_5$

Fig. 5.3 Inhibitors of adenosine kinase.

adenosine kinase (Fig. 5.3) are important for their potential usefulness in pharmacological and physiological investigations of the role of adenosine in mammalian systems (Davies *et al.* 1984), and in the study of the inter-action of adenosine with adenosine receptors and the role that these receptors play in biological systems (Lin *et al.* 1988). Although it has been suggested that adenosine kinase alone is not a suitable therapeutic target (Bhaumik and Datta 1988), the enzyme is involved in the initial activation of several biologically active compounds. These include anti-coccidial agents

(Miller *et al.* 1982; Gupta *et al.* 1985), antiviral agents (Nord *et al.* 1988), and anticancer agents (Mehta and Gupta 1986; Lin *et al.* 1988). Thus the design of therapeutically useful agents that must first be phosphorylated to their mono-, di-, or triphosphates, for expression of activity must take into account whether such compounds will serve as substrates and/or inhibitors of adenosine kinase or other related cellular kinases.

4-Amino-5-bromopyrrolo[2,3]pyrimidine (**20**) is a natural product isolated from a marine organism (Kazlauskas *et al.* 1983) that has potent broncho-dilator activity and, at 100 μM, inhibits 80 per cent of the adenosine kinase activity in rat brain (Davies *et al.* 1984). This compound also inhibits adenosine uptake in rat brain. Similarly, 5'-deoxy-5-iodotubercidin (**21**) is also a potent inhibitor of adenosine uptake (displaying inhibition an order of magnitude greater than that seen with 5-iodotubercidin), and at 10 μM inhibits 90 per cent of the activity of partially purified rat brain adenosine kinase. It has been suggested that **21**, because it is not a substrate for adenosine kinase, may be useful as a selective inhibitor of this enzyme (Davies *et al.* 1984).

A series of α, ω-di(adenosine-N^6-yl)alkanes in which two adenosine residues are linked by alkyl bridges of varying length have been investigated as inhibitors of rat liver adenosine kinase (Agathocleous *et al.* 1988, 1990; Prescott *et al.* 1989). Such compounds are analogous to the Ap_nA type of inhibitors that have been used previously as inhibitors of adenylate kinase (Lienhard and Secemski 1973). Of these, 1,12-di(adenosin-N^6-yl)-dodecane (**22**) was the most potent, with a K_i value of 75 nM. These compounds are competitive inhibitors with respect to adenosine and non-competitive with respect to ATP, and thus it is not clear whether they are acting as true bisubstrate inhibitors. In addition, Ap_4A and Ap_5A are inhibitors of adenosine kinase with K_i values of 30 nM and 73 nM respectively (Bone *et al.* 1986a). Inhibition by these two compounds is competitive with respect to ATP but non-competitive with respect to adenosine.

Lin *et al.* (1988) investigated the inhibition of purified human placental adenosine kinase by several adenosine analogues. 5'-N-ethylcarboxamido-5'-deoxyadenosine (**23**) and 5'-methylthio-5'-deoxyadenosine (**24**) are inhibitors with IC_{50} values of 25 μM and 250 μM respectively at a fixed concentration of 0.5 μM adenosine. They are not substrates for the enzyme. N^6-cyclohexyladenosine (**25**) and N^6-L-phenylisopropyladenosine (**26**) are inhibitors with IC_{50} values of 220 μM and 200 μM respectively. Together with 2-chloroadenosine, they are also substrates for the enzyme with K_m values of 1 μM (N^6-cyclohexyladenosine), 330 μM (N^6-L-phenylisopropyl-adenosine), and 205 μM (2-chloroadenosine). These compounds also activate adenosine kinase at adenosine concentrations above 1 μM. It has been proposed (Lin *et al.* 1988) that they interact with the enzyme at both the active site and a regulatory site. In addition, 6-methylmercaptopurine riboside inhibits the enzyme with an IC_{50} value of 10 μM at 0.5 μM adenosine, but does not activate the enzyme at high adenosine concentrations and thus may not bind to the proposed regulatory site.

5.5 Pyruvate kinase

Pyruvate kinase (EC 2.7.1.40) catalyses the transfer of a phosphoryl group from phosphoenolpyruvate (PEP) to ADP, yielding pyruvate and ATP. The enzyme is a tetramer, of relative molecular mass 250 kDa, and requires K^+ and either Mg^{2+} or Mn^{2+} for activity. Pyruvate kinase plays a central role in the metabolism of glucose to pyruvate in glycolysis. As a result, selective inhibitors of pyruvate kinase and other PEP-utilizing enzymes (Fig. 5.4) are of potential value in physiological and pharmacological studies, as well as in mechanistic investigations. The kidney isozyme is found in elevated levels in rat hepatoma tissue (Yanagi et al. 1974) and is the major isozyme in meningiomas and malignant gliomas (van Veelen et al. 1978). It has been suggested that selective inhibition of this isozyme may be an attractive strategy in the design of antineoplastic agents (Hai et al. 1982a).

Rabbit muscle pyruvate kinase is known to be inhibited by several PEP analogues bearing different substituents at the 3-position (Stubbe and Kenyon 1971, 1972). Several additional analogues have recently been investigated, some of which also serve as substrates for the enzyme. They include (Z)-3-chloro-PEP (27) (K_i = 0.039 μM, K_m = 2.2 μM) (Liu et al. 1990), (E)-3-cyano-PEP (28) (K_i = 0.76 μM, K_m = 4 μM) (Wirsching and O'Leary 1985), and phosphoenolthiopyruvate (29) (K_m = 230 μM, K_i = 110 μM) (Sikkema and O'Leary 1988). (Z)-3-fluoromethyl-PEP (30) (Wirsching and O'Leary 1988a) and 1-carboxyallenyl phosphate (31) (Wirsching and O'Leary 1988b) both irreversibly inactivate rabbit muscle pyruvate kinase, presumably in each case as a result of the formation of 2-oxo-3-butenoate (from 3-fluoromethyl-PEP by elimination of fluoride and from 1-carboxylallenyl phosphate by protonation of the allenolate generated after enzyme-catalysed phosphoryl transfer). The amino acid residue that is modified in each case has not been determined; however, the inactivation does not appear to occur at the active site and, in solution, 2-oxo-3-butenoate is relatively specific for sulphydryls (Wirsching and O'Leary 1988b). In an extension of previous studies (Stubbe and Kenyon 1971, 1972), Duffy and Nowak (1984) prepared (Z)- and (E)-3-fluoro-PEP and (Z)-3-bromo-PEP and studied the stereoselectivities of their interactions with rabbit muscle pyruvate kinase and several other PEP-utilizing enzymes. Both the (E)- and (Z)-isomers of 3-fluoro-PEP are substrates for pyruvate kinase, but with less than 1 per cent of the V_{max} of PEP. However, only the (Z)-isomer was a substrate for phosphoenolpyruvate carboxykinase and pyruvate phosphate dikinase. The K_i values of these compounds, along with that of 2-phosphoenolbutyrate

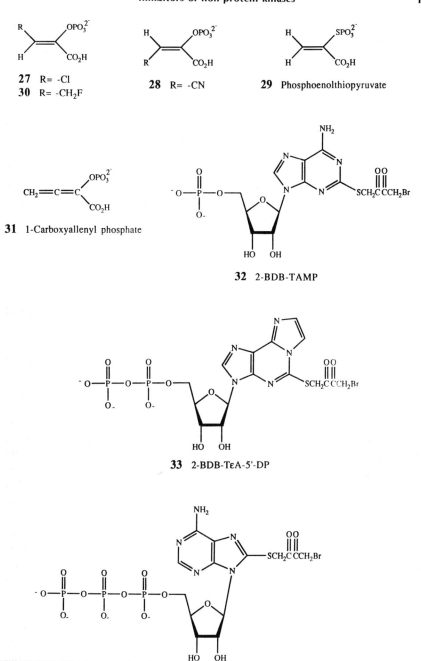

27 R= -Cl
30 R= -CH₂F

28 R= -CN

29 Phosphoenolthiopyruvate

31 1-Carboxyallenyl phosphate

32 2-BDB-TAMP

33 2-BDB-TεA-5'-DP

34 8-BDB-TA-5'-TP

Fig. 5.4 Inhibitors of pyruvate kinase.

(Duffy *et al.* 1982), parallel the van der Waals radii of the substituent at the 3-position.

Colman and colleagues have designed and synthesized several new ATP-based affinity labels as probes of the active sites of pyruvate kinase and other nucleotide-utilizing enzymes. These include 2-[(4-bromo-2,3-dioxobutyl)thio]adenosine 5'-monophosphate (2-BDB-TAMP, **32**) (Kapetanovic *et al.* 1985), 2-[(4-bromo-2,3-dioxobutyl)thio]-1, N^6-ethenoadenosine (2-BDB-TεA-5'-DP, **33**) (DeCamp and Colman 1989), and 8-[(4-bromo-2,3-dioxobutyl)thio]adenosine 5'-triphosphate (8-BDB-TA-5'-TP, **34**) (DeCamp *et al.* 1988; Vollmer and Colman 1990). Presumably, the bromo-dioxobutyl group of these compounds will be reactive towards amino acid residues in the purine binding region of nucleotide binding sites; the bromo-keto group may react with a variety of nucleophilic groups, and the dioxo group may be reactive towards arginine residues (Kapetanovic *et al.* 1985). Each of these affinity labels modifies pyruvate kinase with a stoichiometry of 2 mol of reagent per mol enzyme subunit. 8-BDB-TA-5'-TP modifies Cys-151 of rabbit muscle pyruvate kinase, which is known to be near the active site, and Cys-164, which is not thought to be essential (Stuart *et al.* 1979). 2-BDB-TεA-5'-DP modifies Tyr-147 in the PEP binding site and also Cys-164. The identities of the residues labelled by 2-BDB-TAMP are not known. Tomich and Colman (1985) have also found that cysteine and histidine residues of rabbit muscle pyruvate kinase are modified by 5'-*p*-fluorosulphonylbenzoyl-1, N^6-ethenoadenosine.

Finally, Hai *et al.* (1982a), in an attempt to design selective inhibitors of different pyruvate kinase isozymes, have prepared several derivatives of adenosine 5'-diphosphate with substituents of one to four atoms at several positions of the purine and the sugar rings. All these compounds are inhibitors of rat pyruvate kinases and show varying degrees of selectivity for the muscle, liver, and kidney isozymes. Most were also substrates for the enzyme.

5.6   Hexokinase

Hexokinase (EC 2.7.1.1) catalyses the phosphorylation of the 6-hydroxyl of glucose using the γ-phosphate of MgATP. Hexokinase plays a central role in glucose utilization and as a result has been the subject of numerous mechanistic and structural investigations. There are four major forms of the dimeric mammalian enzyme: types I, II, III, and IV. In rapidly growing rat hepatoma AS-30D cells, hexokinase levels are elevated 100-fold and the major isozyme in these cells has characteristics of the type II enzyme (Nakashima *et al.* 1988). Although this has not yet been extensively investigated with this enzyme, selective targeting of isozymes that are differentially expressed in cancer tissue can form the basis of an approach to chemotherapy (Fig. 5.5).

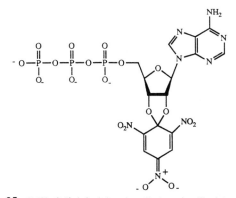

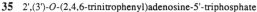

35 2',(3')-O-(2,4,6-trinitrophenyl)adenosine-5'-triphosphate

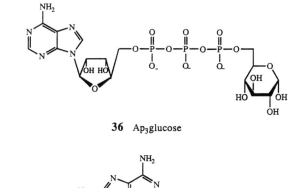

36 Ap₃glucose

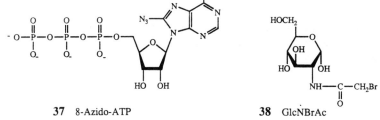

37 8-Azido-ATP   **38** GlcNBrAc

Fig. 5.5 Inhibitors of hexokinase.

The X-ray structure of hexokinase from yeast has been determined (Steitz *et al*. 1977). The yeast enzyme is a homodimer of 50 kDa subunits and is folded into a structure with two lobes that are divided by a central cleft. When glucose binds in this cleft, the smaller of the two lobes rotates and closes down over the bound glucose (Steitz *et al*. 1977; Anderson *et al*. 1978). The nucleotide binding site has been modelled into the yeast enzyme, starting with the structure of the open (no bound sugar) form of the enzyme complexed with 8-bromoadenosine monophosphate (Shoham and Steitz 1980). This site is located on the surface of the large lobe and places the γ-phosphate of ATP ca. 6 Å from the 6-hydroxyl of glucose. Presumably, significant conformational changes must occur upon formation of the closed form of the enzyme to bring these two reacting groups closer together. Putative nucleotide and sugar binding sites have been identified in several mammalian hexokinases based upon homology with the yeast enzyme and with protein kinases (e.g. Andreone *et al.* 1989). The nucleotide binding sites predicted from these homology studies are situated in the smaller lobe of the yeast enzyme and do not correspond to the region predicted from the X-ray studies. Tamura *et al.* (1988) have labelled a lysine residue (Lys-111) of the yeast enzyme with adenosine diphospho-pyridoxal (15). This residue (and regions near it in the sequence) show significant homology among the hexokinases and with the proposed nucleotide binding site of cAMP-dependent protein kinase (Andreone *et al.* 1989). Lys-111 is located in the smaller lobe of the enzyme and again is not close to the nucleotide binding site predicted from the X-ray structure of the open form of the enzyme. Possibly, the conformational changes that occur upon formation of the enzyme–glucose–ATP ternary complex are sufficient to place this residue in proximity to bound ATP (Shoham and Steitz 1980; Tamura *et al.* 1988).

The possibility that the ATP binding site is in the smaller lobe of yeast hexokinase has been further investigated by Arora *et al.* (1990) who synthesized a 50-amino acid fragment of the enzyme that contains a region of the smaller lobe that is homologous among several hexokinases and contains Lys-111. This peptide binds the fluorescent ATP analogue 2′,(3′)-O-(2,4,6-trinitrophenyl)adenosine-5′-triphosphate (35) in a manner similar to the native enzyme. ATP prevents binding of the analogue to both the peptide and the native enzyme but glucose has no effect. Although not conclusive, these results support the proposal that the smaller lobe of hexokinase is involved in nucleotide binding.

The interaction of hexokinase with multisubstrate analogues (Danenberg and Danenberg 1977) has been extended to mammalian brain hexokinase (Hampton *et al.* 1982b; Manning and Wilson 1984). In contrast with the results typically seen with dinucleotide inhibitors (see above), P^1-(adenosine-5′)-P^3-glucose-6-triphosphate (Ap$_3$glucose, 36) and the corresponding Ap$_4$glucose are not potent inhibitors of either yeast or brain hexokinase. The relatively high K_i values of Ap$_3$glucose and Ap$_4$glucose (1.4 mM and 3.5 mM respectively (Hampton *et al.* 1982b)) for the mammalian enzyme may be explained by the observation that they appear to bind as ATP analogues and not as true bisubstrate analogues (Danenberg and Danenberg 1977; Hampton *et al.* 1982b; Manning and Wilson 1984).

The photolabile nucleotide analogue 8-azido-ATP (37) is a substrate for rat brain hexokinase and, upon irradiation of its complex with the enzyme, labels a 40 kDa C-terminal structural domain of the enzyme (Nemat-Gorgani and Wilson 1986). The reactive glucose analogue N-(bromoacetyl)-D-glucosamine (GlcNBrAc, **38**), multiply labels rat brain hexokinase at three cysteines that are located in this C-terminal region (Schirch and Wilson 1987a,b). Two of these peptides are homologous to the active site region of the yeast enzyme, particularly to the proposed glucose binding site. This region in the yeast enzyme does not contain any cysteine residues and thus it is unlikely that cysteines play an essential role in catalysis (Schirch and Wilson 1987a). Labelling of the third peptide is not protected by substrates and it shows no appreciable homology to the yeast enzyme.

5.7   Creatine kinase

Creatine kinase (EC 2.7.3.2) catalyses the reversible transfer of a phosphoryl group from MgATP to creatine, yielding phosphocreatine and MgADP. There are two known cytosolic creatine kinase subunits: brain (B) and muscle (M), each of relative molecular mass ca. 43 kDa. These subunits associate to form the muscle (MM), brain (BB), and heterodimer (MB) isozymes. In addition to the three cytosolic isozymes, there is also an isozyme associated with the inner mitochondrial membrane. The majority of the enzymological and biochemical studies have been performed with enzyme from rabbit muscle. Much of this work, including structure–activity relationships of substrate analogues, has been reviewed previously (Kenyon and Reed 1983).

Creatine kinase is important in maintaining cellular levels of 'high energy phosphate' in the form of phosphocreatine. Specific inhibitors of creatine kinase (Fig. 5.6) are of potential value in investigations of the bioenergetics of ATP utilization in many cellular energy-requiring processes including muscle contraction. A number of creatine and nucleotide analogues have been investigated as substrates or inhibitors of creatine kinase (Kenyon and Reed 1983). Of these, 1-carboxymethyl-2-iminoimidazolidine (cyclocreatine, **39**) (Rowley et al. 1971) is an excellent substrate for the enzyme, with a V_{max} 90 per cent of that of creatine itself (McLaughlin et al. 1972). This compound has been used extensively in physiological and biochemical studies of ATP utilization and the regulation of ATP levels during ischaemia in muscle, brain, and heart tissue (Griffiths and Walker 1976; Annesley and Walker 1980). It has recently been demonstrated that cyclocreatine accumulates in the breast muscle of chickens that have been fed a diet high in cyclocreatine (Turner and Walker 1987). This tissue is able to maintain high ATP levels following ischaemia for substantially longer periods than obtained with control tissue. It has been suggested that this system may be useful in elucidating the biochemical basis of the protective effect of ATP in ischaemic tissue (Turner and Walker 1987). The *in vitro* equilibrium constant for the reaction catalysed by creatine kinase with

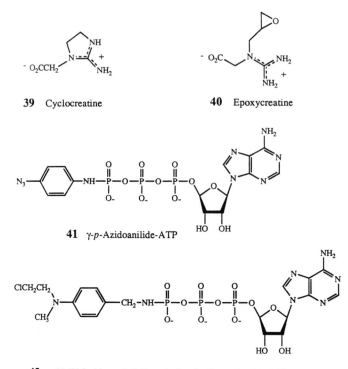

39   Cyclocreatine   **40**   Epoxycreatine

41   γ-*p*-Azidoanilide-ATP

42   γ-[4-(*N*-2-chloroethyl-*N*-methyl)amino]benzylamide-ATP

Fig. 5.6   Inhibitors of creatine kinase.

cyclocreatine as a substrate has been determined by ^{31}P NMR (LoPresti and Cohn 1989). Comparison of this value with that obtained with creatine as a substrate indicates that at equilibrium phosphocyclocreatine is favoured over phosphocreatine by a factor of 26. β-Guanidinopropionic acid is a second analogue of creatine that has proved to be useful in studies of cellular ATP utilization (Shoubridge and Radda 1984; Meyer *et al.* 1986; Moerland and Kushmerick 1987). This compound is a poor substrate for creatine kinase (Fitch *et al.* 1974) but competes effectively with creatine for transport into cells (Fitch *et al.* 1968). It has recently been of use in investigations of the physiological function of creatine kinase using *in vivo* NMR spectroscopy (Shoubridge and Radda 1984; Holtzman *et al.* 1989). *N*-methyl-3-guanidinopropionate and *N*-ethylguanidinoacetate are other analogues of creatine that have also been used in physiological investigations of the creatine kinase–ATP system (Roberts and Walker 1985).

The creatine-based affinity label *N*-(2,3-epoxypropyl)-*N*-amidinoglycine (epoxycreatine, **40**) irreversibly inactivates rabbit muscle creatine kinase

(Marletta and Kenyon 1979). Mass spectrometry, including collision-induced dissociation analysis, of the peptides resulting from tryptic digestion of enzyme affinity labelled with [^{14}C]epoxycreatine was used to identify the site of labelling as Cys-282 (Buechter *et al.* 1991). This residue is known to be near the active site of the enzyme (Cohn *et al.* 1971), although its exact location with respect to bound substrates and the role that it plays in catalysis are controversial. The affinity labelling results suggest that it is either in or near the creatine binding site and within striking distance of the oxirane ring of enzyme-bound epoxycreatine. This same sulphydryl is believed to be labelled upon photolysis of a mixture of the enzyme and γ-p-azidoanilide ATP (**41**) (Vandest *et al.* 1980). Although the results of this work suggest that Cys-282 is near the phosphate groups of ATP, it is reasonable to expect that the arylnitrene group of γ-p-azidoanilide ATP could overlap into the creatine binding site. A similar ATP analogue, γ-[4-(N-2-chloroethyl-N-methyl)amino]benzylamide adenosine triphosphate (**42**), was found to label an aspartic acid residue (Asp-335) of mitochondrial creatine kinase from chicken heart (James *et al.* 1990). The authors suggest that this aspartic acid is either within the creatine binding site or near the metal binding region of the mitochondrial enzyme and may correspond to the carboxylate residue in rabbit muscle creatine kinase that has been implicated from the pH−rate profile as being involved in catalysis (Cook *et al.* 1981). However, there is no evidence that protein ligands are involved in the binding of the metal ion to the rabbit muscle enzyme (Reed and Leyh 1980). Whether this ATP analogue acts as an affinity label of the enzyme from rabbit muscle is not known.

5.8   Miscellaneous enzymes and inhibitors

Young *et al.* (1990) have examined several purine derivatives as inhibitors of human phosphatidylinositol 4-kinase (EC 2.7.1.67) (Fig. 5.7). The reaction catalysed by this enzyme is one of the first steps in the extra-cellular signal-induced generation of diacylglycerol and D-*myo*-inositol 1,4, 5-trisphosphate (IP$_3$) from phosphatidylinositol. These two compounds are important intracellular messengers which mediate a variety of physiological responses (Berridge and Irvine 1984; Nishizuka 1984). The purine derivatives investigated by Young and coworkers were chosen so as to bind to the nucleotide binding site of the kinase and inhibit it competitively with respect to ATP. A purine or related ring system was found to be a minimum requirement for inhibitory activity. In particular, derivatives of adenine substituted at the 9-position were found to be the best inhibitors. 9-Cyclohexyladenine (**43**) was the most potent with a K_i value of 3.7 μM. Whether these compounds would be able to achieve any specificity for phosphatidylinositol kinase was not addressed. In another attempt to develop inhibitors to manipulate the diacylglycerol−IP$_3$ system, Hirata

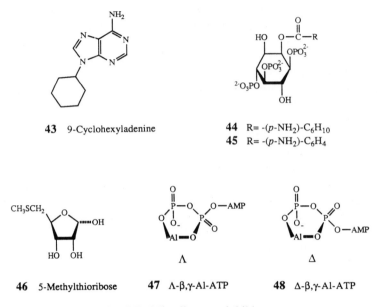

43   9-Cyclohexyladenine

44   R= -(p-NH$_2$)-C$_6$H$_{10}$
45   R= -(p-NH$_2$)-C$_6$H$_4$

46   5-Methylthioribose

47   Λ-β,γ-Al-ATP

48   Δ-β,γ-Al-ATP

Fig. 5.7   Miscellaneous inhibitors.

et al. (1989, 1990) examined several analogues of D,L-inositol 1,4,5-triphosphate for their ability to inhibit D-inositol 1,4,5-triphosphate 3-kinase. The D-isomers of 2-(4-aminocyclohexylcarbonyl)-inositol 1,4,5-triphosphate **(44)** and the corresponding 2-(4-aminobenzoyl) derivative **(45)** were found to be of comparable potency in inhibition of the phosphorylation of D-[^{3}H]IP$_3$ by the enzyme from rat brain. The L-isomers were considerably less potent. Only the D-isomer of the 4-aminocyclohexylcarbonyl analogue was a substrate for the enzyme, and inhibition is presumably the result of this property.

Gianotti *et al.* (1990) have demonstrated that 5-trifluoromethylthioribose **(46)** is a potent inhibitor (K_i = 7.1 μM) of 5-methylthioribose kinase (EC 2.7.1.100) from *Klebsiella pneumoniae*. This enzyme is essential for methionine salvage in lower organisms but is not present in humans. 5-Trifluoromethylthioribose has an IC$_{50}$ value of only 40 nM towards *K. pneumoniae*, but, at concentrations 1000-fold greater than its IC$_{50}$ value, it had no apparent effect on mammalian cells. This inhibitor is also a substrate for the kinase, and it is not clear whether the toxicity towards *K. pneumoniae* is the result of direct inhibition of 5-methylthioribose kinase or of the metabolism of **46** via the methionine salvage pathway to toxic metabolites.

Al-ATP is a potent inhibitor of several kinases and ATP-utilizing enzymes (Furumo and Viola 1989b). Al-ATP has K_i values in the micromolar range for hexokinase and glycerokinase and in the several hundred micromolar range for creatine kinase, acetate kinase, and arginine kinase. However, several kinases, including phosphofructokinase and 3-phosphoglycerate kinase, are not appreciably inhibited by it. Subsequently, Al-ATP was found to be a substrate for creatine kinase with a V_{max} of 0.6 per cent that of MgATP (Furumo and Viola 1989a). However, the complex cannot be utilized as a substrate by either hexokinase or glycerokinase. It was suggested that those enzymes that utilize the Λ screw sense isomer of the metal–nucleotide complex (47) are inhibited by Al-ATP, whereas those that use the Δ-isomer (48) are not (Furumo and Viola 1989b). It is not known whether these results are significant with respect to the association of aluminum with Alzheimer's disease and other conditions. In related work, the Λ- and Δ-isomers of the tetraaquarhodium(III) complex with ADP have been synthesized and also found to inhibit a range of kinases (Shorter et al. 1987). With the exception of arginine and creatine kinase, which bind the Δ-isomer considerably more tightly than the Λ-isomer, there was little difference in the inhibition constants of the two isomers for the kinases examined.

Acknowledgement

Generous financial support from the National Institute of Athritis, Metabolism, and Digestive Diseases, Grant AR17323, is gratefully acknowledged.

References

Agathocleous, D. C., Cosstick, R., Galpin, I. J., McLennan, A. G., Page, P. C. B., and Prescott, M. (1988). Biological activity of (N^6-N^6)-bridged diadenosines. *Biochemical Society Transactions*, 16, 756–7.

Agathocleous, D. C., Page, P. C. B., Cosstick, R., Galpin, I. J., McLennan, A. G., and Prescott, M. (1990). Synthesis of bridged dinucleosides. *Tetrahedron*, 46, 2047–58.

Anderson, C. M., Stenkamp, R. E., and Steitz, T. A. (1978). Sequencing a protein by X-ray crystallography. II. Refinement of yeast hexokinase B co-ordinates and sequence at 2.1 Å resolution. *Journal of Molecular Biology*, 123, 15–33.

Andreone, T. L., Printz, R. L., Pilkis, S. J., Magnuson, M. A., and Granner, D. K. (1989). The amino acid sequence of rat liver glucokinase deduced from cloned cDNA. *Journal of Biological Chemistry*, 264, 363–9.

Annesley, T. M. and Walker, J. B. (1980). Energy metabolism of skeletal muscle containing cyclocreatine phosphate. *Journal of Biological Chemistry*, 255, 3924–30.

Arora, K. K., Shenbagamurthi, P., Fanciulli, M., and Pedersen, P. L. (1990). Glucose phosphorylation. Interaction of a 50-amino acid peptide of yeast hexokinase with trinitrophenyl ATP. *Journal of Biological Chemistry*, 265, 5324–8.

Ashton, W. T., Meurer, L. C., Tolman, R. L., Karkas, J. D., Liou, R., Perry, H. C., et al. (1989). A potent, selective, non-substrate inhibitor of HSV-1 thymidine kinase: (±)-9-[[(Z)-2-(hydroxymethyl)cyclohexyl]methyl]guanine and related compounds. *Nucleosides and Nucleotides*, 8, 1157–8.

Baker, B. R. and Neenan, J. P. (1972). Irreversible enzyme inhibitors. 195. Inhibitors of thymidine kinase from Walker 256 carcinoma derived from thymidine 5'-acetate. *Journal of Medicinal Chemistry*, **15**, 940–4.

Balzarini, J., De Clercq, E., Verbruggen, A., Ayusawa, D., and Seno, T. (1985). Highly selective cytostatic activity of (*E*)-5-(2-bromovinyl)-2'-deoxyuridine derivatives for murine mammary carcinoma (FM3A) cells transformed with the herpes simplex virus type 1 thymidine kinase gene. *Molecular Pharmacology*, **28**, 581–7.

Barrie, S. E., Davies, L. C., Stock, J. A., and Harrap, K. R. (1984). A reappraisal of the effect upon thymidine kinase of thymidine derivatives carrying large groups at the 5'-position. *Journal of Medicinal Chemistry*, **27**, 1044–7.

Berridge, M. J. and Irvine, R. F. (1984). Inositol trisphosphate, a novel second messenger in cellular signal transduction. *Nature, London*, **312**, 315–21.

Bhaumik, D. and Datta, A. K. (1988). Reaction kinetics and inhibition of adenosine kinase from *Leishmania donovani*. *Molecular and Biochemical Pharmacology*, **28**, 181–8.

Bone, R., Cheng, Y.-C., and Wolfenden, R. (1986a). Inhibition of adenosine and thymidylate kinases by bisubstrate analogs. *Journal of Biological Chemistry*, **261**, 16410–13.

Bone, R., Cheng, Y.-C., and Wolfenden, R. (1986b). Inhibition of thymidine kinase by P^1-(adenosine-5')-P^5-(thymidine-5')-pentaphosphate. *Journal of Biological Chemistry*, **261**, 5731–5.

Buechter, D. D., Medzihradszky, K. F., Burlingame, A. L., and Kenyon, G. L. (1991). Identification by mass spectrometry of the site of modification of creatine kinase by the affinity label epoxycreatine. In *Techniques in protein chemistry II* (ed. J. J. Villafranca), pp. 537–42. Academic Press, San Diego, CA.

Busson, R., Colla, L., Vanderhaeghe, H., and De Clercq, E. (1981). Synthesis and antiviral activity of some sugar-modified derivatives of (*E*)-5-(2-bromovinyl)-2'-deoxyuridine. *Nucleic Acids Research, Symposium Series*, **9a**, 49–52.

Cheng, Y.-C. (1977). A rational approach to the development of antiviral chemotherapy: Alternative substrates of herpes simplex virus type 1 (HSV-1) and type 2 (HSV-2) thymidine kinase (TK). *Annals of the New York Academy of Sciences*, **284**, 594–8.

Cheng, Y.-C. (1978). Strategy for the development of selective antiherpes virus agents based on the unique properties of viral induced enzymes–thymidine kinase, DNase and DNA polymerase. In *Antimetabolites in biochemistry, biology and medicine* (ed. J. Skoda and P. Langen), pp. 263–74. Pergamon Press, Oxford.

Chuan, H., Lin, J., and Wang, J. H. (1989). 8-Azido-2'-*O*-dansyl-ATP. A fluorescent photoaffinity reagent for ATP-binding proteins and its application to adenylate kinase. *Journal of Biological Chemistry*, **264**, 7981–8.

Coen, D. M., Kosz-Vnenchak, M., Jacobson, J. G., Leib, D. A., Bogard, C. L., Schaffer, P. A., *et al.* (1989). Thymidine kinase–negative herpes simplex virus mutants establish latency in trigeminal ganglia but do not reactivate. *Proceedings of the National Academy of Sciences of the United States of America*, **86**, 4736–40.

Cohn, M., Diefenbach, H., and Taylor, J. S. (1971). Magnetic resonance studies of the interaction of spin-labeled creatine kinase with paramagnetic manganese-substrate complexes. *Journal of Biological Chemistry*, **246**, 6037–42.

Cook, P. F., Kenyon, G. L., and Cleland, W. W. (1981). Use of pH studies to elucidate the catalytic mechanism of rabbit muscle creatine kinase. *Biochemistry*, **20**, 1204–10.

Crivellone, M. D., Hermodson, M., and Axelrod, B. (1985). Inactivation of muscle adenylate kinase by site-specific destruction of tyrosine 95 using potassium ferrate. *Journal of Biological Chemistry*, **260**, 2657–61.

Danenberg, P. V. and Danenberg, K. D. (1977). Inhibition of hexokinase by multisubstrate analogs *Biochimica et Biophysica Acta*, **480**, 351–6.

Darby, G., Field, H. J., and Salisbury, S. A. (1981). Altered substrate specificity of herpes simplex virus thymidine kinase confers acyclovir-resistance. *Nature, London*, **289**, 81–3.

Davies, L. C., Stock, J. A., Barrie, S. E., Orr, R. M., and Harrap, K. R. (1988). Dinucleotide analogues as inhibitors of thymidine kinase, thymidylate kinase, and ribonucleotide reductase. *Journal of Medicinal Chemistry*, **31**, 1305–8.

Davies, L. P., Jamieson, D. D., Baird-Lambert, J. A., and Kazlauskas, R. (1984). Halogenated pyrrolopyrimidine analogues of adenosine from marine organism: pharmacological activities and potent inhibition of adenosine kinase. *Biochemical Pharmacology*, **33**, 347–55.

DeCamp, D. and Colman, R. F. (1989). 2-[(4-Bromo-2,3-dioxobutyl)thio]-1, N[6]-ethenoadenosine 5′-diphosphate. A new fluorescent affinity label of a tyrosyl residue in the active site of rabbit muscle pyruvate kinase. *Journal of Biological Chemistry*, **264**, 8430–41.

DeCamp, D. L., Lim, S., and Colman, R. (1988). Reaction of pyruvate kinase with the new nucleotide affinity labels 8-[(4-bromo-2,3-dioxobutyl)thio]adenosine 5′-diphosphate and 5′-triphosphate. *Biochemistry*, **27**, 7651–8.

De Clercq, E., Descamps, J., De Somer, P., Barr, P. J., Jones, A. S., and Walker, R. T. (1979). (E)-5-(2-bromovinyl)-2′-deoxyuridine: a potent and selective anti-herpes agent. *Proceedings of the National Academy of Sciences of the United States of America*, **76**, 2947–51.

Dreusicke, D., Karplus, P. A., and Schulz, G. E. (1988). Refined structure of porcine cytosolic adenylate kinase at 2.1 Å resolution. *Journal of Molecular Biology*, **199**, 359–71.

Duffy, T. H. and Nowak, T. (1984). Stereoselectivity of interaction of phosphoenolpyruvate analogues with various phosphoenolpyruvate-utilizing enzymes. *Biochemistry*, **23**, 661–70.

Duffy, T. H., Saz, H. J., and Nowak, T. (1982). Stereospecificity of (E)- and (Z)-phosphoenol-α-ketobutyrate with chicken liver phosphoenol carboxykinase and related phosphoenolpyruvate-utilizing enzymes. *Biochemistry*, **21**, 132–9.

Egner, U., Tomasselli, A. G., and Schulz, G. E. (1987). Structure of the complex of yeast adenylate kinase with the inhibitor P[1],P[5]-di(adenosine-5′)pentaphosphate at 2.6 Å resolution. *Journal of Molecular Biology*, **195**, 649–58.

Elwell, L. P., Ferone, R., Freeman, G. A., Fyfe, J. A., Hill, J. A., Ray, P. H., et al. (1987). Antibacterial activity and mechanism of action of 3′-azido-3′-deoxythymidine (BW A509U). *Antimicrobial Agents and Chemotherapy*, **31**, 274–80.

Field, H. J. and Darby, G. (1980). Pathogenicity in mice of strains of herpes simplex virus which are resistant to acyclovir *in vitro* and *in vivo*. *Antimicrobial Agents and Chemotherapy*, **17**, 209–16.

Fischer, P. H., Murphy, D. G., and Kawahara, R. (1983). Preferential inhibition of 5′-trifluoromethyl-2′-deoxyuridine phosphorylation by 5′-amino-5′-de-oxythymidine in uninfected versus herpes simplex virus-infected cells. *Molecular Pharmacology*, **24**, 90–6.

Fitch, C. D., Shields, R. P., Payne, W. F., and Dacus, J. M. (1968). Creatine metabolism in skeletal muscle. III. Specificity of the creatine entry process. *Journal of Biological Chemistry*, **243**, 2024–7.

Fitch, C. D., Jellinek, M., and Mueller, E. J. (1974). Experimental depletion of creatine and phosphocreatine from skeletal muscle. *Journal of Biological Chemistry*, **249**, 1060–3.

Focher, F., Hildebrand, C., Freese, S., Ciarrocchi, G., Noonan, T., Sangalli, S., et al. (1988). N^2-phenyldeoxyguanosine: a novel selective inhibitor of herpes simplex thymidine kinase. *Journal of Medicinal Chemistry*, **31**, 1496–1500.

Fry, D. C., Kuby, S. A., and Mildvan, A. S. (1985). NMR studies of the MgATP binding site of adenylate kinase and of a 45-residue peptide fragment of the enzyme. *Biochemistry*, **24**, 4680–94.

Furumo, N. C. and Viola, R. E. (1989a). Aluminum-adenine nucleotides as alternate substrates for creatine kinase. *Archives of Biochemistry and Biophysics*, **275**, 33–9.

Furumo, N. C. and Viola, R. E. (1989b). Inhibition of phosphoryl-transferring enzymes by aluminum-ATP. *Inorganic Chemistry*, **28**, 820–823.

Gianotti, A. J., Tower, P. A., Sheley, J. H., Conte, P. A., Spiro, C., Ferro, A. J., et al. (1990). Selective killing of *Klebsiella pneumoniae* by 5-trifluoro-methylthioribose. *Journal of Biological Chemistry*, **265**, 831–7.

Griffiths, G. R. and Walker, J. B. (1976). Accumulation of analog of phospho-creatine in muscle of chicks fed 1-carboxymethyl-2-iminoimidazolidine (cyclo-creatine). *Journal of Biological Chemistry*, **251**, 2049–54.

Gupta, R. S., Singh, B., and Stetsko, D. K. (1985). Inhibition of metabolic co-operation by phorbol esters in a cell culture system based on adenosine kinase deficient mutants of V79 cells. *Carcinogenesis*, **6**, 1359–66.

Hai, T. T., Abo, M., and Hampton, A. (1982a). Species- or isozyme-specific enzyme inhibitors. 9. Selective effects in inhibitions of rat pyruvate kinase isozymes by adenosine 5′-diphosphate derivatives. *Journal of Medicinal Chemistry*, **25**, 1184–8.

Hai, T. T., Picker, D., Abo, M., and Hampton, A. (1982b). Species- or isozyme-specific enzyme inhibitors. 7. Selective effects in inhibitions of rat adenylate kinase isozymes by adenosine 5′-phosphate derivatives. *Journal of Medicinal Chemistry*, **25**, 806–12.

Hampton, A., Chawla, R. R., and Kappler, F. (1982a). Species- or isozyme-specific enzyme inhibitors. 5. Differential effects of thymidine substituents on affinity for rat thymidine kinase isozymes. *Journal of Medicinal Chemistry*, **25**, 644–649.

Hampton, A., Hai, T. T., Kappler, F., and Chawla, R. R. (1982b). Species- or isozyme-specific enzyme inhibitors. 6. Synthesis and evaluation of two-substrate condensation products as inhibitors of hexokinases and thymidine kinases. *Journal of Medicinal Chemistry*, **25**, 801–5.

Hampton, A., Kappler, F., and Picker, D. (1982c). Species- or isozyme-specific enzyme inhibitors. 4. Design of a two-site inhibitor of adenylate kinase with isozyme selectivity. *Journal of Medicinal Chemistry*, **25**, 638–44.

Hildebrand, C., Sandoli, D., Focher, F., Gambino, J., Ciarrocchi, G., and Spadari, S. (1990). Structure–activity relationships of N^2-substituted guanines as inhibitors of HSV1 and HSV2 thymidine kinase. *Journal of Medicinal Chemistry*, **33**, 203–6.

Hirata, M., Watanabe, Y., Ishimatsu, T., Ikebe, T., Kimura, Y., Yamaguchi, K., Ozaki, S., and Koga, T. (1989). Synthetic inositol triphosphate analogs and their effects on phosphatase, kinase, and the release of Ca^{2+}. *Journal of Biological Chemistry*, **264**, 20303–8.

Hirata, M., Yanaga, F., Koga, T., Ogasawara, T., Watanabe, Y., and Ozaki, S. (1990). Stereospecific recognition of inositol 1,4,5-trisphosphate analogs by the phosphatase, kinase, and binding proteins. *Journal of Biological Chemistry*, **265**, 8404–7.

Holtzman, D., McFarland, E., Moerland, T., Koutcher, J., Kushmerick, M. J., and Neuringer, L. J. (1989). Brain creatine phosphate and creatine kinase in mice fed an analogue of creatine. *Brain Research*, **483**, 68–77.

Humphrey, S. M., Holliss, D. G., and Cartner, L. A. (1986). The influence of inhibitors of the ATP degradative pathway on recovery of function and high energy phosphate after transient ischemia in the rat heart. *Journal of Molecular and Cellular Cardiology*, **18**, (Suppl. 4), 55–9.

James, P., Wyss, M., Lutsenko, S., Wallimann, T., and Carafoli, E. (1990). ATP binding site of mitochondrial creatine kinase. Affinity labelling of Asp-335 with CIRATP. *Federation of European Biochemical Societies Letters*, **273**, 139–43.

Kapetanovic, E., Bailey, J. M., and Colman, R. F. (1985). 2-[(4-Bromo-2, 3-dioxobutyl)thio]adenosine 5′-monophosphate, a new nucleotide analogue that acts as an affinity label of pyruvate kinase. *Biochemistry*, **24**, 7586–93.

Kappler, F., Hai, T. T., Abo, M., and Hampton, A. (1982). Species- or isozyme-specific enzyme inhibitors. 8. Synthesis of disubstituted two-substrate condensation products as inhibitors of rat adenylate kinases. *Journal of Medicinal Chemistry*, **25**, 1179–84.

Kazlauskas, R., Murphy, P. T., Wells, R. J., Baird-Lambert, J. A., and Jamieson, D. D. (1983). Halogenated pyrrolo[2,3-*d*]pyrimidine nucleosides from marine organisms. *Australian Journal of Chemistry*, **36**, 165–70.

Kenyon, G. L. and Garcia, G. A. (1987). Design of kinase inhibitors. *Medicinal Research Reviews*, **7**, 389–416.

Kenyon, G. L. and Reddick, R. E. (1984). Design of kinase inhibitors. Conformational and mechanistic considerations. In *Conformationally directed drug design* (ed. J. A. Vida and M. Gordon), pp. 189–209. American Chemical Society Symposium Series, American Chemical Society, Washington, DC.

Kenyon, G. L. and Reed, G. H. (1983). Creatine kinase: structure–activity relationships. *Advances in Enzymology and Related Areas in Molecular Biology*, **54**, 367–426.

Kit, S. (1976). Thymidine kinase, DNA synthesis and cancer. *Molecular and Cellular Biochemistry*, **11**, 161–82.

Lai, M.-H. T. and Weber, G. (1983). Increased concentration of thymidine kinase in rat hepatomas. *Biochemical and Biophysical Research Communications*, **111**, 280–7.

Leib, D. A., Ruffner, K. L., Hildebrand, C., Schaffer, P. A., Wright, G. E., and Coen, D. M. (1990). Specific inhibitors of herpes simplex virus thymidine kinase diminish reactivation of latent virus from explanted murine ganglia. *Antimicrobial Agents and Chemotherapy*, **34**, 1285–6.

Lienhard, G. E., and Secemski, I. I. (1973). P^1,P^5-Di(adenosine-5'pentaphosphate, a potent multisubstrate inhibitor of adenylate kinase. *Journal of Biological Chemistry*, **248**, 1121–3.

Lin, B. B., Hurley, M. C., and Fox, I. H. (1988). Regulation of adenosine kinase by adenosine analogs. *Molecular Pharmacology*, **34**, 501–5.

Liu, J., Peliska, J. A., and O'Leary, M. H. (1990). Synthesis and study of (Z)-3-chlorophosphoenolpyruvate. *Archives of Biochemistry and Biophysics*, **277**, 143–8.

LoPresti, P. and Cohn, M. (1989). Direct determination of creatine kinase equilibrium constants with creatine or cyclocreatine as substrate. *Biochimica et Biophysica Acta*, **998**, 317–20.

McDonald, G. G., Cohn, M., and Noda, L. (1975). Proton magnetic resonance spectra of porcine muscle adenylate kinase and substrate complexes. *Journal of Biological Chemistry*, **250**, 6947–54.

McLaughlin, A. C., Cohn, M., and Kenyon, G. L. (1972). Specificity of creatine kinase for guanidino substrates. *Journal of Biological Chemistry*, **247**, 4382–8.

Manning, T. A. and Wilson, J. E. (1984). Inhibition of brain hexokinase by a multisubstrate analog results from binding to a discrete regulatory site. *Biochemical and Biophysical Research Communications*, **118**, 90–6.

Marletta, M. A. and Kenyon, G. L. (1979). Affinity labeling of creatine kinase by *N*-(2,3-epoxypropyl)-*N*-amidinoglycine. *Journal of Biological Chemistry*, **254**, 1879–86.

Martin, J. A., Duncan, I. B., Hall, M. J., Wong-Kai-In, P., Lambert, R. W., and Thomas, G. J. (1989). New potent and selective inhibitors of herpes simplex virus thymidine kinase. *Nucleosides and Nucleotides*, **8**, 753–64.

Mehta, K. D. and Gupta, R. S. (1986). Novel mutants of CHO cells resistant to adenosine analogs and containing biochemically altered form of adenosine kinase in cell extracts. *Somatic Cell and Molecular Genetics*, **12**, 21–31.

Meyer, R. A., Brown, T. R., Krilowicz, B. L., and Kushmerick, M. J. (1986). Phosphagen and intracellular pH changes during contraction of creatine-depleted rat muscle. *American Journal of Physiology*, **250**, C264–74.

Miller, R. L., Adamczyk, D. L., Rideout, J. L., and Krenitsky, T. A. (1982). Purification, characterization, substrate and inhibitor specificity of adenosine kinase from several *Eimeria* species. *Molecular and Biochemical Parasitology*, **6**, 209–23.

Miwa, I., Hara, H., Matsunaga, H., and Okuda, J. (1984). Inhibition of glucokinase in hepatocytes by alloxan. *Biochemistry International*, **9**, 595–602.

Moerland, T. S. and Kushmerick, M. J. (1987). Metabolic adaptation in the skeletal muscle of mice intoxicated with a poorly-metabolized analogue of creatine. *Biophysical Journal*, **51**, 478a.

Nakashima, R. A., Paggi, M. G., Scott, L. J., and Pedersen, P. L. (1988). Purification and characterization of a bindable form of mitochondrial bound hexokinase from the highly glycolytic AS-30D rat hepatoma cell line. *Cancer Research*, **48**, 913–19.

Neenan, J. P. and Rohde, W. (1973). Inhibition of thymidine kinase from Walker 256 carcinoma by thymidine analogs. *Journal of Medicinal Chemistry*, **16**, 580–1.

Nemat-Gorgani, M. and Wilson, J. E. (1986). Rat brain hexokinase: location of the substrate nucleotide binding site in a structural domain at the C-terminus of the enzyme. *Archives of Biochemistry and Biophysics*, **251**, 97–103.

Nishizuka, Y. (1984). The role of protein kinase C in cell surface signal transduction and tumor promotion. *Nature, London*, **308**, 693–8.

Nord, L. D., Willis, R. C., Smee, D. F., Riley, T. A., Revankar, G. R., and Robins, R. K. (1988). Inhibition of orotidylate decarboxylase by 4(5H)-oxo-1-beta-D-ribofuranosylpyrazolo[3,4-d]pyrimidine-3-thiocarboxamide (APR-TC) in B lymphoblasts. Activation by adenosine kinase. *Biochemical Pharmacology*, **37**, 4697–705.

Nutter, L. M., Grill, S. P., Dutschman, G. E., Sharma, R. A., Bobek, M., and Cheng, Y.-C. (1987). Demonstration of viral thymidine kinase inhibitor and its effect on deoxynucleotide metabolism in cells infected with herpes simplex virus. *Antimicrobial Agents and Chemotherapy*, **31**, 368–74.

Orr, R. M., Davies, L. C., Stock, J. A., Taylor, G. A., Powles, R. L., and Harrap, K. R. (1988). Inhibition of human leukaemic thymidylate kinase and L1210 ribonucleotide reductase by dinucleotides of adenosine and thymidine and their phosphonate analogues. *Biochemical Pharmacology*, **37**, 673–7.

Pai, E. F., Sachsenheimer, W., Schirmer, R. H., and Schulz, G. E. (1977). Substrate positions and induced-fit in crystalline adenylate kinase. *Journal of Molecular Biology*, **114**, 37–45.

Prescott, M., McLennan, A. G., Agathocleous, D. C., Page, P. C. B., Cosstick, R., and Galpin, I. J. (1989). The inhibition of adenosine kinase by a, ω-di(adenosin-N^8-yl)alkanes. *Nucleosides and Nucleotides*, **8**, 297–303.

Reed, G. H. and Leyh, T. S. (1980). Identification of the six ligands to manganese(II) in transition-state-analogue complexes of creatine kinase: oxygen-17 superhyperfine coupling from selectively labeled ligands. *Biochemistry*, **19**, 5472–80.

Reeves, R. E., South, D. J., Blytt, H. J., and Warren, L. G. (1974). Pyrophosphate: D-fructose 6-phosphate 1-phosphotransferase. *Journal of Biological Chemistry*, **249**, 7737–41.

Roberts, J. J. and Walker, J. B. (1985). Higher homolog and N-ethyl analog of creatine as synthetic phosphagen precursors in brain, heart, and muscle, repressors of liver amidinotransferase, and substrates for creatine catabolic enzymes. *Journal of Biological Chemistry*, **260**, 13502–8.

Rowley, G. L., Greenleaf, A. L., and Kenyon, G. L. (1971). On the specificity of creatine kinase. New glycocyamines and glycocyamine analogs related to creatine. *Journal of the American Chemical Society*, **93**, 5542–51.

Schirch, D. M. and Wilson, J. E. (1987a). Rat brain hexokinase: amino acid sequence at the substrate hexose binding site is homologous to that of yeast hexokinase. *Archives of Biochemistry and Biophysics*, **257**, 1–12.

Schirch, D. M. and Wilson, J. E. (1987b). Rat brain hexokinase: location of the substrate hexose binding site in a structural domain at the C-terminus of the enzyme. *Archives of Biochemistry and Biophysics*, **254**, 385–96.

Schulz, G. E., Elzinga, M., Marx, F., and Schirmer, R. H. (1974). Three-dimensional structure of adenyl kinase. *Nature, London*, **250**, 120–3.

Shoham, M., and Steitz, T. A. (1980). Crystallographic studies and model building of ATP at the active site of hexokinase. *Journal of Molecular Biology*, **140**, 1–14.

Shorter, A. L., Haromy, T. P., Scalzo-Brush, T., Knight, W. B., Dunaway-Mariano, D., and Sundaralingam, M. (1987). Structural and biochemical properties of bidentate tetraaquarhodium(III) complexes of inorganic pyrophophate and adenosine 5′-diphosphate. *Biochemistry*, **26**, 2060–6.

Shoubridge, E. A. and Radda, G. K. (1984). A ^{31}P-nuclear magnetic resonance study of skeletal muscle metabolism in rats depleted of creatine with the analogue β-guanidinopropionic acid. *Biochimica et Biophysica Acta*, **805**, 79–88.

Sikkema, K. D. and O'Leary, M. H. (1988). Synthesis and study of phosphoenol-thiopyruvate. *Biochemistry*, **27**, 1342.

Sim, I. S., Picton, C., Cosstick, R., Jones, A. S., Walker, R. T., and Chamiec, A. J. (1988). Inhibition of the herpes simplex virus thymidine kinase by 5′-substituted thymidine analogues. Comparison of the types 1 and 2 enzymes. *Nucleosides and Nucleotides*, **7**, 129–35.

Smith, G. M. and Mildvan, A. S. (1982). Nuclear magnetic resonance studies of the nucleotide binding sites of porcine adenylate kinase. *Biochemistry*, **21**, 6119–23.

Steitz, T. A., Anderson, W. F., Fletterick, R. J., and Anderson, C. M. (1977). High resolution crystal structures of yeast hexokinase complexes with substrates, activators, and inhibitors. *Journal of Biological Chemistry*, **252**, 4494–500.

Stuart, D. I., Levine, M., Muirhead, H., and Stammers, D. K. (1979). Crystal structure of cat muscle pyruvate kinase at a resolution of 2.6 Å. *Journal of Molecular Biology*, **134**, 109–42.

Stubbe, J. and Kenyon, G. L. (1971). Analogs of phosphoenolpyruvate. On the specificity of pyruvate kinase from rabbit muscle. *Biochemistry*, **10**, 2669–77.

Stubbe, J. and Kenyon, G. (1972). Analogs of phosphoenolpyruvate. Substrate specificities of enolase and pyruvate kinase from rabbit muscle. *Biochemistry*, **11**, 338–345.

Tagaya, M., Yagami, T., and Fukui, T. (1987). Affinity labeling of adenylate kinase with adenosine diphosphopyridoxal. Presence of Lys^{21} in the ATP-binding site. *Journal of Biological Chemistry*, **262**, 8257–61.

Tamura, J. K., LaDine, J. R., and Cross, R. L. (1988). The adenine nucleotide binding site on yeast hexokinase PII. Affinity labeling of Lys-111 by pyridoxal 5′-diphospho-5′-adenosine. *Journal of Biological Chemistry*, **263**, 7907–12.

Tenser, R. B., Hay, K. A., and Edris, W. A. (1989). Latency-associated transcript but not reactivatable virus is present in sensory ganglion neurons after inoculation of thymidine kinase-negative mutants of herpes simplex virus type 1. *Journal of Virology*, **63**, 2861–5.

Tian, G., Sanders, C. R. I., Kishi, F., Nakazawa, A., and Tsai, M.-D. (1988). Mechanism of adenylate kinase. Histidine-36 is not directly involved in catalysis, but protects cysteine-25 and stabilizes the tertiary structure. *Biochemistry*, **27**, 5544–52.

Tian, G., Yan, H., Jiang, R.-T., Kishi, F., Nakazawa, A., and Tsai, M.-D. (1990). Mechanism of adenylate kinase. Are the essential lysines essential? *Biochemistry*, **29**, 4296–04.

Tomich, J. M. and Colman, R. F. (1985). Reaction of 5′-*p*-fluorosulfonyl-benzoyl-1, N^6-ethenoadenosine with histidine and cysteine residues in the active site of rabbit muscle pyruvate kinase. *Biochimica et Biophysica Acta*, **827**, 344–57.

Tsai, M.-D. and Yan, H. (1991). Mechanism of adenylate kinase: site-directed mutagenesis versus X-ray and NMR. *Biochemistry*, **30**, 6806–18.

Turner, D. M. and Walker, J. B. (1987). Enhanced ability of skeletal muscle containing cyclocreatine phosphate to sustain ATP levels during ischemia following β-adrenergic stimulation. *Journal of Biological Chemistry*, **262**, 6605–9.

Vandest, P., Labbe, J.-P., and Kassab, R. (1980). Photoaffinity labeling of arginine kinase and creatine kinase with a γ-p-substituted arylazido analogue of ATP. *European Journal of Biochemistry*, **104**, 433–42.

van Veelen, W. M. C., Verbiest, H., Vlug, A. M. C., Gert, R., and Staal, G. E. J. (1978). Isozymes of pyruvate kinase from human brain, meningiomas, and malignant gliomas. *Cancer Research*, **38**, 4681–7.

Vollmer, S. H. and Colman, R. F. (1990). Cysteinyl peptides of rabbit muscle pyruvate kinase labeled by the affinity label 8-[(4-bromo-2,3-dioxobutyl)thio]-adenosine 5'-triphosphate. *Biochemistry*, **29**, 2495–501.

Washtien, W. L. and Santi, D. V. (1982). Mechanism of action of 5-nitro-2'-deoxyuridine. *Journal of Medicinal Chemistry*, **25**, 1252–5.

Weber, G., Ichikawa, S., Nagai, M., and Natsumeda, Y. (1990). Azidothymidine inhibition of thymidine kinase and synergistic cytotoxicity with methotrexate and 5-fluorouracil in rat hepatoma and human colon cancer cells. *Cancer Communications*, **2**, 129–33.

Wirsching, P. and O'Leary, M. H. (1985). (*E*)-3-cyanophosphoenolpyruvate, a new inhibitor of phosphoenolpyruvate-dependent enzymes. *Biochemistry*, **24**, 7602–6.

Wirsching, P. and O'Leary, M. H. (1988a). (*Z*)-3-(Fluoromethyl)phosphoenolpyruvate: synthesis and enzymatic studies. *Biochemistry*, **27**, 1348–55.

Wirsching, P. and O'Leary, M. H. (1988b). 1-Carboxyallenyl phosphate, an allenic analogue of phosphoenolpyruvate. *Biochemistry*, **27**, 1355–60.

Yagami, T., Tagaya, M., and Fukui, T. (1988). Adenosine di-, tri- and tetra-phosphopyridoxals modify the same lysyl residue at the ATP-binding site in adenylate kinase. *Federation of European Biochemical Societies Letters*, **229**, 261–4.

Yanagi, S., Makiura, S., Arai, M., Matsumura, K., Hirao, K., Ito, N., and Tanaka, T. (1974). Isozyme patterns of pyruvate kinase in various primary liver tumors induced during the process of hepatocarcinogenesis. *Cancer Research*, **34**, 2283–9.

Young, R. C., Jones, M., Milliner, K. J., Rana, K. K., and Ward, J. G. (1990). Purine derivatives as competitive inhibitors of human erythrocyte membrane phosphatidylinositol 4-kinase. *Journal of Medicinal Chemistry*, **33**, 2073–80.

Zou, F. C., Dutschman, G. E., De Clercq, E., and Cheng, Y.-C. (1984). Differential binding affinities of sugar modified derivatives of (*E*)-5-(2-bromovinyl)-2'-deoxyuridine for herpes simplex virus-induced and human cellular deoxythymidine kinases. *Biochemical Pharmacology*, **33**, 1797–1800.

6

Enzyme targets as an approach to therapy for HIV infections

Section 6A

Potential chemotherapeutic targets in the replicative cycle of HIV

Erik De Clercq, Anne-Mieke Vandamme, Dominique Schols, and Zeger Debyser

6A.1   Introduction

The life-cycle of human immunodeficiency virus (HIV) begins with the binding of the viral envelope glycoprotein (gp120) to the CD4 receptor of the host cells. Fusion between the viral envelope and the cell membrane follows, whereupon the viral nucleocapsid gains entry into the cell. After entry, uncoating of the nucleocapsid takes place. Once it has been released (at least partially) from its core (group-specific antigen (*gag*)) proteins, the genomic RNA is converted into double-stranded (proviral) DNA by reverse transcriptase (RT). The proviral DNA then migrates to the nucleus where it is integrated into the host genome by integrase. Both integrase and RT (and hence associated ribonuclease H) are encoded by the viral polymerase (*pol*) gene. The first part of the HIV replicate cycle ends with its integration into the host genome (Fig. 6A.1) where it remains indefinitely. It can be silent or actively expressed into progeny virus. Viral gene expression starts from the upstream HIV long terminal repeat (LTR) region, following interaction of the LTR (consisting of U3, R, and

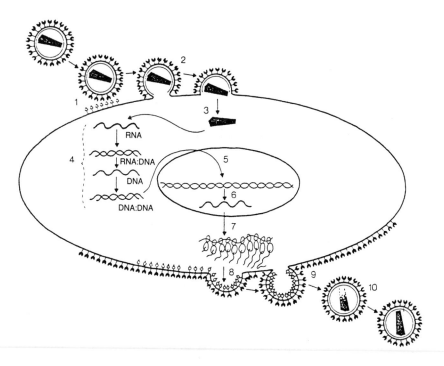

Fig. 6A.1 Life-cycle of HIV-1.

U5 regions) with cellular transcriptional factors. Of the RNA molecules thus transcribed some serve as mRNA for viral precursor protein synthesis and others as RNA genomes to be packaged into progeny virions. Viral precursor proteins need to be processed through proteolytic cleavage (which, for the *gag* and *pol* proteins, requires the intervention of a protease that is itself encoded by the *pol* gene), glycosylation (required for the viral envelope glycoproteins encoded by the viral *env* gene), and myristoylation (attachment of myristic acid at aminoterminal end of the *gag* and *gag–pol* precursor proteins). Assembly of the viral RNA genomes with the core (*gag*) proteins occurs at the inner surface of the cell membrane, and as soon as the viral envelope glycoproteins have accumulated on the outer cell surface, assembly is completed and HIV virions are released from the cell (Fig. 6A.1).

The life-cycle of HIV thus reveals a variety of specific events, from the initial virus adsorption step to the eventual release (budding) of virions from the cell, which could be considered as potential targets for chemotherapeutic intervention. Along with the structural genes (*gag*, *pol*, and *env*), the HIV genome contains several accessory genes which encode regulatory proteins imparting either stimulatory or inhibitory effects on the HIV life-cycle (Fig. 6A.2): *trans*-activator (*tat*), which ensures high level expression, primarily through transcriptional activation of all viral genes; regulator of virion protein expression (*rev*), which differentially regulates the splicing of different viral mRNAs; negative factor (*nef*), which has originally been assumed to downgrade HIV gene expression; viral protein R (*vpr*) which can act as a *trans*-activator; viral protein U (*vpu*) which would facilitate assembly and release of the virus particles; virion infectivity factor (*vif*) which increases infectivity of the virus particles; viral protein T (*vpt*) with

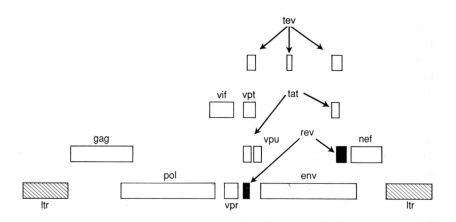

Fig. 6A.2 Genomic structure of HIV-1.

unknown function; *tat-env-rev* fusion protein (*tev*) which is a chimeric protein with both *tat* and *rev* activities. Of these regulatory gene products, *tat* in particular has been envisaged as a chemotherapeutic target because it is the master switch for the expression of all viral genes.

6A.2   CD4–gp120 interaction as a target for anti-HIV therapy

The CD4 molecule is a T-cell surface glycoprotein which interacts with major histocompatibility complex (MHC) class II molecules on the surface of antigen-presenting cells to mediate an efficient cellular immune response (Doyle and Strominger 1987; Gay *et al*. 1987). The mature 55 kDa CD4 protein consists of a 372 amino acid extracellular segment composed of four tandem immunoglobulin-like domains, a 23 amino acid transmembrane domain, and a 38 amino acid C-terminal cytoplasmic tail (Fig. 6A.3) (Maddon *et al*. 1985, 1986, 1987). The first domain (D1) shares several features with immunoglobulin variable domains, but the sequence similarities between immunoglobulins and the other extracellular domains (D2, D3, and D4) are more remote.

6A.2.1   Natural role of CD4

The CD4 receptor is not expressed only on T-lymphocytes but also, to a lesser extent, on B-cells (Montagnier *et al*. 1984), monocytes/macrophages (Wood *et al*. 1983), dendritic cells (Patterson and Knight 1987), eosinophils (Lucey *et al*. 1989), and megakaryocytes (Basch *et al*. 1990). Originally, $CD4^+$ T-cells have been assigned the role of helper/inducer cells, indicating their function in providing activating signals to B-cells or inducing T-lymphocytes to become cytotoxic/suppressor cells ($CD8^+$ T-cells) (Golstein *et al*. 1982). However, it is incorrect to call $CD4^+$ T-cells 'helper' cells and $CD8^+$ T-cells 'cytotoxic/suppressor' cells. $CD4^+$ T-cells recognize foreign antigens in the context of MHC class II molecules (HLA-D in humans), while $CD8^+$ T-cells recognize foreign antigens in the context of MHC class I antigens (HLA-A, HLA-B, and HLA-C in humans). Because most cells, and also most virus-infected cells, are MHC class I^+ and MHC class II^-, the great majority of cytotoxic T-cells eliminating intracellular infections by target cell lysis are $CD8^+$. Similarly, most antigen-presenting cells and B-cells (the targets of helper T-cell action) are MHC class II^+, and therefore a significant fraction of helper T-cells are $CD4^+$. However, $CD4^+$ cytotoxic cells exist (Thomas *et al*. 1981), and it should be evident that these cells could play unique and crucial roles in the elimination of MHC class II^+ HIV-infected cells such as monocytes, macrophages, and Langerhans cells (McCune 1991).

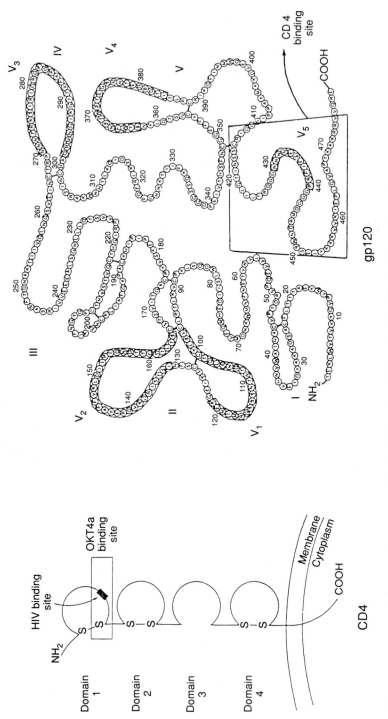

Fig. 6A.3 Structure of the CD4 and gp120 molecules. For further explanation see text.

6A.2.2   Role of CD4 as the receptor for HIV

A number of observations have suggested that CD4 also serves as an HIV receptor in humans. CD4$^+$ helper/inducer T-cells decrease in AIDS patients (Gottlieb et al. 1981), probably because HIV has a specific tropism for CD4$^+$ T-cells (Klatzmann et al. 1984). Also, in AIDS patients CD4$^+$ T-cell counts decrease in parallel with the number of CD4$^+$ monocytes (Lucey et al. 1991). Only certain CD4-specific monoclonal antibodies (mAbs) (i.e. OKT4A, anti-Leu3a) prevent binding and infectivity of HIV for CD4$^+$ cells (Dalgleish et al. 1984; McDougal et al. 1985, 1986a; Sattentau et al. 1986; Lyerly et al. 1987). Human cells that are CD4 antigen negative and refractory to infection with HIV acquire the ability to bind virus and become permissive for infection with HIV following transfection with cloned CD4 cDNA (Maddon et al. 1986). In immunoprecipitation experiments, CD4 coprecipitates with the viral glycoprotein gp120 as a single complex (McDougal et al. 1986b). HIV−cell binding, HIV replication, and HIV-induced syncytium formation can be prevented by soluble CD4 molecules (referred to as sCD4, rCD4, or rsCD4) (Smith et al. 1987; Deen et al. 1988; Fisher et al. 1988; Hussey et al. 1988; Traunecker et al. 1988; Byrn et al. 1989). Monoclonal anti-idiotypic antibodies (anti-anti-Leu3a) bind to gp120 and partially neutralize HIV infection of human T-cells (Chanh et al. 1987). CD4 molecules linked with toxins selectively kill HIV-infected cells expressing viral envelope glycoproteins (Chaudhary et al. 1988; Till et al. 1988; Berger et al. 1989, 1990; Capon et al. 1989). Aurintricarboxylic acid, which specifically binds to the OKT4A epitope, also prevents the binding of HIV to CD4$^+$ cells (Schols et al. 1989, 1991). Not only HIV-1 but also HIV-2 and simian immunodeficiency virus (SIV) bind to the same site at CD4, which thus points to CD4 as the specific and universal receptor for HIV and SIV (McClure et al. 1987; Sattentau et al. 1988). Conserved regions of the HIV-1 envelope protein gp120 bind to the N-terminal domain of CD4 with high affinity ($K_d = 10^{-9}$ M) (Lasky et al. 1987; Sattentau et al. 1989).

Various efforts have been made to define the HIV binding site on the CD4 molecule. The first studies, using mAb panels to different portions of the CD4 molecule (Sattentau et al. 1986) and synthetic peptides prepared from the CD4 protein sequence or antisera raised against these peptides (Jameson et al. 1988), showed that OKT4A mAb is a potent inhibitor of HIV binding and infection. Thus it was proposed that the HIV binding site is located very closely to the epitope defined by OKT4A mAb which binds to a peptide residue of 32−47 in the first domain of CD4 (Fig. 6A.3) (Jameson et al. 1988).

Later, more sophisticated techniques, e.g. saturation mutagenesis followed by negative selection by antibody binding and complement fixation (Peterson and Seed 1988), chimaeric recombinant molecules between human CD4 and mouse CD4 (L3T4) (Clayton *et al.* 1988; Landau *et al.* 1988), single- and double-substitution mutations (Arthos *et al.* 1989; Bowman *et al.* 1990), insertion mutations (Mizukami *et al.* 1988) and synthesis of over-lapping peptides of CD4 (Lifson *et al.* 1988; Kalyanaraman *et al.* 1990) demonstrated that the most important region for HIV binding is contained within the first domain of CD4 and probably spans the peptide segment from amino acid residues 30 to 60.

Recently, several groups have obtained crystals of recombinant soluble CD4 derivatives. Those representing the four-domain species diffract rela-tively poorly (Davis *et al.* 1990; Kwong *et al.* 1990). In contrast, crystals of the N-terminal two-domain products (D1D2), diffract with high reso-lution (Ryu *et al.* 1990; Wang *et al.* 1990). The recombinant fragment consisting of residues 1−183 is as active as the whole soluble CD4 molecule in binding to gp120 (Ryu *et al.* 1990; Wang *et al.* 1990). Many of the amino acid residues that are assumed to interact with gp120 lie between positions 38 and 52. There may also be additional contacts: for example, at residues 77 (Ashkenazi *et al.* 1990) and 87 (Camerini and Seed 1990) in D1, and at residues 122 and 164 in D2 (Clayton *et al.* 1988; Mizukami *et al.* 1988).

Synthetic CD4 peptide derivatives have been tested for their ability to inhibit HIV infection and HIV-induced syncytium formation (Lifson *et al.* 1988; Hayashi *et al.* 1989; Nara *et al.* 1989). Their mode of action can obviously be attributed to inhibition of the binding of HIV gp120 to intact CD4 molecules on the surface of the CD4$^+$ target cells. Soluble rCD4 has a very short terminal half-life (15 min in rabbits). Therefore hybrid mole-cules have been created by genetically combining CD4 with the constant heavy-chain domains of immunoglobulins (rCD4-Ig) (Byrn *et al.* 1989; Capon *et al.* 1989; Traunecker *et al.* 1989). Such constructs have been termed CD4-immunoadhesins. These hybrid molecules retain their activity against HIV-1, comparable with that of soluble rCD4 in T-cells and macro-phages. Because of the presence of the immunoglobin heavy-chain domains, the CD4-immunoadhesins possess a much longer plasma half-life (7−48 h) and a capacity to cross the placenta. Soluble rCD4 can also be linked to toxins, such as ricin or *Pseudomonas exotoxin*, and may be expected to kill HIV-infected cells expressing gp120 (Chaudhary *et al.* 1988; Till *et al.* 1988, 1989; Berger *et al.* 1989; Capon *et al.* 1989; Tsubota *et al.* 1990). Such toxin−rCD4 hybrid molecules can be considered as rCD4 immuno-toxins. They are able to destroy and thus eliminate persistently HIV-infected cells (i.e. macrophages) which otherwise may go on producing HIV virions for ever.

Fresh HIV-1 isolates appear to be less susceptible than the laboratory III-B strain of HIV-1 to sCD4 *in vitro* (Daar *et al.* 1990). HIV-2 strains are also less susceptible than HIV-1 strains to the inhibitory effects of soluble rCD4 (Looney *et al.* 1990). Recently, it has been shown that sCD4 may even enhance SIV infection *in vitro* (Werner *et al.* 1990). Also, sCD4 fails to inhibit HIV-2-induced syncytium formation (Sekigawa *et al.* 1990), possibly because of the lower affinity of CD4 for HIV-2 glycoproteins (Moore 1990). As recently demonstrated (Schols *et al.* 1992), the effect of sCD4 on HIV-induced formation is dependent not only on the virus strain but also on the target cell type.

Novel anti-CD4 mAbs that are not reactive with the first and second domain of CD4 but inhibit steps, subsequent to virus binding, which are critical for HIV infection and virus−cell fusion have recently been described. These mAbs do not interfere with the binding of recombinant gp120 or virus but block infection and syncytium formation (Celada *et al.* 1990; Healey *et al.* 1990). These findings indicate that, in addition to its role in virus binding, CD4 also plays an active role in virus−cell membrane fusion.

6A.2.3   Characteristics of HIV gp120

The *env* gene of HIV-1 encodes a 160 kDa precursor glycoprotein which is processed to the external 120 kDa and membrane-associated 41 kDa glycoproteins (Veronese *et al.* 1985). Both the precursor and the mature cleavage products are glycosylated. Almost half the total molecular weight of gp160 and gp120 can be attributed to asparagine-linked carbohydrate (Veronese *et al.* 1985). The glycoproteins gp120 and gp41 give rise to the spikes observed on the surface of newly released HIV-1 virions (Gelderblom *et al.* 1987). The amino acid sequence of gp120 contains five relatively conserved domains interspersed with five hypervariable domains (Fig. 6A.3) (Modrow *et al.* 1987; Willey *et al.* 1988, 1989; Leonard *et al.* 1990). The hypervariable domains contain extensive amino acid substitutions, insertions, and deletions. Glycosylation of the envelope glycoproteins takes place in the rough endoplasmatic reticulum and Golgi apparatus. Newly synthesized gp160 contains mannose-rich oligosaccharides which are required for the association of gp160 with the endoplasmic reticulum. These oligosaccharide portions will be trimmed by specific carbohydrate-modifying enzymes after gp160 has been transported from the endoplasmic reticulum to the Golgi apparatus, where gp160 is cleaved to gp120 and gp41. The carbohydrate portions of both gp120 and gp41 are further modified by the addition of galactose, fucose, and sialic acid residues (Dewar *et al.* 1989). The endo-proteolytic processing of gp160 to gp120 and gp41 is essential for the production of infectious virions (McCune *et al.* 1988).

Since gp120 is heavily glycosylated, the glycosylation process of gp120 could be envisaged as a target for chemotherapeutic intervention, as glycosylation inhibitors may be expected to affect viral replication, virus infectivity, or virus-induced syncytium formation. Thus the following have been evaluated: inhibitors of the transfer of N-linked oligosaccharides to protein (tunicamycin), inhibitors of the processing of N-linked oligosaccharides (e.g. inhibitors of the trimming enzymes, glucosidases I and II (castanospermine and its derivatives, 1-deoxynojirimycin and its derivatives; see also Section 6D), mannosidase I (1-deoxymannojirimycin), mannosidase II (swainsonine), and inhibitors of protein transport from the endoplasmic reticulum to the Golgi apparatus (monensin) (De Clercq 1991). Thus the glycosylation of HIV glycoproteins depends entirely on cellular enzymes. To achieve any selectivity in their anti-HIV activity, glycosylation inhibitors have to rely on quantitative differences in the demands of glycosylation between cellular and viral glycoproteins.

6A.2.4   Functional regions of HIV gp120

Monoclonal antibodies capable of blocking the gp120–CD4 interaction react with a conserved region (amino acids 413–456) of gp120 (Lasky *et al.* 1987). *In vitro* mutagenesis, deletion of 12 amino acids (426–437) from this region, or substitution of amino acid 433 results in a reduction of the binding to CD4 (Lasky *et al.* 1987). The 44 carboxy terminal amino acids are necessary for the specific binding of gp120 with CD4 (Linsley *et al.* 1988), but a mAb to this region has no effect on the gp120–CD4 interaction (McKeating and Willey 1989), suggesting that the carboxy-terminal end may be necessary for correct folding of gp120. In addition, some hyperconserved regions of gp120 may be essential for proper binding of gp120 with CD4 (Cordonnier *et al.* 1989). Thus the primary sequences of those gp120 regions that are involved in the interaction with CD4 may be distantly located, while their tertiary structure brings them in close contact.

Murine mAbs against the CD4 binding region of gp120 have been generated, and all of them neutralize the infectivity of different isolates of HIV-1 and inhibit HIV-1 binding to CD4$^+$ cells (Sun *et al.* 1989). An immunological or chemical intervention directed towards the CD4 binding region of gp120 may be a promising therapeutic or prophylactic approach since, in principle, all HIV isolates that use CD4 as receptor should be blocked in this way. Also, the amino acid 413–456 region of HIV-1 gp120 shares significant homology with the corresponding region in the HIV-2 gp120 glycoprotein. However, symptomatic and asymptomatic HIV-infected persons lack antibodies to this epitope, suggesting that the CD4 binding site of gp120 is immunorecessive in humans (Sun *et al.* 1989), possibly because of the cleft structure of this site (Lasky *et al.* 1987)

The HIV-1 gp120 domain recognized by neutralizing antibody corresponds to the loop region located near the middle of gp120 (Goudsmit *et al.* 1988a,b; Palker *et al.* 1988; Rusche *et al.* 1988; Skinner *et al.* 1988a). This loop is located in the variable region 3 (V_3). It is formed by a disulphide bridge between Cys residues 266 and 301 (Fig. 6A.3) (Leonard *et al.* 1990). Although most of the amino acids of the V_3 loop are highly variable among different strains of HIV-1, a Gly-Pro-Gly-Arg sequence at the tip of the loop is highly conserved. This epitope corresponds to the binding site for neutralizing antibodies (which block HIV-1 infection and syncytium formation) (Matsushita *et al.* 1988; Palker *et al.* 1988; Rusche *et al.* 1988; Skinner *et al.* 1988a; Javaherian *et al.* 1989; Scott *et al.* 1990; Schols *et al.* 1991b). Although HIV-infected individuals possess these neutralizing antibodies, it is not known under what circumstances they are protective against viral infection. Antibodies to this domain do not block gp120–CD4 interactions but neutralize the virus at a post-CD4 binding stage (Skinner *et al.* 1988b). From a recent study (Devash *et al.* 1990), it appears that the presence of anti-V_3 loop antibodies in HIV-1-infected women correlates with a significantly lower rate of HIV transmission to fetuses *in utero*.

Single amino acid changes in the tip of the V_3 loop completely abolish or greatly reduce the ability of HIV-1 to induce cell fusion (Freed *et al.* 1991), which points to the V_3 loop as a fusion domain. Monoclonal antibodies to the V_3 loop block HIV-1 infection of several cell types (McKeating and Willey 1989). This proves that the V_3 loop still has an important function in the life-cycle of HIV, even if it is not involved in the binding of gp120 to CD4. Thus antibodies or chemical agents targeted at this loop could be the basis of an effective anti-HIV immunotherapy- or chemotherapy (Schols *et al.* 1990; Emini *et al.* 1992).

Other regions within the amino terminal half of gp120 have also been implicated in events occuring post-CD4 binding (Willey *et al.* 1988, 1989). Thus the HIV glycoproteins should not be considered in terms of well-defined domains with specific functions, but rather as a collection of epitopes whose interactions with one another contribute to the functional integrity of the whole HIV envelope.

6A.3 Synthesis and integration of proviral DNA as targets for anti-HIV therapy

6A.3.1 Key role of HIV-1 RT

Reverse transcriptase (RT) is a key enzyme of the replication cycle of HIV. It is responsible for transcription of the single-stranded viral RNA to double-stranded proviral DNA (Temin and Baltimore 1972). RT is a multifunctional enzyme displaying RNA-dependent DNA polymerase (RDDP) activity, ribonuclease H (degradation of RNA of the RNA:DNA hybrid) activity, and DNA-dependent DNA polymerase (DDDP) activity. RT appears to be the only non-organellar polymerase present in the cytoplasm of HIV-infected cells. It is the target enzyme for a number of $2',3'$-dideoxy-nucleosides such as AZT, DDC, and DDI, which are currently used in the treatments of AIDS (De Clercq 1991), and for a series of specific HIV-1 RT inhibitors belonging to widely differing chemical classes such as HEPT (Baba *et al.* 1991), TIBO, α-APA (Pauwels *et al.* 1990, 1993; Debyser *et al.*

1991), and dipyridodiazepinone (Merluzzi *et al.* 1990). (For a review see De Clercq 1993; see also Section 6C.)

6A.3.2   Structure of HIV RT

HIV-1 RT, as present in virions and infected cells, is a heterodimer consisting of two tightly associated chains of 66 and 51 kDa (Veronese *et al.* 1986). Similarly, HIV-2 RT consists of two chains of 68 and 55 kDa respectively (De Vico *et al.* 1989). Monomeric p66 displays two enzymatic activities. The DNA polymerase function of the enzyme resides in the amino-terminal part, while the 15 kDa carboxy-terminal end displays ribonuclease (RNase) H activity (Hansen *et al.* 1988). Monomeric p51 lacks RNase H activity. The two enzymatic functions of monomeric p66 cannot be completely separated, as has been shown by the observation that carboxy-terminal site-directed mutagenesis also affects amino-terminal DNA polymerase activity (Tisdale *et al.* 1988). The three-dimensional structure of HIV-1 RT and its RNase H has recently been resolved (Davies *et al.* 1991; Kohlstaedt *et al.* 1992; Jacobo-Molina *et al.* 1993). Resolution of the total structure of HIV-1 RT should help in designing compounds that fit into the active site(s) of the molecule.

6A.3.3   Function of HIV RT

Reverse transcription is a complicated process (Fig. 6A.4) which requires several successive steps catalysed by the same enzyme. The polymerization is initiated by a tRNA^{Lys}, annealed to the 5' primer binding site (PBS) of the viral RNA genome. After elongation of the primer by RDDP and formation of so-called '(−) strand strong stop' DNA, the 5' direct repeat of the RNA template is degraded by ribonuclease H, enabling the newly formed DNA to anneal to the homologous 3' direct repeat, a process referred to as 'first jump'. After this switch, further elongation of the (−) DNA strand can occur. The synthesis of (+) strand DNA (DDDP) requires specific cleavage of ribonuclease H at a polypurine tract of the RNA template. The primer is elongated, using the minus strand DNA as template, to form another short DNA product called '(+) strand strong stop'. The tRNA^{Lys} is then removed by RNase H. This allows the PBS segment of the (−)DNA strand to pair with the PBS segment of the (+) DNA strand, whereupon the (+) DNA strand is extended to its full length. The final double-stranded proviral DNA product is characterized by long terminal repeats (LTRs) at both ends, resulting from the extension of both strong stop DNAs.

Reverse transcriptase is pivotal for retrovirus replication. The lack of proof-reading capacity, the low fidelity of nucleotide incorporation, as has been shown in particular for HIV-1 RT (Ricchetti and Buc 1990), and the recombination between different RNA copies (Hu and Temin 1990) by

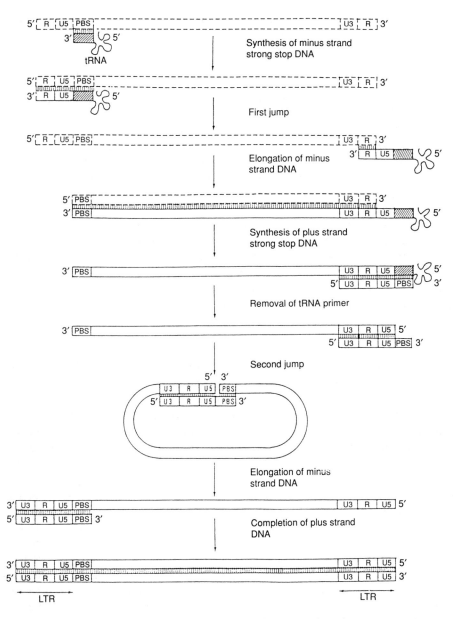

Fig. 6A.4 Functioning of HIV RT. For further explanation see text.

template switching ensure a high variability of the viral RNA genome. This high variability may represent a major challenge in the development of RT inhibitors.

6A.3.4   Integrase as a target for anti-HIV therapy

Cleavage of the carboxy terminal end of the *gag−pol* polyprotein results in the formation of a 32 kDa protein which catalyses the integration of double-stranded DNA into the host chromosome. This protein is called integrase (IN). Following integration, the proviral genome is passed on as a stable element of the host genome. Integration of the proviral DNA into the host cell genome can be considered as an attractive target for anti-HIV chemotherapy. *In vitro* integration assays have recently been established (Bushman and Craigie 1991; Fesen *et al.* 1993). The proviral DNA precursor for integration is the linear form. Integration occurs without apparent specificity for the target host DNA sequence. The integrated proviral DNA is directly flanked by a five-base pair duplication of the target DNA site and is further characterized by the loss of two base pairs from the long terminal repeats. The only HIV protein required for proviral DNA integration is IN, which has been overexpressed in insect cells and partially purified (Bushman *et al.* 1990).

6A.4   Regulatory proteins as targets for anti-HIV therapy

6A.4.1   *Trans*-activation by the *tat* protein

Following integration of proviral DNA into the host cell genome, the virus can remain latent for an indefinite period of time. Initiation of transcription appears to rely mainly on the presence in the viral *ltr* of binding sites for cellular transcription factors such as NF-κB (Nabel *et al.* 1988; Clark *et al.* 1990) and SP1 (Jones *et al.* 1986). Several factors, i.e. various virus gene products (Gendelman *et al.* 1986; Mosca *et al.* 1987; Ensoli *et al.* 1989), UV light (Nabel *et al.* 1988; Stein *et al.* 1989; Valerie and Rosenberg 1990), mitogens, antigens, and cytokines, can activate cellular enhancer binding proteins like NF-κB (Folks *et al.* 1987; Nabel *et al.* 1988) and in this way promote viral transcription (Rosenberg and Fauci 1990).

The earliest viral product made following initiation of expression of the proviral DNA is the *tat* protein (Kim *et al.* 1989a). In most cell types *tat* is essential for the HIV life-cycle (Dayton *et al.* 1986; Fisher *et al.* 1986). The HIV *tat* protein is responsible for the *trans*-activation process which involves the interaction of *tat* with a specific sequence of approximately 60 bases in the R region of the *ltr*, which is known as the *trans*-activation region (TAR) (Feng and Holland 1988). The *trans*-activation process requires the interplay of the *tat* protein, TAR RNA, promotor DNA sequences including TAR DNA, and a number of cellular proteins (Fig. 6A.5). Binding of the *tat* protein to the TAR RNA would increase the stability of the stem−loop structure of TAR RNA (Feng and Holland 1988; Garcia *et al.* 1989; Selby *et al.* 1989; Roy *et al.* 1990), thereby preventing its degradation

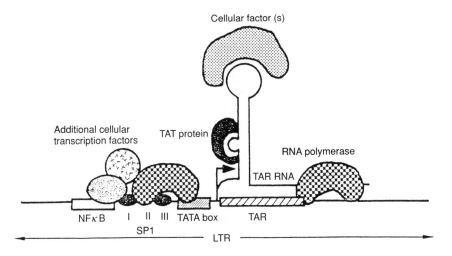

Fig. 6A.5 *Trans*-activation of HIV-1 transcription.

(Schröder *et al.* 1990) and facilitating its interaction with a number of cellular proteins (Gaynor *et al.* 1989; Hart *et al.* 1989), among which is the TAR RNA binding protein (Gatignol *et al.* 1991). *Trans*-activation has a stimulatory effect on several processes, including initiation of transcription, elongation of nascent RNAs, RNA transport, and the efficiency of RNA translation to viral proteins (Okamoto and Wong-Staal 1986; SenGupta *et al.* 1990; Southgate *et al.* 1990).

6A.4.2   Functional regions of the *tat* protein

Based on site-directed mutagenesis, deletion mutagenesis, and studies with synthetic peptide segments, a number of critical regions have been identified within the *tat* protein. The proline-rich amino-terminal domain has no clear function. The cysteine-rich region (amino acids 21–38) has metal-chelatlng potential (Frankel *et al.* 1988; Kubota *et al.* 1989). The HIV-1 *tat* protein forms a metal-linked dimer in the presence of Zn^{2+}, Ca^{2+}, and other divalent cations (Frankel *et al.* 1988). If this dimerization is necessary for the functioning of *tat* protein, it could be a suitable target for antiviral therapy. The stretch of basic amino acid residues (49–57) is well conserved among different HIV isolates. They are required for TAR RNA binding and nucleolar localization of the *tat* protein (Hauber *et al.* 1989; Kuppuswamy *et al.* 1989; Ruben *et al.* 1989; Calnan *et al.* 1991). The exact role of the amino acid stretch 58–72 is not known. According to some authors, the 58–72 amino acid stretch should have an enhancing effect on *trans*-activation (Green and Lowenstein 1988;

Kuppuswamy *et al.* 1989). The function of the region encoded by the second exon (amino acids 72–86) is not essential for *trans*-activation, as synthetic peptides corresponding to the 1–72 amino acid region exert full *trans*-activation capacity (Green and Lowenstein 1988). However, the second exon contains the Arg-Gly-Asp (RGD) sequence, which is typical for integrin-mediated cell adhesion (Brake *et al.* 1990) and may allow the *tat* protein to act on adjacent cells (Ensoli *et al.* 1993). Structural studies of the *tat* TAR interaction are in progress (Puglisi *et al.* 1992; Loret *et al.* 1992).

Screening of '*tat* inhibitors' has begun, using *trans*-activation systems, whereby a reporter gene monitors HIV-1 LTR activity. The *tat* inhibitors reported so far (Hsu *et al.* 1991; Witvrouw *et al.* 1992) seems to inhibit the interaction of the *tat* protein and/or TAR RNA with an essential cellular factor. Some anti-sense oligonucleotides (Zaia *et al.* 1988; Rhodes and James 1990) and ribozyme constructs directed against TAR RNA have also been shown to inhibit HIV replication (James *et al.* 1991; Jayasena and Johnston 1992). *Tat* inhibitors might have therapeutic potential in the treatment of Kaposi's sarcoma in AIDS patients since the *tat* protein seems to stimulate the growth of these tumours (Ensoli *et al.* 1990).

6A.4.3   Regulatory role of the *rev* protein

Transport of the viral mRNAs to the cytoplasm and translation to proteins are controlled, at least in part, by the regulator of virion production (*rev*) protein, a 19 kDa phosphorylated tetrameric product of the *rev* gene (Feinberg *et al.* 1986; Sodroski *et al.* 1986b; Cochrane *et al.* 1989a; Nalin *et al.* 1990), The *rev* protein starts off by upregulating the production of regulatory proteins (i.e. *tat*) at an early phase. Through *trans*-activation, the *rev* protein attains levels which, on the one hand, stimulate expression of the *gag* and *pol* proteins and, on the other hand, inhibit the expression of regulatory proteins (Malim *et al.* 1988; Arrigo *et al.* 1989). The *rev* protein interacts with a *cis*-acting sequence of about 240 nucleotides in the *rev* RNA, referred to as the *rev* responsive element (RRE) (Daly *et al.* 1989; Hadzopoulou-Cladaras *et al.* 1989; Hammarskjold *et al.* 1989). Recent data indicate that RRE consists of multiple elements (Daly *et al.* 1989; Nalin *et al.* 1990; Kjems *et al.* 1991) and that the minimal 'responsive' sequence of such an element should be 13 nucleotides long (Huang *et al.* 1991; Tiley *et al.* 1992).

The early regulatory proteins like *tat*, *rev* and *nef* are all encoded by extensively spliced short mRNAs, while the RRE motif is only present in late long mRNAs encoding the structural proteins.

The *rev* protein stimulates the nuclear export of unspliced viral mRNA (Malim *et al.* 1989a) and appears to interact with a particular carrier protein, thereby facilitating the translocation of RRE-containing RNAs through the nuclear pore (Emerman *et al.* 1989; Hadzopoulou-Cladaras *et al.* 1989; Malim *et al.* 1989a; Lu *et al.* 1990; Holland 1991; Müller *et al.* 1991).

6A.4.4 Functional regions of the *rev* protein

Mutational analysis of the *rev* gene has revealed a number of functional regions within the *rev* protein. A highly basic domain is located between amino acid residues 35 and 51. This region contains 10 arginine residues, and is necessary for nucleolar localization (Cochrane *et al.* 1989b; Perkins *et al.* 1989; Hope *et al.* 1990). The 35–51 amino acid region is also involved in the binding to RRE (Daly *et al.* 1989; Zapp and Green 1989; Olsen *et al.* 1990; Halim and Cullen 1991). The 78–84 portion of the protein contains the Leu-Glu-Arg-Leu-Thr-Leu-Asp sequence which may, at least in part, function as a minimal activation domain (Malim *et al.* 1989b). Just like *tat*, *rev* protein also seems to interact with a cellular protein, but it is not clear if this interaction is important for its function (Vaishnav *et al.* 1991).

As the structural determinants for *rev* *trans*-activation become clear, it should be possible to tailor inhibitors of this function. Malim *et al.* (1989b) and Baltimore (1988) have described an intracellular immunization approach to inhibit *rev* function by co-transfection with *trans*-dominant negative mutants. Anti-sense RNAs and ribozymes directed against RRE represent another approach designed to interfere with HIV production at the *rev* level (Matsukura *et al.* 1989).

6A.4.5 Other regulatory proteins

Nef protein is a 27 kDa protein which can be myristoylated and phosphorylated (Ahmad and Venkatesan 1988; Rimsky *et al.* 1988; Kaminchik *et al.* 1991). The role of *nef* is rather controversial and probably depends on the interplay with cellular factors. Terwilliger *et al.* (1986) and Luciw *et al.* (1987) reported that the *nef* protein inhibits HIV-1 replication, but others did not see any inhibition (Hammes *et al.* 1989; Kim *et al.* 1989b; Kim *et al.* 1989b) and De Ronde *et al.* (1991) even found a positive regulatory effect on viral replication. New developments strengthen the role of *nef* in HIV pathogenesis (Kestler *et al.* 1991).

The protein products of *vif* and *vpr* have not yet been characterized. *Vif* mutants show reduced infectivity in some cell lines (Sodroski *et al.* 1986a; Strebel *et al.* 1987), and *vpr* mutants grow more slowly than wild type viruses (Ogawa *et al.* 1989; Cohen *et al.* 1990a). The *vpu* protein is a non-glycosylated 16 kDa polypeptide. *vpu* mutants show a decrease in the number of virus particles released from the cells (Terwilliger *et al.*

1989). *Vif*, *vpu*, and *vpr* are not essential for viral replication and therefore they do not seem attractive targets for therapy. Until the role of the recently identified *vpt* and *tev* proteins in the viral life-cycle (Benko *et al.* 1990; Cohen *et al.* 1990b; Salfeld *et al.* 1990) is established, it is too early to assess their suitability as targets for anti-HIV therapy.

6A.5   HIV protease as target for anti-HIV therapy

6A.5.1   Role of HIV protease

The *gag* and *gag–pol* genes are expressed as polyproteins $Pr55^{gag}$ and $Pr160^{gag–pol}$ that then need proteolytic processing by HIV protease. This processing is essential in the final maturation step of the viral life-cycle (Kohl *et al.* 1988; Gheysen *et al.* 1989; Ashorn *et al.* 1990). Blocking the protease activity results in the formation of immature virions which are non-infectious.

The *gag* and *pol* genes of most retroviruses occur in different reading frames. The *pol* proteins of HIV-1 are expressed when approximately one in every 20 *gag* translation products is extended into the *pol* region via a -1 translational frameshift. This allows readthrough of the entire *pol* gene, producing a 160 kDa *gag–pol* precursor (Jacks *et al.* 1988; Wilson *et al.* 1988; Hatfield and Oroszlan 1990). This frameshift may be considered as a suitable site of chemotherapeutic attack since, in the absence of such frameshift, the *pol* enzymes (protease, RT, ribonuclease H, and integrase) would not be expressed (Hatfield and Oroszlan 1990). The HIV protease, which is autocatalytically cleaved from its precursor, cleaves the $Pr55^{gag}$ precursor protein to the core proteins p24, p17, p9 (p7), p6, and p1 and the *pol* precursor protein to reverse transcriptase, ribonuclease H (p15), and integrase. In contrast, the envelope precursor glycoprotein gp160 is proteolytically processed to gp120 and gp41 by a host protease with trypsin-like specificity (McCune *et al.* 1988). Inhibition of this host protease may not be attractive as a therapeutic target, as this cellular enzyme could have an important role in cellular processes.

6A.5.2   Nature of the HIV protease

HIV protease belongs to the aspartyl protease family and shows significant sequence homology with cellular aspartyl proteases (Pearl and Taylor 1987). Aspartyl proteases have been extensively characterized over the past years. The vast knowledge of their biosynthesis, kinetics, amino acid sequence, and three-dimensional structure (Davies 1990) has been most useful in establishing the characteristics of the HIV proteases. With the aid of the information gathered for cellular aspartyl proteases, a computer-aided three-dimensional model has been developed (Pearl and Taylor 1987) and has recently shown to be similar to that derived from crystallography (Lapatto *et al.* 1989; Navia *et al.* 1989; Wlodawer *et al.* 1989). Cellular aspartyl proteases consist of a single chain with an internal pseudodyad symmetry, while HIV-1 protease is a dimer with two separate identical chains. Miller *et al.* (1989) determined the structure of HIV-1 protease complexed with several inhibitory substrate analogues. From comparison with the structure of the native enzyme, it appeared that ligand binding led to large conformational changes. The conformational shifts of HIV-1 protease upon interaction with substrates (or inhibitors) are of crucial importance in the design of protease inhibitors.

6A.5.3 Transition state mimetics

The main principle that has guided the development of HIV protease inhibitors is based on the transition state mimetic concept (Fig. 6A.6). The protease inhibitors are conceived such that they mimic the transition stage of the peptide bond recognized as the substrate. Instead of the scissile peptide bond, however, protease inhibitors contain a non-scissile bond, resembling the transition state of the peptide bond, so that, once it has been bound to its 'false' substrate, the HIV protease should remain bound and hence become unavailable for interaction with its genuine substrate.

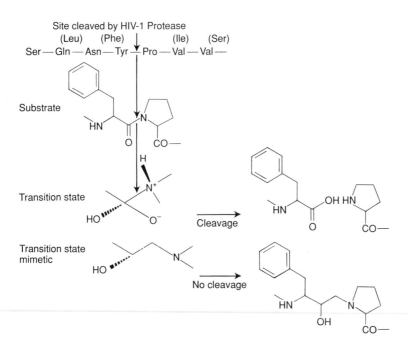

Fig. 6A.6 Transition state mimetic inhibition of HIV-1 protease.

Various HIV protease inhibitors have been designed according to this concept (e.g. Dreyer *et al*. 1989; McQuade *et al*. 1990; Meek *et al*. 1990; Roberts *et al*. 1990) (see also Section 6B). In recent reviews Tomasselli *et al*. (1991) and Debouck (1992) described more than 20 such HIV protease inhibitors.

6A.5.4   Post-translational modifications

In addition to proteolytic cleavage, post-translational modifications such as myristoylation, glycosylation, and phosphorylation could be considered as targets for chemotherapeutic intervention. These modifications are required for the processing of the precursor proteins to mature viral proteins and thus are essential for production of infectious viral progeny.

Thus the HIV protease inhibitors, as well as any other compounds that interfere with post-translational processes, block the HIV life-cycle after the proviral DNA has been integrated into the host cell genome. Such compounds may be expected to reduce viral infectivity owing to a block in the maturation of the viral proteins. Hence their primary usefulness would lie in the treatment of chronic HIV infections and, as they reduce the infectivity of any newly formed virus particles, they may also prevent recruitment of new cells by the infection and thus help in curbing the spread of the disease.

References

Ahmad, N. and Venkatesan, S. (1988). *Nef* protein of HIV-1 is a transcriptional repressor of HIV-1 LTR. *Science*, **241**, 1481–5.

Arrigo, S. J., Weitsman, S., Rosenblatt, J. D., and Chen, I. S. (1989). Analysis of rev gene function on human immunodeficiency virus type 1 replication in lymphoid cells by using a quantitative polymerase chain reaction method. *Journal of Virology*, **63**, 4875–81.

Arthos, J., Deen, K. C., Chaikin, M. A., Fornwald, J. A., Sathe, G., Sattentau, Q. J., *et al*. (1989). Identification of the residues in human CD4 critical for the binding of HIV. *Cell*, **57**, 469–81.

Ashkenazi, A., Presta, L. G., Marsters, S. A., Camerato, T. R., Rosenthal, K. A., Fendly, B. M., and Capon, D. J. (1990). Mapping the CD4 binding site for human immunodeficiency virus by alanine-scanning mutagenesis. *Proceedings of the National Academy of Sciences of the United States of America*, **87**, 7150–4.

Ashorn, P., McQuade, T. J., Thaisrivongs, S., Tomasselli, A. G., Tarpley, W. G., and Moss, B. (1990). An inhibitor of the protease blocks maturation of human and simian immunodeficiency viruses and spread of infection. *Proceedings of the National Academy of Sciences of the United States of America*. **87**, 7472–6.

Baba, M., De Clercq, E., Tanaka, H., Ubasawa, M., Takashima, H., Sekiya, K., *et al*. (1991). Potent and selective inhibition of human immunodeficiency virus type 1 (HIV-1) by 5-ethyl-6-phenylthiouracil derivatives through their interaction with the HIV-1 reverse transcriptase. *Proceedings of the National Academy of Sciences of the United States of America*, **88**, 2356–60.

Baltimore D. (1988). Intracellular immunization. *Nature, London*, **335**, 395–6.

Basch, R. S., Kouri, Y. H., and Karpatkin, S. (1990). Expression of CD4 by human megakaryocytes. *Proceedings of the National Academy of Sciences of the United States of America*, **87**, 8085–9.

Benko, D. M., Schwartz, S., Pavlakis, G. N., and Felber, B. K. (1990). A novel human immunodeficiency virus type 1 protein, tev, shares sequences with tat, env and rev proteins. *Journal of Virology*, **64**, 2505–18.

Berger, E. A., Clouse, K. A., Chaudhary, V. K., Chakrabarti, S., FitzGerald, D. J., Pastan, and Moss, B. (1989). CD4-*Pseudomonas exotoxin* hybrid protein blocks the spread of human immunodeficiency virus infection *in vitro* and is active against cells expressing the envelope glycoproteins from diverse primate immuno-deficiency retro-viruses. *Proceedings of the National Academy of Sciences of the United States of America*, **86**, 9539–43.

Berger, E. A., Chaudhary, V. K., Clouse, K. A., Javaquemada, D., Nicholas, J. A., Rubino, K. L., *et al.* (1990) Recombinant CD4-*Pseudomonas exotoxin* hybrid protein displays HIV-specific cytotoxicity without affecting MHC class II-dependent functions. *AIDS Research and Human Retroviruses,* **6**, 795–803.

Bowman, M. R., McFerrin, K. D., Schreibe, S. L., and Burakoff, S. J. (1990). Identification and structural analysis of residues in the V1 region of CD4 involved in interaction with human immunodeficiency virus envelope glyco-protein gp120 and class II major histocompatibility complex molecules. *Proceedings of the National Academy of Sciences of the United States of America*, **87**, 9052–6.

Brake, D. A., Debouck, C., and Biesecker, G. (1990). Identification of an Arg-Gly-Asp (RGD) cell adhesion site in human immunodeficiency virus type 1 trans-activation protein, *tat*. *Journal of Cell Biology*, **111**, 1275–81.

Bushman, F. D., Fujiwara, T., and Craigie, R. (1990). Retroviral DNA integration directed by HIV integration protein *in vitro*. *Science*, **249**, 1555–8.

Bushman, F. D. and Craigie, R. (1991). Activities of human immunodeficiency virus (HIV) integration protein *in vitro*: specific cleavage and integration of HIV DNA. *Proceedings of the National Academy of Sciences of the United States of America*, **88**, 1339–43.

Byrn, R. A., Sekigawa, I., Chamow, S. M., Johnson, J. S., Gregory, T. J., Capon, D. J., and Groopman, J. E. (1989). Characterization of *in vitro* inhibition of human immunodeficiency virus by purified recombinant CD4. *Journal of Virology*, **63**, 4370–5.

Calnan, B. J., Tidor, B., Biancalana, S., Hudson, D., and Frankel, A. D. (1991). Arginine-mediated RNA recognition: the arginine fork. *Science*, **252**, 1167–71.

Camerini, D. and Seed, B. (1990). A CD4 domain important for HIV-mediated syncytium formation lies outside the virus binding site. *Cell*, **60**, 747–54.

Capon, D. J., Chamow, S. M., Mordenti, J., Marsters, S. A., Gregory, T., Mitsuya, H., *et al.* (1989). Designing CD4 immunoadhesins for AIDS therapy. *Nature, London*, **337**, 525–31.

Celada, F., Cambiaggi, C., Maccari, J., Burastero, S., Gregory, T., Patzer, E., *et al.* (1990). Antibody raised against soluble CD4-rgp120 complex recognizes the CD4 moiety and blocks membrane fusion without inhibiting CD4-gp120 binding. *Journal of Experimental Medicine*, **172**, 1143–50.

Chanh, T. C., Dreesman, G. R., and Kennedy, R. C. (1987). Monoclonal anti-idiotypic antibody mimics the CD4 receptor and binds human immunodeficiency virus. *Proceedings of the National Academy of Sciences of the United States of America*, **84**, 3891.

Chaudhary, V. K., Mizukami, T., Fuerst, T. R., FitzGerald, D. J., Moss, B., Pastan, I., and Berger, E. A. (1988). Selective killing of HIV-infected cells by recombinant human CD4-*Pseudomonas exotoxin* hybrid protein. *Nature, London*, **335**, 369–72.

Clark, L., Matthews, J. R., and Hay, R. T. (1990). Interaction of enhancer-binding protein EBP1 (NF-κB) with the human immunodeficiency virus type 1 enhancer. *Journal of Virology*, **64**, 1335–44.

Clayton, L. K., Hussey, R. E., Steinbrich, R., Ramachandran, H., Husain, Y., and Reinherz, E. L. (1988). Substitution of murine for human CD4 residues identifies amino acids critical for HIV-gp120 binding. *Nature, London*, **335**, 363–6.

Cochrane, A., Golub, E., Volsky, D., Ruben, S., and Rosen, C. A. (1989a). Functional significance of phosphorylation to the human immunodeficiency virus rev protein. *Journal of Virology*, **63**, 4438–40.

Cochrane, A., Kramer, R., Ruben, S., Levine, J., and Rosen C. A. (1989b). The human immunodeficiency virus *rev* protein is a nuclear phosphoprotein. *Virology*, **171**, 264–6.

Cohen, E. A., Dehni, G., Sodroski, J. G., and Haseltine, W. A. (1990a). Human immunodeficiency virus *vpr* product is a virion-associated regulatory protein. *Journal of Virology* **64**, 3097–9.

Cohen, E. A., Lu, Y., Gottlinger, H., Dehni, G., Jalinoos, Y., Sodroski, J., and Haseltine W. (1990b). The T open reading frame of human immunodeficiency virus type 1. *Journal of Acquired Immune Deficiency Syndromes*, **3**, 601–8.

Cordonnier, A., Rivière, Y., Montagnier, L., and Emerman, M. (1989). Effects of mutations in hyperconserved regions of the extracellular glycoprotein of human immunodeficiency virus type 1 on receptor binding. *Journal of Virology*, **63**, 4464–8.

Daar, E. S., Li, X. L., Moudgil, T., and Ho, D. D. (1990). High concentrations of recombinant soluble CD4 are required to neutralize primary human immunodeficiency virus type 1 isolates. *Proceedings of the National Academy of Sciences of the United States of America*, **87**, 6574–8.

Dalgleish, A. G., Beverley, P. C. L., Clapham, P. R., Crawford, D. H., Greaves, M. F., and Weiss, R. A. (1984). The CD4 (T4) antigen is an essential component of the receptor for the AIDS retrovirus. *Nature, London*, **312**, 763–7.

Daly, T. J., Cook, K. S., Gray, G. S., Maione, T. E., and Rusche, J. R. (1989). Specific binding of HIV-1 recombinant Rev protein to the Rev-responsive element *in vitro*. *Nature, London*, **342**, 816–19.

Davies D. R. (1990). The structure and function of the aspartic proteinases. *Annual Review of Biophysics and Biophysical Chemistry*, **19**, 189–215.

Davies, J. F., Hostomska, Z., Hostomsky, Z., Jordan, S. R., and Matthews, D. A. (1991). Crystal structure of the ribonuclease H domain of HIV-1 reverse transcriptase. *Science*, **252**, 88–95.

Davis, S. J., Brady, R. L., Barclay, A. N., Harlos, K., Dodson, G. G., and Williams, A. F. (1990). Crystallization of a soluble form of the rat T-cell surface glycoprotein CD4 complexed with Fab from the W3/25 monoclonal antibody. *Journal of Molecular Biology*, **213**, 7–10.

Dayton, A., Sodroski, J. G., Rosen, C. A., Goh, W. C., and Haseltine, W. A. (1986). The *trans*-activator gene of the human T cell lymphotropic virus type III is required for replication. *Cell*, **44**, 941–7.

Debouck, C. (1992). The HIV-1 protease as a therapeutic target for AIDS. *AIDS Research and Human Retroviruses*, **8**, 153–64.

Debyser, Z., Pauwels, R., Andries, K., Desmyter, J., Kukla, M., Janssen, P. A. J., and De Clercq, E. (1991). An antiviral target on reverse trancriptase of human immunodeficiency virus type 1 revealed by tetrahydroimidazo[4,5,1-*jk*][1,4]-benzo-diazepin-2(1H)-one and -thione derivatives. *Proceedings of the National Academy of Sciences of the United States of America*, **88**, 1451–5.

De Clercq, E. (1991). Basic approaches to anti-retroviral treatment. *Journal of Acquired Immune Deficiency Syndromes*, **4**, 207–18.

De Clercq, E. (1993). HIV-1-Specific RT inhibitors: highly selective inhibitors of human immunodeficiency virus type 1 that are specifically targeted at the viral reverse transcriptase. *Medicinal Research Reviews*, **13**, 229–58.

Deen, K. C., McDougal, J. S., Inacker, R., Folena-Wasserman, G., Arthos, J., Rosenberg, J., *et al.* (1988). A soluble form of CD4 (T4) protein inhibits AIDS virus production. *Nature, London*, **331**, 82–4.

De Ronde, A., Klaver, B., Keulen, W., and Goudsmit, J. (1991). Natural HIV-1 3′orf acts as a positive regulator for viral replication in primary human lymphocytes. *Abstracts of the 7th International Conference on AIDS*, 16–21 June 1991, Florence, p. 94, M.A.1208.

Devash, Y., Calvelli, T. A., Wood, D. G., Reagan, K. J., and Rubinstein, A. (1990). Vertical transmission of human immunodeficiency virus is correlated with the absence of high-affinity/avidity maternal antibodies to the gp120 principal neu-tralizing domain. *Proceedings of the National Academy of Sciences of the United States of America*, **87**, 3445–9.

De Vico, A. L., Copeland, T. D., Di Marzo-Véronese, F., Oroszlan, S., Gallo, R. C., and Sarngadharan, M. G. (1989). Purification and partial characterization of human immunodeficiency virus type 2 reverse transcriptase. *AIDS Research and Human Retroviruses*, **5**, 51–60.

Dewar, R. L., Vasudevachari, M. B., Natarajan, V., and Salzman, N. P. (1989). Biosynthesis and processing of human immunodeficiency virus type 1 envelope glycoproteins: effects of monensin on glycosylation and transport. *Journal of Virology*, **63**, 2452–6.

Doyle, C. and Strominger, J. L. (1987). Interaction between CD4 and class II MHC molecules mediates cell adhesion. *Nature, London*, **330**, 256–9.

Dreyer, G. B., Metcalf, B. W., Tomaszek, T. A. Jr., Carr, T. J., Chandler, A. C. III, Hyland, L., *et al.* (1989). Inhibition of human immunodeficiency virus 1 protease *in vitro*: rational design of substrate analogue inhibitors. *Proceedings of the National Academy of Sciences of the United States of America*, **86**, 9752–6.

Emerman, M., Vazeux, R., and Peden, K. (1989). The *rev* gene product of the human immunodeficiency virus affects envelope-specific RNA localization. *Cell*, **57**, 1155–65.

Emini, E. A., Schleif, W. A., Nunberg, J. H., Conley, A. J., Eda, Y., Tokiyoshi, S., *et al.* (1992). Prevention of HIV-1 infection in chimpanzees by gp120 V3 domain-specific monoclonal antibody. *Nature, London*, **355**, 728–30.

Ensoli, B., Lusso, P., Schachter, F., Josephs, S. F., Rappaport, J., Negro, F., Gallo, R. C., and Wong-Staal, F. (1989). Human herpes virus-6 increases HIV-1 expression in co-infected T cells via nuclear factors binding to the HIV-1 enhancer. *EMBO Journal*, **8**, 3019–27.

Ensoli, B., Barillari, G., Salahuddin, S. Z., Gallo, R. C., and Wong-Staal, F. (1990). Tat protein of HIV-1 stimulates growth of cells derived from Kaposi's sarcoma lesions of AIDS patients. *Nature, London*, **345**, 84–6.

Ensoli, B., Buonaguro, L., Barillari, G., Fiorelli, V., Gendelman, R., Morgan, R. A., *et al.* (1993). Release, uptake, and effects of extracellular human immunodeficiency virus type 1 tat protein on cell growth and viral transactivation. *Journal of Virology*, **67**, 277–87.

Feinberg, M. B., Jarrett, R. F., Adovini, A., Gallo, R. C., and Wong-Staal, F. (1986). HTLV-III expression and production involve complex regulation at the levels of splicing and translation of viral RNA. *Cell*, **46**, 807–17.

Feng, S. and Holland, E. C. (1988). HIV-1 *tat trans*-activation requires the loop sequence within *tar*. *Nature, London*, **334**, 165–7.

Fesen, M. R., Kohn, K. W., Leteurtre, F., and Pommier, Y. (1993). Inhibitors of human immunodeficiency virus integrase. *Proceedings of the National Academy of Sciences of the United States of America*, **90**, 2399–403.

Fisher, A. G., Feinberg, M. B., Josephs, S. F., Harper, M. E., Marselle, L. M., Reyes, G., *et al.* (1986). The *trans*-activator gene of HTLV-III is essential for virus replication. *Nature, London*, **320**, 367–70.

Fisher, R. A., Bertonis, J. M., Meier, W., Johnson, V. A., Costopoulos, D. S., Liu, T., *et al.* (1988). HIV infection is blocked *in vitro* by recombinant soluble CD4. *Nature, London*, **331**, 76–8.

Folks, T. M., Justement, J., Kinter, A., Dinarello, C. A., and Fauci, A. S. (1987). Cytokine-induced expression of HIV-1 in a chronically infected promonocyte cell line. *Science*, **238**, 800–2.

Frankel, A. D., Bredt, D. S., and Pabo, C. O. (1988). *Tat* protein from human immunodeficiency virus forms a metal-linked dimer. *Science*, **440**, 70–3.

Freed, E. O., Myers, D. J., and Risser, R. (1991). Identification of the principal neutralizing determinant of human immunodeficiency virus type 1 as a fusion domain. *Journal of Virology*, **65**, 190–4.

Garcia, J. A., Harrich, D., Soultanakis, E., Wu, F., Mitsuyasu, R., and Gaynor, R. B. (1989). Human immunodeficiency virus type 1 LTR TATA and TAR region sequences required for transcriptional regulation. *EMBO Journal*, **8**, 765–78.

Gatignol, A., Buckler-White, A., Berkhout, B., and Jeang, K.-T. (1991). Characterization of a human TAR RNA-binding protein that activates the HIV-1 LTR. *Science*, **251**, 1597–1600.

Gay, D., Maddon, P., Sekaly, R., Talle, M. A., Godfrey, M., Long, E., *et al.* (1987). Functional interaction between human T-cell protein CD4 and the major histocompatibility complex HLA-DR antigen. *Nature, London*, **328**, 626–9.

Gaynor, R. B., Soultanakis, E., Kuwabara, M., Garcia, J., and Sigmon, D. S. (1989). Specific binding of a HeLa cell nuclear protein to RNA sequences in the human immunodeficiency virus transactivation region. *Proceedings of the National Academy of Sciences of the United States of America*, **86**, 4858–62.

Gelderblom, H. R., Hausmann, E. H. S., Özel, M., Pauli, G., and Koch, M. A. (1987). Fine structure of human immunodeficiency virus (HIV) and immunolocalization of structural proteins. *Virology*, **156**, 171–6.

Gendelman, H. E., Phelps, W., Feigenbaum, L., Ostrove, J. M., Adachi, A., Howley, P. M., *et al.* (1986). *Trans*-activation of the human immunodeficiency virus long terminal repeat sequence by DNA viruses. *Proceedings of the National Academy of Sciences of the United States of America*, **83**, 9759–63.

Gheysen, D., Jacobs, E., de Foresta, F., Thiriart, C., Francotte, M., Thines, D., and De Wilde, M. (1989). Assembly and release of HIV-1 precursor Pr55^{gag} virus-like particles from recombinant baculovirus-infected insect cells. *Cell*, **59**, 103–12.

Golstein, P., Goridis, C., Schmitt-Verhulst, A.-M., Hayot, B., Pierres, A., Van Agthoven, A., *et al.* (1982). Lymphoid cell surface interaction structures detected using cytolysis-inhibiting monoclonal antibodies. *Immunological Reviews*, **68**, 5–42.

Gottlieb, M. S., Schroff, R., Schanker, H. M., Weisman, J. D., Fan, P. T., Wolf, R. A., and Saxon A. (1981). *Pneumocystis carinii* pneumonia and mucosal candidiasis in previously healthy homosexual men. Evidence of a new acquired cellular immunodeficiency. *New England Journal of Medicine*, **305**, 1425–31.

Goudsmit, J., Debouck, C., Meloen, R. H., Smit, L., Bakker, M., Asher, D. M., *et al.* (1988a). Human immunodeficiency virus type 1 neutralization epitope with conserved architecture elicits early type-specific antibodies in experimentally infected chimpanzees. *Proceedings of the National Academy of Sciences of the United States of America*, **85**, 4478–82.

Goudsmit, J., Boucher, C. A. B., Meloen, R. H., Epstein, L. G., Smit, L., Van der Hoek, L., and Bakker, M. (1988b). Human antibody response to a strain-specific HIV-1 gp120 epitope associated with cell fusion inhibition. *AIDS*, **2**, 157–64.

Green, M. and Loewenstein, P. M. (1988). Autonomous functional domains of chemically synthesized human immunodeficiency virus Tat *trans*-activator protein. *Cell*, **55**, 1179–88.

Hadzopoulou-Cladaras, M., Felber, B. K., Cladaras, C., Athanassopoulos, A., Tse, A., and Paulakis, G. N. (1989). The rev/art protein of human immuno-deficiency virus type 1 affects viral mRNA and protein expression via a *cis*-acting sequence in the *env* region. *Journal of Virology*, **63**, 1265–74.

Hammarskjold, M., Heimer, J., Hammarskjold, B., Sangwan, I., Albert, L., and Rekosh, D. (1989). Regulation of human immunodeficiency virus *env* expression by the *env* gene product. *Journal of Virology*, **63**, 1959–66.

Hammes, S. R., Dixon, E. P., Malim, M. H., Cullen, B. R., and Green, W. C. (1989). Nef protein of human immunodeficiency virus type 1: evidence against its role as a transcriptional silencer. *Proceedings of the National Academy of Sciences of the United States of America*, **86**, 9549–53.

Hansen, J., Schultze, T., Mellert, W., and Moelling, K. (1988). Identification and characterization of HIV-specific RNase H by monoclonal antibody. *EMBO Journal*, **7**, 239–43.

Hart, C. E., Ou, C.-Y., Galphin, J. C., Moore, J., Bacheler, L. T., Wasmuth, J. J., *et al.* (1989). Human chromosome 12 is required for elevated HIV-1 expression in human-hamster hybrid cells. *Science*, **246**, 488–91.

Hatfield, D. and Oroszlan, S. (1990). The where, what and how of ribosomal frameshifting in retroviral protein synthesis. *Trends in Biochemical Sciences*, **15**, 186–90.

Hauber, J., Malim, M. H., and Cullen, B. R. (1989). Mutational analysis of the conserved basic domain of human immunodeficiency virus *tat* protein. *Journal of Virology*, **63**, 1181–7.

Hayashi, Y., Ikuta, K., Fujii, N., Ezawa, K., and Kato, S. (1989). Inhibition of HIV-1 replication and syncytium formation by synthetic CD4 peptides. *Archives of Virology*, **105**, 129–35.

Healey, D., Dianda, L., Moore, J. P., McDougal, J. S., Moore, M. J., Estess, P., *et al.* (1990). Novel anti-CD4 monoclonal antibodies separate human immunodeficiency virus infection and fusion of CD4$^+$ cells from virus binding. *Journal of Experimental Medicine*, **172**, 1233–42.

Holland, S. M. (1991). Structural and functional analysis of interactions of HIV-1 REV responsive element RNA with REV and putative host factors. *7th International Conference on AIDS*, 16–21 June 1991, Florence, p. 189, TH.A.6.

Hope, T., Huang, J. X., McDonald, D., and Parslow, T. G. (1990). Steroid-receptor fusion of the human immunodeficiency virus type 1 Rev transactivator: mapping cryptic functions of the arginine-rich motif. *Proceedings of the National Academy of Sciences of the United States of America*, **87**, 7787–91.

Hsu, M.-C., Schutt, A. D., Holly, M., Slice, L. W., Sherman, M. I., Richman, D. D., *et al.* (1991). Inhibition of HIV replication in acute and chronic infections in vitro by a tat antagonist. *Science*, **254**, 1799–802.

Hu, W.-S. and Temin, H. N. (1990). Retroviral recombination and reverse transcription. *Science*, **250**, 1227–33.

Huang, X., Hope, T. J., Bond, B. L., McDonald, D., Grahl, K., and Parslow, T. G. (1991). Minimal Rev-response element for type 1 human immunodeficiency virus. *Journal of Virology*, **65**, 2131–4.

Hussey, R. E., Richardson, N. E., Kowalski, M., Brown, N. R., Chang, H. C., Siliciano, R. F., *et al.* (1988). A soluble CD4 protein selectively inhibits HIV replication and syncytium formation. *Nature, London*, **331**, 78–81.

Jacks, T., Power, M. D., Masiarz, F. R., Luciw, P. A., Barr, P. J., and Varmus, H. E. (1988). Characterization of ribosomal frameshifting in HIV-1 *gag–pol* expression. *Nature, London*, **331**, 280–3.

Jacobo-Molina, A., Ding, J., Nanni, R. G., Clark, A. D. Jr., Lu, X., Tantillo, C., *et al.* (1993). Crystal structure of human immunodeficiency virus type 1 reverse transcriptase complexed with double-stranded DNA at 3.0 Å resolution shows bent DNA. *Proceedings of the National Academy of Sciences of the United States of America*, **90**, 6320–4.

James, W., Rhodes, A., and Crisell, P. (1991). Inhibition of HIV replication in cell culture by endogenously synthesized antisense RNA and mRNA cleaving ribozymes. *Abstracts of the 7th International Conference on AIDS*, 16–21 June 1991, Florence, p. 202, W.A.1009.

Jameson, B. A., Rao, P. E., Kong, L. I., Hahn, B. H., Shaw, G. M., Hood, L. E., and Kent, S. B. H. (1988). Location and chemical synthesis of a binding site for HIV-1 on the CD4 protein. *Science*, **240**, 1335–9.

Javaherian, K., Langlois, A. J., McDanal, C., Ross, K. L., Eckler, L. I., Jellis, C. L., *et al.* (1989). Principal neutralizing domain of the human immunodeficiency virus type 1 envelope protein. *Proceedings of the National Academy of Sciences of the United States of America*, **86**, 6768–72.

Jayasena, S. D. and Johnston, B. H. (1992). Site-specific cleavage of the transactivation response site of human immunodeficiency virus RNA with a tat-based chemical nuclease. *Proceedings of the National Academy of Sciences of the United States of America*, **89**, 3526–30.

Jones, K. A., Kadonaga, J. T., Luciw, P. A., and Tjian, R. (1986). Activation of the AIDS retrovirus promoter by the cellular transcription factor SP1. *Science*, **232**, 755–9.

Kalyanaraman, V. S., Rausch, D. M., Osborne, J., Padgett, M., Hwang, K. M., Lifson, J. D., and Eiden, L. E. (1990). Evidence by peptide mapping that the region CD4(81–92) is involved in gp120/CD4 interaction leading to HIV infection and HIV-induced syncytium formation. *Journal of Immunology*, **145**, 4072–8.

Kaminchik, J., Bashan, N., Itach, A., Sarver, N., Gorecki, M., and Panet, A. (1991). Genetic characterization of human immunodeficiency virus type 1 Nef gene products translated *in vitro* and expressed in mammalian cells. *Journal of Virology*, **65**, 583–8.

Kestler, H. W. III, Ringler, D. J., Mori, K., Panicali, D. L., Sehgal, P. K., Daniel, M. D., and Desrosiers, R. C. (1991). Importance of the *nef* gene for maintenance of high virus loads and for development of AIDS. *Cell*, **65**, 651–62.

Kim, S., Byrn, R., Groopman, J., and Baltimore, D. (1989a). Temporal aspects of DNA and RNA synthesis during human immunodeficiency virus infection: evidence for differential gene expression. *Journal of Virology*, **63**, 3708–13.

Kim, S. Y., Ikeuchi, K., Byrn, R., Groopman, J., and Baltimore, D. (1989b). Lack of a negative influence on viral growth by the *nef* gene of human immunodeficiency virus type 1. *Proceedings of the National Academy of Sciences of the United States of America*, **86**, 9544–8.

Kjems, J., Brown, M., Chang, D. D., and Sharp, P. A. (1991). Structural analysis of the interaction between the human immunodeficiency virus Rev protein and the Rev response element. *Proceedings of the National Academy of Sciences of the United States of America*, **88**, 683–7.

Klatzmann, D., Champagne, E., Chamaret, S., Gruest, J., Guetard, D., Hercend, T., et al. (1984). T-lymphocyte T4 molecule behaves as the receptor for human retrovirus LAV. *Nature, London*, **312**, 767–8.

Kohl, N. E., Emini, E. A., Schleif, W. A., Davis, L. J., Heimbach, J. C., Dixon, R. A. F., et al. (1988). Active human immunodeficiency virus protease is required for viral infectivity. *Proceedings of the National Academy of Sciences of the United States of America*, **85**, 4686–90.

Kohlstaedt, L. A., Wang, J., Friedman, J. M., Rice, P. A., and Steitz, T. A. (1992). Crystal structure at 3.5 Å resolution of HIV-1 reverse transcriptase complexed with an inhibitor. *Science*, **256**, 1783–90.

Kubota, S., Endo, S., Maki, M., and Hatanaka, M. (1989). Role of the cysteine-rich region of HIV tat protein on its trans-activational ability. *Virus Genes*, **2**, 113–8.

Kuppuswamy, M., Subramanian, T., Srinivasan, A., and Chinnadurai, G. (1989). Multiple functional domains of Tat, the trans-activator of HIV-1, defined by mutational analysis. *Nucleic Acids Research*, **17**, 3551–61.

Kwong, P. D., Ryu, S., Hendrickson, W. A., Axel, R., Sweet, R. M., Folena-Wasserman, G., et al. (1990). Molecular characteristics of recombinant human CD4 as deduced from polymorphic crystals. *Proceedings of the National Academy of Sciences of the United States of America*, **87**, 6423–7.

Landau, N. R., Warton, M., and Littman, D. R. (1988). The envelope glycoprotein of the human immunodeficiency virus binds to the immunoglobulin-like domain of CD4. *Nature, London*, **334**, 159–62.

Lapatto, R., Blundell, T., Hemmings, A., Overington, J., Wilderspin, A., Wood, S., et al. (1989). X-ray analysis of HIV-1 proteinase at 2.7 Å resolution confirms structural homology among retroviral enzymes. *Nature, London*, **342**, 299–302.

Lasky, L. A., Nakamura, G., Smith, D. H., Fennie, C., Shimasaki, C., Patzer, E., et al. (1987). Delineation of a region of the human immunodeficiency virus type 1 gp120 glycoprotein critical for interaction with the CD4 receptor. *Cell*, **50**, 975–85.

Leonard, C. K., Spellman, M. W., Riddle, L., Harris, R. J., Thomas, J. N., and Gregory, T. J. (1990). Assignment of intrachain disulfide bonds and characterization of potential glycosylation sites of the type 1 recombinant human immunodeficiency virus envelope glycoprotein (gp120) expressed in chinese hamster ovary cells. *Journal of Biological Chemistry*, **265**, 10363–82.

Lifson, J. D., Hwang, K. M., Nara, P. L., Fraser, B., Padgett, M., Dunlop, N. M., and Eiden, L. E. (1988). Synthetic CD4 peptide derivatives that inhibit HIV infection and cytopathicity. *Science*, **241**, 712–16.

Linsley, P. S., Ledbetter, J. A., Kinney-Thomas, E., and Hu, S. (1988). Effects of anti-gp120 monoclonal antibodies on CD4 receptor binding by the *env* protein of human immunodeficiency virus type 1. *Journal of Virology*, **62**, 3695–702.

Looney, D. J., Hayashi, S., Nicklas, M., Redfield, R. R., Broder, S., Wong-Staal, F., and Mitsuya, H. (1990). Differences in the interaction of HIV-1 and HIV-2 with CD4. *Journal of Acquired Immune Deficiency Syndromes*, **3**, 649–57.

Loret, E. P., Georgel, P., Johnson, W. C. Jr., and Ho, P. S. (1992). Circular dichroism and molecular modeling yield a structure for the complex of human immunodeficiency virus type 1 trans-activation response RNA and the binding region of tat, the trans-acting transcriptonal activator. *Proceedings of the National Academy of Sciences of the United States of America*, **89**, 9734–8.

Lu, X., Heimer, J., Rekosh, D., and Hammarskjöld, M.-L. (1990). U1 small nuclear RNA plays a direct role in the formation of a Rev-regulated human immunodeficiency virus *env* mRNA that remains unspliced. *Proceedings of the National Academy of Sciences of the United States of America*, **87**, 7598–602.

Lucey, D. R., Dorsky, D. I., Nicholson-Weller, A., and Weller, P. F. (1989). Human eosinophils express CD4 protein and bind human immunodeficiency virus 1 gp120. *Journal of Experimental Medicine*, **169**, 327–32.

Lucey, D. R., Hensley, R. E., Ward, W. W., Butzin, C. A., and Boswell, R. N. (1991). CD4$^+$ monocyte counts in persons with HIV-1 infection: an early increase is followed by a progressive decline. *Journal of Acquired Immune Deficiency Syndromes*, **4**, 24–30.

Luciw, P. A., Cheng-Mayer, C., and Levy, J. A. (1987). Mutational analysis of the human immunodeficiency virus: the orf-B region down-regulates virus replication. *Proceedings of the National Academy of Sciences of the United States of America*, **84**, 1434–8.

Lyerly, H. K., Matthews, T. J., Langlois, A. J., Bolognesi, D. P., and Weinhold, K. J. (1987). Human T-cell lymphotropic virus III$_B$ glycoprotein (gp120) bound to CD4 determinants on normal lymphocytes and expressed by infected cells serves as target for immune attack. *Proceedings of the National Academy of Sciences of the United States of America*, **84**, 4601–5.

McClure, M. O., Sattentau, Q. J., Beverley, P. C. L., Hearn, J. P., FitzGerald, A. K., Zuckerman, A. J., and Weiss, R. A. (1987). HIV infection of primate lymphocytes and conservation of the CD4 receptor. *Nature, London*, **330**, 487–9.

McCune, J. M. (1991). HIV-1: the infective process *in vivo*. *Cell*, **64**, 351–63.

McCune, J. M., Rabin, L. B., Feinberg, M. B., Lieberman, M., Kosek, J. C., Reyes, G. R., and Weissman, I. L. (1988). Endoproteolytic cleavage of gp160 is required for the activation of human immunodeficiency virus. *Cell*, **53**, 55–67.

McDougal, J., Mawle, A., Cort, S. P., Nicholson, J. K. A., Cross, G. D., Scheppler-Campbell, J. A., *et al.* (1985). Cellular tropism of the human retrovirus HTLV-III/LAV. *Journal of Immunology*, **135**, 3151–62.

McDougal, J., Nicholson, J., Cross, G., Cort, S., Kennedy, M., and Mawle, A. (1986a). Binding of the human retrovirus HTLV-III/LAV/ARV/HIV to the CD4 (T4) molecule: conformation dependence epitope mapping antibody inhibition and potential for idiopathic mimicry. *Journal of Immunology*, **137**, 2937–44.

McDougal, J., Kennedy, M. S., Sligh, J. M., Cort, S. P., Mawle, A., and Nicholson, K. A. (1986b). Binding of HTLV-III/LAV to T4$^+$ T cells by a complex of the 110 K viral protein and the T4 molecule. *Science*, **231**, 382–5.

McKeating, J. A. and Willey, R. L. (1989). Structure and function of the HIV envelope. *AIDS*, **3**, S35–41.

McQuade, T. J., Tomasselli, A. G., Liu, L., Karacostas, V., Moss, B., Sawyer, T. K., *et al.* (1990). A synthetic HIV-1 protease inhibitor with antiviral activity arrests HIV-1 like particle maturation. *Science*, **247**, 454–6.

Maddon, P. J., Littman, D. R., Godfrey, M., Maddon, D. E., Chess, L., and Axel, R. (1985). The isolation and nucleotide sequence of a cDNA encoding the T cell surface protein T4: a new member of the immunoglobulin gene family. *Cell*, **42**, 93–104.

Maddon, P. J., Dalgleish, A. G., McDougal, J. S., Clapham, P. R., Weiss, R. A., and Axel, R. (1986). The T4 gene encodes the AIDS virus receptor and is expressed in the immune system and the brain. *Cell*, **47**, 333–48.

Maddon, P. J., Molineaux, S. M., Maddon, D. E., Zimmerman, K. A., Godfrey, M., Alt, F. W., *et al.* (1987). Structure and expression of the human and mouse T4 genes. *Proceedings of the National Academy of Sciences of the United States of America*, **84**, 9155–9.

Malim, M. H. and Cullen, B. R. (1991). HIV-1 Structural gene expression requires the binding of multiple Rev monomers to the viral RRE: implications for HIV-1 latency. *Cell*, **65**, 241–8.

Malim, M. H., Hauber, J., Fenrick, R., and Cullen, B. R. (1988). Immunodeficiency virus rev trans-activator modulates the expression of the viral regulatory genes. *Nature, London*, **335**, 181–3.

Malim, M. H., Hauber, J., Le, S. Y., Maizel, J. V., and Cullen, B. R. (1989a). The HIV-1 rev *trans*-activator acts through a structured target sequence to activate nuclear export of unspliced viral mRNA. *Nature, London* **338**, 254–7.

Malim, M. H., Bohnlein, S., Hauber, J., and Cullen, B. R. (1989b). Functional dissection of the HIV-1 *rev* transactivation: derivation of a *trans*-dominant repressor of *rev* function. *Cell*, **58**, 205–14.

Matsukura, M., Zon, G., Shinozuka, K., Robert-Guroff, M., Shimada, T., Stein, C. A., *et al.* (1989). Regulation of viral expression of human immunodeficiency virus *in vitro* by an antisense phosphorothioate oligodeoxynucleotide against *rev* (*art*/*trs*) in chronically infected cells. *Proceedings of the National Academy of Sciences of the United States of America*, **86**, 4244–8.

Matsushita, S., Robert-Guroff, M., Rusche, J., Koito, A., Hattori, T., Hoshino, H., *et al.* (1988). Characterization of a human immunodeficiency virus neutralizing monoclonal antibody and mapping of the neutralizing epitope. *Journal of Virology*, **62**, 2107–14.

Meek, T. D., Lambert, D. M., Dreyer, G. B., Carr, T. J., Tomaszek, T. A., Jr, Moore, M. L., *et al.* (1990). Inhibition of HIV-1 protease in infected T-lymphocytes by synthetic peptide analogues. *Nature, London*, **343**, 90–2.

Merluzzi, V. J., Hargrave, K. D., Labadia, M., Grozinger, K., Skoog, M., Wu, J. C., *et al.* (1990). Inhibition of HIV-1 replication by a nonnucleoside reverse transcriptase inhibitor. *Science*, **250**, 1411–13.

Miller, M., Schneider, J., Sathyanarayana, B. K., Toth, M. V., Marshall, G. R., Clawson, L., *et al.* (1989). Structure of complex of synthetic HIV-1 protease with a substrate-based inhibitor at 2.3 Å resolution. *Science*, **246**, 1149–52.

Mizukami, T., Fuerst, T. R., Berger, E. A., and Moss, B. (1988). Binding region for human immunodeficiency virus (HIV) and epitopes for HIV-blocking monoclonal antibodies of the CD4 molecule defined by site-directed mutagenesis. *Proceedings of the National Academy of Sciences of the United States of America*, **85**, 9273–7.

Modrow, S., Hahn, B. H., Shaw, G. M., Gallo, R. C., Wong-Staal, F., and Wolf, H. (1987). Computer-assisted analysis of envelope protein sequences of seven human immunodeficiency virus isolates: prediction of antigenic epitopes in conserved and variable regions. *Journal of Virology*, **61**, 570–8.

Montagnier, L., Gruest, J., Chamaret, S., Dauguet, C., Axler, C., Guétard, D., *et al.* (1984). Adaptation of lymphadenopathy associated virus (LAV) to replication in EBV-transformed B lymphoblastoid cell lines. *Science*, **225**, 63–6.

Moore, J. P. (1990). Simple methods for monitoring HIV-1 and HIV-2 gp120 binding to soluble CD4 by enzyme-linked immunosorbent assay: HIV-2 has a 25-fold lower affinity than HIV-1 for soluble CD4. *AIDS*, **4**, 297–305.

Mosca, J. D., Bednarik, D. P., Raj, N. B. K., Rosen, C. A., Sodroski, J. G., Haseltine, W. A., and Pitha, P. M. (1987). Herpes simplex virus type 1 can reactivate transcription of latent human immunodeficiency virus. *Nature, London*, **325**, 67–70.

Müller, W. E. G., Rytik, P. G., Okamoto, T., Pfeifer, K., Merz, H., and Schroder, H. C. (1991). Increase of prion gene expression caused by the HIV-1 transactivator protein *tat* in human astrocytes. *Abstracts of the 7th International Conference on AIDS*, 16–21 June 1991, Florence, p. 195, TH.A.69.

Nabel, G. J., Rice, S. A., Knipe, D. M., and Baltimore, D. (1988). Alternative mechanisms for activation of human immunodeficiency virus enhancer in T cells. *Science*, **239**, 1299–302.

Nalin, C. M., Purcell, R. D., Antelman, D., Mueller, D., Tomchak, L., Wegrzynski, B., *et al.* (1990). Purification and characterization of recombinant Rev protein of human immunodeficiency virus type 1. *Proceedings of the National Academy of Sciences of the United States of America*, **87**, 7593–7.

Nara, P. L., Hwang, K. M., Rausch, D. M., Lifson, J. D., and Eiden, L. E. (1989). CD4 antigen-based antireceptor peptides inhibit infectivity of human immunodeficiency virus *in vitro* at multiple stages of the viral life cycle. *Proceedings of the National Academy of Sciences of the United States of America*, **86**, 7139–43.

Navia, M. A., Fitzgerald, P. M. D., McKeever, B. M., Leu, C.-T., Heimbach, J. C., Herber, W. K., *et al.* (1989). Three-dimensional structure of aspartyl protease from human immunodeficiency virus HIV-1. *Nature, London*, **337**, 615–20.

Ogawa, K., Shibata, R., Kiyomasu, T., Higuchi, I., Kishida, Y., Ishimoto, A., and Adachi, A. (1989). Mutational analysis of the human immunodeficiency virus *vpr* open reading frame. *Journal of Virology*, **63**, 4110–4.

Okamoto, T. and Wong-Staal, F. (1986). Demonstration of virus-specific transcriptional activator(s) in cells infected with HTLV-III by an *in vitro* cell-free system. *Cell*, **47**, 29–35.

Olsen, H. S., Cochrane, A. W., Dillon, P. J., Nalin, C. M., and Rosen, C. A. (1990). Interaction of the human immunodeficiency virus type 1 Rev protein with a structured region in env mRNA is dependent on multimer formation mediated through a basic stretch of amino acids. *Genes Development*, **4**, 1357–64.

Palker, T. J., Clark, M. E., Langlois, A. J., Matthews, T. J., Weinhold, K. J., Randall, R. R., *et al.* (1988). Type-specific neutralization of the human immunodeficiency virus with antibodies to *env*-encoded synthetic peptides. *Proceedings of the National Academy of Sciences of the United States of America*, **85**, 1932–6.

Patterson, S. and Knight, S. (1987). Susceptibility of human peripheral blood dendritic cells to infection by human immunodeficiency virus. *Journal of General Virology*, **68**, 1177–83.

Pauwels, R., Andries, K., Desmyter, J., Schols, D., Kukla, M. J., Breslin, H. J., *et al.* (1990). Potent and selective inhibition of HIV-1 replication *in vitro* by a novel series of TIBO derivatives. *Nature, London*, **343**, 470–4.

Pauwels, R., Andries, K., Debyser, Z., Van Daele, P., Schols, D., Stoffels, P., De Vreese, K., Woestenborghs, R., Vandamme, A.-M., Janssen, C. G. M., Anné, J., Cauwenbergh, G., Desmyter, J., Heykants, J., Janssen, M. A. C., De Clercq, E., and Janssen P. A. J. (1993). Potent and highly selective human immunodeficiency virus type 1 (HIV-1) inhibition by a series of a-anilinophenylacetamide derivatives targeted at HIV-1 reverse transcriptase. *Proceedings of the National Academy of Sciences of the United States of America*, **90**, 1711–15.

Pearl, L. H. and Taylor, W. R. (1987). A structural model for the retroviral proteases. *Nature, London*, **329**, 351–4.

Perkins, A., Cochrane, A. W., Ruben, S. M., and Rosen, C. A. (1989). Structural and functional characterization of the human immunodeficiency virus *rev* protein. *Journal of the Acquired Immune Deficiency Syndromes*, **2**, 256–63.

Peterson, A. and Seed, B. (1988). Genetic analysis of monoclonal anti-body and HIV binding sites on the human lymphocyte antigen CD4. *Cell*, **54**, 65–72.

Puglisi, J. D., Tan, R., Calnan, B. J., Frankel, A. D., and Williamson, J. R. (1992). Conformation of the tar RNA-arginine complex by NMR spectroscopy. *Science*, **257**, 76–80.

Rhodes, A. and James, W. (1990). Inhibition of human immunodeficiency virus replication in cell culture by endogenously synthesized antisense RNA. *Journal of General Virology*, **71**, 1965–74.

Ricchetti, M. and Buc, H. (1990). Reverse transcriptases and genomic variability: the accuracy of DNA replication is enzyme specific and sequence dependent. *EMBO Journal*, **9**, 1583–93.

Rimsky, L., Hauber, J., Dukovich, M., Malim, M. H., Langlois, A., Cullen, B. R., and Green, W. C. (1988). Functional replacement of the HIV-1 *rev* protein by the HTLV-1 rex protein. *Nature, London*, **335**, 738–40.

Roberts, N. A., Martin, J. A., Kinchington, D., Broadhurst, A. V., Craig, J. C., Duncan, I. B., *et al.* (1990). Rational design of peptide-based HIV proteinase inhibitors. *Science*, **248**, 358–61.

Rosenberg, Z. F. and Fauci, A. S. (1990). Activation of latent HIV infection. *Journal of the National Institutes of Health Research*, **2**, 41–5.

Roy, S., Parkin, N. T., Rosen, C., Itovitch, J., and Sonenberg, N. (1990). Structural requirements for *trans* activation of human immunodeficiency virus type 1 long terminal repeat-directed gene expression by *tat*: importance of base pairing, loop sequence, and bulges in the *tat*-responsive sequence. *Journal of Virology*, **64**, 1402–6.

Ruben, S., Perkins, A., Purcell, R., Joung, K., Sia, R., Burghoff, R., *et al.* (1989). Structural and functional characterization of human immunodeficiency virus *tat* protein. *Journal of Virology*, **63**, 1–8.

Rusche, J. R., Javaherian, K., McDanal, C., Petro, J., Lynn, D. L., Grimaila, R., *et al.* (1988). Antibodies that inhibit fusion of human immunodeficiency virus-infected cells bind a 24-amino acid sequence of the viral envelope, gp120. *Proceedings of the National Academy of Sciences of the United States of America*, **85**, 3198–202.

Ryu, S. E., Kwong, P. D., Truneh, A., Porter, T. G., Arthos, J., Rosenberg, M., *et al.* (1990). Crystal structure of an HIV-binding recombinant fragment of human CD4. *Nature, London*, **348**, 419–26.

Salfeld, J., Gottlinger, H. G., Sia, R. A., Park, R. E., Sodroski, J. G., and Haseltine, W. A. (1990). A tripartite HIV-1 tat-env-rev fusion protein. *EMBO Journal*, **9**, 965–70.

Sattentau, Q. J., Dalgleish, A. G., Weiss, R. A., and Beverley, P. C. L. (1986). Epitopes of the CD4 antigen and HIV infection. *Science*, **234**, 1120–3.

Sattentau, Q. J., Clapham, P. R., Weiss, R. A., Beverley, P. C. L., Montagnier, L., Alhalabi, M. F., *et al.* (1988). The human and simian immunodeficiency viruses HIV-1, HIV-2 and SIV interact with similar epitopes on their cellular receptor, the CD4 molecule. *AIDS*, **2**, 101–5.

Sattentau, Q. J., Arthos, J., Deen, K., Hanna, N., Healey, D., Beverley, P. C. L., *et al.* (1989). Structural analysis of the human immunodeficiency virus-binding domain of CD4. Epitope mapping with site-directed mutants and anti-idiotypes. *Journal of Experimental Medicine*, **170**, 1319–34.

Schols, D., Baba, M., Pauwels, R., Desmyter, J., and De Clercq, E. (1989). Specific interaction of aurintricarboxylic acid with the human immunodeficiency virus/ CD4 cell receptor. *Proceedings of the National Academy of Sciences of the United States of America*, **86**, 3322–6.

Schols, D., Pauwels, R., Desmyter, J., and De Clercq, E. (1990). Dextran sulfate and other polyanionic anti-HIV compounds specifically interact with the viral gp120 glycoprotein expressed by T-cells persistently infected with HIV-1. *Virology*, **175**, 556–61.

Schols, D., Wutzler, P., Klöcking, R., Helbig, B., and De Clercq, E. (1991). Selective inhibitory activity of polyhydroxycarboxylates derived from phenolic compounds against human immunodeficiency virus replication. *Journal of Acquired Immune Deficiency Syndromes*, **4**, 677–85.

Schols, D., Pauwels, R., Desmyter, J., and De Clercq, E. (1992). Differential activity of polyanionic compounds and castanospermine against HIV replication and HIV-induced syncytium formation depending on virus strain and cell type. *Antiviral Chemistry and Chemotherapy*, in press.

Schröder, H. C., Ugarkovic, D., Wenger, R., Reuter, P., Okamoto, T., and Müller, W. E. G. (1990). Binding of Tat protein to TAR region of human immunodeficiency virus type 1 blocks TAR-mediated activation of (2′-5′)oligoadenylate synthetase. *AIDS Research and Human Retroviruses*, **6**, 659–72.

Scott, C. F., Jr, Silver, S., Profy, A. T., Putney, S. D., Langlois, A., Weinhold, K., and Robinson, J. E. (1990). Human monoclonal antibody that recognizes the V3 region of human immunodeficiency virus gp120 and neutralizes the human T-lymphotropic virus type III$_{MN}$ strain. *Proceedings of the National Academy of Sciences of the United States of America*, **87**, 8591–601.

Sekigawa, I., Chamow, S. M., Groopman, J. E., and Byrn, R. A. (1990). CD4 immunoadhesin but not recombinant soluble CD4 blocks syncytium formation by human immunodeficiency virus type 2-infected lymphoid cells. *Journal of Virology*, **64**, 5194–8.

Selby, M. J., Bain, E. S., Luciw, P. A., and Peterlin, B. M. (1989). Structure sequence and position of the stem-loop in *tar* determine transcriptional elongation by *tat* through the HIV-1 long terminal repeat. *Genes Development*, **3**, 547–58.

SenGupta, D. N., Berkhout, B., Gatignol, A., Zhou, A. M., and Silverman, R. H. (1990). Direct evidence for translational regulation by leader RNA and TAT protein of human immunodeficiency virus type 1. *Proceedings of the National Academy of Sciences of the United States of America*, **87**, 7492–6.

Skinner, M. A., Ting, R., Langlois, A. J., Weinhold, K. J., Lyerly, H. K., Javaherian, K., and Matthews, T. J. (1988a). Characteristics of a neutralizing monoclonal antibody to the HIV envelope glycoprotein. *AIDS Research and Human Retroviruses*, **4**, 187–97.

Skinner, M. A., Langlois, A. J., McDanal, C. B., McDougal, J. S., Bolognesi, D. P., and Matthews, T. J. (1988b). Neutralizing antibodies to an immunodominant envelope sequence do not prevent gp120 binding to CD4. *Journal of Virology*, **62**, 4195–200.

Smith, D. H., Byrn, R. A., Marsters, S. A., Gregory, T., Groopman, J. E., and Capon, D. J. (1987). Blocking of HIV-1 infectivity by a soluble secreted form of the CD4 antigen. *Science*, **238**, 1704–7.

Sodroski, J., Goh, W. C., Rosen, C., Tartar, A., Portetelle, D., Burny, A., and Haseltine, W. (1986a). Replicative and cytopathic potential of HTLV-III/LAV with *sor* gene deletions. *Science*, **231**, 1549–53.

Sodroski, J., Goh, W. C., Rosen, C., Dayton, A., Terwilliger, E., and Haseltine, W. (1986b). A second post-transcriptional *trans*-activator gene required for HTLV-III replication. *Nature, London*, **321**, 412–17.

Southgate, C., Zapp, M. L., and Green, M. R. (1990). Activation of transcription by HIV-1 Tat protein tethered to nascent RNA through another protein. *Nature, London*, **345**, 640–2.

Stein, B., Rahmsdorf, H. J., Steffen, A., Litfin, M., and Herrlich, P. (1989). UV-induced DNA damage is an intermediate step in UV-induced expression of human immunodeficiency virus type collagenase c-*fos*, and metallothionein. *Molecular and Cellular Biology*, **9**, 5169–81.

Strebel, K., Daugherty, D., Clouse, K., Cohen, D., Folks, T., and Martin, M. A. (1987). The HIV 'A' (*sor*) gene product is essential for virus infectivity. *Nature, London*, **328**, 728–30.

Sun, N., Ho, D. D., Sun, C. R. Y., Liou, R., Gordon, W., Fung, M. S. C., et al. (1989). Generation and characterization of monoclonal antibodies to the putative CD4-binding domain of human immunodeficiency virus type 1 gp120. *Journal of Virology*, **63**, 3579–85.

Temin, H. N. and Baltimore, D. (1972). RNA-directed DNA synthesis and RNA tumor viruses. *Advances in Virus Research*, **17**, 129–86.

Terwilliger, E., Sodroski, J. G., Rosen, C. A., and Haseltine, W. A. (1986). Effects of mutations within the 3' *orf* open reading frame region of human T-cell virus type III (HTLV-III/LAV) on replication and cytopathogenicity. *Journal of Virology*, **60**, 754–60.

Terwilliger, E. F., Cohen, E. A., Lu, Y., Sodroski, J. G., and Haseltine, W. A. (1989). Functional role of human immunodeficiency virus type 1 *vpu*. *Proceedings of the National Academy of Sciences of the United States of America*, **86**, 5163–7.

Thomas, Y., Rogozinski, L., Irigoyen, O. H., Friedman, S. M., Kung, P. C., Goldstein, G., and Chess, L. (1981). Functional analysis of human T cell, subsets defined by monoclonal antibodies. IV. Induction of suppressor cells within the OKT4$^+$ population. *Journal of Experimental Medicine*, **154**, 459–67.

Tiley, L. S., Brown, P. H., Le, S.-Y., Maizel, J. V., Clements, J. E., and Cullen, B. R. (1990). Visna virus encodes a post-transcriptional regulator of viral structural gene expression. *Proceedings of the National Academy of Sciences of the United States of America*, **87**, 7497–501.

Tiley, L. S., Malim, M. H., Tewary, H. K., Stockley, P. G., and Cullen, B. R. (1992). Identification of a high-affinity RNA-binding site for the human immunodeficiency virus type 1 Rev protein. *Proceedings of the National Academy of Sciences of the United States of America*, **89**, 758–62.

Till, M. A., Ghetie, V., Gregory, T., Patzer, E. J., Porter, J. P., Uhr, J. W., *et al.* (1988). HIV-infected cells are killed by rCD4-ricin A chain. *Science*, **242**, 1166–8.

Till, M. A., Zolla-Pazner, S., Gorny, M. K., Patton, J. S., Uhr, J. W., and Vitetta, E. S. (1989). Human immunodeficiency virus-infected T cells and monocytes are killed by monoclonal human anti-gp41 antibodies coupled to ricin A chain. *Proceedings of the National Academy of Sciences of the United States of America*, **86**, 1987–91.

Tisdale, M., Ertl, P., Larder, B. A., Purifoy, D. J. M., Darby, G., and Powell, K. L. (1988). Characterization of human immunodeficiency virus type 1 reverse transcriptase by using monoclonal antibodies: role of the C terminus in antibody reactivity and enzyme function. *Journal of Virology*, **62**, 3662–7.

Tomasselli, A. G., Howe, W. J., Sawyer, T. K., Wlodawer, A., and Heinrikson, R. L. (1991). The complexities of AIDS: an assessment of the HIV protease as a therapeutic target. *Chimica Oggi*, May 6–27.

Traunecker, A., Lucke, W., and Karjalainen, K. (1988). Soluble CD4 molecules neutralize human immunodeficiency virus type 1. *Nature, London*, **331**, 84–6.

Traunecker, A., Schneider, J., Kiefer, H., and Karjalainen, K. (1989). Highly efficient neutralization of HIV with recombinant CD4-immunoglobulin molecules. *Nature, London*, **339**, 68–73.

Tsubota, H., Winkler, G., Meade, H. M., Jakubowski, A., Thomas, D. W., and Letvin, N. L. (1990). CD4-*Pseudomonas exotoxin* conjugates delay but do not fully inhibit human immunodeficiency virus replication in lymphocytes *in vitro*. *Journal of Clinical Investigation*, **86**, 1684–9.

Vaishnav, Y. N., Vaishnav, M., and Wong-Staal, F. (1991). Identification and characterization of a nuclear factor that specifically binds to the Rev response element (RRE) of human immunodeficiency virus type 1 (HIV-1). *New Biology*, **3**, 142–50.

Valerie, K. and Rosenberg, M. (1990). Chromatin structure implicated in activation of HIV-1 gene expression by ultraviolet light. *New Biology* **2**, 812–18.

Veronese, F. D., DeVico, A. L., Copeland, T. D., Oroszlan, S., Gallo, R. C., and Sarngadharan, M. G. (1985). Characterization of gp41 as the transmembrane protein coded by the HTLV-III/LAV envelope gene. *Science*, **229**, 1402–5.

Veronese, F. D., Copeland, T. D., DeVico, A. L., Rahman, R., Oroszlan, S., Gallo, R. C., and Sarngadharan, M. G. (1986). Characterization of highly immunogenic p66/p51 as the reverse transcriptase of HTLV-III/LAV. *Science*, **231**, 1289–91.

Wang, J., Yan, Y., Garrett, T. P. J., Liu, J., Rodgers, D. W., Garlick, R. L., *et al.* (1990). Atomic structure of a fragment of man CD4 containing two immunoglobulin-like domains. *Nature, London*, **348**, 411–18.

Werner, A., Winskowsky, G., and Kurth, R. (1990). Soluble CD4 enhances simian immunodeficiency virus SIV$_{agm}$ infection. *Journal of Virology*, **64**, 6252–6.

Willey, R. L., Smith, D. H., Lasky, L. A., Theodore, T. S., Earl, P. L., Moss, B. (1988). *In vitro* mutagenesis identifies a region within the envelope gene of the human immunodeficiency virus that is critical for infectivity. *Journal of Virology*, **62**, 139–47.

Willey, R. L., Ross, E. K., Buckler-White, A. J., Theodore, T. S., and Martin, M. A. (1989). Functional interaction of constant and variable domains of human immunodeficiency virus type 1 gp120. *Journal of Virology*, **63**, 3595–600.

Wilson, W., Braddock, M., Adams, S. E., Rathjen, P. D., Kingsman, S. M., and Kingsman, A. J. (1988). HIV expression strategies: ribosomal frameshifting is directed by a short sequence in both mammalian and yeast systems. *Cell*, **55**, 1159–69.

Witvrouw, M., Pauwels, R., Vandamme, A.-M., Schols, D., Reymen, D., Yamamoto, N., *et al.* (1992). Cell type-specific anti-human immunodeficiency virus type 1 activity of the transactivation inhibitor Ro5–3335. *Antimicrobial Agents and Chemotherapy*, **36**, 2628–33.

Wlodawer, A., Miller, M., Jaskólski, M., Sathyanavayana, B. K., Baldwin, E., Weber, I. T., *et al.* (1989). Conserved folding in retroviral proteases: crystal structure of a synthetic HIV-I protease. *Science,* **245**, 616–21.

Wood, G. S., Warner, N. L., and Warnke, R. A. (1983). Anti-Leu-3/T4 antibodies react with cells of monocyte/macrophage and Langerhans lineage. *Journal of Immunology*, **131**, 212–16.

Zaia, J. A., Rossi, J. J., Murakawa, G. J., Spallone, P. A., Stephens, D. A., Kaplan, B. E., *et al.* (1988). Inhibition of human immunodeficiency virus by using an oligonucleoside methylphosphonate targeted to the *tat*-3 gene. *Journal of Virology*, **62**, 3914–17.

Zapp, M. L. and Green, M. R. (1989). Sequence-specific RNA binding by the HIV-1 rev protein. *Nature, London*, **342**, 714–16.

Section 6B
HIV protease inhibitors
Jed F. Fisher, W. Gary Tarpley, and Suvit Thaisrivongs

6B.1   Introduction

Life is a fragile possession. This simple instruction is taught to each new generation by the unexpected intervention of catastrophe, war, or pandemic. For many of this generation—from the indigent African to the affluent American—the instructor of this lesson is the pandemic of the human immunodeficiency virus (HIV). From the uncertain time of its appearance this century in the human species to its recognition by the medical community as a pandemic about 12 years ago, the understanding of this virus has progressed to the point that it may fairly be claimed that HIV is, at the molecular level, the best understood human viral pathogen. It is now recognized as one of the genomically more complex members of the lentivirus class of the retroviruses (Ratner *et al*. 1985; Haseltine 1991). Although there is now considerable understanding of the life history of this retrovirus, neither a knowledge of the viral genome nor an awareness of the stratagems by which the viral RNA genome is ultimately integrated into the host DNA offer in and of themselves a cure. While there is no doubt that HIV is indeed the disease contagion, there is much to be learned as to the serpentine connection between the initial infection of permissive cells of the host and the complete collapse of the host immune response years later. However, the available knowledge does identify strategy. Many of the respects in which this virus differs from its human host at the molecular level are now established, and each point of difference offers a potentially viable strategy for the delivery of a selective and lethal chemotherapeutic agent (De Clercq 1990; Mitsuya *et al.* 1990, 1991; Arnold and Arnold 1991; Richman 1991). The focus of this chapter is on one such target—the aspartyl protease of this virus.

The evaluation of each target—here, the protease—is made through the answers to three questions.

Is the target essential? The folly of choosing a target for which the answer is negative is self-evident. Yet few questions in science are satisfactorily answered with unqualified positive or negative responses, and HIV is a case in point. While the evidence that its protease is essential to the cellular synthesis of infectious virions by infected cells is compelling, we are less certain of the full relationship of infectious virion synthesis to the eventual clinical outcome of the disease. The choice of this protease as a chemotherapeutic target is made on the basis of its proven role as the temporal catalyst of virion maturation, and the expectation that an agent which delays the synthesis of the infectious virion (and hence the progression of viral infection) will enable the host immune surveillance to operate and thus ameliorate the disease progression. For the moment, however, this expectation remains a matter of faith.

Is the target suggestive of a defined chemical strategy with respect to its compromise? *Is the target unique*? If either question is answered in the negative, then regardless of the target's essentialness, the promise of intervention at that point is devalued. For example, the rapid antigenic diversification by this virus may preclude the stable epitope necessary for vaccine recognition. Regardless of our ability to identify individual epitopes (the target), their potential instability in the face of a chemical agent (the vaccine) incapable of adjusting to this change reduces confidence in the strategy. This is not to say that such approaches are unworthy (indeed, resistance is the inevitable fate of every chemotherapeutic weapon), but rather that those targets for which a defined chemical strategy is articulated are those for which inhibitor design is facilitated and focused. Two approaches identify the chemical structure by which a strategy is made tangible. The first—empirical discovery of a lead—is the traditional method. A recent example is the identification of a specific inhibitor of the HIV *tat* protein (Hsu *et al.* 1991). The effort to identify HIV protease inhibitors illustrates (primarily) the second method. Here, it is the accrued knowledge of established strategies for protease inhibitor design which has engendered the structural leads. These aspects have been summarized in numerous reviews, including those describing the HIV aspartyl protease structure function (Krausslich and Wimmer 1988; Blundell and Pearl 1989; Hellen *et al.* 1989; Skalka 1989; Kay and Dunn 1990; Navia and McKeever

1990; Oroszlan and Luftig 1990; von der Helm *et al*. 1990; Fitzgerald and Springer 1991; Scharpe *et al*. 1991; Wlodawer *et al*. 1992; Griffiths *et al*. 1992); the assay of its catalytic activity (Billich *et al*. 1991; Tyagi and Carter 1992); and the promise of its inhibitors as therapeutic agents (Debouck and Metcalf 1990; Korant 1990; Meek *et al*. 1990a; Stewart 1990; Baboonian and Dalgleish 1991; Huff 1991; Hui *et al*. 1991; Norbeck and Kempf 1991; Petteway *et al*. 1991; Tomasselli *et al*. 1991c, 1992). The first aim of this chapter is to provide a brief account of the protease as an essential component of the HIV life-cycle. This requires no deeper understanding than that provided by the simplest definition of the word 'protease': a protein catalyst for peptide bond hydrolysis. The full role of this protease in the HIV life-cycle and the task of fashioning an effective inhibitor requires more detailed knowledge. Here, the protease must be recognized as an *aspartyl* protease, named for the vicinal aspartic acid pair flanking the scissile amide. By this identification the intimacy requisite to inhibitor design is obtained. Finally, inhibitor design—a task of enormous breadth and rigour—is considered. Not only must the understanding of the protease as an enzyme allow a potent inhibitory molecular entity to be identified, but this entity must meet the demanding criteria of the practical therapeutic agent. These include accessible synthesis, acceptable means of delivery, satisfactory pharmacodynamics, and proven safety and efficacy. Thus the three criteria requisite for all therapeutic agent design—essentiality, strategy, and execution—comprise the organizational framework of this chapter.

6B.2   Essentiality: the HIV aspartyl protease as a catalyst for virion maturation

The placing of this proteolytic enzyme within the natural history of this virus begins with the relationship of the *gag* and *gag-pol* elements of the HIV genome to the mature infectious HIV virion. The HIV genome of some 9200 nucleotides is dominated by the three large open reading frames (*gag*, *pol*, and *env*) characteristic of the retroviruses (Cullen 1991). In addition, several smaller reading frames are found corresponding to the essential regulatory proteins *rev* and *tat*, to a second pair of proteins (*vif*, *vpu*), also essential to the maturation and release of the infective virion, and to two proteins of uncertain (and possibly non-essential) function (*vpr* and *nef*). The *gag* reading frame is the first encountered at the 5′ end, and follows the long terminal repeat at the beginning of the genome and a transactivation response element. The key structural proteins of the mature virus are made from the *gag* gene (Wills and Craven 1991; Henderson *et al*. 1992). These are the matrix protein (MA or p17), forming the structural shell on the inner viral membrane face, the capsid protein (CA or p24) obtained by proteolysis of the p25 precursor (Ehrlich *et al*. 1990), forming the exterior of the RNA-containing core within the capsid envelope, the nucleocapsid proteins (NC or p9), which coat the two genomic RNA molecules within each core, and the proline-rich p6 protein found at the *gag-pol* overlap which although unique to the HIV, has an essential role in enabling the occurrence of virion budding and release from the infected cell (Gottlinger *et al*. 1991). The *gag* gene is expressed as the single contiguous union of these four proteins (the p55 polyprotein) of overall structure H_2N-p17-p24-p1-p9-p6-CO_2H. This ordering MA-CA-NC is the same for all retroviral *gag* genes. The HIV aspartyl protease liberates each separate protein from this single polyprotein during the process of virion maturation.

In contrast to the proteins of the *gag* gene, *gag-pol* also encodes enzymes. During *gag* translation, a sequence-dependent -1 frameshift at UUA leucine codon, resulting in the formation of the p160 *gag-pol* polyprotein, occurs with a 5–10 per cent efficiency (Jacks *et al*. 1988; Park and Morrow 1991). This polyprotein contains, in addition to the *gag* structural proteins of MA-CA-NC (but not p6), three *pol* enzymes. These are the protease (PR) monomer (frame-shifted throughout the p6 reading frame), the reverse transcriptase (RT) monomer, and the integrase (IN). Release of these three enzymes is also protease dependent. However, since the protease is active as the catalyst only when existing as the homodimer (the non-covalent association of two monomers), prior to autoproteolytic release of itself (and the other components), two *gag-pol* polyproteins must engage the natured domains of their own protease monomers (see below).

Both the *gag* and *gag-pol* polyproteins are co-translationally modified by the addition of myristic acid to their N-terminus glycine residues (Bryant and Ratner 1990). The ability of this fatty acid to penetrate the inner membrane of the infected cell ultimately allows the congregation of all polyproteins at a membrane nucleating site (Gottlinger *et al*. 1989; Kaplan and Swanstrom 1991a; Ross *et al*. 1991). Moreover, this modification is essential to virion formation; prevention of myristoylation (for example, as by substitution of the glycine terminus by an alanine) results in the cytoplasmic accumulation of HIV gene products (Kaplan and Swanstrom 1991b; Park and Morrow 1991). The aggregation of polyproteins at the plasma membrane is the first step in virion formation. Even in the absence of the *gag-pol* polyprotein (and hence in the absence of a functional protease), the natured MA domain of the *gag* polyprotein commences the self-association process by which it forms a spherical shell, carrying forward the host cell membrane as its exterior ('budding'). In the HIV-infected cell, copious budding and release of immature virion occur continuously. The morphological appearance of the immature virion is that of a sphere, approximately 100–140 nm in diameter, with a hollow centre (Gelderblom 1991; Hoglund *et al*. 1992). Such an appearance is indicative of the close congregation of the intact polyproteins, still held to the inner membrane face by the myristoylated MA protein end. Immediately upon release, protease-dependent maturation of the immature virion commences. Proteo-lytic fragmentation of the polypeptide (leaving the myristoylated matrix protein still attached to the inner membrane face) permits the migration of protein mass to the virion centre, where the dense cone-shaped core assembles. This core is made of a capsid protein envelope, surrounding and protecting the pair of NC-RNA complexes. The products of the *env* gene also require proteolytic liberation, although not by the HIV aspartyl pro-tease. A cellular protease separates the *env* polypeptide into the membrane-embedded glycoprotein gp41 and the exterior glycoprotein gp120. As the mobile and now mature (hence infectious) virion travels, it is the ability of its exterior gp120 'knob' to form a non-covalent complex with recognition structures on the exterior of uninfected cells (Phillips 1991) which permits the first step of the infection cycle. Following gp120 recognition, structure binding is by membrane fusion and entry of the core into the cell. Dis-solution of the capsid structure releases the RNA which, by reverse tran-scription and integration, inserts as a permanent viral DNA addition to the cell's genome. Expression of the HIV genome provides the gene products (*gag*, *gag-pol*, *env*, *rev*, *tat*, . . .) and recommences immature virion synthesis. The release of these progeny completes the viral life-cycle.

The preceding summary has implied that the protease is *the* single catalyst of the temporal maturation of the HIV virion by an innate deconvolution of the *gag* and *gag-pol* polyproteins of the budding virion. This conclusion is inescapable from the experimental evidence, which falls almost seamlessly into place in a chronological narrative of experiment and observation. Initial recognition of a protease as a requisite catalyst for the retroviruses was established by deletion experiments within the protease gene of the related murine leukaemia virus (Crawford and Goff 1985; Katoh *et al.* 1985). Accordingly, having the sequenced HIV genome, Ratner *et al.* (1985) predicted that a protease would be found among the entities coded for by the HIV reading frames. Upon inspection of the HIV sequence, Toh *et al.* (1985) identified the constant active site amino acid triplet -AspThr(Ser)-Gly- of the aspartyl proteases (Yasunaga *et al.* 1986). However, a problem remained with respect to the identity of this triplet with an HIV aspartyl protease. All known aspartyl proteases are eukaryotic and comprise approximately 200 amino acids organized into two homologous domains, each contributing one of the two catalytic active site aspartyls (Blundell *et al.* 1990; Cooper *et al.* 1990; James *et al.* 1990; Sielecki *et al.* 1990; Veerapandian *et al.* 1990). However, the HIV open reading frame con-taining this triplet coded for only a 99 amino acid protein. A resolution of this dilemma was provided by Pearl and Taylor (1987), who predicted (correctly) that the viral aspartyl protease is a non-covalent dimer of the 99 amino acid protein. In this C_2-symmetric homodimer each half con-tributes one of the two active-site aspartate residues. Evidence in support of this hypothesis was provided by several self-consistent experiments, many

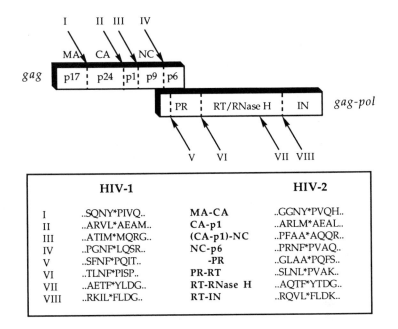

Fig. 6B.1 A schematic summary of the primary protease cleavage points in the HIV-1 and HIV-2 *gag* and *gag–pol* polyproteins.

of which were performed virtually simultaneously in several laboratories. These experiments begin with the heroic isolation of a protein from the virus itself (albeit without catalytic activity) with the predicted amino acid sequence (Lilehoj *et al.* 1988). Catalytic activity with respect to protease-dependent processing (or peptide cleavage) was found to be abolished by pepstatin, the classic aspartyl protease inhibitor (Katoh *et al.* 1987; Darke *et al.* 1988; Giam and Boros 1988; Hansen *et al.* 1988; Krausslich *et al.* 1988; Nutt *et al.* 1988; Schneider and Kent 1988; Seelmeier *et al.* 1988; Meek *et al.* 1989; Richards *et al.* 1989a,b; von der Helm *et al.* 1989; Grinde *et al.* 1990). Substitution for the active site Asp25 within the PR gene blocks proteolytic activity (Kohl *et al.* 1988; Le Grice *et al.* 1988; Seelmeier *et al.* 1988; Darke *et al.* 1989; Guenet *et al.* 1989) while the native enzyme (prepared by either recombinant or synthetic means) recombinant *gag* (or *gag-pol*) polyprotein proteolysis occurs (see Fig. 6B.1) (Crawford and Goff 1985; Kramer *et al.* 1986; Debouck *et al.* 1987; Darke *et al.* 1988; Giam and Boros 1988; Graves *et al.* 1988; Hansen *et al.* 1988; Kohl *et al.* 1988, 1991; Krausslich *et al.* 1988; Mous *et al.* 1988; Seelmeier *et al.* 1988; Krausslich *et al.* 1989; Meek *et al.* 1989; Peng *et al.* 1989; Strickler *et al.* 1989; Vlasuk *et al.* 1989; Overton *et al.* 1990; Pichuantes *et al.* 1990;

Wu *et al.* 1990; Moosmayer *et al.* 1991; Nitschko *et al.* 1991; Ross *et al.* 1991; Tritch *et al.* 1991).

Experimental determination gives the molecular mass of the active protease as that of the dimer (Darke *et al.* 1989; Hostomsky *et al.* 1989; Meek *et al.* 1989; Tomasselli *et al.* 1990a; Holzman *et al.* 1991; Zhang *et al.* 1991a). Manipulation of the PR gene to effect monomer duplication and fusion into a single contiguous protein retains catalytic activity (Boutelje *et al.* 1990; Cheng *et al.* 1990a; Di Ianni *et al.* 1990; Burstein *et al.* 1991; Krausslich 1991; Louis *et al.* 1991). Finally, in the most aesthetically pleasing and interpretatively unambiguous experiments, the X-ray visualization of the protease reveals the dimeric organization (Lapatto *et al.* 1989; McKeever *et al.* 1989; Weber *et al.* 1989; Gustchina and Weber 1990; Weber 1990; Rao *et al.* 1991; Spinneli *et al.* 1991) and positioning of inhibitors (see below). The sense imparted by these efforts is a remarkably rapid maturity of the HIV aspartyl protease from a notional component of the virus machinery to a mature target, ripe for chemotherapeutic dispatch.

The unambiguous association of impaired protease activity (by deleterious modification of the protease gene) and loss of viral infectivity—the element of essentiality—was an early accomplishment (Katoh *et al.* 1985; Kohl *et al.* 1988). Proof that this correlation would remain when impairment was effected by the presence of a specific protease inhibitor required the development of more potent inhibitors than pepstatin. Although pepstatin presents, in its central statine amino acid the requisite structural feature for inhibition, it is a poor inhibitor of the HIV aspartyl protease relative to other aspartyl proteases (Katoh *et al.* 1987; Krausslich *et al.* 1988; Dreyer *et al.* 1989; Billich *et al.* 1990). The availability of potent protease inhibitors (K_i in the nanomolar range) permitted detailed addressing of this question, following the suggestive experiments of Seelmeier *et al.* (1988). For quite understandable reasons, all these experiments use noninfectious virus constructs in appropriate cell cultures or isolated lymphocytes. Addition of a moderately potent protease inhibitor (Upjohn U-81749, $K_i = 70$ nM) to lymphocytes immediately following virus addition significantly diminished proteolytic processing (usually measured by p24 immunoassay) and viral RNA synthesis in a dose-dependent manner (McQuade *et al.* 1990). However, removal of the inhibitor from the medium permitted a recovery of proteolytic processing. An identical set of observations was reported simultaneously by Meek *et al.* (1990b). In the presence of moderately potent inhibitors (but not pepstatin) proteolytic maturation in chronically infected lymphocytes was arrested and the resulting infectivity of the virions was significantly attenuated. The correlation of this lack of infectivity with morphological virion immaturity was proved by Ashorn *et al.* (1990) with a more potent inhibitor (Upjohn U-75875, $K_i = 1$ nM) (**Figs. 6B.2** and **6B.3**). Moreover, the suppression of proteolytic processing by this inhibitor was functionally irreversible, although whether this

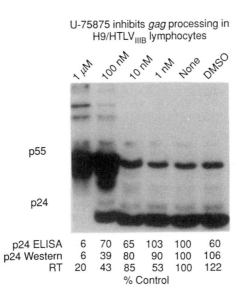

U-75875 inhibits *gag* processing in
H9/HTLV$_{\text{IIIB}}$ lymphocytes

	1 µM	100 nM	10 nM	1 nM	None	DMSO
p24 ELISA	6	70	65	103	100	60
p24 Western	6	39	80	90	100	106
RT	20	43	85	53	100	122

% Control

Fig. 6B.2 H9/HTLV$_{\text{IIIB}}$ cells were cultured in the presence of U-75875; the control contained no U-75875 (none) or 0.02 per cent dimethyl sulphoxide (DMSO). The supernatants were harvested, the HIV-1 particles were dissociated, and the proteins were electrophoresed on a 10 per cent polyacryamide gel, transferred onto nitrocellulose, and incubated with anti-serum from an HIV-infected patient. Relative amounts of p24 in each sample, as quantified by an antigen-capture ELISA and densitometric analysis of the Western blot, and the relative RT activity are shown. (From Ashorn *et al.* 1990.)

irreversibility arose from an innately greater potency of the inhibitor or from an intrinsic aspect of its structure was not determined. In further studies, addition of a potent inhibitor (Roche Ro 31–8959) to acutely infected cells blocked viral spread and host cell cytotoxicity (Craig *et al.* 1991). This inhibitor retained efficacy even during late-stage (syncytia-forming) infection. Virus antigen, virus particles, and virus cytopathic effects were largely cleared upon exposure to the inhibitor from 3 to 6 days after viral infection. With chronically infected cells, these same authors observed a transformation from released maturing virion to released immature virion which occurred 24 h after addition of 10–100 nM inhibitor. The velocity of viral gene expression in chronically infected cells, in the presence and absence of a protease inhibitor (E. Merck EMD 57.464), was examined by Schatzl *et al.* (1991). Whereas there was only a small decrease in overall viral protein production in the presence of the inhibitor, the expected

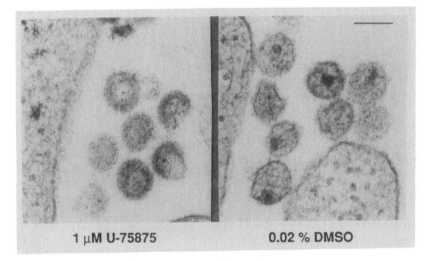

1 µM U-75875   0.02 % DMSO

Fig. 6B.3 H9/HTLV$_{IIIB}$ cells were cultured in the presence of 1 μM U-75875 or dimethyl sulphoxide (DMSO) alone. Washed cells were pelleted, fixed, embedded, sectioned, and examined using a transmission electron microscope (bar represents 100 nm) for analysis of the HIV-1 particles. (From Ashorn *et al.* 1990.)

morphological arrest at the non-infectious immature virion was seen. The protease does not prevent viral gene translation in these cells, but intervenes within the virion at the point of polyprotein maturation. Without this maturation, the released virions are not infectious.

An important issue is the sequence of bond cleavages in the maturation process. This has proved to be an almost intractable experimental question as the processing sequence is almost certainly vector dependent (Moosmayer *et al.* 1991, and references cited therein) and there is no assurance that the processing steps observed in a recombinant system are mirrored in the HIV-infected lymphocyte (or any other cell for that matter). However, there is no doubt that there are protease-dependent processing nuances. The present consensus with respect to *gag* processing is summarized from Erickson-Viitanen *et al.* (1989) and Tritch *et al.* (1991). The first bond cleaved is the met*met bond of the ..ATIM*MQRG.. sequence dividing the immature p25 capsid from the p15 C-terminus end of the polyprotein. The next cleavages occur much more slowly, at the ..SQNY*PIVQ sequence, dividing the p17 MA (which remains embedded in the membrane) and the released immature p25 CA protein, and dividing the p15 into the p9 NC protein and p6. This latter cleavage appears to be the most unpredictable (vector dependent). The final, and slowest, step is maturation of p25 to the mature p24 capsid by hydrolysis at an ..ARVL*AEAM.. sequence (Mervis *et al.* 1988). Bennett *et al.* (1991) have also observed late proteolytic maturation (post-budding) of the capsid in the related Rous sarcoma virus to two slightly less massive forms. It is tempting to speculate that a continuing proteolysis of the capsid protein by this protease may be important to the disruption of the capsid, so as to facilitate release of the NC-coated viral RNA from the core following virion internalization. With respect to the *pol* portion, much attention has focused on the role of the protease in the maturation of the reverse transcriptase from the released p66–p66 homodimer to the p66–p51 heterodimer found within the virion. The specifics of this transformation are discussed below as a practical illustration of the enzyme capability of the protease.

The presentation of the protease as primarily the temporal catalyst for *gag* and *gag-pol* maturation is a reflection of the limits of our present understanding, rather than a full understanding of its purpose. This phenomenon is the most visible of the protease's roles and hence has received the preponderance of early scrutiny. One answer with respect to polyprotein processing—the suppression of the protease during nucleation and assembly of the virion, and its liberation within the virion—eludes us. A partial solution derives from the need for two *gag-pol* polyproteins to aggregate, and thus each to contribute to dimer formation (Navia and McKeever 1990). Aggregation occurs only upon the migration and nucleation of the myristoylated polyproteins at the plasma membrane. Within the cell, the polyproteins are dispersed in a three-dimensional space, but at the membrane surface they are constrained and ordered into a two-dimensional aggregate allowing dimer formation. While it is reasonable to believe that this is a portion of the final answer, it is no longer seriously considered as the full answer (Wills and Craven 1991). The source of this difficulty is that the polyproteins are as proximal within the nascent shell as they are in the released immature virion, yet the experimental evidence is that proteolytic maturation is delayed until budding. A deeper explanation is demanded. A possible answer (or partial answer) may be found in the HIV-unique p6. It has previously been noted that removal of this protein from the *gag* terminus results in a loss of budding capability (Gottlinger *et al.* 1991) or the release of aberrant (and presumably non-functional) virions (Mergener *et al.* 1992). A molecular explanation may be provided by the experiments of Partin *et al.* (1991). As the p6 and the protease coincide with the *gag-pol* frameshift region, it is reasonable to believe that these polyprotein regions spatially abut in the nascent virion shell at the plasma membrane. In addition to the p6, found in its entirety at the end of the more abundant *gag* polyprotein, there is a related 68 amino acid upstream region (termed p6*) preceding the protease in the *gag-pol*. Might protease activity be attenuated by a *trans* p6-PR or *cis* p6*-PR association? In the construct described by Partin *et al.* (1991), with a p6* deletion and slightly modified PR structure, an increase in proteolytic activity was seen despite a quantitatively less capable (relative to wt) protease. The suggestion provided by these authors to account for this apparent contradiction is an increased accessibility of the protease upon p6* removal. A sequence comparison of the p6* to the proenzyme fragment of pepsinogen is suggestive but not remarkable. The possibility that release of an inhibitory p6*–protease interaction, induced by an alteration in the *gag–gag-pol* environment at the point of capsid–membrane closure to the spherical immature virion, triggers both the budding and maturation process remains speculative.

Regardless of the precise molecular basis for the temporal control of protease catalytic activity, there is no doubt that the control mechanism is delicate. There are several stratagems by which this control has been abrogated, resulting in intracellular proteolysis and the concomitant appearance of cellular toxicity. The simultaneous enhancement of proteolytic activity, observation of premature polyprotein processing, and appearance of cellular toxicity is sufficient proof for an intimate association of these phenomena. Further, the evidence is strong (although circumstantial) that the cytotoxicity is a consequence of HIV proteolytic degradation of essential cellular proteins. Various aspects of this relationship are discussed in a number of papers (Baum *et al.* 1990; Shoeman *et al.* 1990, 1991; Tomasselli *et al.* 1990c, 1991a,b; Wallin *et al.* 1990; Craig *et al.* 1991; Kaplan and Swanstrom 1991b; Krausslich 1991, 1992; Montgomery *et al.* 1991; Oswald and von der Helm 1991; Park and Morrow 1991; Schatzl *et al.* 1991; Mergener *et al.* 1992). Indeed, one of the early difficulties in the recombinant expression of the protease was its intrinsic toxicity toward the cellular vector. Among the methods for the disruption of protease control is the expression in the same gene of linked protease monomers, giving rise to a single protein species, which has been shown by several groups to secure high proteolytic specific activity (Boutelje *et al.* 1990; Cheng *et al.* 1990a; Di Ianni *et al.* 1990; Burstein *et al.* 1991; Krausslich 1991; Patterson *et al.* 1992). Expression of the linked dimer as a component of a polyprotein, by an *in vitro* translation system, gave rapid proteolysis (in contrast with the wt polyprotein); likewise, transfection with the linked dimer gene effected premature processing and prevention of virion formation (Krausslich 1991). Alternatively, positioning of the *gag* and *pol* into the same reading frame prevents normal budding, and results in the intracellular accumulation and extracellular release (possibly by cell death and lysis) of the (proteolysed) polyprotein fragments (Park and Morrow 1991; Mergener *et al.* 1992). Evidence for the protease as the causative agent of the cytotoxicity is the amelioration of this effect by potent protease inhibitors. Both Craig *et al.* (1991) and Schatzl *et al.* (1991) observed increased cell viability in the presence of a protease inhibitor. In a comprehensive study of polyprotein expression, containing a linked protease gene insertion, Krausslich (1992) observed a remarkable dependence of several phenomena with respect to the presence of the protease inhibitor Ro 31–8959. Without inhibitor (as noted above) there is rapid intracellular processing of the polyprotein and hence prevention of virion assembly (which requires a minimum length *gag* polyprotein) (Gottlinger *et al.* 1991; Hoshikawa *et al.* 1991; Wills and Craven 1991). At 10 nM concentration of this potent protease inhibitor, cytotoxicity was abolished but intracellular processing continued; at 100 nM inhibitor, release of partially processed particles is observed; at 1000 nM inhibitor, polyprotein processing is significantly slowed and the poly-protein is deposited as an insoluble aggregate. Given the specificity of the inhibitor, a conclusion that the intracellular HIV aspartyl protease is potentially cytotoxic is justified.

However, is the cytotoxic effect fortuitous, or is it indirect evidence of a necessary role for the protease (apart from polyprotein maturation within the virion) within the infected cell? A starting point for discussion is the list of cellular proteins which are proteolysed by this enzyme. This list is brief but increasing. However, it remains only suggestive with respect to enquiries regarding cytotoxicity and broadened catalytic role. Among the proteins acting as intracellular protease substrates are ribonuclease A (Hui *et al.* 1990), a_2-macroglobulin (Meier *et al.* 1991), fibronectin (Oswald and von der Helm 1991), NF-κB (Riviere *et al.* 1991), the intermediate filament proteins vimentin, desmin, and fibrillary acidic protein (Shoeman *et al.* 1990), actin, a-actinin, spectrin, and tropomyosin (Shoeman *et al.* 1991), Ca^{2+}-free (but not Ca^{2+}-containing) calmodulin (Tomasselli *et al.* 1991a), actin, troponin C, Alzheimer amyloid precursor protein, and inter-leukin 1β (Tomasselli *et al.* 1991b), and the microtubule-associated proteins 1 and 2 (Wallin *et al.* 1990). Attention has focused on the NF-κB regulatory protein and the cytoskeletal protein cleavages as potentially essential, or useful, to HIV propagation by protease-dependent cleavage. The NF-κB protein is a well-known inducible transcription factor binding to regulatory sites in the HIV enhancer sequence to effect viral transcription after T-cell activation whose action is induced by the virus (Bachelerie *et al.* 1991; Englund *et al.* 1991) and possibly regulated by protease-dependent cleavage so as to enhance viral gene transcription (Nabel 1991; Riviere *et al.* 1991). Clearly, the degradation of the cytoskeleton proteins would diminish cellular viability (Shoeman *et al.* 1990, 1991; Wallin *et al.* 1990; Tomasselli *et al.* 1991b), although there are no data which even suggest that this degradation may contribute to the observed (eukaryotic) cellular toxicity. The fact that the protease is quite toxic to the bacterial vectors would indicate (at least for these cells) other essential targets. Mergener *et al.* (1992) have speculated that cytoskeletal degradation may assist in the targeting of the polyproteins to the membrane assembly site, based on their observation that impairment of the protease results in substantial budding into intracellular vacuoles, as also reported by Peng *et al.* (1989). Baboonian *et al.* (1991) reported an intriguing experiment for which some new accounting of the protease is required. Addition of a potent protease inhibitor (Pfizer UK-88,947) to H9 cells 1 h prior to infection blocked the appearance of cytoplasmic and nuclear viral DNA, whereas simultaneous addition at the time of infection, or delayed addition, permitted viral DNA appearance although at reduced levels. AZT produced an identical effect. The implication of this observation is an essential role for the protease at a point between virus binding to the cellular surface receptors and reverse transcription. While this encompasses an almost limitless number of possibilities, Oroszlan and colleagues (Roberts and Oroszlan 1989; Copeland *et al.* 1990; Roberts *et al.* 1991) have directed attention to the RNA-associated nucleocapsid protein. Using the related equine infectious anaemia virus as an HIV model, they found (not unexpectedly) that the viral cores contained equal quantities of the NC and CA proteins, and the IN, RT, and PR enzymes. (The quantity and distribution of the PR within the virion remains largely unknown; a priori, the protease must be within the virion but, apart from the suggestion given below, there are no experimental data which compel its presence with the core.) The nucleocapsid protein sequence identifies two Cys-His zinc-finger motifs (EIAV sequence: ...C_{24}YXCXXPGHXSXQCRXXXXXC$_{43}$-FXCXXPGHXSXQCR...) which are indeed occupied by Zn^{2+} (South *et al.* 1990; Summers *et al.* 1990; Roberts *et al.* 1991; Bess *et al.* 1992). Upon removal of the Zn^{2+} ion, the fingers collapse into an extended conformation capable of protease cleavage at the ..$TC_{24}*Y_{25}N$.. and $VC_{43}*F_{44}K$.. sites (Roberts *et al.* 1991). This cleavage may represent an important transformation in the early stages of infection by this virus and, by analogy, by HIV as well. Furthermore, the recent observations that the HIV protease is inhibited by Zn^{2+} (Zhang *et al.* 1991b) and other metals (Karlstrom and Levine 1991) lead to the speculation that intracellular dissociation of Zn^{2+} may simultaneously activate the protease and render the nucleocapsid protein permissive to protease degradation. An essential PR-NC cleavage alone justifies the protease as a chemotherapeutic target.

These experiments establish this protease as a worthy opponent. This point has been attained with no more than the simple recognition of the enzyme as a protease; its identity as an aspartyl protease has been useful only in facilitating the understanding of several experiments. However, inhibitor design requires an intimate understanding.

6B.3   Strategy: the HIV protease as a molecular catalyst

The enzyme inhibitor is perfected through the iterative application to a lead structure of enzyme mechanism, structure, and substrate recognition. The lead structure itself is identified by empirical screening of microbial fermentations, mechanistic inference, and empirical evaluation (by either direct or indirect (computational) screening) of synthetic chemical libraries. Extensive HIV protease inhibitors exemplify each approach, although at this time the most potent are peptidomimetics with the naturally occurring dipeptide 'transition state' mimic, pepstatin, as an antecedent. As such they represent a fusion of the first two approaches, focused upon this aspartyl protease by knowledge of its mechanism, structure, and substrate specificity. It is the revelation of these characteristics which enables a specific potent inhibitor to be designed.

6B.3.1   Mechanism

The fundamental mechanistic distinction of the amide-hydrolysing enzyme catalysts is the division between those which use a sequential general base hydrolysis via an acyl enzyme intermediate and those which do not. The aspartyl proteases are included in the latter category (Blum *et al.* 1991). Although the history leading to this conclusion is long and difficult, a consensus now exists. From structural studies of the aspartyl protease class (see below) it is seen that the scissile amide juxtaposes between the aspartic acid pair, with one aspartate operating as a general base to deliver a nucleophilic water and the second operating as a general acid with respect to the incipient negative charge on the amide carbonyl oxygen. The confounding aspect of this catalysis from the experimentalist's viewpoint is that the bond-making and bond-breaking steps are not rate limiting for any of the aspartyl proteases. In the case of penicillopepsin, the rate-limiting step involves a reorganization of protein structure associated with proton movement (Cunningham *et al.* 1990); likewise, in the case of pepsin, the rate-limiting step occurs after amide bond cleavage and first product release, and is also associated with proton movement (Rebholz and Northrop 1991). The latter authors suggest that the proton movement involves protonation adjustment of the active-site carboxylates, and suggest that an identical rate-limiting step is encountered for renin (the second aspartyl protease, with the HIV, has a pH optimum only just below neutrality). The applicability of these studies to the HIV protease is uncertain. This aspartyl protease, although similar to renin in its pH optimum, differs from all other aspartyl proteases in its C_2 homodimer symmetry. In contrast with the other aspartyl proteases, where the aspartyls are diastereotopic and the role of basic and acidic catalyst is individually assigned, the aspartyls in the HIV aspartyl protease are enantiotopic. Therefore the need for a protonation adjustment at the completion of catalysis is obviated. Fortunately, the critical mechanistic investigations of the HIV protease are complete (Hyland *et al.* 1991a,b). On the basis of ^{18}O exchange experiments, the intervention of an acyl enzyme during turnover is excluded. The enzyme exhibits a bell-shaped V/K versus pH plot, having (depending on the substrate) an acidic (aspartic) pK_a of 3.4–3.7 and a basic (aspartate) pK_a of 5.5–6.5. The analysis of log V versus pH indicates a competence for substrate binding only by the HIV protease form with one of the aspartyls protonated. These data, coupled with extensive solvent kinetic isotope studies, led Hyland and coworkers to suggest, for most substrates, a two-proton involvement in the rate-limiting step which is proposed to be the collapse of the enzyme-bound amide hydrate resulting from water addition to the scissile amide.

These studies are relevant to inhibitor design. The chemical strategies for blocking catalysis in hydrolytic enzymes can be divided into those which divert a covalent intermediate (in the case of many hydrolases, an acyl enzyme) by competitive fragmentation, and those which achieve an energetic duplication (in a stable structure) of what is loosely referred to as the 'transition state' (Rich 1985). Given the proven absence of the acyl enzyme for all enzymes of the aspartyl class, the only strategy for successful peptidomimetic intervention at these enzymes is the transition state mimic.

6B.3.2   Enzyme structure

The importance of structure to the postulated development with respect to this enzyme cannot be overemphasized. The revelation of its homodimeric organization has impacted on thinking with respect to the temporal control of virus maturation, proton reorganization during the catalytic cycle, and inhibitor design. Experimental vindication of Pearl and Taylor's leap of faith followed rapidly with reports from the Merck group (McKeever et al. 1989; Navia et al. 1989) indicating a dimeric arrangement (albeit with a missed tracing of the peptide termini). Confirmation of the general features of this model, but with the correct backbone trace, was suggested by Weber et al. (1989) based on the related Rous sarcoma retroviral aspartyl protease (Miller et al. 1989a, Jaskolski et al. 1990) and confirmed by the same group (Wlodawer et al. 1989) and other workers (Lapatto et al. 1989) shortly thereafter (Fig. 6B.4).

With the addition of these structures to those already known for this protease class (Blundell et al. 1990; Cooper et al. 1990; Gilliland et al. 1990; James et al. 1990; Veerapandian et al. 1990; Newman et al. 1991; Rahuel et al. 1991; Rao et al. 1991) the aspartyl proteases constitute an enzymatic family for which the study of enzyme structure function is possible at an unprecedented level. One of the most intriguing issues is whether, as first predicted by Tang et al. (1978), the HIV protease constitutes an evolutionary antecedent of the eukaryotic aspartyl proteases. Speculation on this point is more facile than experimental solution; it must suffice to acknowledge the trenchant (and proper) rebuke of such anthropomorphic prejudices by Rao and colleagues (Rao and Wlodawer 1990; Rao et al. 1991). As discussed by these authors, the objective interpretation of the evidence favours the viral enzyme as a descendant of the eukaryotic enzymes (aspartyl proteases have not, as yet been found among the prokaryotes) cleaved in half by the demand of viral genetic economy.

There are several aspects of the unoccupied dimeric enzyme that are unusual with respect to the eukaryotic aspartyl protease enzymes which

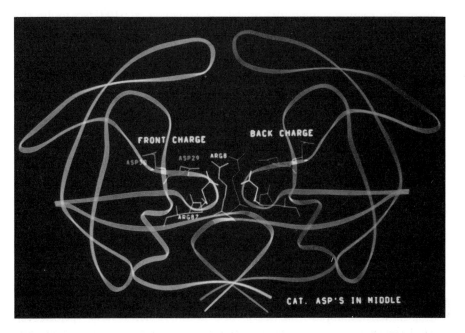

Fig. 6B.4 Ribbon representation or the crystal structure of the homodimeric HIV-1 protease showing the two catalytically essential aspartic acid residues at the active site. An extended anti-parallel β-sheet of the first and last four amino acids at the floor of the enzyme constitutes the most important structural feature by which the dimer is stabilized. The flap at the ceiling of the enzyme is a pair of six amino acids covering the active-site cavity.

have been studied for longer. One feature which has already been mentioned is the main-chain location of the amino and carboxy termini of each 99 amino acid protease monomer. These ends, through the formation of an extended anti-parallel β-sheet of the first and last four amino acids, constitute the most important structural feature by which the dimer is stabilized (Wlodawer *et al.* 1989; Weber 1990). This conclusion derives from mutational analysis of the protease structural domains (Loeb *et al.* 1989a,b) and the remarkable observation that the single deletion of the C-terminus phenylalanine of each monomer is sufficient to prevent monomer association (Hostomsky *et al.* 1989). Not unexpectedly, the suggestion (Weber 1990) that effective inhibition of the protease can be attained by prevention of dimer formation, by a competitor for β-sheet hydrogen-bonding, has already been proved correct (see below). The quantitative assessment of dimer stability has proved difficult, with the dissociation constant estimated in the low nanomolar range (Zhang *et al.* 1991a), the moderate nanomolar range (Cheng *et al.* 1990a), and low micromolar (with inhibitor) to high micromolar (without inhibitor) range (Holzman *et al.* 1991). Presumably this discrepancy is related to differences in experimental conditions, which have also resulted in divergent substrate catalytic values among different laboratories. A second stabilizing (and unprecedented) structural feature of the retroviral proteases is the ..$G_{86}R_{87}N_{88}$.. (or ..GRD..) triad (Rao *et al.* 1991). This triad's importance is again attested to by mutational analysis (Guenet *et al.* 1989; Loeb *et al.* 1989b; Louis *et al.* 1991; Wondrak *et al.* 1991b). The role of the central arginine, as visualized by X-ray studies, is structural. It is in electrostatic and hydrogen-bond contact with two amino acids, D29 in its own chain and R8′ of the opposing monomer. However, conservative replacement of the arginine (R87K) yields a dimeric protein, capable of pepstatin binding but utterly without catalytic capability (Louis *et al.* 1991; Wondrak *et al.* 1991b). This behaviour may be directly related to the observation, discussed in the next section, that this enzyme requires full occupancy of its active site for hydrolytic competence. Thus it is possible that small alterations in the presentation of the peptide may strongly influence the ability of the enzyme to attain the requisite transition-state stability for catalysis. A crystallographic study of this mutant would be most interesting.

An understanding of the difference in active-site acidity (pepsin and fungal aspartyl protease have pH optima of 2−4, whereas both renin and the HIV protease are maximally active at pH 4−6) has also been gained from studies of the crystallographic structure. Although this displacement in the optimal pH has been known for some time for renin, its crystal structures have only recently become available (Rahuel *et al.* 1991, and references cited therein) and generally have neither the quality nor the scope of those of the viral enzyme. Ido *et al.* (1991) have suggested, as a structural rationale, a difference in hydrogen-bonding of the active site aspartyls (see also Goldblum 1990). In pepsin, one of the aspartyl residues is hydrogen-bonded to the hydroxyl of a serine and, similarly, the second aspartic residue is also hydrogen-bonded to the hydroxyl of a threonine. The amino acid of the viral protease found at the ser/thr positions is a conserved alanine, however, and no hydrogen bond is possible. For this reason, the A28S viral enzyme mutant was prepared (the natural amino acid at position 28, alanine, was replaced with the amino acid serine), its pH behaviour was evaluated, and the predicted alteration was observed. Although its magnitude is not large enough to attribute the entire effect to the A28S change, it is significant (aspartic pK_i values of 5.1 and 6.9 for the wt enzyme and the enzyme−substrate complex respectively, and of 4.3 and 5.6 for the A28S enzyme and the enzyme−substrate complex respectively). This is not to say that the mutant is the more accomplished enzyme; as measured by V/K, the A28S mutant is nearly 100-fold poorer. Ido *et al.* (1991) suggest that there may be an unfavourable alteration in hydrogen bond strength between substrate and mutant enzyme. It is necessary to look beyond the

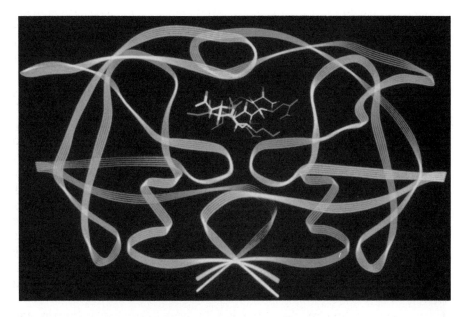

Fig. 6B.5 Ribbon representation of the crystal structure of an HIV–inhibitor complex showing the ligand in the active site. The inhibitor is secured via hydrophobic interaction and hydrogen-bonding by a closing motion of the flap across a distance of approximately 1.5 nm. As the flap shuts, a single water molecule is trapped so as to participate directly in the enzyme–ligand hydrogen-bonding.

static picture of the extensively hydrogen-bonded enzyme–inhibitor complex, discussed below, to the ethereal vision of the enzyme–substrate complex. In the former the hydrogen bonds are static but in the latter they are fluid, so as to permit the formation of a substrate complex and dissociation from the product complex, on a catalytically meaningful time-scale.

In addition to the native enzyme, the structures of a number of enzyme–inhibitor complexes (Fig. 6B.5) are now in hand (Miller *et al.* 1989b; Erickson *et al.* 1990; Fitzgerald *et al.* 1990; Swain *et al.* 1990; Bone *et al.* 1991; Jaskolski *et al.* 1991; Krohn *et al.* 1991; Thanki *et al.* 1992) (see Fig. 6B.6 and 6B.7). Two noteworthy structural features, the substrate binding flap and the tetrahedrally enzyme–inhibitor hydrogen-bonded water, are encountered. Both are involved in the correct positioning of the protease inhibitor (substrate?). Whereas the flap is precedented in the eukaryotic aspartyl proteases (Blundell *et al.* 1990; Veerapandian *et al.* 1990), the water is not. The protease flap (see Fig. 6B.4) is a pair of six amino acids (sequence ...IGGIGG...) covering the active site cavity. It is essential to catalysis (Loeb *et al.* 1989a,b). The enzyme flap is open in an encounter

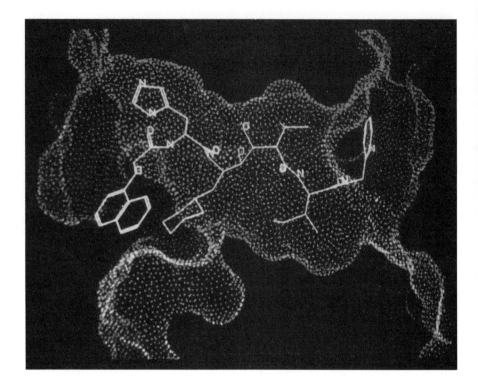

Fig. 6B.6 Conformation of the inhibitor U-75875 in the crystal structure of the HIV-1–inhibitor complex. The two hydroxyl groups at the cleavage-site dipeptide mimic of the inhibitor are positioned to form hydrogen bonds with the two catalytic aspartic acid residues of the enzyme. Side-chains of residues from P_2 to $P_{2'}$ are found in relatively well-defined binding pockets of the enzyme. (From Thanki *et al.* 1992.)

with a substrate (at the minimum, an extended oligopeptide at least six or seven amino aids long with a central pair presenting a suitable dipeptide (see below)). The substrate is then secured, via hydrogen-bonding, by a closing motion of the flap across a distance of approximately 1.5 nm (Fig. 6B.5) (Miller *et al.* 1989a,b; Fitzgerald *et al.* 1990; Gustchina and Weber 1990; Harte *et al.* 1990). As the flap shuts, a single water molecule is trapped so as to participate directly in the enzyme–substrate hydrogen-bonding. The hydrogen-bonding pattern among these three cooperating entities, taken by inference from the protease–inhibitor X-ray structures, is shown in Fig. 6B.8. Given this unprecedented revelation of the structural machinery used during catalysis, there is a temptation to expound on the implications with respect to the enzyme's evolutionary origins (difficult),

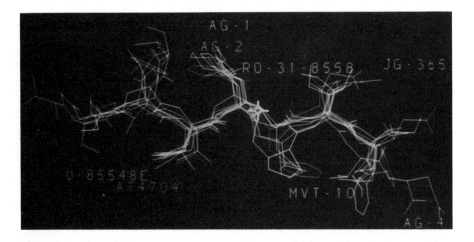

Fig. 6B.7 Overlay of conformations of eight representative inhibitors in the crystal structures of HIV-1–inhibitor complexes. With different amino acid compositions and utilizing a variety of dipeptide mimics at the cleavage site, these inhibitors exhibit a uniform and general conformation with an extensive hydrogen-bonding scheme along the active-site surface of the enzyme and with complementary side-chains to the binding pockets. (From Tomasselli *et al.* 1991c.)

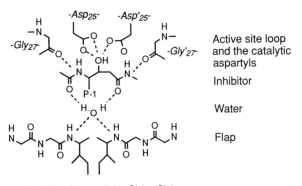

Fig. 6B.8 Hydrogen bond organization around the transition state insert core derived from the X-ray structure of the protease–acetyl pepstatin complex. (From Fitzgerald *et al.* 1990.)

the catalytic benefit (no less difficult), and the relevance to inhibitor design (straightforward in comparison).

Given the intention of this chapter, and for parenthetical opinion, discussion here is restricted to the last topic as it relates to peptidomimetics. The superficial interpretation of the extensive hydrogen-bonding interaction between enzyme and substrate is that these interactions are energetically favourable and, as such, must be replicated in inhibitor design. In the broadest sense, however, this interpretation is not correct. One point bears repeating. To a first approximation, the hydrogen-bonding process is energetically neutral (each new bond made compensates for one lost to solvent) and kinetically fluid, so as to permit the repetitive process of catalysis. As the substrate (inhibitor) is shortened by deleting the amino acid segments on each side of the scissile amide, hydrogen bonds are expended. The energetic cost of their loss need not be large, however, as hydrogen-bonded water remains. In fact, the number of necessary hydrogen bonds is small, and correspond to those key contacts which permit positioning of the inhibitor so as to allow a truly energetically favourable process—the displacement of the water barrier between mutual hydrophobic surfaces. With regard to the practical matter of HIV protease inhibitors, the identification of which hydrogen bonds are necessary and which are superfluous is done by experiment. It is found that the practical peptidomimetic HIV protease inhibitors (K_i in the nanomolar range) are ersatz di- and tripeptides with suitable aryl amino and carboxy terminus 'caps'. The effective size for a protease inhibitor is approximately half that of a protease substrate. As is noted below in the discussion of HIV protease substrates, there are few data to indicate the relevance of the substrate structure–activity relationships to that for inhibitors. In the particular example of the popular hydroxyethyl 'transition state' replacement ($\psi[CH(OH)CH_2]$) for the scissile amide, the necessary hydrogen bonds provided by the inhibitor are the insert hydroxyl (Ferguson *et al.* 1991; Krohn *et al.* 1991; Rich *et al.* 1991), the leading amide bond to the amino terminus end of the insert, and the trailing amide bond of the carboxy terminus end of the insert. While additional hydrogen bonds are useful with respect to improving potency, in effect they remain expendable in the optimization process with respect to the other objectives of inhibitor design (solubility, deliverability, and so forth).

6B.3.3   Enzyme specificity in substrate recognition

This introduces two interrelated issues. First, what are the differences in specificity between the HIV protease enzymes? Second, within each HIV protease class, what is the intrinsic preference in substrate recognition? The specific topic of protease recognition of structure is both challenging and important. If we are correct in our perception of the protease as a temporal coordinator of virus maturation, we are assigning to this enzyme the responsibility for the discrete and ordered assembly of the viral components. Not only must the protease recognize and cleave at disparate structural recognition sites (promiscuity), but this must be done in the prescribed order such that, for example, essential components are not prematurely lost to the interior of the infected cell (fidelity). Our present knowledge does not reconcile this paradox. However, the sense remains that this enzyme, in order to retain both attributes, may be less susceptible than other viral targets to the selection of resistant mutations. Given the recognition of the rather sloppy nature of the replication of this virus associated with its ability to diversify to more pathogenic (Englund *et al.* 1991) and resistant progeny, there is the hope that this optimism will be vindicated in time.

The first topic is the plurality of protease enzymes. There are two recognized HIV species, sharing approximately 40 per cent sequence identity, termed HIV-1 and HIV-2. HIV-1 dominates among infected individuals in the Western world, while a more balanced situation between the two exists elsewhere. HIV-2 has a close sequence homology to the simian immunodeficiency virus (SIV), and all three bear a discernible relationship to other retroviral proteases with respect to protease structure (Lapatto *et al.* 1989; Wlodawer *et al.* 1989; Gustchina and Weber 1990; Jaskolski *et al.* 1990; Weber 1990; Rao *et al.* 1991) but not with respect to the organization of the protease gene (Henderson *et al.* 1988; Bennett *et al.* 1991; Craven *et al.* 1991; Stewart and Vogt 1991). Despite clear sequence and recognition differences among these aspartyl proteases, the three most closely related (HIV-1, HIV-2, and SIV) are capable of an identical processing of the *gag* polyprotein (Pichuantes *et al.* 1990; Wu *et al.* 1990; Grant *et al.* 1991). The HIV-1 and HIV-2 proteases have been compared directly with a number of oligopeptide substrates (Richards *et al.* 1989a; Tomasselli *et al.* 1990b; Blaha *et al.* 1991; Tozser *et al.* 1991a,b) and polypeptide substrates (Tomasselli *et al.* 1991a), with the consensus that the two have more similarities than differences (Poorman *et al.* 1991). The primary point of difference between the two is a preference for rather smaller amino acid side-chains (particularly at the scissile P1*P-1' position) by the HIV-2 enzyme, which can be rationalized by a structural model of the active sites (Gustchina and Weber 1991). The tolerance of enzymatic activity with respect to structure has been put to what may be the ultimate test by Patterson *et al.* (1992) who have prepared the HIV-1—HIV-2 heterodimer and found it to possess remarkably similar catalytic properties to the two separate homodimers (however, see Babe *et al.* 1991). Differences exist between these two and the SIV enzyme (Grant *et al.* 1991) and (understandably) an even greater difference exists with respect to the other retroviral proteases (Kotler *et al.* 1989; Tomasselli *et al.* 1990c). Experiment has shown that the effective peptidomimetic inhibitor of this enzyme is the ersatz blocked tripeptide (R-(P-2)-(P-1 ψ[insert] P-2)-R' or R-(P-1 ψ[insert] P-2)-(P-2')-R', or dipeptide (R-(P-1 ψ[insert] P-2)-R'). Given the extraordinary limitations of peptidomimetics as practical pharmaceuticals, the inhibitor can have no larger mass than that necessary to achieve the requisite antiviral potency. With a consensus HIV-1−HIV-2 inhibitor as a goal (Poorman *et al.* 1991), a second question arises: What is the common HIV-1−HIV-2 di- and tripeptide recognition across the (P-2)-(P-1)-(P-1′)-(P-2′) binding site domain?

This question has been addressed through the study of the natural *gag* and *gag-pol* cleavage points (see Fig. 6B.1), cleavage point mutations within these polyproteins, and the competence of oligopepticle substrates. Early investigations of this issue produced inconsistent data. To a certain extent this is still true, but with improved vectors for the production, recovery, and renaturation of recombinant protease (Debouck *et al.* 1987; Hansen *et al.* 1988; Darke *et al.* 1989; Hostomsky *et al.* 1989; Krausslich *et al.* 1989; Meek *et al.* 1989; Strickler *et al.* 1989; Billich *et al.* 1990; Boutelje *et al.* 1990; Cheng *et al.* 1990b; Di Ianni *et al.* 1990; Hirel *et al.* 1990; Pichuantes *et al.* 1990; Rittenhouse *et al.* 1990; Tomasselli *et al.* 1990a; Goobar *et al.* 1991; Ido *et al.* 1991; Kohl *et al.* 1991; Louis *et al.* 1991; Margolin *et al.* 1991; Montgomery *et al.* 1991; Wondrak *et al.* 1991b) and, as importantly, a better sense of the enzyme itself, there is increasingly better agreement. Among the problems encountered with this enzyme were significant autoproteolysis (Babe *et al.* 1991; Grant *et al.* 1991), irreversible loss of activity with dilution or pH $\geqslant 7$ (Cheng *et al.* 1990a), a sensitivity to cysteine modification (for the HIV-1 enzyme) (Mous *et al.* 1988; Strickler *et al.* 1989; Karlstrom and Levine 1991; Montgomery *et al.* 1991; Zhang *et al.* 1991b), substrate-dependent pH optima (Billich *et al.* 1991; Hostomska *et al.* 1991; Hyland *et al.* 1991b; Ido *et al.* 1991; Newman *et al.* 1991), and a pronounced effect of salt concentration on substrate K_m (Kotler *et al.* 1989; Billich et al; 1990; Cheng *et al.* 1990a; Montgomery *et al.* 1991; Wondrak *et al.* 1991a). The salt effect (less correctly referred to as the ionic strength effect (Leberman 1991)) improves the enzyme's catalytic ability by a decrease in the substrate K_m and may be interpreted by a simple salting out phenomenon, or may reflect an effect on the oligopeptide conformation which improves its presentation to the active site (Kotler *et al.* 1989; Wondrak *et al.* 1991a; Tropea *et al.* 1992). Nevertheless the interpretative sense of these studies is that the amino acids found at the natural cleavage sites indeed display complementarity to the protease active site. Particular attention is called to the unusual P-1*P-1′ cleavage sites of ..F*P.. and ..Y*P.. which, because of the presence of the proline, can reasonably be thought of as specific to this protease (although pepsin also accepts a P-1′ proline (Kotler *et al.* 1989)). Not surprisingly, a preliminary sorting of the protease cleavage points divided these between the ..F(Y)*P.. classes and the other cleavage points exemplified by the ..L*A.., ..M*M.., ..F*L.., and ..L*F.. pairs (Henderson *et al.* 1988). The predilection for a P-2′ glu or gln, suggested by the natural cleavage points, is also borne out by the oligopeptide and protein substrates, and also inhibitors, for this enzyme (Hui *et al.* 1990; Tomasselli *et al.* 1990b,

1991a,b; Urban *et al.* 1992). Further discussion of substrate recognition is beyond the scope of this review, if for no other reason than the behaviour of this enzyme defies simple generalizations beyond a preference (not absolute) for certain hydrophobic amino acids (with the exception of the P-2′ E or Q) at the important ..(P-2)-(P-1)*(P-1′)-(P-2′).. positions (Kotler *et al.* 1989; Parkin *et al.* 1990; Konvalinka *et al.* 1990; Margolin *et al.* 1990; Richards *et al.* 1990; Billich and Winkler 1991; Blaha *et al.* 1991; Jupp *et al.* 1991; Tozser *et al.* 1991a,b). For example, arginine (Tomasselli *et al.* 1990c, 1991a,b; Shoeman *et al.* 1991), carboxymethyl cysteine (Tomasselli *et al.* 1991b), and asparagine (Shoeman *et al.* 1990) are tolerated at ..(P-1)*(P-1′) if presented in a suitable peptide. A disinterested statistical perspective has been provided by Poorman *et al.* (1991), from which the importance of the P-1 residue in dictating the overall recognition can be seen. In summary, the image of the stereotypical protease substrate is that of an extended hydrophobic peptide capable of the β-strand-like hydrogen-bonding of the active site, which is capable of both fully occupying the six to seven binding subsites of the active site (Tozser *et al.* 1991b) and presenting a tolerated pair of ..(P-1)*(P-1′).. residues for the central scissile dipeptide (Partin *et al.* 1990).

The proteolysis of the reverse transcriptase homodimer to the mature form is illustrative (Mous *et al.* 1988). Although this transformation is not necessarily typical, it has received extraordinary scrutiny, given the importance of the reverse transcriptase to the virus (and to viral chemotherapy). As proteolysis alters the breadth of activities present in this enzyme (which include RNA- and DNA-directed DNA synthesis, heteroduplex separation (RNase H), primer endonuclease, and $tRNA^{Lys}$ binding and hydrolysis; see Davies *et al.* (1991), Evans *et al.* (1991), Ben-Artzi *et al.* (1992), and Boyer *et al.* (1992), for summaries), the catalytic properties of the initially synthesized p61 homodimer, the p66:p51 mature heterodimer actually present in the virions (Becerra *et al.* 1991), and the liberated p15 piece have been evaluated (not always with the same conclusion). To begin with, there is the question of why the p66−p66 homodimer is cleaved in only one domain. At the present time, there is a consensus that the primary cleavage is between a phenylalanine and tyrosine bond in the sequence ..$AETF_{440}*Y_{441}VD$.., as reported by Graves *et al.* (1990) and Becerra *et al.* (1990). The proteolysis liberates the 120 amino acid 'RNase H' domain from the carboxy terminus of one subunit. A crystallographic analysis of a larger carboxy terminus domain (although lacking in enzymatic activity (Becerra *et al.* 1990; Davies *et al.* 1991; Boyer *et al.* 1992; however, see Hafkemeyer *et al.* 1991; Schulze *et al.* 1991), encompassing amino acids $Y_{427}...L_{560}$, shows full protein structure with the ..$F_{440}*Y_{441}$.. cleavage point as a component of a long central β-sheet strand (Davies *et al.* 1991). Separation of the amino terminus to expose this bond must be possible, however, as treatment of this construct with the protease results in cleavage at this point (Becerra *et al*. 1990). The troubling absence of enzymatic activity has been identified by Evans *et al*. (1991) as resulting from the absence of some 20–30 amino acids, presumably required for productive binding and orientation of the RNA-DNA duplex, upstream from this cleavage point. The catalytic function of the p15 domain, if indeed there is one, in the HIV life-cycle remains unresolved. The circumstances of the protease cleavage of the p66 homodimer remain a less controversial focus. Using recombinant peptides Becerra *et al*. (1991) have determined that proteolytic cleavage to the p66–p51 heterodimer results in a more stable dimer ($K_a = 5 \times 10^5$ M^{-1}) than the p66 homo-dimer ($K_a = 5 \times 10^4$ M^{-1}); the p51 alone does not dimerize and is functionally incompetent (Peng *et al*. 1991; Schulze *et al*. 1991). Although the ..F*Y.. bond is known to be in a proteolytically sensitive region (Graves *et al*. 1990; Hostomska *et al*. 1991), the image of this junction being recognized by the protease as a suitable ..(P-1)*(P-1′).. in the midst of a flexible peptide tether has been demonstrated to be overly simplistic (Hostomska *et al*. 1991). Protease treatment of the p66–p66 homodimer results in rapid cleavage to p66–p51; further cleavage is exceedingly slow but occurs if dimer protein structure is disrupted by sodium dodecylsulphate (Schulze *et al*. 1991). These authors also report a fourfold increase in reverse transcriptase, and 1.5-fold increase in RNase H activity resulting from the proteolysis. In contrast, Hostomska *et al*. (1991) observed pre-ferential protease cleavage, in a p66 fusion protein construct, within the fusion protein linker at a ..LDA*YAS.. sequence. Modification of the linker to abolish this cleavage diverts the protease to permit slow proteolysis at the expected ..F*Y.. or dual proteolysis to the p51 monomers. An analogous diversion to other cleavage points by amino acid substitution is also observed in oligopeptides with the p51:p15 cleavage segment sequence (Jupp *et al*. 1991). Clearly, the ..AETF*YVD.. sequence is not fortuitous. It fulfils the demand of the protease for recognition and the demand of the reverse transcriptase–RNase p66–p51 for structural stability, presumably accomplished by a structural reorganization that sequesters the remaining ..F*Y.. from further hydrolysis. The study of this cleavage leads to the conclusion that protease recognition is not simply sequence dependent but is also dictated, in an as yet unknown fashion, by the protein structure itself. The capricious appearance of 'unusual' amino acids within observed cleavages supports this conclusion (Poorman *et al*. 1991). The interrelation-ship of peptide sequence and structure in protease recognition remains an inscrutable aspect of this enzyme's catalytic abilities.

Yet it is precisely this understanding that the designer of a protease inhibitor covets, and since it is not available inhibitor design remains em-pirical. Although (as will be evident from the following section) empirical design is hardly impotent, it is a statement of fact that peptidomimetic inhibitor design has been driven by a strategy to insert a 'transition state' between two amino acids which mimic substrates (most frequently ..Fψ-[insert]F.. , ..Fψ[insert]Y.. and ..Fψ[insert]P..). Of course this strategy is rationalized by the expectation that the choice of these structural segments as substrate mimetics will yield inhibitors that at least bind. The alternative strategy is one that complements the binding strength of the insert with flanking structures that synergize its binding; whether or not this corresponds to the 'substrate peptidomimetic' requires a more eclectic exploration of the flanking structures than is now being reported. Only the simple experiment of Tozser *et al.* (1991b), who observed that the tetrapeptide YPIV binds ($K_i = 0.15$ mM) but is not hydrolysed, is needed to remind us that protease recognition of substrates and of inhibitors is divergent.

6B.4   Execution: the HIV protease inhibitors

6B.4.1   Peptidic structures

The nonapeptide H-Val-Ser-Gln-Asn-Tyr-Pro-Ile-Val-Gln-NH$_2$ has been shown to be a good substrate for the HIV-1 protease and is cleaved at the expected site between the P$_1$ Tyr and P$_1$' Pro residues (Tomasselli *et al.* 1990b). Replacing L-proline with L-pipecolic acid (Pip) resulted in the substrate analogue peptide 1 (Table 6B.1), which inhibited the enzyme with an IC$_{50}$ value of 1.4 μM (Copeland *et al.* 1990). Pepstatin A (peptide 2), which is a naturally occurring general aspartyl protease inhibitor, was shown to inhibit HIV-1 protease with a K_i value of 0.36 μM (Tomasselli *et al.* 1990a). The more soluble acetyl pepstatin (peptide 3) was found to be more active, with a K_i value of 0.035 μM (Richards *et al.* 1989b). Previous investigations of inhibitors of aspartyl proteases have successfully relied on the 'transition-state analogue' concept in the design of highly potent enzyme inhibitors (Rich 1985). The logic of this concept is based on the fact that enzymes accelerate chemical reactions by possessing much higher binding affinity to the transition states of reaction pathways than to substrates or products. Chemical entities that are designed to mimic metastable structures of transition states will also have high binding affinity to the enzymes. For example, pepstatin A contains the unusual amino acid statine (4S-amino-3S-hydroxy-6-methylheptanoic acid), the hydroxyl group of which is assumed to mimic the tetrahedral hydrated amide which is a high energy species along the reaction pathway of amide bond hydrolysis. Design of aspartyl protease inhibitors containing statine (Boger *et al.* 1983) or other transition state analogues of the dipeptide cleavage site has resulted in a variety of very potent enzyme inhibitors (Greenlee 1990). More recently, these findings have been applied successfully to the preparation of HIV protease inhibitors with very high binding affinity.

A series of compounds based upon the substrate sequence and incorporating the statine residue at the cleavage site have been shown to exhibit

Table 6B.1 Statine containing inhibitors

#									NH$_2$	K_i (µM)
1	H	Val	Ser	Gln	Asn	Tyr-Pip	Ile	Val	Gln	1.4
2			Iva	Val	Val	Sta	Ala	Sta	OH	0.36
3			Ac	Val	Val	Sta	Ala	Sta	OH	0.035
4	H	Val	Ser	Gln	Asn	Sta	Ile	Val	OH	3.7
5		Ac	Ser	Leu	Asn	Sta	Ile	Val	OMe	1.1
6		Ac	Ser	Gln	Asn	pSta	Val	Val	NH$_2$	39
7		Ac	Ser	Leu	Asn	pSta	Ile	Val	OMe	8
8		H	Ser	Ala	Ala	pSta	Val	Val	OMe	0.81
9		Boc	Ser	Ala	Ala	pFSta	Val	Val	OMe	0.16
10		H	Ser	Ala	Ala	pPSta	Val	Val	OMe	4.5

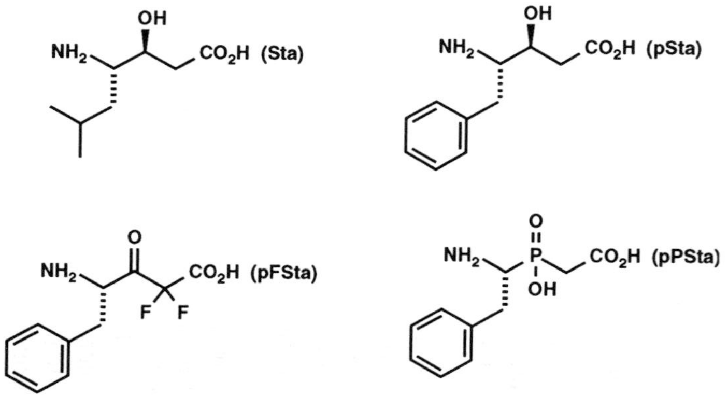

NH_2 · OH · CO_2H (Sta)

NH_2 · OH · CO_2H (pSta)

NH_2 · O · F F · CO_2H (pFSta)

NH_2 · P=O · OH · CO_2H (pPSta)

inhibitory activity (Table 6B.1). For example, peptides **4** (Tomasselli *et al.* 1990a) and **5** (Rich *et al.* 1990), with statine in place of the dipeptide Tyr-Pro in the substrate, were shown to inhibit HIV-1 protease at micromolar concentrations (K_i values of 3.7 μM and 1.1 μM respectively). Since Phe is among the preferred residues at the P_1 site of the substrates, the corresponding phenylmethyl analogue of statine (4S-amino-3S-hydroxy-5-phenylpentanoic acid) was also evaluated. Peptides **6** (Moore *et al.* 1989), **7** (Rich *et al.* 1990), and **8** (Dreyer *et al.* 1989) did not show enhancement of inhibitory activity and they exhibited inhibitory activity in the micromolar range. It is interesting to note that small changes in substitutions (compare peptides **6** and **8**) led to a significant difference in the observed inhibitory activity.

The congeneric peptide **9** (Dreyer *et al.* 1989) contains the corresponding difluoroketone analogue of statine (4S-amino-2,2-difluoro-3-oxo-5-phenyl-pentanoic acid) at the cleavage site. Previous work has demonstrated that the carbonyl function at C3 of the difluoroketone analogue of statine is readily hydrated, and the resulting tetrahedral species can function as a mimic of the hydrated amide of peptide bond hydrolysis. Very potent inhibitors of aspartyl proteases can readily be prepared utilizing the difluorostatone dipeptide mimic (Gelb *et al.* 1985; Thaisrivongs *et al.* 1985). In the present case, compound **9**, with $K_i = 0.16$ μM, was shown to be slightly more active than compound **8**. Congeneric peptide **10** (Dreyer *et al.* 1989) contains (carboxymethyl)(1′R-amino-phenethyl)phosphinic acid, the phosphinate analogue of statine, at the cleavage site. The tetrahedral phosphinate functional group has previously been shown to be an effective mimic of the hydrated amide, and potent aspartyl protease inhibitors containing the phosphastatine can be prepared (Bartlett and Kezer 1984). In this case however, compound **10** with a phosphastatine analogue showed only moderate binding affinity, with $K_i = 4.5$ μM.

Although the statine analogues have been shown to function as dipeptide mimics of the cleavage site, they contain one fewer carbon atom in the peptide backbone when compared with a dipeptide unit. With the exception of a few 2-substituted statine analogues (Greenlee 1990), this dipeptide mimic also lacks a side-chain at the $P_1{}'$ site. A number of transition state analogues at the dipeptide cleavage site have been designed to reflect the positioning of the P_1 and $P_1{}'$ sites more accurately. Among the first dipeptide mimics to be evaluated was the reduced-bond isostere in which the carbonyl group of the amide bond is replaced by a methylene unit (Szelke *et al.* 1982). For HIV protease inhibitors, the Phe-Pro dipeptide cleavage site of the substrate is replaced by the corresponding reduced bond. Incorporation of this insert into a number of substrate templates (Table 6B.2) led to compounds with moderate inhibitory activity as exemplified by peptides **11** (Tomasselli *et al.* 1990a), **12** (Rich *et al.* 1990), and **13** (Dreyer *et al.* 1989), with K_i values in the high micromolar range. Peptide **14** (Rich *et al.* 1990),

Table 6B.2 Inhibitors containing reduced-bond isosteres

									K_i (μM)
11	H	Val	Ser	Gln	Asn	PheRPro	Ile	Val	OH	3.5
12		Ac	Ser	Gln	Asn	PheRPro	Val	Val	NH$_2$	13
13		H	Ser	Ala	Ala	PheRPro	Val	Val	NH$_2$	19
14			Ac	Thr	Ile	NleRNle	Gln	Arg	NH$_2$	0.79

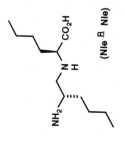

(Phe ^R Pro)

(Nle ^R Nle)

with the reduced-bond isostere of norleucylnorleucine, was shown to be rather more active with $K_i = 0.79 \ \mu M$.

As described above, compound **10** containing the phosphinate analogue of statine is not a highly effective HIV protease inhibitor. The phosphinate analogues (Table 6B.3) of the dipeptide Phe-Gly and Phe-Pro were equally disappointing, and peptides **15** (Dreyer *et al.* 1989) and **16** (Grobelny *et al.* 1990) also showed only moderate inhibitory activity in the micromolar range. Interestingly, pipecolic acid at the P_1' site (which was previously used as a substrate analogue in peptide **1**) in the phosphinate dipeptide analogue was shown to be much more effective. Peptide **17** (Grobelny *et al.* 1990), with $K_i = 50$ nM, is about 50 times more active than the direct congener **16** containing proline at the P_1' site. More potent inhibitors still were prepared when phenylalanine was placed at the P_1' site. Peptide **18** was shown to be 25 times more active than the congeneric peptide **17** with pipecolic acid at the P_1' site. Peptide **19**, with this phosphinate analogue of Phe-Phe dipeptide, is highly potent, with $K_i = 0.4$ nM (Grobelny *et al.* 1990). Replacing the N-terminal portion of peptide **19** with a simple *tert*-butyloxycarbonyl group resulted in peptide **20** (Huff 1991) which maintained very high binding affinity with $IC_{50} = 9$ nM. Phosphonamidates and phosphonamidate esters as HIV-1 protease inhibitors have also been described (McLeod *et al.* 1991).

A transition state analogue that has been studied extensively in the preparation of very potent aspartyl protease inhibitors is the hydroxyethylene isostere. This insert has also been applied to the design of HIV protease inhibitors (Table 6B.4). Very interestingly, this type of isostere bearing the side-chains of the Phe-Pro cleavage site proved ineffective, as exemplified by peptide **21** (Dreyer *et al.* 1989; Prasad and Rich 1991) with relatively poor binding affinity. Replacing Pro at the P_1' site with the simplest amino acid Gly resulted in peptides **22** and **23** (Meek *et al.* 1990b) with significant enhancement of inhibitory activity. Tyr at P_1, as in peptide **24**, was shown to be equally effective. In congeneric peptides **25** and **26** (Huff *et al.* 1990; Moore *et al.* 1990) in which Gly in peptides **22** and **23** was replaced by Ala, the resulting peptides, with a methyl group at the P_1' site, showed more than 50-fold enhancement in binding affinity with inhibitory activity in the nanomolar range. Increasing the sizes of the P_1' side-chain to the isopropyl and phenylmethyl group (peptides **27** and **28** respectively) showed only marginal enhancement of binding affinity over peptide **25**.

Compound **29** (Vacca *et al.* 1991) (Table 6B.5), with the hydroxyethylene isostere of phenylalanylphenylalanine dipeptide, incorporated a simple N-terminal *tert*-butyloxycarbonyl group and still maintained very high binding affinity with an IC_{50} value of 0.6 nM. Replacing the P_3' Phe in compound **29** with a benzyl amide resulted in compound **30** with maintenance of nanomolar potency. Among compounds that have been optimized for inhibitory potency, compound **31**, with a 3-phenyl-2-propenyl side-chain

Table 6B.3 Phosphinate containing inhibitors

								K_i (nM)
15	H	Ser	Ala	Ala	PhePGly	Val	Val	OMe	4400
16				Cbz	PhePPro	Val	Val	NH$_2$	2400
17				Cbz	PhePPip	Val	Val	NH$_2$	50
18				Bz	PhePPhe	Val	Val	NH$_2$	2
19		Boc	Val	Val	PhePPhe	Val	Val	NH$_2$	0.4
20				Boc	PhePPhe	Leu	Phe	NH$_2$	9

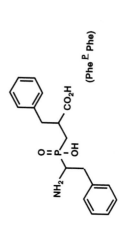

(Phe ^{P} Pro)

(Phe ^{P} Phe)

Table 6B.4 Inhibitors containing hydroxyethylene isosteres

								K_i (nM)
21	H	Ser	Ala	Ala	PheOHPro	Val	Val	OMe	500
22		Cbz	Ala	Ala	PheOHGly	Val	Val	OMe	48
23			Cbz	Ala	PheOHGly	Val	Val	OMe	120
24	Boc	Ser	Ala	Ala	TyrOHGly	Val	Val	OMe	180
25		Cbz	Ala	Ala	PheOHAla	Val	Val	OMe	0.7
26			Cbz	Ala	PheOHAla	Val	Val	OMe	2.2
27			Cbz	Ala	PheOHVal	Val	Val	OMe	0.2
28			Cbz	Ala	PheOHPhe	Val	Val	OMe	0.5

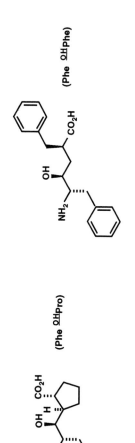

(Phe OHPro)   (Phe OHPhe)

Table 6B.5 Inhibitors containing hydroxyethylene isosteres

						K_i (nM)
29	Boc	Phe**OH**Phe	Leu	Phe	NH$_2$	0.6
30	Boc	Phe**OH**Phe	Leu	NH	Bn	1.4
31	Boc	Phe**OH**Ppg	Ile	Amb		0.03
32	Boc	Phe**OH**Phe	Ahi			0.3
33	Boc	Phe**OH**Met	Ahi			0.45
34	Boc	Met**OH**Phe	Ahi			0.55
35	Boc	Met**OH**Met	Ahi			1.9

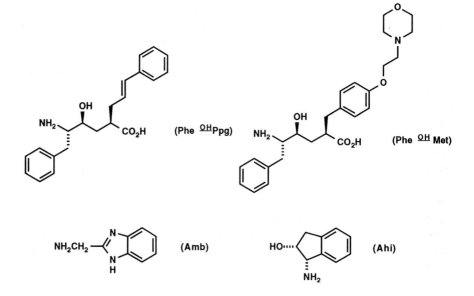

at the P_1' site and a 2-aminomethyl-benzimidazole C-terminus, showed exceedingly potent binding affinity with an IC$_{50}$ value of 0.03 nM (de Solms *et al.* 1991). Significant further advance in the discovery of small and less peptidic compound was realized in a series of compounds exemplified by compound **32** (Lyle *et al.* 1991) with 1S-amino-2R-hydroxyindane at the C-terminus. This is the smallest compound yet reported with inhibitory activity in the subnanomolar range. Interest in enhancing water solubility and influencing the pharmacokinetic property of these compounds has led to the preparation of analogues with substitutions at the *para* position of Phe at the P_1' site. Molecular modelling has suggested that substituents at this position extended into a channel at the active site and would not interfere with proper ligand binding (Thompson 1992). Compound **33**, with the 2-morpholino-ethoxy-phenylmethyl group at the P_1' site, maintained potent inhibitory activity with $IC_{50} = 0.45$ nM. Since the HIV protease is a C_2 symmetric homodimer, the 2-morpholino-ethoxy-phenylmethyl group can equally be added to Phe at the P_1 site and resulted in compound **34** with essentially the same binding affinity as compound **33**. Additionally, the 2-morpholino-ethoxy-phenylmethyl group can be simultaneously added to both Phe residues and resulted in compound 35 with nanomolar inhibitory activity ($IC_{50} = 1.9$ nM).

Previous work on inhibitors of the aspartyl protease renin has utilized the hydroxyethylene isostere of the Leu-Val dipeptide cleavage site of human angiotensinogen as a transition state mimic for the preparation of potent inhibitors (Thaisrivongs *et al.* 1986). Replacing the Tyr-Pro cleavage site of the nonapeptide H-Val-Ser-Gln-Asn-Tyr-Pro-Ile-Val-Gln-NH$_2$ substrate of HIV protease with this insert generated peptide **36** (Tomasselli *et al.* 1990b) (Table 6B.6) with very high inhibitory activity and a K_i value of less than 1 nM. Interestingly, many active renin inhibitors based upon the amino acid sequence of angiotensinogen have also been proved to be effective inhibitors of HIV protease. Peptide **37** (Richards *et al.* 1989b) and the smaller peptide **38** (Ashorn *et al.* 1990), both of which are very potent renin inhibitors, inhibited HIV protease with K_i values of 15 nM and 28 nM respectively. Further reduction in size (Sawyer *et al.* 1992, 1993; Tomasselli *et al.* 1990a) of the N-terminus of peptide **38** provided peptide **39** with improvement in binding affinity and a K_i value of 1.5 nM. The corresponding simple N-acetylated peptide **40** maintained respectable inhibitory potency with a K_i value of 70 nM. Replacing the isobutyl P_1 side-chain of peptide **40** with the cyclohexylmethyl group provided peptide **41** with about a 10-fold enhancement of binding affinity. The larger N-terminal *tert*-butylacetyl group in peptide **42** (McQuade *et al.* 1990) led to a decrease in inhibitory potency. However, the N-terminal carbamate *tert*-butyloxycarbonyl proved more effective, and peptide **43** inhibited HIV protease with a K_i value of 8 nM (Sawyer *et al.* 1992, 1993).

A closely related dipeptide transition state analogue of the hydroxyethylene isostere is the corresponding dihydroxyethylene isostere (Thaisrivongs *et al.* 1987). In a template derived from inhibitor **38**, a series of congeneric peptides containing dihydroxyethylene isosteres (Table 6B.7), which differ in the composition of side-chains at the P_1 and P_1' sites, were examined as HIV protease inhibitors (Thaisrivongs *et al.* 1991). Because of the C_2 symmetric nature of the enzyme dimer, a number of inserts with identical side-chains at the P_1 and P_1' sites were evaluated. Peptides **44**, **45**, and **46**, which contain the dihydroxyethylene isosteres of Leu-Leu, Phe-Phe, and Cha-Cha respectively, proved to be active inhibitors. Increasing the size of the two side-chains from isobutyl to phenylmethyl to cyclohexylmethyl

Table 6B.6 Inhibitors containing hydroxyethylene isosteres

										K_i (nM)
36	H	Val	Ser	Gln	Asn	Leu**OH**Val	Ile	Val	**OH**	< 1
37	Boc	His	Pro	Phe	His	Leu**OH**Val	Ile	His	**OH**	15
38			Boc	Phe	His	Leu**OH**Val	Ile	Amp		28
39				Ac	Val	Leu**OH**Val	Ile	Amp		1.5
40					Ac	Leu**OH**Val	Ile	Amp		70
41					Ac	Cha**OH**Val	Ile	Amp		8
42					Tba	Cha**OH**Val	Ile	Amp		74
43					Boc	Cha**OH**Val	Ile	Amp		8

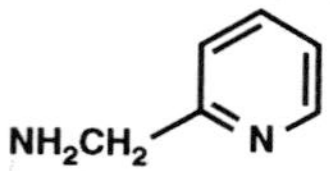

(Amp)

$(CH_3)_3CCH_2CO_2H$ (Tba)

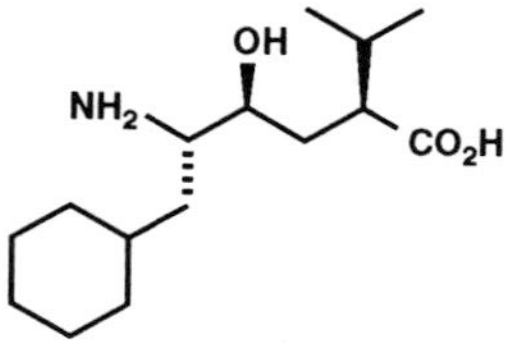

(Cha OH Val)

Table 6B.7   Inhibitors containing dihydroxyethylene isosteres

						K_i (nM)
44	Noa	His	Leu**dOH**Leu	Ile	Amp	7
45	Noa	His	Phe**dOH**Phe	Ile	Amp	12
46	Noa	His	Cha**dOH**Cha	Ile	Amp	26
47	Noa	His	Leu**dOH**Val	Ile	Amp	<10
48	Noa	His	Cha**dOH**Val	Ile	Amp	<1

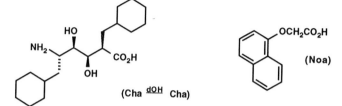

(Cha $\underline{dOH}$ Cha)   (Noa)

led to a correspondingly small erosion of binding affinity. Peptides **47** and **48**, with non-identical side-chains at the P_1 and P_1' sites, proved to be much more potent, with inhibitory activity in the subnanomolar range.

The hydroxyethylamine transition state insert previously described has been applied to the design of HIV protease inhibitors with Pro at the P_1' site (Rich *et al*. 1990) (Table 6B.8). In a substrate template and with Leu at the P_1 site, peptide **49** was shown to be an active inhibitor with a K_i value of 11 nM. The direct congeneric peptide **50**, with Phe at the P_1 site, turned out to be a very potent inhibitor with a K_i value of 0.66 nM. In a study with simple C-terminal groups, as exemplified by peptides **51**, **52**, and **53** (Roberts *et al*. 1990), it was found that increasing the size of the P_1' group from proline to pipecolic acid to decahydroisoquinoline carboxylic acid led to significant and steady improvement of binding affinity. Peptide **53** was shown to be a highly potent HIV protease inhibitor with an IC_{50} value of less than 0.4 nM. The absolute stereochemistry at the carbinol centre of the dipeptide transition state insert as in peptide **53** was shown to be *R* which is opposite to the expected *S* stereochemistry existing in peptide **50** (Rich *et al*. 1991). With the availability of crystallographic data of enzyme-bound inhibitors for both types of peptides, it became apparent that the presence of the bulky decahydroisoquinoline carboxylic acid at the P_1' site of peptide **53** (Thomas 1991) resulted in a binding conformer that proved different from that of an extended peptide. This resulted in the preference of the *R* stereochemistry at the carbinol centre for proper interaction with the aspartic acid residues at the enzyme active site.

Table 6B.8 Inhibitors containing hydroxyethylamine isoteres

									K_i (nM)
49	Ac	Ser	Leu	Asn	LeuHEAPro	Ile	Val	OMe	11
50	Ac	Ser	Leu	Asn	PheHEAPro	Ile	Val	OMe	0.66
51			Qnc	Asn	PheHEAPro	O	Bu^t		23
52			Qnc	Asn	PheHEAPip	NH	Bu^t		2
53			Qnc	Asn	PheHEADiq	NH	Bu^t		< 0.4

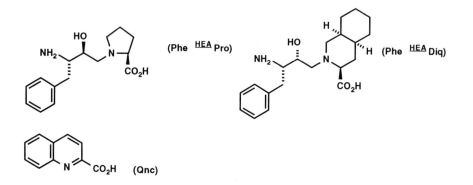

There has also been considerable interest in the design of inhibitors with C_2 symmetry to take advantage of the same symmetry in the HIV protease homodimer. A number of dipeptide mimics of the cleavage site have been designed and have proved useful in the preparation of very active inhibitors (Table 6B.9). Peptide **54** (Erickson *et al.* 1990; Kempf *et al.* 1990), with the 2*S*,4*S*-diamino-3-hydroxy-1,5-diphenylpentane dipeptide insert, is a potent inhibitor with an IC$_{50}$ value of 3 nM. Peptide **55** with the N-acetyl group in place of the benzyloxycarbonyl group was also shown to be an effective inhibitor with an IC$_{50}$ value of 12 nM. With the dihydroxy homo-logue insert as shown in peptides **56** and **57** (Kempf *et al.* 1990), there are two possible symmetric inserts when the two phenylmethyl side-chains maintain the *S* stereochemistry of Phe. Both the 3*R*,4*R* and the 3*S*,4*S* dihydroxy inserts in peptides **56** and **57** respectively were shown to be equally effective in this template. These peptides are highly potent inhibitors with activity in the subnanomolar range. The remaining possible diastereomer for the dihydroxy insert is shown in peptide **58**, again maintaining the *S* stereochemistry of Phe. This last insert is not C_2 symmetric, although the corresponding peptide was also shown to be a potent inhibitor with an IC$_{50}$ value of 0.22 nM. These initial compounds exhibited extremely poor water solubility, however, and additional analogues were prepared. For example, peptide **59** (Kempf *et al.* 1991) was found to have significant

Table 6B.9 Inhibitors with C_2 symmetry

								K_i (nM)
54		Cbz	Val	Phe**A**Phe	Val	Cbz		3
55		Ac	Val	Phe**A**Phe	Val	Ac		12
56		Cbz	Val	Phe**B**Phe	Val	Cbz		0.22
57		Cbz	Val	Phe**C**Phe	Val	Cbz		0.38
58		Cbz	Val	Phe**D**Phe	Val	Cbz		0.22
59		Mpc	Val	Phe**D**Phe	Val	Mpc		<1
60		Cbz	Val	Phe**E**Phe	Val	Cbz		0.1
61		Qnc	Cda	Phe**F**Phe	Cda	Qnc		1
62	MeO	Val	Val	Nle**F**Nle	Val	Val	OMe	1
63			Ahi	Phe**F**Phe	Ahi			0.67

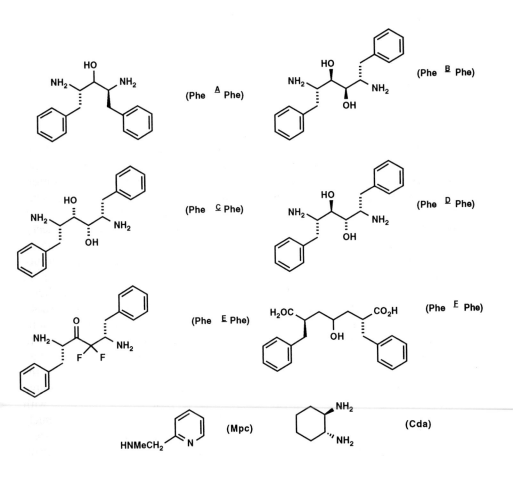

Table 6B.10 Antiviral activity *in vitro*: compound **33** (L-689,502, Boc-PheOHMet-Ahi)

Virus strain	Cell line	MIC_{100} (nM)
HIV-1$_{IIIB}$	MT4	25
HIV-1$_{IIIB}$	PBL	> 0.78
HIV-1$_{SF162}$	Monocyte/macrophage	50
HIV-1$_{IIIB}$	H9	6–25
HIV-1$_{RF}$	H9	50
HIV-1$_{MN}$	H9	50
HIV-1$_{WMJ-2}$	H9	12
HIV-1$_{RUTZ}$	H9	12
SIV$_{mac251}$	H9	800

Data from Thompson 1991.

improvement in water solubility (0.2 mg ml^{-1} at pH 7.4) while maintaining very high inhibitory activity. Another related insert, which is also not C_2 symmetric and is based upon the difluoroketone moiety (Sham *et al.* 1991a,b), is shown in peptide **60**. As anticipated, it is a very potent HIV protease inhibitor with a K_i value of 0.1 nM. A series of C_2 symmetric inserts, based upon the design of 2,6-disubstituted-4-hydroxy-1,7-dioic acid, were also evaluated as useful transition state inserts for HIV protease inhibitors (Babine 1992). Peptide **61**, with phenylmethyl side-chains at the 2 and 6 positions of the insert and the substituted 1,2-diaminocyclohexyl terminus, was shown to be a potent inhibitor with $K_i = 1$ nM. Peptide **62**, with simple butyl side-chains at the 2 and 6 positions of the insert, was also shown to be highly effective with $K_i = 1$ nM. Using peptide **32** as a template, rotation of the C-terminal half around the central hydroxyl-bearing carbon led to the design of the C_2 symmetric peptide **63**. This peptide inhibits HIV protease with an IC_{50} value of 0.67 nM (Bone *et al.* 1991).

Tables 6B.10–6B.13 show some selected examples of HIV protease inhibitors which exhibit potent antiviral activities in cells *in vitro*. For each compound, data from the references indicated above are included for the specific viral isolate and the type of cell used in the assay, as well as for the antiviral concentration.

6B.4.2   Lead inhibitors with non-peptidic structures

There are increasing numbers of examples of non-peptidic HIV protease inhibitors which are neither naturally occurring peptides, such as pepstatins (a-MAPI (Stella *et al.* 1991)), nor synthetic peptides based upon the

Table 6B.11 Antiviral activity *in vitro*: compound **48** (U-75875, Noa-His-ChadOHVal-Ile-Amp)

Virus strain	Cell line	Assay	IC$_{50}$ (nM)
HIV-1$_{IIIB}$	PBL	p24 antigen, HIV RNA	<10
HIV-1$_{LAV}$	MT2	p24 antigen	30
HIV-1$_{IIIB}$	H9	p24 antigen	<1000
HIV-1$_{LAV}$	PBMC	p24, RT	<1000
HIV-1$_{LAV}$	CEM × 174	CPE, RT	<1000
SIV$_{mac251}$	CEM × 174	CPE, RT	<1000
SIV$_{delta670}$	PBL	p24 antigen	<1000
HIV (primary isolate A)	PBMC	p24 antigen	<2
HIV (primary isolate B)	PBMC	p24 antigen	<20

Data from Ashorn *et al.* 1990.

Table 6B.12 Antiviral activity *in vitro*: compound **53** (Ro 31-8959, Qnc-Asn-PheHEADiq-NHBu^t)

Virus strain	Cell line	Assay	IC$_{50}$ (nM)
HIV-1$_{RF}$	C8166	p24 antigen	2
HIV-1$_{GB8}$	JM	Syncytia	2.5
HIV-1$_{RF}$	H9	infectivity	<10,000
HIV-1$_{IIIB}$	CEM	p24 antigen	1–10
SIV$_{mac251}$	C8166	p27 antigen	10.5

Data from Roberts *et al.* 1990.

substrate templates. At present, the inhibitory potencies of these non-peptidic compounds are low (Table 6B.14). The antifungal–antibiotic cerulenin (Blumenstein *et al.* 1989; Moelling *et al.* 1990) (compound **64**), with a reactive epoxide functional group, has been shown to have weak inhibitory activity (IC$_{50}$ = 2.5 nM). A number of compounds containing charged groups have been evaluated for HIV protease inhibitory activity (Brinkworth *et al.* 1991). It was proposed that the simple docosanedioic acid (compound **65**) interacted with the charged residues (Arg 8 and Arg 108) located at each end of the active site groove. This compound was found to have an IC$_{50}$ value of 12 μM. Light Green SF Yellowish (compound **66**), a dye of a different chemical structure with separated sulphonic acid charged groups, inhibited the HIV protease with an IC$_{50}$ value of 12 μM. Pyronin B (compound **67**), with separated cationic amines, was also found to inhibit

Table 6B.13 Antiviral activity *in vitro*: compound **59** (A-77003, Mpc-Val-PheDPhe-Val-Mpc)

Virus strain	Cell line	Assay	EC_{50} (μM)
HIV-1$_{IIIB}$	H9	p24 antigen	0.15
HIV-1$_{IIIB}$	CEM	p24 antigen	0.07
HIV-1$_{MN}$	CEM	p24 antigen	0.03
HIV-1$_{RF}$	CEM	p24 antigen	0.055
HIV-1$_{CDC451}$	CEM	p24 antigen	0.07
HIV-1$_{SF}$	H9	p24 antigen	0.30
HIV-2$_{ROD}$	MT4	p24 antigen	0.27
HIV-1$_{IIIB}$	MT4	CPE	0.20
HIV-1$_{MN}$	MT4	CPE	0.12
LAV	MT4	CPE	0.24
LAV	CEM	CPE	0.15
HIV-2$_{MS}$	MT4	CPE	0.24
HIV-1$_{IIIB}$	PBL	p24 antigen	0.06
HIV (primary isolate)	PBL	p24 antigen	0.03
HIV-1$_{A018}$H112-2 pre-AZT isolate	MT2	CPE	0.12
HIV-1$_{A018}$G910-6 post-AZT isolate	MT2	CPE	0.21

Data from Kempf *et al.* 1991.

the enzyme with an IC_{50} value of 17 μM. Preliminary data suggested that these last three compounds are likely to be non-competitive inhibitors. A mechanism-based natural product screen identified inhibitory activity from the magenta ascidian *Didemnum* sp. collected at Auluptagel Island, Palau (Potts *et al.* 1991). Isolation and purification of these materials led to the identification of two linear heptaprenoids, didemnaketal A (compound **68**) and didemnaketal B (compound **69**), which inhibited HIV protease with IC_{50} values of 2 μM and 10 μM respectively. It was stated that the lability of esters under physiological conditions would probably preclude further development of these compounds.

A computer-assisted search of the structures of compounds in the Cambridge Crystallographic Database which sought steric complementarity with the HIV-1 protease active site identified bromperidol as a lead structure. Testing of additional compounds led to the discovery of the known antipsychotic agent haloperidol (compound **70**) as a weak inhibitor with a K_i value of 100 μM (Des Jarlais *et al.* 1990). In another study (Bures *et al.* 1992), a computer-assisted three-dimensional substructure search in a number of large databases was based upon the crystallographic structure of HIV-1 protease bound inhibitor (compound **54**). The patterns of selected

Table 6B.14 Non-peptidic inhibitors

		IC$_{50}$ (μM)
64	Cerulenin	2500
65	Docosanedioc acid	12
66	Light Green SF Yellowish	12
67	Pyronin B	17
68	Didemnaketal A	2
69	Didemnaketal B	10
70	Haloperidol	100
71	Substituted benzophenone	11

64

65 $HO_2C\text{-}(CH_2)_{20}\text{-}CO_2H$

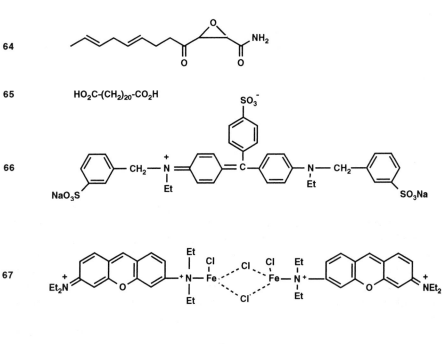

66

67

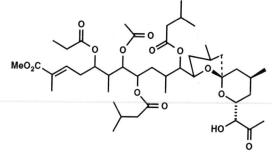

68

Table 6B.14 (*continued*)

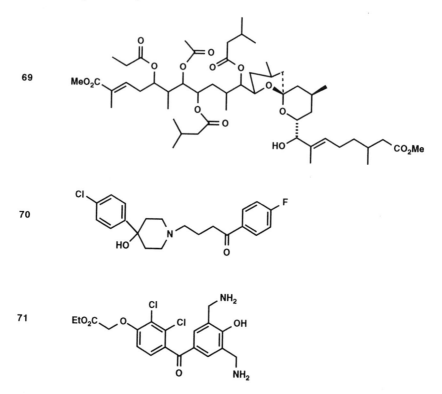

important atoms which are related by specific geometric constraints were constructed based upon the detailed interactions between compound **54** and the enzyme active site. The databases consist of (1) Abbott Laboratories compound file with 70 000 structures, (2) Fine Chemicals Directory (Molecular Design Limited, San Leandro, CA) with 50 000 structures, and (3) compounds with log P values (Daylight Chemical Information Systems, New Orleans, LA) with 20 000 structures. Approximate three-dimensional structures for these compounds were generated using the program CONCORD (Tripos Associates, St. Louis, MO). Selected compounds from the search were tested for HIV inhibitory activity and three structurally related non-peptidic compounds were identified. Compound **71** was found to be the most active and inhibited HIV protease with an IC$_{50}$ value of 11 μM.

6B.4.3 Dimerization inhibitors

A competent HIV protease is an obligatory dimer, and the equilibrium constant at pH 5 (0.1 M acetate + 1 M NaCl + 1 mM EDTA buffer, 37 °C) was determined to be 3.6 nM (Zhang *et al.* 1991a). A dimerization inhibitor offers another mechanism by which the protease can be inactivated. Much of the stability of the dimeric enzyme is due to the interaction between the two monomeric units in the β-sheet comprising the N- and C-terminal segments, and the intermolecular interaction involves a number of critical hydrogen bonds (Weber 1990). Two inhibitory peptides, Ac-Pro-Gln-Ile-Thr-Leu-Trp-Gln-Arg-NH$_2$ and Ac-Gln-Ile-Gly-Met-Thr-Leu-Asn-Phe-NH$_2$, were derived from the N- and C-termini respectively of HIV-1 protease (Schramm *et al.* 1991). The C-terminal tetrapeptide Ac-Thr-Leu-Asn-Phe—OH was shown by kinetic analysis to bind the inactive monomer and prevent the dimerization of the enzyme (Zhang *et al.* 1991a). The dissociation constant for the monomer–inhibitor complex was determined to be 45 μM. These inhibitors offer another design strategy. It has the added benefit of being highly specific for these viral dimeric enzymes compared with other aspartyl proteases which do not function by this obligatory dimer mechanism. This type of inhibitor also has a unique advantage in an ability to bind to the monomeric unit present in the *gag-pol* protein, and it can be concentrated into the budding virions along with viral polyproteins.

6B.4.4 Inhibition of HIV protease by cations

Enzymes that possess metal cation binding sites are susceptible to inactivation by metal-catalysed oxidation. Aspartyl proteases do not require metals for catalytic activity and are generally not known to be inhibited by divalent cations. However, in studies of the susceptibility of HIV-1 protease to metal-catalysed oxidation, it was found that, among a large number of cations studied, micromolar concentrations of copper(II) and mercury(II) caused marked inhibition of the enzyme (Karlstrom and Levine 1991). The inactivation was rapid, not oxygen dependent, and not reversed by subsequent addition of EDTA or dithiothreitol. The monomer of HIV-1 protease has two cysteine residues; Cys[67] lies on the surface while Cys[95] is involved in the dimeric interface. Direct inhibition by copper(II) requires the presence of these residues since a competent synthetic protease lacking cysteine residues was not inactivated in the presence of copper(II). The addition of dithiothreitol as an exogenous thiol rendered this synthetic protease sensitive to copper(II) inhibition. The mechanism by which copper(II) inactivates HIV-1 protease remained unresolved.

In the analysis of fractions from the venom of the American copperhead snake, zinc(II) was identified as a renin inhibitory component. It was also found to be an effective inhibitor of HIV-1 protease and, depending on substrates, the inhibition can be either competitive or non-competitive (Zhang *et al.* 1991b). The observed K_i values are strongly pH dependent and optimal in the range of 20 μM at or above pH 7. The inhibition is reversed by

EDTA, and available data suggest that the inhibitory effect is not due to the disruption of the dimer but, rather, is a consequence of the binding of zinc(II) at or near the active-site aspartic acid residues. It is suggested that a ligand could be designed to incorporate binding to both zinc(II) and the enzyme to create a tight-binding specific inhibitor.

6B.5 Assessment: the practical HIV protease inhibitor

The staggering number of HIV protease inhibitors (most of which are undisclosed) belie the immaturity of the medicinal effort. An objective evaluation of these exposes shortcomings. Many of the non-peptidic inhibitors possess charged functional groups, which are poorly tolerated with respect to antiviral activity, and all have K_i values in the micromolar range, at least two orders of magnitude removed from viable antiviral potency. The non-peptidic inhibitors are the less developed of the two classes. However, although non-peptidic inhibitors may be dismissed out of hand for the moment, they may well be the future of protease inhibition. Their potency *will* be improved, and yield structures which are less expensive to prepare and have better formulation, deliverability, and clearance than the peptidomimetics. Although the shortcomings of the peptidomimetics in these respects are well known (Plattner and Norbeck 1989), it is appropriate here to give a brief assessment of their impact on the peptidomimetic protease inhibitors. The degree to which this causes problems depends on the objective. The immediate but less ambitious objective is the validation of the protease as a chemotherapeutic target. No matter how compelling the circumstantial arguments, a continuing effort towards practical protease inhibitors will depend on a positive outcome to this question. The entity chosen for this validation need not be the final candidate, as the smaller scale of the studies permits the experimental design to work around particular shortcomings. Nevertheless, for a disease like AIDS where there is no directly appropriate animal model, even for the validation, an entity must be chosen of sufficient quality that the experimental outcome is unambiguous. This concept probing is now being carried out with potent peptidomimetic inhibitors, even with their obvious deficiencies, by Abbott, Roche, and possibly other pharmaceutical companies.

What are the virtues and shortcomings of the peptidomimetics? At the most fundamental level the peptidomimetics are no different from any other chemotherapeutic agent, and the lead structures which have been disclosed have attained many of the basic criteria of practical therapeutics. They are efficacious and not cytotoxic, as determined from the lymphocyte and cell culture antiviral assays. There is no evidence of metabolic instability, although this is one of the last and most unpredictable criteria to meet. Generally speaking, the experience with other peptidomimetics is that achieving metabolic stability is an easier objective than those which follow.

They are HIV aspartyl protease selective. There are several human aspartyl proteases, involved in digestion, lysosomal degradation, and blood pressure regulation, which must be transparent to the inhibitor. Meeting this objective appears to have been easier than might first have been supposed, and it is possible that the design process has benefited serendipitously from the distinctive homodimeric structure of the viral enzyme. In brief, the structures possess *most* of the basic criteria for safety and efficacy, although there are two caveats with respect to efficacy. First, many of the inhibitors have been optimized with respect to the HIV-1 protease, notably those with large (P-1), (P-1 ') side-chain pairings (such as phe-phe and cha-val). However, since there are two HIV viruses which present structural divergence but functional identity, it would appear imperative that the clinical candidate encompass both activities so as to minimize the rate at which resistant phenotypes emerge. The second caveat is related to deliverability and pharmacokinetics, and is discussed below.

Thus the difficulty with the peptidomimetics is not primarily safety and efficacy, but the associated issues of formulation, deliverability, and pharmacokinetics. The particular challenge faced in formulation is the insolubility of the most potent peptidomimetics. The best antiviral activity is seen with those compounds presenting an almost complete lipophilic veneer and hence have an aqueous insolubility that makes routine screening, pathology and toxicology evaluation, and formulation painstaking. Although the chemical strategy in optimizing peptidomimetics is always to identify the superfluous peptidic elements and then remove or replace them, the end product often cannot disguise its ancestry. A compound with a linear amide-bond-containing backbone from which project hydrophobic appendages is deemed a peptide by our physiology and treated accordingly. This has two important consequences. The peptidomimetics generally have unsatisfactory oral availability ($\leqslant 20$ per cent). Although AIDS is a life-threatening disease and, in principle, other delivery means are possible, the reality is that this disease requires a chemotherapeutic agent capable of chronic use in the ill immune-compromised patient, preferably without the use of a syringe or health practitioner's assistance. Furthermore, a biliary transporter in the liver sequesters and eliminates that portion of the peptidomimetic which is absorbed with ruthless efficiency. The consequence of these dual barriers, intended to prevent our exposure to information-containing xenobiotics, is that high serum blood levels are not maintained. Whether the levels which can be maintained are adequate to deliver an effective dose to the mobile HIV virion or HIV-infected cell is, short of the clinical study, an almost impossible question to answer. Although the effort to discover patterns for which these rules are exempted, or to identify singular (empirical) exceptions, continues (Plattner and Norbeck 1989; Burton *et al.* 1991; Dutta 1991; Matthews 1991; Nellens 1991; Ward 1991), the effort thus far has been mostly unrewarding.

The information at hand to address in detail the applicability of these concerns to specific inhibitors remains, at this time, almost completely proprietary. However, two recent disclosures do provide optimism. Black *et al.* (1991) have evaluated the ability of peptidomimetic protease inhibitors to block the spread of Rauscher murine leukaemia virus in mice by 14 days of twice daily intraperitoneal inhibitor administration. The peptidomimetics were non-toxic, and reduced viraemia in a dose-dependent manner, providing a first demonstration of *in vivo* antiviral activity. A complete pharmacokinetic evaluation of several inhibitors from Abbott Laboratories, one of which is presently undergoing collaborative concept testing (with the National Institutes of Health) have been reported by Kempf *et al.* (1991). One of the C_2-symmetric inhibitors (A-77003, see above) possessed broad-spectrum activity (HIV-1 and HIV-2) against infected transformed, and primary, human cell lines, including one which was AZT resistant. Although the oral activity of this particular compound was low, a 5 mg kg^{-1} intravenous bolus resulted in plasma concentrations which exceeded the antiviral ED_{50} for several hours. This is sufficient, as noted by Kempf *et al.* (1991), for an assessment of the clinical potential of protease inhibition using an intravenous delivery.

6B.6   Envoi

At the present time, the HIV protease is merely one of many opportunities for AIDS chemotherapy. It is hoped that the extraordinary interest in this enzyme is in true proportion to its promise. In a remarkably short period of time, the integrated experimental study of the AIDS virus has brought forward the protease as an essential viral catalyst, identified strategies for inhibitor design, and guided the execution of these strategies to non-toxic inhibitors with potent *ex vivo* lymphocyte and cell culture anti-viral activity. The entities now in hand fulfil a sufficient number of the criteria for the practical inhibitor and should soon yield a suggestive (at least) answer as to their merit. However, there must be no misunderstanding of the further effort to transform suggestive promise to proven value. None of the disclosed entities comes close to the breadth of criteria believed to be appropriate to clinical antiviral capability. The medical need of the human immunodeficiency virus will demand that the first-generation inhibitors necessarily reflect compromise, at first without the understanding of where compromise is most easily extracted or of where the sacrifice in one criterion has been more than offset by the gain in a second. At least, the most serious shortcomings of the present leads are obvious. The peptidomimetics possess potency, but lack deliverability; the non-peptidics offer a likelihood of deliverability, but are impotent. The refinement of each strategy will continue, driven by the fervent anticipation that one strategy will ultimately secure success.

References

Arnold, E. and Arnold, G. F. (1991). HIV structure: implications for antiviral design. *Advances in Virus Research* **39**, 1–87.

Ashorn, P., McQuade, T. J., Thaisrivongs, S., Tomasselli, A. G., Tarpley, W. G., and Moss, B. (1990). An inhibitor of the protease blocks maturation of human and simian immunodeficiency viruses and spread of infection. *Proceedings of the National Academy of Sciences of the United States of America*, **87**, 7472–6.

Babe, L. M., Pichuantes, S., and Craik, C. S. (1991). Inhibition of HIV protease by heterodimer formation. *Biochemistry*, **30**, 106–11.

Babine, R., Zhang, N., Jurgers, A. R., Schow, S. R., Desai, P. R., James, J. C., and Semmelhack, M. F. (1992). Use of HIV-1 protease structure in inhibitor design. *Biol. Med. Chem. Lett.*, **2**, 541–6.

Baboonian, C. and Dalgleish, A. (1991). Proteinase inhibitors. *Molecular Aspects of Medicine*, **12**, 329–40.

Baboonian, C., Dalgleish, A., Bountiff, L., Gross, J., Oroszlan, S., Rickett, G., Smith-Burchnell, C., Troke, P., and Merson, J. (1991). HIV-1 protease is required for synthesis of pro-viral DNA. *Biochemical and Biophysical Research Communications*, **179**, 17–24.

Bachelerie, F., Alcami, J., Arenzana-Seisdedos, F. and Virelizier, J.-L. (1991). HIV enhancer activity perpetuated by NF-κB induction on infection of monocytes. *Nature, London*, **350**, 709–12.

Bartlett, P. A. and Kezer, W. B. (1984). Phosphinic acid dipeptide analogs: potent, slow-binding inhibitors of aspartic peptidases. *Journal of the American Chemical Society*, **106**, 4282–3.

Baum, E. Z., Bebernitz, G. A., and Gluzman, Y. (1990). Isolations of mutants of HIV protease based on the toxicity of the enzyme in *E. coli*. *Proceedings of the National Academy of Sciences of the United States of America*, **87**, 5573–7.

Becerra, S. P., Clore, G. M., Angela, M., Gronenborn, A. M., Karlstrom, A. R., Stahl S. J., *et al*. (1990). Purification and characterization of the RNase H domain of HIV-1 reverse transcriptase expressed in *E. coli*. *Federation of European Biochemical Societies Letters*, **270**, 76–80.

Becerra, S. P., Kumar, A., Lewis, M. S., Widen, S. G., Abbotts, J., and Wilson, S. H. (1991). Protein–protein interactions of HIV-1 reverse transcriptase: implication of central and C-terminal regions in subunit binding. *Biochemistry*, **30**, 11707–19.

Ben-Artzi, H., Zeelon, E., Gorecki, M., and Panet, A. (1992). Double-stranded RNA-dependent RNase activity associated with HIV-1 reverse transcription. *Proceedings of the National Academy of Sciences of the United States of America*, **99**, 927–31.

Bennett, R. P., Rhee, S., Craven, R. C., Hunter, E., and Wills, J. W. (1991). Amino acids encoded downstream of *gag* are not required by Rous sarcoma virus protease during *gag*-mediated assembly. *Journal of Virology*, **65**, 272–80.

Bess, J. W., Jr., Powell, P. J., Issaq, H. J., Schumack, L. J., Grimes, M. K., Henderson, L. E., and Arthur, L. O. (1992). Tightly bound zinc in HIV-1, human T-cell leukemia virus type 1, and other retroviruses. *Journal of Virology*, **66**, 840–7.

Billich, A. and Winkler, G. (1991). Analysis of subsite preferences of HIV-1 protease using MA/CA junction peptides substituted at the P3-P1′ positions. *Archives of Biochemistry and Biophysics*, **290**, 186–90.

Billich, A., Hammerschmid, F., and Winkler, G. (1990). Purification, assay, and kinetic features of HIV-1 protease. *Biological Chemistry* Hoppe Seyler, **371**, 265–72.

Billich, A., Billich, S., and Rosenwirth, B. (1991). Assay systems for HIV-1 proteinase and their use for evaluation of inhibitors. *Antiviral Chemistry and Chemotherapy*, **2**, 65–73.

Black, P. L., Ussery, M. A., Downs, M. B., Lewis, M. G., Bell, R. C., Baldoni, J., *et al.* (1991). Antiviral activity *in vivo* of HIV protease inhibitors in a murine model of AIDS. Presented at 4th International Conference of the NCDDG Groups; Frontiers in HIV Therapy, San Diego, CA.

Blaha, I., Nemec, J., Tozser, J., and Oroszlan, S. (1991). Synthesis of homologous peptides as analogs of an HIV proteinase substrate. *International Journal of Peptide and Protein Research*, **38**, 453–8.

Blum, M., Cunningham, A., Pang, H., and Hofmann, T. (1991). Mechanism and pathway of penicillopepsin-catalzed transpeptidation and evidence for non-covalent trapping of amino acid and peptide intermediates. *Journal of Biological Chemistry*, **266**, 9501–7.

Blumenstein, J. J., Copeland, T. D., Oroszlan, S., and Michejda, C. J. (1989). Synthetic non-peptide inhibitors of HIV protease. *Biochemical and Biophysical Research Communications*, **163**, 980–7.

Blundell, T. and Pearl, L. (1989). A second front against AIDS. *Nature, London*, **337**, 596–7.

Blundell, T. L., Jenkins, J. A., Sewell, B. T., Pearl, L. H., Cooper, J. B., Tickle, I. J., *et al.* (1990). X-ray analysis of aspartic proteinases. Endothiapepsin at 0.21 nm. *Journal of Biological Chemistry*, **211**, 919–41.

Boger, J., Lohr, N. S., Ulm, E. H., Poe, M., Blaine, E. H., Fanelli, G. M., *et al.* (1983). Novel renin inhibitors containing the amino acid statine. *Nature, London*, **303**, 82–4.

Bone, R., Vacca, J. P., Anderson, P. S., and Holloway, M. K. (1991). X-ray structure of the HIV-1 protease complex with L-700,417: an inhibitor with pseudo C_2 symmetry. *Journal of the American Chemical Society*, **113**, 9382–4.

Boutelje, J., Karlstrom, A. R., Hartmanis, M. G. N., Holmgren, E., Sjoegren, A., and Levine, R. L. (1990). HIV protease is catalytically active as a fusion protein: characterization of the fusion and native enzymes produced in *E. coli*. *Archives of Biochemistry and Biophysics*, **283**, 141–9.

Boyer, P. L., Ferris, A. L., and Hughes, S. H. (1992). Cassette mutagenesis of the reverse transcriptase of HIV-1. *Journal of Virology*, **66**, 1031–9.

Brinkworth, R. I., Woon, T. C., and Fairlie, D. P. (1991). Inhibition of HIV-1 protease by non-peptide carboxylates. *Biochemical and Biophysical Research Communications*, **176**, 241–6.

Bryant, M. and Ratner, L. (1990). Myristoylation-dependent replication and assembly of HIV-1. *Proceedings of the National Academy of Sciences of the United States of America*, **87**, 523–7.

Bures, M. G., Hutchins, C. W., Maus, M., Kohlbrenner, W., Kadam, S., and Erickson, J. W. (1992). Using three-dimensional substructure searching to identify novel, non-peptidic inhibitors of HIV-1 protease *Tetrahedron Computer Methodology*, **3**, 673–80.

Burstein, H., Bizub, D., and Skalka, A. M. (1991). Assembly and processing of avian retroviral *gag* polyproteins containing linked protease dimers. *Journal of Virology*, **65**, 6165–72.

Burton, P. S., Conradi, R. A., and Hilgers, A. R. (1991). Mechanisms of peptide and protein absorption: transcellular mechanism of peptide and protein absorption, passive aspects. *Advances in Drug Delivery Reviews*, **7**, 365–86.

Cheng, Y.-S. E., Yin, F. H., Foundling, S., Blomstrom, D., and Kettner, C. A. (1990a). Stability and activity of the HIV protease: comparison of the natural dimer with a homologous, single chain tethered dimer. *Proceedings of the National Academy of Sciences of the United States of America*, **87**, 9660–4.

Cheng, Y.-S. E., McGowan, M. H., Kettner, C. A., Schloss, J. V., Erickson-Viitanen, S., and Yin, F. H. (1990b). High-level synthesis of recombinant HIV protease and the recovery of active enzyme from inclusion bodies. *Gene*, **87**, 243–8.

Cooper, J. B., Khan, G., Tickle, I. J., and Blundell, T. L. (1990). X-ray analysis of aspartic proteases. Porcine pepsin at 0.23 nm resolution. *Journal of Molecular Biology*, **214**, 199–222.

Copeland, T. D., Wondrak, E. M., Tozser, J., Roberts, M. M., and Oroszlan, S. (1990). Substitution of proline with pipecolic acid at the scissile bond converts a peptide substrate of the HIV protease into a selective inhibitor. *Biochemical and Biophysical Research Communications*, **169**, 310–14.

Craig, J. C., Duncan, I. D., Hockley, D., Grief, C., Roberts, N. A., and Mills, J. S. (1991). Antiviral properties of Ro31–8959, an inhibitor of the HIV protease. *Antiviral Research*, **16**, 295–305.

Craven, R. C., Bennett, R. P., and Wills, J. W. (1991). Role of the avian retroviral protease in the activation of reverse transcriptase during virion assembly. *Journal of Virology*, **65**, 6205–17.

Crawford, S. and Goff, S. P. (1985). A deletion in the 5′ part of the *pol* gene of Moloney murine leukemia virus blocks proteolytic processing of the *gag* and *pol* polyproteins. *Journal of Virology*, **53**, 899–907.

Cullen, B. R. (1991). Regulation of gene expression in HIV-1. *Advances in Virus Research*, **40**, 1–17.

Cunningham, A., Hofmann, M. I., and Hofmann, T. (1990). Rate-determining steps in penicillopepsin-catalzed reactions. *Federation of European Biochemical Societies Letters*, **276**, 119–22.

Darke, P. L., Nutt, R. F., Brady, S. F., Garsky, V. M., Ciccarone, T. M., Leu, C.-T., *et al.* (1988). HIV-1 protease specificity of peptide cleavage is sufficient for processing of *gag* and *pol* polyproteins. *Biochemical and Biophysical Research Communications*, **156**, 297–303.

Darke, P. L., Leu, C.-T., Davis, L. J., Heimbach, J. C., Diehl, R. E., Hil, W. S., *et al.* (1989). HIV-1 protease: bacterial expression and characterization. *Journal of Biological Chemistry*, **264**, 2307–12.

Davies, J. F., II, Hostomska, Z., Hostomsky, Z., Jordan, S. R., and Matthews, D. A. (1991). Crystal structure domain of the ribonuclease H domain of HIV-1 reverse transcriptase. *Science*, **252**, 88–95.

De Clerq, E. (1990). Targets and strategies for the antiviral chemotherapy of AIDS. *Trends in Pharmacological Sciences*, **11**, 198–205.

Debouck, C. and Metcalf, B. W. (1990). HIV protease: a target for AIDS therapy. *Drug Development Research*, **21**, 1–17.

Debouck, C., Gorniak, J. G., Strickler, J. E., Meek, T. D., Metcalf, B. W., and Rosenberg, M. (1987). HIV protease expressed in *E. coli* exhibits autoprocessing and specific maturation of the *gag* precursor. *Proceedings of the National Academy of Sciences of the United States of America*, **84**, 8903–6.

Des Jarlais, R. L., Seibel, G. L., Kuntz, I. D., Furth, P. S., Alverez, J. C., Ortiz de Montellano, P. R., *et al.* (1990). Structure-based design of nonpeptide inhibitors specific for the HIV-1 protease. *Proceedings of the National Academy of Sciences of the United States of America*, **87**, 6644–8.

de Solms, S. J., Giuliani, E. A., Guare, J. P., Vacca, J. P., Sanders, W. M., Graham, S. L., *et al.* (1991). Design and synthesis of HIV protease inhibitors. Variations of the carboxy terminus of the HIV inhibitor L-682,679. *Journal of Medicinal Chemistry*, **34**, 2852–7.

Di Ianni, C. L., Davis, L. J., Holloway, M. K., Herber, W. K., Darke, P. L., Kohl, N. E., and Dixon, R. A. F. (1990). Characterization of an active single polypeptide form of the HIV-1 protease. *Journal of Biological Chemistry*, **265**, 17348–54.

Dreyer, G. B., Metcalf, B. W., Tomaszek, T. A., Carr, T. J., Chandler, A. C., Hyland, L., *et al.* (1989). Inhibition of HIV-1 protease *in vitro*: rational design of substrate analog inhibitors. *Proceedings of the National Academy of Sciences of the United States of America*, **86**, 9752–6.

Dutta, A. S. (1991). Design and therapeutic potential of peptides. *Advances in Drug Research* **21**, 145–280.

Ehrlich, L. S., Krausslich, H.-G., Wimmer, E., and Carter, C. A. (1990). Expression in *E. coli* and purification of HIV-1 capsid protein p24. *AIDS Research and Human Retroviruses*, **6**, 1169–76.

Englund, G., Hoggan, M. D., Theodore, T. S., and Martin, M. A. (1991). A novel HIV-1 isolate containing alterations affecting the NF-κB element. *Virology*, **181**, 150–7.

Erickson, J., Neidhart, D. J., VanDrie, J., Kempf, D. J., Wang, X. C., Norbeck, D. W., *et al.* (1990). Design, activity, and 0.28 nm crystal structure of a C_2-symmetric inhibitor complexed to the HIV-1 protease. *Science*, **249**, 527–3.

Erickson-Viitanen, S., Manfredi, J., Viitanen, P., Tribe, D. E., Tritch, R., Hutchison, C. A., *et al.* (1989). Cleavage of HIV-1 *gag* polyprotein synthesized *in vitro*: sequential cleavage by the viral proteinase. *AIDS Research and Human Retroviruses*, **5**, 577–91.

Evans, D. B., Brawn, K., Deibel, M. R., Jr., Tarpley, W. G., and Sharma, S. K. (1991). A recombinant ribonuclease H domain of HIV-1 reverse transcriptase that is enzymatically active. *Journal of Biological Chemistry*, **266**, 20583–5.

Ferguson, D. M., Radmer, R. J., and Kollman, P. A. (1991). Determination of the relative binding free energies of peptide inhibitors to the HIV-1 protease. *Journal of Medicinal Chemistry*, **34**, 2654–9.

Fitzgerald, P. M. D. and Springer, J. P. (1991). Structure and function of retroviral proteases. *Annual Review of Biophysics and Biophysical Chemistry*, **20**, 299–320.

Fitzgerald, P. M. D., McKeever, B. M., VanMiddlesworth, J. F., Springer, J. P., Heimbach, J. C., Leu, C. T., *et al.* (1990). Crystallographic analysis of a complex between HIV-1 protease and acetylpepstatin. *Journal of Biological Chemistry*, **265**, 14209–19.

Gelb, M. H., Svaren, J. P., and Abeles, R. H. (1985). Fluoroketone inhibitors of hydrolytic enzymes. *Biochemistry*, **24**, 1813–17.

Gelderblom, H. R. (1991). Assembly and morphology of HIV: potential effect of structure on viral function. *AIDS*, **5**, 617–38.

Giam, C.-Z. and Boros, I. (1988). *In vitro* and *in vivo* autoprocessing of HIV protease expressed in *E. coli*. *Journal of Biological Chemistry*, **263**, 14617–20.

Gilliland, G. L., Winborne, E. L., Nachman, J., and Wlodawer, A. (1990). The three-dimensional structure of recombinant bovine chymosin at 0.23 nm resolution. *Proteins*, **8**, 82–101.

Goldblum, A. (1990). Modulation of the affinity of aspartic proteases by mutated residues in active site models. *Federation of European Biochemical Societies Letters*, **261**, 241–4.

Goobar, L., Danielson, U., Brodin, P., Grundstroem, T., Oeberg, B., and Norrby, E. (1991). High-yield purification of HIV-1 protease expressed by a synthetic gene in *E. coli*. *Protein Expression and Purification*, **2**, 15–23.

Gottlinger, H. G., Sodroski, J. G., and Haseltine, W. A. (1989). Role of capsid precursor processing and myristoylation in morphogenesis and infectivity of HIV-1. *Proceedings of the National Academy of Sciences of the United States of America*, **86**, 5781–5.

Gottlinger, H. G., Dorfman, T., Sodroski, J. G., and Haseltine, W. A. (1991). Effect of mutations affecting the p6 *gag* protein on HIV particle release. *Proceedings of the National Academy of Sciences of the United States of America*, **88**, 3195–9.

Grant, S. K., Deckman, I. C., Minnich, M. D., Culp, J., Franklin, S., Dreyer, G. B., *et al.* (1991). Purification and biochemical characterization of recombinant SIV protease and comparison to HIV-1 protease. *Biochemistry*, **30**, 8424–34.

Graves, M. C., Lim, J. J., Heimer, E. P., and Kramer, R. A. (1988). An 11-kDa form of HIV protease expressed in *E. coli* is sufficient for enzymatic activity. *Proceedings of the National Academy of Sciences of the United States of America*, **85**, 2449–53.

Graves, M. C., Meidel, M. C., Pan, Y.-C. E., Manneberg, M., Lahm, H. W., and Grueninger-Leitch, F. (1990). Identification of a HIV-1 protease cleavage site within the p66 subunit of reverse transcriptase. *Biochemical and Biophysical Research Communications*, **168**, 30–6.

Greenlee, W. J. (1990). Renin inhibitors. *Medicinal Research Reviews*, **10**, 173–236.

Griffiths, J. T., Phylip, L. H., Konvalinka, J., Strop, P., Gustchina, A., Wlodaver, A. *et al.* (1992). Different requirements for productive interaction between the active site of HIV-1 protease and substrates containing hydropholic or aromatic *a* pro cleavage sites. *Biochemistry*, **31**, 193–200.

Grinde, B., Hungnes, O., and Tjoetta, E. (1990). Modified oligopeptides designed to interact with the HIV-1 proteinase inhibit viral replication. *Archives of Virology*, **114**, 167–73.

Grobelny, D., Wondrak, E. M., Galardy, R. E., and Oroszlan, S. (1990). Selective phosphinate transition-state analog inhibitors of the HIV protease. *Biochemical and Biophysical Research Communications*, **169**, 1111–16.

Guenet, C., Leppik, R. A., Pelton, J. T., Moelling, K., Lovenberg, W., and Harris, B. A. (1989). HIV-1 protease: mutagenesis of asn 88 indicates a domain required for dimer formation. *European Pharmacology, Molecular Pharmacology Section* **172**, 443–51.

Gustchina, A. and Weber, I. T. (1990). Comparison of inhibitor binding in HIV-1 protease and in non-viral aspartic proteases. *Federation of European Biochemical Societies Letters*, **269**, 269–72.

Gustchina, A. and Weber, I. T. (1991). Comparative analysis of the sequences and structures of HIV-1 and HIV-2 proteases. *Proteins*, **10**, 325–39.

Hafkemeyer, P., Ferrari, E., Brecher, J., and Huebscher, U. (1991). The p15 carboxy-terminal proteolysis product of the HIV-1 reverse transcriptase p66 has DNA polymerase activity. *Proceedings of the National Academy of Sciences of the United States of America*, **88**, 5262–6.

Hansen, J., Billich, S., Schulze, T., Sukrow, S., and Moellling, K. (1988). Partial purification and substrate analysis of bacterially expressed HIV protease. *EMBO Journal*, **7**, 1785–91.

Harte, W. E., Jr., Swaminathan, S., Mansuri, M., Martin, J. C., Rosenberg, I. E., and Beveridge, D. L. (1990). Domain communication in the dynamical structure of of HIV-1 protease. *Proceedings of the National Academy of Sciences of the United States of America*, **87**, 8864–8.

Haseltine, W. A. (1991). Molecular biology of the human-immunodeficiency virus type 1. *FASEB Journal*, **5**, 2349–60.

Hellen, C. U. T., Krausslich, H.-G., and Wimmer, E. (1989). Proteolytic processing of polyproteins in the replication of RNA virus. *Biochemistry*, **28**, 9881–90.

Henderson, L. E., Benveniste, R. E., Sowder, R., Copeland, T. D., Schultz, A. M., and Oroszlan, S. (1988). Molecular characterization of *gag* proteins from SIV $_{mne}$. *Journal of Virology*, **62**, 2587–95.

Henderson, L. E., Bowers, M. A., Sowder, R. C., Serabyn, S. A., Johnson, D. G., Bess, J. W., *et al.* (1992). *Gag* Proteins of the highly replicative MN strain of HIV-1 post-translational-modifications, proteolytic processing, and complete amino acid sequence. *Journal of Virology*, **66**, 1856–65.

Hirel, P.-H., Parker, F., Boizian, J., Jung, G., Outerovitch, D., Dugue, A., *et al.* (1990). HIV-1 aspartic protease: high level production and automated fluorometric screening assay of inhibitors. *Antiviral Chemistry and Chemotherapy*, **1**, 9–15.

Hoglund, S., Ofverstedt, L.-G., Nilsson, A., Lundquist, P., Gelderblom, H., Ozel, M., and Skoglund, U. (1992). Spatial visualization of the maturing HIV-1 core and its linkage to the envelope. *AIDS*, **8**, 1–7.

Holzman, T. F., Kohlbrenner, W. E., Weig, D., Rittenhouse, J., Kempf, D., and Erickson, J. (1991). Inhibitor stabilization of HIV-2 proteinase dimer formation. *Journal of Biological Chemistry*, **266**, 19217–20.

Hoshikawa, N., Kojima, A., Yasuda, A., Takayashiki, E., Masuko, S., Chiba, J., *et al.* (1991). Role of the *gag* and *pol* genes of HIV in the morphogenesis and maturation of retrovirus-like particles expressed by recombinant vaccinia virus: an ultrastructural study. *Journal of Virology*, **72**, 2509–17.

Hostomska, Z., Matthews, D. A., Davies, J. F., Nodes, B. R., and Hostomsky, Z. (1991). Proteolytic release and crystallization of the RNase H domain of HIV-1 reverse transcriptase. *Journal of Biological Chemistry*, **266**, 14697–702.

Hostomsky, Z., Appelt, K., and Ogden, R. C. (1989). High level expression of self-processed HIV-1 protease in *E. coli* using a synthetic gene. *Biochemical and Biophysical Research Communications*, **161**, 1056–63.

Hsu, M. T., Schutt, A., Holly, M., Slice, L. W., Sherman, M. I., Richman, D. D., *et al.* (1991). Inhibition of HIV replication in acute and chronic infections *in vitro* by a tat inhibitor. *Science*, **254**, 1799–1802.

Huff, J. R. (1991). HIV protease: a novel chemotherapeutic target for AIDS. *Journal of Medicinal Chemistry*, **34**, 2305–14.

Huff, J. R., Anderson, P. S., Britcher, S. F., Drake, P., de Solms, S. J., Dixon, R. A. F., *et al.* (1990). The design and synthesis of HIV protease inhibitors. Presented at Ortho-UCLA Colloquium on Synthetic Peptides: Approaches to Biological Problems, Frisco, CO.

Hui, J. O., Tomasselli, A. G., Zurcher-Neely, H. A., and Heinrikson, R. L. (1990). Ribonuclease A as a substrate of the HIV-1 protease. *Journal of Biological Chemistry*, **265**, 21386–9.

Hui, K. Y., Manetta, J. V., Gygi, T., Bowdon, B. J., Keith, K. A., Shannon, W. M., and Lai, M. H. T. (1991). A rational approach in the search for potent inhibitors against HIV proteinase. *FASEB Journal*, **5**, 2606–10.

Hyland, L. J., Tomaszek, T. A., Roberts, G. D., Carr, S. A., Magaard, V. W., Bryan, H. L., *et al.* (1991a). HIV-1 protease 1. Initial velocity studies and kinetic characterization of reaction intermediates by ^{18}O isotope exchange. *Biochemistry*, **30**, 8441–53.

Hyland, L. J., Tomaszek, T. A., and Meek, T. D. (1991b). HIV-1 protease. 2. Use of pH rate studies and solvent kinetic isotope effects to elucidate details of the chemical mechanism. *Biochemistry*, **30**, 8454–63.

Ido, E., Han, H.-P., Kezdy, F. J., and Tang, J. (1991). Kinetic studies of HIV-1 protease and its active site H-bond A28S mutant. *Journal of Biological Chemistry*, **266**, 24359–66.

Jacks, T., Power, M. D., Masiarz, F. R., Luciw, P. A., Barr, P. J., and Varmus, H. E. (1988). Characterization of ribosomal frameshifting in HIV-1 *gag-pol* expression. *Nature, London*, **331**, 280–3.

James M. N. G., Sielecki, A. R., Fraser, M., Fedorov, A. A., and Andreeva, N. S. (1990). Crystal structure studies of fungal, mammalian, and viral aspartic proteases. In *Frontiers in Drug Research (Alfred Benzon Symposium 28)* (ed. B. Jensen, F. S. Jorggensen, and H. Kofod), pp. 300–21. Munksgaard, Copenhagen.

Jaskolski, M., Miller, M., Rao, J. K. M., Leis, J., and Wlodawer, A. (1990). Structure of the aspartic protease from Rous sarcoma retrovirus refined at 0.2 nm resolution. *Biochemistry*, **29**, 5889–98.

Jaskolski, M., Tomasselli, A. G., Sawyer, T. K., Staples, D. G., Heinrikson, R. L., Schneider, J., *et al.* (1991). Structure at 0.25 nm resolution of chemically synthesized HIV-1 protease complexed with a hydroxyethylene-based inhibitor. *Biochemistry*, **30**, 1600–9.

Jupp, R. A., Phylip, L. H., Mills, J. S., Le Grice, S. F. J., and Kay, J. (1991). Mutating P2 and P1 residues at cleavage junctions in the HIV-1 *pol* protein. *Federation of European Biochemical Societies Letters* **283**,, 180–4.

Kaplan, A. H. and Swanstrom, R. (1991a). HIV-1 *gag* proteins are processed in two cellular compartments. *Proceedings of the National Academy of Sciences of the United States of America*, **88**, 4528–32.

Kaplan, A. H. and Swanstrom, R. (19921b). HIV-1 *gag* precursor is processed via two pathways: implications for cytotoxicity. *Biochimica et Biophysica Acta*, **50**, 647–53.

Karlstrom, A. R. and Levine, R. L. (1991). Copper inhibits the protease from HIV-1 by both cysteine-dependent and cysteine-independent mechanisms. *Proceedings of the National Academy of Sciences of the United States of America*, **88**, 5552–6.

Katoh, I., Yoshinaka, Y., Rein, A., Shibuya, M., Odaka, T., and Oroszlan, S. (1985). Murine leukemia virus maturation: protease region is required for conversion from immature to mature core form and for virus infectivity. *Virology*, 145, 280–92.

Katoh, I., Yasunaga, T., Ikawa, Y., and Yoshinaka, Y. (1987). Inhibition of retrovirus protease activity by an aspartyl proteinase inhibitor. *Nature, London*, 329, 654–7.

Kay, J. and Dunn, B. M. (1990). Viral proteinases: weakness is strength. *Biochimica et Biophysica Acta*, 1048, 1–18.

Kempf, D. J., Norbeck, D. W., Codacovi, L. M., Wang, X. C., Kohlbrenner, W. E., Wideburg, N. E., *et al.* (1990). Structure based C_2-symmetric inhibitors of HIV protease. *Journal of Medicinal Chemistry*, 33, 2687–9.

Kempf, D. J., Marsh, K. C., Paul, D. A., Knigge, M. F., Norbeck, D. W., Kohlbrenner, W. E., *et al.* (1991). Antiviral and pharmokinetic properties of C_2-symmetric inhibitors of the HIV-1 protease. *Antimicrobial Agents and Chemotherapy Journal*, 35, 2209–14.

Kohl, N. E., Emini, E. A., Schleif, W. A., Davis, L. J., Heimbach, J. C., Dixon, R. A. F., *et al.* (1988). Active protease is required for viral infectivity. *Proceedings of the National Academy of Sciences of the United States of America*, 85, 4686–90.

Kohl, N. E., Diehl, R. E., Randa, E., Davis, L. J., Hanobik, M. G., Wolanski, B., and Dixon, R. A. F. (1991). Expression of active HIV-1 protease by non-infectious chimeric virus particles. *Journal of Virology*, 65, 3007–14.

Konvalinka, J., Strop, P., Velek, J., Cerna, V., Kostka, V., Phylip, L. H., Richards, A. D., Dunn, B. M., and Kay, J. (1990). Sub-site preferences of the aspartic proteinase from the HIV-I virus. *Federation of European Biochemical Societies Letters*, 268, 35–8.

Korant, B. D. (1990). Strategies to inhibit viral polyprotein cleavages. *Annals of the New York Academy of Sciences*, 616, 252–7.

Kotler, M., Danho, W., Katz, R. A., Leis, J., and Skalka, A. M. (1989). Avian retroviral protease and cellular aspartic proteases are distinguished by activities on peptide substrates. *Journal of Biological Chemistry*, 264, 3428–35.

Kramer, R. A., Schraber, M. D., Skalka, A. M., Ganguly, K., Wong-Staal, F., and Reddy, E. P. (1986). HTLV-III *gag* protein is processed in yeast cells by the virus *pol* protease. *Science*, 231, 1580–4.

Krausslich, H.-G. (1991). Human immunodeficiency virus proteinase dimer as a component of the viral polypeptide prevents particle assembly and viral infectivity. *Proceedings of the National Academy of Sciences of the United States of America*, 88, 3213–17.

Krausslich, H.-G. (1992). Specific inhibitor of HIV proteinase prevents cytotoxic effects of a single chain proteinase dimer and restores particle formation. *Journal of Virology*, 66, 567–72.

Krausslich, H.-G. and Wimmer, E. (1988). Viral proteinases. *Annual Review of Biochemistry*, 57, 701–54.

Krausslich, H.-G., Schneider, H., Zybarth, G., Carter, C. A., and Wimmer, E. (1988). Processing of *in vitro* synthesized *gag* precursor proteins of HIV-1 by HIV proteinase generated in *E. coli*. *Journal of Virology*, 62, 4393–7.

Krausslich, H.-G., Ingraham, R. H., Skoog, M. T., Wimmer, E., Pallai, P. V., and Carter, C. A. (1989). Activity of purified biosynthetic protease of HIV on natural substrates and synthetic peptides. *Proceedings of the National Academy of Sciences of the United States of America*, **86**, 807–11.

Krohn, A., Redshaw, S., Ritchie, J. C., Graves, B. J., and Hatada, M. H. (1991). Novel binding mode of potent HIV-protease inhibitors incorporating the *R*-hydroxyethylamine isostere. *Journal of Medicinal Chemistry*, **34**, 3340–2.

Lapatto, R., Blundell, T., Hemmings, A., Overington, J., Wilderspin, A., Wood, S., *et al.* (1989). X-ray analysis of HIV-1 proteinase confirms structural homology among retroviral enzymes. *Nature, London*, **342**, 299–302.

Leberman R. (1991). The Hofmeister series and ionic strength. *Federation of European Biochemical Societies Letters*, **284**, 293–4.

Le Grice, S. F. J., Mills, J., and Mous, J. (1988). Active site mutagenesis of the AIDS virus protease and its alleviation by *trans* complementation. *EMBO Journal*, **7**, 2547–53.

Lilehoj, E. P., Salazar, F. H. R., Mervis, R. J., Raum, M. G., Chan, H. W., Ahmad, N., and Venkatesan, S. (1988). Purification and structural characterization of the putative *gag-pol* protease of HIV. *Journal of Virology*, **63**, 3053–8.

Loeb. D. D., Hutchinson, C. A., Edgell, M. H., Farmerie, W. G., and Swanstrom, R. (1989a). Mutational analysis of HIV-1 protease suggests functional homology with aspartic proteases. *Journal of Virology*, **63**, 111–21.

Loeb, D. D., Swanstrom, R., Everitt, L., Manchester, M., Stamper, S. E., and Hutchison, C. A. (1989b). Complete mutagenesis of the HIV-1 protease.*Nature, London*, **340**, 397–400.

Louis, J. M., McDonald, R. A., Nashed, N. T., Wondrak, E. M., Jerina, D. M., Oroszlan, S., and Mora, P. T. (1991). Autoprocessing of the HIV-1 protease using purified wt and mutated fusion proteins expressed at high levels in *E. coli*. *European Journal of Biochemistry*, **199**, 361–9.

Lyle, T. A., Wiscount, C. M., Guare, J. P., Thompson, W. T., Anderson, P. S., Darke, P. L., *et al.* (1991). Bicycloalkyl amines as novel C-termini for HIV protease inhibitors. *Journal of Medicinal Chemistry*, **34**, 1228–30.

McKeever, B. M., Navia, M. A., Fitzgerald, P. M. D., Springer, J. P., Leu, C.-T., Heimbach, J. C., *et al.* (1989). Crystallization of the aspartyl protease from HIV-1 virus. *Journal of Biological Chemistry*, **264**, 1919–21.

McLeod, D. A., Brinkworth, R. I., Ashley, J. A., Janda, K. D., and Wirsching, P. (1991). Phosphonamidates and phosphonamidate esters as HIV-1 protease inhibitors. *Bioorganic and Medicinal Chemistry Letters*, **1**, 653–8.

McQuade, T. J., Tomasselli, A. G., Liu, L., Karacostas, V., Moss, B., Sawyer, T. K., *et al.* (1990). A synthetic HIV-1 protease inhibitor with antiviral activity arrests HIV-like particle maturation. *Science*, **247**, 454–6.

Margolin, N., Heath, W., Osborne, E., Lai, M., and Vlahos, (1990). Substitutions at the P2′ site of *gag* p17-p24 affect cleavage efficiency by HIV-1 protease. *Biochemical and Biophysical Research Communications*, **167**, 554–60.

Margolin, N., Dee, A., Lai, M., and Vlahos, C. (1991). Purification of recombinant HIV-1 protease. *Preparative Biochemistry*, **21**, 163–73.

Matthews, D. M. (1991). *Protein Absorption: development and present state of the subject*. Wiley-Liss, New York.

Meek, T. D., Dayton, B. D., Metcalf, B. W., Dreyer, G. B., Strickler, J. E., Gorniak, J. G., *et al.* (1989). HIV-1 protease expressed in *E. coli* behaves as a dimeric protease. *Proceedings of the National Academy of Sciences of the United States of America*, **86**, 1841–5.

Meek, T. D., Lambert, D. M., Metcalf, B. W., and Petteway, S. R. (1990a). HIV-1 protease as a target for potential anti-AIDS drugs. *Pharmacochemistry Library*, **14**, 225–56.

Meek, T. D., Lambert, D. M., Dreyer, G. B., Carr, T. J., Tomaszek, T. A., Morre, M. L., *et al*. (1990b). Inhibition of HIV-1 protease in infected T-lymphocytes by synthetic peptide analogs. *Nature, London*, **343**, 90–2.

Meier, U.-C., Billich, A., Mann, K., Schramm, H. J., and Schramm, W. (1991). (α2-Macroglobulin is cleaved by HIV-1 protease in the bait region but not in the C-terminal interdomain region. *Biological Chemistry Hoppe Seyler*, **372**, 1051–6.

Mergener, K., Facke, M., Welker, R., Brinigmann, V., Gelderblom, H. R., and Krausslich, H.-G. (1992). Analysis of HIV particle formation using transient expression of subviral constructs in mammalian cells. *Virology*, **186**, 25–39.

Mervis, R. J., Ahmad, N., Lillehoj, E. P., Raum, M. G., Salazar, F. H. R., Chan, H. W., and Venkatesan, S. (1988). The *gag* gene products of HIV-1: alignment within the *gag* open reading frame, identification of post-translational modifications, and evidence, for alternative *gag* precursors. *Journal of Virology*, **63**, 3993–4002.

Miller, M., Jaskolski, M., Rao, J. K. M., Leis, J., and Wlodawer, A. (1989a). Crystal structure of retroviral protease proves relationship to aspartic acid family. *Nature, London*, **337**, 576–9.

Miller, M., Schneider, J., Sathyanarayana, B. K., Toth, M. V., Marshall, G. R., Clawson, L., *et al*. (1989b). Structure of a complex of synthetic HIV-1 protease with a substrate-based inhibitor at 0.23 nm resolution. *Science*, **246**, 1149–52.

Mitsuya, H., Yarchoan, R., and Broder, S. (1990). Molecular targets for AIDS chemotherapy. *Science*, **249**, 1533–44.

Mitsuya, H., Yarchoan, R., Kageyama, S., and Broder, S. (1991). Targeted therapy of HIV-related disease. *FASEB Journal*, **5**, 2369–81.

Moelling, K., Schulze, T., Knoop, M.-T., Kay, J., Jupp, R., Nicolaou, G., and Pearl, L. H. (1990). *In vitro* inhibition of HIV-1 proteinase by cerulenin. *Federation of European Biochemical Societies Letters*, **261**, 373–7.

Montgomery, D. S., Singh, O. M. P., Gray, N. M., Dykes, C. W., Weir, M. P., and Hobden, A. N. (1991). Expression of an autoprocessing cat-HIV-1 protease fusion protein: purification to homogeneity of the 99 residue protease. *Biochemical and Biophysical Research Communications*, **175**, 784–94.

Moore, M. L., Bryan, W. M., Fakhoury, S. A., Magaard, V. W., Huffman, W. F., Dayton, B. D., *et al*. (1989). Peptide substrates and inhibitors of the HIV-1 protease. *Biochemical and Biophysical Research Communications*, **159**, 420–5.

Moore, M. L., Bryan, W. M., Fakhoury, S. A., and Huffman, W. F. (1990). Structure–activity studies on inhibitors of recombinant HIV-1 protease. Presented at Ortho-UCLA Colloquium on Synthetic Peptides: Approaches to Biological Problems, Frisco, CO.

Moosmayer, D., Reil, H., Ausmeier, M., Scharf, J. G., Hauser, H., Jentsch, K. D., and Hunsmann, G. (1991). Expression and frameshifting but extremely inefficient proteolytic processing of the HIV-1 *gag* and *pol* gene products in stably transfected rodent cell lines. *Virology*, **183**, 215–24.

Mous, J., Heimer, E. P., and Le Grice, S. F. J. (1988). Processing protease and reverse transcriptase from HIV-1 polyprotein in *E. coli*. *Journal of Virology*, **62**, 1433–6.

Nabel, G. J. (1991). Tampering with transcription. *Nature, London*, **350**, 658.

Navia, M. A. and McKeever, B. M. (1990). A role of the aspartyl protease from HIV-1 in the orchestration of virus assembly. *Annals of the New York Academy of Sciences*, **616**, 73–85.

Navia, M. A., Fitzgerald, P. M. D., McKeever, B. M., Leu, C. T., Heimbach, J. C., Herber, W. K., *et al.* (1989). Three-dimensional structure of aspartyl protease from HIV-1. *Nature, London*, **337**, 615–20.

Nellens, H. N. (1991). Mechanisms of peptide and protein absorption: paracellular intestinal transport and modulation of absorption. *Advances in Drug Delivery Reviews*, **7**, 339–64.

Newman, M., Safro, M., Frazad, C., Khan, G., Zdanov, A., Tickle, I. J., *et al.* (1991). X-ray analysis of aspartyl proteinases IV. Structure and refinement at 0.22 nm resolution of bovine chymosin. *Journal of Molecular Biology*, **221**, 1295–1309.

Nitschko, H., Schatzl, H., Oswald, M., and von der Helm, K. (1991). Inhibition of the retroviral HIV-proteinase impairs maturation to infectious virus. *Biochimica et Biophysica Acta*, **50**, 655–8.

Norbeck, D. W. and Kempf, D. J. (1991). HIV protease inhibitors. *Annual Reports of Medicinal Chemistry*, **26**, 141–50.

Nutt, R. F., Brady, S. F., Darke, P. L., Ciccarone, T. M., Colton, C. D., Nutt, E. M. (1988). Chemical synthesis and enzymatic activity of a 99-residue peptide with the HIV protease sequence. *Proceedings of the National Academy of Sciences of the United States of America*, **85**, 7129–33.

Oroszlan, S. and Luftig, R. B. (1990). Retroviral proteinases. *Current Topics in Microbiology and Immunology*, **157**, 158–85.

Oswald, M. and von der Helm, K. (1991). Fibronectin is a non-viral substrate for the HIV protease. *Federation of European Biochemical Societies Letters*, **292**, 298–300.

Overton, H. A., McMillan, D. J., Gridley, S. J., Brenner, J., Redshaw, S., and Mills, J. S. (1990). Effect of two novel inhibitors of the HIV protease on the maturation of the HIV *gag* and *gag-pol* polyproteins. *Virology*, **179**, 508–11.

Park, J. and Morrow, C. D. (1991). Overexpression of the *gag-pol* precursor from HIV-1 proviral genomes results in efficient proteolytic processing in the absence of virion production. *Journal of Virology*, **65**, 5111–17.

Partin, K., Krausslich, H.-G., Ehrlich, L., Wimmer, E., and Carter, C. (1990). Mutational analysis of native substrate of the HIV-1 proteinase. *Journal of Virology*, **64**, 3938–47.

Partin, K., Zybarth, G., Ehrlich, L., DeCrombrugghe, M., Wimmer, E., and Carter, C. (1991). Deletion of sequences upstream of the protease improves the proteolytic processing of HIV-1 virus. *Proceedings of the National Academy of Sciences of the United States of America*, **88**, 4776–80.

Patterson, C. E., Seetharam, R., Kettner, C. A., and Cheng, Y.-S. E. (1992). HIV-I and HIV-2 protease monomers are functionally interchangeable in the dimeric enzymes. *Journal of Virology*, **66**, 1228–31.

Pearl, L. H. and Taylor, W. R. (1987). A structural model for the retroviral proteases. *Nature, London*, **329**, 351–4.

Peng, C., Ho, B. K., Chang, T. W., and Chang, N. T. (1989). Role of HIV-1 protease in core protein maturation and viral infectivity. *Journal of Virology*, **63**, 2550–6.

Peng, C., Chang, N. T., and Chang, T. W. (1991). Identification and characterization of HIV-1 *gag-pol* fusion protein in transfected mammalian cells. *Journal of Virology*, **65**, 2751–6.

Petteway, S. R., Lambert, D. M., and Metcalf, B. W. (1991). The chronically infected cell as a target for the treatment of HIV infection and AIDS. *Trends in Pharmacological Sciences*, **12**, 28–34.

Phillips, R. E. (1991). Molecular interactions between HIV and the T lymphocyte. *Biochimica et Biophysica Acta*, **1096**, 10–13.

Pichuantes, S., Babe, L. M., Barr, P. J., DeCamp, D. L., and Craik, C. S. (1990). Recombinant HIV-2 protease processes HIV-1 Pr53 *gag* and analogous junction peptides *in vitro*. *Journal of Biological Chemistry*, **265**, 13890–8.

Plattner, J. J. and Norbeck, D. W. (1989). Obstacles to drug development from peptide leads. In *Drug discovery technologies* (ed. C. R. Clark and W. R. Moos), pp. 92–128. Ellis Horwood, Chichester.

Poorman, R. A., Tomasselli, A. G., Heinrikson, R. L., and Kezdy, F. J. (1991). A cumulative specificity model for HIV-1 and HIV-2 proteases inferred from statistical analysis of an extended substrate data base. *Journal of Biological Chemistry*, **266**, 14554–61.

Potts, B. C. M., Faulkner, D. J., Chan, J. A., Simolike, G. C., Offen, P., Hemling, M. E., and Francis, T. A. (1991). Didernnaketals A and B, HIV-1 protease inhibitors. *Journal of the American Chemical Society*, **113**, 6321–2.

Prasad, J. V. N. V. and Rich, D. H. (1991). Synthesis of hydroxyethylene dipeptide isosteres that mimic a P-1′ cyclic amino acid. *Tetrahedron Letters*, **32**, 5857–60.

Rahuel, J., Prieszle, J. P., and Grutter, M. G. (1991). Crystal structures of recombinant glycosylated human renin alone and in complex with a transition state analog inhibitor. *Journal of Structural Biology*, **107**, 227–36.

Rao, J. K. and Wlodawer, A. (1990). Is the pseudo-dyad in retroviral protease monomers structural or evolutionary? *Federation of European Biochemical Societies Letters*, **260**, 201–5.

Rao, J. K. M., Erickson, J. W., and Wlodawer, A. (1991). Structural and re-volutionary relationships between retroviral and eukaryotic aspartic proteinases. *Biochemistry*, **30**, 4663–71.

Ratner, L., Haseltine, W. H., Patarca, R., Livak, K. J., Starcich, B., Josephs, S. F., *et al.* (1985). Complete nucleotide sequence of the AIDS HTLV-III Virus. *Nature, London*, **313**, 277–84.

Rebholz, K. L. and Northrop, D. B. (1991). Slow step after bond-breaking by porcine pepsin identified using solvent ^{2}H isotope effects. *Biochemical and Biophysical Research Communications*, **176**, 65–9.

Rich, D. H. (1985). Pepstatin-derived inhibitors of aspartic proteinases. A close look at an apparent transition-state analogue inhibitor. *Journal of Medicinal Chemistry*, **28**, 263–73.

Rich, D. H., Green, J., Toth, M. V., Marshall, G. R., and Kent, S. B. H. (1990). Hydroxyethylamine analogs of the p17/p24 substrate cleavage site are tight-binding inhibitors of HIV protease. *Journal of Medicinal Chemistry*, **33**, 420–5.

Rich, D. H., Sun, C.-Q., Prasad, J. V. N. V., Pathiasseril, A., Toth, M. V., Marshall, G. R., *et al.* (1991). Effect of hydroxyl group configuration in hydroxy-ethylamine dipeptide isosteres on HIV protease inhibition. Evidence for multiple binding modes. *Journal of Medicinal Chemistry*, **34**, 1222–5.

Richards, A. D., Broadhurst, A. V., Ritchie, A. J., Dunn, B. M., and Kay, J. (1989a). Inhibition of the aspartic proteinases from HIV-2. *Federation of European Biochemical Societies Letters*, **253**, 214–16.

Richards, A. D., Roberts, R., Dunn, B. M., Graves, M. C., and Kay, J. (1989b). Effective blocking of HIV-1 proteinase activity by characteristic inhibitors of aspartic proteinases. *Federation of European Biochemical Societies Letters*, **247**, 113–17.

Richards, A. D., Phylip, L. H., Farmerie, W. G., Scarborough, P. E., Alvarez, A., Dunn, B. M., *et al.* (1990). Sensitive, soluble chromogenic substrates for HIV-1 protease. *Journal of Biological Chemistry*, **265**, 7733–6.

Richman, D. D. (1991). Therapy-HIV. In *Control of virus diseases* (ed. N. J. Dimmock, P. D. Griffiths, and C. R. Madeley), pp. 261–313. Cambridge University Press.

Rittenhouse, J., Turon, M. C., Helfrich, R. J., Albrecht, K. S., Weigl, D., Simmer, R. L., *et al.* (1990). Affinity purification of HIV-1 and HIV-2 proteases from recombinant *E. coli* strains using pepstatin-agarose. *Biochemical and Biophysical Research Communications*, **171**, 60–6.

Riviere, Y., Blank, V., Kourilsky, P., and Israel, A. (1991). Processing of the precursor of NF-κB by the HIV-1 protease during acute infection. *Nature, London*, **350**, 625–6.

Roberts, M. M. and Oroszlan, S. (1989). Preparation and biochemical characterization of intact capsids of equine infectious anemia virus. *Biochemical and Biophysical Research Communications*, **160**, 486–94.

Roberts, M. M., Copeland, T. D., and Oroszlan, S. (1991). *In situ* processing of a retroviral nucleocapsid protein by the viral protease. *Protein Engineering*, **4**, 695–700.

Roberts, N. A., Martin, J. A., Kinchington, D., Broadhurst, A. V., Craig, J. C., Duncan, I. B., *et al.* (1990). Rational design of peptide-based HIV proteinase inhibitors. *Science*, **248**, 358–61.

Ross, E. K., Fuerst, T. R., Orenstein, J. M., O'Neill, T., Martin, M. A., and Venkatesan, S. (1991). Maturation of HIV particles from the *gag* precursor protein requires *in situ* processing by *gag-pol* protease. *AIDS Research and Human Retroviruses*, **7**, 475–83.

Sawyer, T. K., Staples, D. J., Liu, L., Tomasselli, A. G., Hui, J. O., O'Connell, K., Schostarez, H., Hester, J. B., Moon, J., Howe, W. J., Smith, C. W., Decamp, D. L., Craik, C. S., Dunn, B. M., Lowther, W. T., Harris, J., Poorman, R. A., Wlodawer, A., Jaskolski, M., and Heinrikson, R. L. (1992). HIV Protease inhibitor structure–activity-selectivity, and active site molecular modeling of high affinity LeuY[CH(OH)CH2]Val modified viral and nonviral substrate analogs. *Int. J. Pept. Protein Res.*, **40**, 274–81.

Sawyer, T. K., Fisher, J. F., Hester, J. B., Smith, C. W., Tomasselli, A. G., Tarpley, W. G., Burton, P. S., Hui, J. O., McQuade, T. J., Conradi, R. A., Bradford, V. S., Liu, L., Kinner, J. H., Tustin, J., Alexander, D. L., Harrison, A. W., Emmert, D. E., Staples, D. J., Maggiora, L. L., Zhang, Y. Z., Poorman, R. A., Dunn, B. M., Rao, C., Scarborough, P. E., Lowther, W. T., Craik, C., Moon, J., Howe, W. J., Heinrikson, R. L. (1993). *Bioorg. Med. Chem. Lett.*, **3**, 819–24.

Scharpe, S., De Meester, I., Hendriks, D., Vanhoff, G., van Sande, M., and Vriend, G. (1991). Proteases and their inhibitors: today and tomorrow. *Biochemie*, **73**, 121–6.

Schatzl, H., Gelderblom, H. R., Nitschko, H., and von der Helm, K. (1991). Analysis of non-infectious HIV particles produced in the presence of an HIV proteinase inhibitor. *Archives of Virology*, **120**, 71–81.

Schneider, J. and Kent, S. B. H. (1988). Enzymatic activity of a synthetic 99-residue protein corresponding to the putative HIV-1 protease. *Cell*, **54**, 363–8.

Schramm, H. J., Nakashima, H., Schramm, W., Wakayama, H., and Yamamoto, N. (1991). HIV-1 reproduction is inhibited by peptides derived from the N- and C-termini of HIV-1 protease. *Biochemical and Biophysical Research Communications*, **179**, 847–51.

Schulze, T., Nawrath, M., and Moelling, K. (1991). Cleavage of the HIV-1 p66 reverse transcriptase/RNase H by the p9 protease *in vitro* generates active p15 RNase H. *Archives of Virology*, **18**, 179–88.

Seelmeier, S., Schmidt, H., Turk, V., and von der Helm, K. (1988). HIV virus has an aspartyl protease that can be inhibited by pepstatin A. *Proceedings of the National Academy of Sciences of the United States of America*, **85**, 6612–16.

Sham, H. L., Wideburg, N. E., Spanton, S. G., Kohlbrenner, W. E., Betebenner, D. A., Kempf, D. J., *et al.* (1991a). Synthesis of (2S, 5S, 4R)-2, 5-diamino-3, 3-difluoro-1,6-diphenylhydroxyhexane: the core unit of a potent HIV proteinase inhibitor. *Journal of the Chemical Society, Chemical Communications*, 110–12.

Sham, H. L., Betebenner, D. A., Wideburg, N. E., Saldivar, A. C., Kohlbrenner, W. E., Vasasanonda, S., *et al.* (1991b). Potent HIV-1 protease inhibitors with antiviral activity *in vitro*. *Biochemical and Biophysical Research Communications*, **175**, 175, 914–19.

Shoeman, R. L., Hoener, B., Stoller, T. J., Kesselmeier, C., Miedel, M. C., and Traub, P. (1990). HIV-1 protease cleaves the intermediate filament proteins vimentin, desmin, and gilial fibrillary acidic protein. *Proceedings of the National Academy of Sciences of the United States of America*, **87**, 6336–40.

Shoeman, R. L., Kesselmeier, C., Mothes, E., Hoener, B., and Traub, P. (1991). Non-viral cellular substrates for HIV-1 protease. *Federation of European Biochemical Societies Letters*, **278**, 199–203.

Sielecki, A. R., Federov, A. A., Andreeva, N. S., and James, M. N. G. (1990). Molecular and crystal structures of monoclinic porcine pepsin refined at 0.18 nm resolution. *Journal of Molecular Biology*, **214**, 143–70.

Skalka, A. M. (1989). Retroviral proteases: first glimpses at the anatomy of a processing machine. *Cell*, **56**, 911–13.

South, T. L., Blake, P. R., Sowder, R. C., Arthur, L. O., Henderson, L. E., and Summers, M. F. (1990). The nucleocapsid protein isolated from HIV-1 particles binds zinc and forms retroviral-type zinc fingers. *Biochemistry*, **29**, 7786–9.

Spinneli, S., Liu, Q. Z., Alzari, P. M., and Poljak, R. J. (1991). The three-dimensional structure of the aspartyl protease from the HIV-1 isolate BRU. *Biochemie*, **73**, 1391–6.

Stella, S., Saddler, G., Sarubbi, E., Colombo, L., Stefanelli, S., Denaro, M., and Selva, E. (1991). Isolation of α-MAPI from fermentation broths during a screening program for HIV-1 protease inhibitors. *Journal of Antibiotics*, **44**, 1019–22.

Stewart, K. (1990). New shapes in HIV protease inhibitors. *Protein Engineering*, **4**, 1–2.

Stewart, L. and Vogt, V. M. (1991). *trans*-Acting viral protease is necessary and sufficient for activation of avian leukosis virus reverse transcriptase. *Journal of Virology*, **65**, 6218–31.

Strickler, J. E., Gorniak, J., Dayton, B., Meek, T., Moore, M., Magaard, V., *et al.* (1989). Characterization and autoprocessing of precursor and mature forms of HIV-1 protease from *E. coli. Proteins*, **6**, 139–54.

Summers, M. F., South, T. K., Kim, B., and Hare, D. R. (1990). High resolution structure of an HIV zinc finger-like domain via a new NMR-based distance geometry approach. *Biochemistry*, **29**, 329–40.

Swain, A. L., Moller, M. M., Green, J., Rich, D. H., Schneider, J., Kent, S. B. H., and Wlodawer, A. (1990). X-ray crystallographic structure of a complex between a synthetic protease of HIV-1 and a substrate-based hydroxyethylamine inhibitor. *Proceedings of the National Academy of Sciences of the United States of America*, **87**, 8805–9.

Szelke, M., Leckie, B., Hallett, A., Jones, D. M., Sueiras, J., Atrash, B., and Lever, A. F. (1982). Potent new inhibitors of human renin. *Nature, London*, **299**, 555–7.

Tang, J., James, M. N. G., Hsu, I. N., Jenkins, J. A., and Blundell, T. L. (1978). Structural evidence for gene duplication in the evolution of the aspartyl proteases. *Nature, London*, **271**, 618–21.

Thaisrivongs, S., Pals, D. T., Kati, W. M., Turner, S. R., and Thomasco, L. M. (1985). Difluorostatine- and difluorostatone-containing peptides as potent and specific renin inhibitors. *Journal of Medicinal Chemistry*, **28**, 1553–5.

Thaisrivongs, S., Pals, D. T., Harris, D. W., Kati, W. M., and Turner, S. R. (1986). Design and synthesis of a potent and specific renin inhibitor with a prolonged duration of action *in vivo. Journal of Medicinal Chemistry*, **29**, 2088–93.

Thaisrivongs, S., Pals, D. T., Kroll, L. T., Turner, S. R., and Han, F.-S. (1987). Design of angiotensinogen transition state analogues containing novel (2R, 3R, 4R, 5S)-amino-3,4-dihydroxy-2-isopropyl-7-methyloctanoic acid. *Journal of Medicinal Chemistry*, **30**, 2344–56.

Thaisrivongs, S., Tomasselli, A. G., Moon, J. P., Hui, J. O., McQuade, T. J., Turner, S. R., *et al.* (1991). Inhibitors of the HIV protease: design and modeling of a compound containing a dihydroxyethylene isostere insert with high binding affinity and effective antiviral activity. *Journal of Medicinal Chemistry*, **34**, 2344–56.

Thanki, N., Rao, J. K. M., Foundling, S. I., Howe, W. J., Moon, J. B., Hui, J.-O., *et al.* (1992). Crystal structure of a complex of HIV-1 protease with a dihydroxyethylene-containing inhibitor: comparisons with molecular modeling. *Protein Science*, **1**, 1061–72.

Thomas, G. J. (1991). The design and synthesis of inhibitors of HIV protease. Presented at 32nd Annual Medicinal Chemistry Symposium, State University of New York at Buffalo.

Thompson, W. J., Fitzgerald, P. M. D., Holloway, M. K., Ennini, E. A., Darke, P. L., McKeever, B. M., *et al.* (1992). Synthesis and antiviral activity of a series of HIV-1 protease inhibitors with functionality tethered to the P-1 or P-1′ phenyl substituents: X-ray crystal structure assisted design. *Journal of Medicinal Chemistry*, **35**, 1685–701.

Toh, H., Ono, M., Saigo, K., and Miyata, T. (1985). Retroviral protease-like sequence in the yeast transposon Tyl. *Nature, London*, **315**, 691.

Tomasselli, A. G., Olsen, M. K., Hui, J. O., Sawyer, T. K., Heinrikson, R. L., and Tomich, C.-S. C. (1990a). Substrate analog inhibition and active site titration of purified recombinant HIV-1 prolease. *Biochemistry*, **29**, 264–9.

Tomasselli, A. G., Hui, J. O., Sawyer, T. K., Staples, D. J., Bannow, C., Reardon, I. M., *et al.* (1990b). Specificity and inhibition of proteases from HIV-1 and HIV-2. *Journal of Biological Chemistry*, **265**, 14675–83.

Tomasselli, A. G., Hui, J. O., Sawyer, T. K., Staples, D. J., Bannow, C. A., Reardon, I. M., *et al.* (1990c). Proteases from HIV and avian myeloblastosis show distinct specificities in hydrolysis of multidomain protein substrates. *Journal of Virology*, **64**, 3157–61.

Tomasselli, A. G., Howe, W. J., Hui, J. O., Sawyer, T. K., Reardon, I. M., DeCamp, D. L., and Craik, C. S. (1991a). Calcium-free calmodulin is a substrate of HIV-1 and HIV-2 proteases. *Proteins*, **10**, 1–9.

Tomasselli, A. G., Hui, J. O., Adams, L., Chosay, J., Lowery, D., Greenberg, B., *et al.* (1991b). Actin, troponin C, Alzheimer amyloid precursor protein and pro-interleukin 1β as substrates of the HIV-1 protease. *Journal of Biological Chemistry*, **266**, 14548–53.

Tomasselli, A. G., Howe, W. J., Sawyer, T. K., Wlodawer, A., and Heinrikson, R. L. (1991c). The complexities of AIDS: an assessment of the HIV protease as a therapeutic target. *Chimica Oggi*, **5**, 1–22.

Tomasselli, A. G., Hui, J. O., Sawyer, T. K., Thaisrivongs, S., Hester, J. B., Jr., and Heinrikson, R. L. (1992). The evaluation of non-viral substrates of the HIV protease as leads in the design of inhibitors for AIDS therapy. In *Structure and function of the aspartic proteinases: genetics, structure, and mechanism* (ed. B. Dunn), pp. 469–81. Plenum Press, New York.

Tozser, J., Blaha, I., Copeland, T. D., Wondrak, E. M., and Oroszlan, S. (1991a). Comparison of the HIV-1 and HIV-2 proteinases using oligopeptide substrates representing cleavage sites in *gag* and *gag-pol* polyproteins. *Federation of European Biochemical Societies Letters*, **281**, 77–80.

Tozser, J., Gustchina, A., Weber, I. T., Blaha, I., Wondrak, E. M., and Oroszlan, S. (1991b). Studies on the role of the S4 substrate binding site of HIV proteases. *Federation of European Biochemical Societies Letters*, **279**, 356–60.

Tritch, R. J., Cheng, Y.-S. E., Yin, F. H., and Erickson-Viitanen, S. (1991). Mutagenesis of protease cleavage sites in the HIV-1 *gag* polyprotein. *Journal of Virology*, **65**, 922–30.

Tropea, J. E., Nashed, N. T., Louis, J. M., Sayer, J. M., and Jerina, D. M. (1992). Effect of salt on the kinetic parameters of retroviral and mammalian aspartic acid proteases. *Bioorganic Chemistry*, **20**, 67–76.

Tyagi, S. C. and Carter, C. A. (1992). Continuous assay of the hydrolytic activity of HIV-1 protease. *Analytical Biochemistry*, **200**, 143–8.

Urban, J., Konvalinka, J., Stehlikova, J., Gregorova, E., Majer, P., Soucek, M., *et al.* (1992). Reduced-bond light-binding inhibitors of HIV-1 protease. *Federation of European Biochemical Societies Letters*, **298**, 9–13.

Vacca, J. P., Guare, J. P., de Solms, S. J., Sanders, W. M., Giuliani, E. A., Young, S. J., *et al.* (1991). L-687,908, a potent hydroxyethylene-containing HIV protease inhibitor. *Journal of Medicinal Chemistry*, **34**, 1225–8.

Veerapandian, B., Cooper, J. B., Sali, A., and Blundell, T. L. (1990). X-ray analysis of aspartic proteinases. III. Structure of endothiapepsin complexed with a transition state isostere inhibitor at 0.16 nm resolution. *Journal of Molecular Biology*, **216**, 1017–29.

Vlasuk, G. P., Waxman, L., Davis, L. J., Dixon, R. A. F., Schultz, L. D., Hofmann, K. J., *et al.* (1989). Purification and characterization of HIV core precursor p55 expressed in *S. cerevisiae*. *Journal of Biological Chemistry*, **264**, 12106–12.

von der Helm, K., Gurtler, L., Eberle, J., and Deinhardt, F. (1989). Inhibition of HIV replication in cell culture by the aspartic protease inhibitor pepstatin A. *Federation of European Biochemical Societies Letters*, **247**, 349–52.

von der Helm, K., Seelmeier, S., and Junker, U. (1990). Characterization and inhibition of the retroviral HIV-proteinase. *Biological Chemistry Hoppe Seyler*, **371**, 277–81.

Wallin, M., Deinum, J., Goobar, L., and Danielson, U. H. (1990). Proteolytic cleavage of microtubule-associated proteins by retroviral proteinases. *Journal of Virology*, **71**, 1985–91.

Ward, D. J. (1991). Introduction to peptide pharmaceuticals. In *Peptide pharmaceuticals. Approaches to the design of novel drugs* (ed. D. J. Ward), pp. 1–17. Elsevier, London.

Weber, I. T. (1990). Comparison of the crystal structures and intersubunit interactions of HIV and Rous sarcoma virus proteases. *Journal of Biological Chemistry*, **265**, 10492–6.

Weber, I. T., Miller, M., Jaskolski, M., Leis, J., Skalka, A. M., and Wlodawer, A. (1989). Molecular modeling of the HIV-1 protease and its substrate binding site. *Science*, **243**, 928–30.

Wills, J. W. and Craven, R. C. (1991). Form, function, and use of retroviral *gag* proteins. *AIDS*, **5**, 639–54.

Wlodawer, A., Miller, M., Jaskolski, M., Sathyanarayana, B. K., Baldwin, E., Weber, I. T., *et al.* (1989). Conserved folding in retroviral proteases: crystal structure of a synthetic HIV-1 protease. *Science*, **245**, 616–21.

Wondrak, E. M., Louis, J. M. and Oroszlan, S. (1991a). The effect of salt on the Michaelis–Menten constant of the HIV-1 protease correlates with the Hofmeister series. *Federation of European Biochemical Societies Letters*, **280**, 344–6.

Wondrak, E. M., Louis, J. M., Mora, P. T., and Oroszlan, S. (1991b). Purification of HIV-1 protease and characterization of proteolytically inactive HIV-1 protease mutants by pepstatin A affinity column. *Federation of European Biochemical Societies Letters*, **280**, 347–50.

Wu, J. C., Carr, S. F., Jarnagin, K., Kirsher, S., Barnett, J., Chow, J., *et al.* (1990). Synthetic HIV-2 protease cleaves *gag* precursor of HIV-1 with the same specificity as HIV-1 protease. *Archives of Biochemistry and Biophysics*, **277**, 306–11.

Yasunaga, T., Sagata, N., and Ikawa, Y. (1986). Protease gene structure and *env* gene variability of the AIDS virus. *Federation of European Biochemical Societies Letters*, **199**, 145–50.

Zhang, Z.-Y., Poorman, R. A., Maggiora, L. L., Heinrikson, R. L., and Kezdy, F. J. (1991a). Dissociative inhibition of dimeric enzymes: kinetic characterization of HIV-1 protease by its COOH-terminal tetrapeptide. *Journal of Biological Chemistry*, **266**, 1559–4.

Zhang, Z.-Y., Reardon, I. M., Hui, J. O., O'Connell, K. L., Poorman, R. A., Tomaselli, A. G., and Heinrikson, R. L. (1991b). Zinc inhibition of renin and the HIV-1 protease. *Biochemistry*, **30**, 8717–21.

Section 6C

Reverse transcriptase as a target for AIDS therapy

Barry Anderson and Hiroaki Mitsuya

6C.1   Introduction

An outbreak of unusual infections, particularly *Pnueumocystis carinii* pneumonia and Kaposi's sarcoma, in hitherto healthy young men, first described in the United States in 1981 (Gottlieb *et al.* 1981; Masur *et al.* 1981), brought about a significant redirection in basic science and clinical research efforts world-wide. In 1983, a human retrovirus, now referred to as the human immunodeficiency virus (HIV), was discovered to be the infectious pathogenic agent which caused the clinical entity later designated acquired immunodeficiency disease or AIDS (Barre-Sinoussi *et al.* 1983). Since the discovery of HIV, a major international effort has been made to understand and control AIDS and its related diseases.

HIV is classified as a lentivirus in the retroviridae and its replicative cycle includes the reverse transcription of its RNA genome to DNA, which is mediated by the virally encoded reverse transcriptase, and the subsequent integration of the viral double-stranded DNA (proviral DNA) into the host genome. This family of viruses causes a persistent infection of the host with a variable but continual rate of viral reproduction (Narayan and Clements 1989). These lentiviruses adroitly escape from and ultimately destroy the host immune defence system. Both primary viral pathology and consequent secondary immunopathology are believed to lead to the death of the host.

HIV is known to mutate its genome rapidly within the host, and many variants of the virus can be isolated from a single patient. Isolated HIV strains demonstrate different rates of replication, selective cellular tropisms, variable cytopathic effects, and different susceptibility to neutralization by antibodies (Klatzmann *et al*. 1984; Wong-Staal and Gallo 1985; Gartner *et al*. 1986; Nicholson *et al*. 1986). For example, an antigenic site of the viral surface glycoproteins (e.g. the V-3 loop) is particularly variable. This makes it difficult for the host immune system to neutralize certain variants and has frustrated the effort to develop anti-HIV vaccines. However, in recent years HIV has revealed enough of its replicative cycle to allow development of a variety of therapeutic strategies, and some of these have already yielded practical success (Mitsuya *et al*. 1991b; De Clercq 1992).

In this chapter we discuss the central role which the virally encoded reverse transcriptase (RT) plays in the HIV replicative cycle and the strategies attacking this enzyme which have proved to be successful in AIDS therapy. In particular, certain dideoxynucleoside analogues which inhibit this enzyme are described in terms of their laboratory and clinical development. We shall also discuss different classes of antiretroviral drugs which target the RT and the future role that RT inhibitors may play in the treatment of HIV infection.

6C.2   Reverse transcriptase as a target for antiretroviral therapy

The RT enzyme of HIV is the target of the two currently available anti-retroviral prescription drugs, 3′-azido-2′,3′-dideoxythymidine (AZT or zidovudine) and 2′,3′-dideoxyinosine (ddI or didanosine). While many aspects of the HIV replicative cycle are potentially exploitable for the purposes of blocking viral replication and consequent host pathology (De Clercq 1991; Mitsuya *et al*. 1991a) (see Chapter 6A), the strategy which inhibits proper functioning of the HIV RT enzyme has indeed provided the first antiretroviral drugs, and the RT molecule will probably continue to be among the prime targets for developing antiretroviral agents for at least the next decade.

6C.2.1   Formation of reverse transcriptase

By definition, retroviruses replicate through a DNA intermediate. RT is an enzyme which catalyses the synthesis of double-stranded proviral DNA using viral genomic RNA as a template (Baltimore 1970; Temin and Mizutani 1970). RT is one of three proteins encoded by the retroviral *pol* gene (Fig. 6C.1). The other two proteins include viral integrase, an endo-

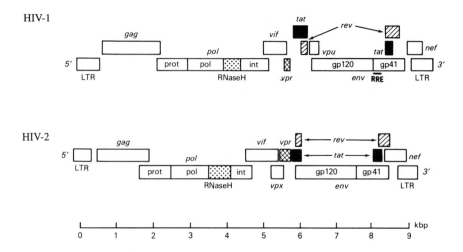

Fig. 6C.1 Genetic organization of HIV-1 and HIV-2. Three lanes in each panel represent three different reading frames where each gene is located. LTR, long terminal repeat; *gag*, group-specific antigen; *pol*, reverse transcriptase; prot, protease; int, integrase (endonuclease); *vif*, viral infectivity factor; *vpr*, viral protein R; *env*, envelope glycoprotein; *vpu*, viral protein U; *tat*, *trans*-activator protein; *rev*, regulator of expression of virion proteins; *nef*, negative regulator factor; *vpx*, viral protein X. Within the LTR are three elements: U5, R, and U3 (not shown). Some sequences upstream of R in the transcript appear to be required for efficient polyadenylation; therefore polyadenylation is brought about by only the 3′LTR. The *rev*-responsive element (RRE) is located in the *env* of HIV-1.

nuclease which mediates the integration of the proviral DNA into the host genome, and viral protease, which catalyses post-translational cleavage of the viral gene products (Fujiwara and Mizuuchi 1988; Skalka 1989). The *pol* gene is transcribed along with the preceding *gag* gene, which encodes viral structural proteins, and translated as a gag-pol fusion protein. However, the *gag* and *pol* genes lie in different translational reading frames within the transcribed mRNA. This reading frame differential allows an HIV-1 genetic regulatory mechanism based on ribosomal frame-shifting (Jacks and Varmus 1985; Ratner *et al.* 1985; Jack *et al.* 1988; Wilson *et al.* 1988; Hatfield and Oroszlan 1990). The *gag* and *pol* gene reading frames overlap at the 3′ end of the *gag* gene and the 5′ end of the *pol* gene. The translation of the *gag* gene usually stops at a termination codon located in this overlapping region. In the event that the ribosome slips back in the negative direction while translating in this overlap region, the ribosome frame-shifts into *pol* mRNA translation. This frame-shifting event occurs in 5–10 per cent of translational episodes and creates the *gag-pol* fusion protein (Jacks *et al.* 1988, Panganiban 1988; Brierley *et al.* 1989). This translational control mechanism is known to yield a ratio of *gag* to *gag-pol* protein of about 8:1 (Jacks *et al.* 1988). The *gag-pol* polyprotein is then transported to the cell membrane inner surface for inclusion in virion assembly.

The virally coded aspartyl protease enzyme is required for subsequent cleavage of the *gag-pol* polyprotein (Yoshinaka and Luftig 1977; Crawford and Goff 1985). The protease is also a component of the polyprotein (Fig. 6C.1); however, it probably undergoes an autocatalytic excision reaction so that the mature fully functional protease can then act on the remaining *gag-pol* protein structure. The uncleaved *gag-pol* polyprotein is capable of 10–50 per cent of the polymerase activity of the mature RT enzyme (Gottlinger *et al.* 1989; Peng *et al.* 1991). Based on information largely from electron microscopy, the final stages of maturation, including the post-translational cleavage, generally appear to occur extracellularly. In fact, viral genomes with an inactive protease (generated through site-specific mutagenesis) have been shown to produce and release virion particles (Crawford and Goff 1985; Katoh *et al.* 1985; Gottlinger *et al.* 1989). Such protease mutant virions contain uncleaved *gag* and *gag-pol* poly-proteins. Hence it would appear that cleavage modification occurs during or after viral budding, and this polyprotein modification is not required for assembly and budding of virions. However, it is also true that the mature p24 *gag* protein can be detected in the lysates of infected cells as assessed by immunoprecipitation (Kageyama and Mitsuya, unpublished observation). The timing of the post-translational modification remains to be further defined.

The mature RT molecule is generated by cleavage of the 66 kDa RT domain from the 160 kDa *gag-pol* precursor polyprotein (Farmerie *et al.* 1987; Hansen *et al.* 1988; Mous *et al.* 1988). Half the resultant 66 kDa protein (p66) products are then further proteolytically trimmed near their COOH-terminal to create a 51 kDa protein (p51). The ribonuclease (RNase) H activity resides within the COOH-terminal of p66 while DNA polymerase activity maps to the NH_2-terminal (Fig. 6C.2) (Hansen *et al.* 1988; Hizi *et al.* 1988; Tisdale *et al.* 1988; Prasad and Goff 1989; Davies *et al.* 1991). After protease cleavage of the p66 molecule, the p51 molecule displays no RNase H activity (Hizi *et al.* 1988; Lori *et al.* 1988; Tisdale *et al.* 1988; Prasad and Goff 1989). The catalytic sites for the two enzymatic activities, the polymerase activity and the RNase H activity, are separated by approximately one helical turn in the p66 monomer (Oyama *et al.* 1989). The p66 and p51 proteins combine to create the mature form of the RT enzyme, a p66–p51 heterodimer (Fig. 6C.2), although the p66 monomer exists in equilibrium with the p66–p66 homodimer (Muller *et al.* 1989; Restle *et al.* 1990; Rowley *et al.* 1990). *In vitro* treatment of single full-length p66 chains with protease, apparently of cellular origin, results in a heterodimeric molecule similar to the natural viral p66–p51 product

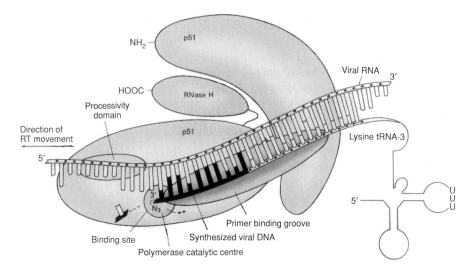

Fig. 6C.2 The structure of reverse transcriptase and chain-termination of viral DNA by AZT. The mature RT is a heterodimer with subunit molecular masses of 51 and 66 kDa. The larger peptide (p66) contains a COOH-terminal sequence (approximately 15 kDa) that has a RNase H active site. The active moiety of AZT (5′-triphosphate or other forms of AZT) can terminate the synthesis of viral DNA, as shown in this figure. RT, in the cytoplasm of the cell, binds to the viral RNA copy and to lysine tRNA-3, which provides the starting point for reverse transcription (see Fig. 6C.3). The growing viral DNA transcript is held in the primer binding groove. When the (−) strand DNA transcript is generated, RNase H digests the template viral RNA in an orderly manner so that a (+) strand DNA transcript can subsequently be formed in its place (the synthesis of the (+) strand DNA transcript is also catalysed by the viral RT. Natural deoxynucleosides such as thymidine are anabolically phosphorylated by a series of cellular enzymes, as are nucleoside analogues such as AZT. Normally, the RT then cleaves off two of the phosphates, and the remaining phosphate forms a phosphodiester linkage to the hydroxyl group at the 3′ end of the growing DNA chain. However, if AZT-5′-triphosphate is incorporated in place of thymidine-5′-triphosphate, no further nucleotides can be added because the azido (N_3) group of AZT cannot form the phosphodiester linkage. Consequently, viral DNA synthesis is terminated.

(Mous *et al.* 1988; Mizrahi *et al.* 1989). Further proteolytic cleavage of the mature heterodimeric RT molecule does not occur, suggesting that a significant conformational change results from the initial p66 cleavage which blocks protease access to the cleavage site on the remaining p66 chain. Although monomers of p66 or p51 demonstrate low levels of polymerizing ability, the p66–p66 and p66–p51 dimers have significantly greater polymerase efficiency, with the greatest activity demonstrated by the heterodimer (Lowe *et al.* 1988). A theoretical model of the interaction between the two RT chains suggests that the polymerization grooves (primer binding groove) of the two chains interact in the RT dimer (Fig. 6C.2) (Arnold and Arnold 1991). The contact between the two chains is thought to enhance the enzymatic polymerase activity by stabilizing and better localizing the active polymerization sites. The p66–p51 heterodimer is also known to display a tighter association than the p66–p66 homo-dimer (Hizi *et al.* 1988; Lowe *et al.* 1988; Tisdale *et al.* 1988). It has been suggested that the second RNase H domain of the p66–p66 homodimer does not allow optimal contact of the polymerase domains, which may explain the superiority of the heterodimer polymerase activity (Arnold *et al.* 1989).

6C.2.2   Reverse transcrption of the viral RNA genome

The HIV virion enters the host cell after contact between the viral gp120 molecule and the cellular CD4 molecule, although the CD4 molecule is not the only receptor for viral entry (Harouse *et al.* 1991). After subsequent viral fusion with the cell membrane, viral penetration of the host cell and shedding of the viral envelope take place. The virus then generates a double-stranded DNA (proviral DNA) copy of its RNA genome. The synthesis of this proviral DNA copy is catalysed by the virally encoded RT which is packaged into the mature virion and is thus readily available to the HIV RNA genome in the newly infected host cell (Arnold and Arnold 1991).

Within the HIV-1 ribonucleoprotein core are two (+) strand viral RNA copies linked as a dimer, and probably multiple molecules of the RT and integrase enzymes (Panet *et al.* 1975; Bender and Davidson 1976). The viral RNA strand is capped with 7-methylguanosine-5′-triphosphate at the 5′ end and polyadenylated at the 3′ end (Furuichi *et al.* 1975). Each RNA strand also has a lysine tRNA-3 ($tRNA_{lys}$) bound near its 5′ terminus at the 'primer binding site' P which functions as a DNA synthesis primer (Fig. 6C.2 and 6C.3). HIV-1 RT has a specific binding affinity for $tRNA_{lys}$, showing preference for it even in the presence of 100-fold excess of other tRNAs (Barat *et al.* 1989). Retroviruses are believed to encapsidate their specific tRNA primer selectively from tRNAs of an infected cell during virion assembly (Peters and Glover 1980). A cooperative interaction between the p66 and p51 subunits apparently creates the single tRNA binding site since neither subunit has been shown to bind to the primer (Barat *et al.* 1989). Cross-linking studies have shown the RT enzyme to bind at the tRNA anticodon loop (Barat *et al.* 1989). These charac-teristics of the RT–$tRNA_{lys}$ interaction suggest that tRNA primer binding is both structure and sequence dependent (Abbotts *et al.* 1991). Each p51 subunit is believed to contain a template binding groove which surrounds

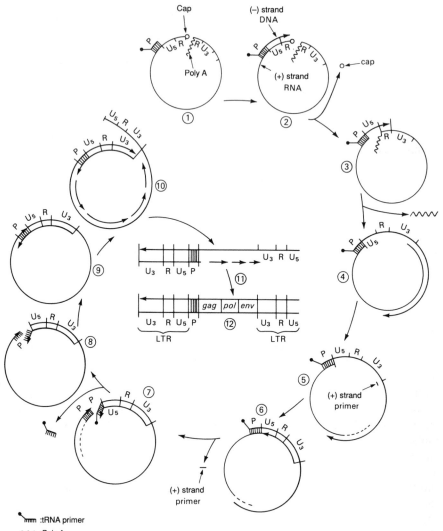

Fig. 6C.3 Proviral DNA synthesis mediated by RT. Reverse transcription of the viral RNA begins at the tRNA$_{lys}$ primer site from which synthesis of (−) strand viral DNA (1) proceeds to the 5′ end of the viral RNA and elongation stops ((−) strand strong stop DNA) (2). The RNA segment (U5-R) is digested by RNase H activity of the RT molecule and the cap structure is released. The R segment of the newly synthesized (−) strand DNA transcript is complementary to the R segment located at the 3′ end of the viral RNA. These complementary R segments anneal and (−) strand DNA synthesis continues (first jump) (3). As DNA synthesis continues, the 3′ end viral RNA is degraded by RNase H and poly A is subsequently

Fig. 6C.3 (*continued*)

released (3, 4). RNase H degradation of the viral RNA template spares a specific RNA segment which subsequently functions as the primer site for (+) strand DNA synthesis (5). The synthesis of (+) strand DNA stops at the 5 ′ end of U5 of the (−) strand DNA transcript ((+) strand strong stop DNA) (6). The primer RNA portion is dissociated from the RNA–DNA hybrid by RNase H activity and the synthesis of (+) strand DNA extends beyond U5 to the P portion. Subsequently, tRNA primer is released (7). The synthesis of (−) strand DNA extends to the P segment of the viral RNA template (7). (+) strand DNA also extends to the P region and, following RNase H removal of the tRNA primer, it anneals to the complementary (−) strand P region to allow further (+) strand DNA elongation (8,9). This is the second DNA jump. The synthesis of (+) strand DNA continues, using the (−) strand strong stop DNA as a template, and is completed at the 5 ′-end of U5 of the (−) strand DNA transcript. (−) strand DNA elongation is completed by 'strand displacement' of the 5 ′ end of the (−) strand DNA (10). Fragments of (+) strand DNA transcripts are finally ligated and a complete double-strand DNA containing LTR comprising U3, R, and U5 is formed (11, 12). This model is based on the review by Tsuchida and Sakuma (1985) and studies by Taylor (1977) and Gilboa *et al.* (1979).

the template–primer segment and directs the template through the polymerization domain of the enzyme (Fig. 6C.2).

RNA-dependent DNA polymerase activity of RT begins synthesis of the (−) strand DNA copy from the viral RNA template by initially binding at the tRNA primer site (Figs 6C.2 and 6C.3 (1)). The DNA copy is elongated along the short distance of the U5 and homologous repeat (R) sequence to the 5 ′ terminus of the RNA template resulting in '(−) strand strong stop DNA' (Fig. 6C.3 (2)). (Haseltine *et al.* 1976; Taylor 1977; Gilboa *et al.* 1979). As the process has reached a template terminus, further replication requires that RT switch templates (Gilboa *et al.* 1979). To accomplish the switch, the capping and R sequence at the 5 ′ end of the RNA template are removed by RNase H-catalysed degradation, exposing the strong stop DNA (Fig. 6C.3 (3)) (Collett *et al.* 1978; Friedrich and Moelling 1979; Luo and Taylor 1990). The homologous repeat sequence (R), which is also found at the 3 ′ RNA terminus, allows the strong stop DNA (containing a complementary R sequence) to pair with the 3 ′ homologous R sequence of the RNA template. This DNA movement is referred to as an interstrand 'jump' between the two different viral RNA strands (Fig. 6C.3 (3)) (Panganiban 1988). The RT enzyme remains attached to the (−) strand strong stop DNA and is believed to guide the DNA fragment through the interstrand DNA jump (DeVico and Sarngadharan 1992). Other viral proteins may also be involved in this process as integrity of the viral ribonucleoprotein core is essential to successful template switching *in vitro* (Arnold and Arnold 1991; DeVico and Sarngadharan 1992).

Once template switching by the (−) strand strong stop DNA is achieved, elongation of the (−) strand DNA is accompanied by RNase H degradation of the hybridized RNA template (Fig. 6C.3 (4)) (Darlix *et al.* 1977; Mitra *et al.* 1979). This RNase H activity includes an initial endonucleolytic cleavage around a polypurine site adjacent to the U3 region that will later serve as the primer for (+) strand DNA synthesis also mediated by RT (Fig. 6C.3 (5)). The loss of the 3′ poly-A tail is also believed to occur by an early endonucleolytic action of the RNase H (Gilboa *et al.* 1979; Mitra *et al.* 1979, Smith *et al.* 1984; Olsen and Watson 1985). Further RNase H degradation of hybridized RNA results from 3′→ 5′ exonucleolytic activity of the enzyme, but the polypurine primer site is spared. Recent work has demonstrated that although a single RT molecule is capable of both polymerase and RNase H activity, once it becomes involved in DNA synthesis it cleaves the RNA template only intermittently (DeStefano *et al.* 1991). The activity of multiple RT molecules is believed to be necessary for the complete removal of the RNA template (DeVico and Sarngadharan 1992). This degradative activity results in RNA oligomer structures 7–13 nucleotides in length which corresponds to the approximate distance (one turn of the double helix) between the polymerase and RNase H domains (Oyama *et al.* 1989; Arnold and Arnold 1991).

As mentioned above, before (+) strand DNA synthesis can be initiated, the RNA template−(−) strand DNA hybrid molecule is selectively cleaved by RNase H to create an RNA primer (Fig. 6C.3 (5)) (Gilboa *et al.* 1979; Mitra *et al.* 1979; Omer *et al.* 1984; Smith *et al.* 1984). Further degradation of the RNA template allows (+) strand DNA synthesis to procede by extension from the primer. As the RT enzyme progresses towards the 5′-terminus of the (−) strand DNA (Fig. 6C.3 (6)), it copies the first approximately 18 bases of the tRNA template molecule to yield a copy of the primer binding site P, at which point elongation stops. This short DNA sequence is called (+) strand strong stop DNA. Further (+) strand DNA synthesis requires a template switch to the 3′ end of the (−) strand DNA (Fig. 6C.3 (7)–(9)) (Gilboa *et al.* 1979). The tRNA molecule is removed by RNase H endonucleolytic action (Omer and Faras 1982) and the template switch occurs through re-annealing between the (+) and (−) strand P regions. Thus the second switch mechanism involves intrastrand transfer with subsequent creation of a circular molecule (Fig. 6C.3 (9)) (Gilboa *et al.* 1979; Boone and Skalka 1981).

At this point, both the (+) and (−) DNA strands are completed by RT in opposing directions. The final elongation of the (−) DNA strand requires that the 5′ tail of the (−) strand be moved aside (Fig. 6C.3 (10)). This clearance of the hybrid DNA strand is accomplished by the 'strand displacement synthesis' activity of the RT polymerase rather than the template degradation method used for displacing the RNA of the RNA–DNA hybrid (Boone and Skalka 1981). As the double-stranded DNA synthetic sequence includes two separate DNA jumping episodes, the final linear DNA product is longer (Fig. 6C.3 (11), (12)) than the original RNA template molecule with a copy of the U3−R−U5 regions at the 5′ and 3′ termini of the DNA strand. These redundant termini are termed the long terminal repeats (LTRs).

The double stranded proviral DNA thus formed is then transported from the cytoplasm to the cellular nucleus by an as yet unknown mechanism. It is integrated within the nucleus through the catalytic activity of the viral integrase protein. With integration, the virus establishes persistent infection of the host cell.

6C.2.3   DNA polymerase activity of the RT enzyme

As noted above, the RT enzyme proceeds through DNA synthesis in an orderly manner. The free RT binds the template−primer complex into the RT polymerization groove via a recognition process controlled by the primer (Fig. 6C.2), as indicated by studies showing that the primer sequence alone binds to RT as readily as the template−primer complex (Majumdar et al. 1988, 1989). Subsequently, nucleoside-5′-triphosphates bind to RT and proper incorporation occurs depending on the RNA or DNA template. Both RNA- and DNA-dependent DNA syntheses are believed to involve the same polymerization groove and triphosphate addition sites at the structural and enzymatic locales within the RT molecule (Arnold et al. 1989). DNA synthesis on the RNA template is processive in nature with over 300 nucleotides comprising the longest primer extensions (Majumdar et al. 1988). Initiation and elongation of nucleotide incorporation appear to occur through distinct kinetic mechanisms (Majumdar et al. 1988). One study shows that the dissociation constant K_d for the initial reaction step is approximately 1000-fold greater than that for the subsequent elongation of the DNA strand and, once initiated, DNA strand elongation procedes with much greater efficiency (Kedar et al. 1990). Termination of polymerization occurs approximately 20-fold more often after the initial nucleotide base incorporation than with subsequent nucleotide additions (Majumdar et al. 1988). DNA-dependent DNA synthesis appears to proceed in a distributive fashion, and much smaller average primer extensions, approximately 50 nucleotides long, develop before termination of synthesis (Huber et al. 1989).

6C.2.4   Infidelity of reverse transcriptase in DNA synthesis

The RT enzyme lacks 3′ to 5′ exonuclease activity, thus preventing the enzyme from proof-reading its DNA synthesis errors (Roberts et al. 1988). HIV-1 RT is very prone to misincorporate nucleotides and is particularly tolerant of G−A mispairs. This misincorporation has been studied using a poly(rA) · oligo(dT) system (Abbotts et al. 1991). When the dTTP substrate is substituted with dCTP, the RT continues to extend primer by 10 or fewer nucleotides (Abbotts *et al.* 1991). In contrast, when dGTP is used as substrate, HIV-1 RT extends primers by 100 or more nucleotides. Interestingly, the inappropriate inclusion of dGMP continues even when dGTP and dTTP are simultaneously available to the RT enzyme, resulting in over 0.5 per cent incorrect single-base substitutions (Abbotts *et al.* 1991).

Similarly, the study of DNA 'bypass' synthesis by Abbots *et al.* (1991), in which continued DNA chain elongation using a ϕX174 single-stranded DNA template is monitored during omission of individual dNTPs from the available substrate mixture, has demonstrated that HIV-1 RT readily continues DNA synthesis in the absence of the correct nucleotides. Only the lack of dGTP halted RT polymerase nucleotide misincorporation (Abbotts *et al.* 1991). DNA-dependent DNA synthesis by HIV-1 RT also demonstrated mutation during synthesis through single-base frame-shifts at homopolymer 'hot spots'. This frame-shift is proposed to occur by slippage between the template and the primer sequence during DNA strand elongation (Bebenek *et al.* 1989).

Because of the combination of single-base misincorporation and elongation at mispaired 3'-termini, the HIV-1 RT demonstrates a mutation frequency one order of magnitude greater than that of other reverse transcriptases studied, including avian myeloblastosis and murine leukaemia virus (Preston *et al.* 1988; Roberts *et al.* 1988; Tekeuchi *et al.* 1988). Indeed, using M13mp2-based fidelity assays, the error rate has been estimated at 1 per 1700 bases incorporated (Roberts *et al.* 1988). The extreme inaccuracy and lack of proof-reading ability of HIV RT are believed to cause the hypermutability of HIV-1 which is important when the development of drug resistance by this virus is considered. This issue will be discussed in greater detail later.

6C.3   Inhibitors of reverse transcriptase as therapeutics for AIDS

HIV RT has been a central target in the development of anti-retroviral therapy for HIV-infected individuals. In fact, the first agents demonstrated to inhibit HIV replication in culture (suramin) and in patients with AIDS (AZT) both targeted the RT molecule. This is, in part, because the amount of information regarding RT has increased enormously during the past two decades of study of retroviruses.

6C.3.1   2',3'-Dideoxynucleoside analogues as RT inhibitors

In 1985, a large family of nucleoside analogues containing a 2',3'-dideoxyribose moiety was found to inhibit the *in vitro* infectivity and replication of various HIV-1 strains during the early years of anti-HIV

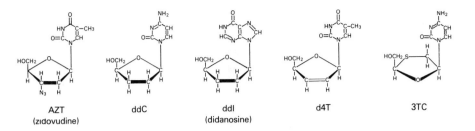

Fig. 6C.4 Selected nucleoside analogues active against HIV under preclinical and clinical development. Structures of 3′-azido-2′,3′-dideoxythymidine (AZT or zidovudine), 2′,3′-dideoxycytidine (ddC), 2′,3′-dideoxyinosine (ddI or didanosine), 2′,3′-didehydro-2′,3′-dideoxythymidine (2′,3′-dideoxythymidinene or d4T), and 2′,3′-dideoxy-3′-thiacytidine (3TC) are shown.

drug development at the National Cancer Institute (Mitsuya *et al*. 1985; Mitsuya and Broder 1986). This group of agents included 3′-azido-2′,3′-dideoxythymidine (AZT or zidovudine), 2′,3′-dideoxycytidine (ddC), 2′,3′-dideoxyadenosine (ddA), 2′,3′-dideoxyinosine (ddI or didanosine), and 2′,3′-dideoxyguanosine (ddG) (Fig. 6C.4). These nucleoside analogues demonstrated the ability to inhibit the infectivity and replication of HIV at drug levels that caused minimal interference with cellular growth. Since the discovery of the antiretroviral activity of these compounds in 1985 a variety of related 2′,3′-dideoxynucleoside agents have been identified as inhibitors of HIV replication.

Three dideoxynucleosides, AZT, ddI, and ddA, are known to diffuse passively into the cell without active transport, while ddC appears to require active transport for its entry into the cell. These compounds are then converted to their putatively active 5′-triphosphate form (see following discussion regarding mechanisms of activity) by cellular kinases in the cytoplasm (Cooney *et al*. 1986, 1987; Furman *et al*. 1986; Ahluwalia *et al*. 1988). The process of anabolic phosphorylation and subsequent intracellular metabolism is different for each of the dideoxynucleoside analogues (Fig. 6C.5) (Yarchoan *et al*. 1989b). Thus it is not surprising that each compound demonstrates a unique pattern of activity and toxicity *in vitro* and *in vivo* (Mitsuya *et al*. 1991a). Therefore each compound should be considered individually despite their apparently common structures and occasional similarities of biochemistry.

The dideoxynucleosides lack the 3′-ribose hydroxy (—OH) group that is common to the natural deoxynucleosides. Instead, the 3′-ribose site of the dideoxynucleoside analogues is substituted with a hydrogen or other molecular groups such as the azide (N_3) of AZT. Without the hydroxyl group the necessary 3′,5′-phosphodiester internucleotide linkage in a

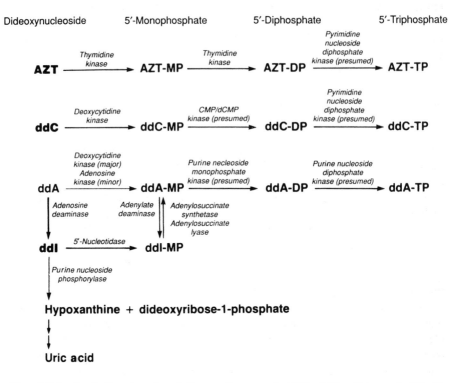

Fig. 6C.5 Anabolic phosphorylation pathways of AZT, ddC, ddA, and ddI. It should be noted that each dideoxynucleoside has its own metabolic pathway. MP, monophosphate; DP, diphosphate; TP, triphosphate. (Modified and reprinted with permission from Yarchoan *et al.* 1989a.)

growing DNA strand cannot be formed and further elongation of the DNA molecule is blocked. As mentioned, the HIV polymerase lacks an excisional repair mechanism; hence the 2′,3′-dideoxynucleosides are presumed to inhibit viral replication by causing premature termination of viral DNA synthesis. As these dideoxynucleosides are analogues of the natural deoxynucleosides, they may also act as competitive inhibitors of the binding of natural substrates to the enzyme. In fact, it has been found that AZTTP has a binding affinity for RT which is approximately 100-fold greater than that of dTTP (Kedar *et al.* 1990). The K_i for inhibition of dTTP incorporation by AZTTP (20 nM) is substantially lower than the K_m for incorporation of dTTP (2.9 μM) (Majumdar *et al.* 1988). Thus the competitive binding of AZTTP to the RT–template complex may also operate as a mechanism of inhibition of HIV replication by AZT (Kedar *et al.* 1990). Additionally, owing to the stability of the dideoxynucleotide–RT enzyme–template complex (Muller *et al.* 1991), the RT is apparently prevented from initiating other polymerization reactions, and the quantity of RT enzyme available for further viral DNA synthesis is significantly diminished. Thus dideoxynucleoside analogues appear to inhibit HIV replication by more than one mechanism.

It is important to note that minor alterations of the chemical composition of these agents can drastically alter their activity against HIV replication. Invoking AZT again, it has been demonstrated that the simple substitution of the azide group by an amino group (thus generating 3'-amino-2',3'-dideoxythymidine) nullifies the potent antiviral activity of AZT (Mitsuya *et al.* 1987). However, if 5'-triphosphorylated, 3'-amino-2',3' dideoxythymidine-5'-triphosphate (3'-amino-ddTTP) apparently exerts a potent inhibitory activity against RT, interacting with the RT molecule differently than AZTTP (Kedar *et al.* 1990). The resulting DNA strands obtained with these two agents were found to differ such that increasing concentrations of AZTTP caused shorter DNA strands to be synthesized while the 3'-amino-ddTTP analogue caused a generalized decrease in the quantity of DNA molecules produced without decreasing the length of the DNA strands (Kedar *et al.* 1990).

Recent studies have questioned whether it is AZTTP or some other metabolite(s) of AZT which is the active form of the nucleoside analogue (Tan *et al.* 1991). The intracellular conversion of AZT to its 5'-triphosphate form appears to require the activity of thymidine kinase, thymidylate kinase, and pyrimidine nucleoside diphosphate kinase (Yarchoan *et al.* 1986; Mitsuya and Broder 1987). While AZTTP is known to be active against the RNA-dependent DNA polymerase activity of HIV RT, the intracellular conversion of AZT to AZTMP by thymidine kinase is much more efficient than the conversion of AZTMP to AZTDP by thymidylate kinase (Furman *et al.* 1986; Furman and Barry 1988). This circumstance leads to the intracellular presence of millimolar amounts of AZTMP, some 100–1000 times the available intracellular concentration of AZTTP. Tan *et al.* (1991) have investigated the relative effect of the nucleoside-5'-monophosphates on the RNase-H- and RNA-dependent DNA polymerase functions of the HIV RT. AZTMP was found to inhibit RNase H activity by 50 per cent at a concentration of 0.05 mM. This inhibition was reversible on increasing the concentration of the RNase H substrate, poly(rA) · poly(dT), suggesting that AZTMP may compete with the substrate for the active binding site of RNase H. AZTMP caused only minimal inhibition of the RNA-dependent DNA polymerase activity and, although it did not directly compete with the natural substrate dTTP, the binding of AZTMP at the RNase H site may interfere with subsequent binding of dTTP to the binding site for DNA polymerase activity (Tan *et al.* 1991). Since AZTTP inhibits the activity of the HIV-1 RT at nanomolar concentrations, AZTTP (or its metabolites) would appear to play a major role in the antiviral effect of AZT. However, AZTMP inhibition of RNase H activity may also be a component of the sensitivity of HIV-1 to AZT, although its role may not be predominant.

6C.3.2   Clinical features of AIDS and therapy with dideoxynucleoside analogues

Individuals infected with HIV-1 develop a variety of clinical symptoms, with the delay between initial infection and subsequent progression to AIDS symptoms averaging from 8 to 10 years for adults (Fauci 1988; Munoz et al. 1989) and from months to several years for children (Krasinski et al. 1989). The patient's cellular immune system is the main casualty of HIV infection. The HIV virion primarily infects a subset of T-lymphocytes (known as helper T-cells) which express the CD4 surface glycoprotein (Dalgleish et al. 1984; KIatzmann et al. 1984). These lymphocytes are important in initiating and promoting the immune system's response to bacterial, fungal, viral, and oncological challenge. Through mechanisms that remain unclear, HIV infection results in a dramatic decline in the number of $CD4^+$ lymphocytes, thus leading to overall immune dysfunction (Gottlieb et al. 1981; Masur et al. 1981). HIV is also known to cause a prolonged productive infection of the host's monocyte/macrophage lineage, and this results in further viral dissemination and damage to the body's immunological capability (Gartner et al. 1986). As the immune system undergoes continued decline, the patient becomes increasingly susceptible to opportunistic infections such as Pneumocystis carinii pneumonia, Candida oesophagitis, pulmonary or systemic infection by Mycobacterium avium intracellulare, and Cytomegalovirus retinitis. Some patients suffer from a dramatically increased incidence of an aggressive form of Kaposi's sarcoma (Rabkin and Goedert 1990) and non-Hodgkin's lymphoma (Ziegler et al. 1984).

During the incubation or latent period, HIV apparently undergoes only low levels of replication. Because patients typically display few significant symptoms during this latent stage, it is desirable to be able to detect progression of the underlying HIV disease without relying on a patient's obvious symptomatic decline. As viral replication increases an increased number of viral components can be detected in the serum of some patients. For example, the level of viral replication can be measured through quantification of HIV p24, a major viral capsid antigen, by enzyme-linked immunoadsorption assay or radio-immunoassay. The decline of CD4 cell numbers in the peripheral blood also appears to be indicative of disease progression (Yarchoan et al. 1991). Parameters such as p24 antigen level and CD4 cell counts are used as surrogate markers to assess the patient's disease status or clinical activity of antiviral chemotherapy, but these measures are not always useful for certain patients. For example, a substantial number of patients with AIDS do not have measurable p24 antigen levels. In this regard, research efforts to develop other means of quantifying HIV viral load are now under way through the exploitation of recent technical advances such as the polymerase chain reaction (Aoki *et al.* 1990; Holodiny *et al.* 1991; Aoki-Sei *et al.* 1992).

6C.3.2.1 *AZT*

AZT was the first antiretroviral drug administered to HIV-1 infected patients. Five months after the initial observation by Mitsuya, Broder, and coworkers (Mitsuya *et al.* 1985; Mitsuya and Broder 1986) of the inhibitory effect of AZT on *in vitro* HIV replication, a phase I clinical trial was initiated at the National Cancer Institute (NCI) and Duke University Medical Center. Results from this trial demonstrated an increase in CD4 counts, HIV p24 antigen reduction, weight gain, and reports of increased energy in patients with AIDS or AIDS-related complex (ARC) receiving the drug (Yarchoan *et al.* 1986). Patients with HIV-associated dementia also showed improved neurological function (Yarchoan *et al.* 1987; Pizzo *et al.* 1988; Schmitt *et al.* 1988). Subsequent phase II trials demonstrated similar clinical findings as well as a lower incidence of opportunistic infections and decreased mortality among the AZT-treated patients. In March 1987, AZT was approved as the first prescription drug for HIV-infected patients with *Pneumocystis carinii* pneumonia or with CD4 cell counts below 200 mm^{-3}. Subsequent studies have found that lower AZT doses can provide equivalent clinical benefit with a diminution of the side-effects noted in the patients receiving a full dose of AZT (Fischl *et al.* 1990).

The side-effects of AZT therapy include bone marrow suppression, with commonly occurring macrocytic anaemia and neutropenia, as well as occasional thrombocytopenia (Gill *et al.* 1987; Richman *et al.* 1987). Patients also suffer from nausea, vomiting, myalgias, myositis, headaches, and/or liver function abnormalities. Some of these toxicities, particularly the suppression of early bone marrow components, may result from the interference with cellular β- and γ-DNA polymerases by AZT (Furman *et al.* 1986; Cheng *et al.* 1987). AZT-associated myositis is believed to be caused by AZT's inhibition of mitochondrial γ-DNA polymerase and subsequent muscle mitochondrial dysfunction (Dalakos *et al.* 1990). Interference with normal cell division may also occur through the diminished availability of thymidine-5′-triphosphate, mainly because of the competition for thymidylate kinase by AZTMP (Furman *et al.* 1986).

6C.3.2.2 *ddC*

2′,3′-Dideoxycytidine (ddC or zalcitabine) was the second dideoxynucleoside administered to patients with HIV-1 infection. *In vitro* studies suggested that ddC was more potent than AZT on a molar basis and less toxic to bone marrow precursor cells (Mitsuya and Broder 1986; Du *et al.* 1989).

Patients with advanced AIDS or ARC treated with oral ddC in a phase I study at NCI demonstrated diminished HIV replication and improvement of certain clinical symptoms (Yarchoan *et al.* 1988). However, continued use of ddC was limited in many patients owing to a severe, but mostly reversible, sensory–motor peripheral neuropathy. As painful peripheral neuropathy was not a common adverse effect of AZT therapy, trials of AZT and ddC on alternating weekly schedules were employed in an effort to avoid the side-effects of each drug (Yarchoan *et al.* 1988). Recent data show a favourable clinical effect of the combination use of AZT and ddC over AZT monotherapy. Paediatric trials of ddC alone or in an alternating schedule with AZT have also demonstrated decreased p24 antigen levels and improved CD4 cell counts in children with AIDS or ARC without severe painful neuropathy (Pizzo *et al.* 1990).

6C.3.2.3   *ddI*

In 1985 2',3'-dideoxyinosine (ddI) and 2',3'-dideoxyadenosine (ddA) were also found to inhibit *in vitro* HIV-1 replication (Mitsuya and Broder 1986). It is believed that ddI is phosphorylated by cytoplasmic 5'-nucleo-tidase to yield ddIMP and converted to ddAMP by adenylosuccinate synthase-lyase (Fig. 6C.5) (Ahluwalia *et al.* 1987). ddAMP subsequently undergoes phosphorylation with purine nucleoside mono- and diphosphate kinases and is ultimately converted to ddATP. ddA can be directly phosphorylated to ddAMP, but can also be deaminated to ddI by cellular adenosine deaminase and subsequently undergoes phosphorylation to ddATP (Fig. 6C.5). Because ddA is known to form an insoluble metabolite, 2,8-dihydroxyadenine, which is associated with possible renal failure, ddI was the drug of greater interest for clinical application. The first trials of ddI began in July 1988 at the NCI (Yarchoan *et al.* 1990a). ddATP is known to have an intracellular half-life of 12–24 h, much longer than AZT and ddC (both with half-lives of about 3 h). Thus ddI was successfully administered, with effective drug levels attained, on a less frequent dosing schedule than AZT or ddC (twice a day compared with six times daily for AZT) (Starnes and Cheng 1987; Ahluwalia *et al.* 1988; Yarchoan *et al.* 1990a). ddI is acid labile; thus concomitant antacid administration was necessary for effective use of the drug. In studies of both adult and paediatric patients with AIDS or ARC, clinical and immunological improvements, as well as anti-viral activity, have been noted (Yarchoan *et al.* 1989c; Butler *et al.* 1991). Significantly, patients whose HIV disease had apparently become resistant to the anti-viral effects of AZT still showed a decrease in viral load with ddI therapy, although these patients did not demonstrate a significant improvement in their CD4 cell count values. Associated with these initial trials of ddI were side-effects such as painful peripheral neuropathy (less severe than with ddC) and acute pancreatitis (Yarchoan *et al.* 1990b). However, there were few cases of bone marrow suppression (Lambert *et al.* 1990).

Because of the accelerated programme of drug development now in effect in the United States, ddI received conditional approval in October 1991 for use in those with AIDS or ARC whose disease is refractory to AZT treatment or who cannot tolerate AZT owing to its associated side-effects.

6C.3.2.4   *Other dideoxynucleoside analogues active against HIV*

Although the dideoxynucleosides appear to be structurally closely related, individual drugs within this class exert different anti-viral activity and/or adverse effects probably because of variations in dideoxynucleoside metabolism or differential effects on target organs. Moreover, minor changes in the stereochemistry of a compound's component structure can drastically alter its biological activities. Such changes can influence the practical use of the drug, as seen, for example, in the acid lability of ddI and ddA. Simply substituting a β-fluorine atom at the $2'$ carbon of di-deoxypurine nucleosides such as ddI, which are otherwise acid labile, can produce acid stability (Marquez *et al.* 1987). The range of clinical useful-ness of a drug may also be altered. AZT, perhaps in part because of its relative lipophilicity, penetrates well into the central nervous system, while ddI and ddC are significantly less lipophilic and this may limit the pene-tration of these drugs into the central nervous system. In fact, ddI appears to be less efficacious in improving HIV-associated encephalopathy (Pizzo *et al.* 1988; Yarchoan *et al.* 1989d). With these findings in mind, several $2',3'$-dideoxypurine nucleosides with a halogen atom substituted at the 6-position have been synthesized and found to have increased lipophilicity without reducing anti-retroviral activity (Fig. 6C.6) (Shirasaka *et al.* 1990a; Murakami *et al.* 1991). Once taken up by cells, these compounds are acted upon by adenosine deaminase and converted to ddI or ddG in the cyto-plasm. Preclinical studies of these compounds are now underway.

Other dideoxynucleoside analogues under clinical trial include the ddC analogues $2',3'$-dideoxy-$3'$-thiacytidine (3TC) (Chen *et al.* 1992) (Fig. 6C.4) and $2'$-β-fluoro-$2',3'$-dideoxycytidine ($2'$-threo-F-ddC) (Siddiqui *et al.* 1992), currently undergoing phase I clinical trials in both adults and paediatric patients with the hope that they will display the high antiretro-viral potency observed with ddC but with reduced toxicity.

$2',3'$-Didehydro-$2',3'$-dideoxythymidine ($2',3'$-dideoxythymidinene or d4T) (Fig. 6C.4) and $3'$-azido-$2',3'$-dideoxyuridine (AZddU) are two other pyrimidine dideoxynucleoside analogues currently under clinical investi-gation. d4T has a good anti-HIV activity *in vitro* (Hamamoto *et al.* 1987) and, unlike AZT, its $5'$-monophosphate form apparently does not inhibit thymidylate kinase. Phase I data on d4T treatment of patients with AIDS or ARC have demonstrated an early rise in CD4 cell counts, a decrease in p24 serum antigen levels, and improved constitutional symptoms (Browne 1990). Peripheral neuropathy, anaemia, and hepatitis have been identified as dose-limiting toxicities for d4T.

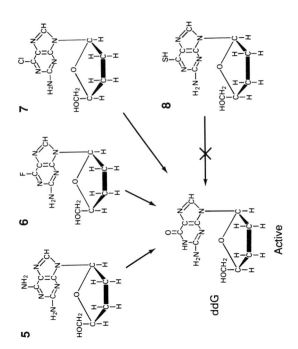

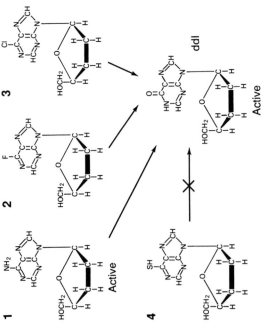

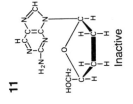

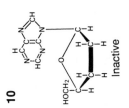

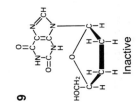

Fig. 6C.6 Structures and *in vitro* anti-retroviral activity of selected 2′,3′-dideoxypurine nucleoside analogues. The antiretroviral activity of each compound was assessed under conditions of high multiplicities of infection (MOI) using ATH8 cells, H9 cells, normal clonal CD4$^+$ T-cells, MT-2 cells, and/or normal unfractionated peripheral blood mononuclear cells, based on the inhibition of the cytopathic effect of HIV, suppression of *gag* protein production, and/or suppression of HIV viral DNA or RNA synthesis. Compounds which can give almost complete inhibition (80–100 per cent) of the infectivity and cytopathic effect of HIV at concentrations which do not significantly affect the growth of target cells are defined as *active*. Compounds which give less than 30 per cent inhibition are defined as *inactive*. **1** 2′,3′-dideoxyadenosine (ddA); **2** 6-fluoro-2′,3′-dideoxypurine ribofuranoside; **3** 6-chloro-2′,3′-dideoxypurine ribofuranoside; **4** 6-mercapto-2′,3′-dideoxypurine ribofuranoside; **5** 2,6-diamino-2′,3′-dideoxypurine ribofuranoside; **6** 2-amino-6-fluoro-2′,3′-dideoxypurine ribofuranoside; **7** 2-amino-6-chloro (or fluoro)-2′,3′-dideoxypurine ribofuranoside; **8** 2-amino-6-mercapto-2′,3′-dideoxypurine ribofuranoside; **9** 2′,3′-dideoxyxanthosine; **10** 2′,3′-dideoxypurine ribofuranoside; **11** 2-amino-2′,3′-dideoxypurine ribofuranoside. Compounds **1–3** and **5–7** are enzymatically hydrolysed by a ubiquitous enzyme adenosine deaminase, converted to ddI and ddG respectively, and exert a potent antiretroviral activity against HIV. Compound **1** is active without deamination, while compounds **2**, **3**, **6**, and **7** require deamination to be active against the virus. Requirement of deamination for the activity of compound **5** is not clear. Compounds **4** and **8** are not a substrate for adenosine deaminase and do not work against the virus.

AZddU has reportedly demonstrated a wider therapeutic index *in vitro* than AZT (Schinazi and Ahn 1987). Its antiretroviral activity is also increased in the presence of Granulocyte/Macrophage-Colony Stimulating Factor (GM-CSF) *in vitro* (Perno *et al.* 1989). However, certain HIV strains isolated from patients on long-term AZT treatment have been found to be cross-resistant to AZddU *in vitro* (Richman 1990). This finding may indicate a limitation to the the potential utility of AZddU (see following discussion of drug resistance).

Finally, phosphonylmethoxyethyladenine (PMEA) is an acyclic nucleoside which shows inhibition of a variety of DNA and RNA viruses, including HIV (Pauwels *et al.* 1988). PMEA is believed to act via the viral reverse transcriptase, despite its lack of the 2',3'-dideoxyribose moiety. PMEA is also at the preclinical stage of development.

6C.3.2.5   *Development of drug resistance*

The development of drug resistance can be seen in antibacterial and oncological therapy. Antiviral therapy has also led to viral drug resistance in certain human infections such as influenza A virus, herpes simplex virus, varicella zoster virus, cytomegalovirus, and rhinovirus infections. The ability to provide effective long-term antiretroviral therapy of AIDS using a single agent became a complex issue when Larder, Darby, and Richman reported the isolation of AZT-resistant HIV-1 variants from patients who had received prolonged anti-retroviral therapy with AZT (Larder *et al.* 1989; Richman *et al.* 1990). Although pretherapy viral isolates have a sensitivity to AZT in a low relatively narrow concentration range, post-therapy HIV-1 strains isolated from patients treated with AZT for more than 6 months often demonstrate the acquisition of resistance to AZT (Richman 1992). One to five mutations within the *pol* gene region of the HIV genome, which cause amino acid substitutions (Met41 → Leu, Asp67 → Asn, Lys70 → Arg, Thr215 → Phe or Tyr, and Lys219 → Gln), have been commonly identified in such AZT-resistant variants (Kellam *et al.* 1992; Larder and Kemp 1989). *In vitro* assays of drug sensitivity using these viral mutants demonstrated the virus to be up to 500 times less sensitive to AZT, with partial resistance measured in those strains displaying only a subgroup of these amino acid substitutions. While the AZT-resistant strains are not cross-resistant to other dideoxynucleosides such as ddC, ddI, and d4T, they do show cross-resistance to other 3'-azido-containing nucleosides such as AZddU, 3'-azido-2',3'-dideoxyguanosine (AZG) and 3'-azido-2',3'-dideoxyadenosine (AZA) (Larder *et al.* 1990; Shirasaka *et al.* 1990b).

More recently, Shirasaka *et al.* (1992) have demonstrated that patients receiving a combination therapy of alternating AZT and ddC still developed AZT resistant variants. Such AZT-resistant variants contained more than one of the four AZT-related genotypic changes found by Larder *et al.* (1990). Thus the addition of ddC does not seem to prevent the development of AZT resistance, although whether this combination therapy delayed the onset of AZT resistance remains to be defined. The influence of the combined administration of AZT and other antiretroviral agents on the development of AZT resistance is also the topic of future study. St Clair *et al.* (1991) have recently reported that patients with AIDS receiving 6–12 months of ddI therapy after long-term AZT treatment had HIV-1 variants that were 6- to 26-fold less sensitive to ddI than viral strains isolated previous to ddI therapy. The viral strains isolated from these patients continued to display the AZT-associated amino acid substitutions at residue 215, but an additional mutation of Leu → Val at residue 74 was also identified. St. Clair *et al.* reported that the acquisition of the 74 Val substitution rendered the 215 substitution-carrying AZT-resistant variant to be sensitive to AZT. However, studies by Shirasaka *et al.* (1992) have shown that, in five patients with AIDS or ARC, no appreciable resistance to ddI was identified for up to 29 months after initiating ddI therapy, although some post-therapy strains had the 74 Val substitution.

The clinical significance of these mutant viruses is as yet unclear. While the improvement in patient CD4 counts is often transient in nature and apparently AZT-resistant variants are isolated more readily when CD4 counts begin to decline, no definitive clinical evidence of an association of the emergence of AZT-resistant variants with deterioration of the clinical status has been demonstrated despite continuous AZT therapy. In fact, a recent study which monitored the ordered appearance of AZT-resistant mutations in patients receiving AZT for 2 years suggests that HIV-1 variants which acquired one or two of the four reported amino acid substitutions showed relatively lower levels of resistance to AZT than those acquiring all four of the substitutions (Boucher *et al.* 1992). Nevertheless, no clear relationship between the occurrence of partial resistance and disease progression has been identified as yet.

Paradoxically, the RT enzyme isolated from the AZT-resistant HIV-1 variants does not demonstrate a decreased sensitivity to AZTTP when assayed in a cell-free enzymatic assay (Larder *et al.* 1989). This may suggest that the *in vitro* RT assay conditions do not sufficiently mimic the intracellular circumstances under which *in vitro* HIV replication occurs, or that AZTTP may not be the major form of the active moiety of AZT but that some other metabolites of AZT may be responsible for the anti-viral activity. Much more in-depth research is required to elucidate the mechanism(s) of HIV-1 drug resistance development.

6C.3.3 Non-nucleoside RT inhibitors

As discussed above, a few years after the seminal discovery of HIV-1 as the causative agent for AIDS, the RT molecule proved to be a successful target for the development of antiretroviral agents. Hence in recent

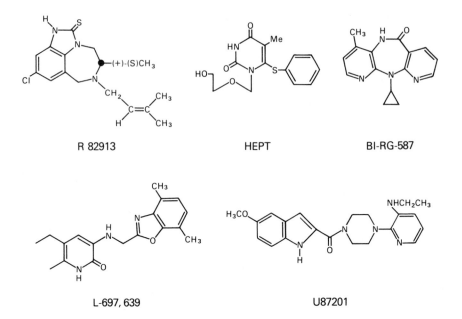

Fig. 6C.7 Selected non-nucleoside HIV RT inhibitors. Structures of a TIBO analogue (R 82913), HEPT, a dipyridodiazepinone derivative (BI-RG-587), a pyridinone derivative (L-697,639), and a bis(heteroaryl)piperazine derivative (U87201) are shown.

years, an intense research effort has focused on the search for novel and more effective inhibitors of the RT enzyme. Thus at the beginning of the 1990s, a number of non-nucleoside RT inhibitors were identified, mostly with the involvement of major pharmaceutical firm researchers. These compounds include tetrahydro-imidazo(4,5,1-jk)(1,4)-benzo-diazepin-2(1H)-one and -thione (TIBO) derivatives (Pauwels *et al.* 1990), dipyridodiaze-pinone analogues (Merluzzi *et al.* 1990), pyridinone derivatives (Goldman *et al.* 1991), and certain bis(heteroaryl)piperazines (Romero *et al.* 1991) (Fig. 6C.7). Although the structures of these compounds are apparently unrelated, they are all active against HIV-1 only and are inert against other retroviruses including HIV-2, simian immunodeficiency viruses (SIVs), and other animal retroviruses. In this regard, a series of antiretroviral nucleo-sides, 1-((2-hydroxyethoxy)methyl)-6-(phenylthio)-thymine(HEPT) (Fig. 6C.7) and its analogues, appear to fall into the same category as non-nucleoside reverse transcriptase inhibitors. HEPT analogues exert antiviral activity against HIV-1 but not against HIV-2 or animal retroviruses (Baba *et al.* 1989). In addition, unlike dideoxynucleoside analogues, HEPT analogues do not require phosphorylation to exert their antiretroviral effect. Therefore, in this chapter, HEPT analogues are discussed as members of non-nucleoside RT inhibitors.

6C.3.3.1   TIBO derivatives

In 1990, Pauwels, De Clercq, and their coworkers (Pauwels *et al.* 1990) reported a series of TIBO derivatives as a new class of selective inhibitors of HIV-1 replication. TIBO derivatives inhibited a wide spectrum of HIV-1 strains *in vitro* in nanomolar concentration levels that were 10^4-10^5 times lower than their cytotoxic concentration. The antiviral activity of TIBO derivatives against HIV-1 seems to be mediated by its inhibitory effect on the HIV-1 RT enzymatic activity (Debyser *et al.* 1991). However, unlike AZTTP and other dideoxynucleoside 5'-triphosphates that are almost equally effective against RTs of a variety of human and animal retroviruses, TIBO compounds do not show activity against the RT of HIV-2 or other animal retroviruses.

The inhibition of HIV-1 RT by TIBO compounds is demonstrated with different template primers (i.e. both poly(rA) · oligo(dT) and poly (rC) · oligo(dG)) and is not reversed by increasing concentrations of deoxynucleotides (Debyser *et al.* 1991, 1992). This contrasts with the dideoxynucleotides which inhibit RT activity only with the complementary homopolymer as template (e.g. AZTTP with poly(rA) · oligo(dT)). These findings indicate that TIBO derivatives probably interact with RT at a site distant from the template–primer binding site or nucleotide binding sites of the RT molecule. These characteristics of TIBO derivatives are shared by four other groups of non-nucleoside RT inhibitors (Fig. 6C.7). As will be discussed later, it has been reported that HIV-1 developed an extremely high level of resistance after only one to three serial passages in the presence of a pyridinone inhibitor (nevirapine) *in vitro* (Numberg *et al.* 1991). Furthermore, such pyridinone-resistant HIV-1 variants were cross-resistant to the potent antiretroviral TIBO compound R82150 (Numberg *et al.* 1991). These findings have posed a serious concern for this class of RT inhibitors regarding the emergence of drug-resistant HIV-1 variants as a consequence of antiviral therapy with any of the non-nucleoside RT inhibitors.

Recently, one of the most potent TIBO derivatives, R82913 (Fig. 6C.7), was intravenously administered to 22 patients with AIDS or ARC in a dose-escalating pilot study in Paris and London, and some pharmacokinetic and antiviral data have been reported (Pialoux *et al.* 1991). In this study, daily doses of 10–300 mg were well tolerated for up to 50 weeks, with no haematological or biochemical evidence of toxicity. However, patients did not have significant increases in CD4$^+$ cells and showed no striking clinical improvement, although serum p24 levels reportedly showed a statistically significant decrease. It should be noted that this pilot study was not designed to assess the efficacy of R82913 in patients (Pialoux *et al.* 1991).

6C.3.3.2   HEPT and its analogues

HEPT and its analogues represent a new class of 6-substituted acyclouridine derivatives (Fig. 6C.7) (Baba et al. 1989). These compounds can inhibit the replication of HIV-1 at nanomolar concentrations without affecting the growth of target cells in vitro; however, like TIBO compounds, they have no activity against the replication of other retroviruses including HIV-2, SIV, and murine retroviruses in vitro. HEPT analogues inhibit RT activity in a competitive fashion with regard to dTTP when poly(rA) · oligo(dT) is used as template–primer (Baba et al. 1991). However, when dGTP is used as substrate with poly(rC) · oligo(dG) as template–primer, non-competitive inhibitory activity is displayed. These findings suggest that the HEPT compounds interact with different sites on the RT enzyme as a function of available template primers. Structurally, HEPT compounds belong to the acyclic nucleosides, and, unlike dideoxynucleosides and certain antiretroviral acyclic analogues (e.g. adenallene and cytallene (Hayashi 1990) and PMEA (Pauwels et al. 1988)), HEPT compounds do not require intracellular metabolic processing or phosphorylation to exert their antiretroviral activity. In this context, the HEPT compounds resemble other non-nucleoside RT inhibitors, which implies that HEPT compounds may also easily allow the emergence of HIV-1 drug resistance. Indeed, Richman et al. (1991b) have recently reported that HIV-1 variants resistant to nevirapine (BI-RG-587) (Fig. 6C.7) also showed a high level of resistance to two HEPT derivatives. HEPT compounds may have an advantage when compared with other non-nucleoside RT inhibitors in that HEPT compounds are relatively easy to synthesize; however, more studies are required to define the usefulness of the HEPT compounds for therapy of AIDS.

6C.3.3.3   Dipyridodiazepinone derivatives

The dipyridodiazepinones represent tricyclic compounds originally designed as possible muscarinic receptor antagonists. Some of these compounds showed potent antiviral activity against HIV-1 in vitro. One such compound, nevirapine (BI-RG-587) (Fig. 6C.7), had a K_i of 200 nM for inhibition of HIV-1 RT and exerted extremely potent antiviral activity against HIV-1 at nanomolar concentrations (Merluzzi et al. 1990). Nevirapine, like TIBO derivatives and HEPT compounds, fails to suppress the replication of other retroviruses including HIV-2 and several animal retroviruses. The inhibition of RT activity by nevirapine appears to be non-competitive with respect to dGTP, and this compound has been shown to bind to a site of RT that is not adjacent to the natural substrate binding site (Merluzzi et al. 1990). Although its binding to RT competes with the TIBO compounds, nevirapine shows partial inhibition of HIV-1 RNase-H activity, unlike the TIBO compounds (Merluzzi et al. 1990); therefore the binding site of nevirapine may be slightly different from that of the TIBO compounds.

Recent data show that nevirapine interacts at the highly conserved tyrosine residues at positions 181 and 188 in the RT molecule. Richman *et al.* (1991a) have demonstrated that HIV-1 variants highly resistant to nevirapine emerge after just a few passages in cell culture in the presence of the drug. These variants had a substitution of cysteine for the tyrosine at position 181. Introduction of this substitution at residue 181 into a wild-type HIV-I viral genome conferred a similar resistance to nevirapine. The data on drug resistance have raised a serious concern that HIV-1 may readily develop resistance to nevirapine when the drug is administered to patients.

6C.3.3.4   *Pyridinone derivatives*

In 1991, derivatives of pyridinones were first shown to inhibit HIV-1 RT activity and block the replication of a variety of HIV-1 strains without an appreciable effect on other retroviral or cellular polymerases (Goldman *et al.* 1991). The analogue L-697,639 inhibits the infectivity of HIV-1 by at least 95 per cent at concentrations of 12–200 nM. Synergism between L-697,639 and AZT has also been demonstrated in cell culture (Goldman *et al.* 1991). Based on the specificity for HIV-1 RT, template–primer dependence, and ability to displace ^{3}H-radiolabelled L-697,639, the pyridinones appear to inhibit RT activity by the same mechanism as TIBO compounds and dipyridodiazepinone derivatives. Indeed, HIV-1 variants resistant to a pyridinone derivative are cross-resistant to a TIBO compound (R82150) and nevirapine (Numberg *et al.* 1991).

6C.3.3.5   *Bis(heteroaryl)piperazines*

Certain bis(heteroaryl)piperazines (BHAPs) inhibit HIV-1 RT at concentrations two to four orders of magnitude lower than that which inhibits the activity of cellular DNA polymerases (Romero *et al.* 1991). BHAPs block the replication of laboratory and clinical HIV-1 isolates in primary cultures of human peripheral blood mononuclear cells without cytotoxicity. However, like other non-nucleoside RT inhibitors, the BHAPs do not inhibit the replication of HIV-2, SIV, or other animal retroviruses. Evaluation of a BHAP (U87201) (Fig. 6C.7) in HIV-1-infected SCID mice (severe combined immunodeficient mice implanted with human haemato-lymphoid organs) showed that the compound could block HIV replication *in vivo*. Synthesis of the BHAPs is relatively easy. In laboratory animals the BHAPs reportedly exhibit good oral bioavailability, and drug serum levels in great excess of those required for *in vitro* antiviral activity are maintained for prolonged periods. It is not yet known whether the BHAPs use similar or distinct mechanisms to inhibit HIV-1 RT compared with other non-nucleoside RT inhibitors.

6C.3.3.6 *Prospects for non-nucleoside RT inhibitors*

All the non-nucleoside RT inhibitors described above have demonstrated a high therapeutic index as their anti-retroviral activity and cytotoxicity were measured *in vitro*. They are currently in various stages of preclinical or clinical development. As noted above, preliminary clinical testing of the first non-nucleoside RT inhibitor, the TIBO derivative R82913, has demonstrated good tolerance of the drug; unfortunately, the clinical impact of the drug was not evident (Pialoux *et al.* 1991). More problematically, HIV-1 has been shown readily to develop significant *in vitro* resistance to four of the compounds of this class: TIBO derivatives, HEPT derivatives, pyridinone derivatives, and dipyridodiazepinone derivatives. Since, unlike other known antiretroviral agents such as the dideoxynucleoside analogues and certain HIV protease inhibitors, all these non-nucleoside reverse transcriptase inhibitors are active against HIV-1 but *not* against HIV-2, the lack of activity against HIV-2 and other animal retroviruses in a given drug may predict that the particular drug will allow the rapid development of drug resistance by HIV-1.

These initial findings regarding several of the non-nucleoside RT inhibitors are quite frustrating in view of the fact that other classes of antiretroviral drugs acting through antiviral mechanisms which differ from those of dideoxynucleoside analogues are urgently needed. It is probable that all five non-nucleoside RT inhibitors described here possess the same or similar antiviral mechanisms and may readily allow the emergence of HIV-1 variants cross-resistant to these drugs. Currently ongoing clinical trials administering these non-nucleoside RT inhibitors should help to determine the clinical usefulness of these drugs shortly. The non-nucleoside class of specific HIV-1 inhibitors may prove to be a beneficial component in the antiretroviral repertoire, possibly in a combination therapeutic strategy if not in a single-agent chemotherapeutic regimen. It is worth noting that none of the non-nucleoside RT inhibitors interferes with human DNA polymerases. In any event, these compounds will be useful in further elucidation of the structure–activity relationship between the RT enzyme and its various inhibitors, thus enabling the development of more effective drugs targeted against the RT molecule.

6C.3.4   RNase H as a target for AIDS therapy

The RNase H domain of the mature RT enzyme is vital to successful viral replication, and therefore RNase H can also serve as a new legitimate target for therapeutic intervention. Although significantly less research activity has been focused on the possible use of RNase H as a target in the past, with recent success in crystallization of the RNase H domain of HIV-1 RT (Davies *et al.* 1991), knowledge in this area is growing rapidly.

For example, Hafkemeyer *et al.* (1991) have recently identified a degradation product of the cephalosporin ceftazidim (HP 0.35) that has a specific inhibitory effect on the RNase H activity of RTs isolated from HIV-1 and feline immunodeficiency virus (FIV) at concentrations that did not affect the DNA polymerizing activity of the RTs. Cellular or bacterial RNase H activity was much less affected by HP 0.35. Although this compound reportedly inhibits the replication of FIV in cat CD4$^+$ lymphocytes, no anti-HIV-1 data have been reported yet. Captan, an inhibitor of RNA and DNA polymerases, has been shown to inhibit avian myeloblastosis virus RT polymerase and RNase H activity (Freeman-Wittig *et al.* 1986). Certain sulphated polyanions also preferentially block HIV-1 RNase H activity rather than RT polymerase (Moelling *et al.* 1989). Others have suggested the use of non-dissociable DNA · RNA heteroduplexes in order to engage and then permanently block the RNase H enzymatic binding site (Arnold and Arnold 1991). All these compounds appear to be interesting; however, none have been extensively investigated as to whether they are sufficiently active against HIV-1 to merit possible preclinical or clinical development. The previously mentioned work of Tan *et al.* (1991), in which the possible RNase H inhibitory role of AZT was investigated, also indicates that this enzymatic domain of the RT molecule may be involved in the activity of other anti-HIV-1 compounds for which a mechanism of action has not been defined. Further work in these areas should be encouraged.

6C.3.5   Other RT inhibitors

Other non-nucleoside compounds which have been shown to have an activity against HIV-1 RT and the *in vitro* infectivity of HIV-1 include suramin (Mitsuya *et al.* 1984), phosphonoformate (Sandstrom *et al.* 1985), phosphorothioate oligodeoxynucleotides (Matsukura *et al.* 1987), and rifabutin (Anand *et al.* 1986).

Suramin was the first drug shown to have an activity against the infectivity and replication of HIV-1 *in vitro* (Mitsuya *et al.* 1984). Its inhibitory activity on the RTs of animal retroviruses had been demonstrated by De Clercq and the anti-viral activity of suramin against HIV-1 was believed to be due to an inhibition of the HIV-1 RT activity (De Clercq 1979). However, given its polyanionic character, this compound may also interfere with the adsorption of the virus by target cells, similar to dextran sulphate (Mitsuya *et al.* 1988; Baba *et al.* 1989). Based on *in vitro* data, suramin was first administered to patients with AIDS or ARC in 1984. It was shown to be somewhat virustatic in patients; however, no changes in clinical parameters were observed. Furthermore, long-term treatment regimens were complicated by its toxicities, including fever, erythematous rashes, and proteinuria in nearly all the patients receiving this drug.

Phosphonoformate (PFA), a pyrophosphate analogue originally developed for its anti-herpes activity, had also been shown to suppress retroviral RT by Sundquist and Oberg (1979) before the outbreak of AIDS in the United States. PFA proved to be a potent inhibitor of HIV RT and suppressed the infectivity of HIV-1 at about 100 μM *in vitro* without suppressing cellular growth (Sandstrom *et al*. 1985). Although this drug concentration is attainable in patients, no significant antiviral activity against HIV-1 has been observed. Instead, PFA has been used for treatment of cytomegalovirus infection, and has recently been approved as a prescription drug for cytomegalovirus retinitis in patients with HIV-1 infection.

Recent studies by Matsukura *et al*. (1987) have demonstrated that nuclease-resistant phosphorothioate oligomers (oligodeoxynucleotides which contain a sulphur atom in place of one of the two non-bridging inter-nucleotide oxygens) can exert a potent antiviral activity against HIV-1 *in vitro*. One such oligomer, a 28-mer homo-oligomer of deoxycytidine (S-dC$_{28}$), showed a potent inhibitory activity against HIV-1 RT (Majumdar *et al*. 1989) and the infectivity of the virus *in vitro* (Matsukura *et al*. 1987). Given its polyanionic character, this compound may also interfere with the adsorption of the virus in target cells, similar to suramin and dextran sulphate. However, formidable obstacles to the clinical development of modified oligomers relate to the cost and technical difficulty of large-scale synthesis for therapy.

Rifampin derivatives have been recognized in the past as inhibitors of RTs of animal retroviruses (Yang *et al*. 1972). One derivative, rifabutine (ansamycin), was reported to suppress the replication of HIV-1 *in vitro* (Anand *et al*. 1986). Based on these *in vitro* data, rifabutine was administered to patients with AIDS or ARC; however, no clinical indication of antiviral activity against HIV-1 has been observed.

6C.4   Combination therapy

As more agents become available, the possibility of combining treatment strategies in the therapy of HIV infection becomes an important issue. Decades of clinical research in anticancer chemotherapy, in particular in the treatment of certain types of lymphomas, and therapy of certain infectious diseases such as tuberculosis have demonstrated the superior effectiveness of multiple agents given in combination rather than single-agent therapy. It is probable that, in the therapy of AIDS, a possible synergistic action between drugs for enhanced direct antiviral effect may be attained by employing different targets of the HIV replicative cycle simultaneously, and the onset of drug resistance may also be delayed. Indeed, synergistic activity has been demonstrated *in vitro* for dipyridamole (DPM), a coronary vasodilator and antithrombotic agent, and AZT or ddC (Szebeni *et al*. 1989). DPM appears to inhibit monocyte/macrophage uptake and phosphorylation of thymidine but not AZT, thus providing a selective advantage for AZT. AZT has also been used in combination with acyclovir which has been shown to enhance AZT activity *in vitro* (Mitsuya and Broder 1987). A combination regimen of AZT and acyclovir has generated favourable clinical results in several pilot studies (Surbone *et al.* 1988). Trials are also being considered to combine AZT with probenecid in an attempt to boost the circulatory half-life of AZT (Kornhauser *et al.* 1989).

However, not all combinations of anti-retroviral agents have a synergistic or additive effect. Drug combinations can sometimes be antagonistic, as has been demonstrated by the combination of ribavirin and AZT. Ribavirin has been reported to suppress HIV-1 replication, presumably by blocking the capping of viral RNA (McCormick *et al.* 1984). However, this compound blocks AZT phosphorylation if used together with AZT in culture (Vogt *et al.* 1987), thus diminishing the anti-HIV activity of AZT. In contrast, ribavirin can increase the phosphorylation of dideoxypurine nucleosides such as ddI *in vitro* (Baba *et al.* 1987; Hartman *et al.* 1991). Although no clinical benefit was detected during clinical trials of ribavirin as a single agent (Roberts *et al.* 1990; Spanish Retroviral Trial Group 1991), coadministration of ribavirin with dideoxynucleosides may be theoretically useful.

Combined therapy may also allow the use of decreased doses of individual drugs compared with single-agent therapy. This may be significant, particularly when drugs with severe, but differing, toxicity profiles are employed in this manner, since a decrease in overall drug-related toxicity of therapy can often be achieved. Indeed, as noted earlier, recent studies involving a combination of AZT with ddC (Yarchoan *et al.* 1988; Merigan *et al.* 1989) have found substantially more favourable anti-HIV effect in adults and children with decreased toxicity. In order to obtain a greater clinical effect, the dideoxynucleosides have been used *in vitro* and/or *in vivo* in combination with agents such as interferon a (IFNa), which is believed to affect the budding process of the virus as well as several late events in the replicative cycle (Hartshorn *et al.* 1987; Poli *et al.* 1989; Johnson and Hirsch 1990), non-nucleoside RT inhibitors (Richman *et al.* 1991), or protease inhibitors (Kageyama *et al.* 1992). Some of these combinations have demonstrated synergism in the inhibition of HIV replication, at least *in vitro*; however, it should be noted that the combined use of antiretroviral drugs may lead to decreased antiviral activity and even enhanced toxicity (Vogt *et al.* 1987; Hedaya and Sawchuk 1989). Therefore such experimental co-administration should take place only in the setting of a clinical trial.

Despite the apparent effectiveness of current antiretroviral therapy, significant and sustained recuperation of the patient's immune system has not been evident with currently available antiviral therapies for AIDS. The clinical investigation of immunostimulatory agents such as insulin-like growth factor-1 (IGF-1) and other cytokines, such as granulocyte colony-stimulating factor (G-CSF) or bioactive agents, is under way in an attempt to boost the patient's immune system recovery while controlling viral replication through anti-RT agents.

6C.5   Conclusions

The urgent need to discover and implement effective therapy against HIV disease has resulted in rapid progress in the development and testing of potential new drugs for clinical use. Through efforts over the past decade, multiple therapeutic agents which can be used for the treatment of HIV-associated opportunistic infections have also been developed. Drugs which target the HIV-1 RT enzyme have provided the major therapeutic treatments currently available, and continued research targeting the polymerase and RNase H activity of the RT molecule is expected to bring about further insights into more effective control of HIV-related diseases. The RT enzyme will probably remain a major focus in the development of anti-HIV-1 therapy for at least another decade, although other modalities, such as protease inhibitors, may also come into play in the near future. During future drug development, the avoidance of drug toxicity takes on added significance as therapy will probably require continuous life-long administration of antiretroviral drugs. These advances, together with improvements in managing the clinical care of HIV infected individuals, have already extended patient life expectancy. For the immediate future, further progress with inhibitors of the HIV-1 RT is probable; however, if combined with other classes of agents that affect multiple stages in the replicative cycle of the virus, antiretroviral therapy of AIDS will exert major effects against the morbidity and mortality caused by HIV.

References

Abbotts, J., Jaju, M., and Wilson, S. H. (1991). Thermodynamics of A:G mismatch poly(dG) synthesis by human immunodeficiency virus 1 reverse transcriptase. *Journal of Biological Chemistry*, **266**, 3937−43.

Ahluwalia, G., Cooney, D. A., Mitsuya, H., Fridland, A., Flora, K. P., Hao, Z., *et al.* (1987). Initial studies on the cellular pharmacology of 2′,3′-dideoxyinosine, an inhibitor of HIV infectivity. *Biochemical Pharmacology*, **36**, 3797−800.

Ahluwalia, G., Johnson, M. A., Fridland, A., Cooney, D. A., Broder, S., and Johns, D. G. (1988). Cellular pharmacology of the anti-HIV agent 2′,3′-dideoxyadenosine. *Proceedings of the American Association for Cancer Research*, New Orleans, LA, p. 349. American Association for Cancer Research Inc.

Anand, R., Moore, J., Feorino, P., Curran, J., and Srinivasan, A. (1986). Rifabutine inhibits HTLV-III. *Lancet*, **i**, 97−8.

Aoki, S., Yarchoan, R., Thomas, R., Pluda, J., Marczyk, K., Broder, S., and Mitsuya, H. (1990). Quantitative analysis of HIV-1 proviral DNA in peripheral blood mononuclear cells from patients with AIDS or ARC: decrease of proviral

DNA content following treatment with 2′,3′-dideoxyinosine (ddI). *AIDS Research and Human Retroviruses*, **6**, 1331–9.

Aoki-Sei, S., Yarchoan, R., Kageyama, S., Hoekzema, D., Pluda, J., Wyvill, K., *et al.* (1992). Plasma HIV-1 viremia in HIV-1 infected individuals assessed by polymerase chain reaction. *AIDS Research and Human Retroviruses*, **8**, 1263–70.

Arnold, E. and Arnold, G. F. (1991). Human immunodeficiency virus structure: implications for antiviral design. *Advances in Virus Research*, **39**, 1–87.

Arnold, E., Arnold, G. F., Clark, A., Jacobo-Molina, A., Nanni, R., Paidhungat, M. M., and Zemaitis, G. (1989). Structural studies of HIV RT. Presented at Meeting of Groups Studying the Structure of AIDS-Related Systems and Their Application to Targeted Drug Design, NIGMS, Bethesda, MD.

Baba, M., Pauwels, R., Balzarini, J., Herdewijn, P., DeClercq, E., and Desmyter, J. (1987). Ribavirin antagonizes inhibitory effects of pyrimidine 2′,3′-dideoxy-nucleosides but enhances inhibitory effects of purine 2′,3′-dideoxynucleosides on replication of human immunodeficiency virus *in vitro*. *Antimicrobial Agents and Chemotherapy*, **31**, 1613–17.

Baba, M., Tanaka, H., DeClercq, E., Pauwels, R., Balzarini, J., Schols, D., Nakashima, H., *et al.* (1989). Highly specific inhibition of human immuno-deficiency virus type 1 by a novel 6-substituted acyclouridine derivative. *Biochemical and Biophysical Research Communications*, **165**, 1375–81.

Baba, M., De Clercq, E., Hiromichi, T., Ubasawa, M., Takashima, H., Sekiya, K., *et al.* (1991). Potent and selective inhibition of human immunodeficiency virus type 1 (HIV-1) by 5-ethyl-6-phenylthiouracil derivatives through their interaction with the HIV-1 reversed transcriptase. *Proceedings of the National Academy of Sciences of the United States of America*, **88**, 2356–60.

Baltimore, D. (1970). RNA-dependent DNA polymerase in virions of RNA tumor viruses. *Nature, London*, **27**, 1209–11.

Barat, C., Lullien, V., Schatz, O., Keith, G., Nugeyre, M. T., Gruninger-Leitch, F., *et al.* (1989). HIV-1 reverse transcriptase specifically interacts with the anticodon domain of its cognate primer tRNA. *EMBO Journal*, **8**, 3279–85.

Barre-Sinoussi, F., Cherman, J. C., and Rey, F. (1983). Isolation of a T-lym-photropic retrovirus from a patient at risk for acquired immunodeficiency syndrome (AIDS). *New England Journal of Medicine*, **220**, 868–71.

Bebenek, K., Abbotts, J., Roberts, J. D., Wilson, S. H., and Kunkel, T. A. (1989). Specificity and mechanism of error-prone replication by human immunodeficiency virus-1 reverse transcriptase. *Journal of Biological Chemistry*, **264**, 16948–56.

Bender, W. and Davidson, N. (1976). Mapping of poly(A) sequences in the electron microscope reveals unusual structure of type C oncornavirus RNA molecules. *Cell*, **7**, 595–607.

Boone, L. R. and Skalka, A. M. (1981). Viral DNA synthesized *in vitro* by avian retrovirus particles permeabilized with melittin. II. Evidence for a strand dis-placement mechanism in plus-strand synthesis. *Journal of Virology*, **37**, 117–26.

Boucher, C. A., O'Sullivan, E., Mulder, J. W., Ramautarsing, C., Kellam, P., Darby, G., *et al.* (1992). Ordered appearance of zidovudine resistance mutations during treatment of 18 human immunodeficiency virus-positive subjects. *Journal of Infectious Diseases*, **165**, 105–10.

Brierley, I., Digard, P., and Inglis, S. C. (1989). Characterization of an efficient coronavirus ribosomal frameshifting signal: requirement for an RNA pseudoknot. *Cell*, **57**, 537–47.

Browne, M. J. (1990). Phase I study of 2′,3′-didehydro-2′,3′-dideoxythymidine (d4T) in patients with AIDS or ARC, Proceedings of the 6th International Conference on AIDS, San Francisco, CA, p. 200. University of California, San Francisco.

Butler, K. M., Husson, R. N., Balis, F. M., Brouwer, P., Eddy, J., El-Amin, D., *et al.* (1991). Dideoxyinosine (ddI) in symptomatic HIV-infected children: a phase I-II study. *New England Journal of Medicine*, **324**, 137–44.

Chen, M. S., Suttmann, R. T., Wu, J. C., and Prisbe, E. J. (1992). Metabolism of 4′-azidothymidine: a compound with potent and selective activity against the human immunodeficiency virus. *Journal of Biological Chemistry*, **267**, 257–60.

Cheng, Y.-C., Dutschman, G., Bastow, K., Sarngadharan, M., and Ting, R. (1987). Human immunodeficiency virus reverse transcriptase: general properties and its interactions with nucleoside triphosphate analogs. *Journal of Biological Chemistry*, **262**, 2187–9.

Collett, M. S., Dierks, P., Parsons, J. T., and Faras, A. J. (1978). RNase H hydrolysis of the 5′ terminus of the avian sarcoma virus genome during reverse transcription. *Nature, London*, **272**, 181–4.

Cooney, D. A., Dalal, M., Mitsuya, H., McMahon, J. B., Nadkarni, M., Balsarini, J., *et al.* (1986). Initial studies on the cellular pharmacology of 2′,3′-dideoxy-cytidine, an inhibitor of HTLV-III infectivity. *Biochemical Pharmacology*, **35**, 2065–8.

Cooney, D. A., Ahluwalia, G., Mitsuya, H., Fridland, A., Johnson, M., Hao, Z., *et al.* (1987). Initial studies on the cellular pharmacology of 2′,3′-dideoxyadeno-sine, an inhibitor of HTLV-III infectivity. *Biochemical Pharmacology*, **36**, 1765–8.

Crawford, S. and Goff, S. P. (1985). A deletion mutation in the 5′ part of the pol gene of Moloney murine leukemia virus blocks proteolytic processing of the gag and pol polyproteins. *Journal of Virology*, **53**, 899–907.

Dalakos, M. C., Illa, I., Pezeshkpour, G. H., Laukaitis, J. P., Cohen, B., and Griffin, J. L. (1990). Mitochondrial myopathy caused by long-term zidovudine therapy. *New England Journal of Medicine*, **322**, 1098–1105.

Dalgleish, A. G., Beverley, P. C., Clapham, P. R., Crawford, D. H., Greaves, M. F., and Weiss, R. A. (1984). The CD4 (T4) antigen is an essential component of the receptor for the AIDS retrovirus. *Nature, London*, **312**, 763–7.

Darlix, J. L., Bromley, P. A., and Spahr, P. F. (1977). Extensive *in vitro* tran-scription of Rous sarcoma virus RNA by avian myeloblastosis virus DNA poly-merase and concurrent activation of the associated RNase H. *Journal of Virology*, **23**, 659–68.

Davies, J., Hostomska, Z., Hostomsky, Z., Jordan, S., and Matthews, D. (1991). Crystal structure of the Ribonuclease H domain of HIV-1 reverse transcriptase. *Science*, **252**, 88–95.

Debyser, Z., Pauwels, R., Andries, K., Desmyter, J., Kukla, M., Janssen, P. A. J., and De Clercq, E. (1991). An antiviral target on reverse transcriptase of human immunodeficiency virus type 1 revealed by tetrahydroimidazo[jk}[1,4]benzodia-zepin-2(1H)-one and -thione compounds. *Proceedings of the National Academy of Sciences of the United States of America*, **88**, 1451–5.

Debyser, Z., Pauwels, R., Andries, K., and De Clercq, E. (1992). Specific HIV-1 reverse transcriptase inhibitors. *Journal of Enzyme Inhibition*, **6**, 47–53.

De Clercq, E. (1979). Suramin: a potent inhibitor of the reverse transcriptase of RNA tumor viruses. *Cancer Letters*, **8**, 9–22.

De Clercq, E. (1991). Basic approaches to anti-retrovirus treatment. *Journal of Acquired Immune Deficiency Syndrome*, **4**, 207–18.

De Clercq, E. (1992). HIV inhibitors targeted at the reverse transcriptase. *AIDS Research and Human Retroviruses*, **8**, 119–34.

DeStefano, J., Buiser, R., Mallaber, L., Myers, T., Bambara, R., and Fay, P. (1991). Polymerization and RNase H activities of the reverse transcriptases from avian myeloblastosis, human immunodeficiency, and Moloney murine leukemia viruses are functionally uncoupled. *Journal of Biological Chemistry*, **266**, 7423–31.

De Vico, A. L. and Sarngadharan, M. G. (1992). Reverse transcriptase-a general discussion. *Journal of Enzyme Inhibition*, **6**, 9–34.

Du, D. L., Volpe, D. A., Murphy, M. J., and Griehaber, C. K. (1989). *In vitro* myelotoxicity of new anti-HIV drugs (2′,3′-dideoxynucleosides) on human hematopoietic progenitor cells *in vitro*. *Experimental Hematology*, **18**, 832–6.

Farmerie, W. G., Loeb, D. D., Casavant, N. C., Hutchison, C. A., Edgell, M. H., and Swanstrom, R. (1987). Expression and processing of the AIDS virus reverse transcriptase in *Escherichia coli*. *Science*, **236**, 305–8.

Fauci, A. S. (1988). The human immunodeficiency virus: infectivity and mechanisms of pathogenesis. *Science*, **239**, 617–22.

Fischl, M., Parker, C., Pettinelli, C., Wulfsohn, M., Hirsch, M. S., Collier, A. C., *et al.* (AIDS Clinical Trial Group) (1990). A randomized controlled trial of a reduced daily dose of zidovudine in patients with acquired immunodeficiency syndrome. *New England Journal of Medicine*, **323**, 1009–15.

Freeman-Wittig, M. J., Vinocour, M., and Lewis, R. A. (1986). Differential effects of captan on DNA polymerase and ribonuclease H activities of avian myeloblastosis virus reverse transcriptase. *Biochemistry*, **25**, 3050–5.

Friedrich, R. and Moelling, K. (1979). Effect of viral RNase H on the avian sarcoma viral genome during early transcription *in vitro*. *Journal of Virology*, **31**, 630–8.

Fujiwara, T. and Mizuuchi, K. (1988). Retroviral DNA integration: structure of an integration intermediate. *Cell*, **54**, 497–504.

Furman, P. A. and Barry, D. W. (1988). Spectrum of antiviral activity and mechanism of action of zidovudine. An overview. *American Journal of Medicine*, **85** (Suppl. 2A), 176–81.

Furman, P. A., Fyfe, J. A., St. Clair, M., Weinhold, K., Rideout, J. L., Freeman, G. A., *et al.* (1986). Phosphorylation of 3′-azido-3′-deoxythymidine and selective interaction of the 5′-triphosphate with human immunodeficiency virus reverse transcriptase. *Proceedings of the National Academy of Sciences of the United States of America*, **83**, 8333–7.

Furuichi, Y., Shatkin, A. J., Stavenezer, E., and Bishop, J. M. (1975). Blocked, methylated 5′-terminal sequence in avian sarcoma virus RNA. *Nature, London*, **257**, 618–20.

Gartner, S., Markovits, P., Markovitz, D. M., Kaplan, M. H., and Gallo, R. C. (1986). The role of mononuclear phagocytes in HTLV-III/LAV infection. *Science*, **233**, 215–19.

Gilboa, E., Mitra, S. W., Goff, S., and Baltimore, D. (1979). A detailed model of reverse transcription and tests of crucial aspects. *Cell*, **18**, 93–100.

Gill, P., Rarick, M., Byrnes, R. K., Causey, D., Loureiro, C., and Levine, A. M. (1987). Azidothymidine associated with bone marrow failure in the acquired immunodeficiency syndrome (AIDS). *Annals of Internal Medicine*, **107**, 502–5.

Goldman, M. E., Ninberg, J. H., O'Brien, J. A., Quintero, J. C., Schleif, W. A., Freund, K. F., *et al*. (1991). Pyridinone derivatives: specific human immunodeficiency virus type 1 reverse transcriptase inhibitors with antiviral activity. *Proceedings of the National Academy of Sciences of the United States of America*, **88**, 6863–7.

Gottlieb, M. S., Schroff, R., Schanker, H. M., Weisman, J. D., Thim Fan, P., Wolf, R. A., and Saxon, A. (1981). *Pneumocystis carinii* pneumonia and mucosal candidiasis in previously healthy homosexual men: evidence of a new acquired cellular immunodeficiency. *New England Journal of Medicine*, **305**, 1425–31.

Gottlinger, H. G., Sodroski, J. G., and Haseltine, W. A. (1989). Role of capsid precursor processing and myristoylation in morphogenesis and infectivity of human immunodeficiency virus type 1. *Proceedings of the National Academy of Sciences of the United States of America*, **86**, 5781–5.

Hafkemeyer, P., Neftel, K., Hobi, R., Pfaltz, A., Lutz, H., Luthi, K., *et al*. (1991). HP 0.35, a cephalosporin degradation product is a specific inhibitor of lentiviral RNAses H. *Nucleic Acids Research*, **19**, 4059–65.

Hamamoto, Y., Nakashioma, H., Matsui, T., Matsuda, A., Ueda, T., and Yamamoto, N. (1987). Inhibitory effect of 2′,3′-didehydro-2′,3′-dideoxynucleosides on infectivity, cytopathic effects, and replication of human immunodeficiency virus. *Antimicrobial Agents and Chemotherapy*, **31**, 907–10.

Hansen, J., Schulze, T., Mellert, W., and Moelling, K. (1988). Identification and characterization of HIV-specific RNase H by monoclonal antibody. *EMBO Journal*, **239**, 239–43.

Harouse, J., Bhat, S., Spitalnik. S., Laughlin, M., Stefano, K., Silberberg, D., and Gonzalez-Scarano, F. (1991). Inhibition of entry of HIV-1 in neural cell lines by antibodies against galactosyl ceramide. *Science*, **253**, 320–3.

Hartman, N., Ahluwalia, G., Cooney, D., Mitsuya, H., Kageyama, S., Fridland, A., *et al*. (1991). Inhibitors of IMP dehydrogenase stimulate the phosphorylation of the anti-human immunodeficiency virus nucleosides 2′,3′-dideoxyadenosine and 2′,3′-dideoxyinosine. *Molecular Pharmacology*, **40**, 118–24.

Hartshorn, K. L., Vogt, M. W., Chou, T.-C., Blumberg, R. S., Byington, R., Schooley. R. T., and Hirsch, M. S. (1987). Synergistic inhibition of human immunodeficiency virus *in vitro* by azidothymidine and recombinant alpha A interferon. *Antimicrobial Agents and Chemotherapy*, **31**, 168–72.

Haseltine, W. A., Kleid, D. G., Panet, A., Rothenberg, E., and Baltimore, D. (1976). Ordered transcription of RNA tumor virus genomes. *Journal of Molecular Biology*, **106**, 109–31.

Hatfield, D. and Oroszlan, S. (1990). The where, what and how of ribosomal frameshifting in retroviral protein synthesis. *Trends in Biochemical Science*, **15**, 186–90.

Hayashi, S., Fine, R. L., Chou, T.-C., Currens, M. J., Broder, S., and Mitsuya, H. (1990) *In vitro* inhibition ot the infectivity and replication of human immunodeficiency virus type 1 by combination of antiretroviral 2′,3′-dideoxynucleosides and virus-binding inhibitors. *Antimicrobial Agents and Chemotherapy*, **34**, 82–8.

Hedaya, M. A. and Sawchuk, R. J. (1989). Effect of probenecid on the renal and nonrenal clearances of zidovudine and its distribution into cerebrospinal fluid in the rabbit. *Journal of Pharmaceutical Science*, **78**, 716–22.

Hizi, A., McGill, C., and Hughes, S. H. (1988). Expression of soluble, enzymatically active, human immunodeficiency virus reverse transcriptase in *Escherichia coli* and analysis of mutants. *Proceedings of the National Academy of Sciences of the United States of America*, **85**, 1218–22.

Holodiny, M., Katzenstein, D., and Sengupta, S. (1991). Detection and quantitation of human immunodeficiency virus RNA in patient serum by use of the polymerase chain reaction. *Journal of Infectious Diseases*, **163**, 862–6.

Huber, H. E., McCoy, J. M., Seehra, J. S., and Richardson, C. C. (1989). Human immunodeficiency virus 1 reverse transcriptase. Template binding, processivity, strand displacement synthesis, and template switching. *Journal of Biological Chemistry*, **264**, 4669–78.

Jacks, T. and Varmus, H. E. (1985). Expression of the Rous sarcoma virus *pol* gene by ribosomal frameshifting. *Science*, **230**, 1237–42.

Jacks, T., Power, M. D., Masiarz, F. R., Luciw, P. A., Barr, P. J., and Varmus, H. E. (1988). Characterization of ribosomal frameshifting in HIV-1 *gag-pol* expression. *Nature, London*, **331**, 280–3.

Johnson, V. A. and Hirsch, M. S. (1990). New developments in combination chemotherapy of anti-human immunodeficiency virus drugs. *Annals of the New York Academy of Science*, **616**, 318–27.

Kageyama, S., Weinstein, J. N., Shirasaka, T., Kempf, D. J., Norbeck, D. W., Plattner, J. J., et al. (1992). *In vitro* inhibition of HIV-1 replication by C_2 symmetry-based HIV-1 protease inhibitors as single agents or in combinations. *Antimicrobial Agents and Chemotherapy*, **36**, 926–33.

Katoh, I., Yoshinaka, Y., Rein, A., Shibuya, M., Odaka, T., and Oroszlan, S. (1985). Murine leukemia virus maturation: protease region required for conversion from "immature" to "mature" core form and for virus infectivity. *Virology*, **145**, 280–92.

Kedar, P. S., Abbotts, J., Kovacs, T., Lesiak, K., Torrence, P., and Wilson, S. H. (1990). Mechanism of HIV reverse transcriptase:enzyme-primer interaction as revealed through studies of a dNTP analogue, 3′-azido-dTTP. *Biochemistry*, **29**, 3603–11.

Kellam, P., Boucher, C. A. B., and Larder, B. A. (1992). Fifth mutation in human immunodeficiency virus type 1 reverse transcriptase contributes to the development of high-level resistance to zidovudine. *Proceedings of the National Academy of Sciences of the United States of America*, **89**, 1934–8.

Klatzmann, D., Barre-Sinoussi, F., and Nugeyre, M. T. (1984). Selective tropism of lymphadenopathy associated virus (LAV) for helper–inducer T lymphocytes. *Science*, **225**, 59–63.

Kornhauser, D. M., Petty, B. G., Hendrix, C. W., Woods, A. S., Nerhood, L. J., Bartlet, J. G., and Lietman, P. S. (1989). Probenecid and zidovudine metabolism. *Lancet*, **ii**, 473–75.

Krasinski, K., Borkowsky, W., and Holzman, R. S. (1989). Prognosis of human immunodeficiency virus infection in children and adolescents. *Pediatric Infectious Disease Journal*, **8**, 216–20.

Lambert. J. S., Seidin, M., Reichman, R. C., Plank, C. S., Laverty, M., Morse, G. D., et al. (1990). 2′,3′-Dideoxyinosine (ddI) in patients with the acquired immunodeficiency syndrome or the AIDS-related complex. A phase I trial. *New England Journal of Medicine*, **322**, 1333–40.

Larder, B. A. and Kemp, S. D. (1989). Multiple mutations in HIV-I reverse transcriptase confer high-level resistance to zidovudine (AZT). *Science*, **246**, 1155–8.

Larder, B. A., Darby, G., and Richman, D. D. (1989). HIV with reduced sensitivity to zidovudine (AZT) isolated during prolonged therapy. *Science*, **243**, 1731–4.

Larder, B. A., Chesebro, B., and Richman, D. D. (1990). Susceptibilities of zidovudine-susceptible and -resistant human immunodeficiency virus isolates to antiviral agents determined by using a quantitative plaque reduction assay. *Antimicrobial Agents and Chemotherapy*, **34**, 436–41.

Lori, F., Scovassi, A. I., Zella, D., Achilli, G., Cattaneo, E., Casoli, C., and Bertazzoni, U. (1988). Enzymatically active forms of reverse transcriptase of the human immunodeficiency virus. *AIDS Research and Human Retroviruses*, **4**, 393–8.

Lowe, D. M., Aitken, A., Bradley, C., Darby, G. K., Larder, B. A., Powell, K. L., *et al.* (1988). HIV-1 reverse transcriptase: crystallization and analysis of domain structure by limited proteolysis. *Biochemistry*, **27**, 8884–9.

Luo, G. X. and Taylor, J. (1990). Template switching by reverse transcriptase during DNA synthesis. *Journal of Virology*, **64**, 4321–8.

McCormick, J., Getchell, J., Mitchell, S., and Hicks, D. (1984). Ribavirin suppresses replication of lymphadenopathy-associated virus in cultures of human adult T lymphocytes. *Lancet*, **ii**, 1367–9.

Majumdar, C., Abbotts, J., Broder, S., and Wilson, S. H. (1988). Studies on the mechanism of human immunodeficiency virus reverse transcriptase. Steady-state kinetics, processivity, and polynucleotide inhibition. *Journal of Biological Chemistry*, **263**, 15657–65.

Majumdar, C., Stein, C. A., Cohen, J. S., Broder, S., and Wilson, S. H. (1989). Stepwise mechanism of HIV reverse transcriptase: primer function of phosphorothioate oligodeoxynucleotide. *Biochemistry* **28**, 1340–6.

Marquez, V. E., Tseng, C. K., Driscoll, J. S., Mitsuya, H., Broder, S., Roth, J. S., and Kelley, J. A. (1987). 2′,3′-Dideoxy-2′-b-fluoro-adenosine, an acid-stable purine nucleoside active against human immunodeficiency virus (HIV). *Biochemical Pharmacology*, **36**, 2719–22.

Masur, H., Michelis, M. A., Greene, J. B., Onorato, I., Vande Stouwe, R. A., Holzman, R. S., *et al.* (1981). An outbreak of community-acquired *Pneumocystis carinii* pneumonia: initial manifestations of cellular immune dysfunctions. *New England Journal of Medicine*, **305**, 1431–8.

Matsukura, M., Shinozuka, K., Zon, G., Mitsuya, H., Reitz, M., and Cohen. J. (1987). Phosphorothioate analogs of oligodeoxynucleotides: inhibitors of replication and cytopathic effects of human immunodeficiency virus. *Proceedings of the National Academy of Sciences of the United States of America*, **84**, 7706–10.

Merigan, T. C., Skowron, G., Bozzette, S. A., Richman, D., Uttamchandani, R., Fischl, M., *et al.* (1989). Circulating p24 antigen levels and responses to dideoxycytidine in human immunodeficiency virus (HIV) infections. A phase I and II study. *Annals of Internal Medicine*, **110**, 189–94.

Merluzzi, V. J., Hargrave, K. D., Labadia, M., Grozinger, K., Skoog, M., Wu, J. C., *et al.* (1990). Inhibition of HIV-1 replication by a nonnucleoside reverse transcriptase inhibitor. *Science*, **250**, 1411–1413.

Mitra, S. W., Goff, S., Gilboa, E., and Baltimore, D. (1979). Synthesis of a 600-nucleotide-long plus-strand DNA by virions of Moloney murine leukemia, virus. *Proceedings of the National Academy of Sciences of the United States of America*, **76**, 4355–9.

Mitsuya, H. and Broder, S. (1986). Inhibition of the *in vitro* infectivity and cyto-pathic effect of human T-lymphotropic virus type III/lymphadenopathy virus-associated virus (HTLV-III/LAV) by 2′,3′-dideoxynucleosides. *Proceedings of the National Academy of Sciences of the United States of America*, **83**, 1911–1915.

Mitsuya, H. and Broder, S. (1987). Strategies for antiviral therapy in AIDS. *Nature, London*, **325**, 773–778.

Mitsuya, H., Popovic, M., Yarchoan, R., Matsushita, S., Gallo, R., and Broder, S. (1984). Suramin protection of T cells *in vitro* against infectivity and cytopathic effect of HTLV-III. *Science*, **226**, 172–4.

Mitsuya, H., Weinhold, K. J., Furman, P. A., St. Clair, M. H., Nusiniff-Lehrman, S., Gallo, R. C., *et al.* (1985). 3′-Azido-3′-deoxythymidine (BW A509U): an antiviral agent that inhibits the infectivity and cytopathic effect of human T-lymphotropic virus type III/lymphadenopathy-associated virus *in vitro*. *Proceedings of the National Academy of Sciences of the United States of America*, **82**, 7096–100.

Mitsuya, H., Matsukura, M., and Broder, S. (1987). Rapid *in vitro* systems for assessing activity of agents against HTLV-III/LAV. In *AIDS: modern concepts and therapeutic challenges* (ed. S. Broder), pp. 303–33. Marcel Dekker, New York.

Mitsuya, H., Looney, D., Kuno, S., Keno, S., Wong-Staal, F., and Broder, S. (1988). Dextran sulfate suppression of viruses in the HIV family: inhibition of virion binding to CD4+ cells. *Science*, **240**, 646–9.

Mitsuya, H., Yarchoan, R., and Broder, S. (1991a). Molecular targets for AIDS therapy. *Science*, **249**, 1533–44.

Mitsuya, H., Yarchoan, R., Kageyama, S., and Broder, S. (1991b). Targeted therapy of human immunodeficiency virus-related disease. *FASEB Journal*, **5**, 2369–81.

Mizrahi, V., Lazarus, G. M., Miles, L. M., Meyers, C. A., and Debouck, C. (1989). Recombinant HIV-1 reverse transcriptase: purification, primary structure, and polymerase/ribonuclease H activities. *Archives of Biochemistry and Biophysics*, **273**, 347–58.

Moelling, K., Schulze, T., and Diringer, H. (1989). Inhibition of human immuno-deficiency virus type I RNase H by sulfated polyanions. *Journal of Virology*, **63**, 5489–91.

Mous, J., Heimer, E. P., and Le Grice, S. F. (1988). Processing protease and reverse transcriptase from human immunodeficiency virus type I polyprotein in *Escherichia coli*. *Journal of Virology*, **62**, 1433–6.

Muller, B., Restle, T., Weiss, S., Gaute, M., Sczakiel. G., and Goody, R. S. (1989). Coexpression of the subunits of the heterodimer of HIV-1 reverse tran-scriptase in *Escherichia coli*. *Journal of Biological Chemistry*, **264**, 13975–8.

Muller, B., Restle, T., Reinstein, J., and Goody, R. S. (1991). Interaction of fluorescently labeled dideoxynucleotides with HIV-1 reverse transcriptase. *Bio-chemistry*, **30**, 3709–15.

Munoz, A., Wang, M. C., and Bass, S. (1989). Acquired immunodeficiency syn-drome (AIDS)-free time after human immunodeficiency virus type 1 (HIV-1) seroconversion in homosexual men. Multicenter AIDS Cohort Study Group. *American Journal of Epidemiology* **130**, 530–9.

Murakami, K., Shirasaka, T., Yoshioka, H., Kojima, E., Aoki, S., Ford, H., *et al.* (1991). *Escherichia coli* mediated biosynthesis and *in vitro* anti-HIV activity of lipophilic 6-halo-2′,3′-dideoxypurine nucleosides. *Journal of Medicinal Chemistry*, **34**, 1606–12.

Narayan, O. and Clements, J. E. (1989). Biology and pathogenesis of lentiviruses. *Journal of General Virology*, **70**, 1617–39.

Nicholson, J. K., Cross, G. D., Callaway, C. S., and McDougal, J. S. (1986). *In vitro* infection of human monocytes with human T lymphotropic virus type III/lymphadenopathy-associated virus (HTLV-III/LAV). *Journal of Immunology*, **137**, 323–9.

Numberg, J. H., Schleif, W. A., Boots, E. J., O'Brien, J. A., Quintero, J. C., Hoffman, J. M., *et al.* (1991). Viral resistance to human immunodeficiency virus type 1-specific pyridinone reverse transcriptase inhibitors. *Journal of Virology*. **65**, 4887–92.

Olsen, J. C. and Watson, K. F. (1985). RNase H-mediated release of the retrovirus RNA polyadenylate tail during reverse transcription. *Journal of Virology*, **53**, 324–9.

Omer, C. A. and Faras, A. J. (1982). Mechanism of release of the avian rotavirus tRNATrp primer molecule from viral DNA by ribonuclease H during reverse transcription. *Cell*, **30**, 797–805.

Omer, C. A., Resnick, R., and Faras, A. J. (1984). Evidence for involvement of an RNA primer in initiation stop plus DNA synthesis during reverse transcription *in vitro*. *Journal of Virology*, **50**, 465–70.

Oyama, F., Kikuchi, R., Croucy, R. J., and Uchida, T. (1989). Intrinsic properties of reverse transcriptase in reverse transcription. *Journal of Biological Chemistry*, **264**, 18808–17.

Panet, A., Baltimore, D., and Hanafusa, T. (1975). Quantitation of avian RNA tumor virus reverse transcriptase by radioimmunoassay. *Journal of Virology*, **16**, 146–52.

Panganiban, A. T. (1988). Retroviral *gag* gene amber codon suppression is caused by an intrinsic cis-acting component of the viral mRNA. *Journal of Virology*, **62**, 3574–80.

Pauwels, R., Balzarini, J., Schols, D., Baba, M., Desmyter, J., Rosenberg, I., *et al.* (1988). Phosphonylmethoxyethyl purine derivatives, a new class of anti-human immunodeficiency virus agents. *Antimicrobial Agents and Chemotherapy*, **32**, 1025–30.

Pauwels, R., Andries, K., Desmyter, J., Schols, D., Kukla, N. J., Breslin, H. S., *et al.* (1990). Potent and selective inhibition of HIV-1 replication *in vitro* by a novel series of TIBO derivatives. *Nature, London*, **343**, 470–4.

Peng, C., Chang, N. T., and Chang, T. W. (1991). Identification and characterization of human immunodeficiency virus type 1 *gag-pol* fusion protein in transfected mammalian cells. *Journal of Virology*, **65**, 2751–6.

Perno, C.-F., Yarchoan, R., Cooney, D. A., Hartman, N. R., Webbs, D. S., Hao, Z., *et al.* (1989). Replication of human immunodeficiency virus in monocytes. Granulocytes/macrophages colony-stimulating factor (GM-CSF) potentiates viral production yet enhances the antiviral effect mediated by 3'-azido-2',3'-dideoxythymidine (AZT) and other dideoxynucleoside congeners of thymidine. *Journal of Experimental Medicine*, **169**, 933–51.

Peters, G. and Glover, C. (1980). tRNA's and priming of RNA-directed DNA synthesis in mouse mammary tumor virus. *Journal of Virology*, **35**, 31–40.

Pialoux, G., Youle, M., Dupont, B., Gazzard, B., Cauwenbergh, G., Stoffels, P., *et al.* (1991). Pharmacokinetics of R82913 in patients with AIDS or AIDS-related complex. *Lancet*, **i**, 140–3.

Pizzo, P. A., Eddy, J., Falloon, J., Balis, F. M., Murphy, R. F., Moss, H., *et al.* (1988). Effect of continuous intravenous infusion of zidovudine (AZT) in children with symptomatic HIV infection. *New England Journal of Medicine*, **319**, 889–96.

Pizzo, P. A., Butler, K., Balis, F., Brouwers, P., Hawkine, M., Eddy, J., *et al.* (1990). Dideoxycytidine alone and in an alternating schedule with zidovudine (AZT) in children with symptomatic human immunodeficiency virus infection. *Journal of Pediatrics*, **117**, 799–808.

Poli, G., Orenstien, J. M., Kinter, A., Folks, T. M., and Fauci, A. S. (1989). Interferon-*a* but not AZT supresses HIV expression in chronically infected cell lines. *Science*, **244**, 575–7.

Prasad, V. R. and Goff, S. P. (1989). Linker insertion mutagenesis of the human immunodeficiency virus reverse transcriptase expressed in bacteria: definition of the minimal polymerase domain. *Proceedings of the National Academy of Sciences of the United States of America*, **86**, 3104–8.

Preston, B. D., Poiesz, B. J., and Loeb, L. A. (1988). Fidelity of HIV-1 reverse transcriptase. *Science*, **242**, 1168–71.

Rabkin, C. S. and Goedert, J. J. (1990). Risk of non-Hodgkin's lymphoma and Kaposi's sarcoma in homosexual men. *Lancet*, **ii**, 248.

Ratner, L., Haseltine, W., Patarca, R., Livak, K. J., Starcich, B., and Josephs, S. F. (1985). Complete nucleotide sequence of the AIDS virus, HTLV-III. *Nature, London*, **313**, 277–84.

Restle, T., Muller, B., and Goody, R. S. (1990). Dimerization of human immunodeficiency virus reverse transcriptase. *Journal of Biological Chemistry*, **265**, 8986–8.

Richman, D. D., Shih, C.-K., Lowy, I., Rose, J., Prodanovich, P., Goff, S., and Griffin, J. (1991a). Human immunodeficiency virus type 1 mutants resistant to nonnucleoside inhibitors of reverse transcriptase arise in tissue culture. *Proceedings of the National Academy of Sciences of the United States of America*, **88**, 11241–45.

Richman, D. D. (1990). Zidovudine resistance of human immunodeficiency virus. *Review of Infectious Diseases*, **12**, S507–12.

Richman, D. D. (1992). Emergence of mutant HIV reverse transcriptase conferring resistance to AZT. *Journal of Enzyme Inhibition*, **6**, 55–64.

Richman, D. D., Fischl, M. A., Grieco, M. H., Gottlieb, M. S., Volberding, P. A., Laskin, O. L., *et al.* (1987). The toxicity of azidothymidine (AZT) in the treatment of patients with AIDS and AIDS-related complex: A double-blind, placebo-controlled trial. *New England Journal of Medicine*, **317**, 192–7.

Richman, D. D., Grimes, J., and Lagakos, S. (1990). Effect of stage of disease and drug dose on zidovudine susceptibilities of isolates of human immunodeficiency virus. *Journal of Acquired Immune Deficiency*, **3**, 743–6.

Richman, D. D., Rosenthal, A. S., Skoog, M., Eckner, R. J., Chou, T.-C., Sabo, J. P., and Merluzzi, V. J. (1991b). BI-RG-587 is active against zidovudine-resistant human immunodeficiency virus type 1 and synergistic with zidovudine. *Antimicrobial Agents and Chemotherapy*, **35**, 305–8.

Roberts, J. D., Bebenek, K., and Kunkel, T. A. (1988). The accuracy of reverse transcriptase from HIV-I. *Science*, **242**, 1171–3.

Roberts, R. B., Jurica, K., Meyer, W. A., Paxton, H., and Makuch, R. W. (1990). A phase I study of ribavirin in human immunodeficiency virus-infected patients. *Journal of Infectious Diseases*, **162**, 638–42.

Romero, D. L., Busso, M., Tan, C.-K., Reusser, F., Palmer, J. R., Poppe, S. M., et al. (1991). Non nucleoside reverse transcriptase inhibitors that potently and specifically block human immunodeficiency virus type 1 replication. *Proceedings of the National Academy of Sciences of the United States of America*, **88**, 8806–10.

Rowley, G. L., Ma, Q.-F., Bathurst, I. C., Barr, P. J., and Kenyon, G. L. (1990). Stabilization and activation of recombinant human immunodeficiency virus-1 reverse transcriptase-p66. *Biochemical and Biophysical Research Communications*, **167**, 673–9.

St. Clair, M. H., Martin, J. L., Tudor-Williams, G., Bach, M. C., Vavro, C. L., King, D. M. *et al.* (1991). Resistance to ddI and sensitivity to AZT induced by a mutation in HIV-I reverse transcription. *Science*, **253**, 1557–1559.

Sandstrom, E., Kaplan, J., Byington, R., and Hirsch, M. (1985). Inhibition of human T-cell lymphotropic virus type III *in vitro* by phosphonoformate. *Lancet*, **i**, 1480–2.

Schinazi, R. F. and Ahn, M. K. (1987). Selective *in vitro* inhibition of human immunodeficiency virus (HIV) replication by 3′-azido-2′,3′-dideoxythymidine (CS-87). *Journal of Clinical Biochemistry*, **11D** (Suppl), 74.

Schmitt, F. A., Bigley, J. W., McKinnis, R., Logue, P. E., Evans, R. W., Drucker, J. L., et al. (1988). Neuropsychological outcome of zidovudine (AZT) treatment of patients with AIDS and AIDS-related complex. *New England Journal of Medicine*, **319**, 1573–8.

Shirasaka, T., Murakami, D., Ford, H., Kelley, J. A., Yoshioka, H., Kojima, E., et al. (1990a). Lipophilic halogenated congeners of 2′,3′-dideoxypurine nucleosides active against human immunodeficiency virus *in vitro*. *Proceedings of the National Academy of Sciences of the United States of America*, **87**, 9426–30.

Shirasaka, T., Yarchoan, R., Aoki, S., Ford, H., DeVico, A., Sarngadharan, M. G., et al. (1990b). *In vitro* study of drug-sensitivity of HIV strains isolated from patients with AIDS or ARC before and after therapy with AZT and/or 2′,3′-dideoxycytidine., International Conference on AIDS, San Francisco, CA, p. 185, University of California, San Francisco.

Shirasaka, T., Yarchoan, R., O'Brien, M. C., Husson, R. N., Anderson, B. D., Kojima, E., et al. (1993). Changes in drug sensitivity of human immunodeficiency virus type I during therapy with azidothymidine, dideoxycytidine and dideoxyinosine. *Proceedings of the National Academy of Sciences of the United States of America*, **90**, 562–6.

Siddiqui, M., Driscoll, J., Kelley, J., Roth, J., Mitsuya, H., Shirasaka, T., et al. (1992). Chemistry and anti-HIV properties of 2′-fluoro-2′,3′-dideoxyarabino-furanosyl pyrimidines. *Journal of Medicinal Chemistry*, **35**, 2195–201.

Skalka, A. M. (1989). Retroviral proteases: first glimpse at the anatomy of a processing machine. *Cell*, **56**, 911–13.

Smith, J. K., Cywinski, A., and Taylor, J. M. (1984). Initiation of plus-strand DNA synthesis during reverse transcription of an avian retrovirus genome. *Journal of Virology*, **49**, 200–4.

Spanish Retroviral Trial Group (1991). Comparison of ribavirin and placebo in CDC group III human immunodeficiency virus infection. *Lancet*, **i**, 6–9.

Starnes, M. C. and Cheng, Y.-C. (1987). Cellular metabolism of 2′,3′-dideoxy-cytidine a compound active against human immunodeficiency virus *in vitro*. *Journal of Biological Chemistry*, **262**, 988–991.

Sundquist, B. and Oberg, B. (1979). Phosphonoformate inhibits reverse transcriptase. *Journal of General Virology*, **45**, 273–81.

Surbone, A., Yarchoan, R., McAtee, N., Blum, M. R., Maha, M., and Allain, J. P. (1988). Treatment of the acquired immunodeficiency syndrome (AIDS) and AIDS-related complex with a regimen of 3′-azido-2′,3′-dideoxythymidine (azidothymidine or zidovudine) and acyclovir. *Annals of Internal Medicine*, **108**, 534–40.

Szebeni, J., Wahl, S. M., Popovic, M., Wahl, L. M., Gartner, S., Fine, R. L., *et al.* (1989). Dipyridamole potentiates the inhibition of 3′-azido-3′-deoxythymidine and other dideoxynucleosides of human immunodeficiency virus replication in monocyte-macrophages. *Proceedings of the National Academy of Sciences of the United States of America*, **86**, 3842–6.

Tan, C.-K., Civil, R., Mian, A. M., So, A. G., and Downey, K. M. (1991). Inhibition of the RNase H activity of HIV reverse transcriptase by azidothymidylate. *Biochemistry*, **30**, 4831–43.

Taylor, J. M. (1977). An analysis of the role of tRNA species as primers for the transcription into DNA of RNA tumor virus genomes. *Biochimica et Biophysica Acta*, **473**. 57–71.

Taylor, J. (1979). DNA intermediates of ovian RNA tumour viruses. *Current Topics in Microbiology and Immunology,* **87**, 23–41.

Tekeuchi, Y., Nagumo, T., and Hoshino, H. (1988). Low fidelity of cell-free DNA synthesis by reverse transcriptase of human immunodeficiency virus genomes. *Journal of Virology*, **62**, 3900.

Temin, H. M. and Mizutani, S. (1970). RNA-dependent DNA polymerase in virions of Rous sarcoma virus. *Nature, London*, **226**, 1211–13.

Tisdale, M., Ertl, P., Larder. B. A., Purifoy. D. J., Darby, G., and Powell, K. L. (1988). Characterization of human immunodeficiency virus type 1 reverse transcriptase by using monoclonal antibodies: role of the C terminus in antibody reactivity and enzyme function. *Journal of Virology*, **62**, 3662–7.

Tsuchida, N. and Sakuma, S. (1985). Replication of retroviruses. *Metabolism*, **22**, 1357–68.

Vogt, M. W., Hartshorn, K. L., Furman, P. A., Chou, T.-C., Fyfe, J. A., Coleman, L. A., *et al.* (1987). Ribavirin antagonizes the effect of azidothymidine on HIV replication. *Science*, **235**, 1376–9.

Wilson, W., Braddock, M., Adams, S. E., Rajthen, P. D., Kingsman, S. M., and Kingsman, A. J. (1988). HIV expression strategies: ribosomal frameshifting is directed by a short sequence in both mammalian and yeast systems. *Cell*, **55**, 1159–69.

Wong-Staal, F. and Gallo, R. C. (1985). Human T-lymphotropic viruses. *Nature, London*, **317**, 395–7.

Yang, S., Herrera, F., Smith, R., Reitz, M., Lancini, G., Ting, R., and Gallo, R. (1972). Rifamycin antibiotics: inhibitors of Rauscher murine leukemia virus reverse transcriptase and of purified DNA polymerases from human normal and leukemic lymphoblasts. *Journal of the National Cancer Institute*, **49**, 7–25.

Yarchoan, R., Klecker, R. W., Weinhold, K. J., Markham P. D., Lyerly, H. K., Durack, D. T., *et al.* (1986). Administration of 3′-azido-3′deoxythymidine, an inhibitor of HTLV-III/LAV replication, to patients with AIDS or AIDS-related complex. *Lancet*, **i**, 575–80.

Yarchoan, R., Berg, G., Brouwers, P., Fischl, M. A., Spitzer, A. R., Wichman, A.

(1987). Response of human-immunodeficiency-virus-associated neurological disease to 3'-azido-3'-deoxythymidine. *Lancet*, **i**, 132–5.

Yarchoan, R., Perno, C. F., Thomas, R. V., Klecker, R. W., Allain, J.-P., McAtee, N., *et al*. (1988). Phase I studies of 2',3'-dideoxycytidine in severe human immunodeficiency virus infection as a single agent and alternating with zidovudine (AZT). *Lancet*, **i**, 76–81.

Yarchoan, R., Mitsuya, H., Myers, C. E., and Broder, S. (1989a). Antiretroviral therapy of HIV infection: clinical pharmacology of 3'-azido-2', 3'-dideoxythymidine (AZT) and related dideoxynucleosides. *New England Journal of Medicine*, **321**, 726–39.

Yarchoan, R., Mitsuya, H., Myers, C. E., and Broder, S. (1989b). Clinical pharmacology of 3'-azido-2',3'-dideoxythymidine (zidovudine) and related dideoxynucleosides. *New England Journal of Medicine*, **321**, 726–38.

Yarchoan, R., Mitsuya, H., Thomas, R. V., Pluda, J. M., Hartman, N. R., Perno, C.-F., *et al*. (1989c). *In vivo* activity against HIV and favorable toxicity profile of 2',3'-dideoxyinosine. *Science*, **245**, 412–15.

Yarchoan, R., Thomas, R., Pluda, J. M., Perno, C. F., Mitsuya, H., Marczyk, K. S., *et al*. (1989d). Phase I study of the administration of recombinant soluble CD4 (rCD4) by continuous infusion to patients with AIDS or ARC. 5th International Conference on AIDS, Montreal, p. 212. International Development Research Centre.

Yarchoan, R., Mitsuya, H., Pluda, J., Marczyl, K. S., Thomas, R. V., Hartman, N. R., *et al*. (1990a). The National Cancer Institute phase I study of ddI administration in adults with AIDS or AIDS-related complex: Analysis of activity and toxicity profiles. *Review of Infectious Diseases*, **12**, S522–33.

Yarchoan, R., Pluda, J. M., Thomas, R. V., Mitsuya, H., Brouwers, P., Wyvill, K. M., *et al*. (1990b). Long-term toxicity/activity profile of 2',3'-dideoxyinosine in AIDS or AIDS-related complex. *Lancet*, **ii**, 526–9.

Yarchoan, R., Venzon, D., Pluda, J. M., Lietzav, J., Wyvill, K. M., Tsiatis, A. A., *et al*. (1991). CD4 count and the risk for death in patients infected with HIV receiving antiretroviral therapy. *Annals of Internal Medicine*, **115**, 184–9.

Yoshinaka, Y. and Luftig, R. B. (1977). Properties of a P70 proteolytic factor of murine leukemia viruses. *Cell*, **12**, 709–19.

Ziegler, J. L., Beckstead, J., Volberding, P. A., Abrams, D. I., Levine, A. M., Lukes, R. J., *et al*. (1984). Non-Hodgkin's lymphoma in 90 homosexual men. Relation to generalized lymphadenopathy and the acquired immunodeficiency syndrome. *New England Journal of Medicine*, **311**, 565–70.

6D.1   Introduction

It has been recognized that viruses utilize the host cell machinery for many of the post-translational modifications which are needed to produce a fully functional viral protein. Much recent work has concentrated on the glycosylation events surrounding maturation of viral encoded glyco-proteins essential for the life-cycle of a virus. In addition, viruses may direct the synthesis of both glycosylated and non-glycosylated infected cell-specific proteins, some of which are later incorporated into the virion cell membrane. These membrane-bound proteins will have many different roles, such as mediating cell tropism and subsequent fusion.

Glycosylation has been shown to be important, with specific reference to HIV-1, in the following areas (see Ratner *et al.* 1991, and references cited therein). First, the glycans or the effect of glycosylation on protein structure have been shown to be important in the binding of the HIV-1 envelope to its receptor CD4. Second, the glycans themselves may be important for virus uptake after CD4 binding. Third, viral envelope formation, including folding, oligomerization, cleavage, and/or transport to the cell surface, are dependent on oligosaccharide addition and subsequent pro-cessing. In addition, glycosylation may be important in determining the interactions with antibody, particularly neutralizing antibody to peptide domains.

It could be argued that, since the virus is using host cell enzymes for carrying out these tasks, targeting drugs to inhibit the glycosylation pathway will also result in host-cell morbidity. While the presence of a therapeutic window could be envisaged, as a general strategy, drug design via inhi-bitors of the glycosylation processing pathway does appear flawed. One theoretical way around this dilemma would be to develop compounds

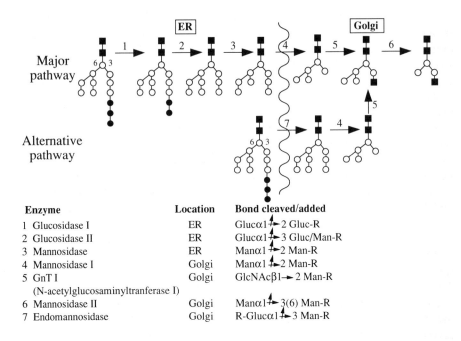

Enzyme	Location	Bond cleaved/added
1 Glucosidase I	ER	Glucα1→2 Gluc-R
2 Glucosidase II	ER	Glucα1→3 Gluc/Man-R
3 Mannosidase	ER	Manα1→2 Man-R
4 Mannosidase I	Golgi	Manα1→2 Man-R
5 GnT I (N-acetylglucosaminyltranferase I)	Golgi	GlcNAcβ1→2 Man-R
6 Mannosidase II	Golgi	Manα1→3(6) Man-R
7 Endomannosidase	Golgi	R-Glucα1→3 Man-R

Fig. 6D.1 Biosynthetic pathway for N-glycosylation of viral proteins: ■ *N*-acetyl-glucosamine; ○ mannose; ● glucose. For a detailed description of the enzymes involved in the main pathway, see Kornfeld and Kornfeld (1985) and references cited therein. For those involved in the alternative pathway see Lobas and Spiro (1987).

which are activated or active only in virally infected host cells. As a general strategy for antiviral drug design, this must await a further description of viral encoded enzymes. To date, no viral encoded glycosyltransferases or glycosidases have been reported, with the exception of neuraminidases which are ubiquitous.

The N-glycosylation of proteins is a cotranslational event (Kornfeld and Kornfeld 1985) (see Fig. 6D.1). All other glycosylations are post-translational, i.e. glycosylphosphatidylinositol (GPI) anchor addition, O-glycosylation. The enzyme oligosaccharyl transferase catalyses the *en bloc* addition of a glucosylated oligomannose glycan to asparagine residues from a lipid (dolichol-pyrophosphate) donor. This oligosaccharide is then remodelled in the endoplasmic reticulum and Golgi apparatus. The degree of processing and remodelling is tailored for each glycoprotein, and it is thought that the peptide sequence, as well as the secondary and tertiary structures, determines the final oligosaccharide structure at each glycosylation site (Rademacher *et al.* 1988). Glycoprotein can have from one to over 20 sites glycosylated. In addition, each site will not contain a single structure but will be heterogeneous. Therefore glycoproteins are not single unique structures but a single peptide chain diversified into hundreds of structures differing in oligosaccharide structure. A set of glycoforms constitutes a glycoprotein. The processing of an oligosaccharide can stop at any step of the pathway. In general, cell surface and circulating glycoproteins contain oligosaccharides which are processed such that the terminal residues of the oligosaccharide are sialic acid. If the processing of an oligosaccharide is inhibited (e.g. glucosidase I by 1-deoxynojirimycin (DNJ)), then a glycoprotein containing a glucosylated oligomannose structure will be synthesized. Consequently this glycoprotein (a) may not be secreted from the cell, (b) may be secreted but not bioactive, or (c) may be secreted and bioactive but with its half-life reduced due to clearance by circulating or cell-surface-associated mannose-specific carbohydrate-binding protein (e.g. lectins).

The therapeutic targets would be vast, if it were not for the caveat that the host also requires the same biosynthetic machinery for its own survival. To date, little is known concerning the actual carbohydrate structures present on viral cell surfaces taken from patients. However, all indications are that the oligosaccharides present are representative of the 'current' glycosylation capacity of the cell, and that no 'embryonic' (silent linkages) are present to give a 'viral-specific' handle. (For HIV gp120 carbohydrate structures from a variety of cell lines, see Abel et al. (1987), Geyer et al. (1988), Mizouchi et al. (1988) and Hansen et al. (1989)).

In addition to the vast targets glycosylation affords, various synthetic strategies for sugar derivatives, such as amino sugars, have been developed (see Fleet et al. (1988), and references cited therein) and hundreds of modifications of monosaccharides and oligosaccharides can be produced. Most inhibitors have been directed at the exoglycosidases, and some recent work has been focused on inhibitors of the glycosyltransferases.

6D.2 Amino sugar derivatives

Polyhydroxylated indolizidines, piperidines, pyrrolidines, and pyrrolizidines (see Winchester and Fleet (1992) for a review of the chemical structures of these compounds) extracted from plants and micro-organisms have been found to have a number of biological activities which, in many cases, can probably be ascribed to their acting as glycosidase inhibitors. Many of these alkaloids can be considered as analogues of monosaccharides in which the ring oxygen is replaced by nitrogen as shown in Fig. 6D.2. It has been found that some of these alkaloids inhibit α-glucosidase I and II, enzymes present in the endoplasmic reticulum and used in the trimming phase of oligosaccharide biosynthesis of N-linked glycosylated proteins (see Fig. 6D.1 and Table 6D.1).

Table 6D.1 Compounds with anti-HIV activity

Compound	Target	Reference
Compounds believed to act via inhibition of enzymes involved in glycosylation		
Castanospermine	Glucosidase I	Merkle *et al.* 1985; Lifson *et al.* 1986; Grukers *et al.* 1987; Tyms *et al.* 1987; Walker *et al.* 1987; Fleet *et al.* 1988; Karpas *et al.* 1988; Montefiori *et al.* 1988, 1989; Müller *et al.* 1988; Johnson *et al.* 1989
Swainsonine	Mannosidase II	Merkle *et al.* 1985; Robinson *et al.* 1987; Fleet *et al.* 1988; Montefiori *et al.* 1988, 1989; Pal *et al.* 1989a
1-deoxynojirimycin (DNJ)	Glucosidase I	Gruters *et al.* 1987; Fennie *et al.* 1989; Fleet *et al.* 1989; Karpas *et al.* 1989; Montefiori *et al.* 1988, 1989; Müller *et al.* 1988; Pal *et al.* 1989a,b; Fenouillet *et al.* 1991
N-methyldeoxynojirimycin (MeDNJ)	Glucosidase I	Fleet *et al.* 1988; Karpas *et al.* 1988
N-ethyldeoxynojirimycin (EtDNJ)	Glucosidase I	Fleet *et al.* 1988; Karpas *et al.* 1988
N-butyldeoxynojirimycin (BuDNJ)	Glucosidase I and II	Fleet *et al.* 1988; Karpas *et al.* 1988; Dedera *et al.* 1990; Ratner *et al.* 1991
1,4 dideoxy-1, 4-imino-L-arbinitol (LAB)	Glucosidase (I and II)?	Fleet *et al.* 1988; Karpas *et al.* 1988
N-(5-carboxymethyl-1-pentyl) 1,5-imino-L-fucitol (LFT)	Fucosidase	Fleet *et al.* 1988; Karpas *et al.* 1988
Bryostatin I	CD4 glycosylation	Boto *et al.* 1991
Bromoconduritol	Glucosidase II	Montefiori *et al.* 1988, 1989
Deoxymannojirimycin	Mannosidase I	Fleet *et al.* 1988; Montefiori *et al.* 1988, 1989; Fennie *et al.* 1989; Pal *et al.* 1989a; Offner *et al.* 1990

Table 6D.1 (*continued*)

Compound	Target	Reference
Compounds believed to act via inhibition of enzymes involved in glycosylation (*continued*)		
2,6-Dideoxy-2,6-imino-7-*O*-D-(β-D-glucopyranosyl)-D-glycero-L-gulohepitol (MDL)	Glucosidase II	Kaushal *et al.* 1988
Compounds believed to act by blocking carbohydrate-mediated adhesion of intact virus to host cell		
Sodium pentosan polysulphate	gp120	Baba *et al.* 1988; Anand *et al.* 1990
Anti-carbohydrate monoclonal antibodies	gp120	Hansen *et al.* 1990
Gerardia savaglia lectin (D-mannose specific)	gp120	Müller *et al.* 1988
Conconavalin A	gp120	Lifson *et al.* 1986; Hansen *et al.* 1989
Sulphated gangliosides	gp120	Handa *et al.* 1991
Conglutinin (C-type lectin, *N*-acetyl-D-glucosamine specific)	gp120	Anderson *et al.* 1991
Mannose binding protein (C-type lectin)	gp120	Ezekowitz *et al.* 1989
Compounds affecting glycosylation but mechanism unknown		
Chloroquine	Terminal glycosylation in trans-Golgi apparatus	Tsai *et al.* 1990
Monensin	Endoproteolytic cleavage gp160, glycosylation	Dewar *et al.* 1989
2-deoxy-D-glucose	Glycosylation	Blough *et al.* 1986
β-hydroxynorvaline	Glycosylation	Blough *et al.* 1986

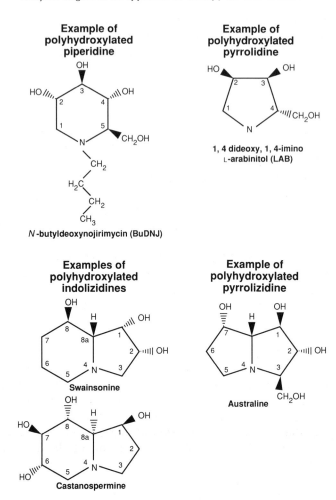

Fig. 6D.2 Examples of amino sugar glycosidase inhibitors. The polyhydroxylated piperidines and the polyhydroxylated pyrrolidines are analogues of pyranose sugars and furanose sugars respectively. The polyhydroxylated indolizidines are a fused piperidine and pyrrolidine and the pyrrolizidines are two fused pyrrolidines (Winchester and Fleet 1992). The carbohydrate ring numbering systems for pyranose and furanose sugars are used for the piperidine and pyrrolidine rings respectively.

Work by three groups of workers (Gruters *et al.* 1987; Tyms *et al.* 1987; Walker *et al.* 1987) have demonstrated that members of this class of compound, in particular castanospermine and DNJ, exhibited anti-HIV activity (see Fig. 6D.2 for structures). The most comprehensive survey of both synthetic and naturally occurring plant alkaloids and anti-HIV activity was performed by Fleet *et al.* (1988). In that study, 47 different compounds, many novel, were synthesized or isolated from natural sources and screened for both anti-HIV activity and host cell cytotoxicity.

6D.3   Anti-HIV activity versus cell cytotoxicity

Table 6D.1 lists the compounds which have been shown to have anti-HIV activity. In the vast majority of cases, these are not viral-specific effects. Many of the 'hit' compounds screened in these studies were eventually shown to have antiviral activity by virtue of cell morbidity. The comprehensive study by Fleet *et al.* (1988) supports the view that inhibition of the sugar processing pathway leads to cell morbidity and that, in general, the antiviral effects are secondary to this toxicity. In a subsequent study, the compounds LAB, LFT and BuDNJ (see Table 6D.1 and Fig. 6D.2 for structures) were found to have antiviral activity at non-cytotoxic concentrations (Karpas *et al.* 1988). In addition, in long-term growth of infected T-45 cells in the presence of BuDNJ the proportion of infected cells gradually decreased, leading to eventual elimination of HIV from culture. While these compounds could be shown to inhibit glycosidases *in vitro*, no evidence has yet been put forward that their *in vitro* antiviral activity relates to inhibition of the processing of glycoproteins. A recent study by Platt *et al.* (1992) suggests that the compound BuDNJ inhibits the up-expression of the cell surface transferrin receptor (TfR) while not affecting its constitutive expression. The up-expression of the TfR has previously been linked to tumour transformation. In the study, the effect of BuDNJ on the expression of the cell-surface TfR appears selective. For example, no change in the cell surface expression of CD3, CD4, or CD5 was found. The mechanism of reduced membrane expression of the TfR in response to BuDNJ was shown not to be caused at the level of receptor transcription, translation, or recycling.

The importance of the above studies lies not so much in the proposed mechanism of action of *N*-BuDNJ, but as a reminder that carbohydrate-mediated events are ubiquitous in cells. For example, it is now recognized that many proteins are anchored to the membrane with GPI membrane anchors (see Thomas *et al.* 1990, and references cited therein). The biosynthesis of these anchors involves exoglycosidases, endoglycosidases, and glycosyltransferases (Urakaze *et al.* 1991, and references cited therein). Furthermore, large numbers of cytoplasmic and nuclear lectins of the S-type family have been described over the last few years. While their precise biological roles are not completely defined, the results from some studies are intriguing. For example, the L-35 or MAC-2 lectin has recently been shown to be part of the RNA splicing complex, and the human placental 14 kDa β-galactosidase binding lectin can suppress experimental auto-immune encephalomyelitis (Offner *et al.* 1990). It has been proposed that a family of intracellular glycosyl-phosphatidylinositols are present in the cell and act as second messengers. Insulin, (Romero *et al.* 1988) nerve growth factor, (Chan *et al.* 1989), and interleukin-2 (IL-2) (Eardley and Koshland 1991) are now believed to utilize such second messengers. Their structures are under intense investigation, and the composition of these putative messengers includes galactose, mannose, and glucosamine, the same residues as found on glycosylated proteins.

6D.4 *In vivo* activity, side effects and contraindications

Few data exist in the public domain concerning the *in vivo* HIV activity of these compounds or their side-effects. However it is known that glycosidase inhibitors will affect the activity of both intestinal glycosidases and the resident bacterial flora. Flatulence and diarrhoea have been reported to be common side-effects of these drugs (see Jacob *et al.* 1993, and references cited therein; Winchester and Fleet 1992, and references cited therein). Various strategies can be used to overcome these intestinal problems. The most obvious is oral administration of inactive derivatives, which are metabolized to an active compound after absorption into the blood stream. Common derivatizations include esterification or phosphorylation. For example, *N*-BuDNJ-6-phosphate is only a weak inhibitor of the intestinal disaccharidases (sucrase and maltase), in contrast with the non-phosphorylated parent compound (Scudder *et al.* 1992). After absorption, serum phosphatases are able to convert the phosphorylated compound to an active compound. Some amino sugar derivatives are currently undergoing clinical trial and it will be of interest to see whether their *in vivo* efficacy correlates with the *in vitro* studies.

Acknowledgements

The Glycobiology Institute is supported by Monsanto. The author wishes to thank Daryl Fernandes for help with the literature search and Raymond Dwek for his support. T. W. R.'s present address is Department of Molecular Pathology, University College London Medical School, London W1P 6DB.

References

Abel, C. A., Noble, E. L., Raymond, W. W., Mielke, C. H., and Klock, J. C. (1987). The envelope glycoproteins of the human immunodeficiency virus contain different types of oligosaccharides. *Federation Proceedings. Federation of American Societies for Experimental Biology*, **46**, 1318.

Anand, R., Nayyar, S., Galvin, T. A., Merril, C. R., and Bigelow, L. B. (1990). Sodium pentosan polysulfate (PPS), and anti-HIV agent, a also exhibits synergism with AZT, lymphoproliferative activity, and virus enhancement. *AIDS Research and Human Retroviruses*, **6**, 679–89.

Andersen, O., Sorenson, A. M., Svehag, S. E., and Fenouillet, E. (1991). Con-glutinin binds the HIV-1 envelope glycoprotein gp 160 and inhibits its inter-action with cell membrane CD4. *Scandinavian Journal of Immunology*, **33**, 81–8.

Baba, M., Nakajima, M., Schols, D., Pauwels, R., Balzarini, J., and De Clercq, E. (1988). Pentosan polysulfate, a sulfated oligosaccharide, is a potent and selective-anti-HIV agent *in vitro*. *Antiviral Research* **9**, 335–43.

Blough, H. A., Pauwels, R., De Clercq, E., Cogniaux, J., Sprecher-Goldberger, S., and Thiry, L. (1986). Glycosylation inhibitors block the expression of LAV/ HTLV-III (HIV) glycoproteins. *Biochemical and Biophysical Research Communi-cations*, **141**, 33–8.

Boto, W. M., Brown. L., Chrest, J., and Adler, W. H. (1991). Distinct modulatory effects of bryostatin 1 and staurosporine on the biosynthesis and expression of the HIV receptor protein (CD4) by T cells. *Cell Regulation*, **2**, 95–103.

Chan, B. L., Chao, M. V., and Saltiel, A. R. (1989). Nerve growth factor sti-mulates the hydrolysis of glycosyl-phosphatidylinositol in PC12 cells: a mechanism of protein kinase C regulation. *Proceedings of the National Academy of Sciences of the United States of America*, **86**, 1756–60.

Dedera, D., Vander Heyden, N., and Ratner, L. (1990). Attenuation of HIV-1 infectivity by an inhibitor of oligosaccharide processing. *AIDS Research and Human Retroviruses*, **6**, 785–94.

Dewar, R. L., Vasudevachari, M. B., Natarajan, V., and Salzman, N. P. (1989). The biosynthesis and processing of human immunodeficiency virus type 1 envelope glycoproteins: effects of monensin on glycosylation and transport. *Journal of Virology*, **63**, 2452–6.

Eardley, D. D., and Koshland, M. E. (1991), Glycosylphosphatidylinositol: a candidate system for interleukin-2 signal transduction. *Science*, **251**, 78–81.

Ezekowitz, A., Kuhlmann, M., Groopman, J. E., and Bryn, R. A. (1989). A human serum mannose-binding protein inhibits *in vitro* infection by the human immuno-deficiency virus. *Journal of Experimental Medicine*, **169**, 185–96.

Fennie, C. and Lasky, L. A. (1989). Model for intracellular folding of the human immunodefiency virus type 1 gp120. *Journal of Virology*, **63**, 639–46.

Fenouillet, E. and Gluckman, J. C. (1991). Effect of a glucosidase inhibitor on the bioactivity and immunoreactivity of human immunodeficiency virus type 1 envelope glycoprotein. *Journal of General Virology*, **72**, 1919–26.

Fleet, G. W. J., Kalpas, A., Dwek, R. A., Fellows, L. E., Tyms, A. S., Petursson, S., *et al.* (1988). Inhibition of HIV replication by amino-sugar derivatives. *Federation of European Biochemical Societies Letters*, **237**, 128–32.

Geyer, H., Holschbach, C., Hunsmann, G., and Schneider, J. (1988). Carbohydrates of human immunodeficiency virus: structure of oligosaccharides linked to the envelope glycoprotein 120. *Journal of Biological Chemistry*, **11**, 760–7.

Gruters, R. A., Neefjes, J. J., Tersmette, M., de Goede, R. E. Y., Tulp, A., Huisman, H. G., *et al.* (1987). Interference with HIV-induced syncytium formation and viral infectivity by inhibitors of trimming glucosidase. *Nature, London*, **330**, 74–7.

Handa, A., Hoshino, H., Nakajima, K., Adachi, M., Ikeda, K., Achiwa, K., *et al.* (1991). Inhibition of infection with human immunodeficiency virus type 1 by sulfated gangliosides. *Biochemical and Biophysical Research Communications*, **175**, 1–9.

Hansen, J. E. S., Nielsen, C. M., Nielsen, C., Heegaard, P., Mathiesen. L. R., and Nielsen, J. O. (1989). Correlation between carbohydrate structures on the envelope glycoprotein gp120 of HIV-1 and HIV-2 and syncytium inhibition with lectins. *AIDS*, **3**, 635–41.

Hansen J. E. S., Clausen, H., Nielson, C., Tegbjaerg, L. S., Hansen, L. L., Nielson, C. M., *et al.* (1990). Inhibition of human immunodeficiency virus (HIV) infection *in vitro* by anticarbohydrate monoclonal antibodies: peripheral glycosylation of HIV envelope glycoprotein gp120 may be a target for virus neutralization. *Journal of Virology*, **64**, 2833–40.

Jacob, G. S., Scudder, P., Butters, T. D., Jones, I., and Tiemeier, D. C. (1993). Aminosugar attenuation of HIV infection. In *Natural products as antiviral agents* (ed. C. K. Chu and H. G. Cutler). Plenum Press, New York.

Johnson, V. A., Walker, B. D., Barlow, M. A., Paradis, T. J., Chou, T. C., and Hirsch, M. S. (989). Synergistic inhibition of human immunodeficiency virus type 1 and type 2 replication *in vitro* by castanospermine and 3′-azido-3′ deoxythymidine. *Antimicrobial Agents and Chemotherapy*, **33**, 53–7.

Karpas, A., Fleet, G. W., Dwek, R. A., Petursson, S., Namgoong, S. K., Ramsden, N. G., *et al.* (1988). Aminosugar derivatives as potential anti-human immunodeficiency virus agents. *Proceedings of the National Academy of Sciences of the United States of America*, **85**, 9229–33.

Kaushal, G. P., Pan, Y. T., Tropea, J. E., Mitchell, M., Liu, P., and Elbein, A. D. (1988). Selective inhibition of glycoprotein-processing enzymes. Differential inhibition of glucosidases I and II in cell culture. *Journal of Biological Chemistry*, **263**, 17278–83.

Kornfeld, R. and Kornfeld, S. (1985). Assembly of asparagine-linked oligosaccharides. *Annual Review of Biochemistry*, **54**, 631–64.

Lifson, J., Coutre, S., Huang, E., and Engleman, E. (1986). Role of envelope glycoprotein carbohydrate in human immunodeficiency virus (HIV) infectivity and virus-induced cell fusion. *Journal of Experimental Medicine*, **164**, 2101–6.

Lobas, W. A., Spiro, R. G. (1987). Golgi endo-alpha D-mannosidase from rat liver, a novel N-linked carbohydrate unit processing enzyme. *Journal of Biological Chemistry*, **263**, 3990–8.

Merkle, R. K., Elbein, A. D., and Heifetz, A. (1985). The effect of swainsonine and castanospermine on the sulfation of the oligosaccharide chains of N-linked glycoproteins. *Journal of Biological Chemistry*, **260**, 1083–9.

Mizouchi, T., Spellman, M. W., Larkin, M., Solomon, J., Basa, L., and Feizi, T. (1988). Carbohydrate structures of the human immunodeficiency-virus (HIV) recombinant envelope glycoprotein gp120 produced in Chinese-hamster ovary cells. *Biochemical Journal*, **254**, 599–603.

Montefiori, D. C., Robinson, W. E., Jr, and Mitchell, W. M. (1988). Role of protein N-glycosylation in pathogenesis of human immunodeficiency virus type 1. *Proceedings of the National Academy of Sciences of the United States of America*, **85**, 9248–52.

Montefiori, D. C., Robinson, W. E., Jr, and Mitchell, W. M. (1989). Antibody-independent, complement-mediated enhancement of HIV-1 infection by mannosidase I and II inhibitors. *Antiviral Research*, **11**, 137–46.

Müller, W. E., Renneisen, K., Kreuter, M. H., Schroder, H. C., and Winkler, I. (1988). The D-mannose-specific lectin from *Gerardia savaglia* blocks binding of human immunodeficiency virus type I to H9 cells and human lymphocytes *in vitro*. *Journal of Acquired Immune Deficiency Syndromes*, **1**, 453–8.

Offner, H., Celnik, B., Bringman, T. S., Casentini-Borocz, D. M., Nedwin, G. E., and Vandenbark, A. A. (1990). Recombinant human β-galactoside binding lectin suppresses clinical and histological signs of experimental autoimmune encephalomyelitis. *Journal of Neuroimmunology*, **28**, 177–84.

Pal, R., Hoke, G. M., and Sarngadharan, M. G. (1989a). Role of oligosaccharides in the processing and maturation of envelope glycoproteins of human immunodeficiency virus type 1. *Proceedings of the National Academy of Sciences of the United States of America*, **86**, 3384–8.

Pal, R., Kalyanaraman, V. S., Hoke, G. M., and Sarngadharan, M. G. (1989b). Processing and secretion of envelope glycoproteins of human immunodeficiency virus type 1 in the presence of trimming glucosidase inhibitor deoxynojirimycin. *Intervirology*, **30**, 27–35.

Platt, F. M., Karlsson, G. B., and Jacob, G. S. (1992). Modulation of cell-surface transferrin receptor by the imino sugar *N*-butyldeoxynojirimycin. *European Journal of Biochemistry*, **208**, 187–93.

Radenmacher, T. W., Parekh, R. B., and Dwek, R. A. (1988). Glycobiology. *Annual Review of Biochemistry*, **57**, 785–838.

Ratner, L., Heyden N. C., and Dedera, D. (1991). Inhibition of HIV and SIV infectivity by blockade of α-glucosidase activity. *Virology*, **181**, 180–92.

Robinson, W. E., Jr, Montefiori, D. C., and Mitchell, W. M. (1987). Evidence that mannosyl residues are involved in human immunodeficiency virus type 1 (HIV-1) pathogenesis. *AIDS Research and Human Retroviruses*, **3**, 265–82.

Romero, G., Lutrell, A., Rogol, A., Zeller, K., Hewlett, E., and Larner, J. (1988). Phosphatidylinositol-glycan anchors of membrane proteins: potential precursors of insulin mediators. *Science*, **240**, 509–11.

Scudder, P. R., Dwek, R. A., Rademacher, T. W., and Jacob, G. S. (1992). Compound, *N*-butyl-deoxynojirimycin-6-phosphate. United States Patent 5,103,008.

Thomas, J. R., Dwek, R. A., and Rademacher, T. W. (1990). Structure, biosynthesis, and function of glycosylphosphatidylinositols. *Biochemistry*, **29**, 5413–22.

Tsai, W. P., Nara, P. L., Kung, H. F., and Oroszlan, S. (1990). Inhibition of human immunodeficiency virus infectivity by chloroquine. (1990). *AIDS Research and Human Retroviruses*, **6**, 481–9.

Tyms, A. S., Berrie, E. M., Ryder, T. A., Nash, R. J., Hegarty, M. P., Taylor, T. L., *et al.* (1987). Castanospermine and other plant alkaloid inhibitors of glucosidase activity block the growth of HIV. *Lancet*, **i**, 1025.

Urakaze, M., Kamitani, T., DeGasperi, R., Sugiyama, E., Chang, H. M., Warren, C., and Yeh, E. T. H. (1991). Identification of a missing link in glycosylphosphatidylinositol anchor biosynthesis in mammalian cells. *Journal of Biological Chemistry*, **267**, 6459–62.

Walker, B. D., Kowalski, M., Goh, W. C., Kozarsky, K., Krieger, M., Rosen, C., *et al.* (1987). Inhibition of human immunodeficiency virus syncytium formation and virus replication by castanospermine. *Proceedings of the National Academy of Sciences of the United States of America*, **84**, 8120–4.

Winchester, B. and Fleet, G. W. J. (1992). Amino-sugar glycosidase inhibitors: versatile tools for glycobiologists. *Glycobiology*, **2**, 199–210.

Inhibitors of viral DNA polymerase

Scott A. Foster and Yung-chi Cheng

7.1 Introduction

Viral DNA polymerase offers an attractive target for the development of anti-viral agents. Many DNA viruses encode a DNA polymerase. Examples include adenoviruses (AdV) (Challberg and Kelly 1989), poxviruses such as vaccinia virus (Moss 1986), and herpes viruses such as herpes simplex virus types 1 and 2 (HSV-1 and HSV-2), human cytomegalovirus (CMV), varicella-zoster virus (VZV), and Epstein−Barr virus (EBV) (Roizman, and Batterson 1986). The DNA polymerase of these viruses is a key enzyme for their replication. Further, the viral DNA polymerases often differ enough from the host DNA polymerases to allow some degree of selective inhibition of the viral enzyme over the host DNA polymerases. In addition to the inherent differences between the viral and host DNA polymerases, specificity in inhibiting the viral DNA polymerase over the host enzymes can be achieved through the exploitation of other biochemical differences between infected and uninfected cells. Such differences could include membrane changes associated with the viral infection that allow anti-viral agents to penetrate infected cells more easily or metabolic changes that allow the selective activation of pro-drugs in infected cells. In this chapter, we focus on the herpes simplex virus (HSV) DNA polymerase (EC 3.1.11), although the strategies for inhibiting the enzyme should apply to other viral DNA polymerases as well.

7.2   Role of HSV DNA polymerase in viral replication

Infection of cells with HSV was first shown to induce DNA polymerase activity by Keir and Gold (1963). This DNA polymerase activity was subsequently shown to be distinct from that of host DNA polymerases in several respects, including a requirement for high concentrations of salt for maximal activity and high sensitivity to inhibition by phosphonoacetic acid (Keir *et al.* 1966; Weissbach *et al.* 1973; Ostrander and Cheng 1980). Further studies resulted in the purification of the enzyme and its genetic mapping on the HSV genome (Schaffer *et al.* 1973; Jofre *et al.* 1977; Powell and Purifoy 1977; Purifoy *et al.* 1977). Physical mapping followed, and later the HSV DNA polymerase gene was fully sequenced (Chartrand *et al.* 1979; Parris *et al.* 1980; Coen *et al.* 1984; Gibbs *et al.* 1985; Quinn and McGeoch 1985).

The HSV DNA polymerase is essential for viral replication, as demonstrated by studies of temperature-sensitive and drug-resistant mutants. Mutants with temperature-sensitive lesions in the DNA polymerase gene are defective for viral replication and fail to synthesize viral DNA at the non-permissive temperature (Schaffer *et al.* 1973; Purifoy *et al.* 1977). Mutants selected for resistance to various compounds that inhibit HSV DNA replication have been shown to induce altered DNA polymerases that are resistant to inhibition by the active metabolite of the compound that they were selected against (Derse *et al.* 1982; Larder and Darby 1985). Thus HSV DNA polymerase is a critical enzyme for viral replication. Any compound that can selectively interfere with the function of HSV DNA polymerase could be considered as a potential anti-HSV agent.

7.3   HSV DNA polymerase

HSV-1 DNA polymerase is encoded by the HSV-1 gene designated UL30 by McGeoch and other workers (Gibbs *et al.* 1985; McGeoch *et al.* 1988). The polymerase is a polypeptide with a molecular weight of approximately 136 kDa, as estimated from the predicted amino acid sequence (Gibbs *et al.* 1985; McGeoch *et al.* 1988). This value is in reasonable agreement with estimates from SDS-PAGE (Powell and Purifoy 1977; Derse *et al.* 1982; Weisshart and Knopf 1988).

The HSV DNA polymerase has several intrinsic activities, including a DNA polymerase activity, a 3',5'-exonuclease activity, and 5',3'-exonuclease activity which also acts as an RNase H activity (Crute and Lehman 1989). The 3',5'-exonuclease is believed to act as a proof-reading function, while the 5´,3´-exonuclease–ribonuclease (RNase H) activity may remove the RNA primers generated during replication of the lagging strand of DNA (Crute and Lehman 1989).

Associated with the 136 kDa polypeptide is a double-stranded DNA-binding protein encoded by the HSV-1 UL42 gene (Gottlieb *et al.* 1990). A similar association occurs between the polymerase of HSV-2 and an HSV DNA-binding protein (Vaughan *et al.* 1985). In HSV-1, the UL42 DNA-binding protein increases the processivity of the polymerization reaction *in vitro* (Gottlieb *et al.* 1990).

The primary amino acid sequence of HSV-1 DNA polymerase as determined from the DNA sequence, has been compared with other DNA viruses and the human DNA polymerase *a*. Six conserved regions, designated I–VI (Fig. 7.1), were shared among the DNA polymerases from HSV, EBV, vaccinia virus, CMV, AdV, and human DNA polymerase *a* (Gibbs *et al.* 1988; Wong *et al.* 1988). In addition, another conserved region, designated A, was reported among HSV, EBV, and vaccinia virus DNA polymerases (Gibbs *et al.* 1988). Mutations that confer altered sensitivity to various HSV DNA polymerase inhibitors are clustered within several of these conserved regions. For example, regions II and III are proposed to interact directly with substrates and drugs, since a cluster of mutations conferring alterations in drug sensitivity occurs in each of them (Gibbs *et al.* 1988). In addition, regions II and III share a high degree of sequence similarity among viral and human DNA polymerase *a*. Several mutations affecting sensitivity to HSV DNA polymerase inhibitors were found in region A (Gibbs *et al.* 1988). This region shares sequence similarity with some viral DNA polymerases, but not with human DNA polymerase *a*. It has been proposed that this region interacts with certain drugs, such as

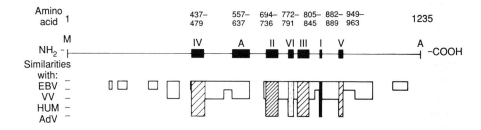

Fig. 7.1 Amino acid sequence similarity between HSV DNA polymerase and other DNA polymerases. Shown at the top is the HSV-1 (KOS) DNA polymerase with solid boxes indicating conserved regions. Below, regions of sequence similarity are shown by boxes with the degree of similarity indicated by the degree of shading. EBV, Epstein–Barr virus; VV, vaccinia virus; HUM, human polymerase *a*; AdV, adenovirus. (Modified from Gibbs *et al.* 1988.)

phosphonoacetic acid (PAA), acyclovir (ACG) triphosphate, and ganciclovir (DHPG) triphosphate in a way that permits selective inhibition of the viral DNA polymerase over DNA polymerase a (Gibbs *et al.* 1988). Other regions, such as I, IV, and VI, did not contain mutations conferring altered drug sensitivity but had a high degree of sequence similarity among viral and human DNA polymerase (Gibbs *et al.* 1988). Thus these may represent regions that do not interact directly with the drugs but still contribute to the formation of a substrate binding site. A more complete understanding of the interactions between the HSV DNA polymerase, its substrates, and its inhibitors will be useful in the design of more selective inhibitors.

7.4   Inhibitors of HSV DNA polymerase

7.4.1   Selectivity in inhibiting HSV DNA polymerase

It is not difficult to inhibit DNA polymerases in practice; a wide array of inhibitors already exist, including nucleotide derivatives, pyrophosphate analogues, and other structures. In terms of therapeutics, the problem is selectivity. Since both HSV and human cells rely on DNA polymerases to replicate their genetic material, any compound that interferes with HSV DNA polymerase is at risk for inhibiting the DNA replication of uninfected host cells. Inhibition of host cell DNA synthesis is often manifested as bone marrow suppression, and the potential mutagenic effects of disturbing host cell DNA synthesis cannot be dismissed. Thus selectivity in the inhibition of HSV DNA polymerase is of critical importance.

There are several approaches to inhibiting the HSV DNA polymerase in a selective manner. The simplest approach is to use HSV DNA polymerase inhibitors or alternative substrates that do not inhibit or serve as alternative substrates for cellular DNA polymerases at the concentrations used. Several important antiviral agents have this as one mechanism for selectively inhibiting viral replication.

Another approach to achieving selective inhibition of the HSV DNA polymerase is to take advantage of the biochemical differences between HSV-infected cells and uninfected cells. For example, HSV encodes a viral thymidine kinase gene that has a different substrate specificity to that of corresponding host nucleoside kinases (Cheng 1976; Lee and Cheng 1976). Thus HSV-infected cells can phosphorylate certain nucleoside analogues to their monophosphate forms, whereas uninfected cells cannot. Once at the monophosphate level, host nucleoside mono- and diphosphate kinases further phosphorylate the compound to the triphosphate form, which is a substrate of the viral DNA polymerase. The antiviral nucleoside analogue acyclovir owes a large part of its selectivity against HSV to its ability to be phosphorylated by the HSV thymidine kinase. Although HSV thymidine kinase has been very important in the development of selective antiviral agents, the use of other biochemical differences between infected and uninfected cells can be entertained.

A third approach is to utilize differences in plasma membrane permeability of infected cell to allow for greater uptake of antiviral agents in infected cells. It is well known that infection of cells with various viruses causes changes in the plasma membrane. Thus it has been proposed that antiviral agents might be developed to take advantage of the increased membrane leakiness of virally infected cells (Carrasco 1978). For example, it has been shown that hygromycin B, a translation inhibitor that is impermeable to uninfected cells, selectively inhibits protein synthesis in HSV-infected cell (Lacal and Carrasco 1983). In addition to the increased membrane permeability of virally infected cells, some antiviral compounds appear to bind to virions and to be internalized with them. For example, heparin, which has anti-HSV activity in cell culture, appears to bind to the HSV virions and be internalized with the viral particles (Gonzalez and Carrasco 1987). A similar interaction occurs between HSV-2 and the phosphorothioate oligonucleotide S-(dC)28, an inhibitor of HSV-2 DNA polymerase (Gao *et al*. 1990b). Thus increased cellular uptake of compounds as a result of interaction with the virions or alterations in the plasma membrane during or subsequent to the viral infection can be used as a mechanism to increase the selectivity of antiviral agents, including viral DNA polymerase inhibitors.

7.4.2   Approaches to inhibiting HSV DNA polymerase

A mechanism for the DNA polymerization reaction has been proposed (Leinbach *et al*. 1976; Cheng *et al*. 1979). The basic reaction is believed to occur by a modified ordered bi-bi mechanism, as shown in Fig. 7.2. Initially, the enzyme binds to the DNA template-primer. Following this, binding of the appropriate deoxyribonucleoside triphosphates (dNTP) occurs.

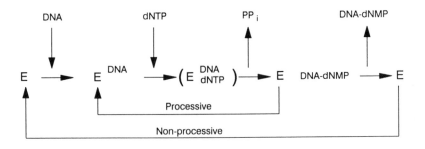

Fig. 7.2 General reaction scheme for DNA polymerase. (Redrawn from Cheng *et al*. 1979.)

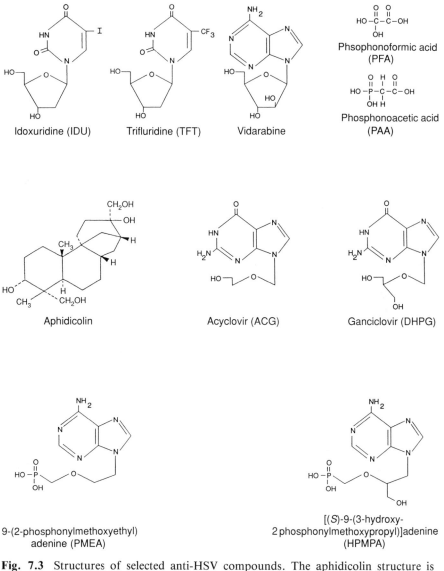

Idoxuridine (IDU)   Trifluridine (TFT)   Vidarabine

Phsophonoformic acid (PFA)

Phosphonoacetic acid (PAA)

Aphidicolin   Acyclovir (ACG)   Ganciclovir (DHPG)

9-(2-phosphonylmethoxyethyl) adenine (PMEA)

[(S)-9-(3-hydroxy-2 phosphonylmethoxypropyl)]adenine (HPMPA)

Fig. 7.3 Structures of selected anti-HSV compounds. The aphidicolin structure is modified from Spadari *et al.* (1982).

The enzyme then catalyses the hydrolysis of the dNTP and addition of the resulting nucleotide monophosphate to the growing DNA chain with the release of pyrophosphate.

This mechanism suggests several possible ways of inhibiting the enzyme. Some of the strategies for inhibiting the HSV DNA polymerase and some of the compounds that inhibit these aspects of the DNA polymerase function are discussed below. The structures of the various compounds are shown in Fig. 7.3.

7.4.3   Nucleoside analogues and compounds that compete with dNTPs

The most fruitful approach to inhibiting the HSV DNA polymerase so far has been to use compounds that interfere with utilization of the natural dNTP by the polymerase. Most of the compounds in this class are nucleoside analogues that require activation inside the cell by phosphorylation to their triphosphate forms, although some non-nucleoside inhibitors of this type exist. In addition to simple inhibition of the enzyme, at least some of the nucleoside analogue triphosphates can be incorporated into the viral DNA where they can have additional inhibitory and/or mutational effects.

7.4.3.1   *Idoxuridine and trifluridine*

Idoxuridine (5-iodo-2′-deoxyuridine, IDU) was reported as the first useful anti-HSV compound in 1962 (Kaufman *et al*. 1962). Trifluridine (trifluoro-thymidine, TFT) was originally synthesized as an anti-cancer agent but was shown to have activity against HSV (Kaufman and Heidelberger 1964). Both IDU and TFT are phosphorylated to the monophosphate form by HSV thymidine kinase, as well as by host nucleoside kinases (Heidelberger 1975; Prusoff and Goz 1975). Host enzymes then further phosphorylate the monophosphates to the triphosphate forms. The triphosphates of IDU and TFT are inhibitors of viral and host DNA polymerases and both can be incorporated into DNA (Heidelberger 1975; Prusoff and Goz 1975; Lehrman 1988). However, the fact that both compounds can be anabolized to the triphosphate form in uninfected cells and that neither of the tri-phosphates are particularly selective inhibitors of the viral DNA polymerase limits their utility. Thus, in each case, considerable toxicity in the form of bone marrow suppression is observed when the compounds are given systemically (Lehrman 1988). Although they have largely been replaced by newer more selective antivirals agents, as discussed below, both compounds have been useful therapeutically, simply by limiting their use to topical application for herpes keratitis (Chou and Merigan 1986; Lehrman 1988).

7.4.3.2   *Vidarabine*

Vidarabine 1-(β-D-arabinofuranosyl)adenine, (Ara-A) was originally de-veloped as an anticancer agent but was shown to have anti-HSV activity (Miller *et al*. 1968). Ara-A preferentially inhibits viral DNA polymerase over host DNA polymerase after its phosphorylation to the triphosphate form, making it less toxic than either IDU or TFT (Lehrman 1988). Since Ara-A is less toxic than IDU or TFT, it can be used systemically for herpes simplex encephalitis or disseminated neonatal HSV infections (Chou and Merigan 1986; Lehrman 1988). Since poor water solubility has been a problem with Ara-A, Ara-A monophosphate has also been used for systemic applications.

7.4.3.3   *Acyclovir*

Acyclovir (ACG) was first reported to have selective anti-HSV activity in 1977 (Elion *et al.* 1977). The discovery of ACG wag particularly exciting because it is considerably less toxic than the previous compounds, while retaining a potent anti-HSV activity. The selectivity of ACG as an anti-HSV agent occurs in two steps. First, the initial phosphorylation of ACG to its monophosphate form is catalysed by the HSV thymidine kinase; mammalian nucleoside kinases or 5'-nucleotidases phosphorylate ACG very slowly, if at all (Elion *et al.* 1977). Once at the monophosphate level, ACG monophosphate is further phosphorylated to the di- and triphosphate forms by cellular kinases (Miller and Miller 1980, 1982). Thus formation of the active triphosphate form of ACG is dependent upon its initial phosphorylation to a monophosphate by HSV thymidine kinase. The second level of selectivity occurs at the DNA polymerase itself. HSV DNA polymerase is more sensitive than cellular DNA polymerases to inhibition by ACG triphosphate (Elion *et al.* 1977; Derse *et al.* 1981). The low toxicity of ACG has allowed the use of the drug not only for life-threatening conditions such as herpes simplex encephalitis and neonatal herpes simplex, but also for conditions such as recurrent genital herpes (Tilson 1988).

The mechanism of HSV DNA polymerase inhibition by ACG triphosphate has been studied for some years. The kinetics of inhibition follow a competitive pattern, with ACG triphosphate competing with dGTP for binding to the DNA polymerase (Furman *et al.* 1979; Derse *et al.* 1981). In addition, ACG triphosphate can serve as a substrate for HSV DNA polymerase and be incorporated into the DNA as ACG monophosphate (Furman *et al.* 1979; Derse *et al.* 1981). The product of this reaction, DNA terminated with an ACG monophosphate residue, cannot be elongated further because it lacks a 3'-hydroxyl group. Thus ACG triphosphate is considered to be a chain-terminating compound. This ACG-terminated DNA itself inhibits the DNA polymerase reaction (Derse *et al.* 1981). Further mechanistic studies of inhibition of HSV DNA polymerase by ACG triphosphate revealed that binding of the next nucleotide after ACG monophosphate incorporation traps the enzyme in a dead-end complex (Reardon and Spector 1989).

7.4.3.4   *Ganciclovir*

Following the discovery of ACG, a number of ACG derivatives were tested for antiviral activity. The anti-HSV activity of one ACG derivative, ganciclovir (DHPG), was first described in 1982 (Ashton *et al.* 1982; Smith *et al.* 1982). This compound is similar in structure to ACG, except that DHPG contains a 3′ carbon and hydroxyl group (Ashton *et al.* 1982; Smith *et al.* 1982; Martin *et al.* 1983). Like ACG, DHPG is phosphorylated by the HSV thymidine kinase to its monophosphate form and can be further phosphorylated by host enzymes (Ashton *et al.* 1982; Cheng *et al.* 1983a). The triphosphate form of DHPG is an inhibitor of HSV DNA polymerase *in vitro* (Germershausen *et al.* 1983; Frank *et al.* 1984a) and treatment of cells with DHPG inhibits viral DNA synthesis (Cheng *et al.* 1984).

Although similar in many respects, there are important differences between DHPG and ACG. First, the metabolism of DHPG to its phosphorylated forms in HSV-infected cells is more efficient than for ACG (Germershausen *et al.* 1983). In part, this is due to the fact that DHPG is a better substrate than ACG for the HSV thymidine kinase (Ashton *et al.* 1982). In addition, DHPG is phosphorylated to a greater extent than ACG in CMV-infected cells (Germershausen *et al.* 1983; Biron *et al.* 1985). Thus, DHPG is active against CMV while ACG shows weak anti-CMV activity (Cheng *et al.* 1983b). DHPG may also be different from ACG in terms of its mechanism of action. Unlike ACG, incorporation of DPHG into viral DNA is not necessarily a chain-terminating event, since DHPG contains a 3′ hydroxyl group from which DNA chain elongation could occur. In addition, mutant HSVs that are resistant to ACG by virtue of DNA polymerase alterations are fully sensitive to DHPG (Cheng *et al.* 1983b). This observation is particularly interesting because the purified DNA polymerases from these ACG-resistant viruses are resistant to DHPG triphosphate (Frank *et al.* 1984a). This raises the possibility that DHPG may have a site of action in addition to or instead of the viral DNA polymerase.

7.4.3.5   *Phosphonate derivatives*

Over the past few years a new class of antiviral agents has emerged (Holy and Rosenberg 1987a,b; Rosenberg and Holy 1987). Structurally, these compounds are similar to other acyclic nucleoside analogues in that the 'sugar' moiety of the molecule does not form a complete ring. However, what makes these compounds unique is that they contain a phosphonate residue on what would be the sugar moiety of the molecule. This contrasts with a normal nucleotide in which a phosphate residue is attached to the 5′ carbon. Thus they can be considered as acyclic nucleotide analogues (Holy and Rosenberg 1987a).

The phosphonate residue is designed to be resistant to dephosphorylation and allows these compounds to be phosphorylated to the diphosphate form by the action of cellular enzymes (Holy and Rosenberg 1987a; Votruba *et al.* 1987; Merta *et al.* 1990b; Balzarini *et al.* 1991). The diphosphate forms, which are analogous to a nucleoside triphosphate, are inhibitors of HSV DNA polymerase. Since activation by viral thymidine kinase is not required for antiviral activity, these compounds have activity against viruses that do not induce a thymidine kinase. While this feature has the potential to decrease the antiviral selectivity of the compound, several structures of this type appear to have relatively low toxicity.

Some of these phosphonyl nucleoside analogues show activity against DNA viruses. PMEA has activity against HSV-1, HSV-2, EBV and also retroviruses including HIV (Lin *et al.* 1987; Pauwels *et al.* 1988; De Clercq *et al.* 1989). As noted above, the diphosphate of PMEA is an inhibitor of HSV DNA polymerase and studies have confirmed that HSV DNA polymerase is indeed the antiviral target of PMEA in cell culture (Merta *et al.* 1990a; Foster *et al.* 1991). PMEA can be incorporated into DNA *in vitro* by the HSV DNA polymerase, where it acts as a chain terminator since it lacks a 3′ hydroxyl group from which to extend the DNA chain (Foster *et al.* 1991). HPMPA differs from PMEA in that a hydroxymethyl group is present on the alkyl side-chain (Holy and Rosenberg 1987b). This modification alters the spectrum of antiviral activity for HPMPA; it is active against a broad spectrum of DNA viruses including HSV-1, HSV-2, EBV, VZV, CMV, vaccinia virus, and adenovirus (De Clercq *et al.* 1986) but it is not active against retroviruses. The presence of the hydroxymethyl group opens the possibility that HPMPA may not be a chain-terminating compound. Preliminary results from this laboratory indicate that HPMPA diphosphate can serve as a substrate for HSV DNA polymerase *in vitro*, and that DNA chain termination occurs several nucleotides after HPMPA incorporation. Although HPMPA diphosphate is an inhibitor of HSV DNA polymerase and is similar in structure to PMEA, a PMEA-resistant variant of HSV-1 is more sensitive than the parent virus to HPMPA (Vonka *et al.* 1990; Foster *et al.* 1991). However, the DNA polymerase from the PMEA-resistant HSV is slightly resistant to HPMPA diphosphate *in vitro* (Foster *et al.* 1991). This suggests the possibility that HPMPA may have an alternative site of action instead of or in addition to the HSV DNA polymerase. It is intriguing to note that the relationship between PMEA and HPMPA has certain parallels to the ACG−DHPG relationship, as discussed above. In both cases, viruses resistant to the DNA chain-terminating compound (ACG or PMEA) are sensitive to the corresponding compound containing a 3′ carbon and hydroxyl group from which DNA chain elongation could occur (DHPG or HPMPA). Also, the difference in sensitivity observed in tissue culture systems is not reflected in studies of the purified DNA polymerases in either case. Thus it will be interesting to determine the exact mechanism of action for HPMPA and DHPG.

HPMPC is similar in structure to HPMPA except that it is a derivative of cytosine rather that adenosine. Whereas the anti-HSV activity of HPMPC is similar to that of HPMPA, its anti-CMV activity is much more selective (Snoeck *et al.* 1988). In addition, the anti-CMV effect of HPMPC in cell culture is longer lasting than that of the currently used drug DHPG (Neyts *et al.* 1990). This long-lasting antiviral activity may be due to a long half-life of the phosphonate type analogues inside the cell, as has been shown for PMEA (Cerny *et al.* unpublished results).

7.4.3.6   *Aphidicolin*

Aphidicolin is a tetracyclic diterpenoid compound that inhibits HSV DNA polymerase as well as human DNA polymerase α (Spadari *et al.* 1982). Although its structure appears very different from that of nucleotides, nevertheless, it does inhibit HSV DNA polymerase in a competitive mode with dCTP, dATP, and dTTP (Frank *et al.* 1984b). In contrast, aphidicolin is an inhibitor of DNA polymerase α by competing with dCTP only. Thus the interaction of aphidicolin with human polymerase α is quite different from that with HSV DNA polymerase (Frank *et al.* 1984b).

Therefore it is possible that aphidicolin derivatives could be selective against HSV DNA polymerase (Frank *et al.* 1984b).

7.4.4   Compounds that compete with the DNA template

Some compounds can inhibit HSV DNA polymerase by competing with the DNA template for access to the enzyme. Compounds in this class include modified oligonucleotides as well as some ribonucleotide monophosphates. While none of the compounds in this class have been used clinically, some of the nucleoside analogues discussed above that can be incorporated into DNA may actually owe part of their anti-viral action to this type of mechanism.

7.4.4.1   *Ribonucleoside monophosphates*

The ribonucleotide monophosphates 5'-GMP, 5'-AMP, and 5'-IMP can inhibit HSV DNA polymerase by competing with the DNA template-primer (Frank and Cheng 1986). Thus inhibition occurs when the amount of template-primer is rate limiting. In contrast with the HSV DNA polymerase, human polymerase α is not inhibited by GMP under the same conditions (Frank and Cheng 1986). In addition, ribonucleoside monophosphates can inhibit the 3'-5'-exonuclease activity of HSV DNA polymerase in a non-competitive manner (Frank and Cheng 1986). These results suggest that some nucleoside monophosphate analogues might act as selective inhibitors of HSV DNA polymerase without first being converted to the triphosphate form (Frank and Cheng 1986).

7.4.4.2   *ACG-terminated DNA*

As discussed above, acyclovir is a widely used nucleoside analogue anti-viral agent. Although it is clear that the mechanism of antiviral action is through inhibition of HSV DNA polymerase (Elion *et al.* 1977: Furman *et al.* 1979), the exact mechanism of inhibition has been debated. While

ACGTP is a competitive inhibitor of HSV DNA polymerase (Furman *et al.* 1979), it is also apparent that DNA with ACG residues incorporated at the 5′ ends can inhibit HSV DNA polymerase activity non-competitively *in vitro* (Derse *et al.* 1981). Since it is known that ACG residues are incorporated into the DNA of HSV-infected cells (Elion *et al.* 1977; Furman *et al.* 1979), the possibility is raised that the DNA containing terminally incorporated ACG residues contributes to the antiviral activity of ACG by inhibiting HSV DNA polymerase (Derse *et al.* 1981). Further investigation has revealed that the mechanism by which ACG-terminated DNA inhibits HSV DNA polymerase involves the binding of the next nucleotide to the HSV DNA polymerase–DNA–ACG complex (Reardon and Spector 1989). This results in the formation of a dead-end complex. Because of the continued presence of the next nucleotide, a potent inhibition of DNA polymerizing activity results (Reardon and Spector 1989).

On the basis of these results, it is possible that oligonucleotides with altered nucleotides at the 5′ ends could act as selective antiviral agents. It is also possible that other chain-terminating nucleoside analogues could have similar mechanisms of action.

7.4.4.3   *Phosphorothioate oligonucleotides*

In the last few years, a new class of HSV DNA polymerase inhibitors has emerged. It has been shown that some phosphorothioate oligonucleotides can inhibit HSV DNA polymerase (Gao *et al.* 1989). This inhibition is competitive with the primer-template and can be selective for the viral DNA polymerase, depending on the sequence and length of the oligonucleotide (Gao *et al.* 1989). The oligonucleotide S-(dC)28 is an inhibitor of both HSV-2 DNA polymerase *in vitro* and HSV-2 replication in cell culture (Gao *et al.* 1989, 1990a). In contrast, S-(dC)28 is a weaker inhibitor of HSV-1 DNA polymerase and does inhibit HSV-1 replication in cell culture (Gao *et al.* 1989, 1990a). Gao and coworkers proposed that the mechanism of the anti-HSV-2 action of S-(dC)28 involves inhibition of the ability of the viral particles to infect the cell, as well as inhibition of the viral DNA polymerase (Gao *et al.* 1990b). The selectivity of S-(dC)28 against HSV-2 appears to be quite good, since it was not significantly inhibitory to cell growth at 50 μM and completely inhibited HSV-2 plaque formation at 10 μM (Gao *et al.* 1990a). The observation that HSV-2 infection stimulates the uptake of S-(dC)28 may partially explain its selectivity (Gao *et al.* 1990b).

7.4.5   Compounds that interact at the pyrophosphate exchange site

Compounds that inhibit DNA polymerization by interacting with the polymerase at the pyrophosphate release site are analogues of pyrophosphate. While only PFA has been used clinically, new analogues are being tested for anti-viral activity.

The pyrophosphate analogue phosphonoacetic acid (PAA) was first shown to inhibit HSV DNA replication in cell culture in 1974 (Overby *et al.* 1974) and subsequently to inhibit HSV DNA polymerase (Mao *et al.* 1975). The mechanism of inhibition of HSV DNA polymerase by PAA involves its interaction at the pyrophosphate exchange site as shown by work with DNA polymerase induced by herpes virus of turkeys (Leinbach *et al.* 1976). The mode of inhibition is linear non-competitive with respect to the four dNTPs and the activated DNA template (Leinbach *et al.* 1976). PAA is a competitive inhibitor with respect to the pyrophosphate of the HSV DNA polymerase catalysed dNTP−pyrophosphate exchange reaction (Leinbach *et al.* 1976).

Since the discovery of PAA, phosphonoformic acid (PFA) has been shown be a more potent and less toxic inhibitor of HSV DNA polymerase (Alenius *et al.* 1978; Helgstrand 1978; Revio *et al.* 1978; Cheng *et al.* 1981). Its lower toxicity has allowed PFA to be used for the treatment of acyclovir-resistant HSV-2 infections (Erlich *et al.* 1989). While PFA is less toxic than PAA, it does have significant toxicity, including alterations in calcium metabolism and acute renal failure with systemic use (Cacoub *et al.* 1988; Jacobson *et al.* 1991). Thiophosphonoformate (TPFA), a derivative of PFA, has recently been synthesized (McKenna *et al.* 1990). TPFA is a somewhat less potent inhibitor of HSV DNA polymerase, but it is hoped that the toxicity of TPFA or other PFA derivatives will be reduced.

One interesting aspect of viruses selected for resistance to PFA is that they tend to be hypersensitive to inhibition by aphidicolin (Bastow *et al.* 1983). Thus mutations in the HSV DNA polymerase that confer PFA resistance, presumably by altering the charge distribution of the active site of the DNA polymerase, appear to increase the affinity of the polymerase for aphidicolin. Thus a combination approach with PFA and aphidicolin may reduce the possibility of selecting resistant mutants (Derse *et al.* 1982).

7.5 Summary and conclusions

In this chapter we have focused on strategies for inhibiting HSV DNA polymerase, but the principles formulated should also apply to other viral DNA polymerases. HSV encodes its own DNA polymerase which is an essential enzyme for viral replication. In addition, differences in the viral DNA polymerase compared with host DNA polymerases allow for selective inhibition of the viral enzyme. Additional selectivity can be achieved by taking advantage of biochemical differences between infected and un-infected cells. Thus the HSV DNA polymerase is an attractive target for anti-viral therapy. Within the last 20 years, selective antiviral agents have been developed which selectively inhibit HSV DNA polymerase or are selectively metabolized to their active metabolites in virally infected cells or both. Although several potent and selective anti-HSV compounds exist, resistance to these compounds can occur (Freifeld and Ostrove 1991). Thus additional HSV DNA polymerase inhibitors are always welcomed. In addition, it is of interest to develop compounds that are active and selective antiviral agents in the absence of HSV thymidine kinase, since this selective metabolic activation is not always available in virally infected cells. Further research may uncover additional viral DNA polymerase inhibitors that will be useful in treating viral diseases.

References

Alenius, S., Dinter, Z., and Oberg, B. (1978). Therapeutic effect of trisodium phosphonoformate on cutaneous herpesvirus infection in guinea pigs. *Antimicrobial Agents and Chemotherapy*, **14**, 408–13.

Ashton, W. T., Karkas, J. D., Field, J. K., and Tolman, R. L. (1982). Activation by thymidine kinase and potent antiherpetic activity of 2′-nor-2′-deoxyguanosine (2′NDG). *Biochemical and Biophysical Research Communications*, **108**, 1716–21.

Balzarini, J., Hao, Z., Herdewijn, P., Johns, D. G., and De Clercq, E. (1991). Intracellular metabolism and mechanism of anti-retrovirus action of 9-(2-phosphonylmethoxyethyl)adenine, a potent anti-human immunodeficiency virus compound. *Proceedings of the National Academy of Sciences of the United States of America*, **88**, 1499–1503.

Bastow, K. F., Derse, D. D., and Cheng, Y.-C. (1983). Susceptibility of phosphonoformic acid-resistant herpes simplex virus variants to arabinosylnucleotides and aphidicolin *Antimicrobial Agents and Chemotherapy*, **23**, 914–17.

Biron, K. K., Stanat, S. C., Sorrell, J. B., Fyfe, J. A., Keller, P. M., Lambe, C. U., and Nelson, D. J. (1985). Metabolic activation of the nucleoside analog 9-[(2-hydroxy-1-(hydroxymethyl)ethoxy)methyl]guanine in human diploid fibroblasts infected with human cytomegalovirus. *Proceedings of the National Academy of Sciences of the United States of America*, **82**, 2473–77.

Cacoub, P., Deray, G., Baumelou, A., Le Hoang, P., Rozenbaum, W., Gentilini, M., *et al.* (1988). Acute renal failure induced by foscarnet: 4 cases. *Clinical Nephrology*, **29**, 315–18.

Carrasco, L. (1978). Membrane leakiness after viral infection and a new approach to the development of antiviral agents. *Nature, London*, **272**, 694–9.

Challberg, M. D. and Kelly, T. J. (1989). Animal virus DNA replication. *Annual Review of Biochemistry*, **58**, 671–717.

Chartrand, P., Stow, N. D., Timbury, M. C., and Wilkie, N. M. (1979). Physical mapping of paar mutations of herpes simplex virus type 1 and type 2 by intertypic marker rescue. *Journal of Virology*, **31**, 265–76.

Cheng, Y.-C. (1976). Deoxythymidine kinase induced in HeLa TK-cells by herpes simplex virus type I and type II. *Biochimica et Biophysica Acta*, **452**, 370–81.

Cheng, Y.-C., Ostrander, M., Derse, D., and Chen, J.-Y. (1979). Development of antiherpes virus agents on the basis of virus induced enzymes. In *Nucleoside analogues* (ed. R. T. Walker, E. De Clercq, and F. Eckstein), pp. 319–35. Plenum Press, New York.

Cheng, Y.-C., Grill, S., Derse, D., Chen, J.-Y., Caradonna, S. J., and Connor, K. (1981). Mode of action of phosphonoformate as an anti-herpes simplex virus agent. *Biochimica et Biophysica Acta*, **652**, 90–8.

Cheng, Y.-C., Huang, E.-S., Lin, J.-C., Mar, E.-C., Pagano, J. S., Dutschman, G. E., and Grill, S. P. (1983a). Unique spectrum of activity of 9-[(1,3-dihydroxy-2-propoxy)methyl]-guanine against herpesviruses *in vitro* and its mode of action against herpes simplex virus type 1. *Proceedings of the National Academy of Sciences of the United States of America*, **80**, 2767–70.

Cheng, Y. C., Grill, S. P., Dutschman, G. E., Nakayama, K., and Bastow, K. F. (1983a). Metabolism of 9-(1,3-dihydroxy-2-propoxymethyl)guanine, a new anti-herpes virus compound in herpes simplex virus-infected cells. *Journal of Biological Chemistry*, **258**, 12460–4.

Cheng, Y.-C., Grill, S. P., Dutschman, G. E., Frank, K. B., Chiou, J.-F., Bastow, K. F., and Nakayama, K. (1984). Effects of 9-(1,3-dihydroxy-2-propoxymethyl)-guanine, a new antiherpesvirus compound, on synthesis of maromolecules in herpes simplex virus-infected cells. *Antimicrobial Agents and Chemotherapy*, **26**, 283–8.

Cheng, Y.-C., Ostrander, M., Derse, D., Chen, J.-Y. (1979). Development of anti-herpes virus agents on the basis of virus induced enzymes. In *Nucleoside analogues* (ed. R. T. Walker, E. De Clercq, and F. Eckstein), pp. 319–35. Plenum Press, New York.

Chou, S. and Merigan, T. C. (1986). Antiviral chemotherapy. In *Fundamental virology* (ed. B. N. Fields, D. M. Knipe, R. M. Chanock, J. L. Melnick, B. Roizman, and R. E. Shope), pp. 309–34. Raven Press, New York.

Coen, D. M., Aschman, D. P., Gelep, P. T., Retondo, M. J., Weller, S. K., and Schaffer, P. A. (1984). Fine mapping and molecular cloning of mutations in the herpes simplex virus DNA polymerase locus. *Journal of Virology*, **49**, 236–47.

Crute, J. J. and Lehman, I. R. (1989). Herpes simplex-1 DNA polymerase identification of an intrinsic 5′-3′ exonuclease with ribonuclease H activity. *Journal of Biological Chemistry*, **264**, 19266–70.

De Clercq, E., Holy, A., Rosenberg, I., Sakuma, T., Balzanni, J., and Maudgal, P. C. (1986). A novel selective broad-spectrum anti-DNA virus agent. *Nature, London*, **323**, 464–7.

De Clercq, E., Holy, A., and Rosenberg, I. (1989). Efficacy of phosphonyl-methoxyalkyl derivatives of adenine in experimental herpes simplex virus and vaccinia virus infections *in vivo*. *Antimicrobial Agents and Chemotherapy*, **33**, 185–91.

Derse, D., Cheng, Y.-C., Furman, P. A., St. Clair, M. H., and Elion, G. B. (1981). Inhibition of purified human and herpes simplex virus-induced DNA polymerases by 9-(2-hydroxyethoxymethyl)guanine triphosphate: effects on primer-template function. *Journal of Biological Chemistry*, **256**, 11447–51.

Derse, D., Bastow, K. F., and Cheng, Y.-C. (1982). Characterization of the DNA polymerases induced by a group of herpes simplex virus type I variants selected for growth in the presence of phosphonoformic acid. *Journal of Biological Chemistry*, **257**, 10251–60.

Elion, G. B., Furman, P. A., Fyfe, J. A., De Miranda, P., Beauchamp, L., and Schaeffer, H. J. (1977). Selectivity of action of an antiherpetic agent 9-(2-hydroxyethoxymethyl)guanine. *Proceedings of the National Academy of Sciences of the United States of America*, **74**, 5716–20.

Erlich, K. S., Jacobson, M. A., Koehler, J. E., Follansbee, S. E., Drennan, D. P., Gooze, L., *et al.* (1989). Foscarnet therapy for severe acyclovir-resistant herpes simplex virus type-2 infections in patients with the acquired immunodeficiency syndrome (AIDS): an uncontrolled trial. *Annals of Internal Medicine*, **110**, 710–13.

Foster, S. A., Cerny, J., and Cheng, Y.-C. (1991). Herpes simplex virus-specified DNA polymerase is the target for the antiviral action of 9-(2-phosphonylmethoxy-ethyl)adenine *Journal of Biological Chemistry*, **266**, 238–44.

Frank, K. B. and Cheng, Y.-C. (1986). Inhibition of herpes simplex virus DNA polymerase by purine ribonucleoside monophosphates. *Journal of Biological Chemistry*, **261**, 1510–13.

Frank, K. B., Chiou, J.-F., and Cheng, Y.-C. (1984a). Interaction of herpes simplex virus-induced DNA polymerase with 9-(1,3-dihydroxy-2-propoxymethyl)-guanine triphosphate. *Journal of Biological Chemistry*, **259**, 1566–9.

Frank, K. B., Derse, D. D., Bastow, K. F., and Cheng, Y.-C. (1984b). Novel interaction of aphidicolin with herpes simplex virus DNA polymerase and polymerase-associated exonuclease. *Journal of Biological Chemistry*, **259**, 13282–6.

Freifeld, A. G. and Ostrove, J. M. (1991). Resistance of viruses to antiviral drugs. *Annual Review of Medicine*, **42**, 247–59.

Furman, P. A., St. Clair, M. H., Fyfe, J. A., Rideout, J. L., Keller, P. M., and Elion, G. B. (1979). Inhibition of herpes simplex virus-induced DNA polymerase activity and viral DNA replication by 9-(2-hydroxyethoxymethyl)guanine and its triphosphate. *Journal of Virology*, **32**, 72–7.

Gao, W., Stein, C. A., Cohen, J. S., Dutschman, G. E., and Cheng, Y.-C. (1989). Effect of phosphorothioate homo-oligodeoxynucleotides on herpes simplex virus type 2-induced DNA polymerase. *Journal of Biological Chemistry*, **264**, 11521–6.

Gao, W.-Y., Hanes, R. N., Vazquez-Padua, M. A., Stein, C. A., Cohen, J. S., and Cheng, Y.-C. (1990a). Inhibition of herpes simplex virus type 2 growth by phosphorothioate oligonucleotides. *Antimicrobial Agents and Chemotherapy*, **34**, 808–12.

Gao, W.-Y., Jaroszewski, J. W., Cohen, J. S., and Cheng, Y.-C. (1990b). Mechanisms of inhibition of herpes simplex virus type 2 growth by 28-mer phosphorothioate oligodeoxycytidine. *Journal of Biological Chemistry*, **265**, 20172–8.

Germershausen, J., Bostedor, R., Field, A. K., Perry, H., Liou, R., Bull, H., *et al.* (1983). A comparison of the antiviral agents 2′-nor-2′-deoxyguanosine and acyclovir uptake and phosphorylation in tissue culture and kinetics of *in vitro* inhibition of viral and cellular DNA polymerases by their respective triphosphates. *Biochemical and Biophysical Research Communications*, **116**, 360–7.

Gibbs, J. S., Chiou, H. C., Hall, J. D., Mount, D. W., Retondo, M. J., Weller, S. K., and Coen, D. M. (1985). Sequence and mapping analyses of the herpes simplex virus DNA polymerase gene predict a C-terminal substrate binding domain. *Proceedings of the National Academy of Sciences of the United States of America*, **82**, 7969–73.

Gibbs, J. S., Chiou, H. C., Bastow, K. F., Cheng, Y.-C., and Coen, D. M. (1988). Identification of amino acids in herpes simplex virus DNA polymerase involved in substrate and drug recognition. *Proceedings of the National Academy of Sciences of the United States of America*, **85**, 6672–6.

Gonzalez, M. E. and Carrasco, L. (1987). Animal virus promote the entry of polysaccharides with antiviral activity into cells. *Biochemical and Biophysical Research Communications*, **146**, 1303–10.

Gotttieb, J., Marcy, A. I., Coen, D. M., and Challberg, M. D. (1990). The herpes simplex virus type 1 UL42 gene product: a subunit of DNA polymerase that functions to increase processivity. *Journal of Virology*, **64**, 5976–87.

Heidelberger, C. (1975). On the molecular mechanism of the antiviral activity of trifluorothymidine. *Annals of the New York Academy of Sciences*, **255**, 317–25.

Helgstrand, E., Eriksson, B., Johansson, N. G., Lannero, B., Larsson, A., Misiorny, A., *et al*. (1978). Trisodium phosphonoformate, a new antiviral compound. *Science*, **201**, 819–21.

Holy, A. and Rosenberg, I. (1987a). Synthesis of 9-(2-phosphonylmethoxyethyl)-adenine and relate compounds. *Collection of Czechoslovak Chemical Communications*, **52**, 2801–9.

Holy, A. and Rosenberg, I. (1987b). Synthesis of isomeric and enantiomeric O-phosphonylmethyl derivatives of 9-(2,3-dihydroxypropyl)adenine. *Collection of Czechoslovak Chemical Communications*, **52**, 2775–91.

Jacobson, M. A., Gambertoglio, J. G., Aweeka, F. T., Causey, D. M., and Portale, A. A. (1991). Foscarnet-induced hypocalcemia and effects of foscarnet on calcium metabolism. *Journal of Clinical Endocrinology and Metabolism*, **72**, 1130–5.

Jofre, J. T., Schaffer, P. A., and Parris, D. S. (1977). Genetics of resistance to phosphonoacetic acid in strain KOS of herpes simplex virus type 1. *Journal of Virology*, **23**, 833–6.

Kaufman, H. E., and Heidelberger, C. (1964). Therapeutic antiviral action of 5-trifluoromethyl-2′-deoxyuridine in herpes simplex keratitis. *Science*, **145**, 585–6.

Kaufman, H. E., Nesburn, A. B., and Maloney, E. D. (1962). IDU therapy of herpes simplex. *Archives of Ophthalmology*, **67**, 583–9.

Keir, H. M. and Gold, E. (1963). Deoxyribonucleic acid nucleotidyltransferase and deoxyribonuclease from cultured cells infected with herpes simplex virus. *Biochimica et Biophysica Acta*, **72**, 263–76.

Keir, H. M., Hay, J., Morrison, J. M., and Subak-Sharpe, H. (1966). Altered properties of deoxyribonucleic acid nucleotidyltransferase after infection of mammalian cells with herpes simplex virus. *Nature, London*, **210**, 369–71.

Lacal, J. C. and Carrasco, L. (1983). Antiviral effects of Hygromycin B, a translation inhibitor nonpermeant to uninfected cells. *Antimicrobial Agents and Chemotherapy*, **24**, 273–5.

Lader, B. A. and Darby, G. (1985). Selection and characterisation of acyclovir-resistant herpes simplex virus type 1 mutants inducing altered DNA polymerase activities. *Virology*, **146**, 262–71.

Lee, L. S. and Cheng, Y.-C. (1976). Human deoxythymidine kinase II: substrate specificity and kinetic behavior of the cytoplasmic and mitochondrial enzymes derived from blast cells of acute myelocytic leukemia. *Biochemistry*, **15**, 3686–90.

Lehrman, S. N. (1988). Herpesviruses. In *Virology* (3rd edn) (ed. W. K. Joklik), pp. 168–79. Appleton and Lange, Norwalk, CT.

Leinbach, S. S., Reno, J. M., Lee, L. F., Isbell, A. F., and Boezi, J. A. (1976). Mechanism of phosphonoacetate inhibition of herpesvirus-induced DNA polymerase. *Biochemistry*, **15**, 426–30.

Lin, J.-C., De Clercq, E., and Pagano, J. S. (1987). Novel acyclic adenosine analogs inhibit Epstein–Barr virus replication. *Antimicrobial Agents and Chemotherapy*, **31**, 1431–3.

McGeoch, D. J., Dalrymple, M. A., Davison, A. J., Dolan, A., Frame, M. C.,

McNab, D., *et al.* (1988). The complete DNA sequence of the long unique region in the genome of herpes simplex virus type 1. *Journal of General Virology*, **69**, 1531–74.

McKenna, C. E., Ye, T.-G., Levy, J. N., Wen, T., Bongartz, J.-P., Cheng, Y.-C., *et al.* (1990). Sodium thiophosphonoformate, a selective HIV inhibitor: facile synthesis and effects in HIV-infected cell culture. *Annals of the New York Academy of Sciences*, **616**, 569–71.

Mao, J. C.-H., Robishaw, E. E., and Overby, L. R. (1975). Inhibition of DNA polymerase from herpes simplex virus-infected Wi-38 cells by phosphonoacetic acid. *Journal of Virology*, **15**, 1281–3.

Martin, J. C., Dvorak, C. A., Smee, D. F., Matthews, T. R., and Verheyden, J. P. H. (1983). 9-[(1,3-dihydroxy-2-propoxy)methyl]guanine: a new potent and selective antiherpes agent. *Journal of Medicinal Chemistry*, **26**, 759–61.

Merta, A., Vesely, J., Votruba, I., Rosenberg, I., and Holy, A. (1990). Phosphorylation of acyclic nucleotide analogues HPMPA and PMEA in L1210 mouse leukemic cell extracts. *Neoplasma*, **37**, 111–20.

Merta, A., Votruba, I., Rosenberg, I., Otmar, M., Hrebabecky, H., Bernaerts, R., and Holy, A. (1990a). Inhibition of herpes simplex virus DNA polymerase by diphosphates of acyclic phosphonylmethoxyalkyl nucleotide analogues. *Antiviral Research*, **13**, 209–18.

Miller, W. H. and Miller, R. L. (1980). Phosphorylation of acyclovir (acycloguanosine) monophosphate by GMP kinase. *Journal of Biological Chemistry*, **255**, 7204–7.

Miller, W. H. and Miller, R. L. (1982). Phosphorylation of acyclovir diphosphate by cellular enzymes. *Biochemical Pharmacology*, **31**, 3879–84.

Miller, F. A., Dixon, G. J., Ehrlich, J., Sloan, B. J., and McLean, I. W., Jr (1968). Antiviral activity of 9-β-D-arabinofuranosyladenine: I. cell culture studies. *Antimicrobial Agents and Chemotherapy*, **1**, 136–47.

Moss, B. (1986). Replication of poxviruses. In *Fundamental virology* (ed. B. N. Fields, D. M. Knipe, R. M. Chanock, J. L. Melnick, B. Roizman, and R. E. Shope), pp. 637–55. Raven Press, New York.

Neyts, J., Snoeck, R., Schols, D., Balzarini, J., and De Clercq, E. (1990). Selective inhibition of human cytomegalovirus DNA synthesis by (*S*)-1-(3-hydroxy-2-phosphonylmethoxypropyl)cytosine [(*S*)-HPMPC] and 9-(1,3-dihydroxy-2-propoxymethyl)guanine (DHPG). *Virology*, **179**, 41–50.

Ostrander, M. and Cheng, Y.-C. (1980). Properties of herpes simplex virus type 1 and type 2 DNA polymerase. *Biochimica et Biophysica Acta*, **609**, 232–5.

Overby, L. R., Robishaw, E. E., Schleicher, J. B., Reuter, A., Shipkowitz, N. L., and Mao, J. C.-H. (1974). Inhibition of herpes simplex virus replication by phosphonoacetic acid. *Antimicrobial Agents and Chemotherapy*, **6**, 360–5.

Parris, D. S., Dixon, R. A. F., and Schaffer, P. A. (1980). Physical mapping of herpes simplex virus type 1 ts mutants by marker rescue: correlation of the physical and genetic maps. *Virology*, **100**, 275–87.

Pauwels, R., Balzarini, J., Schols, D., Baka, M., Desmyter, J., Rosenberg, I., *et al.* (1988). Phosphonylmethoxyethyl purine derivatives, a new class of anti-human immunodeficiency virus agents. *Antimicrobial Agents and Chemotherapy*, **32**, 1025–30.

Powell, K. L. and Purifoy, D. J. M. (1977). Nonstructural proteins of herpes simplex virus I. Purification of the induced DNA polymerase. *Journal of Virology*, **24**, 618–26.

Prusoff, W. H. and Goz, B. (1975). Halogenated pyrimidine deoxyribonucleotides. In *Antineoplastic and immunosuppressive agents II* (ed. A. C. Sartorelli and D. G. Johns), pp. 272–347. Springer-Verlag, New York.

Purifoy, D. J. M., Lewis, R. B., and Powell, K. L. (1977). Identification of the herpes simplex virus DNA polymerase gene. *Nature, London*, **269**, 621–3.

Quinn, J. P. and McGeoch, D. J. (1985). DNA sequence of the region in the genome of herpes simplex virus type 1 containing the genes for DNA polymerase and the major DNA binding protein. *Nucleic Acids Research*, **13**, 8143–63.

Reardon, J. E. and Spector, T. (1989). Herpes simplex virus type 1 DNA polymerase. Mechanism of inhibition by acyclovir triphosphate. *Journal of Biological Chemistry*, **264**, 7405–11.

Reno, J. M., Lee, L. F., and Boezi, J. A. (1978). Inhibition of herpesvirus replication and herpesvirus-induced deoxyribonucleic acid polymerase by phosphonoformate. *Antimicrobial Agents and Chemotherapy*, **13**, 188–92.

Roizman, B. and Batterson, W. (1986). Herpesviruses and their replication. In *Fundamental virology* (ed. B. N. Fields, D. M. Knipe, R. M. Chanock, J. L. Melnick, B. Roizman, and R. E. Shope), pp. 607–36. Raven Press, New York.

Rosenberg, I. and Holy, A. (1987). Synthesis of potential prodrugs and metabolites of 9-(S)-(3-hydroxyl-2-phosphonylmethoxypropyl)adenine. *Collection of Czechoslovak Chemical Communications*, **52**, 2792–800.

Schaffer, P. A., Aron, G. M., Biswal, N., and Benyesh-Melnick, M. (1973). Temperature-sensitive mutants of herpes simplex virus type 1: isolation, complementation and partial characterization. *Virology*, **52**, 57–71.

Smith, K. O., Galloway, K. S., Kennell, W. L., Ogilvie, K. K., and Radatus, B. K. (1982). A new nucleoside analog, 9-[[2-hydroxyl-1-(hydroxymethyl)ethoxy]-methyl]guanine, highly active *in vitro* against herpes simplex virus types 1 and 2. *Antimicrobial Agents and Chemotherapy*, **22**, 55–61.

Snoeck, R., Sakuma, T., De Clercq, E., Rosenberg, I., and Holy, A. (1988). (S)-1-(3-hydroxy-2-phosphonylmethoxypropyl)cytosine, a potent and selective inhibitor of human cytomegalovirus replication. *Antimicrobial Agents and Chemotherapy*, **32**, 1834–44.

Spadari, S., Sala, F., and Pedrali-Noy, G. (1982). Aphidicolin: a specific inhibitor of nuclear DNA replication in eukaryotes. *Trends in Biochemical Sciences*, **7**, 29–32.

Tilson, H. H. (1988). Monitoring the safety of antivirals: the example of the acyclovir experience. *American Journal of Medicine*, **85** (2A), 116–22.

Vaughan, P. J., Purifoy, D. J. M., and Powell, K. L. (1985). DNA-binding protein associated with herpes simplex virus DNA polymerase. *Journal of Virology*, **53**, 501–8.

Vonka, V., Anisimova, E., Cerny, J., Holy, A., Rosenberg, I., and Votruba, I. (1990). Properties of 9-(2-phosphonylmethoxyethyl)adenine (PMEA) resistant herpes simplex type 1 virus. *Antiviral Research*, **14**, 117–22.

Votruba, I., Bernaerts, R., Sakuma, T., De Clercq, E., Merta, A., Rosenberg, I., and Holy, A. (1987). Intracellular phosphorylation of broad spectrum anti-DNA virus agent (S)-9-(3-hydroxy-2-phosphonylmethoxypropyl)adenine and inhibition of viral DNA synthesis. *Molecular Pharmacology*, **32**, 524–9.

Weissbach, A., Hong, S. L., Aucker, J., and Muller, R. (1973). Characterization of herpes simplex viris-induced deoxyribonucleic acid polymerase. *Journal of Biological Chemistry*, **248**, 6270–7.

Weisshart, K. and Knopf, C. W. (1988). The herpes simplex virus type 1 DNA polymerase. Polypeptide structure and antigenic domains. *European Journal of Biochemistry*, **174**, 707–16.

Wong, S. W., Wahl, A. F., Yuan, P.-M., Arai, N., Pearson, B. E., Arai, K., *et al.* (1988). Human DNA polymerase α gene expression is cell proliferation dependent and its primary structure is similar to both prokaryotic and eukaryotic replicative DNA polymerases. *EMBO Journal*, **7**, 37–47.

8

Fungal enzyme targets

Section 8A

Inhibitors of sterol 14-α-demethylase, Δ^{14}-reductase, and $\Delta^8 \rightarrow \Delta^7$-isomerase

Dieter Berg and Manfred Plempel

8A.1 Summary

The therapeutic situation in the treatment of fungal diseases changed dramatically with the development of the sterol biosynthesis inhibitors (SBIs). The imidazoles and 1,2,4,-triazoles that are already on the market are highly effective topical and vaginal antimycotics, and oral administration has become possible in the case of some of these compounds. The azoles, originating from the chemical classes of imidazoles, 1,2,4-triazoles, pyridines, or pyrimidines, interfere with the biosynthesis of fungal sterols by inhibiting the demethylation at C14. The C14-α-demethylase is a monooxygenase of the cytochrome P450 type which is inhibited by direct interference with the prosthetic group, i.e. an iron porphyrin moiety. A double bond is formed as an intermediate during the C14 demethylation reaction, and its reduction is inhibited by several morpholines or piperidines, i.e. Δ^{14}-reductase inhibitors. As some morpholines also affect the isomerization from Δ^8 to Δ^7, this late step in sterol biosynthesis is also considered in this chapter. The chemistry, biochemistry, and therapeutic use of inhibitors of 14-α-demethylase, Δ^{14}-reductase, and $\Delta^8 \rightarrow \Delta^7$-isomerase are discussed.

8A.2 Introduction

After the development of clotrimazole and miconazole in 1968 (Godefroi et al. 1969; Büchel et al. 1972) understanding of sterol biosynthesis in mammals, plants, and fungi was greatly improved. This topic has been and still is the subject of intensive study, which has been facilitated by the availability of a series of antifungal sterol biosynthesis inhibitors as tools (Berg and Plempel 1988). Consequently, studies at the molecular level have become practical (Vanden Bossche 1988).

A selective and incomplete set of examples of sterol biosynthesis inhibitors is given in Fig. 8A.1 to demonstrate the heterogeneity of the chemical classes that have been developed. As an aid to our discussion of the various targets of these compounds, a short description of fungal ergosterol biosynthesis is given below.

Terpenoid biosynthesis starts from 3-hydroy-3-methyl-glutaryl-CoA by generating mevanolate and subsequently isopentenylpyrophosphate (IPP) which then reacts with its isomer dimethyl-allyl-pyrophosphate (DMAPP) to build a C10 unit geranyl-pyrophosphate (GPP); by adding another C5 unit, farnesyl pyrophosphate (FPP) is synthesized. A tail-to-tail reaction of two FPP molecules leads to squalene which, after epoxidation, cyclizes to lanosterol. The epoxidation is the target of a group of antimycotics, the allylamines, which will be discussed in Section 8B.

In contrast with cholesterol synthesis in mammals, ergosterol synthesis in fungi requires side-chain methylation at C24, which is usually performed at the lanosterol stage. Thus 24-methylene-dihydrolanosterol as an intermediate has been found in many fungi such as various *Candida* species (Fryberg et al. 1975; Vanden Bossche et al. 1978; Berg et al. 1984a), *Ustilago maydis* (Ragsdale 1975), and in numerous filamentous fungi (Goulston et al. 1967; Leroux and Gredt 1978). However, 24-methylene-hydrolanosterol has not been found in *Saccharomyces cerevisiae* (Mercer 1984) or *Saccharomycopsis lipolytica* (Berg et al. 1987), as in these yeasts side-chain alkylation proceeds with $\Delta^{8,24}$ cholesterol as substrate. The side-chain-alkylating enzymes require S-adenosylmethionine (SAM) as the donor of the 24-methyl group. Regardless of whether side-chain methylation proceeds first or subsequently, either lanosterol or 24-methylene-dihydrolanosterol are oxidatively demethylated at C14 in the next step. The mechanism of oxidative removal of the C14 methyl group will be discussed in detail later.

The subsequent C14 demethylations remove the two methyl groups as CO_2 and are followed by $\Delta^8 \rightarrow \Delta^7$ isomerization which starts with protonation of the Δ^8 double bond and ends with elimination of a C7 proton. Again, this reaction will be discussed in greater detail later. Δ^5 desaturation leads to the 5,7-diene in ring B and saturation of the $\Delta^{24(28)}$ double bond, and formation of a double bond in the Δ^{22} position concludes ergosterol synthesis.

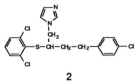

1

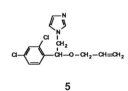

2

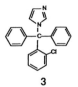

3

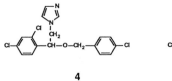

4

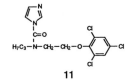

5

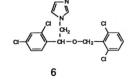

6

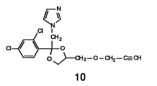

7

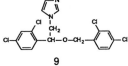

8

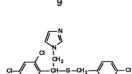

9

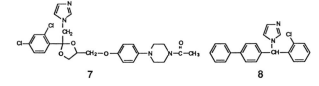

10

11

12

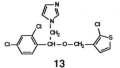

13

1 Bifonazole	**2** Butaconazole	**3** Clotrimazole
4 Econazole	**5** Imazalil	**6** Isoconazole
7 Ketoconazole	**8** Lombazole	**9** Miconazole
10 Parconazole	**11** Prochlorazole	**12** Sulconazole
	13 Tioconazole	

(a)

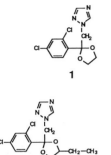

1

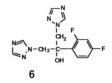

2

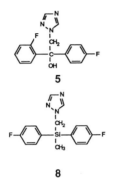

3

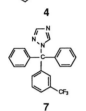

4

5

6

7

8

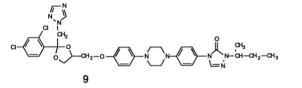

9

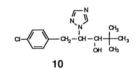

10

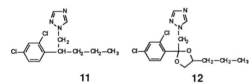

11

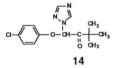

12

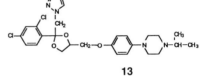

13

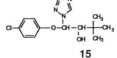

14

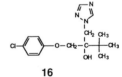

15

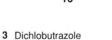

16

1 Azaconazole	**2** Bitertanol	**3** Dichlobutrazole
4 Etaconazole	**5** Flutriafol	**6** Fluconazole
7 Flutrimazole	**8** Flusilazole	
9 Itraconazole	**10** Paclobutrazole	
11 Penconazole	**12** Propionazole	**13** Terconazole
14 Triadimefon	**15** Triadimenol	**16** Vibunazole

(b)

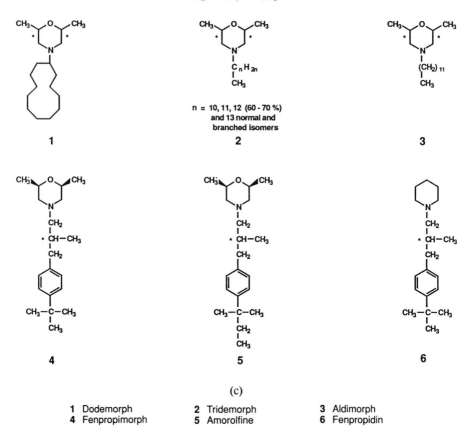

(c)

1 Dodemorph   2 Tridemorph   3 Aldimorph
4 Fenpropimorph   5 Amorolfine   6 Fenpropidin

Fig. 8A.1 Chemical structures of (a) imidazole antifungal agents, (b) triazole antifungal agents, and (c) morpholine and piperidine antifungal agents.

The reason why sterol biosynthesis inhibitors exhibit intense effects as fungicides has been discussed fully in the literature (Nes 1984; Dahl and Dahl 1985). The main question was whether the lack of the sterol end-product or an accumulation of non-planar sterol precursors leads to the fungicidal effect. Up till the present time, it has not been possible to provide a clear answer to this question as the function of sterols in fungal membranes is not as simple as had originally been thought. This function has often been described as a contribution to membrane topology. Nowadays, however, at least four distinct functions need to be discussed. The contribution to membrane topology by interaction with phospholipids, thus stabilizing the membrane, is called the bulk function (Rodriguez and Parks 1983). This function requires sterol concentrations of about 15 μg ml^{-1}. Studies of sterol auxotrophic yeasts showed that sparking by minute amount

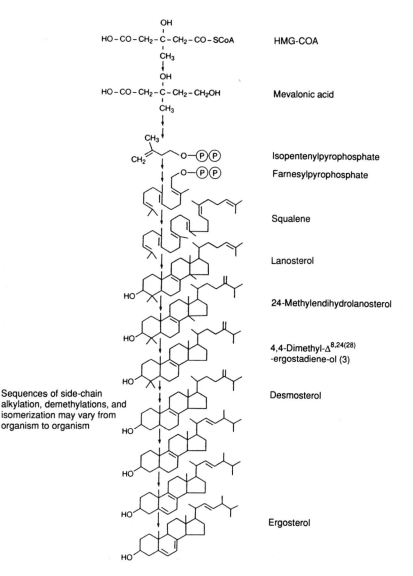

Fig. 8A.2 Scheme of ergosterol biosynthesis in fungi.

of ergosterol, in the region of $1-10$ ng ml^{-1}, is necessary to induce growth (Rodriguez *et al.* 1985). A slightly higher concentration (100 ng ml^{-1}) is required for sterol supply to certain limited areas. This function is called the critical domain function (Taylor and Parks 1980). Finally, at concentrations of about $0.56-1$ μg ml^{-1}, ergosterol prevents detectable changes in properties of lipids possessing a domain function (Thompson and Parks 1974).

After application of antifungal sterol biosynthesis inhibitors, various abnormalities can be observed (Yamaguchi and Osumi 1988), including irregularities of the cell membrane, disappearance or deformation of membrane invaginations, accumulation of lomasome-like vesicles, deformation of buds, apparent thickening of cell walls, and incomplete septa formation, leading to an impaired separation of budding cells, finally resulting in chains of interconnecting cells.

8A.3   Inhibition of C14 demethylation

Demethylation at C14 proceeds via stepwise oxidation of the methyl group. The enzyme responsible is a mono-oxygenase of cytochrome P450 type. The first step leads by oxidation to the alcohol, second reaction and loss of water produces the corresponding aldehyde, and the carboxylic acid is obtained in the third mono-oxygenase reaction (Fig. 8A.3). The carboxylic acid is removed by withdrawing a proton from the 15-position. Thus formic acid is eliminated, building a Δ^{14} double bond as an intermediate. This Δ^{14} double bond is finally reduced by a $NADPH/H^+$-dependent reaction which is discussed in detail in connection with the morpholine inhibitors.

In mammalian systems, e.g. liver, a single cytochrome is responsible for both this oxidation sequence and the lyase activity (Trzaskos et al. 1986a). Its apparent molecular weight after SDS polyacrylamide gel electrophoresis is 51 kDa. In the case of the yeast S. cerevisiae, which, like the mammalian system, uses lanosterol as substrate, it has also been found that one isozyme is responsible for the whole oxidation sequence. The yeast cytochrome P450 has an apparent molecular weight of 58 kDa (Trzaskos et al. 1986).

Studies of the mode of action of sterol biosynthesis inhibitors are normally performed by gas chromotography-mass spectroscopy analysis of sterol patterns, comparing the patterns obtained after treatment with those of untreated controls. A typical example is shown in Table 8A.1, with vibunazole as a representative azole.

A dose-dependent accumulation of lanosterol is observed in S. lipolytica, whereas in filamentous fungi side-chain alkylation proceeds prior to C14 demethylation so that 24-methylene-dihydrolanosterol and sometimes other 14-α-methylsterols, such as obtusifoliol, are detected. This accumulation clearly indicates that the cytochrome P450 involved in the oxidative removal of the C14 methyl group is inhibited. Thus cytochrome P450 has been isolated from various sources, including mammalian livers, and a series of spectroscopic studies of azole interactions have been performed. Vanden Bossche (1988) has recently compared interactions of azole derivatives with cytochrome P450 isozymes from yeast, plant, and mammalian cells. The principle of interaction is always the same, with the free-electron pair of

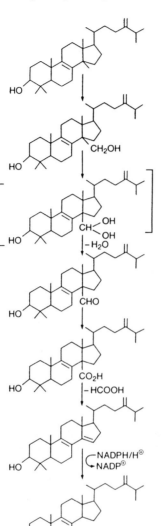

Fig. 8A.3 Cytochrome-P450-dependent demethylation at C14.

the heterocyclic nitrogen in the 3-position in imidazoles, or the 4-position in 1,2,4,-triazoles, binding directly to the iron atom of the iron-porphyrin complex of the cytochrome system (Fig. 8A.4).

The interaction of azoles with the prosthetic group of the cytochrome P450 system yields a type II difference binding spectrum (Fig. 8A.5). This interaction is distinct from that of the barbiturates, which exhibit

Table 8A.1 Sterol distribution in *Candida albicans* after application of vibunazole racemate (Bay n7133), (+)vibunazole (Bay r2303), and (−)vibunazole (Bay r2302)

	Steroid (%)			
	Control	Bay n7133 racemate (1 ppm)	Bay r2303 (1 ppm)	Bay r2302 (1 ppm)
ergosterol	100	–	14.5	–
14-methyl-$\Delta^{8,24(28)}$-ergostadien-ol (3)	–	9.7	8.6	9.2
4,14-dimethyl-$\Delta^{8,24(28)}$-ergostadien-ol (3)	–	24.2	18.5	24.1
lanosterol	–	12.3	10.3	13.3
24-methylenedihydro-lanosterol	–	28.7	28.0	36.4
$\Delta^{8,24(28)}$ergostadien-diol (3,6)	–	25.1	20.1	17.0
Total sterols ($\mu g/ml^{-1}$)	27.1	6.8	16.7	4.8

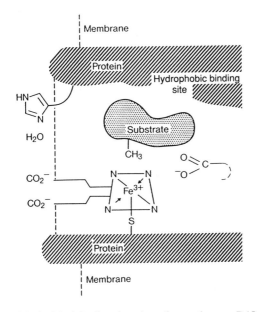

Fig. 8A.4 Model of active site of cytochrome P450.

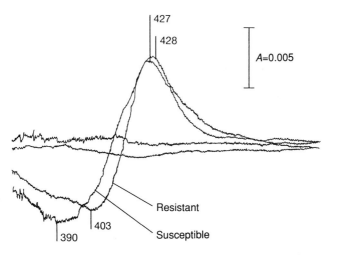

Fig. 8A.5 Difference spectra for cytochromes P450 of susceptible and resistant *S. lipolytica* with triadimenol as ligand.

type I difference binding spectra. The azoles compete with, for example, carbon monoxide for binding to the sixth coordination position of the reduced haeme iron in the prosthetic group. Even stereochemical implications for the fungicidal efficacy of fungicide isomers can be evaluated on this basis (Berg *et al.* 1988). Titration of cytochrome P450 14-α-demethylase with azoles indicates stoichiometric binding of the fungicides to the protein (Yoshida and Aoyama 1986). Variations with respect to binding systems have also been found with enzyme systems from other sources (Shaw *et al.* 1987), but additional aspects responsible for selectivity as well as binding capacity also have to be considered as an explanation for the *in vivo* activity of antifungal azoles. These differences are mainly caused by uptake, translocatlon, metabolism, etc. As mentioned earlier, the C14 demethylation sequence involves, as a final step, an NADPH/H$^+$-dependent reduction of the Δ^{14} double bond which is formed simultaneously with the loss of formic acid. Morpholine inhibitors may serve as promoters of this reaction.

8A.4   Inhibition of sterol-Δ^{14}-reductase

Discussion of the mode of action of morpholines became quite controversial some years ago when Kato *et al.* (1980) described an inhibition of $\Delta^8 \rightarrow \Delta^7$-isomerase in *Botryis cinerea* by the morpholine derivative tridemorph. At about the same time Kerkenaar *et al.* (1979) reached a different conclusion in studies of sterol synthesis in *Ustilago maydis*. As the latter workers were able to support their data using ^{1}H-NMR and UV spectroscopy, they showed convincingly that, at least in *U. maydis*, ignosterol and other $\Delta^{8,14}$ sterols accumulate after tridemorph administration.

Later, Baloch *et al.* (1984) demonstrated that these apparent discrepancies could easily be explained when they compared the effects of tridemorph and fenpropimorph (Fig. 8A.1(c)) on sterol synthesis in *S. cerevisiae* and *U. maydis*. These compounds inhibit both $\Delta^8 \rightarrow \Delta^7$-isomerase and sterol Δ^{14}-reductase, but to different degrees.

Kerkenaar *et al.* (1984) also showed that fenpropimorph inhibits sterol-Δ^{14}-reductase in *Penicillium italicum* as indicated by accumulation of ignosterol. Additionally, it was confirmed using the rice blast fungus *Pyricularia oryzae* that fenpropimorph leads to ignosterol accumulation and that tridemorph is a more potent inhibitor of sterol $\Delta^8 \rightarrow \Delta^7$-isomerase (Berg *et al.* 1984b). More recently, fenpropidine has been developed as an agricultural fungicide, and studies by Baloch and Mercer (1987) confirmed that the piperidine moiety of the molecule behaves similar to the dimethylmorpholines fenpropimorph and tridemorph.

To explain the inhibitory effect of the morpholines on the two enzymes at a molecular level, Benveniste (1986) invoked a structural similarity of the protonized morpholinium cations to the carbocationic high energy intermediates generated in the two different reactions. This is in agreement with the concept of transition state analogue as potent enzyme inhibitors.

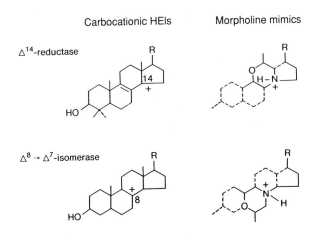

Carbocationic HEIs   Morpholine mimics

Δ^{14}-reductase

$\Delta^8 \rightarrow \Delta^7$-isomerase

Fig. 8A.6 High energy intermediates (HEIs) of Δ^{14}-reductase and $\Delta^8 \rightarrow \Delta^7$ isomerase and hypothetical interactions of inhibitors.

Amorolfine has been found useful as an antimycotic, although only topical application seems to be possible (Polak 1988).

8A.5   General aspects

Most of the compounds currently under development will serve as orally administered antimycotics or will be used in combined oral and topical treatments. Apart from improved compliance by the patient, the advantage of oral systemic compounds is the opportunity that they provide for treating organ mycoses such as those caused by dimorphic and opportunistic fungi. However, satisfactory treatments of such opportunistic infections have not yet been developed.

References

Baloch, R. I. and Mercer, E. I. (1987). Inhibition of sterol $\Delta^8 \rightarrow \Delta^7$-isomerase and Δ^{14}-reductase by fenpropimorph, tridemorph and fenpropidin in cell-free enzyme systems from *Saccharomyces cerevisiae*. *Phytochemistry*, **26**, 663–8.

Baloch, R. I., Mercer, E. I., Wiggins, T. E., and Baldwin, B. C. (1984). Inhibition of ergosterol biosynthesis in *Saccharomyces cerevisiae* and *Ustilago maydis* by tridemorph, fenpropimorph and fenpropidin. *Phytochemistry*, **23**, 2219–26.

Benvenste, P. (1986). Sterol biosynthesis. *Annual Review of Plant Physiology*, **37**, 275–308.

Berg, D. and Plempel, M. (ed.) (1988). *Sterol biosynthesis inhibitors*, VCH, Weinheim.

Berg, D., Krämer, W., Regel, E., Büchel, K. H., Holmwood, G., Plempel, M., and Scheinpflug, H. (1984b). Mode of action of fungicides: Studies on ergosterol biosynthesis inhibitors. *Proceedings of British Crop Protection Conference. Pest and Diseases*, 3, 887–92.

Berg, D., Regel, E., Harenberg, H.-E., and Plempel, M. (1984a). Bifonazole and clotrimazole. Their mode of action and the possible reason for the fungicidal behaviour of bifonazole. *Arzneimittel-Forschung*, 34, 139–46.

Berg, D., Born, L., Büchel, K. H., Holmwood, G., and Kaulen, J. (1987). HWG 1608—chemistry and biochemistry of a new azole fungicide. *Pflanzenschutz Nachrichten Bayer*, 40, 111–32.

Berg, D., Plempel, M., Büchel, K. H., Holmwood, G., and Stroech, K. (1988). Sterol biosynthesis inhibitors. Secondary effects and enhanced *in vivo* efficacy. *Annals of the New York Academy of Sciences*, 544, 338–47.

Büchel, K. H., Draber, W., Regel, E., and Plempel, M. (1972). Synthesis and properties of clotrimazole and other antimycotic 1-triphenylmethyl imidazoles. *Drugs Made In Germany*, 15, 208–9.

Dahl, J. S. and Dahl, C. E. (1985). Stimulation of cell proliferation and poly-phosphoinositide metabolism in *Saccharomyces cerevisiae* GL7 by ergosterol. *Biochemical and Biophysical Research Communications*, 133, 844–50.

Fryberg, M., Oehlschlager, A. C., and Unrau, A. M. (1975). Sterol biosynthesis in antibiotic sensitive and resistant *Candida*. *Archives of Biochemistry and Biophysics*, 173, 171–7.

Godefroi, E. F., Heeves, J., van Cutsem, J., and Janssen, P. A. J. (1969). The preparation and antimycotic properties of derivatives of 1-phenylethylimidazole. *Journal of Medicinal Chemistry*, 12, 784–91.

Goulston, G., Goad, L. J., and Goodwin, T. W. (1967). Sterol biosynthesis in fungi. *Biochemical Journal*, 102, 15c–17c.

Kato, T., Shoami, M., and Kawase, Y. (1980). Comparison of tridemorph with buthiobate in antifungal mode of action. *Journal of Pesticide Science*, 5, 69–79.

Kerkenaar, A., Barug, D., and Kaars-Sijpesteijn, A. (1979). On the antifungal mode of action of tridemorph. *Pesticide Biochemistry and Physiology*, 12, 195–204.

Kerkenaar, A., van Rossum, J. M., Versluis, G. G., and Marsman, J. W. (1984). Effect of fenpropemorph and imazalil on sterol biosynthesis in Penicillium italicum. *Pesticide Science*, 15, 177–87.

Leroux, P. and Gredt, M. (1978). Effect of imazalil [1-(2-(2,4-dichlorophenyl)-2-(2-propanyloxy) ethyl)-IH-imidazole] on ergosterol biosynthesis in *Penicillium expansum* link. *Comptes Rendus Hebdomadaire des Séances de l'Académie des Sciences*, 286, 427–9.

Mercer, E. I. (1984). The biosynthesis of ergosterol. *Pesticide Science*, 15, 133–55.

Nes, W. R. (1984). Uniformity vs. diversity in the structure, biosynthesis and functions of sterols. In *Isopentenoids in plants* (ed. W. D. Nes, G. Fuller, and L.-S. Tsai), pp. 325–47. Dekker, New York.

Polak, A. (1988). Morpholines in clinical use. In *Sterol biosynthesis inhibitors* (ed. D. Berg and M. Plempel), pp. 430–48. VCH, Weinheim.

Ragsdale, N. N. (1975). Specific effects of triarimol on steroid biosynthesis in *Ustilago maydis*. *Biochimica et Biophysica Acta*, 380, 81–96.

Rodriguez, R. J. and Parks, L. W. (1983). Structural and physiological features of sterols necessary to satisfy bulk membrane and sparking requirements in yeast sterol auxotrophs. *Archives of Biochemistry and Biophysics*, 225, 861–71.

Rodriguez, R. J., Low, C., Bottema, C. D. K., and Parks, L. W. (1985). Multiple functions for sterols in *Saccharomyces cerevisiae*. *Biochimica et Biophysica Acta*, **837**, 336–43.

Shaw, J. T. B., Tarbit, M. H., and Troke, P. F. (1987). Cytochrome P-450 mediated sterol synthesis and metabolism: differences in sensitivity to fluconazole and other azoles. In *Recent trends in the discovery, development and evaluation of antifungal agents* (ed. R. A. Fromtling), pp. 125–39. Prous, Barcelona.

Taylor, F. R. and Parks, L. W. (1980). Adaption of *Saccharomyces cerevisiae* to growth on cholesterol: selection of mutants defective in the formation of lanosterol. *Biochemical and Biophysical Research Communications*, **95**, 1437–45.

Thompson, E. D. and Parks, L. W. (1974). The effect of altered sterol composition on cytochrome oxidase and *S*-adenosylmethionine: Δ24 sterol methyltransferase enzymes in yeast mitochondria. *Biochemical and Biophysical Research Communications*, **57**, 1207–13.

Trzaskos, J., Fischer, R. T., and Favata, M. F. (1986b). Mechanistic studies on lanosterol C-32 demethylation. Conditions which promote oxysterol intermediate accumulation during the demethylation process. *Journal of Biological Chemistry*, **261**, 16937–42.

Trzaskos, J., Kawata, S., and Gaylor, J. L. (1986a). Microsomal enzymes of cholesterol biosynthesis. Purification of lanosterol 14a-methyl demethylase cytochrome P-450 from hepatic microsomes. *Journal of Biological Chemistry*, **261**, 14651–7.

Vanden Bossche, H. (1988). Mode of action of pyridine, pyrimidine and azole antifungals. In *Sterol biosynthesis inhibitors* (ed. D. Berg and M. Plempel), pp. 79–119. VCH, Weinheim.

Vanden Bossche, H., Willemsens, G., Cools, W., Lauwers, W. F. J., and Le Jeune, L. (1978). Biochemical effects of miconazole on fungi II. Inhibition of ergosterol biosynthesis in *Candida albicans*. *Chemical and Biological Interactions*, **21**, 59–78.

Vanden Bossche, H., Marichal, P., Gorrens, J., Bellens, D., Verhoeven, H., Coene, M.-C., Lauwers, W., and Janssen, P. A. J. (1984). Molecular basis for the antimycotic and antibacterial activity of N-substituted imidazoles and triazoles: the inhibition of isopenoid biosynthesis. *Pesticide Science*, **15**, 188–205.

Yamaguchi, H. and Osumi, M. (1988). Morphological aspects of azole action. In *Sterol biosynthesis inhibitors* (ed. D. Berg and M. Plempel), pp. 56–78. VCH, Weinheim.

Yoshida, Y. and Aoyama, Y. (1986). Interaction of azole fungicides with yeast cytochrome P-450 which catalyses lanosterol 14a-demethylation. In *In vitro and in vivo evaluation of antifungal agents* (ed. K. Iwata and H. Vanden Bossche), pp. 123–4. Elsevier, Amsterdam.

Section 8B

Inhibitors of squalene epoxidase

Neil S. Ryder, Anton Stuetz, and Peter Nussbaumer

8B.1   Introduction

Squalene epoxidase is a key enzyme in the biosynthetic sequence from acetyl coenzyme A to ergosterol (in fungi) or cholesterol (in mammals) (see Section 8A, Fig. 8A.2). Epoxidation of the long-chain hydrocarbon squalene is a necessary condition for subsequent cyclization to form the rigid tetracyclic sterol structure. Sterols are essential for fungal growth, and appear to have at least four levels of function, including the 'sparking function' (Rodriguez *et al.* 1985) which is highly specific for ergosterol in the nanogram per millilitre range. The importance of ergosterol for fungi is underlined by the fact that the major classes of antifungal agent act by interfering with either its biosynthesis (azoles, allylamines, morpholines) or its function in membranes (polyenes).

Squalene epoxidase has emerged as a major target for antifungal drugs as a result of the recent development of the allylamine class of anti-mycotics (Petranyi *et al.* 1984). Naftifine (**1**, Fig. 8B.1), the prototype of these compounds, was the first specific inhibitor of squalene epoxidase to be reported (Paltauf *et al.* 1982; Ryder *et al.* 1984; Ryder and Dupont 1985). Naftifine has been in clinical use for several years as a topically

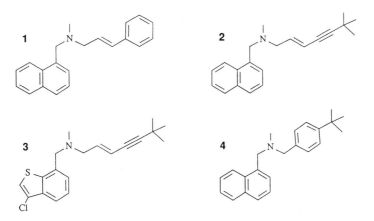

Fig. 8B.1 Structures of naftifine (**1**), terbinafine (**2**), SDZ 87-469 (**3**), and butenafine (**4**).

applied antimycotic. The fungicidal activity of naftifine against a wide range of pathogenic fungi (Georgopoulos *et al.* 1981; Petranyi *et al.* 1987a,b), combined with its novel mode of action, made this compound an attractive lead for the development of more potent drugs. An extensive programme of chemical derivatization (Stuetz and Petranyi 1984; Stuetz *et al.* 1986; Stuetz 1987, 1988) led to the development of terbinafine (**2**), a potent antimycotic (Petranyi *et al.* 1987a, b) which is also effective after oral administration. Terbinafine has been on the market since 1991 as an oral antimycotic which is highly effective against fungal infections of the skin, nails, and hair, and may also be of use in the treatment of some more serious systemic infections (Villars and Jones 1992). The biological and clinical activities of the allylamines have been covered in detail in a recent review (Ryder and Mieth 1991).

The identification of the allylamines as squalene epoxidase inhibitors led to a search for further inhibitors of the enzyme and has also provided a valuable biochemical tool for investigation of the epoxidase. Some other epoxidase inhibitors with well-characterized antifungal activity include SDZ 87−469 (**3**) (Stuetz and Nussbaumer 1989; Nussbaumer *et al.* 1991b) and the benzylamine butenafine (**4**) (Arika *et al.* 1990). Members of a second class of antifungals, the thiocarbamates, have now also been found to inhibit fungal squalene epoxidase, and efforts have also been made to design inhibitors of the enzyme. An interesting and therapeutically valuable property of the antifungal allylamines is that they show high selectivity against the fungal squalene epoxidase and have little effect on the corresponding mammalian enzyme (Ryder and Dupont 1985; Ryder 1988b). However, the mammalian squalene epoxidase itself has recently become of pharmaceutical interest as a potential target for anti-cholesterolaemic drugs.

8B.2   Properties of squalene epoxidase

The 2,3-epoxidation of squalene (Fig. 8B.2) is performed by a microsomal enzyme complex consisting of a flavoprotein with NAD(P)H cytochrome *c* reductase activity and a terminal oxidase, the squalene epoxidase (EC 1.14.99.7). This enzyme was first described by Yamamoto and Bloch (1970) in rat liver extracts. Squalene epoxidase is the first enzyme in the sterol pathway to require molecular oxygen, an aspect which is of considerable evolutionary significance. Virtually all eukaryotic organisms (except insects) have the ability to synthesize sterols and therefore possess squalene epoxidase, but up to now the enzyme has been investigated only in mammalian liver and some yeasts. The detailed enzymology of squalene epoxidase was the subject of a recent review (Ryder 1990a).

8B.2.1   Fungal squalene epoxidase

In fungal ergosterol biosynthesis, squalene epoxidase is of particular significance as the step at which the pathway is regulated by availability of oxygen. There is evidence (M'Baya *et al.* 1989) that, in yeast, squalene epoxidase is a rate-limiting step, permitting regulation by oxygen and by sterol levels in the cell. Klein *et al.* (1967) first demonstrated the conversion of squalene to lanosterol in yeast membrane fractions. Subsequently, microsomal squalene epoxidase has been partially characterized in *Saccharomyces cerevisiae* (M'Baya and Karst 1987) and in the pathogenic

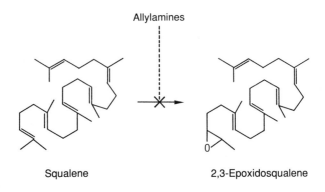

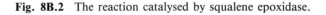

Fig. 8B.2 The reaction catalysed by squalene epoxidase.

yeasts *Candida albicans* (Ryder and Dupont 1984) and *Candida parapsilosis* (Ryder and Dupont 1985).

Fungal squalene epoxidases are membrane-bound enzymes requiring molecular oxygen, FAD, and a reduced pyridine nucleotide. In *Candida* the preferred cofactor is NADH while in yeast it is NADPH, as in the case of the mammalian enzyme. Squalene epoxidase is not an enzyme of the cytochrome P450 superfamily and is unaffected by inhibitors such as carbon monoxide or cyanide (Ryder and Dupont 1984). The epoxidase contains no haeme and appears to have no metal ion requirements. Both thiol reagents and copper ions inhibit the *C. albicans* epoxidase. The distinctive nature of squalene epoxidase has been confirmed by the reported cloning of an epoxidase from *Saccharomyces* (Jandrositz *et al*. 1991), the predicted sequence of which shows no significant homology to any known proteins. The molecular mechanism of squalene epoxidation is currently not well understood. Assuming the epoxidase to be a non-metallic flavoprotein monooxygenase, consistent with its known properties, Oehlschlager and Czyzewska (1992) have postulated a theoretical mechanism involving flavin 4a-hydroperoxide intermediates.

Fungal squalene epoxidases have no requirement for soluble cytoplasmic proteins but are markedly influenced by lipids and detergents. The *C. albicans* epoxidase is strongly inhibited by a range of ionic detergents (Ryder 1990a), including Triton X-100, which has been shown to cause irreversible inactivation of the yeast enzyme (Hata *et al*. 1982). Some nonionic detergents are stimulatory, and a fully soluble enzyme preparation from *Candida* could be made in this way (Ryder 1987). Some fatty acids, particularly long-chain polyunsaturates, also stimulate the enzyme (Ryder 1990a). In this connection, there is evidence that epoxidase activity in yeast may be regulated by membrane fatty acid composition, as a source of unsaturated fatty acids is essential for epoxidase activity in the cells (Buttke *et al*. 1988).

8B.2.2   Mammalian squalene epoxidase

The microsomal squalene epoxidase system from rat liver has been extensively investigated and the components purified (Ono *et al*. 1977, 1982). The purified epoxidase was described as a single 51 kDa polypeptide which required addition of NADPH-cytochrome c reductase, NADPH, FAD, oxygen, and Triton X-100 for reconstitution of activity. As in fungi, the rat epoxidase is clearly distinct from the cytochrome P450 class and does not contain haeme. An interesting difference between the fungal and mammalian microsomal epoxidases is that the latter show an almost complete requirement for the soluble cytoplasmic fraction (Yamamoto and Bloch 1970; Ryder and Dupont 1985). At least two stimulatory protein factors have been isolated from rat liver (reviewed by Ryder (1990a)) but their role *in vivo* is not clear. Although fungal squalene epoxidase shows no requirement for these factors, they appear to be present in both yeast (Dempsey and Meyer 1977) and *Candida* (Ryder 1987). There is good evidence that squalene epoxidase is a secondary site of regulation of cholesterol biosynthesis in rat liver and in the human hepatoma HepG2 cell line, with its activity being modulated by cellular cholesterol levels but not by non-sterol products of mevalonate (Hidaka *et al.* 1990; Satoh *et al.* 1990).

8B.3 Inhibition by allylamines

8B.3.1 Inhibition of fungal squalene epoxidase

Both naftifine and terbinafine are potent dose-dependent inhibitors of *Candida* squalene epoxidase (Ryder and Dupont 1985). In kinetic analysis with *C. albicans* microsomal squalene epoxidase, naftifine and terbinafine both show apparent non-competitive inhibition with respect to the substrate squalene, with K_i values of 1.1 μM and 0.03 μM respectively. Although such results are to be regarded with caution in the case of a water-insoluble substrate and product, this finding is compatible with the fact that the antifungal action is not reversed by the high squalene con-centrations which occur in treated fungal cells. The inhibition is also non-competitive with the cofactors FAD, NADH, and NADPH (Ryder and Dupont 1985). The fully reversible inhibition, with no observable time-dependent effects, rules out a mechanism-based type of inhibition. Similar results have been obtained with the epoxidase from *C. parapsilosis* (Table 8B.1); studies with epoxidase from other fungi have not been performed. Inhibition by terbinafine is unaffected by detergent solubi-lization of the enzyme (Ryder 1987), indicating that the effect is not dependent on membrane integrity.

Table 8B.1 Inhibition of *Candida* microsomal squalene epoxidase by allylamines

Compound	Concentration (μM) for 50% inhibition	
	C. albicans	*C. parapsilosis*
1	1.1	0.34
2	0.03	0.04
3	0.011	0.02

Microsomal squalene epoxidase was assayed as described by Ryder and Dupont (1984).
Data from Ryder and Dupont (1985) and Ryder *et al.* (1992).

8B.3.2   Structure–activity relationships

Well over a thousand compounds of the allylamine class have been synthesized and tested for antifungal activity (Stuetz and Petranyi 1984; Stuetz
et al. 1986; Stuetz 1988; Nussbaumer *et al.* 1991a,b), and about a hundred
of these have been examined biochemically. Representatives of major structural variations are shown in Fig. 8B.3, and their inhibitory potencies
are given in Table 8B.2. These studies indicate that squalene epoxidase
inhibition is required for antifungal activity but, as described later, does
not guarantee it. Penetration of the fungal cell envelope is a further
prerequisite for antifungal activity which is independently influenced by
structural features of the inhibitor. The structural requirements for epoxidase inhibition have been described in detail by Ryder *et al.* (1992).

Considerable modification of the allylamine side-chain is permitted while
retaining epoxidase inhibitory activity. A minimum length of side-chain is
critical for inhibition in the submicromolar range, as seen by comparing
compounds **1**, **2**, and **5**. Compounds with shorter side-chains, including
simple 1-substituted naphthalenes, inhibit the enzyme in the millimolar

Table 8B.2 Inhibition of *C. albicans* squalene epoxidase
by structurally modified allylamine derivatives

Compound	Concentration (μM) for 50% inhibition	
	Epoxidase	Cell-free system
1	1.1	0.59
2	0.03	0.03
3	0.011	0.007
4	0.045	0.05
5	190	–
6	0.04	–
7	–	38.8
8	0.05	–
9	–	0.64
10	–	3.2
11	–	0.24
12	2.16	–
13	3.9	–
14	0.37	–

The test systems employed were microsomal squalene epoxidase
(Ryder and Dupont 1984) and a cell-free ergosterol biosynthesis
system with [^{14}C]mevalonate as substrate (Ryder 1985a).
Data from Ryder *et al.* (1992).

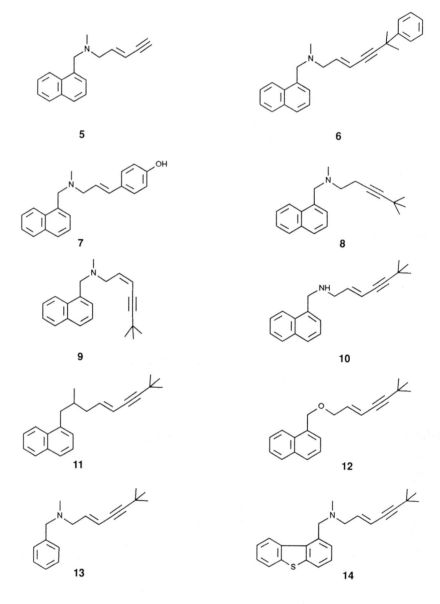

Fig. 8B.3 Structures of modified allylamine derivatives.

range (Ryder *et al.* 1992), implying that the aromatic portion of the molecule alone provides a low affinity binding to the enzyme. The terbinafine side-chain appears to be of optimum length and further extension does not increase activity (compound **6**), whereas addition of a polar group, as in **7**, has a negative influence. The allylamine double bond is not essential for activity (see compounds **4** and **8**), but when present is required to be in the *trans* configuration (compare **2** and **9**). The *N*-methyl group is necessary for high inhibitory potency (compare **2** and **10**) but further extension does not improve activity.

In order to investigate the influence of the amino nitrogen, a series of carbon analogues of allylamines was synthesized (Nussbaumer *et al.* 1991a). This work revealed that the nitrogen is important in providing the correct molecular configuration but is not in itself necessary for epoxidase inhibition, as clearly shown by the activity of compound **11**. This is supported by the significant activity of compound **12** in which the amino nitrogen is replaced by oxygen. However, the tertiary amine appears to be important for penetration of the compound through the fungal cell envelope (Nussbaumer *et al.* 1991a; Ryder *et al.* 1992), thus explaining why the carbon analogues have no significant antifungal activity despite their effective inhibition of squalene epoxidase.

The size of the aromatic ring system is critical for full activity of the allylamines. Neither monocyclic (compound **13**) nor tricyclic (compound **14**) structures can adequately replace the naphthalene ring, but modification of the ring structure is permitted and can lead to increased activity. This is demonstrated by the case of SDZ 87–469 (**3**) which is the most potent inhibitor of the fungal squalene epoxidase to have been identified and is a correspondingly potent antifungal agent (Stuetz and Nussbaumer 1989; Nussbaumer *et al.* 1991b).

8B.3.3 Inhibition of mammalian squalene epoxidase

During the testing and development of terbinafine, the drug was shown to have no significant effect on cholesterol levels or biosynthesis in experimental animals or in patients. Similarly, terbinafine and related compounds showed only very weak inhibitory activity in an *in vivo* cholesterol biosynthesis system from rat liver (Ryder 1985a, 1988b). Subsequent studies revealed that this favourable profile is due to a high degree of selectivity at the enzymatic level (Ryder and Dupont 1985; Ryder 1987, 1990a). Naftifine and terbinafine are only very weak inhibitors of rat liver microsomal squalene epoxidase (Table 8B.3). Inhibition of the rat liver enzyme by terbinafine is reversible and non-competitive with the cofactors FAD and NAD(P)H, but, in contrast with the fungal system, is competitive with respect to the substrate squalene. Unlike its fungal counterpart, the activity of rat liver epoxidase is almost completely dependent on the soluble cytoplasmic protein fraction. This fraction was also found to interact competitively with terbinafine in the epoxidase assay, but not to an extent which would account for the selective action of the drug. Mammalian

Table 8B.3 Selective inhibition of fungal and mammalian squalene epoxidase

Compound	Concentration (μM) for 50% inhibition			
	C. albicans epoxidase	C. albicans cell-free	Rat liver epoxidase	Guinea-pig epoxidase
1	1.1	0.59	144	>137
2	0.03	0.03	77	4
3	0.011	0.007	43	1.2
15	–	34	0.004 *	

Test systems are microsomal squalene epoxidase from *C. albicans*, rat liver, and guinea-pig (Ryder 1987), and a cell-free ergosterol biosynthesis system from *C. albicans* (Ryder 1985a). Data from Ryder *et al.* (1992).

*Value from Horie *et al.* (1990).

squalene epoxidases vary in their sensitivity to allylamines, with the guinea pig enzyme being particularly sensitive (Ryder 1987). The basis for these differences, and for the much greater differences between the fungal and mammalian enzymes, is still not known.

The allylamine derivative NB-598 (**15**, Fig. 8B.4), with a terbinafine-type side-chain and a considerably modified and extended ring system, has been reported as a potent inhibitor of human and mammalian squalene epoxidases both *in vitro* and *in vivo* (Horie *et al.* 1990, 1991). As with terbinafine, NB-598 is also competitive with squalene, but is much more potent (K_i for human microsomal epoxidase of 0.68 nM) (Horie *et al.* 1990). Interestingly, NB-598 is virtually inactive against the fungal epoxidase (Ryder *et al.* 1992) and has no anti-fungal activity (Horie *et al.* 1990), thus displaying a selectivity profile which is exactly the reverse of that of terbinafine (Table 8B.3).

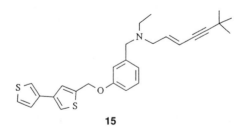

15

Fig. 8B.4 Structure of NB-598 (**15**).

8B.3.4   Mechanism of inhibition

The kinetic properties and the known structural requirements for epoxidase inhibition argue against a mechanism-based irreversible type of inhibition by the allylamines. Amongst other possible targets for inhibition, terbinafine does not inhibit the reductase enzyme, interacts only weakly with the soluble cytoplasmic fraction (mammalian enzyme), and does not require membrane integrity for activity. The high selectivity for the fungal enzyme and the non-competitive kinetics of terbinafine render it unlikely to be a competitor for the squalene substrate. However, the aromatic ring system may interact with the squalene binding site of the enzyme, as suggested by the weak inhibitory activity of 1-substituted naphthalene derivatives (Ryder *et al.* 1992) This may also represent the mechanism of the weak competitive inhibition of mammalian squalene epoxidase by the antifungal allylamines. A number of lipophilic compounds have been reported to inhibit the rat liver epoxidase at high concentrations (Morin and Srikantaiah 1982). The extended structure of NB-598 would have the appropriate length to mimic squalene (or an intermediate of the reaction) and shows high affinity competitive inhibition.

In the case of the fungal epoxidase, the current hypothesis is that the allylamine side-chain interacts with a lipophilic pocket, perhaps a lipid-binding site, adjacent to the active site. Squalene epoxidase is known to require phospholipids for activity, and to be influenced by fatty acids and detergents as described earlier. This lipophilic binding, combined with the interaction of the aromatic ring with the squalene-binding site, would then result in a high affinity of inhibitor for enzyme by the principle of entropic binding (Ryder 1990b, 1991). The requirement for a minimum length of side-chain to act as a rigid bridge between the two binding sites is in agreement with this model, as is the observation that the terbinafine side-chain alone has no inhibitory activity at concentrations up to 1 mM. The selectivity shown by terbinafine, and in the reverse sense by NB-598, can be explained by differences in the configuration of the two postulated binding sites. Nevertheless, this model, although compatible with all the experimental evidence, is still speculative and remains to be confirmed by further studies.

8B.4   Other epoxidase inhibitors

8B.4.1   Thiocarbamates

The topical antimycotic tolnaftate (**16**, Fig. 8B.5), first synthesized by Noguchi *et al.* (1962), shows some structural similarity to naftifine, although the two classes of compound are chemically quite distinct. Tolnaftate also inhibits fungal ergosterol biosynthesis and *Candida* microsomal squalene

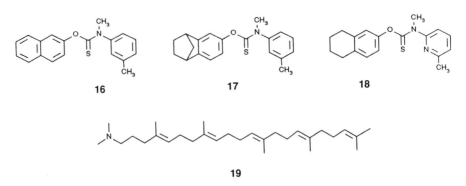

Fig. 8B.5 Structures of tolnaftate (**16**), tolciclate (**17**), piritetrate (**18**), and 2-aza-2,3-dihydrosqualene (**19**).

epoxidase (Morita and Nozawa 1985; Barrett-Bee *et al.* 1986; Ryder *et al.* 1986b; Nozawa and Morita 1992), indicating that the mode of action of this drug is similar to that of the allylamines. Similar results have been found with the closely related compounds tolciclate (**17**) (Ryder *et al.* 1986b) and piritetrate (**18**) (Morita *et al.* 1989). In common with the allyl-amines, the thiocarbamates are selective for the fungal squalene epoxidase (Table 8B.4) and have little effect on the rat liver enzyme (Ryder *et al.* 1986b; Morita *et al.* 1989; Nozawa and Morita 1992). Compounds **16** and **17**, although highly active against dermatophyte fungi, have little activity *in vitro* against *C. albicans*. This was found to be due to poor penetration of the compounds through the *Candida* cell envelope (Ryder *et al.* 1986b).

Table 8B.4 Inhibition of fungal and mammalian sterol biosynthesis and squalene epoxidase by thiocarbamates and azasqualene

Compound	Concentration (μM) for 50% inhibition			
	C. albicans epoxidase	*C. albicans* cell-free	Rat liver epoxidase	Rat liver cell-free
16	1.04	0.42	–	137
17[*]	0.12	0.03	–	124
19[†]	32.9	6.6	2.4	–

The test systems employed are microsomal squalene epoxidase (Ryder and Dupont 1985), and cell-free sterol biosynthesis with mevalonate as substrate (Ryder 1985a).

[*] Data from Ryder *et al.* (1986b).

[†] Data from Ryder *et al.* (1986a).

Detailed mechanistic and kinetic studies with the thiocarbamates have not been reported, and therefore it is not certain whether their mechanism of inhibition is identical with that of the allylamines.

8B.4.2 Squalene derivatives

The squalene derivative 2-aza-2,3-dihydrosqualene (**19**, Fig. 8B.5) is one of a range of compounds synthesized by Cattel and co-workers as potential inhibitors of the 2,3-oxidosqualene cyclase reaction immediately distal to squalene epoxidase in the sterol pathway. Some of these compounds inhibit growth and ergosterol biosynthesis in yeast (Balliano *et al.* 1988). Compound **19** was found to inhibit both squalene epoxidase and the cyclase from *C. albicans* as well as another unidentified step in the pathway (Ryder *et al.* 1986a). However, **19** was much more effective against the rat liver epoxidase (Table 8B.4). Despite the obvious structural similarity of **19** to the substrate squalene, no clear evidence of competitive inhibition could be obtained in kinetic studies. Compound **14** was a weak inhibitor of the cyclase with IC_{50} values of 6.5 μM and 32 μM for the *C. albicans* and rat liver enzyme respectively.

In another approach, a number of synthetic structural variants of squalene have been reported by Prestwich and coworkers as inhibitors of mammalian squalene epoxidase. These include trisnorsqualene cyclopropylamine, a reversible inhibitor with $K_i = 2$ μM (Sen and Prestwich 1989a), trisnorsqualene alcohol, a non-competitive inhibitor with $K_i = 4$ μM (Sen and Prestwich 1989b; Sen *et al.* 1990), and 26-hydroxysqualene, a competitive inhibitor ($K_i = 4$ μM) which also acts as a substrate (Bai *et al.* 1991). Some allenic and acetylenic squalene derivatives with weak activity (in the 0.1 mM range) against rat liver squalene epoxidase have been described by Cattel *et al.* (1989). With the exception of compound **19**, no information is available concerning the effect of these squalene derivatives in fungal systems.

8B.5 Antimycotic efficacy of allylamines

8B.5.1 Basis of fungicidal action

Naftifine and terbinafine are active *in vitro* against a wide range of pathogenic fungi, with a primary fungicidal action in the majority of cases (Georgopoulos *et al.* 1981; Petranyi *et al.* 1987a,b; Ryder and Mieth 1991). There is comprehensive evidence that inhibition of squalene epoxidase is the primary mechanism of these and related anti-fungal allylamines. Among the approximately 100 compounds examined, epoxidase inhibition is a precondition for antifungal activity, and, in general, there is a good correlation between these two parameters, with some exceptions as described previously.

Quantitatively, the inhibition of squalene epoxidase can account for the observed inhibition of cellular ergosterol biosynthesis which has been documented in a number of studies (Ryder *et al.* 1984; Ryder 1985a,b, 1988a). In addition, experiments with cell-free assays for various steps of the ergosterol pathway have failed to find evidence for any significant effect of the allylamines on other enzymes of the pathway (Ryder 1985a, 1988a). Comparison of results from a range of pathogenic fungi also shows good correlation between inhibition of fungal growth and of ergosterol biosynthesis for both naftifine and terbinafine (Ryder 1988a, 1992), although of course physiological differences between fungal species also play an important role in determining susceptibility. Inhibition of squalene epoxidase leads to both ergosterol deficiency and an accumulation of high levels of intracellular squalene. Since ergosterol is essential for fungal growth, the blockade of its biosynthesis would explain the growth-inhibitory fungistatic action of the allylamines. However, the major cause of fungal cell killing by the drug is now thought to be the accumulation of squalene, which has been shown in analytical studies to correlate well with the onset of cell death (Ryder *et al.* 1985; Ryder 1992). The exact mechanism by which this process occurs is still not clear, but is believed to involve progressive loss of intracellular membrane integrity.

8B.5.2   Clinical implications

The specific mechanism of the allylamines is of considerable significance for the clinical application of these drugs. The fungicidal mechanism is a definite advantage, particularly in the case of immunocompromised patients or patients with protracted infections which are difficult to reach, such as in the nails. Oral terbinafine has proved to be a highly effective therapy in nail infections, permitting a significantly shorter period of treatment (Baudraz-Rosselet *et al.* 1992; Goodfield 1992). In addition to its well-established efficacy in dermatology, there is preliminary evidence for clinical application of terbinafine against some more serious systemic fungal infections (Villars and Jones 1992).

Terbinafine is very well tolerated in patients, both systemically and in the skin (Villars and Jones 1992). The high selectivity of the allylamines for fungal squalene epoxidase is of clinical relevance in that no side-effects related to inhibition of human cholesterol biosynthesis are encountered. The more recent discovery of related compounds such as NB-598, with specificity for mammalian squalene epoxidase, may lead to a new class of hypocholesterolaemic drugs.

The apparently unique nature of squalene epoxidase, and in particular its lack of similarity to the cytochrome P_{450} superfamily, is also important in the clinical context. Unlike those antifungal agents which act by inhibition of fungal cytochrome P_{450}, the allylamines have no intrinsic tendency to inhibit this very important class of enzymes, thus avoiding a range of potential side-effects. In human liver, terbinafine binds to, and is metabolized by, only a small proportion (less than 5 per cent) of the total cytochromes P450 (Schuster 1987a). The drug does not inhibit cytochrome P450 types from various human and animal tissues (Schuster 1985, 1987b), neither does it have any influence on the metabolism of other drugs tested (Back *et al.* 1992).

References

Arika, T., Yokoo, M., Hase, T., Maeda, T., Amemiya, K., and Yamaguchi, H. (1990). Effects of butenafine hydrochloride, a new benzylamine derivative, on experimental dermatophytosis in guinea pigs. *Antimicrobial Agents and Chemotherapy*, **34**, 2250–3.

Back, D. J., Tjia, J. F., and Abel, S. M. (1992). Azoles, allylamines and drug metabolism. *British Journal of Dermatology*, **126** (Suppl. 39), 14–18.

Bai, M., Xiao, X., and Prestwich, G. D. (1991). 26-Hydroxysqualene and derivatives: substrates and inhibitors for squalene epoxidase. *Bioorganic and Medicinal Chemistry Letters*, **1**, 227–32.

Balliano, G., Viola, F., Ceruti, M., and Cattel, L. (1988). Inhibition of sterol biosynthesis in *Saccharomyces cerevisiae* by *N,N*-diethylazasqualene and derivatives. *Biochimica et Biophysica Acta*, **959**, 9–19.

Barrett-Bee, K., Lane, A. C., and Turner, R. W. (1986). The mode of action of tolnaftate. *Journal of Medical and Veterinary Mycology*, **24**, 155–60.

Baudraz-Rosselet, F., Rakosi, T., Wili, P. B., and Kenzelmann, R. (1992). Treatment of onychomycosis with terbinafine. *British Journal of Dermatology*, **126** (Suppl. 39), 40–6.

Buttke, T. M., Brint, S. L., and Lowe, M. R. (1988). Regulation of squalene epoxidase activity by membrane fatty acid composition in yeast. *Lipids*, **23**, 68–71.

Cattel, L., Ceruti, M., Balliano, G., Viola, F., Grosa, G., and Schuber, F. (1989). Drug design based on biosynthetic studies: synthesis, biological activity, and kinetics of new inhibitors of 2,3-oxidosqualene cyclase and squalene epoxidase. *Steroids*, **53**, 363–91.

Dempsey, M. E. and Meyer, G. M. (1977). Purification of yeast sterol carrier protein. *Federation Proceedings. Federation of American Societies for Experimental Biology*, **36**, 779.

Georgopoulos, A. G., Petranyi, G., Mieth, H., and Drews, J. (1981). *In vitro* activity of naftifine, a new antifungal agent. *Antimicrobial Agents and Chemotherapy*, **19**, 386–9.

Goodfield, M. J. D. (1992). Short-duration therapy with terbinafine for dermatophyte onychomycosis: a multicentre trial. *British Journal of Dermatology*, **126** (Suppl. 39), 33–5.

Hata, S., Nishino, T., Ariga, N., and Katsuki, H. (1982). Effect of detergents on sterol synthesis in a cell-free system of yeast. *Journal of Lipid Research*, **23**, 803–10.

Hidaka, Y., Satoh, T., and Kamei, T. (1990). Regulation of squalene epoxidase in HepG2 cells. *Journal of Lipid Research*, **31**, 2087–94.

Horie, M., Tsuchiya, Y., Hayashi, M., Iida, Y., Iwasawa, Y., Nagata, Y., et al. (1990). NB-598: a potent competitive inhibitor of squalene epoxidase. *Journal of Biological Chemistry*, **265**, 18075–8.

Horie, M., Sawasaki, Y., Fukuzumi, H., Watanabe, K., Iizuka, Y., Tsuchiya, Y., and Kamei, T. (1991). Hypolipidemic effects of NB-598 in dogs. *Atherosclerosis*, **88**, 183–92.

Jandrositz, A., Turnowsky, F., and Hoegenauer, G. (1991). The gene encoding squalene epoxidase from *Saccharomyces cerevisiae*: cloning and characterization. *Gene*, **107**, 155–160.

Klein, H. P., Volkmann, C. M., and Leaffer, M. A. (1967). Subcellular sites involved in lipid synthesis in *Saccharomyces cerevisiae*. *Journal of Bacteriology*, **94**, 61–5.

M'Baya, B. and Karst, F. (1987). *In vitro* assay of squalene epoxidase of *Saccharomyces cerevisiae*. *Biochemical and Biophysical Research Communications*, **147**, 556–64.

M'Baya, B., Fegueur, M., Servouse, M., and Karst, F. (1989). Regulation of squalene synthetase and squalene epoxidase activities in *Saccharomyces cerevisiae*. *Lipids*, **24**, 1020–3.

Morin, R. J. and Srikantaiah, M. V. (1982). Inhibition of rat liver sterol formation by isoprenoid and conjugated ene compounds. *Pharmacological Research Communications*, **14**, 941–7.

Morita, T. and Nozawa, Y. (1985). Effects of antifungal agents on ergosterol biosynthesis in *Candida albicans* and *Trichophyton mentagraphytes*: differential inhibitory sites of naphthiomate and miconazole. *Journal of Investigative Dermatology*, **85**, 434–7.

Morita, T., Iwata, K., and Nozawa, Y. (1989). Inhibitory effect of a new mycotic agent, piritetrate on ergosterol biosynthesis in pathogenic fungi. *Journal of Medical and Veterinary Mycology*, **27**, 17–25.

Noguchi, T., Kaji, A., Igarashi, Y., Shigematsu, A., and Taniguchi, K. (1962). Antitrichophyton activity of naphthiomates. *Antimicrobial Agents and Chemotherapy*, **2**, 259–67.

Nozawa, Y. and Morita, T. (1992). Biochemical aspects of squalene epoxidase inhibition by a thiocarbamate derivative, naphthiomate-T. In *Recent progress in antifungal chemotherapy* (ed. H. Yamaguchi, G. S. Kobayashi, and H. Takahashi), pp. 53–64. Marcel Dekker, New York.

Nussbaumer, P., Ryder, N. S., and Stuetz, A. (1991a). Allylamine antimycotics: recent trends in structure–activity relationships and syntheses. *Pesticide Science*, **31**, 437–55.

Nussbaumer, P., Petranyi, G., and Stuetz, A. (1991b). Synthesis and structure–activity relationships of benzo[*b*]thienylallylamine antimycotics. *Journal of Medicinal Chemistry*, **34**, 65–73.

Oehlschlager, A. C. and Czyzewska, E. (1992). Rationally designed inhibitors of sterol biosynthesis. In *Emerging targets in antibacterial and antifungal chemotherapy* (ed. J. A. Sutcliffe and N. H. Georgopapadakou), pp. 437–75. Chapman and Hall, New York.

Ono, T., Ozasa, S., Hasegawa, F., and Imai, Y. (1977). Involvement of NADPH-cytochrome *c* reductase in the rat liver squalene epoxidase system. *Biochimica et Biophysica Acta*, **486**, 401–407.

Ono, T., Nakazono, K., and Kosaka, H. (1982). Purification and partial characterization of squalene epoxidase from rat liver microsomes. *Biochimica et Biophysica Acta*, **709**, 84–90.

Paltauf, F., Daum, G., Zuder, G., Hoegenauer, G., Schulz, G., and Seidl, G. (1982). Squalene and ergosterol biosynthesis in fungi treated with naftifine, a new antimycotic agent. *Biochimica et Biophysica Acta*, **712**, 268–73.

Petranyi, G., Ryder, N. S., and Stuetz, A. (1984). Allylamine derivatives: new class of synthetic antifungal agents inhibiting fungal squalene epoxidase. *Science*, **224**, 1239–41.

Petranyi, G., Meingassner, J. G., and Mieth, H. (1987a). Antifungal activity of the allylamine derivative terbinafine *in vitro*. *Antimicrobial Agents and Chemotherapy*, **31**, 1365–8.

Petranyi, G., Stuetz, A., Ryder, N. S., Meingassner, J. G., and Mieth, H. (1987b). Experimental antimycotic activity of naftifine and terbinafine. In *Recent Trends in the Discovery, development and evaluation of antifungal agents* (ed. R. A. Fromtling), pp. 441–450. Prous, Barcelona.

Rodriguez, R. J., Low, C., Bottema, C. D. K., and Parks, L. W. (1985). Multiple functions for sterols in *Saccharomyces cerevisiae*. *Biochimica et Biophysica Acta*, **837**, 336–43.

Ryder, N. S. (1985a). Specific inhibition of fungal sterol biosynthesis by SF 86–327, a new allylamine antimycotic agent. *Antimicrobial Agents and Chemotherapy*, **27**, 252–6.

Ryder, N. S. (1985b). Effect of allylamine antimycotic agents on fungal sterol biosynthesis measured by sterol side-chain methylation. *Journal of General Microbiology*, **131**, 1595–602.

Ryder, N. S. (1987). Squalene epoxidase as the target of antifungal allylamines. *Pesticide Science*, **21**, 281–8.

Ryder, N. S. (1988a). Mode of action of allylamines. In *Sterol biosynthesis inhibitors. Pharmaceutical and agrochemical aspects* (ed. D. Berg and M. Plempel), pp. 151–67. Ellis Horwood, Chichester.

Ryder, N. S. (1988b). Mechanism of action and biochemical selectivity of allylamine antimycotic agents. *Annals of the New York Academy of Sciences*, **544**, 208–20.

Ryder, N. S. (1990a). Squalene epoxidase: enzymology and inhibition. In *Biochemistry of cell walls and membranes in fungi* (ed. P. J. Kuhn, A. P. J. Trinci, M. J. Jung, M. W. Goosey, and L. G. Copping), pp. 189–203. Springer-Verlag, Berlin.

Ryder, N. S. (1990b). Inhibition of squalene epoxidase and sterol side-chain methylation by allylamines. *Biochemical Society Transactions*, **18**, 45–6.

Ryder, N. S. (1991). Squalene epoxidase as a target for the allylamines. *Biochemical Society Transactions*, **19**, 774–6.

Ryder, N. S. (1992). Terbinafine: mode of action and properties of the squalene epoxidase inhibition. *British Journal of Dermatology*, **126** (Suppl 39), 2–7.

Ryder, N. S. and Dupont, M.-C. (1984). Properties of a particulate squalene epoxidase from *Candida* albicans. *Biochimica et Biophysica Acta*, **794**, 466–71.

Ryder, N. S. and Dupont, M.-C. (1985). Inhibition of squalene epoxidase by allylamine antimycotic compounds: a comparative study of the fungal and mammalian enzymes. *Biochemical Journal*, **230**, 765–70.

Ryder, N. S. and Mieth, H. (1991). Allylamine antifungal drugs. In *Current topics in medical mycology*, Vol. 4 (ed. M. Borgers, R. Hay, and M. G. Rinaldi), pp. 158–88. Springer-Verlag, New York.

Ryder, N. S., Seidl, G., and Troke, P. F. (1984). Effect of the antimycotic drug naftifine on growth of and sterol biosynthesis in *Candida albicans*. *Antimicrobial Agents and Chemotherapy*, **25**, 483–7.

Ryder, N. S., Seidl, G., Petranyi, G., and Stuetz, A. (1985). Mechanism of the fungicidal action of SF 86–327, a new allylamine antimycotic agent. In *Recent advances in chemotherapy* (ed. J. Ishigami), pp. 2558–9. University of Tokyo Press.

Ryder, N. S., Dupont, M.-C., and Frank, I. (1986a). Inhibition of fungal and mammalian sterol biosynthesis by 2-aza-2,3-dihydrosqualene. *Federation of European Biochemical Societies Letters*, **204**, 239–42.

Ryder, N. S., Frank, I., and Dupont, M.-C. (1986b). Ergosterol biosynthesis inhibition by the thiocarbarnate antifungal agents tolnaftate and tolciclate. *Antimicrobial Agents and Chemotherapy*, **29**, 858–60.

Ryder, N. S., Stuetz, A., and Nussbaumer, P. (1992). Squalene epoxidase inhibitors: structural determinants for activity and selectivity of allylamines and related compounds. In *Regulation of isopentenoid metabolism* (ed. W. D. Nes and E. J. Parish), pp. 192–204. American Chemical Society, Washington, DC.

Satoh, T., Hidaka, Y., and Kamei, T. (1990). Regulation of squalene epoxidase activity in rat liver. *Journal of Lipid Research*, **31**, 2095–101.

Schuster, I. (1985). The interaction of representative members from two classes of antimycotics—the azoles and the allylamines—with cytochromes P-450 in steroidogenic tissues and liver. *Xenobiotica*, **15**, 529–46.

Schuster, I. (1987a). Metabolic degradation of terbinafine in liver microsomes from man, guinea pig and rat. In *Recent trends in the discovery, development and evaluation of antifungal agents* (ed. R. A. Fromtling), pp. 461–70. Prous, Barcelona.

Schuster, I. (1987b). Potential of allylamines to inhibit cytochrome P-450. In *Recent trends in the Discovery, development and evaluation of antifungal agents* (ed. R. A. Fromtling), pp. 471–8. Prous, Barcelona.

Sen, S. E. and Prestwich, G. D. (1989a). Trisnorsqualene cyclopropylamine: a reversible tight-binding inhibitor of squalene epoxidase. *Journal of the American Chemical Society*, **111**, 8761–3.

Sen, S. E. and Prestwich. G. D. (1989b). Trisnorsqualene alcohol, a potent inhibitor of vertebrate squalene epoxidase. *Journal of the American Chemical Society*, **111**, 1508–10.

Sen, S. E., Wawrzenczyk, C., and Prestwich, G. D. (1990). Inhibition of vertebrate squalene epoxidase by extended and truncated analogues of trisnorsqualene alcohol. *Journal of Medicinal Chemistry*, **33**, 1698–1701.

Stuetz, A. (1987). Allylamine derivatives—a new class of active substances in antifungal chemotherapy. *Angewandte Chemie International Edition in English*, **26**, 320–8.

Stuetz, A. (1988). Synthesis and structure–activity correlations within allylamine antimycotics. *Annals of the New York Academy of Sciences*, **544**, 46–62.

Stuetz, A. and Nussbaumer, P. (1989). SDZ 87–469. *Drugs of the Future*, **14**, 639–42.

Stuetz, A. and Petranyi, G. (1984). Synthesis and antifungal activity of (*E*)-*N*-(6,6-dimethyl-2-hepten-4-ynyl)-*N*-methyl-1-naphthalenemethanamine (SF 86–327) and related allylamine derivatives with enhanced oral activity. *Journal of Medicinal Chemistry*, **27**, 1539–43.

Stuetz, A., Georgopoulos, A. G., Granitzer, W., Petranyi, G., and Berney, D. (1986). Synthesis and structure–activity relationships of naftifine-related allylamine antimycotics. *Journal of Medicinal Chemistry*, **29**, 112–25.

Villars, V. V. and Jones, T. C. (1992). Special features of the clinical use of oral terbinafine in the treatment of fungal diseases. *British Journal of Dermatology*, **129** (Suppl. 39), 61–9.

Yamamoto, S. and Bloch, K. (1970). Studies on squalene epoxidase of rat liver. *Journal of Biological Chemistry*, **245**, 1670–4.

Section 8C

Inhibitors of β(1,3)glucan synthesis

Claude P. Selitrennikoff

8C.1   Introduction

Fungal infections of plants and animals, including humans, present serious medical and agricultural concerns to clinicians and farmers. Agricultural losses are significant; estimates are in the in the range of hundreds of billions of dollars. Infections of humans, particularly immunocompromised patients, often represent life-threatening situations where aggressive intervention is required. However, treatment is significantly hampered by the lack of a safe and effective arsenal of antifungal drugs. Although there are a few new compounds that have recently been approved for clinical use, the general consensus among clinicians is the frequently heard diatribe that safer and more potent therapeutic agents are needed.

Perhaps the most striking difference between fungal and human cells is that fungi are encased in a wall, protecting them from an osmotically and immunologically hostile external environment. The fungal cell wall has a complex structure and function, and has been the subject of a number of recent reviews (see Cabib *et al.* 1988; Wessels 1990). In general, the cell walls of human pathogenic fungi (both yeast and filamentous form*) contain chitin, $\beta(1,3)$glucan, $\beta(1,3;1,6)$glucan, peptides, lipids and a-linked glucans. When viewed using standard electron microscopy techniques, the walls appear trilayered and 150–250 nm thick. Filamentous fungi grow by tip extension (Wessels 1990), a process by which cell-wall assembly occurs only at each hyphal apex. Although the details of cell-wall assembly are only poorly understood, assembly involves at least the *de novo* synthesis of chitin, $\beta(1,3)$glucan, and other polymers, and their subsequent incorporation into the cell wall.

All available data demonstrate that chitin synthase[†] and $\beta(1,3)$glucan synthase activities are essential for growth and viability of a wide variety of fungi, including human pathogens. Cells treated with inhibitors of enzyme activity do not assemble walls normally and either grow poorly or lyse (Mishra and Tatum 1972; Fevre 1978; Taft *et al.* 1988). Since mammalian cells lack chitin and $\beta(1,3)$glucan, the fungal pathways for their syntheses seem to be attractive targets for antifungal drugs. Chitin synthesis as a target has recently been reviewed (Gooday 1990). The exciting recent report that *Pneumocystis carinii* pneumonia had been treated successfully with $\beta(1,3)$glucan synthase inhibitors (Schmatz *et al.* 1990) has greatly stimulated interest in the search for new enzyme inhibitors. In this chapter we focus on the current state of knowledge of fungal $\beta(1,3)$glucan synthesis and the description of known inhibitors of enzyme activity.

8C.2 $\beta(1,3)$Glucan synthase

$\beta(1,3)$Glucan synthase (E.C. 2.4.1.34) (UDP-glucose, 1,3-β-D-glucan 3-β-glucosyl transferase) catalyses the polymerization of glucose ($\beta(1,3)$-linkages) using UDP-glucose as substrate (Quigley *et al.* 1988, and references cited therein). Unfortunately, little is known about the structural requirements and order of binding for catalysis. By analogy with other glucosyl transferases, it is likely that the polymerization reaction involves the substrate being an electrophile while the glucan chain participates as a nucleophile. UDP-glucose is a central metabolite in eukaryotic cell biochemistry (e.g. glycogen metabolism, glycoproteins, etc.) and is synthesized from glucose-6-phosphate by conversion to glucose-1-phosphate by phosphoglucomutase

---

*For example, *Candida albicans* and *Coccidioides immitis* are dimorphic, growing as either yeast or filamentous forms depending on environmental conditions.

[†] There are three chitin synthase (CS) activities in fungi. Present data clearly show that CS I has a repair function. CS II is essential for cell division in yeast and CS II is involved in chitin synthesis during other portions of the life-cycle. Both CS II and CS III are required for cell viability (Shaw *et al.* 1991).

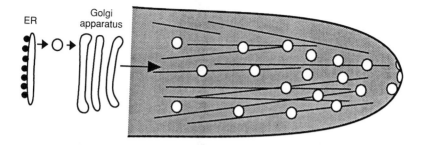

Fig. 8C.1 Targeting of glucan synthase activity. $\beta(1,3)$Glucan synthase is synthesized in the endoplasmic reticulum (ER) and sent to the Golgi apparatus for processing. In the trans-Golgi network, glucan synthase is packaged into transport vesicles and sent to hyphal tips using cytoskeletal elements (shown as straight lines oriented parallel to the long axis of a hyphal tip). Once at the tip, vesicles fuse with the apical tip plasma membrane and polymer synthesis begins.

activity, followed by condensation with UTP to form UDP-glucose and pyrophosphate (uridylyl transferase activity). The pathways in fungal and mammalian cells are identical; however, detailed comparisons of the mammalian and fungal enzymes of this pathway have not been made. Thus it is not known whether any of these reactions have fungal-specific properties that might be exploited as targets for antifungal drugs.

Glucan synthase activity *in vitro* shows a pH optimum between pH 7 and pH 8, has a K_m for UDP-glucose between 0.1 and 5 mM (depending on the enzyme source), does not require a divalent or monovalent metal ion, does not use a lipid-linked intermediate and is not proteolytically activated (Shematek *et al.* 1980; Larriba *et al.* 1981; Cerenius and Soderhall 1984; Quigley and Selitrennikoff 1984). Interestingly, enzyme activity *in vitro* does not require a primer. Disaccharides stimulate enzyme activity but they are not incorporated into glucan chains (Quigley and Selitrennikoff 1987). Disaccharide analogues have not been tested for inhibition of enzyme activity.

Glucan synthase activity *in situ* is localized to the plasma membrane such that the enzymatic site, or more likely the catalytic subunit (see below), for UDP-glucose hydrolysis faces the cytoplasm while the growing glucan chain is vectorially synthesized to the extracytoplasmic face (Jabri *et al.* 1989). The current view is that glucan synthase subunits are synthesized into the endoplasmic reticulum, sent to the Golgi apparatus for processing and assembly, and packaged into vesicles. These 'cell wall' vesicles are sent to hyphal apexes using cytoskeletal elements where they fuse with the apical tip plasma membrane. Vesicle−plasma membrane fusion activates enzyme activity and *de novo* glucan synthesis begins. This process is shown in diagrammatic form in Fig. 8C.1. Unfortunately, direct evidence for this attractive model is very scarce and large gaps in our knowledge exist. For example, none of the targeting signals for the transport of vesicles to apical tips is known, yet it is likely that these will be fungal specific and potentially useful targets for antifungal agents.

8C.2.1   Glucan synthase activity from *Neurospora crassa*

For a number of years work in this laboratory has focused on the bio-chemical and enzymological characterization of $\beta(1,3)$glucan synthase of the filamentous ascomycete *Neurospora crassa*. Using a number of enzyme sources (e.g. disrupted hyphae or protoplasts) we have found that enzyme activity is membrane bound (high speed pellet fractions), has a pH optimum of pH 7.4 in HEPES buffer, and is stabilized by the addition of protease and phosphomonoesterase inhibitors (Quigley *et al.* 1988; Taft *et al.* 1991). Enzyme activity is specific for UDP-glucose with a $K_{m \, app}$ of 0.7 mM. Hill plots for UDP-glucose are linear through eight logarithms of substrate and have a slope of unity, indicating a single substrate binding site per enzyme molecule (Quigley and Selitrennikoff 1984). Glucan synthase does not require a metal ion and is not zymogenic. Recent work has shown that glycerol, GTP, and phospholipids dramatically improve enzyme stabi-lity (half-life of ca. 25 days at 4 °C (Taft *et al.* 1991; Zugel, unpublished results)).

The involvement of a GTP-binding protein in the regulation of glucan synthase activity has been demonstrated by Cabib and coworkers (Kang and Cabib 1986). Our own work, which will be published in detail elsewhere, has confirmed and extended these observations. In agreement with Cabib's group we have been able to obtain conditions where the 'core' glucan synthase enzyme and the GTP-binding protein are separated into different cell-free fractions such that neither fraction has enzyme activity. Glucan synthase activity can be restored by mixing the two fractions. In addition, we have preliminary evidence that there is another regulatory protein, that does not require GTP, which stimulates enzyme activity (Awald, unpublished results). We are currently purifying the GTP-binding regulatory subunit. Since this subunit is required for enzyme activity (at least, *in vitro*), it is an excellent candidate for selective targeting by antifungal drugs. Further work will be needed to test whether this notion is indeed true.

A working model for enzyme activity based on these and other data is presented in Fig. 8C.2. Although this model is, no doubt, an oversimpli-fication of the *in vivo* situation, it is useful in order to stimulate further research. It should be noted that it presents GTP binding to the GTP-binding regulatory subunit prior to its association with the glucan synthase complex (indicated in this model as a large circle) and that both the disaccharide and the non-GTP-binding protein bind and remain attached to the 'core' enzyme complex. However, other possibilities are consistent

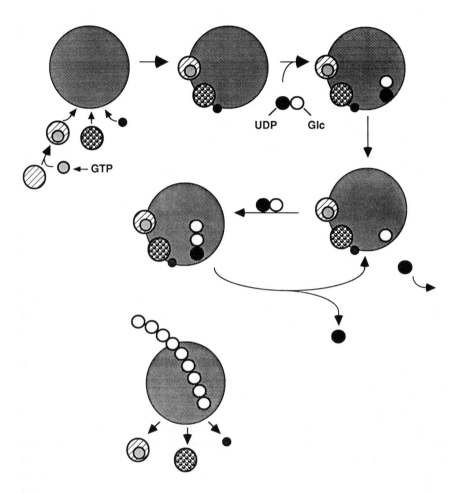

Fig. 8C.2 Model for β(1,3)glucan synthesis. The 'core' glucan synthase enzyme transplasma membrane complex is diagrammatically represented by the large shaded circle oriented so that the intracytoplasmic face is pointing downwards. The GTP-binding protein is represented by the small hatched circle and the GTP-independent protein is shaded with small filled circles. The disaccharide is represented by the smallest shaded circle. In this model, each of the three regulatory components binds to the core enzyme before UDP-glucose. Once a single molecule of substrate is bound, hydrolysis occurs, releasing UDP (dark circle). Another substrate molecule is bound and hydrolysis occurs, forming a β(1,3)-linked disaccharide and UDP. This process occurs repeatedly, forming a glucan chain represented by a series of open circles traversing the glucan synthase complex. Termination is initiated by unknown signals and the three components dissociate from the enzyme. It is not known whether glucan chains remain associated with the glucan synthase complex after termination of synthesis.

with available data. Once these regulatory molecules are bound, hydrolysis
of UDP-glucose occurs, forming a single glucan chain per enzyme molecule that is vectorially synthesized from the cytoplasmic face to the extracytoplasmic face of the plasma membrane, one glucosyl residue at a time.
Termination of synthesis is initiated by intracellular signals that are not
understood. It is probable that several glucan synthase complexes exist in
close proximity, since membrane fragments form microfibrils *in vitro* (Jabri
et al. 1989).

We have been able to solubilize enzyme activity by treatment of proto-
plast lysates or high speed particulate fractions with CHAPS and octyl-
glucoside (Quigley *et al.* 1988). Detergent-solubilized enzyme has essentially
the same kinetic parameters as the particulate enzyme, with one notable
exception described below. Sucrose density centrifugation of solubilized preparations resulted in a four- to sevenfold purification of enzyme activity.
Resulting preparations were very stable and could be useful for mass screening of potential glucan synthase inhibitors (Taft *et al.* 1991). Attempts to
purify enzyme activity further by conventional protein purification techniques
(e.g. column chromatography, precipitation with salts, etc.) have been
uniformly disappointing in that recovery has been extremely poor. However,
very recently we have been able to purify enzyme activity by nearly 300-
fold using the technique of product entrapment (Awald *et al.*). SDS–
polacrylamide gel electrophoresis of the resulting preparations have shown
12 major protein bands (molecular masses of 110 kDa, 90 kDa, 80 kDa,
75 kDa, 67 kDa, 54 kDa, 52 kDa, 43 kDa, 40 kDa, 32 kDa, 31 kDa, and
25 kDa). Although some of these proteins are no doubt contaminants
co-purifing with enzyme activity, we believe that fungal glucan synthase, like
callose synthase (β[1,3]glucan synthase) of plants, exists as a multiprotein
complex. The precise number of proteins and the isolation and characterization of each is a matter of intensive study in our laboratory. Clearly,
much additional work concerning the precise composition of β(1,3)glucan
synthase activity is required. This research is critical for the identification
of novel targets for the inhibition of enzyme activity.

8C.3 β(1,3)Glucan synthase inhibitors

In general, presently available glucan synthase inhibitors fall into the
following classes of compounds: competitive inhibitors, sugars and sugar
analogues, cyclic peptides with fatty acyl side-chains (lipopeptides), lipid-
linked saccharides, and compounds that interfere with hydrogen bonding
of adjacent glucan chains.

8C.3.1   Competitive inhibitors

As shown in Fig. 8C.2, the reaction products of glucan synthase activity
are β(1,3)linked glucan and UDP. Uridine nucleosides (UTP, UDP, UMP)

are competitive inhibitors with $K_{i\ app} \approx 0.2$ mM (Quigley and Selitrennikoff 1984). Surprisingly, glucose had no effect on enzyme activity. In addition, we found that the modified Hill plots were linear, with slopes near unity, confirming that there was one substrate binding site per catalytic subunit (Quigley and Selitrennikoff 1984). Uridine nucleosides are the only competitive inhibitors known for glucan synthase, but it can easily be imagined that a UDP-glucose analogue lacking the correct structure at the 3' position of glucose would be a competitive substrate inhibitor—unfortunately these compounds are currently not available for study. However, since UDP-glucose is a central molecule of intermediary metabolism for most organisms, it is unlikely that a substrate analogue would be therapeutically useful since, in principle, essential reactions requiring UDP-glucose in the host could also be inhibited.

8C.3.2   Sugars and sugar analogues

Previous results from a number of laboratories have shown that sorbose and gluconolactone (structures are shown in Fig. 8C.3) affect fungal growth and morphology (Mishra and Tatum 1972; Fevre 1978). Previous work from our laboratory and by Lopez-Romero and Ruiz-Herrera (1978) has shown that these compounds inhibit $\beta(1,3)$glucan synthase activity *in vitro*, an observation consistent with their *in vivo* effects of altering cell wall glucan levels. Inhibition kinetics showed that both sorbose and gluconolactone were uncompetitive inhibitors (Quigley and Selitrennikoff 1984). Gluconolactone showed complex effects on enzyme activity (stimulated at 1 mM but completely inhibited enzyme activity at 20 mM) while sorbose showed a $K_{i\ app}$ of 18 mM. Mixed inhibitor experiments revealed that sorbose and gluconolactone interact with glucan synthase activity at the same site (Quigley and Selitrennikoff 1984). Unfortunately, the mechanism of action of these sugar analogues is not clear. Since the inhibition constants of these compounds are very high, it is not likely that they will be useful therapeutically although this has not been tested. However, other analogues may prove to be more potent inhibitors of enzyme activity; none of these has been synthesized or tested.

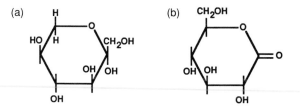

Fig. 8C.3 Structures of (a) sorbose and (b) gluconolactone.

8C.3.3   Lipid-linked saccharides

Papulacandins, chaetiacandin, and L-687,781 are produced by *Papularia sphaerosperma*, *Monochaetia dimorphospora*, and *Dictyochaeta simplex* respectively. They form a group of closely related compounds that have potent *in vitro* and *in vivo* activity against a number of yeast and filamentous fungi (Traxler *et al.* 1977, 1980; Baguley *et al.* 1979; Rommele *et al.* 1983; Bozzola *et al.* 1984; Kopecka 1984a,b; Davila *et al.* 1986; Elorza *et al.* 1987). They contain a diglucoside nucleus (a glucose and galactose moiety connected by a β-1,4 linkage) with two unsaturated fatty acids attached by ester bonds. The diglucoside is connected to an aromatic ring, forming a spirocyclic compound. The structures of the papulacandins and L-687,781 are shown in Fig. 8C.4, and that of chaetiacandin is presented in Fig. 8C.5 (Komori and Itoh 1985; Komori *et al.* 1985). These and derivative compounds were tested by several groups for their biological activity as well as for their abilities to inhibit glucan synthase activity. These results are summarized in Table 8C.1. Several points are noteworthy. First, the galactose and its attached fatty acid are not essential for biological activity and for enzyme inhibition since the removal of these moieties results in papulacandin D (Fig. 8C.6) which is still active. Second, the presence of a long-chain fatty acid is essential for activity since the removal of both fatty acids or of the remaining fatty acid from papulacandin D render the residual compounds inactive. In addition, derivatives of the 6-position of glucose, the *ortho-*, *meta-*, and *para-*positions of the aromatic ring, did not result in compounds with increased activity compared to the parent papulacandin B compound (Rommele *et al.* 1983).

Table 8C.1   Derivatives of various papulacandins

Compound	MIC (μg ml^{-1})	ED$_{50}$ (glucan synthase) (μg ml^{-1})
Papulacandin B	0.1	0.05
L-687,781	1–2	0.45
Papulacandin A	0.2	0.02
Papulacandin C	0.4	0.15
Chaetiacandin	0.2	NR
Papulacandin D	1–2	0.13
Papulacandin D minus fatty acid	>128	>5

Literature values of MICs against *C. albicans* and 50% effective doses against *C. albicans* glucan synthase of the compounds shown. Values obtained from Rommele *et al.* (1983), VanMiddlesworth *et al.* (1991), and Komori *et al.* (1985).

NR, not reported.

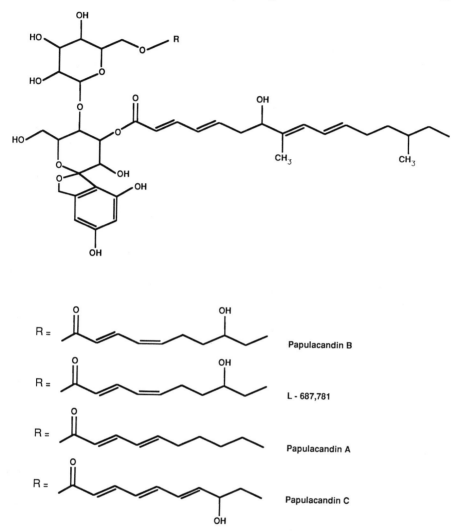

Fig. 8C.4 Structures of papulacandins and L-687,781. Redrawn from Traxler *et al.* (1980), Rommele *et al.* (1983), and VanMiddlesworth (1991).

Papulacandin B is a non-competitive inhibitor of $\beta(1,3)$glucan synthase activity of *Saccharomyces cerevisiae* with $K_{i\ app} = 1.2\ \mu M$, and inhibits enzyme activity of *Schizosaccharomyces pombe* and *Geotrichum lactis* (Perez *et al.* 1981; Varona *et al.* 1983). Another group has reported that L-687,781 inhibits glucan synthase activity of *Candida albicans* (Van Middlesworth *et al.* 1991). Our earlier work with *N. crassa* glucan synthase preparations indicated that papulacandin B is an uncompetitive inhibitor

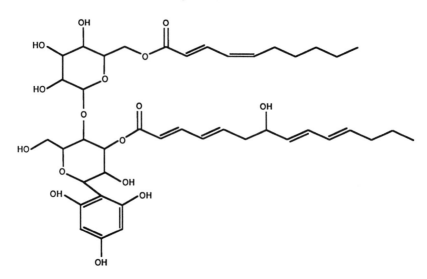

Fig. 8C.5 Structure of chaetiacandin. Redrawn from Komori and Itoh (1985).

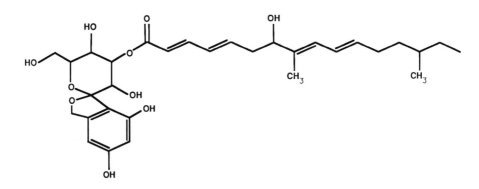

Fig. 8C.6 Structure of papulacandin D. Redrawn from Traxler *et al.* (1980).

of enzyme activity, with $K_{i\ app} \approx 120\ \mu M$ (Quigley and Selitrennikoff 1984). However, more recent data using an optimal *in vitro* assay have revealed that papulacandin B is a non-competitive inhibitor with $K_{i\ app} = 365\ \mu M$ (Taft *et al.* 1991). It is likely that the differences in inhibition type and constants reflect differences in *in vitro* assay conditions.*

---

*This result shows the importance of assay conditions in the determination of inhibition kinetics. Thus results obtained in different laboratories using different organisms and different assay conditions must be compared and interpreted with caution.

It remains to be determined whether these compounds act specifically on the glucan synthase enzyme complex itself or interact with the membrane surrounding the enzyme molecule. Papulacandin B is inactive against chitin synthase (Taft *et al.* 1988), suggesting that, in general, these compounds do not perturb membranes. However, our recent results obtained using detergent solubilized *N. crassa* glucan synthase preparations showed that enzyme activity is five times more sensitive to papulacandin B than preparations without detergents (Taft *et al.* 1991). This suggests that there may be drug–membrane interactions rather than specific drug–enzyme interactions. The observation that the hydrophobic side-chain is required for inhibition is consistent with this idea. Regardless of the precise mechanism of inhibition, kinetic data demonstrate that these compounds do not interact with the UDP-glucose binding site of glucan synthase.

In vivo testing of L-687,781 using an acute *Pneumocystis* rat model showed that intraperitoneal doses of 5 mg kg^{-1} twice daily were effective in reducing the number of *P. carinii* cysts by 80 per cent. However, this same dose was ineffective in treating *C. albicans* infections of rats (VanMiddlesworth *et al.* 1991). The acute toxicity of papulacandins was found to be > 1 g kg^{-1}, and mice infected with *C. albicans* were cured by subcutaneous applications of papulacandin A with an ED$_{50}$ of 180 mg kg^{-1}; however, papulacandin was not orally active, even at doses six times higher (Traxler *et al.* 1977). Thus papulacandins have low acute toxicity with *in vivo* efficacy. It is likely that derivative compounds that are less hydrophobic and orally active can be found. No doubt, these are the object of intense derivatization projects.

8C.3.4 Cyclic peptides (lipopeptides)

The cyclic peptides are a family of compounds that show potent antifungal activity *in vitro* and *in vivo* (Benz *et al.* 1974; Mizoguchi *et al.* 1977; Mizuno *et al.* 1977; Satoi *et al.* 1977; Miyata *et al.* 1980, 1985; Iwata *et al.* 1982; Yamaguchi *et al.* 1982, 1985; Gordee *et al.* 1984; Sawistowka-Schroder *et al.* 1984; Hall *et al.* 1988; Fromtling and Abruzzo 1989; Gordee and Debono 1989; Schwartz *et al.* 1989; Wickmann *et al.* 1989). They comprise a diverse group containing a cyclic peptide core to which a fatty acid side-chain is attached. The structure of several of these compounds is shown in Fig. 8C.7. Aculeacin A is produced by *Aspergillus aculeatus*, echinocandin B by *Aspergillus nidulans*, and L-671,329 by *Zalerion arboricola*. Cilofungin is a semisynthetic derivative of echinocandin while neopeptins are produced by *Streptomyces* sp. and possess a unique (but similar) cyclic peptide ring and the side-chains shown in Fig. 8C.8 (Ubukata *et al.* 1986).

Lipopeptides in general have activity against some yeast species (particularly *C. albicans*) and a few filamentous fungi, including *N. crassa*, but

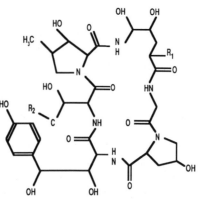

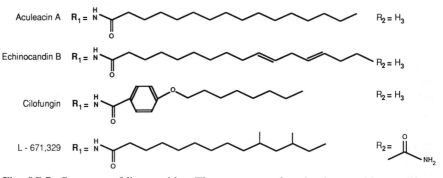

Fig. 8C.7 Structure of lipopeptides. The structures of aculeacin A, echinocandin B, cilofungin, and L-671,329 are shown, redrawn from Keller-Juslen *et al.* (1976), Mizuno *et al.* (1977), Gordee and Debono (1989), Wichmann *et al.* (1989), and Schmatz *et al.* (1990).

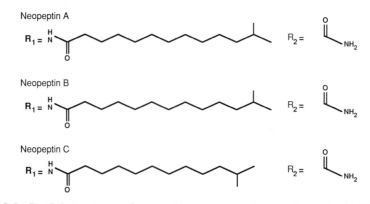

Fig. 8C.8 Partial structures of neopeptin A, neopeptin B and neopeptin C. Only the side-groups are shown and are attached to a central nucleus, similar to that in Fig. 8C.7. (Modified from Ubukata *et al.* 1986.)

have only minimal activity against most other filamentous fungi (Iwata et al. 1982; Yamaguchi et al. 1982; Gordee et al. 1984; Fromtling and Abruzzo 1989; Gordee and Debono 1989). Minimum inhibitory concentrations (MICs) against C. albicans are in the range of 0.625 μg ml^{-1} for echinocandin B and cilofungin, 0.312 μg ml^{-1} for aculeacin, and 0.5μg ml^{-1} for L-671,329. In agar diffusion assays, neopeptins at doses of 4 μg per disc resulted in 20 mm zones of inhibition (Ubukata et al. 1986).

Echinocandin B, cilofungin, and aculeacin A are non-competitive inhibitors of β(1,3)glucan synthase activity from N. crassa with $K_{i\ app}$ of 4 μM, 13 μM, and 24 μM respectively (Taft et al. 1991). Other work using β(1,3)glucan synthase preparations from C. albicans has revealed that cilofungin is a non-competitive inhibitor ($K_{i\ app} = 2.5$ μM) (Taft et al. 1988; Tang and Parr 1991). Neopeptins inhibited glucan synthase activity of S. cerevisiae with an ED_{50} of 300 μg ml^{-1} (ca. 25 μM) (Ubukata et al. 1986). L-671,329 also inhibited C. albicans glucan synthase activity, although the type of inhibition was not reported (Schmatz et al. 1990).

Structure–activity relationship studies have shown that the fatty acid side-chain is essential for inhibition of enzyme activity. For example, the echinocandin B nucleus and the fatty acid of cilofungin did not inhibit enzyme activity separately or when mixed together; only when they were covalently bonded did enzyme inhibition occur (Taft and Selitrennikoff 1990).

Analogues of the fatty acid side-chain of cilofungin revealed that C14–C16 are optimal for biological activity, with MICs increasing with shorter (to C12) and longer (to C22) chains (Debono et al. 1988). As with the papulacandins, it is not clear that the glucan synthase enzyme is the target for lipopeptides. The observation that cilofungin, aculeacin A, and echinocandin B show different inhibition properties between detergent-solubilized and particulate glucan synthase enzyme preparations is consistent with the idea that these compounds inhibit enzyme activity by perturbing the membrane surrounding the enzyme (Taft et al. 1991). As was found for the papulacandins, lipopeptides do not inhibit chitin synthase activity, again showing that these compounds do not perturb membranes in general. The precise mode of action of the lipopeptide family must be determined by additional work.

Mixed inhibitor studies revealed that UDP and sorbose interact with glucan synthase at different sites, a result consistent with their differences in inhibition kinetics (UDP is a competitive inhibitor while sorbose is an uncompetitive inhibitor). Papulacandin B and echinocandin B were found to interact with glucan synthase at the same site (Quigley and Selitrennikoff, 1984). Surprisingly, sorbose and papulacandin B interacted at the same site. This observation remains unexplained, particularly in view of differences in the structures of these compounds.

A number of lipopeptides (and derivatives) have been tested in several *in vivo* infection models. L-671,329 was effective in reducing *P. carinii* cysts by 98 per cent in an acute rat model at doses as low as 0.3 mg kg^{-1} (Schmatz *et al.* 1990). In addition, L-671,329 was effective in reducing the number of *C. albicans* cells in mice with an ED$_{50}$ of 3.38 mg kg^{-1}; the effective dose for aculeacin A in the same study was 6.44 mg kg^{-1} (Fromtling and Abruzzo 1989). Cilofungin was found to be effective at 12.5 mg kg^{-1} in a *C. albicans* mouse model. Long-term (13 weeks) toxicity studies showed that the drug was well tolerated at doses up to 100 mg kg^{-1} (Gordee *et al.* 1984). Unfortunately, these compounds, like the papulacandins, are hydrophobic (poorly water soluble) and must be given intravenously. Programmes designed to modify various positions of the nucleus and the fatty acid chain, and to add hydrophilic moieties (e.g. phosphate groups) to identify compounds that are more potent and water soluble are under way.

8C.3.5   Compounds inhibiting hydrogen bonding

Cell-wall polymer synthases form microfibrils that arise by spontaneous interpolymer hydrogen bonding (Herth 1980). A number of compounds are known to compete for interchain hydrogen bonding, notably Calcofluor white and Congo Red (Herth 1980; Vannini *et al.* 1983; Pancaldi *et al.* 1984). Observations by Fevre and co-workers, among others, revealed that Congo Red resulted in aberrant hyphal morphology of *Saprolegnia monoica* (Nodet *et al.* 1990a,b). Consistent with these observations, they found that Congo Red inhibited *in vitro* glucan synthase activity—50 per cent inhibition at 20 μg ml^{-1} (Nodet *et al.* 1990b). No *in vivo* studies using these compounds have been reported and, to the author's knowledge, the development of compounds that specifically interfere with fungal cell-wall polymer hydrogen bonding has not been explored.

8C.4   New directions and future work

Present glucan synthase inhibitors suffer from poor water solubility, poor bioavailability, and the need to be administered by injection. New delivery systems (e.g. liposomes) may overcome some of these difficulties. The important and exciting observation that glucan synthase inhibitors are effective against *P carinii*, an important opportunistic infection of AIDS patients, should stimulate the much needed search for new compounds and for more active derivatives of existing ones.

The study of glucan synthase is clearly still in its infancy, despite many years of work by a number of laboratories. This is no doubt due to the recent revelation that glucan synthase is a multiprotein complex, rather than a single polypeptide. This would clearly explain the failure of standard protein purification techniques to purify enzyme activity. The use of product entrapment, developed by groups working with plant $\beta(1,3)$glucan synthase, may provide a breakthrough technique for the isolation and eventual characterization of each of the protein components of enzyme activity. To date, none of the genes coding for any polypeptide essential for enzyme activity has been isolated and cloned, although there is a report of *N. crassa* mutants lacking enzyme activity (Phelps *et al.* 1990). We are currently screening a number of gene libraries of *N. crassa* in order to isolate genes which complement glucan-synthase-deficient mutants. This approach would provide a parallel avenue of research to purifying enzyme activity. The first steps towards the understanding of glucan synthase activity must be to catalogue the protein components and to determine the function of each. As our understanding of each of the components of glucan synthase and their functions becomes clear, new targets for intervention by drugs may well be revealed.

Acknowledgements

This work was supported in part by a National Science Foundation award. The author would like to thank Dr C. Enderlin, Paul Awald, and Cathy S. Taft for their comments.

References

Awald, P., Zugel, M., Monks, C., Frost, D., and Selitrennikoff, C. P. (1993). Purification of $\beta(1,3)$glucan synthase activity by product entrapment. *Experimental Mycology* (in press).

Baguley, B. C., Rommele, G., Gruner, J., and Wehrli, W. (1979). Papulacandin B: an inhibitor of glucan synthesis in yeast spheroplasts. *European Journal of Biochemistry*, **97**, 345–51.

Benz, F., Knusel, F., Nuesch, J., Treichler, H., Voser, W., Nyfeler, R., and Keller-Schierlein, W. (1974). Echinocandin B, ein neuartiges Polypeptid-Antibioticum aus *Aspergillus nidulans var. echinulatus*: Isolierung und Bausteine. *Helvetica Chimica Acta*, **57**, 2459–77.

Bozzola, J. J., Mehta, R. J., Nisbet, L. J., and Valenta, J. R. (1984). The effect of aculeacin A and papulacandin B on morphology and cell wall ultrastructure in *Candida albicans*. *Canadian Journal of Microbiology*, **30**, 857–63.

Cabib, E., Bowers, B. Sburtalti, A., and Silverman, S. (1988). Fungal cell wall synthesis. The construction of a biological structure. *Microbiological Sciences*, **5**, 370–5.

Cerenius, L. and Soderhall, K. (1984). Isolation and properties of β-glucan synthetase from the aquatic fungus, *Aphanomyces astaci*. *Physiologia Plantarum*, **60**, 247–52.

Davila, T., San-Blas, G., and San-Blas, F. (1986). Effect of papulacandin B on glucan synthesis in *Paracoccidioides brasiliensis*. *Journal of Medical and Veterinary Mycology*, **24**, 193–202.

Debono, M., Abbott, B., Turner, J., Howard, L., Gordee, R., Hunt, A., et al. (1988). Synthesis and evaluation of LY 121019, a member of a series of semi-synthetic analogues of the antifungal lipopeptide Echinocandin B. Annals of the New York Academy of Sciences, **544**, 141–67.

Elorza, M. V., Murgui, A., Rico, H., Miragall, F., and Sentandreu, R. (1987). Formation of a new cell wall by protoplasts of Candida albicans: effect of papulacandin B, tunicamycin and nikkomycin. Journal of General Microbiology, **133**, 1315–2325.

Fevre, M. (1978). Glucanases, glucan synthases and wall growth in Saprolegnia monoica. In Fungal walls and hyphal growth (ed. J. Burnett and A. P. J. Trinici), pp. 225–63, Cambridge University Press, London.

Fromtling, R. A. and Abruzzo, G. K. (1989). L-671,329, a new antifungal agent III. In vitro activity, toxicity and efficacy in comparison to aculeacin. Journal of Antibiotics, **62**, 174–8.

Gooday, G. W. (1990). Chitin metabolism: a target for antifungal and antiparasitic drugs. In Molecular aspects of chemotherapy (ed. E. Borowski and D. Shugar), pp. 175–85. Pergamon Press, New York.

Gordee, R. and Debono, M. (1989). Cilofungin. Drugs of the Future, **14**, 939–41.

Gordee, R. S., Zeckner, D. J., Ellis, L. F., Thakkar, A. L., and Howard, L. C. (1984). In vitro and in vivo anti-Candida activity and toxicology of LY121019. Journal of Antibiotics, **37**, 1054–65.

Hall, G. S., Myles, C., Pratt, K. J., and Washington, J. A. (1988). Cilofungin (LY121019) an antifungal agent with specific activity against Candida albicans and Candida tropicalis. Antimicrobial Agents and Chemotherapy, **32**, 1331–5.

Herth, W. (1980). Calcofluor white and Congo Red inhbit chitin microfibril assembly of Poterioochromonas: Evidence for a gap between polymerization and micro-fibril formation. Journal of Cell Biology, **87**, 442–50.

Iwata, K., Yamamoto, Y., Yamaguchi, H., and Hiratani, T. (1982). In vitro studies of aculeacin A, a new antifungal antibiotic. Journal of Antibiotics, **35**, 203–9.

Jabri, E., Quigley, D., Alders, M., Hrmova, M., Taft, C., Phelps, P., and Selitrennikoff, C. (1989). (1–3)-β-Glucan synthesis of Neurospora crassa. Current Microbiology, **19**, 153–61.

Kang, M. and Cabib, E. (1986). A guanine nucleotide-binding, proteinaceous component required for activity of 1,3-β-D-glucan synthase. Proceedings of the National Academy of Sciences of the United States of America, **3**, 5808–12.

Keller-Julsen, C., Kuhn, M., Loosli, H., Petcher, T., Wber, H., and VonWartburg, A. (1976). Struktur des Cyclopeptid-Antibiotikum SL 7810 (= Echinocandin B). Tetrahedron Letters, 4147–50.

Komori, T. and Itoh, Y. (1985). Chaetiacandin, a novel papulacandin II. Structure determination. Journal of Antibiotics, **38**, 544–6.

Komori, T., Yamashita M., Tsurumi, Y., and Kohsaka, M. (1985). Chaetiacandin, a novel papulacandin I. Fermentation, isolation and characterization. Journal of Antibiotics, **38**, 455–9.

Kopecka, M. (1984a). Lysis of growing cells of Saccharomyces cerevisiae induced by papulacandin B. Folia Microbiologica, **29**, 115–19.

Kopecka, M. (1984b). Papulacandin B: inhibitor of biogenesis of (1 → 3)-β-D-glucan fibrillar component of the cell wall of Saccharomyces cerevisiae protoplasts. Folia Microbiologica, **29**, 441–9.

Larriba, G., Marales, M., and Ruiz-Herrera, J. (1981). Biosynthesis of β-glucan microfibrils by cell-free extracts from *Saccharomyces cerevisiae*. *Journal of General Microbiology*, **124**, 375–83.

Lopez-Romero, E. and Ruiz-Herrera, J. (1978). Properties of β-glucan synthetase from *Saccaromyces cerevisiae*. *Antonie Van Leeuwenhoek*, **44**, 329–39.

Mishra, N. and Tatum, E. (1972). Effect of L-sorbose on polysaccharide synthetases of *Neurospora crassa*. *Proceedings of the National Academy of Sciences of the United States of America*, **69**, 313–17.

Miyata, M., Kitamura, J., and Miyata, H. (1980). Lysis of growing fission-yeast cells induced by aculeacin A, a new antifungal antibiotic. *Archives of Microbiology*, **127**, 11–16.

Miyata, M., Kanbe, T., and Tanaka, K. (1985). Morphological alterations of the fission yeast *Schizosaccharomyces pombe* in the presence of aculeacin A: spherical wall formation. *Journal of General Microbiology*, **131**, 611–21.

Mizoguchi, J., Saito, T., Mizuno, K., and Hayano, K. (1977). On the mode of action of a new antifungal antibiotic, aculeacin A: inhibition of cell wall synthesis in *Saccharomyces cerevisiae*. *Journal of Antibiotics*, **30**, 308–13.

Mizuno, K., Yagi, A., Satoi, S., Takada, M., Hayashi, M., Asano, K., and Matsuda, T. (1977). Studies on aculeacin. I isolation and characterization of aculeacin A. *Journal of Antibiotics*, **30**, 297–313.

Nodet, P., Capellano, A., and Fevre, M. (1990a). Morphogenetic effects of Congo Red on hyphal growth and cell wall development of the fungus *Saprolegnia monoica*. *Journal of General Microbiology*, **136**, 303–10.

Nodet, P., Girard, V., and Fevre, M. (1990b). Congo Red inhibits *in vitro* β-glucan synthases of *Saprolegnia*. *FEMS Microbiological Letters*, **69**, 225–8.

Pancaldi, S., Poli, F., Dall'Olio, G., and Vannini, G. (1984). Morphological anomalies induced by Congo Red in *Aspergillus niger*. *Archives of Microbiology*, **137**, 185–7.

Perez, P., Varona, R., Garcia-Acha, I., and Duran, A. (1981). Effect of papulacandin B and aculeacin A on β-(1,3) glucan synthase from *Geotrichum lactis*. *Federation of European Biochemical Societies Letters*, **129**, 249–52.

Phelps, P., Stark, T., and Selitrennikoff, C. P. (1990). Cell wall assembly of *Neurospora crassa*: isolation and analysis of cell wall-less mutants. *Current Micobiology*, **21**, 233–42.

Quigley, D. R. and Selitrennikoff, C. P. (1984). β-(1,3)Glucan synthase activity of *Neurospora crassa*: kinetic analysis of negative effectors. *Experimental Mycology*, **8**, 320–33.

Quigley, D. R. and Selitrennikoff, C. P. (1987). β-Linked disaccharides stimulate, but do not act a primer for, β(1–3)glucan synthase activity of *Neurospora crassa*. *Current Microbiology*, **15**, 181–4.

Quigley, D. R., Hrmova, M., and Selitrennikoff, C. P. (1988). β(1–3)Glucan synthase of *Neurospora crassa*: solubilization and partial characterization. *Experimental Mycology*, **12**, 141–50.

Rommele, G., Traxler, P., and Wehrli, W. (1983). Papulacandins—the relationship between chemical structure and effect on glucan synthesis in yeast. *Journal of Antibiotics*, **36**, 1539–42.

Satoi, S., Yagi, A., Asano, K., Mizuno, K., and Watanabe, T. (1977). Studies on aculeacin. II isolation and characterization of aculeacins B, C, D, E, F and G. *Journal of Antibiotics*, **30**, 303–7.

Sawistowska-Schroder, E. T., Kerridge, D., and Perry, H. (1984). Echinocandin inhibition of 1,3-β-D-glucan synthase from *Candida albicans*. *Federation of European Biochemical Societies Letters*, **173**, 134–8.

Schmatz, D. M., Romancheck, M. A., Pittarelli, L. A., Schwartz, R. E., Fromtling, R. A., Nollstadt, K. H., *et al*. (1990). Treatment of *Pneumocystis carinii* pneumonia with 1,3-β-glucan synthesis inhibitors, *Proceedings of the National Academy of Sciences of the United States of America*, **87**, 5950–4.

Schwartz, R. E., Giacobbe, R. A., Bland, J. A., and Monaghan, R. L. (1989). L-671,329, a new antifungal agent I. Fermentation and isolation. *Journal of Antibiotic*, **52**, 163–7.

Shaw, J., Mol, P., Bowers, B., Silverman, S., Valdivieso, M., Duran, A., and Cabib, E. (1991). The function of chitin synthases 2 and 3 in the *Saccharomyces cerevisiae* cell cycle. *Journal of Cell Biology*, **114**, 111–23.

Shematek, E., Braatz, J., and Cabib, E. (1980). Biosynthesis of the yeast cell wall. I. Preparation and properties of β(1-3)glucan synthase. *Journal of Biological Chemistry*, **255**, 888–94.

Taft, C. S. and Selitrennikoff, C. P. (1990). Cilofungin inhibition of (1,3)-β-glucan synthase: the lipophilic side chain is essential for inhibition of enzyme activity. *Journal of Antibiotics*, **43**, 433–7.

Taft, C. S., Stark, T., and Selitrennikoff, C. P. (1988). Cilofungin (LY121019) inhibits *Candida albicans* (1-3)-β-D-glucan synthase activity. *Antimicrobial Agents and Chemotherapy*, **32**, 1901–3.

Taft, C. S., Zugel, M., and Selitrennikoff, C. P. (1991). *In vitro* inhibition of stable 1,3-β-D-glucan synthase activity from *Neurospora crassa*. *Journal of Enzyme Inhibition*, **5**, 41–9.

Tang, J. and Parr, T. R., Jr (1991). W-1 solubilization and kinetics of inhibition by cilofungin of *Candida albicans* (1,3)-β-D-glucan synthase. *Antimicrobial Agents and Chemotherapy*, **35**, 99–103.

Traxler, P., Gruner, J., and Auden J. A. L. (1977). Papulacandins, a new family of antibiotics with antifungal activity I. Fermentation, isolation, chemical and biological characterization of papulacandins A, B, C, D and E. *Journal of Antibiotics*, **30**, 289–96.

Traxler, P., Fritz, H., Fuhrer, H., and Richter, W. J. (1980). Papulacandins, a new family of antibiotics with antifungal activity Structures of papulacandins A, B, C and D. *Journal of Antibiotics*, **33**, 967–78.

Ubukata, M., Uramoto, M., Uzawa, J., and Isono K. (1986). Structure and biological activity of neopeptins A, B and C, inhibitors of fungal cell wall glycan synthesis. *Agricultural Biological Chemistry*, **50**, 357–65.

VanMiddlesworth, F., Omstead, N. M., Schmatz, D., Bartizal, K., Fromtling, R., Bills, G., *et al*. (1991). L-687,781, a new member of the papulacandin family of β-1,3-D-glucan synthesis inhibitors I. Fermentation, isolation, and biological activity. *Journal of Antibiotics*, **44**, 45–51.

Vannini, G., Poli, F., Donini A., and Pancaldi, S. (1983). Effects of Congo Red on wall synthesis and morphogenesis in *Saccharomyces cerevisiae*. *Plant Science Letters*, **31**, 9–17.

Varona, R., Perez, P., and Duran, A. (1983). Effect of papulacandin B on β-glucan synthesis in *Schizosaccharomyces pombe*. *FEMS Microbiological Letters*, **20**, 243–7.

Wessels, J. G. H. (1990). Role of cell wall architecture in fungal tip growth generation. In *Tip growth in plant and fungal cells* (ed. I. B. Heath), pp. 1–29. Academic Press, San Diego, CA.

Wichmann, C. F., Liesch, J. M., and Schwartz, R. E. (1989). L-671,329, a new antifungal agent II. Structure determination. *Journal of Antibiotics*, **62**, 168–72.

Yamaguchi, H., Hiratani, T., Iwata, K., and Yamamoto, Y. (1982). Studies on the mechanism of antifungal action of aculeacin A. *Journal of Antibiotics*, **35**, 210–19.

Yamaguchi, H., Hiratani, T., Baba, M., and Osumi, M. (1985). Effect of Aculeacin A, a wall-active antibiotic, on synthesis of the yeast cell wall. *Microbiology and Immuniology*, **29**, 609–23.

9

Steroidogenesis pathway enzymes

Section 9A

Introduction

Angela Brodie

9A.1 Introduction

The enzymes involved in the biosynthesis of cholesterol and steroid hormones are proving to be major targets for therapeutic intervention. Inhibitors of several of these enzymes have established clinical efficacy and are proving to be important in the treatment of disease. The most important of these enzymes and their inhibitors will be reviewed in the following sections. Figure 9A.1 of this chapter shows an abbreviated version of the biosynthetic sequence of cholesterol and steroid hormones from the three carbon units of mevalonate which are mediated by these enzymes.

Inhibitors of aromatase (oestrogen synthetase) and 5α-reductase have gained much attention in recent years in the treatment of steroid-hormone-related disorders. Aromatase is an enzyme complex consisting of a cytochrome P450 haemoprotein and a ubiquitous electron-donating flavoprotein, NADPH-cytochrome P450 reductase. The C19 androgen substrates androstenedione and testosterone bind to the P450 aromatase (P450 arom) which catalyses the aromatization of the androgen A ring and the loss of the C19 methyl group to yield oestrone and oestradiol (Cole and Robinson 1990). Oestrogens have an important role in the growth of hormone-

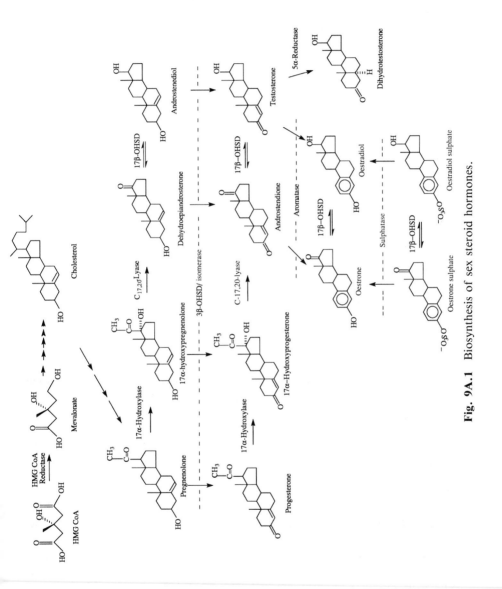

Fig. 9A.1 Biosynthesis of sex steroid hormones.

dependent breast cancer, and inhibitors of oestrogen biosynthesis offer a rational therapeutic strategy for this disease (Brodie *et al*. 1977, 1990). 5*a*-Reductase mediates the conversion of testosterone to dihydrotesto- sterone (DHT), the active androgen in the male reproductive tract and skin. Production of this steroid promotes the growth of the prostate (Bruchovsky and Wilson 1968). Thus inhibitors of 5*a*-reductase reduce the production of DHT and are now being evaluated in patients for the treatment of benign prostatic hypertrophy (BPH) (Gormley and Stoner 1992). There is a logical possibility for their use in the treatment of prostatic cancer (Gormley 1991).

Aromatase and 5*a*-reductase are both excellent targets for inhibition as both are rate limiting and the last step in the biosynthesis of hormones essential for specific tissue growth. Although it does not appear from current information that there is any abnormality in the regulation of these enzymes which results in overproduction of hormone in breast and prostate cancer patients, reduction in normal levels of the hormones leads to amelioration of these diseases.

9A.2 Aromatase

Reduction in oestrogen levels by aromatase inhibitors in post-menopausal breast cancer patients leads to significant tumour regression (Santan *et al*. 1982; Coombes *et al*. 1984). Since the initial publication concerning selective aromatase inhibitors in 1973 (Schwarzel *et al*. 1973), a large number of potent compounds of this type have been reported in recent years and are discussed in more detail in Section 9B. A few of them have already been shown to be of value in the treatment of post-menopausal patients with advanced breast cancer and are becoming available in the United Kingdom and Europe. Several more are now in clinical trials. Current aromatase inhibitors can be categorized into two classes of compound. One consists of steroid analogues which compete with the substrate for the enzyme's active site. Some of these compounds are mechanism-based inhibitors which, on interaction with the enzyme, cause its inactivation (Brodie *et al*. 1981; Metcalf *et al*. 1981). The second group of inhibitors consists of compounds which bind to the haeme of cytochrome P450 arom. Many of them are non-steroidal compounds, but are selective as they also bind to moieties close to the substrate binding site (VanWauwe and Janssen 1989).

It has recently been reported that the anti-oestrogen, tamoxifen, which blocks the action of oestrogen at the receptor site in the tumour, improves long-term survival as well as reducing disease recurrence (Early Breast Cancer Trialists' Collaborative Group 1992). Nevertheless, as with other types of cancer treatment, patients relapse from tamoxifen. Aromatase inhibitors have been found effective in such patients (Coombes *et al*. 1984;

Goss *et al.* 1986). However, it is not yet known whether aromatase inhibitors are more effective than tamoxifen or whether a combination of the two could improve response rates. Aromatase inhibitors offer the possibility of using several different compounds which may contribute significantly to the treatment of breast cancer. This may be particularly useful as development of drug resistance is a frequent cause of patient relapse (Curt *et al.* 1984).

Aromatase inhibitors may also have a role in BPH (Henderson *et al.* 1987). During aging, there is an increase in the ratio of oestrogens to androgens which may have an adverse influence on the prostate (Kozak *et al.* 1982). Several studies suggest that reduction in oestrogens may be a useful approach in treating this disease (Habenich *et al.* 1987), and studies are under way in BPH patients.

9A.3   5α-Reductase

As already discussed, DHT produced by 5α reduction of testosterone, is recognized as the most important mediator of prostatic growth (Bruchovsky and Wilson 1968). Thus a potent inhibitor of 5α-reductase, which reduces DHT levels, may be useful in the treatment of BPH. Testosterone is important for sperm maturation and sexual function. However, blockade of 5α-reductase leads to increases in plasma testosterone concentration. Thus problems of impotence may not be a consequence of treatment with either 5α-reductase or aromatase inhibitors. The first 5α-reductase inhibitor for the treatment of BPH, finasteride (Merck), has recently been approved in the United States (Gormley and Stoner 1992). It remains to be established whether 5α-reductase inhibitors will be useful in the treatment of prostatic cancer, where a reduction in all androgen production is important in preventing tumour growth (Geller *et al.* 1987).

9A.4   17α-Hydroxylase: C-17,20-lyase (P450 17)

As a result of success in the above areas, attention has turned to developing inhibitors of some of the other enzymes involved in steroid biosynthesis. 17α-Hydroxylase: C-17,20-lyase converts progesterone or pregnenolone into the corresponding 17α-hydroxysteroid and then cleaves the C17 side-chain to form C19 androgens (androstanediol, dehydroepiandrosterenedione (DHEA), androstenedione, and testosterone). While this is clearly a key enzyme in regulating androgen production, it is also important in regulating oestrogen production. For example, ovarian aromatase activity is unchanged when oestrogen levels fall following the pro-oestrus surge of gonadotropin in the rat (Banks *et al.* 1991). Thus concentrations of oestrogens closely follow the pattern of changes in androgen concentrations. Inhibitors of 17α-hydroxylase: C-17,20-lyase might be used to reduce androgen levels to normal in women with various forms of infertility, hirsutism, and acne due to hyperandrogenism. As indicated above, inhibition of all androgens and oestrogens might be beneficial for men with prostatic cancer. Ketoconazole, an antifungal imidazole, which inhibits 17α-hydroxylase: C-17,20-lyase, has been used for this purpose with some degree of success (Trachtenberg 1984; Williams *et al.* 1986). However, this compound has significant side-effects. It also is a rather non-specific inhibitor and interacts with 3β-hydroxysteroid dehydrogenase and a number of other cytochrome P450 steroidogenic enzymes (Di Mattina *et al.* 1988). Significant inhibition of 17α-hydroxylase: C-17,20-lyase by ketoconazole results in reduced cortisol production. To date, relatively few attempts have been made to develop more specific inhibitors of this enzyme. Now that 17α-hydroxylase: C-17,20-lyase has been purified and its gene has been cloned, more information about it will become available and may aid development of selective inhibitors. Bifuranol, a compound known to have some antiprostatic activity *in vivo*, and its analogues have been reported to inhibit 17α-hydroxylase: C-17,20-lyase but were rather less active than ketoconazole (Barrie *et al.* 1989). A new imidazole derivative R75251 (liarozole) has recently been reported to reduce testosterone levels in male volunteers and increase plasma 17α-hydroxyprogesterone and progesterone levels (Bruynseels *et al.* 1990). Thus, unlike ketoconazole, this compound does not inhibit cholesterol synthesis. However, it appears to have similar potency to ketoconazole and also reduces cortisol and aldosterone to about the same extent. We have recently investigated a number of C20-substituted pregnene derivatives which have good activity against this enzyme. Several inhibitors have greater potency for C-17,20-lyase than for 17α-hydroxylase and therefore may have limited effects on cortisol production (Li *et al.* 1992). These investigators have also reported that rogletimide (pyridoglutethimide), an analogue of aminoglutethimide, reduces androgen levels in patients while increasing 17α-hydroxyprogesterone (Dowsett *et al.* 1991).

9A.5   Hydroxysteroid dehydrogenases

Other targets for inhibitors able to reduce the production of androgen and estrogens are the hydroxysteroid dehydrogenases. Inhibition of 3β-hydroxysteroid dehydrogenase/isomerase would lead to blockade in the synthesis of testosterone and androstenedione which are converted by this enzyme from their immediate precursors and the less potent androgens DHEA and androstenediol. A disadvantage of this strategy is that inhibition of 3β-hydroxysteroid dehydrogenase/isomerase will impair the production of cortisol and aldosterone. However, in the patient this could be offset with cortisol replacement therapy. A variety of steroidal compounds appear to affect this enzyme. Trilostane, epostane, cyanoketone, and the 5α-reductase inhibitor N,N-diethyl-4-methyl-3-oxo-4-aza-5α-androstan-17β-

carboxamide (4-MA) are all potent inhibitors with K_i values of approximately 50nM. Synthetic progestagens are also potent inhibitors of 3β-hydroxysteroid dehydrogenase/isomerase. For example, the anti-androgen cyproterone acetate, norgestrel, and norethindrone components of the oral contraceptive inhibit with K_i values of 1.5–2.5 μM (Takahashi *et al.* 1990). 3α-Hydroxysteroid dehydrogenase/isomerase is involved in the reduction of DHT to its metabolite 5α-androstan-3,β-17β-diol. Two interesting inhibitors of this enzyme, 1-(4′-nitrophenyl)-2-propen-1-ol and 1-(4′-nitrophenyl)-2-propyn-1-ol, are mechanism based. These compounds are believed to act by generating non-steroidal alkylating agents which inactivate the enzyme (Ricigliano and Penning 1989). These workers have also reported a vinyl ketone (1-(3β-hydroxy-5α-androstan-17β-yl)-2-propen-1-one) as an active-site-directed alkylating agent of 20α-hydroxysteroid dehydrogenase (Ricigliano and Penning 1986). This enzyme plays a key role in progesterone metabolism. Inhibitors have the potential to maintain progesterone levels and, possibly, to prevent miscarriages. Safety would clearly be of crucial importance for such a use.

17β-Hydroxysteroid dehydrogenase (17-HSD) has also been considered as a target for inhibitors. Inhibition of this enzyme would limit the conversion of androstenedione to the more potent androgen testosterone, and of oestrone to the more potent oestradiol. Blockade of 17-HSD would provide more specific inhibition than blockade of 3β-hydroxysteroid dehydrogenase, which is involved in transformation of multiple steroids. Nevertheless, while androstenedione and oestrone are less potent than testosterone and oestradiol, they are bioactive steroids which can produce effects on target tissues. Acetylenic secoestradiol has been reported as a mechanism-based inhibitor of placental 17β,20α-hydroxysteroid dehydrogenase (Auchus and Covey 1986).

9A.6 Sulphatase

As discussed above, aromatase inhibitors have been shown to be effective in breast cancer patients by reducing production of the oestrogens, oestrone and oestradiol. Although these oestrogens are physiologically active, they circulate in relatively low concentrations compared with other steroids. Oestrone sulphate, an inactive conjugate of the oestrogens formed in the liver, circulates in much greater concentrations than the free oestrogens. Plasma oestrone sulphate levels are higher in post-menopausal breast cancer patients than in normal post-menopausal women (Prost *et al.* 1984). At physiological concentrations of substrate, the capacity of the sulphatase to produce oestrone in breast tumours appears to be at least 10 times more important than aromatase (Santen *et al.* 1984). Therefore, this pathway might be important in the production of bioactive oestrogens in the tumour, where the steroid would be in close proximity to oestrogen receptors. While it is expected that aromatase inhibitors would inhibit synthesis of free oestrone and oestradiol prior to conjugation with sulphate, compounds that inhibit the conversion of oestrone sulphate into oestrone may be useful in maximizing suppression of oestrogens. Evidence that this is a useful objective has recently been suggested by the finding that the aromatase inhibitor aminoglutethimide promotes increased clearance of oestrone sulphate in breast cancer patients (Lonning *et al.* 1989). Thus when patients were treated with the aromatase inhibitors 4-hydroandrostenedione followed by aminoglutethimide (AG), there was a greater reduction in plasma oestrogen levels than with treatment by either inhibitor alone. This was attributed to increased clearance of oestrone sulphate (Lonning *et al.* 1993). Evans *et al.* (1991) have investigated several drugs currently used in the treatment of breast cancer as inhibitors of oestrone sulphatase in human breast carcinoma tissue. Tamoxifen, stilboestrol, and the aromatase inhibitors 4-OHA and AG were without effects, but some inhibition was noted with danazol. While inhibition of oestrone sulphatase was only modest (20 per cent with 50 μM), danazol also inhibited the conversion of oestrone to the more potent oestradiol by the 17β-hydroxysteroid dehydrogenase.

9A.7   HMG Co-A reductase

3-Hydroxy-3-methylglutaryl-coenzyme A (HMG Co-A) reductase is involved in an early step in the biosynthesis of cholesterol and has become a very important target for dual action to control cholesterol levels in patients with hypercholesterolaemia. This enzyme converts (HMG Co-A) into mevalonate which forms the key building blocks of several sterols, cholesterol, and steroid hormones. Despite the fact that the enzyme is located several steps away from that producing cholesterol, inhibitors of HMG CoA reductase are proving to be very valuable in controlling cholesterol levels in patients (McKenney 1988). Compactin or lovastatin (formerly mevinolin) are potent HMG CoA reductase inhibitors (Endo 1988). Of particular note is lovastatin, a competitive inhibitor of HMG Co-A reductase which is now being used extensively. It has been proposed that the decalin moiety of compactin acts as a hydrophobic anchor, while the lactonic portion serves as an analogue of mevalonate (Abeles 1987). There is speculation that non-steroidal type II aromatase inhibitors, which contain a similar hydrophobic domain, may bind in the steroid binding pocket, as discussed in Section 9B.

Unlike inhibitors of steroid biosynthesis used for treating hormone-dependent cancer, it is not necessary to achieve total blockade of cholesterol synthesis but only to reduce high levels to the normal range. Inhibition of cholesterol synthesis leads to reduction of the hepatic and peripheral pools of cholesterol. This results in increases in low density lipoprotein (LDL) receptors in the liver, increasing the uptake of LDL particles and thus reducing cholesterol levels in the circulation.

Among the steps in the biosynthetic pathway from mevalonate to cholesterol are several important enzymes which synthesize precursors of basal membrane proteins such as laminin, and the G protein p21*ras* which is involved in conversion of guanosine triphosphate (GTP) to guanosine diphosphate and phosphate. This latter protein appears to act as an 'on–off' signal to regulate the cell cycle by promoting cells to move into the S phase.

In the mutated or oncogenic form of *ras*, the switch appears to set in the 'on' position, thus leading to uncontrolled growth as in cancer. The possibility of inhibiting cell growth by reducing production of p21*ras* with an HMG-CoA reductase inhibitor, such as lovastatin, seemed attractive. However, the drug appears to be toxic in doses sufficient to inhibit cell growth (Sinensky *et al*. 1990). Inhibition of HMG-CoA reductase to control *ras* also lacks specificity and would reduce both normal *ras*, which is essential to cellular function, and oncogenic *ras*. More appropriate targets to control oncogenic forms of *ras* need to be sought. Nevertheless, inhibition of HMG-CoA reductase by lovastatin may provide a useful model for investigating the effects of inhibiting the cell cycle.

In the following sections and Chapter 10 these enzymes are discussed in detail as well as their utility and progress in development of their inhibitors.

References

Abeles, R. H. (1987). Enzyme inhibitors: ground state /transition state analogues. *Drug Development Research*, **10**, 221–34.

Auchus, R. J. and Covey, D. F. (1986). Mechanism-based inactivation of 17β,20α-hydroxysteroid dehydrogenase by an acetylenic secoestradiol. *Biochemistry*, **25**, 7295–300.

Banks, P. K., Meyer, K., and Brodie, A. M. H. (1991). Regulation of ovarian biosynthesis in the rat: Evidence for inhibition of estrogen. *Endocrinology*, **129**, 1295–1304.

Barrie, S. E., Rowlands, M. G., Foster, A. B., and Jarman, M. (1989). Inhibition of 17α-hydroxylase/C17-C20 lyase by bifluranol and its analogues. *Journal of Steroid Biochemistry and Molecular Biology*, **13**, 1191–5.

Brodie, A. M. H., Banks, P. K., Inkster, S. E., Dowsett, M., and Coombes, R. C. (1990). Aromatase inhibitors and hormone-dependent cancers. *Journal of Steroid Biochemistry*, **37**, 327–33.

Brodie, A. M. H., Schwarzel, W. C., Shaikh, A. A., and Brodie, H. J. (1977). The effect of an aromatase inhibitor, 4-hydroxy-4-androstene-3,17-dione, on estrogen-dependent processes in reproduction and breast cancer. *Endocrinology*, **100**, 1684–95.

Brodie, A. M. H., Hendrickson, J. R., Tsai-Morris, C. H., Garrett, W. M., Marcotte, P. A., and Robinson, C. H. (1981). Inactivation of aromatase *in vitro* by 4-OHA and 4-acetoxyandrostenedione and sustained effects *in vivo*. *Steroids*, **38**, 693–702.

Bruchovsky, N. and Wilson, J. D. (1968). The conversion of testosterone to 5α-androstan-17β-ol-3-one by rat prostate *in vitro* and *in vivo*. *Journal of Biological Chemistry*, **243**, 2012–21.

Bruynseels, J., De Coster, R., Van Rooy, P., Wouters, W., Coene, M.-C., Snoeck, E., *et al*. (1990). R 75251, a new inhibitor of steroid biosynthesis. *Prostate*, **16**, 345–57.

Cole, P. A. and Robinson, C. H. (1990). Mechanism and inhibition of cytochrome P-450 aromatase. *Journal of Medicinal Chemistry*, **33**, 2933–42.

Coombes, R. C., Goss, P., Dowsett, M., Gazet, J. C., and Brodie, A. M. H. (1984). 4-Hydroxyandrostenedione treatment of postmenopausal patients with advanced breast cancer. *Lancet*, **ii**, 1237–9.

Curt, G., Clendenin, N. J., and Chabner, B. A. (1984). Drug resistance in cancer. *Cancer Treatment Reports*, **68**, 87–99.

DiMattina. M., Maronian, N., Ashby, H., Loriaux, D. L., and Albertson, B. D. (1988). Ketoconazole inhibits multiple steroidogenic enzymes involved in androgen biosynthesis in the human ovary. *Fertility and Sterility*, **49**, 62.

Dowsett, M., MacNeill, F. Mehta, A., Newton, C., Haynes, B., Jones, A., *et al*. (1991). Endocrine, pharmacokinetic and clinical studies of the aromatase inhibitor 3-ethyl-3-(4-pyridyl)piperidine-2,6-dione(pyridoglutethimide) in postmenopausal breast cancer patients. *British Journal of Cancer*, **74**, 887–94.

Early Breast Cancer Trialists' Collaborative Group. (1992). Systemic treatment of early breast cancer by hormonal, cytotoxic, or immune therapy. *Lancet*, **339**, 1–15.

Endo, A. (1988). Chemistry, biochemist, and pharmacology of HMG-CoA reductase inhibitors. *Klinische Wochenschrift*, **66**, 421–7.

Evans, T. R. J., Rowlans, M. G., Jarman, M., Coombes, R. C. (1991). Inhibition of estrone sulfate enzyme in human placenta and human breast carcinoma. *Journal of Steroid Biochemistry and Molecular Biology*, **62**, 493–9.

Geller, J., Albert, J., and Vik A. (1987). Advantages of total androgen blockade in the treatment of advanced prostate cancer. *Seminars in Oncology*, **15**, 53–61.

Gormley, G. J. (1991). Role of 5α-reductase inhibitors in the treatment of advanced prostatic carcinoma. *Urologic Clinics of North America*, **18**, 93–98.

Gormley, G. J., and Stoner, E. (1992). The role of 5α-reductase inhibitors in the treatment of benign prostatic hyperplasia. *Problems in urology*, Vol. 5, No. 3 (ed. H. Lepor), pp. 436–40. J. B. Lippincott, Philadelphia, PA.

Goss, P. E., Coombes, R. C., Powles, T. J., Dowsett, M., and Brodie, A. M. H. (1986). Treatment of advanced postmenopausal breast cancer with aromatase inhibitor, 4-hydroxyandrostenedione Phase 2 report. *Cancer Research*, **46**, 4823–6.

Habenicht, U-F., Schwarz, K., Neumann, F., and El Etreby, M. F. (1987). Induction of estrogen-related hyperplastic changes in the prostate of the cynomolgus monkey by androstenedione and its antagonism by aromatase inhibitor 1-methyl-1,4-diene-3,17-dione. *Prostate*, **11**, 313–26.

Henderson, D., Habenicht, U. F., Nishino, Y., and El Etreby, M. F. (1987), Estrogens and benign prostatic hypertrophy: the basis for aromatase inhibitor therapy. *Steroids*, **50**, 219–33.

Kozak, I., Bartsch, W., Krieg, M., and Voigt, K. D. (1982). Nuclei of stroma: site of the highest estrogen concentrations in human benign prostatic hyperplasia. *Prostate* **3**, 433–8.

Li J., Li Y., Son., C., Banks, P., and Brodie, A. (1992). 4-Pregnen-3-one-20βcarboxyaldehyde: a potent inhibitor of 17αhydroxylase/lyase and of 5α-reductase. *Journal of Steroid Biochemistry and Molecular Biology*, **42**, 313–21.

Lonning, P. E., Johannessen, D. C., Thorsen, T., and Ekse, D. (1989). Effects of aminoglutethimide on plasma estrone sulfate not caused by aromatase inhibition. *Journal of Steroid Biochemistry and Molecular Biology*, **3**, 541–5.

Lonning, P. E., Dowsett, M., Jones, A., Ekse, D., Jacobs, S., McNeil, F., *et al.* (1993). Aminoglutethimide may further enhance oestrogen suppression and cause tumour regression in breast cancer patients resistant to treatment with the aromatase inhibitor 4-hydroxyandrostenedione. *Cancer Research*, in press.

McKenney, J. M. (1988). Lovastatin: a new cholesterol-lowering agent. *Clinical Pharmacy*, **7**, 21–36.

Metcalf, B. W., Wright, C. L., Burkart, J. P., and Johnston, J. O. (1981). Substrate based inactivation of aromatase by allenic and acetylenic steroids. *Journal of the American Chemical Society*, **103**, 3221.

Prost, O., Turrel, M. O., Dahan, N., Craveur, C., and Adessi, G. L. (1984). Estrone and dehydroepiandrosteredione sulfate activities and plasma estrone sulfate levels in human breast carcinoma *Cancer Research*, **44**, 661–4.

Ricigliano, J. W. and Penning, T. M. (1986). Active-site directed inactivation of rat ovarian 20α-hydroxysteroid dehydrogenase. *Biophysical Journal*, **240**, 717–23.

Ricigliano, J. W. and Penning, T. M. (1989). Synthesis and evaluation of non-steroidal mechanism-based inactivators of 3α-hydroxysteroid dehydrogenase. *Biophysical Journal*, **262**, 139–49.

Santen, R. J., Worgul, T. J., Lipton, A., Harvey, H. A., Boucher, A., Samojlik, E., and Wells, S. A. (1982). Aminoglutethimide as treatment of postmenopausal women with advanced breast carcinoma: correlation of clinical and hormonal responses. *Annals of Internal Medicine*, **96**, 94–101.

Santen, R. J., Leszcynski, D., Tilson-Mallet, N., Feil, P. D., Wright, C., Manni, A., and Santner, S. J. (1984). Enzymatic control of estrogen production in human breast cancer: relative significance of the aromatase versus sulfatase pathway. *Annals of the New York Academy of Sciences*, **464**, 126–37.

Schwarzel, W. C., Kruggel, W., and Brodie, H. J. (1973). Studies on the mechanism of estrogen biosynthesis. VII. The development of inhibitors of the enzyme system in human placenta. *Endocrinology*, **92**, 866–80.

Sinensky, M., Beck, L. A., Leonard, S., and Evans, R. (1990). Differential inhibitory effects of lovastatin on protein isoprenylation and sterol synthesis. *Journal of Biological Chemistry*, **265**, 19937–41.

Takahashi, M., Luu-The, V., and Labrie, F. (1990). Inhibitory effect of synthetic progestins, 4-MA and cyanoketone on human placental 3β-hydroxysteroid de-hydrogenase/5 → 4-ene-isomerase activity. *Journal of Steroid Biochemistry and Molecular Biology*, **37**, 231–6.

Trachtenberg, J. (1984). Ketoconazole therapy in advanced prostatic cancer. *Journal of Urology*, **132**, 61–3.

Van Wauwe, J. P. and Janssen, P. A. J. (1989). Is there a case for P-450 inhibitors in cancer treatment? *Journal of Medicinal Chemistry*, **32**, 2231–9.

Williams, G., Kerle, D. J., Ware, H., Doble, A., Dunlop, H., Smith, C., *et al.* (1986). Objective responses to ketoconazole therapy in patients with relapsed progressive prostatic cancer. *British Journal of Urology*, **58**, 45–51.

9B.1   Introduction

Conversion of C19 androgens to C18 oestrogens is the rate-limiting step in the biosynthesis of oestrogens and is mediated by the enzyme aromatase. Thus this enzyme has a key role in female development and reproduction. In addition, aromatase has important functions in the male. Oestradiol produced in the testis appears to be involved in regulating androgen biosynthesis (Payne 1987). In early development, local production of oestrogens in the brain has been shown to be essential for sexual differentiation of the male phenotype (Naftolin *et al.* 1975). Aromatase is expressed in a number of other structures throughout the body, such as muscle and adipose tissue (Longcope *et al.* 1978). This non-gonadal production of oestrogen increases with age in both sexes and is the main source in post-menopausal women (Hemsell *et al.* 1974).

Oestrogens have a role in a number of disease states, most notably breast and endometrial cancer. There is evidence that, in addition to androgens, oestrogens produced by the testis or peripheral sources have a role in stimulating benign prostatic hypertrophy and possibly prostate cancer (Henderson *et al.* 1987). Production of oestrogens by the prostate itself is unlikely (Brodie *et al.* 1989).

The contribution of oestrogens to the growth of breast cancer has long been recognized (Beatson 1896). However, not all patients have hormone-dependent tumours. In recent years, it has become possible to identify patient who are likely to respond to hormone therapy by measuring concentrations of oestrogen receptor and progesterone receptor in the tumour. Approximately 60 per cent of pre-menopausal patients have hormone-responsive tumours, compared with about 75 per cent of post-menopausal patients (McGuire 1980). In addition, breast cancer is more prevalent in post-menopausal women than in younger women. Oestrogens are produced in many tissues throughout the body. Thus total blockade by systemic methods is likely to be more effective than surgical ovariectomy. Two approaches that have proved to be effective in the form of therapy are inhibition of oestrogen action by anti-oestrogens, which interact with oestrogen receptors, and inhibition of oestrogen production by inhibitors of aromatase. Until recently, all anti-oestrogens were known to be weak or partial agonists, in addition to being antagonists. Inhibitors of aromatase, acting by a different mechanism, may not be associated with oestrogenic activity. Although tamoxifen may not be the optimal anti-oestrogen because of its partial agonist activity, nevertheless it has now been shown to provide better response rates and less toxicity than cytotoxic agents in post-menopausal patients with oestrogen-receptor-positive breast cancer. A recent report indicates that tamoxifen extends the disease-free interval and significantly increases patient survival (Early Breast Cancer Trialists' Collaborative Group 1992). These findings make a strong case for regulating oestrogens as a means of treating this disease.

Despite the benefits of tamoxifen, tumours eventually become resistant to its effect and the disease recurs. A number of patients who responded to tamoxifen initially but later relapsed have been found subsequently to respond to agents which inhibit oestrogen production (Santen et al. 1982; Goss et al. 1986). Thus aromatase inhibitors are providing additional treatment for these women. Because of its low toxicity, tamoxifen can be utilized over an extended period and used as adjuvant therapy. Aromatase inhibitors may have a place as first-line therapy in recurrent disease in these patients. However, it has not yet been determined whether either of these types of agent, alone or in combination, is superior in first-line treatment in terms of rate of response or duration of effectiveness.

The aromatase complex consists of a cytochrome P450 haemoprotein and a flavoprotein, NADPH−cytochrome P450 reductase. The latter is common to most cell types and functions to donate electrons to the cytochrome P450. P450 aromatase (P450 arom) binds the C19 androgen substrates androstenedione and testosterone and catalyses their conversion to oestrone and oestradiol. This reaction appears to involve three steps utilizing 1 molar equivalent of NADPH and oxygen (Thompson and Siiteri 1974). The first step is hydroxylation at C19 of the androgen substrate and appears to be a characteristic cytochrome P450 hydroxylation (Meyer 1955; Morato et al. 1961). This is followed by oxidation to the 19-oxo intermediate and involves stereospecific loss of the C19 pro-R hydrogen. In the third step, there is loss of the angular methyl group at C19 and cis elimination of 1β and 2β hydrogens which results in the aromatization of ring A of the androgens to form the oestrogens. A number of theories have been proposed to explain the mechanisms involved in the last step. Recent evidence (Aktar et al. 1982; Cole and Robinson 1988) supports the possibility that an enzyme-bound ferric peroxide attacks the aldehyde at C19 to form an unstable intermediate which collapses to yield oestrogen and formic acid by hydride shift, proton transfer, or free-radical pathways (Stevenson *et al.* 1985, 1988). Because of high electrophilicity of the aldehyde, normal ferric peroxide breakdown may be circumvented and the normal hydroxylation cycle altered (Cole and Robinson 1990).

Aromatization is unique to oestrogen synthesis. Therefore compounds interfering with this reaction might be selective for aromatase. Furthermore, as aromatization is the last step in the biosynthetic sequence of steroid production (Fig. 9A.1), its blockade should not affect production of other steroids. For these reasons, aromatase is a particularly suitable target for inhibition.

9B.2 Irreversible inhibitors

The first selective aromatase inhibitors reported were a group of C19 steroids (Schwarzel *et al.* 1973). These compounds exhibited properties typical of competitive inhibitors and included 1,4,6-androstatriene-3,17-dione (Brodie *et al.* 1982a), 4-hydroxyandrostenedione (4-OHA) (Brodie *et al.* 1977) and 4-acetoxyandrostenedione (Brodie *et al.* 1978). Interestingly, some of these inhibitors were later found to cause inactivation of the enzyme (Brodie *et al.* 1981). These compounds are believed to function as mechanism-based inhibitors. While not intrinsically reactive, they initially compete rapidly with the enzyme's natural substrate and subsequently interact with the active site of the enzyme, binding to it either very tightly or irreversibly and causing its inactivation (Sjoerdsma 1981). Compounds of this type should have long-lasting effects *in vivo* so that the continued presence of the drug is not required, thus reducing the chance of toxic side-effects. Since these inhibitors interact with the active site of the enzyme, they should be quite specific. Inactivation of aromatase by 4-OHA was demonstrated by pre-incubating the compound for various lengths of time with microsomes of human placenta or rat ovaries in the presence of NADPH (Brodie *et al.* 1981). After removal of the compound, a time-dependent loss of enzyme activity was observed which followed pseudo-first-order kinetics. High concentrations of substrate can protect the enzyme from inactivation. Binding of [6,7-^{3}H]4-OHA to aromatase purified from placenta was prevented by pre-incubation with androstenedione and suggests that the inhibitor interacts with the enzyme's active site. In addition, the interaction appears to be irreversible as the radiolabel was not displaced by excess concentrations of androstenedione (unpublished data). Investigations of the pharmacokinetics of oral administration of 250 mg 4-OHA in breast cancer patients indicate that the half-life of 4-OHA is about 3 hours. However, the initial serum concentrations of 4-OHA were quite high (averaging about 50 ng ml^{-1} for 30−90 minutes) relative to the serum levels of androstenedione (0.5 ng ml^{-1}) (Dowsett *et al.* 1989). These results suggest that endogenous androstenedione concentrations would not be sufficient to protect aromatase from inactivation by 4-OHA. After 24 hours, the plasma concentrations of 4-OHA were found to be almost undetectable (< 0.8 ng ml^{-1}). Nevertheless, progressive suppression of plasma oestradiol levels continued during the first 24 hours of treatment, despite the rapid clearance of 4-OHA from the blood, suggesting that irreversible inhibition of aromatase by 4-OHA may be occurring *in vivo*. A number of other steroidal aromatase inhibitors have also been reported to cause inactivation. In addition to 4-OHA, studies with the mechanism-based inhibitor 10(2-propynlestr)-4-ene-3,17-dione (MDL 18962) have demonstrated that this compound inactivates aromatase (Metcalf *et al.* 1981). In addition, Brueggemeier *et al.* (1987, 1990) have reported that a number of 7a-substituted androstenedione derivatives cause inactivation of aromatase. There are a large number of other steroid analogues that have now been reported to inhibit aromatase. Several of these have demonstrated biological activity. Of note are 1-methylandrosta-1,4-diene-3,17-dione (SH 289) (Henderson *et al.* 1986), 6-methylen-androsta-1,4-diene-3,17-dione (FCE 24304), and 4-aminoandrosta-1,4,6-triene-3,17-dione (FCE 24928) (Guidici 1988), which cause inactivation of aromatase. Following oral administration of FCE 24304 to rats, plasma oestrogen levels remained depressed after 24 hours. The time course of inhibition of ovarian aromatase activity was found to be similar to that of the reduction in plasma oestradiol (E_2) levels suggesting that FCE 24304 inactivates ovarian aromatase *in vivo* (Zaccheo *et al.* 1989, 1991). It was recently reported that 14-hydroxyandrostene-3,6,17-trione also causes inactivation of the enzyme and inhibits ovarian aromatase and oestrogen production in the rat (Bowden *et al.* 1990).

9B.3 Reversible inhibitors

On interaction with the enzyme, most steroids show characteristic type 1 binding spectra due to a difference spectrum with an absorbance maximum at about 420 nm and a minimum at 392 nm. In addition to the steroidal derivatives, aromatase may be inhibited by compounds such as aminoglutethimide (3-(4-aminophenyl)-3-ethylpiperidine-2,6-dione, AG), its analogues, and several imidazole derivatives. These compounds, which have a nitrogen atom possessing a free electron pair, appear to inhibit cytochrome P450 enzymes by interacting as the sixth ligand with the haeme atom. These types of inhibitor exhibit type II binding, characterized by a difference spectrum with an absorption maximum at 429 nm. Interestingly, Kellis *et al.* (1987) and Wright *et al.* (1991) have described strong competitive inhibitors which are steroid analogues with C19 heteroatoms. Based on their binding spectra, these compounds appear to bond with the haeme iron of P450 arom forming hexa-coordinated species.

As the non-steroidal inhibitors interact with the haeme of the cytochrome P450, they may inhibit a number of cytochrome P450 enzymes as well as aromatase, such as those involved in the adrenal production of aldosterone (18-hydroxylase) and cortisol (11β-hydroxylase). AG inhibits several of the steroidogenic steps and for this reason was initially used to produce a medical adrenalectomy in breast cancer patients. Subsequently, it was observed by Samojlik *et al.* (1977) that androstenedione levels were preserved while oestrone levels were reduced in patients treated with AG, possibly because of compensatory increases in ACTH. This finding indicates that the main mechanism of AG in lowering oestrogen levels may be aromatase inhibition. Additional effects of AG in patients appear to be enhanced conversion of Δ^5 to Δ^4 steroids (Badder *et al.* 1983) and reduction of plasma levels of oestrone sulphate by increasing its metabolism (Lonning *et al.* 1987b). This action may occur as a result of induction of hepatic mixed-function oxidases by AG (Lonning *et al.* 1987a). Oestrone sulphate could be an important source of oestrogen within breast tumours (Santen *et al.* 1984). As oestrone sulphate is thought to be derived from circulating oestrone and oestradiol (Ruder *et al.* 1972), aromatase inhibitors would be expected to be effective in inhibiting the production of oestrone prior to its sulphation. However, it is unclear why plasma oestrone and oestradiol levels are reduced by only 50 per cent of pretreatment values by AG, whereas there is almost complete inhibition of peripheral aromatization of androstenedione to oestrone (Santen *et al.* 1982; Dowsett *et al.* 1985). Recently, analogues of AG have been developed. One such compound, pyridoglutethimide, has similar potency to AG but appears to be rather more specific and less toxic (Dowsett *et al.* 1990). Other more potent analogues have been described such as 3-(cyclohexylmethyl)-1-(4-aminophenyl)-3-azabicyclo[3.1.0]hexane-2,4-dione which has a potency more than 140 times greater than that of AG (Stanek *et al.* 1991).

Selectivity for specific cytochrome P450 enzymes can be achieved with inhibitors that interact as the sixth ligand with the haeme atom but which also combine with amino acid residues located near the haeme site (Van Wauwe and Janssen 1989). With this approach in mind, several imidazoles, such as fadrozole [4-(5,6,7,8-tetrahydroimidazo[1,5a]pyridin-5-yl)benzonitrile monohydrochloride (CGS 16949A)], CGS 20267 (Bhatnagar *et al.* 1990), and 6-[(4-chlorophenyl)(1H-1,2,4-triazol-1-yl)methyl]1-methyl-1H-benzotriazole (R 76 713) (Wouters *et al.* 1990), which have much greater potency for aromatase than AG, have been investigated and shown to have much less effect on other cytochrome P450 enzymes. In comparison with AG, CGS 16949A is 1000 times more selective for aromatase than for other cytochrome P450 enzymes (Kochak *et al.* 1990). Studies of the interaction of R76 713 with the enzyme indicate that this triazole derivative not only coordinates with the haeme but that its N-1-substituent also occupies a lipophilic region of the apoprotein moiety of the P450. The reverse type I spectral change which occurs when R76 713 is added to placental microsomes and the kinetic data suggest a competitive component to its inhibition which appears to involve the substrate binding site. This compound appears to have good specificity for cytochrome P450 arom and a low affinity for the 11β-hydroxylase. Therefore it would be expected to have minimal effects on cortisol and aldosterone biosynthesis (Vanden Bossche *et al.* 1990).

9B.4   Biological activity of aromatase inhibitors

A number of studies have been carried out which demonstrate that 4-OHA inhibits oestrogen production *in vivo*. Inhibition of ovarian oestrogen secretion and aromatase activity correlated with marked regression of DMBA-induced hormone-dependent mammary tumours in the rat (Brodie *et al.* 1977, 1982b). In the intact cycling animal, reduction in plasma oestradiol concentrations results in reflex increases in luteinizing hormone (LH) secretion which in turn stimulates ovarian aromatase activity. Several of the steroidal inhibitors, such as 4-OHA, FCE 24304, and MDL 18962, have weak androgenic activity although it is sufficient to block release of LH at certain doses. This activity can result in maintaining ovarian oestrogen suppression and may also contribute to tumour regression in the 'pre-menopausal' DMBA-mammary tumour model. Although initially inhibitory, other inhibitors such as AG (Wing *et al.* 1985), which do not interfere with LH feedback regulation, were found not to be effective in suppressing oestradiol levels in the rat after long-term treatment. In contrast, the non-steroidal inhibitor R76 713, a triazole derivative, maintained suppression of oestradiol levels in the intact rat. This compound appears to be very selective, and was found to be devoid of effects on cholesterol, progesterone, androgen, and mineralocorticoid biosynthesis, and is without oestrogenic or androgenic activity (De Coster *et al.* 1990).

Because of the importance of peripheral aromatase in post-menopausal breast cancer patients, studies have been conducted to determine the effects of inhibitors on production of oestrogens from non-gonadal sources. Unlike the control of aromatase in the gonads, peripheral aromatase is not regulated by gonadotropins (Mahendroo *et al.* 1991). Non-human primates (male cynomolgus or rhesus monkeys or baboons) have been utilized for these studies since most of their oestrogen production is from peripheral sources. Peripheral aromatization is measured using a primed constant infusion of [7^{3}H]androstenedione and [4^{14}C]oestrone. After reaching steady state conditions, blood samples are collected and analysed for plasma radioactivity, as infused, and product steroids (Longcope *et al.* 1978). Early studies with 4-OHA utilized this procedure first and demonstrated marked inhibition of peripheral aromatization (Brodie and Longcope 1980). Similar studies have been carried out with other aromatase inhibitors, such as MDL 18962 (Longcope *et al.* 1988) and R 76 713, both of which were highly effective. Studies with R 76 713 in cynomolgus monkeys demonstrated dose dependent inhibition (Tuman *et al*. 1991). Peripheral aromatization, measured 4–5 hours after injection of R 76 713, was decreased by 87 per cent (10 μg kg^{-1}), 85 per cent (3 μg kg^{-1}), 61 per cent (0.3 μg kg^{-1}), and 33 per cent (0.03 μg kg^{-1}) compared with controls. After 15–16 hours aromatization was still suppressed at 53 ± 11 per cent of control by the 3 μg kg^{-1} dose. The ID$_{50}$ was 0.13 μg kg^{-1}, suggesting that this is a potent inhibitor *in vivo*. Neither the metabolic clearance rates of androstenedione and oestrone, determined in the same experiment, nor the conversion rates between androgens and oestrogens were altered by treatment with R76 713. These findings suggest that the effects were selective for aromatization.

Inhibition of peripheral aromatization by 4-OHA has been confirmed in breast cancer patients (Reed *et al*. 1990; Jones 1991). Aromatase activity in breast tumours of seven patients in the former study (Reed *et al*. 1990) was found to be inhibited in three patients and unchanged in two patients, but in the remaining two aromatase appeared to be resistant to the effects of 4-OHA. A decrease in DNA polymerase a was noted in most tumours in which aromatase activity was inhibited. However, there was no statistically significant correlation between aromatase activity and this marker of proliferation (Reed *et al*. 1990). Other studies have failed to find a correlation between the presence of tumour aromatase and oestrogen receptors (Varela and Dao 1978; Lipton *et al*. 1987). Although there are a number of reports of aromatase activity in breast tumours (Miller *et al*. 1974), the contribution of tumour aromatase to growth stimulation still requires further clarification.

Aromatase activity is at the limit of sensitivity of most assays. We recently evaluated a series of breast tumours utilizing the polymerase chain reaction (PCR) to amplify detection of aromatase mRNA. Aromatase mRNA was detectable in most of the tumours, suggesting the potential for aromatase expression. However, the mRNA aromatase levels were generally very low, except in a few tumours. No correlation was observed between the presence of significant levels of oestrogen receptors and mRNA aromatase in these tumors (Koos *et al*. 1993).

9B.5   Clinical studies with aromatase inhibitors

Several steroidal and non-steroidal aromatase inhibitors are now undergoing clinical trial. Phase 1 trials have been undertaken for MDL 18,962, SH 289, FCE 24304, and R 76 712. In a small group of normal male volunteers, a single oral dose of 5 or 10 mg of R76 713 was found to lower plasma oestradiol levels to 40 pmol l^{-1}, the detection limit of the assay, after 4 and 8 hours. In pre-menopausal women, plasma oestradiol levels fell from 389 pmol l^{-1} to a mean of 149 pmol l^{-1} over 4–24 hours (DeCoster *et al*. 1990). In studies of the imidazole CGS 16949A in postmenopausal patients, maximal suppression of oestradiol levels was achieved with doses of 2–4 mg daily. However, higher doses of 8–16 mg daily appeared to inhibit C11- and C21-hydroxylases and increase ACTH levels, suggesting some inhibition of cortisol biosynthesis (Santen *et al*. 1989a). Inhibition of C11-hydroxylase has been confirmed *in vitro* in isolated adrenal cells (Lamberts *et al*. 1989). At a dose of 16 mg daily CGS 16949A also blocks the corticosterone methyl oxidase type II step, increasing the ratios of plasma 18-hydroxycorticosterone to aldosterone and of urinary tetra-hydro compound A to tetrahydroaldosterone (Demers *et al*. 1990). However, cortrosyn-stimulated aldosterone levels were significantly blunted (Santen *et al*. 1989b). A study of low doses of CGS 16949A, with which relatively selective inhibition of aromatase might be achieved, was carried out in 54 post-menopausal breast cancer patients who were given 1.8–4 mg two or three times daily. Plasma oestrone, oestradiol and oestrone sulphate were equally suppressed and peripheral aromatization was inhibited by 84 per cent. Aldosterone and cortisol did not change over the two week observation period and there was no clinical evidence of mineralocorticoid deficiency, although ACTH-stimulated cortisol concentrations were blunted. Androstenedione and 17a-hydroxyprogesterone tended to be increased. It was concluded that, at these doses, CGS 16949A blocks aromatase but does not produce clinically important inhibition of cortisol and aldosterone production and can be used without supplementation (Santen *et al*. 1991).

4-OHA was the first selective aromatase inhibitor to be studied in patients (Coombes *et al*. 1984; Goss *et al*. 1986). 4-OHA, now known as lenteron (CGS 32349), has been evaluated in three recently completed trials of 465 breast cancer patients (Dowsett and Coombes 1990). The overall results of the three studies indicate that 4-OHA is effective in post-menopausal breast cancer patients with advanced metastatic disease who have relapsed from previous hormonal therapy, usually tamoxifen. The patients received either 500 mg intramuscularly weekly or biweekly, or 250 mg biweekly. Injections of 4-OHA appeared to be well tolerated and had notably less toxicity than AG. Side-effects occurred in 17 per cent of patients and were mostly mild; only 3–5 per cent discontinued treatment. Local reactions, including sterile abscesses, were mainly a feature of the higher injected dose (500 mg) in a small percentage of the patients (< 10 per cent) (Hoffken 1990; Hoffken *et al*. 1990; Stein *et al*. 1990). The response rates were not significantly different between the different doses and frequencies of administration. Overall, 28 per cent of patients experienced complete or partial regression of their tumours, while the disease was stabilized in a further 22 per cent. The disease progressed in the remaining women. These results were similar to earlier reports by these groups when smaller numbers of patients had been studied (Hoffken *et al*. 1990; Pickles *et al*. 1990; Stein *et al*. 1990). The response rates among patients receiving 250 mg daily orally were also similar (Cunningham *et al*. 1987).

Although a significant proportion of the patients in all the studies had unknown receptor status rather than oestrogen-receptor-positive status, the response rate to 4-OHA was similar to that with AG in previously treated patients (Powles *et al.* 1978; Smith *et al.* 1978). All regimens were effective in reducing serum oestradiol levels to a similar extent. Observation of a group receiving 500 mg intramuscularly once a month, studied over a 4 month period, showed that there was no escape from oestradiol suppression (Dowsett *et al.* 1987). Therefore it appears that treatment failure in some patients is more likely to be due to hormone insensitivity than to suboptimal doses of 4-OHA. It is interesting that patients who have relapsed from tamoxifen respond to aromatase inhibitor treatment, and this suggests the possibility that their tumours have become supersensitive to oestrogens. Studies with human breast cancer cell lines treated with tamoxifen have been found to have increased the number of oestrogen receptors (Gottardis and Jordan 1988) or progesterone receptors (Graham *et al.* 1992) in some cell populations.

It is now apparent that 4-OHA, and possibly several newer compounds entering clinical trials, will have a place as second-line treatment in patients relapsing from tamoxifen. Aromatase inhibitors could also be useful as first-line treatment in patients who progress to advanced disease following adjuvant therapy with tamoxifen. How these compounds will compare with one another in view of their different modes of interaction with the enzyme and their different potencies awaits further evaluation. Steroidal inhibitors may have weak biological activities mediated via steroid receptors, while some non-steroidal compounds may interfere with production of other hormones. These actions may affect the optimal doses which can be used to inhibit aromatase. Studies in patients may reveal other activities of a compound which could influence its efficacy and tolerability. Differences between the types of compound which inhibit aromatase offer the possibility that a variety of useful compounds will become available for improving treatment for breast cancer patients.

References

Akhtar, M., Calder, M. R., Corina, D. L., and Wright J. N. (1982). Mechanistic studies on C-19 demethylation in oestrogen biosynthesis. *Biophysical Journal*, **201**, 569–80.

Badder, E. M., Lerman, S., and Santen, R. J. (1983). Aminoglutethimide stimulates extra-adrenal delta-4 androstenedione production. *Journal of Surgical Research*, **34**, 380–7.

Beatson, G. T. (1896). On the treatment of inoperable cases in carcinoma of the mamma: suggestion for new method of treatment with illustrative cases. *Lancet*, **ii**, 104–7.

Bhatnagar, A. S., Hausler, A., Trunet, P., Muller, P., Lang, M., and Bowman, P. (1990). Inhibitors of estrogen biosynthesis: CGS16949A and CGS20267, preclinical and clinical endocrine effects. *Symposium on Aromatase Inhibition—Past, Present and Future*, 15th Cancer Congress, Hamburg, p. 3. Ciba-Geigy, Basel, Switzerland.

Bowden, C. R., Yoshihama, M., Tamura, K., Nakakoshi, M., and Nakamura, J. (1990). 14a-hydroxyandrost-4-ene-3,6,17-trione as a mechanism-based irreversible inhibitor of estrogen biosynthesis. *Chemical and Pharmaceutical Bulletin*, **38**, 2834–7.

Brodie, A. M. H. and Longcope, C. (1980). Inhibition of peripheral aromatization by aromatase inhibitors, 4-hydroxy- and 4-acetoxyandrostenedione. *Endocrinology*, **106**, 19–21.

Brodie, A. M. H., Schwarzel, W. C., Shaikh, A. A., and Brodie, H. J. (1977). The effect of an aromatase inhibitor, 4-hydroxy-4-androstene-3,17-dione, on estrogen-dependent processes in reproduction and breast cancer. *Endocrinology*, **100**, 1684–95.

Brodie, A. M. H., Wu, J. T., Marsh, D. A., and Brodie, H. J. (1978), Aromatase-inhibitors III. Studies on the antifertility effects of 4-acetoxy-4-androstene-3,17-dione. *Biology of Reproduction*, **18**, 365.

Brodie, A. M. H., Hendrickson, J. R., Tsai-Morris, C. H., Garrett, W. M., Marcotte, P. A., and Robinson, C. H. (1981). Inactivation of aromatase *in vitro* by 4-OHA and 4-acetoxyandrostenedione and sustained effects *in vivo*. *Steroids*, **38**, 693–702.

Brodie, A. M. H., Garrett, W., Hendrickson, J. M., Marsh, D. A., and Brodie H. J. (1982a). The effect of 1,4,6-androstatriene-3,17-dione (ATD) on DMBA-induced mammary tumors in the rat and its mechanism of action *in vivo*. *Biochemical Pharmacology*, **31**, 2017–23.

Brodie, A. M. H., Garrett, W. M., Hendrickson, J. R., and Tsai-Morris, C. H. (1982b). Effects of 4-hydroxyandrostenedione and other compounds in the DMBA breast carcinoma model. *Cancer Research*, **42**, 3360s–4s.

Brodie, A. M. H., Son, C., King, D. A., Meyer, K. M., and Inkster, S. E. (1989). Lack of aromatase in human prostatic tissue: effects of 4-OHA and other inhibitors on androgen metabolism. *Cancer Research*, **49**, 6551–5.

Brueggemeier, R. W., Li, P-K., Snider, C. E., Darby, M. V., and Katlic, N. E. (1987). 7a-substituted androstenediones as effective *in vitro* and *in vivo* inhibitors of aromatase. *Steroids*, **50**, 163–78.

Brueggemeier, R. W., Li, P. K., Chen, H. H., Moh, P. P., and Katlic, N. E. (1990). Biochemical pharmacology of new 7-substituted androstenediones as inhibitor of aromatase. *Journal of Steroid Biochemistry*, **37**, 379–85.

Cole, P. A. and Robinson, C. H. (1988). A peroxide model reaction for placental aromatase. *Journal of the American Chemical Society*, **110**, 1284–5.

Cole, P. A. and Robinson, C. H. (1990). Mechanism and inhibition of cytochrome P-450 aromatase. *Journal of Medicinal Chemistry*, **33**, 2933–42.

Coombes, R. C., Goss, P., Dowsett, M., Gazet, J. C., and Brodie, A. M. H. (1984). 4-Hydroxyandrostenedione treatment of postmenopausal patients with advanced breast cancer. *Lancet*, **ii**, 1237–9.

Cunningham, D., Powles, T. J., Dowsett, M., Hutchinson, G., Brodie, A. M. H., Ford, H. T., *et al.* (1987). Oral 4-hydroxyandrostenedione, a new endocrine treatment for disseminated breast cancer. *Cancer Chemotherapy and Pharmacology*, **20**, 253–5.

De Coster, R., Wouters, W., Bowden, C. R., Vanden Bossche, H., Bruynseels, J.,

Tuman, R. W., *et al.* (1990). New non-steroidal aromatase inhibitors: focus on R76713. *Journal of Steroid Biochemistry*, **37**, 335–41.

Demers, L. M., Melby, J. C., Wilson, T. E., Lipton, A., Harvey, H. A., and Santen, R. J. (1990). The effects of CGS 16949A, an aromatase inhibitor on adrenal mineralocorticoid biosynthesis. *Journal of Clinical Endocrinology and Metabolism*, **70**, 1162–6.

Dowsett, M. and Coombes, R. C. (1990). The development of the new aromatase inhibitor 4-OHA. Endocrine and clinical aspects. *Symposium on Aromatase Inhibition—Past, Present and Future, 15th Cancer Congress, Hamburg*, pp. 9–10. Ciba-Geigy, Basel, Switzerland.

Dowsett, M., Harris, A. L., Stuart-Harris, R., Hill, M., Cantwell, B. M., Smith, I. E., and Jeffcoate, S. L. (1985). A comparison of the endocrine effects of low dose aminoglutethimide with and without hydrocortisone in postmenopausal breast cancer patients. *British Journal of Cancer*, **52**, 525.

Dowsett, M., Goss, P. E., Powles, T. J., Brodie, A. M. H., Jeffcoate, S. L., and Coombes, R. C. (1987). Use of aromatase inhibitor 4-hydroxyandrostenedione in post-menopausal breast cancer: optimization of therapeutic dose and route. *Cancer Research*, **47**, 1957–61.

Dowsett, M., Cunningham, D. C., Stein, R. C., Evans, S., Dehennin, L., Hedley, A., and Coombes, R. C. (1989). Dose-related endocrine effects and pharmacokinetics of oral and intramuscular 4-hydroxyandrostenedione in postmenopausal breast cancer patients. *Cancer Research*, **49**, 1306–12.

Dowsett, M., Jarman, M., Mehta, A., Haynes, B., Lonning, P. E., Jones, A., *et al.* (1990). Endocrine pharmacology of a new aromatase inhibitor 3-ethyl-3-(4-pyridyl)piperidine-2,6-dione (PG). *Journal of Steroid Biochemistry*, **36** (Suppl.), Abstr. 336.

Early Breast Cancer Trialists' Collaborative Group. (1992). Systemic treatment of early breast cancer by hormonal, cytotoxic, or immune therapy. *Lancet*, **339**, 1–15.

Goss, P. E., Coombes, R. L., Powles, T. J., Dowsett, M., and Brodie, A. M. H. (1986). Treatment of advanced postmenopausal breast cancer with aromatase inhibitor, 4-hydroxyandrostenedione-Phase 2 report. *Cancer Research*, **46**, 4823–6.

Gottardis, M. M. and Jordan, V. C. (1988). Development of tamoxifen-stimulated growth of MCF-7 tumors in athymic mice after long-term antiestrogen administration. *Cancer Research*, **48**, 5183–7.

Graham, M. L., II, Smith, J. A., Jewett, P. B., and Horwitz, K. B. (1992). Heterogeneity of progesterone receptor content and remodeling by tamoxifen characterize subpopulations of cultured human breast cancer cells: analysis by quantitative dual parameter flow cytometry. *Cancer Research*, **52**, 593–602.

Guidici, D., Ornati, G., Briatico, G., Buzzetti, F., Lombardi, P., and Salle, E. D. (1988). 6-Methylenandrosta-1,4-diene-3,17-dione (FCE 24304): a new irreversible aromatase inhibitor. *Journal of Steroid Biochemistry*, **30**, 391–4.

Hemsell, D. L., Grodin, J., Breuner, P. F., Siiteri, P. K., and MacDonald, P. C. (1974). Plasma precursors of estrogen. II Correlation of the extent of conversion of plasma androstenedione to estrone with age. *Journal of Clinical Endocrinology and Metabolism*, **38**, 476–9.

Henderson, D., Norbirath, G., and Kerb, U. (1986). 1-Methyl-1,4-androstadiene-3,17-dione (SH 489): characterization of an irreversible inhibitor of estrogen biosynthesis. *Journal of Steroid Biochemistry*, **24**, 303–6.

Henderson, D., Habenicht, U. F., Nishino, Y., and El Etreby, M. F. (1987). Estrogens and benign prostatic hypertrophy: the basis for aromatase inhibitor therapy. *Steroids*, **50**, 219–33.

Hoffken, K. (1990). Clinical experience with 4-OHA in the treatment of advanced breast cancer. *Symposium on Aromatase Inhibition—Past, Present and Future. 15th International Cancer Congress, Hamburg*, p. 11. Ciba-Geigy, Basel, Switzerland.

Hoffken, K., Jonat, W., Possinger, K., Kolbel, M., Kunz, T., Wagner, H., *et al.* (1990). Aromatase inhibition with 4-hydroxyandrostenedione in the treatment of postmenopausal patients with advanced breast cancer: a phase II study. *Journal of Clinical Oncology*, **8**, 875–80.

Jones, A. L. (1991). Inhibition of peripheral aromatization by 4-hydroxyandrostenedione: radioactive tracer studies *in vivo*. In *4-Hydroxyandrostenedione— a new approach to hormone-dependent cancer* (ed. R. C. Coombes and M. Dowsett). International Congress and Symposium Series. Royal Society of Medicine Service, London, pp. 29–33.

Kellis, J. T., Childers, W. E., Robinson, C. H., and Vickery, L. E. (1987). Inhibition of aromatase cytochrome P-450 by 10-oxirane and 10-triiane substituted androgens. *Journal of Biological Chemistry*, **262**, 4421–6.

Kochak, G. M., Mangat, S., Mulagha, M. T., Entwistle, E. A., Santen, R. J., Lipton, A., and Demers, L. (1990). The pharmacodynamic inhibition of estrogen synthesis by fadrozole, an aromatase inhibitor, and its pharmacokinetic disposition. *Journal of Clinical Endocrinology and Metabolism*, **71**, 1349–55.

Koos, R. D., Banks, P. K., Inkster, S. E., Yue, W., and Brodie, A. M. H. (1993). Detection of aromatase and keratinocyte growth factor expression using reverse transcription-polymerase chain reaction. *Journal of Steroid Biochemistry and Molecular Biology*, **45**, 217–25.

Lamberts, S. W. J., Bruining, H. A., Marzouk, H., Zuiderwijk, J., Uitterlinden, P., Blijd, J. J., *et al.* (1989). The new aromatase inhibitor CGS-16949A suppresses aldosterone and cortisol production by human adrenal cells *in vitro*. *Journal of Clinical Endocrinology and Metabolism*, **69**, 896–901.

Lipton, A., Santner, S. J., Santen, R. J., Harvey, H. A., Feil, P. D., White-Hershey, D., *et al.* (1987). Aromatase activity in primary and metastatic human breast cancer. *Cancer*, **59**, 779–82.

Longcope, C., Pratt, J. H., Schneider, S. H., and Fineberg, S. E. (1978). Aromatization of androgens by muscle and adipose tissue *in vivo*. *Journal of Clinical Endocrinology and Metabolism*, **46**, 146–52.

Longcope, C., Femino, A., and Johnston, J. O. (1988). Inhibition of peripheral aromatization in baboons by an enzyme-activated aromatase inhibitor (MDL 18,962). *Endocrinology*, **122**, 2007–11.

Lonning, P. E., Kvinnsland, S., and Bakke, O. M. (1987a). Effect of aminoglutethimide on antipyrine, theophylline and digitoxin disposition in breast cancer. *Clinical Pharmacology and Therapeutics*, **36**, 796–802.

Lonning, P. E., Kvinnsland, S., Thoren, T., and Ueland, P. M. (1987b). Alterations in the metabolism of oestrogens during treatment with aminoglutethimide in breast cancer patients: preliminary findings. *Clinical Pharmacokinetics*, **13**, 393–406.

McGuire, W. L. (1980). An update on estrogen and progesterone receptors in prognosis for primary and advanced breast cancer. *Hormones and Cancer* **15**, 337–44.

Mahendroo, M. S., Means, G. D., Mendelson, C. R., and Simpson, E. R. (1991). Tissue-specific expression of human P-459$_{arom}$. *Journal of Biological Chemistry*, **266**, 11276–81.

Metcalf, B. W., Wright, C. L., Burkhart, J. P., and Johnston, J. O. (1981). Substrate-induced inactivation of aromatase by allenic and acetylenic steroids. *Journal of the American Chemical Society*, **103**, 3221–2.

Meyer, A. S. (1955). Conversion of 19-hydroxy-4-androstene-3,17-dione to estrone by endocrine tissue. *Biochimica et Biophysica Acta*, **17**, 441–2.

Miller, W. R., Forrest, A. P. M., and Hamilton, T. (1974). Steroid metabolism by human breast and rat mammary carcinoma. *Steroids*, **23**, 379–95.

Morato, T., Hayano, M., Dorfman, R. I., and Axelrod, L. R. (1961). The intermediate steps in the biosynthesis of estrogens from androgens. *Biochemical and Biophysical Research Communications*, **6**, 334–8.

Naftolin, F., Ryan, K. J., Davis, I. J., Reddy, V. V., Flores, F., Petro, Z., and Kuhn, M. (1975). The formation of estrogen by central neuroendocrine tissues. *Recent Progress in Hormone Research*, **31**, 295–319.

Payne, A. H. (1987). Intratesticular site of aromatase activity and possible function of testicular aromatase. *Steroids*, **50**, 435–48.

Pickles, T., Perry, L., Murray, P., and Plowman, P. (1990). 4-Hydroxyandrostenedione—further clinical and extended endocrine observations. *British Journal of Cancer*, **62**, 309–13.

Powles, T. J., Ashley, S., Ford, H. T., Gazet, J. C., Nash, A. G., Neville, A. M., and Coombes, R. C. (1978). Treatment of disseminated breast cancer with tamoxifen, aminoglutethimide, hydrocortisone and danazol, used in combination or sequentially. *Lancet*, **ii**, 646–9.

Reed, M. J., Lai, L. C., Owen, A. M., Singh, A., Coldham, N. G., Purohit, A., *et al.* (1990). The effect of treatment with 4-hydroxyandrostenedione on the peripheral conversion of androstenedione to oestrone and *in vitro* tumor aromatase activity in postmenopausal women with breast cancer. *Cancer Research*, **50**, 193–96.

Ruder, H., Loriaux, L., and Lambert, M. B. (1972). Estrone sulfate production rates and metabolism in man. *Journal of Clinical Investigation*, **51**, 1021–33.

Samojlik, E., Santen, R. J., and Wells, S. A. (1977). Adrenal suppression with aminoglutethimide II. Differential effects of aminoglutethimide on plasma androstenedione and estrogen levels. *Journal of Clinical Endocrinology and Metabolism*, **45**, 480–7.

Santen, R. J., Worgul, T. J., Lipton, A., Harvey, H. A., Boucher, A., Samojlik, E., and Wells, S. A. (1982). Aminoglutethimide as treatment of postmenopausal women with advanced breast carcinoma: correlation of clinical and hormonal responses. *Annals of Internal Medicine* **96**, 94–101.

Santen, R. J., Leszcynski, D., Tilson-Mallet, N., Feil, P. D., Wright, C., Manni, A., and Santner, S. J. (1984). Enzymatic control of estrogen production in human breast cancer: relative significance of the aromatase versus sulfatase pathway. *Annals of the New York Academy of Sciences*, **464**, 126–37.

Santen, R. J., Demers, L., Lipton, A., Harvey, H. A., Hanagan, J., Mulagha, M., *et al.* (1989a). Phase II study of the potency and specificity of a new aromatase inhibitor—CGS 16949A. *Clinical Research*, **37**, 535A.

Santen, R. J., Demers, L. M., Adlercreutz, H., Harvey, H. A., Santner, S., Sanders, S., and Lipton, A. (1989b). Inhibition of aromatase with CGS-16949A in postmenopausal women. *Journal of Clinical Endocrinology and Metabolism*, **68**, 99–106.

Santen, R. J., Demers, L. M., Lynch, J., Harvey, H., Lipton, A., Mulagha, M., *et al.* (1991). Specificity of low dose fadrozole hydrochloride (CGS 16949 A) as an aromatase inhibitor. *Journal of Clinical Endocrinology and Metabolism*, **73**, 99–106.

Schwarzel, W. C., Kruggel, W., and Brodie, H. J. (1973). Studies on the mechanism of estrogen biosynthesis. VII. The development of inhibitors of the enzyme system in human placenta. *Endocrinology*, **92**, 866–80.

Sjoerdsma, A. (1981). Suicide inhibitors as potential drugs. *Clinical Pharmacology and Experimental Therapeutics*, **30**, 3–22.

Smith, I. E., Fitzharris, B. M., McKinna, J. A., Fahmy, D. R., Nash, A. G., Neville, A. M., *et al.* (1978). Aminoglutethimide in treatment of metastatic breast carcinoma. *Lancet*, **ii**, 646–9.

Stanek, J., Alder, A., Bellus, D., Bhatnagar, A. S., Hausler, A., and Schieweck, K. (1991). Synthesis and aromatase inhibitory activity of novel 1-(4-aminophenyl)-3-azabicyclo[3.1.0]hexane- and -[3.1.1]heptane-2,4-diones. *Journal of Medicinal Chemistry*, **34**, 1329–34.

Stein, R., Dowsett, M., Hedley, A., Davenport, J., Gazet, J. C., Ford, H. T., and Coombes, R. C. (1990). Treatment of advanced breast cancer in postmenopausal women with 4-hydroxyandrostenedione. *Cancer Chemotherapy and Pharmacology*, **26**, 75–8.

Stevenson, D. E., Wright, J. N., and Akhtar, M. (1988). Mechanistic consideration of P-450 dependent enzymatic reactions: studies on oestriol biosynthesis. *Journal of the Chemical Society, Perkin Transactions I*, 2043–52.

Stevenson, D. E., Wright, J. N., and Akhtar, M. (1985). Synthesis of 19-functionalised derivatives of 16a-hydroxytestosterone: Mechanistic studies on oestriol biosynthesis. *Journal of the Chemical Society, Chemical Communications*, 1078–80.

Thompson, E. A. Jr and Siiteri, P. K. (1974). Utilization of oxygen and reduced nicotinamide adenine dinucleotide phosphate by human placental microsomes during aromatization of androstenedione. *Journal of Biological Chemistry*, **249**, 5364–72.

Tuman, R. W., Morris, S. M., Wallace, N. H., and Bowden, C. R. (1991). Inhibition of peripheral aromatization in the male cynomolgus monkey by a novel nonsteroidal inhibitor (R 76713). *Journal of Clinical Endocrinology and Metabolism*, **72**, 755–60.

Vanden Bossche, H., Willemsens, G., Roels, I., Bellens, D., Moereels, H., Coene, M. C., *et al.* (1990). R 76713 and enantiomers: selective nonsteroidal inhibitors of the cytochrome P-450-dependent oestrogen biosynthesis. *Biochemical Pharmacology*, **40**, 170–18.

Van Wauwe, J. P. and Janssen, P. A. J. (1989). Is there a case for P-450 inhibitors in cancer treatment? *Journal of Medicinal Chemistry*, **32**, 2231–9.

Varela, R. M. and Dao, T. L. (1978). Estrogen synthesis and estradiol binding by human mammary tumors. *Cancer Research*, **38**, 2429–33.

Wing, L.-Y., Garrett, W. M., and Brodie, A. M. H. (1985). The effect of aromatase inhibitors, aminoglutethimide and 4-hydroxyandrostenedione in cyclic rats with DMBA-induced mammary tumors. *Cancer Research*, **45**, 2425–8.

Wouters, W., DeCoster, R., Beerens, D., Doolaege, R., Gruwez, J. A., Van Camp, K., *et al.* (1990). Potency and selectivity of the aromatase inhibitor

R 76 713. A study in human ovarian, adipose, stromal, testicular and adrenal cells. *Journal of Steroid Biochemistry*, **36**, 57–65.

Wright, J. N., Slachter, G., and Akhtar, M. (1991). 'Slow-binding' sixth-ligand inhibitors of cytochrome P-450 aromatase. *Biophysical Journal*, **273**, 533–7.

Zaccheo, T., Giudici, D., Lombardi, P., and di Salle, E. (1989). A new irreversible aromatase inhibitor, β-methylandrosta-1,4-diene-3–17-dione (FCE 24304): anti-tumor activity and endocrine effects in rats with DMBA-induced mammary tumors. *Cancer Chemotherapy and Pharmacology*, **23**, 47–50.

Zaccheo, T., Giudici, D., Ornati, G., Panzeri, A., and di Salle, E. (1991). Comparison of the effects of the irreversible aromatase inhibitor exemestane with atamestane and MDL-18962 in rats with DMBA-induced mammary tumors. *European Journal of Cancer*, **27**, 1145–50.

Section 9C

17α-Hydroxylase/17,20-lyase

Hugo Vanden Bossche and Henri Moereels

9C.1   Introduction

In western Europe, prostatic carcinoma is the second most frequent cancer in men (Denis 1991). It has surpassed lung cancer as the most commonly diagnosed cancer in United States males and is the second leading cause of cancer deaths in men (Chiarodo 1991). At present, prostate cancer costs the United States more than a billion dollars annually, requires 250 000 admissions to hospital, and results in more than 28 000 deaths (Chiarodo 1991). Adenocarcinoma of the prostate originates from the prostatic epithelium (Denis 1991). The morphologically distinct stages of prostate cancer range from a latent or hidden form, focal carcinoma (microscopic size), localized nodule to metastatic disease (Chiarodo 1991; Denis 1991).

The prostate gland depends on androgens (particularly 5α-dihydrotesto-sterone (DHT)) both for development within the fetus and for maintenance in the adult (Mooradian *et al.* 1987; Martini *et al.* 1990; Chiarodo 1991). Although the mechanisms that regulate growth of normal and malignant prostate tissue are poorly understood, clinically manifested prostate cancer, like the normal prostate, is androgen dependent at least in part or for a certain period (Pierrepoint *et al.* 1985; Bartsch *et al.* 1990). Studies by Huggins *et al.* (1941) first revealed the impact of androgens on prostatic carcinoma and provided the rationale for the treatment of cases of this condition by androgen deprivation. A number of treatment regimens are available at present, such as surgical and medical castration, androgen blockade, and inhibition of androgen synthesis (Grayhack *et al.* 1987; Denis 1991).

9C.2   Steroids biosynthesis

The steroid hormones are derived from cholesterol (Fig. 9.C.1). The cholesterol side-chain cleavage enzyme (cytochrome P450 scc) catalyses the synthesis of the pregnenolone in the inner mitochondrial membrane of steroidogenic cells. Pregnenolone can be dehydrogenated at the 3β-position by 3β-hydroxysteroid dehydrogenase to form progesterone. Both progesterone and pregnenolone are 17-hydroxylated in the smooth endoplasmic reticulum by the P450 17 [product of the *CYP17* gene (Nebert *et al.* 1991)]. 17α-Hydroxypregnenolone and 17α-hydroxyprogesterone undergo cleavage of the 17,20-carbon bond via the 17,20-lyase reaction to form dehydroepiandrosterone (DHEA) and androstenedione respectively, the precursors of testosterone, dihydrotestosterone (DHT), and the oestrogens oestradiol and oestrone.

9C.3   17α-Hydroxylase/17,20-lyase

Chung *et al.* (1987) called the P450 17 enzyme a key branch point in the system of adrenal steroid hormone synthesis. Indeed, as 17α-hydroxylase, it distinguishes between the synthesis of mineralocorticoids (e.g. aldosterone) and glucocorticoids (cortisol) in the adrenal cortex; as 17,20-lyase, it distinguishes between the synthesis of glucocorticoids and C19 precursors of androgens such as DHEA (Fig. 9C.1).

Studies of bovine adrenocortical cells in culture and of bovine fetal adrenals suggest that the bovine P450 17 gene is predominantly regulated by corticotropin (ACTH) in a cAMP-dependent manner, as evidenced by the inability to detect P450 17 mRNA in the absence of ACTH and by the increase P450 17 mRNA or protein upon treatment with ACTH or cAMP analogues (John *et al.* 1986; Zuber *et al.* 1986b; Lund *et al.* 1988, 1990; Yanase *et al.* 1991). cAMP regulates steroid hydroxylase expression in the adrenal cortex by increasing transcription of the gene and requires ongoing protein synthesis (John *et al.* 1986).

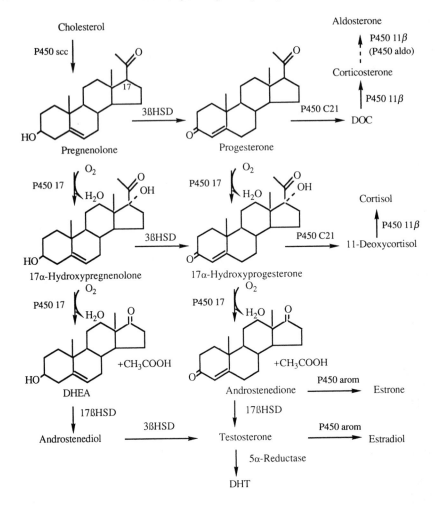

Fig. 9C.1 Biosynthetic pathways for steroids: SCC, side-chain cleavage; 17α, 17α-hydroxylase/17,20-lyase; arom, aromatase; C21, 21-hydroxylase; aldo, aldosterone; 11β, 11β-hydroxylase; 3βHSD, 3β-hydroxysteroid dehydrogenase; 17βHSD, 17β-hydroxysteroid dehydrogenase; DOC, 11-deoxycorticosterone; DHEA, dehydro-epiandrosterone; DHT, dihydrotestosterone.

P450 17 has been observed immunohistochemically in pig adrenal cortex, testis, and ovary (Sasano *et al.* 1989). In the adrenal cortex P450 17 has been found in the zona fasciculata and reticularis but not in the zona glomerulosa (Sasano *et al.* 1989). In the testis, P450 17 was present exclusively in Leydig cells, and in the ovary immunoreactivity was observed exclusively in the theca interna (Sasano *et al.* 1989). Porcine thecal lyase activity increased as the follicle matured, providing more androgen substrate for the production of oestrogen (Tonetta and Hernandez 1989). P450 17 has also been immunolocalized in bovine follicles and found in the cells of the theca interna at or near the time of its differentiation (Rodgers *et al.* 1986). P450 17 is also expressed in the sheep placenta near term, presumably under the control of cortisol production by the fetal adrenal (France *et al.* 1988; Tangalakis *et al.* 1990). In rats, P450 17 is not expressed in the adrenal cortex (Voutilainen *et al.* 1986). P450 17 mRNA has been detected in human fetal adrenals, testis, and ovary, but was undetectable in the human placenta and non-steroidogenic cells (i.e. kidney, liver, spleen, intestine, or muscle) (Voutilainen and Miller 1986). Only miniscule amounts of P450 17 mRNA were found in human granulosa cells (Voutilainen *et al.* 1986).

As mentioned above, P450 17 catalyses two distinct mixed-function oxidase reactions (Fig. 9C.1). Nakajin *et al.* (1981b, 1984) proved that the 17a-hydroxylase and 17,20-lyase activities of pig testicular and adrenal smooth endoplasmic reticulum result from the action of a single P450. Their results also suggest one active site for both hydroxylase and lyase activities (Nakajin *et al.* 1981a). This has been confirmed for guinea-pig adrenal microsomes (Kominami *et al.* 1982; Shinzawa *et al.* 1985). Expression studies of the human (Bradshaw *et al.* 1987), bovine (Zuber *et al.* 1986a), and rat (Fevold *et al.* 1989) P450 17 cDNA clones in COS-1 cells further proved that P450 17 catalyses both 17a-hydroxylation and 17,20-lyase reactions.

The mechanism for the P450 17-catalysed conversion of pregnenolone into DHEA via 17a-hydroxypregnenlone is based on mechanistic studies using $^{18}O_2$ (Miller *et al.* 1991). These studies indicate that the 17a-hydroxyl derives from molecular oxygen and that one atom of oxygen is incorporated into the released acetate (Miller *et al.* 1991).

Slight differences in amino acid sequence have been reported in porcine P450 17 isolated from adrenal and testis (Nakajin *et al.* 1984). Thus it appears that the pig might have two P450 17 isozymes, one expressed in the testis and the other in the adrenal cortex (Miller 1988). However, in man a single gene (6.6 kb long) on chromosome 10 codes for P450 17, which, as expected, is identical in testis and adrenals (Matteson *et al.* 1986; Bradshaw *et al.* 1987; Chung *et al.* 1987; Picado-Leonard and Miller 1987; Kagimoto *et al.* 1988; Miller 1988; Yanase *et al.* 1991). The molecular mass of the human P450 is ± 57 kDa (Yanase *et al.* 1991). As in man, the bovine gene (± 6.2 kb long) consists of eight exons and seven introns, and the locations of the exon–intron boundaries are identical (Bhasker *et al.* 1989). Table 9C.1 shows the correspondence between the available P450 17 sequences.

From sequence comparison, it can be deduced that there are 75 positions where amino acids are the same in bovine and human forms of P450 17

Table 9C.1 Identity and similarity between P450 17 sequences[*]

	Human (508)	Bovine	Rat	Chicken
Bovine (509)	71.1			
	90.7			
Rat (507)	68.4	64.3		
	86.6	86.4		
Chicken (508)	48.4	47.4	48.7	
	76.0	72.8	74.6	
Porcine (423[†])	63.8	72.8	60.0	43.3
	83.2	88.2	80.1	68.8

[*]Calculated using CGEMA (Moereels *et al.* 1990); upper number, percentage identity; lower number, percentage similarity (both relative to the shortest sequence). Numbers in parentheses give the number of amino acids. Sequences taken from the following: human and porcine, Chung *et al.* (1987); bovine, Bhasker *et al.* (1989); chicken, Ono *et al.* (1988); rat, Namiki *et al.* (1988).

[†]Incomplete sequence.

but which differ in the rat enzyme (Fevold *et al.* 1989). This may be the origin of differences in catalytic properties. Indeed, comparison of 17*a*-hydroxylase and 17,20-lyase activities in COS-1 cells transfected with bovine, human, or rat P450 17, shows interesting differences. Although rat, bovine, and human P450 17 can hydroxylate progesterone and pregnenolone at C17 (Lorence *et al.* 1990), only the rat 17,20-lyase is able to convert both 17*a*-hydroxypregnenolone and 17*a*-hydroxyprogesterone into their respective androgens DHEA and androstenedione. The human and bovine enzymes catalyse the conversion of 17*a*-hydroxypregnenolone into DHEA (Fevold *et al.* 1989). Similar results are found after the expression of bovine P450 17 in *Escherichia coli* (Barnes *et al.* 1991). Pregnenolone and progesterone are rapidly converted to their 17*a*-hydroxylated products and only 17*a*-hydroxypregnenolone is converted to DHEA. Following expression in COS-1 cells, P450 17 from bovine and human catalyse the 17*a*-hydroxylation of progesterone more efficiently than the 17*a*-hydroxylation of pregnenolone; the bovine enzyme is two to three times more active than the human form. Furthermore, the bovine enzyme is about four times more efficient at catalysing the 17,20-lyase conversion of 17*a*-hydroxypregnenolone into DHEA. Human P450 17 has also been shown to catalyse 16*a*-hydroxylation of progesterone more than 10 times more efficiently than does the bovine enzyme (Lorence *et al.* 1990), whereas the rat enzyme is unable to carry out this conversion (Fevold *et al.* 1989). Lorence *et al.* (1990) constructed bovine amino terminus–human carboxy terminus and human amino terminus–

bovine carboxy terminus cDNA chimeras and expressed them in COS-1 cells. The chimeras with a bovine amino terminus and a human carboxy terminus catalysed 17α-hydroxylase activities intermediate between wild-type bovine and human levels. 17α-Hydroxylase activity was much less affected than 17,20-lyase activity, which was decreased by 80 per cent or more when compared with wild-type bovine activity and by about 50 per cent when compared with wild-type human activity. 16α-Hydroxylase activity was also 50 per cent lower. The chimeras with a human amino terminus and a bovine carboxy terminus were expressed in the COS-1 cells at the same level as the first group. However, these chimeras were inactive. These results may indicate that the folding pattern initiated by the bovine amino terminus upon anchoring in the endoplasmic reticulum can accommodate human carboxy-terminal sequences without severe steric hindrance, leading to stable functional enzymes with relatively normal 17α-hydroxylase activity. In contrast, the human amino terminus initiates a folding pathway that does not accommodate bovine carboxy-terminal sequences and results in enzymes with little or no 17α-hydroxylase activity. Based on these results, Lorence *et al.* (1990) conclude that the differences between the bovine and the human enzyme may be due to differences in their tertiary structure. Changes in tertiary structure seem to have a greater impact on 17,20-lyase activity.

Bovine adrenocortical P450 17 expressed in COS-1 cells supports 17α-hydroxylation of pregnenolone and progesterone with equal efficiency, but catalyses C17,20-bond scission of 17α-hydroxypregnenolone 4–14.7 times more than that of 17α-hydroxyprogesterone (Zuber *et al.* 1986a). Furthermore, the 17α-hydroxylation reaction occurs at a higher rate than the 17,20-lyase reaction (Zuber *et al.* 1986a). As with other P450 enzymes from the endoplasmic reticulum, activity is supported by a two-electron transfer from the microsomal flavoprotein NADPH–P450 reductase. The second electron may also be provided to the P450 by cytochrome b_5. Results obtained by Onoda and Hall (1982) indicate that the participation of cytochrome b_5 can change the ratio of 17α-hydroxylation to 17,20-lyase activities. Also, the addition of porcine hepatic P450 reductase to microsomes from adrenal and testis increases the activity of lyase relative to hydroxylase until the rates of activity become almost equal. The same effect is obtained when reductase is added to the purified enzymes (Yanagibashi and Hall 1986). As the reductase concentration increases, lyase activity increases relative to hydroxylase activity. Antibodies to reductase, when added to porcine testicular micosomes, inhibit both activities, but lyase is more inhibited than hydroxylase. Furthermore, porcine testicular microsomes contain three to four times more P450 reductase than adrenal microsomes (Yanagibashi and Hall 1986). Thus the ratio of cytochrome b_5 and/or reductase to P450 17 seems to determine whether a steroid will undergo 17,20-bond scission after 17α-hydroxylation. These studies also indicate that, although both 17,20-bond scission and 17-hydroxylation are catalysed at the same site on the polypeptide of P450 17, the 17,20-lyase and 17α-hydroxylase differ in many aspects. These differences may also explain why the 17,20-lyase is more sensitive to some chemical compounds (see below).

Namiki *et al.* (1988) suggest that the P450 17 of rat testis is anchored to the membrane of the endoplasmic reticulum by two transmembrane regions, one at the NH_2 terminal site (amino acids 2–21) and a second from amino acids 169 to 186. The two transmembrane regions are also found in the bovine and human P450s. In addition, four hydrophobic clefts are identified at positions 280–300, 320–360, 400–420, and 465–485 in bovine and human P450 17 (Namiki *et al.* 1988). However, in a more recent study, Edwards *et al.* (1991) collected evidence that supports a model in which the endoplasmic reticular P450s are anchored in the membrane by a single transmembrane N-terminal helix 20–30 residues long, with the globular part of the protein in the cytosol. In their model the haeme lies at or nearly perpendicular to the membrane. Thus the active site of P450 appears to be located at some distance from the endoplasmic reticular membrane. In this model hydrophilic substrates may enter the active site directly from the cytosol. Cytosolic proteins, microsomal proteins, and lipids may form a contiguous hydrophobic phase from which hydrophobic substrates can partition to the hydrophobic active site of P450 without entering the aqueous phase of the system (Edwards *et al.* 1991).

Zuber *et al.* (1986b) analysed a region in the bovine adrenocortical cytochrome P450 17 and human P450 C21 sequences that contains a peptide first described by Ozols *et al.* (1981) as conserved for phenobarbital-inducible P450s. Although an alignment of the complete sequences shows less than 30 per cent identity (Miller 1988), the sequence identity in the extended 'Ozols peptide' is much higher (Fig. 9C.2). These P450s have two substrates in common, progesterone and 17α-hydroxyprogesterone. Therefore this conserved region may be involved in substrate binding and is also found in other steroidogenic P450s (Picado-Leonard and Miller 1988; Nonaka *et al.* 1989; Vanden Bossche *et al.* 1991). It should be noted that the only

17α	346 D R N R L L L L E A T I R E V L R L R P V A P M	(Chung *et al.* 1987)
C-21	338 D R A R L P L L N A T I A E V L R L R P V V P L	(White *et al.* 1986)
SCC	331 M L Q L V P L L K A S I K E T L R L H P I S V T	(Morohashi *et al.* 1987)
11β	334 A T T E L P L L R A A L K E T L R L Y P V G L F	(Mornet *et al.* 1989)
arom	349 D I Q K L K V M E N F I Y E S M R Y Q P V V D L	(Harada 1988)
cam	280 R I P A A C E E L L R R F	(Unger *et al.* 1986)

Fig. 9C.2 Comparison of tentative steroid binding regions in human P450 corresponding to the K helix of P450 cam. The numbers of the two mitochondrial P450s (SCC and 11β) are relative to the NH_2 terminus of mature proteins.

P450 that acts on the A-ring of the steroid, i.e. P450 arom has the least similarity to the consensus sequence (Fig. 9C.2). This may suggest that its substrate androstenedione binds to another region, as proposed by Graham-Lorence *et al*. (1991). The amino acids 346–366 of human P450 17 (encoded by exon 6 of the *CYP17* gene) also identified regions of significant similarity in the sequences of the human, chicken, and rabbit progesterone receptor, the human, mouse, and rat glucocorticoid receptor, and human mineralocorticoid, androgen, and oestrogen receptors. Although the amino acid identity was less than that among the steroidogenic P450s, the similarity remained great (Picado-Leonard and Miller 1988). The suggestion that the proposed region may be involved in steroid binding was tested using molecular modelling and computational chemistry. As a result a convincing complex was obtained between progesterone and the tentative binding region of human P450 17 in a helical conformation (details will be published elsewhere). According to known sequence alignments (Edwards *et al*. 1989; Gotoh and Fuyii-Kuriyama 1989; Nelson and Strobel 1989), this region corresponds to the K helix in P450 cam. In the three-dimensional structure of P450 cam (Poulos *et al*. 1987) this helix, being ± 28 Å away from the haeme, is certainly in a very unfavourable position to be part of the active site, provided that the structure of P450 cam is a good template. From our results and alignments, it could be argued that it is not a good template. Therefore in the structure of P450s other than P450 cam the K helix may have a different spatial position. It is also possible that, after steroid binding to the K helix, a major conformational change is induced, allowing the steroid to slip into a 'P450 cam-like' active site between the haeme group and the I helix. It is clear that site-directed mutagenesis will be of great help in further testing the K helix hypothesis.

The different alignments also agree that the region containing the conserved threonine (252 in P450 cam corresponds to the P450 cam I helix which is well known to be involved in ligand binding. Using the P450 cam structure as a template, this region, which is similar among P450s, may be involved in ligand binding. This idea is supported by the results of molecular modelling of androstenedione with the haeme and the corresponding I helix of human P450 arom (Graham-Lorence *et al*. 1991). In addition Graham-Lorence *et al*. (1991) constructed seven different mutants, that were transfected in COS-1 cells, in this region and examined the activities of the expressed proteins. Changing Glu[302] to Ala, Val, or Gln resulted in proteins devoid of activity, while mutating Pro[308] to Val reduced activity to about one-third of that of the wild type. These observations strongly support the idea that the corresponding I helix in P450 arom is involved in androstenedione binding. Whatever suggestion is made, it is clear that there is a strong need for more experimental three-dimensional structures of P450s.

The study of the molecular bases of 17a-hydroxylase/17,20-lyase deficiencies offers another possibility of revealing structural requirements.

Deficiency of 17α-hydroxylase is a rare cause of congenital adrenal hyperplasia (Bigliery and Kater 1991; Yanase *et al.* 1991). This deficiency is
expressed in the adrenal cortex, testes, and ovary, leading to impaired
production of cortisol and the clinical manifestations of mineralocorticoid excess (hypokalaemia and hypertension) and sex hormone deficiency
(hypogonadism) (Yanase *et al.* 1990; Bigliery and Kater 1991). Closely
related to reduced production of sex steroids are increased height, eunu-
choidism, bone age retardation, and osteoporosis (Yanase *et al.* 1991).
A detailed investigation of a mutant P450 17 protein revealed that the
mutation occurred at the C-terminal side of the haeme binding region
(Kagimoto *et al.* 1988). The mutant sequence is identical with that of the
normal gene, except for the four-base duplication CATC at the position
of codon 479. Consequently, the reading frame is altered at this point in
the mutant gene, leading to a C-terminal sequence which is completely
different from that of the normal P450 17. In the mutant proline 480
is replaced by histidine and, in contrast with the normal P450 17 containing six basic residues between amino acids 480 and 508, it only possesses
one basic residue (arginine) in this region. Kagimoto *et al.* (1988) suggest
that the reduced positive charge at the C terminus of the mutant P450 17
diminishes its ability to interact with P450 reductase, leading to the observed 17α-hydroxylase/17,20-lyase deficiency. A male pseudohermaphrodite
was found to carry two different inherited mutant alleles in the *CYP17*
gene (Yanase *et al.* 1991). One allele contains a stop codon (TGA) in place
of arginine (CGA) at amino acid position 239 in exon 4. The resultant
truncated protein is totally non-functional. The second allele contains a
mis-sense mutation, i.e. the substitution of threonine (ACA) for proline
(CCA) at amino acid position 342 (P450$^{P \rightarrow T(342)}$) in exon 6. This exon
encodes the amino acid sequence which contains the putative steroid binding
place (see above). Both the 17α-hydroxylase and 17,20-lyase activities
expressed in COS-1 cells transfected with the cDNA construct containing
the proline 342 → threonine mutation were reduced by 40–45 per cent
(Yanase *et al.* 1991). Thus these results further support the hypothesis that
the amino acid sequence encoded by exon 6 may be involved in substrate
binding.

9C.4 17α-Hydroxylase/17,20-lyase inhibitors

As discussed earlier, inhibition of androgen synthesis is of therapeutic
importance. Compounds that interfere with the 17,20-lyase activity of
P450 17 and much less with its 17α-hydroxylase activity are of great
interest. Indeed, these compounds will inhibit androgen synthesis in testis,
ovary, and adrenals (the primary source of androgens after orchidectomy)
without cortisol depletion (a feature of 17α-hydroxylase inhibitors).

9C.4.1   Ketoconazole

Ketoconazole (R 41400; Fig. 9C.3) is an imidazole derivative with broad-spectrum oral antifungal activity. Such activity originates from interaction with the P450-dependent demethylation of lanosterol or 24-methylene-dihydrolanosterol, a key step in the synthesis of ergosterol (Vanden Bossche *et al.* 1980, 1989, 1990a). The effective single daily dose of ketoconazole for most fungal infections is 200–400 mg (Graybill 1990). The incidence of side-effects is low. However, gynaecomastia was reported in two patients during treatment with 200 mg ketoconazole daily (De Felice *et al.* 1981) and in a few patients receiving high multiple doses (600–1200 mg daily) (Pont *et al.* 1982). This rare side-effect suggested that ketoconazole affected the oestrogen-to-androgen ratio in these patients (Pont *et al.* 1982).

Ketoconazole is a poor inhibitor of aromatase (Mason *et al.* 1985) and no clear reduction in plasma oestradiol levels at 600 mg ketoconazole daily was seen (Pont *et al.* 1982). However, on measuring testosterone serum levels, a dose-related reversible decrease was observed (Pont *et al.* 1982; Schurmeyer and Nieschlag 1982; Santen *et al.* 1983; De Coster *et al.* 1986; Feldman 1986; Vanden Bossche *et al.* 1987). The finding of a marked but transient decrease in plasma testosterone levels initiated a series of studies to determine the site of action of ketoconazole in the androgen biosynthetic pathway. Testosterone synthesis was studied in a rat testicular subcellular fraction containing cytosol and microsomes (Lauwers *et al.* 1985; Vanden

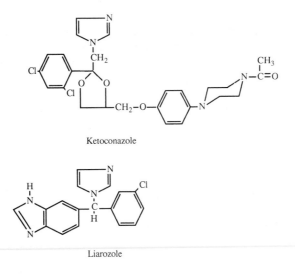

Ketoconazole

Liarozole

Fig. 9C.3 Structures of ketoconazole and liarozole.

Bossche *et al.* 1985a,b). With pregnenolone as substrate, 50 per cent inhibition of androgen synthesis was achieved in the presence of 6 μM ketoconazole. This inhibition coincided with an accumulation of a steroid with a mass spectrum identical with that obtained with pregn-5-ene-3β,-17α,20α-triol (17α-hydroxy-20-dihydropregnenolone), indicating that keto-conazole is an inhibitor of C17,20-bond scission. Table 9C.2 summarizes the results obtained with testicular subcellular fractions from different species. The P450 17 catalysed androgen synthesis from pregnenolone in human testes is much more sensitive than that in rat, boar, and dog testes. Further studies revealed that ketoconazole inhibits the conversion of 17α-hydroxy-20-dihydroprogesterone into androstenedione by rat testi-cular microsomes, with 50 per cent inhibition being achieved at 0.26 μM (Table 9C.2). These studies further prove that ketoconazole is an inhibitor of 17,20-lyase and indicate that 17α-hydroxy,20-dihydroprogesterone is a substrate. Of course, this does not prove that 17α-hydroxy,20-dihydro-progesterone or 17α-hydroxy,20-dihydropregnenolone are obligatory inter-mediates in the conversion of C21 steroids to C19 steroids. It is possible that, under the incubation and extraction conditions used, 17α-hydroxy-progesterone and 17α-hydroxypregnenolone are reduced. Studies by Kan *et al.* (1985), Rajfer *et al.* (1985), and Higashi *et al.* (1987) further prove that the ketoconazole-induced inhibition of androgen synthesis originates from its effects on the 17,20-lyase. In rat testis, the 17,20-lyase was almost four times more sensitive to ketoconazole than the 17α-hydroxylase (Higashi *et al.* 1987).

Imidazole derivatives display high affinity for P450, causing a type II difference spectrum with maxima at 430–432 nm and minima at 393–412 nm. Type II difference spectra obtained when increasing concentrations of ketoconazole were added to piglet testis microsomes consisted of a maximum at about 433 nm, a minimum at 412 nm, and an isosbestic point at 423 nm (Vanden Bossche *et al.* 1985b). This type II spectrum indicates the binding of a ligand to a low spin haemoprotein (Hajek *et al.* 1982). Thus, ketoconazole might exert its inhibitory action on the 17,20-lyase, at least partially, by interacting with the haeme iron of P450 17.

In human ovarian cells (mainly theca cells), ketoconazole also inhibits the production of androstenedione from 17α-hydroxyprogesterone. However, a concentration of 23 μM is needed to achieve 50 per cent inhibition (Weber *et al.* 1991). Ketoconazole inhibits the 17α-hydroxylase and 17,20-lyase in human adrenal microsomes (Couch *et al.* 1987), with the latter being about twice as sensitive (Ayub and Levell 1989). Ketoconazole inhibits androgen synthesis when added to bovine adrenal microsomes (IC_{50} = 0.4 μM) (Table 9C.2). This inhibition coincided with an accumulation of pregnenolone and 11-deoxycorticosterone (Vanden Bossche *et al.* 1987). At higher concentrations, it also inhibited the synthesis of 11-deoxycortisol, coinciding with a further increase in 11-deoxycorticosterone. This again

Table 9C.2 Effects of ketoconazole and liarozole on *in vitro* steroid synthesis [*]

Species and tissue	Subcellular fraction	Substrate	P450	IC$_{50}$ (μM)	
				Ketoconazole	Liarozole [†]
Testes					
Rat	S-10 000	17OH,20	17α(17,20)	0.26	0.22
		pregnenolone	17α	6.00	3.20
Pig				3.00	4.15
Dog				5.41	0.26
Bovine					0.27
Human				0.34	0.26
Adrenal [‡]					
Bovine	Microsomes	Pregnenolone	17α(17-OH)	2.80	0.15
			17α(17-OH + 17,20)	0.40	12.70

[*] Effects on 17,20-lyase (17,20) were studied using an S-10 000 fraction of rat testes and [1,2, 6,7 [³H]]-17-hydroxy-20-dihydroprogesterone (17OH,20) as substrate (products formed from 17-hydroxy-20-dihydroprogesterone are androstenedione and testosterone). Effects on 17-hydroxylase + 17,20-lyase (17α) were studied using [¹⁴C]-pregnenolone as substrate (products formed from pregnenolone are DHEA, androstenedione, androstenediol, and testosterone). Most of the results obtained with ketoconazole are taken from Vanden Bossche *et al.* (1989, 1990a) and unpublished results.

[†] Taken from Vanden Bossche *et al.* (1990b) and unpublished results.

[‡] Effects on adrenal 17α-hydroxylase (17-OH) were studied by measuring the incorporation of radioactivity from [¹⁴C]-pregnenolone into 11-deoxycortisol. The conversion of pregnenolone into 11-deoxycortisol requires 3β-hydroxysteroid dehydrogenase, 17α-hydroxylase, and 21-hydroxylase. However, since under the experimental conditions used more than 10 μM ketoconazole and more than 1 μM liarozole are needed to affect the synthesis of 11-deoxycorticosterone from pregnenolone (requires the presence of 3β-hydroxysteroid dehydrogenase and 21-hydroxylase), a decreased formation of 11-deoxycortisol can be taken as a measure of inhibition of 17α-hydroxylase. Adrenal androgen synthesis (requires both 17α-hydroxylase and 17,20-lyase) was studied by following the incorporation of radioactivity from [¹⁴C]-pregnenolone into androstenedione (17-OH + 17,20).

indicates that the 17α-hydroxylase-catalysed conversion of pregnenolone to 17α-hydroxyprogesterone is less sensitive than that catalysed by 17,20-lyase. The accumulation of 11-deoxycorticosterone indicates that ketoconazole interferes much less with the 21-hydroxylase. A K_i value of 5 μM was found in rat adrenal microsomes (Higashi *et al.* 1987). This is 12.5 times higher than the value found for rat testicular 17,20-lyase. Ketoconazole also had little or no effect on 21-hydroxylase activity in human adrenal microsomes (Couch *et al.* 1987). This is surprising since, as discussed above, P450 17 and P450 C21 shows a well-conserved domain that has been proposed as the putative steroid binding site.

An effect of ketoconazole (400 mg three times daily) on the synthesis of adrenal steroids was also proved in 14 previously untreated patients with stage D metastatic prostate cancer (De Coster *et al*. 1986). In addition to a striking decrease in testosterone plasma levels, a decline in androstenedione and DHEA, which are mainly of adrenal origin, was noted. As expected from the *in vitro* results, the decrease in androgen levels coincided with a rise in 17α-hydroxyprogesterone and progesterone plasma levels. A marked inhibition of the 17,20-lyase and a moderate effect on the 17α-hydroxylase was also found in patients with metastatic prostate carcinoma on long-term high dose ketoconazole therapy. (Trachtenberg and Zadra 1988).

The fact that ketoconazole interferes with testicular as well as adrenal androgen synthesis has made it a candidate for the treatment of androgen-dependent prostate carcinoma (Trachtenberg *et al*. 1983; Denis *et al*. 1985; Heyns *et al*. 1985; Amery *et al*. 1986; Tapazoglou *et al*. 1986; Vanden Bossche *et al*. 1987; Sonino 1987; Lowe and Bamberger 1990). Since androgens are also of causal significance in the aetiology of hirsutism (Neumann 1987), inhibitors of androgen synthesis such as ketoconazole may also be of help in the treatment of this disease (Sonino 1987). Successful therapy with ketoconazole has also been reported in three children with precocious puberty and autonomous Leydig cell hyperactivity who exhibited low basal and gonadotropin-releasing hormone-stimulated gonadotropin levels (Sonino 1987).

The frequent administration of high doses of ketoconazole (400 mg three times daily) produces symptomatic relief of bone pain and sustained clinical remission in the majority of patients with advanced prostate cancer (Trachtenberg and Zadra 1988). However, at the high dose used, the principal side-effect is gastric discomfort with nausea (Amery *et al*. 1986). Thus, although striking clinical improvement is seen in many patients treated with ketoconazole, its use is limited by gastric discomfort and an uncomfortable intake schedule. However, these investigations indicated the therapeutic potential of P450 17 inhibitors in the treatment of prostatic cancer, provided P450 systems to evaluate activity and predict possible toxicity, and triggered a multidisciplinary study to open up new possibilities in medical treatment.

9C.4.2 Liarozole

An early product of these studies is liarozole (R 75251; liarozole fumarate, R85246). In contrast with ketoconazole, this imidazole derivative (Fig. 9C.3) is devoid of antifungal activity and has no effect on cholesterol synthesis or cholesterol side-chain cleavage, but has the same effect as ketoconazole on testicular androgen synthesis from pregnenolone (Bruynseels *et al*. 1990; Vanden Bossche *et al*. 1990b, unpublished results). Testicular androgen synthesis inhibition originates first from an effect on the 17,20-lyase while, at higher concentrations, 17α-hydroxylase activity is inhibited (Vanden Bossche *et al.* 1990b). As shown in Table 9C.2, liarozole and ketoconazole are almost equipotent inhibitors of rat testicular 17,20-lyase and of androgen synthesis from pregnenolone by subcellular fractions from rat and human testes. However, liarozole is a more potent inhibitor of the 17α-hydroxylase/17,20-lyase activity in dog testicular microsomes. In rat testicular cells, testosterone and androstenedione synthesis stimulated by human chorionic gonadotrophin (hCG) is inhibited with IC$_{50}$ values of 2.3 μM and 0.7 μM respectively (Bruynseels *et al.* 1990). In dogs, liarozole at 2.5 mg kg^{-1} reduced plasma testosterone and androstenedione levels to castrate levels for at least 12 h (De Coster, personal communication). In dogs, the reduction of plasma androgen levels coincided with an accumulation of 17α-hydroxyprogesterone and progesterone.

A single oral dose of 300 mg liarozole significantly lowered plasma testosterone levels in human volunteers for 24 hours. A peak suppressive effect on testosterone was reached after 8 hours, with plasma testosterone levels decreasing from 23.6 to 3.3 nM. After 24 hours testosterone levels were still decreased by 40 per cent (Bruynseels *et al.* 1990). These results prove that liarozole is an inhibitor of testicular androgen synthesis both *in vitro* and *in vivo*. Liarozole inhibits (IC$_{50}$ = 0.15 μM) the synthesis of 11-deoxycortisol from pregnenolone in bovine adrenal microsomes, proving that the adrenocortical 17α-hydroxylase activity of P450 17 is also sensitive. However, when compared with its effects on androgen synthesis by bovine testicular microsomes, almost 47 times more liarozole is needed to achieve 50 per cent inhibition of androstenedione synthesis by adrenocortical microsomes (Table 9C.2). This indicates that, in contrast with the 17,20-lyase activity of bovine testicular P450 17, the adrenal enzyme is not a target for liarozole. Since P450 17 is encoded by a single gene, variations in sensitivity may originate from conformational differences.

Both ketoconazole and liarozole clearly suppressed circulating testosterone levels in male volunteers, and ketoconazole also significantly suppressed production of the adrenal androgens DHEA and androstenedione whereas liarozole caused only minor changes (Vanden Bossche *et al.* 1987, Bruynseels *et al.* 1990). Nevertheless, in a pilot study of orchidectomized stage D prostate cancer patients, liarozole (300 mg twice daily) induced both subjective improvement (pain, performance status, and urological complaints) and objective improvement (serum prostatic specific antigen (PSA) level, tumour, and lymph node reduction) (Mahler *et al.* 1989; Denis 1991). Adrenal androgen synthesis was not inhibited in these patients (De Coster *et al.* 1991). Furthermore, liarozole reduced growth of both androgen-dependent (Van Ginckel *et al.* 1990) and androgen-independent (De Coster *et al.* 1992) prostatic adenocarcinoma in rats. These results suggest that the antitumour effects of liarozole may not be related to its inhibitory effects on androgen biosynthesis.

In contrast with ketoconazole, liarozole is a potent inhibitor of the aromatase in human placental microsomes (Vanden Bossche *et al.* 1990b). Fifty per cent inhibition of oestrogen synthesis (oestrone plus oestradiol) is reached at 3.8 nM. In rat granulosa cells, a 50 per cent inhibition of oestradiol synthesis stimulated by follicle-stimulating hormone (FSH) achieved at 0.4 μM (measured by quantifying ^3H_2O released from [^3H]-androstenedione) and oestradiol plasma levels were significantly suppressed after a single oral intake of 300 mg liarozole by male volunteers (Bruynseels *et al.* 1990).

Oestrogens are described as prostatic growth stimulators and may play a role in prostatic pathology (Kaburagi *et al.* 1987; Karr *et al.* 1987; Belanger 1990). Although peripheral aromatization is the primary source of oestrogens in aging men (Kaburagi *et al.* 1987; Karr *et al.* 1987), low aromatase activity is found in rat prostate (Marts *et al.* 1987) and human prostate (Stone *et al.* 1986; Kaburagi *et al.* 1987; Ayub and Levell 1990). Aromatase activity has also been demonstrated in microsomes from Dunning R 3327 H adenocarcinoma (Marts *et al.* 1987). Furthermore, the aromatase inhibitors 4-OHA and 1-methyl-1,4-androstadiene-3,17-dione (SH 489) are able to antagonize androstenedione-induced prostatic hypertrophy in dogs and cynomolgus monkeys respectively (Habenicht *et al.* 1986; Henderson *et al.* 1986). It should be noted that Brodie *et al.* (1989) proved that 4-OHA also inhibits 5a-reductase in both benign prostatic hyperplasia (BPH) and cancer tissue. Thus, the observed antagonism may be due to combined oestrogen and DHT deprivation. The mechanism of the palliative action of 4-OHA in patients with advanced prostatic cancer is also still obscure, but aromatase inhibition may be involved (Shearer *et al.* 1990). Thus the benefit of oestrogen depletion in prostate carcinoma remains to be determined, but the possibility that the effects of liarozole on androgen-dependent and androgen-independent prostatic adenocarcinoma in rats and prostate cancer in men may partly originate from its effects on aromatase cannot be excluded.

Liarozole shares with ketoconazole (Williams and Napoli 1985, 1987; Van Wauwe *et al.* 1988; Vanden Bossche and Willemsens 1991) its *in vitro* inhibitory effects on the P450-dependent 4-hydroxylation of retinoic acid. *In vivo*, liarozole increased the biological half-life of exogenously administered retinoic acid and enhanced its endogenous plasma level (Van Wauwe *et al.* 1990). Increased plasma retinoic acid levels and cutaneous reactions similar to those observed after high doses of vitamin A were observed in orchidectomized stage D prostate cancer patients treated with liarozole (De Coster *et al.* 1991). Retinoids are shown to be of key importance in differentiation and morphogenesis. Retinoic acid induces an attenuation or complete reversal of the malignant phenotype for many cell lines. For example, upon exposure to retinoic acid, F9 mouse teratocarcinoma and HL60 human promyelocytic leukaemia cells differentiate respectively to normal parietal endoderm and functional mature granulocytes (de Thé and Dejean 1991). It has been proved that retinoic acid itself rather than its metabolites mediate differentiation in F9 cells (Williams and Napoli 1985). Since extensive metabolism occurs simultaneously with retinoid-induced differentiation, inhibition of the 4-hydroxylase will prolong the activity of retinoic acid. Liarozole (10 μM) enhanced the effects of retinoic acid in F9 teratocarcinoma cells (De Coster et al. 1992), an effect shared with ketoconazole (Williams and Napoli 1985, 1987).

On the basis of these results, it is tempting to speculate that liarozole's antitumoral action may involve effects on the metabolism of endogenous retinoic acid and aromatase. Pre-clinical and clinical studies are needed to prove or reject this hypothesis. The effects of ketoconazole may originate from its interaction with 17,20-lyase activity and the P450 involved in 4-hydroxylation of retinoic. acid.

9C4.3 Other 17α-hydroxylase/17,20-lyase inhibitors

Pyridylacetic acid derivatives may provide a basis for the design of inhibitors of steroid hormone biosynthesis (Laughton and Neidle 1990; McCague et al. 1990). The most potent inhibitor of rat testicular 17α-hydroxylase (IC$_{50}$ = 0.28 μM) and 17,20-lyase (IC$_{50}$ = 0.26 μM) in this series of derivatives is (1S,2S,3S,5R)-(+)isopinocampheyl 4-pyridylacetic acid ester (McCague et al. 1990). This ester is also a good inhibitor of human placental aromatase (IC$_{50}$ = 0.12 μM). The (1R,2R,3R,5S)-(−)-isopino-campheyl 4-pyridylacetic acid ester is an almost equipotent inhibitor of the aromatase (IC$_{50}$ = 0.096 μM) but a less potent inhibitor of 17α-hydroxylase (IC$_{50}$ = 1.8 μM) and 17,20-lyase (IC$_{50}$ = 1.7 μM). Although the 4-pyridylacetic acid esters have good in vitro activity, their in vivo action may be compromised by metabolic degradation by esterases (McCague et al. 1990). Furthermore, since they are equipotent inhibitors of both 17α-hydroxylase and 17,20-lyase, cortisol depletion can be expected.

9C.5 Concluding remarks

It is evident from the foregoing that P450 17 is an important target for the development of new tools for the treatment of androgen-dependent pathophysiological processes. Although both 17,20-bond scission and 17-hydroxylation are catalysed by a single P450, the 17,20-lyase and 17α-hydroxylase differ in many aspects. These differences may be exploited to develop compounds that preferentially inhibit 17−20 bond cleavage, avoiding effects on cortisol synthesis. Ketoconazole is a more potent inhibitor of adrenal and testicular 17,20-lyase than of 17α-hydroxylase activity.

However, liarozole shows a marked difference in its activity against testicular and adrenal lyase, with the latter being much less sensitive. This suggests distinct tertiary structures in the same P450 from different organs and increases considerably the problems of finding superior and more selective inhibitors.

Although liarozole is the product of a screening programme developed to aid the search for selective androgen biosynthesis inhibitors, it is possible that its beneficial effects in prostate cancer may originate from its inhibitory action on oestrogen synthesis and its capacity to inhibit the catabolism of retinoic acid. The latter effect, together with the inhibition of adrenal and testicular androgen synthesis, may be at the origin of the striking clinical improvement seen in many patients with prostate carcinoma after treatment with ketoconazole.

References

Amery, W. K., De Coster, R., and Caers, I. (1986). Ketoconazole: from an antimycotic to a drug for prostate cancer. *Drug Development Research*, **8**, 299–307.

Ayub, M., and Levell, M. J. (1989). Inhibition of human adrenal steroidogenic enzymes *in vitro* by imidazole drugs including ketoconazole. *Journal of Steroid Biochemistry*, **32**, 515–24.

Ayub, M. and Levell. M. J. (1990). The inhibition of human prostatic aromatase activity by imidazole drugs including ketoconazole and 4-hydroxyandrostenedione. *Biochemical Pharmacology*, **40**, 1569–75.

Barnes, H. J., Arlotto, M. P., and Waterman, M. R. (1991). Expression and enzymatic activity of recombinant cytochrome P450 17α-hydroxylase in *Escherichia coli*. *Proceedings of the National Academy of Sciences of the United States of America*, **88**, 5597–601.

Bartsch, W., Klein, H., Schieman, U., Bauer, H. W., and Voigt, K. D. (1990). Enzymes of androgen formation and degradation in the human prostate. *Annals of the New York Academy of Sciences*, **595**, 53–66.

Bélanger, C., Veilleux, R., and Labrie, F. (1990). Stimulatory effects of androgens, estrogens, progestins, and dexamethasone on the growth of the LNCaP human prostate cancer cells. *Annals of the New York Academy of Sciences*, **595**, 399–402.

Bigliery, E. G. and Kater, C. E. (1991). 17α-Hydroxylation deficiency. *Endocrinology and Metabolism Clinics of North America*, **20**, 257–68.

Bhasker, C. R., Adler, B. S., Dee, A., John, M. E., Kagimoto, M., Zuber, M. X., *et al.* (1989). Structural characterization of the bovine *CYP17* (17α-hydroxylase) gene. *Archives of Biochemistry and Biophysics*, **271**, 479–87.

Bradshaw, K. D., Waterman, M. R., Couch, R. T., Simpson, E. R., and Zuber, M. X. (1987). Characterization of complementary deoxyribonucleic acid for human adrenocortical 17α-hydroxylase: probe for analysis of 17α-hydroxylase deficiency. *Molecular Endocrinology*, **1**, 348–54.

Brodie, A. M. H., Son, C., King, D. A., Meyer, K. M., and Inkster, S. E. (1989). Lack of evidence for aromatase in human prostatic tissues: effects of 4-hydroxyandrostenedione and other inhibitors on androgen metabolism. *Cancer Research*, **19**, 6551–5.

Bruynseels, J., De Coster, R., Van Rooy, P., Wouters, W., Coene, M.-C., Snoeck, E., *et al.* (1990). R 75251, a new inhibitor of steroid synthesis. *Prostate*, **16**, 345–57.

Chiarodo, A. (1991). National Cancer Institute round table on prostate cancer: future research directions. *Cancer Research*, **51**, 2498–505.

Chung, B.-C., Picado-Leonard, J., Haniu, M., Bienkowski, M., Hall, P. F., Shively, J. E., and Miller, W. L. (1987). Cytochrome P450C17 (steroid 17α-hydroxylase/17,20 lyase): cloning of human adrenal and testis cDNAs indicates the same gene is expressed in both tissues. *Proceedings of the National Academy of Sciences of the United States of America*, **84**, 407–11.

Couch, R. M., Muller, J., Perry, Y. S., and Winter, J. S. D. (1987). Kinetic analysis of inhibition of human adrenal steroidogenesis by ketoconazole. *Journal of Clinical Endocrinology and Metabolism*, **65**, 551–4.

De Coster, R., Caers, I., Coene, M.-C., Amery, W., Beerens D., and Haelterman, C. (1986). Effects of high dose ketoconazole therapy on the main plasma testicular and adrenal steroids in previously untreated prostatic cancer patients. *Clinical Endocrinology*, **24**, 657–664.

De Coster, R., Van Ginckel, R., van Moorselaar, R. J. A., Schalken, J. A., De Bruyne, F. M. J., Bruynseels, J., and Denis, L. (1991). Antitumoral effects of R 75251 in prostatic carcinoma: experimental and clinical studies. *Proceedings of the 82nd Meeting of the American Association of Cancer Research*, **32**, 213.

De Coster, R., Wouters W., Van Ginckel, R., End, D., Krekels, M., Coene, M.-C., and Bowden, C. (1992). Experimental studies with liarozole (R 75251): an antitumoral agent which inhibits retinoic acid breakdown. *Journal of Steroid Biochemistry and Molecular Biology*, **43**, 197–201.

De Felice, R., Johnson, D. G., and Galgiani, J. N. (1981). Gynecomastia with ketoconazole, *Antimicrobial Agents and Chemotherapy*, **19**, 1073–4.

Denis, L. J. (1991). Controversies in the management of localised and metastatic prostatic cancer. *European Journal of Cancer*, **27**, 333–41.

Denis, L. J., Chaban, M., and Mahler, Ch. (1985). Clinical application of ketoconazole in prostatic cancer. In *EORTC genitourinary group monograph 2, Part A: Therapeutic principles in metastatic prostatic cancer* (ed. F. H. Schroeder and B. Richards), pp. 319–6. Liss, New York.

de Thé, H. and Dejean, A. (1991). The retinoic acid receptors. In *Retinoids: 10 years on* (ed. J.-H. Saurat), pp. 2–9. Karger, Basel.

Edwards, R. J., Murray, B. P., Boobis, A. R., and Davies, D. S. (1989). Identification and location of α-helices in mammalian cytochromes P450. *Biochemistry*, **28**, 3762–70.

Edwards, R. J., Murray, B. P., Singleton, A. M., and Boobis, A. R. (1991). Orientation of cytochromes P450 in the endoplasmic reticulum. *Biochemistry*, **30**, 71–6.

Feldman, D. (1986). Ketoconazole and other imidazole derivatives as inhibitors of steroidogenesis. *Endocrine Reviews*, **7**, 409–20.

Fevold, H. R., Lorence, M. C., McCarthy, J. L., Trant, J. M., Kagimoto, M., Waterman, M. R., and Mason, J. I. (1989). Rat P450$_{17α}$ from testis: characterization of a full-length cDNA encoding a unique steroid hydroxylase capable of catalyzing both Δ^4- and Δ^5-steroid-17,20-lyase reactions, *Molecular Endocrinology*, **3**, 968–75.

France, J. T., Magness, R. R., Murry, B. A., Rosenfeld, C. R., and Mason, J. I. (1988). The regulation of ovine placental steroid 17α-hydroxylase and aromatase by glucocorticoid. *Molecular Endocrinology*, **2**, 193–9.

Gotoh, O. and Fuyii-Kuriyama, Y. (1989). Evolution and structure, and gene regulation of cytochrome P-450. In *Basis and mechanism of regulation of cytochrome P-450* (ed. K. Ruckpaul and H. Rein), pp. 195–243. Akademie Verlag, Berlin.

Graham-Lorence, S., Khalil, M. W., Lorence, M. C., Mendelson, C. R., and Simpson, E. R. (1991). Structure–function relationships of human aromatase cytochrome P-450 using molecular modeling and site-directed mutagenesis. *Journal of Biological Chemistry*, **266**, 11939–46.

Graybill, J. R. (1990). The modern revolution in antifungal drug therapy. In *Mycoses in AIDS Patients* (ed. H. Vanden Bossche, D. W. R. Mackenzie, G. Cauwenbergh, J. Van Cutsem, E. Drouhet, and B. Dupont), pp. 265–77. Plenum Press, New York.

Grayhack, J. T., Keeler, T. C., and Kozlowski, J. M. (1987). Carcinoma of the prostate. Hormonal therapy. *Cancer*, **60**, 589–601.

Habenicht, U. F., Schwartz, K., Schweikert, H. U., Neumann, F., and El Etreby, M. F. (1986). Development of a model for the induction of estrogen-related prostatic hyperplasia in the dog and its response to the aromatase inhibitor 4-hydroxy-androstene-3,17-dione. *Prostate*, **8**, 81–94.

Hajek, K. K.. Cook, N. I., and Novak, R. F. (1982). Mechanism of inhibition of microsomal drug metabolism by imidazole. *Journal of Pharmacology and Experimental Therapeutics*, **223**, 97–104.

Harada, N. (1988). Cloning of a complete cDNA encoding human aromatase: immunochemical identification and sequence analysis. *Biochemical and Biophysical Research Communications*, **156**, 725–32.

Henderson, D., Habenicht, U. F., Nishino, Y., Kerb, U., and El Etreby, M. F. (1986). Artomatase inhibitors and benign prostatic hyperplasia. *Journal of Steroid Biochemistry*, **25**, 867–76.

Heyns, W., Drochmans, A., vander Schueren, E., and Verhoeven, G. (1985). Endocrine effects of high dose ketoconazole therapy in advanced prostatic cancer. *Acta Endocrinologica*, **110**, 276–83.

Higashi, Y., Omura, M., Suzuki, K., Inano H., and Oshima, H. (1987). Ketoconazole as a possible universal inhibitor of cytochrome P-450 dependent enzymes: its mode of inhibition, *Endocrinology Japan*, **34**, 105–15.

Huggins, C., Stevens, R. E., and Hodges, C. V. (1941). Studies on prostatic cancer. II. Effects of castration on advanced carcinoma of the prostate gland. *Archives of Surgery*, **43**, 209–23.

John, M. E., John, M. C., Boggaram, V., and Simpson, E. R. (1986). Transcriptional regulation of steroid hydroxylase genes by corticotropin. *Proceedings of the National Academy of Sciences of the United States of America*, **83**, 4715–19.

Kaburagi, Y., Marino, M. B., Kirdani, R. Y., Greco, J. P., Karr, J. P., and Sandberg, A. A. (1987). The possibility of aromatization of androgen in human prostate. *Journal of Steroid Biochemistry*, **26**, 739–42.

Kagimoto, M., Winter, J. S. D., Kagimoto, K., Simpson, E. R., and Waterman, M. R. (1988). Structural characterization of normal and mutant human steroid 17α-hydroxylase genes: molecular basis of one example of combined 17α-hydroxylase/17,20 lyase deficiency. *Molecular Endocrinology*, **2**, 564–70.

Kan, P., Hirst, M. A. and Feldman, D. (1985). Inhibition of steroidogenic cytochrome P-450 enzymes in rat testis by ketoconazole and related imidazole antifungal drugs. *Journal of Steroid Biochemistry*, **23**, 1023–9.

Karr, J. P., Kaburagi, Y., Mann, C. F., and Sandberg, A. A. (1987). The potential significance of aromatase in the etiology and treatment of prostatic disease. *Steroids*, **50**, 451–7.

Kominami, S., Shinzawa, K., and Takemori, S. (1982). Purification and some properties of cytochrome P-450 specific for steroid 17α-hydroxylation and 17–20 bond cleavage from guinea pig adrenal microsomes. *Biochemical and Biophysical Research Communications*, **109**, 916–21.

Laughton, C. A. and Neidle, S. (1990). Inhibitors of the P450 enzymes aromatase and lyase. Crystallographic and molecular modeling studies suggest structural features of pyridylacetic acid derivatives responsible for differences in enzyme inhibitory activity. *Journal of Medicinal Chemistry*, **33**, 3055–60.

Lauwers, W. F. J., Le Jeune, L., Vanden Bossche, H., and Willemsens, G. (1985). Identification of 17α,20-dihydroxyprogesterone in testicular extracts after incubation with ketoconazole. *Biomedical Mass Spectometry*, **12**, 296–301.

Lorence, M. C., Trant, J. M., Clark, B. J., Khyatt, B., Mason, J. I., Estabrook, R. W., and Waterman, M. R. (1990). Construction and expression of human/bovine P450$_{17\alpha}$ chimeric proteins: evidence for distinct tertiary structures in the same P450 from different species. *Biochemistry*, **29**, 9819–24.

Lowe, F. C. and Bamberger, M. H. (1990). Indications for use of ketoconazole in management of metastatic prostate cancer. *Urology*, **36**, 511–5.

Lund, J., Faucher, D. J., Ford, S. P., Porter, J. C., and Waterman, M. R. (1988). Developmental expression of bovine adrenocortical steroid hydroxylases. Regulation of P450$_{17\alpha}$ expression leads to episodic fetal cortisol production. *Journal of Biological Chemistry*, **263**, 16195–201.

Lund, J., Ahlgren, R., Wu, D., Kagimoto, M., Simpson, E. R., and Waterman, M. R. (1990). Transcriptional regulation of the bovine *CYP17* (P450$_{17\alpha}$) gene. *Journal of Biological Chemistry*, **265**, 3304–12.

McCague, R., Rowlands, M. G., Barrie, S. E., and Houghton, J. (1990). Inhibition of enzymes of estrogen and androgen biosynthesis by esters of 4-pyridylacetic acid. *Journal of Medicinal Chemistry*, **33**, 3050–5.

Mahler, C., Denis, L., and De Coster, R. (1989). The effects of a new imidazole derivative in advanced prostatic cancer. A preliminary report. In *Therapeutic progress in urological cancers* (ed. G. P. Murphy and S. Khoury), pp. 205–9. Liss, New York.

Martini, L., Celotti, F., Lechuga, M. J., Melcangi, R. C., Motta, M., Negri-Cesi, P., *et al.* (1990). Androgen metabolism in different target tissues. *Annals of the New York Academy of Sciences*, **595**, 184–98.

Marts, S. A., Padilla, G. M., and Petrow, V. (1987). Aromatase activity in microsomes from rat ventral prostate and Dunning R3327H rat prostatic adenocarcinoma. *Journal of Steroid Biochemistry*, **26**, 25–9.

Mason, J. I., Murry, B. A., Olcott, M., and Sheets, J. J. (1985). Imidazole antimycotics: inhibitors of steroid aromatase. *Biochemical Pharmacology*, **34**, 1087–92.

Matteson, K. J., Picado-Leonard, J., Chung, B., Mohandas, T. K., and Miller, W. L. (1986). Assignment of the gene for adrenal P450c17 (17α-hydroxylase/17,20-lyase) to human chromosome 10. *Journal of Clinical Endocrinology and Metabolism*, **63**, 789–91.

Miller, W. L. (1988). Molecular biology of steroid hormone synthesis. *Endocrine Reviews*, **9**, 295–318.

Miller, S. L., Wright, J. N., Corina, D. L., and Akhtar, M. (1991). Mechanistic studies on pregnene side-chain cleavage enzyme (17α-hydroxylase-17,20-lyase) using $^{18}O_2$. *Journal of the Chemical Society, Chemical Communications*, 157–9.

Moereels, H., De Bie, L., and Tollenaere, J. P. (1990). CGEMA and VGAP: a colour graphics editor for multiple alignment using a variable gap penalty. Application to the muscarinic acetylcholine receptor. *Journal of Computer-aided Molecular Design*, **4**, 131–45.

Mooradian, A. D., Morley, J. E., and Korenman, S. G. (1987). Biological actions of androgens. *Endocrine Reviews*, **8**, 1–28.

Mornet, E., Dupont, J., Vitek, A., and White, P. C. (1989). Characterization of two genes encoding human steroid 11β-hydroxylase (P450$_{11\beta}$). *Journal of Biological Chemistry*, **264**, 20961–67.

Morohashi, K., Sogawa, K., Omura, T., and Fujii-Kuriyama, Y. (1987). Gene structure of human cytochrome P-450(SCC), cholesterol desmolase. *Journal of Biochemistry*, **101**, 879–87.

Nakajin, S., Hall, P. F., and Onoda, M. (1981a). Testicular microsomal cytochrome P-450 for C21 steroid side chain cleavage. Spectral and binding studies. *Journal of Biological Chemistry*, **256**, 6134–9.

Nakajin, S., Shively, J. E., Yuan, P.-M., and Hall, P. F. (1981b). Microsomal cytochrome P-450 from neonatal pig testis: two enzymatic activities (17α-hydroxylase/17,20-lyase) associated with one protein. *Biochemistry*, **20**, 4037–42.

Nakajin, S., Shinoda, M., Haniu, M., Shively, J. E., and Hall, P. F. (1984). C_{21} steroid side-chain cleavage enzyme from porcine adrenal microsomes. Purification and characterization of the 17α-hydroxylase/$C_{17,20}$-lyase cytochrome P-450. *Journal of Biological Chemistry*, **259**, 3971–6.

Namiki, M., Kitamura, M., Buczko, E., and Dufau, M. L. (1988). Rat testis P-450$_{17\alpha}$ cDNA: the deduced amino acid sequence, expression and secondary structural configuration. *Biochemical and Biophysical Research Communications*, **157**, 705–12.

Nebert, D. W., Nelson, D. R., Coon, M. J., Estabrook, R. W., Fevereisen, R., Fuyii-Kuriyama, Y., *et al*. (1991). The P450 superfamily: update on new sequences, gene mapping, and recommended nomenclature. *DNA and Cell Biology*, **10**, 1–14.

Nelson, D. R. and Strobel, H. W. (1989). Secondary Structure prediction of 52 membrane-bound cytochrome P450 shows a strong structural simillarity to P450$_{cam}$ *Biochemistry*, **28**, 656–60.

Neumann, F. (1987). Pharmacology and clinical uses of cyproterone acetate. In *Pharmacology and clinical uses of inhibitors of hormone secretion and action* (ed. B. J. A. Furr and A. E. Wakeling), pp. 132–59. Baillière Tindall, London.

Nonaka, Y., Matsukawa, N., Morohashi, K., Omura, T., Ogihara, T., Teraoka, H., and Okamoto, M. (1989). Molecular cloning and sequence analysis of cDNA encoding rat adrenal cytochrome P-450$_{11\beta}$. *Federation of European Biochemical Societies Letters*, **255**, 21–6.

Ono, H., Iwasaki, M., Sakamoto, N., and Mizuno, S. (1988). cDNA cloning and sequence analysis of a chicken gene expressed during the gonadal development and homologous to mammalian cytochrome P-450C17. *Gene*, **66**, 77–85.

Onoda, M. and Hall, P. F. (1982). Cytochrome b_5 stimulates purified microsomal cytochrome P-450 (C_{21} side-chain cleavage). *Biochemical and Biophysical Research Communications*, **108**, 454–60.

Ozols, J., Heinemann, F. S., and Johnson, E. F. (1981). Amino acid sequence of an analogous peptide from two forms of cytochrome P-450. *Journal of Biological Chemistry*, **256**, 11405–8.

Picado-Leonard, J. and Miller, W. L. (1987). Cloning and sequence of the human gene for P450C17 (steroid 17a-hydroxylase/17,20-lyase): similarity with the gene for P450C21. *DNA*, **6**, 439–48.

Picado-Leonard, J. and Miller, W. L. (1988). Homologous sequences in steroidogenic enzymes, steroid receptors and a steroid binding protein suggest a conscensus steroid-binding sequence. *Molecular Endocrinology*, **2**, 1145–50.

Pierrepoint, C. G., Turkes, A. O., Walker, K. J., Harper, M. E., Wilson, D. W., Peeling, W. B., and Griffiths, K. (1985). Endocrine factors in the treatment of prostatic cancer. In *EORTC genitourinary group monograph 2. Part A: Therapeutic principles in metastatic prostatic cancer* (ed. F. H. Schroeder and B. Richards), pp. 51–72. Liss, New York.

Pont, A., Williams, P. L., Azhar, S., and Reirz, R. E. (1982). Ketoconazole blocks testosterone synthesis. *Archives of Internal Medicine*, **142**, 2137–40.

Poulos, T. L., Finzel, B. C., and Howard, A. J. (1987). High-resolution crystal structure of cytochrome P450$_{cam}$. *Journal of Molecular Biology*, **195**, 687–700.

Rajfer, J., Sikka, S., Xie, H. W., and Swerdloff, R. S. (1985). Effect of ketoconazole on steroid production in rat testis, *Steroids*, **46**, 867–81.

Rodgers, R. J., Rodgers, H. F., Hall, P. F., Waterman, M. R., and Simpson, E. R. (1986). Immunolocalization of cholesterol side-chain-cleavage cytochrome P-450 in bovine adrenal follicles. *Journal of Reproduction and Fertility*, **78**, 627–38.

Santen, R. J., Vanden Bossche, H., Symoens, J., Brugmans J., and De Coster, R. (1983). Site of action of low dose ketoconazole on androgen biosynthesis in men. *Journal of Clinical Endocrinology and Metabolism*, **57**, 732–6.

Sasano, H., Mason, J. I., and Sasano, N. (1989). Immunohistochemical analysis of cytochrome P-450 17a-hydroxylase in pig adrenal cortex, testis and ovary. *Molecular and Cellular Endocrinology*, **62**, 197–202.

Schürmeyer, Th. and Nieschlag, E. (1982). Ketoconazole-induced drop in serum and saliva testosterone. *Lancet*, **ii**, 1098–9.

Shearer, R. J., Davies, J. H., Dowsett, M., Malone, P. R., Hedley, A., Cunningham, D., and Coombes. R. C. (1990). Aromatase inhibition in advanced prostatic cancer: preliminary communication. *British Journal of Cancer*, **62**, 275–76.

Shinzawa, K., Kominami, S., and Takemori, S. (1985). Studies on cytochrome P-450 (P-450$_{17a,lyase}$) from guinea pig adrenal microsomes. Dual function of a single enzyme and effect of cytochrome b_5, *Biochimica et Biophysica Acta*, **833**, 151–60.

Sonino, N. (1987). The use of ketoconazole as an inhibitor of steroid production. *New England Journal of Medicine*, **317**, 812–18.

Stone, N. N., Fair, W. R., and Fishman, J. (1986). Estrogen formation in human prostatic tissues from patients with and without benign prostatic hyperplasia. *Prostate*, **9**, 311–18.

Tangalakis, K., Coghlan, J. P., Crawford, R., Hammond, V. E., and Wintour, E. M. (1990). Steroid hydroxylase gene expression in the ovine fetal adrenal gland following ACTH infusion. *Acta Endocrinologica* (Copenhagen), **123**, 371–7.

Tapazoglou, E., Subramanian, M. G., Al-Sarraf, M., Kresge, C., and Decker, D. A. (1986). High-dose ketoconazole therapy in patients with metastatic prostate cancer. *Amencan Journal of Clinical Oncology*, **9**, 369–75.

Tonetta, S. and Hernandez, M. (1989). Modulation of 17α-hydroxylase/17,20-lyase activity in porcine theca cells. *Journal of Steroid Biochemistry*, **33**, 263–70.

Trachtenberg, J. and Zadra, J. (1988). Steroid synthesis inhibition by ketoconazole: sites of action. *Clinical and Investigative Medicine*, **11**, 1–5.

Trachtenberg, J., Halpern N., and Pont, A. (1983). Ketoconazole, a novel and rapid treatment for advanced prostatic cancer. *Journal of Urology*, **130**, 152–3.

Unger, B. P., Gunsalus, I. C., and Sligar, S. G. (1986). Nucleotide sequence of the *Pseudomonas putida* cytochrome P-450$_{cam}$ gene and its expression in *Escherichia coli*. *Journal of Biological Chemistry*, **261**, 1158–63.

Vanden Bossche, H. and Willemsens, G. (1991). Retinoic acid and cytochrome P450. In *Retinoids; 10 years on* (ed. J.-H. Saurat), pp. 79–88. Karger, Basel.

Vanden Bossche, H., Willemsens, G., Cools, W., Cornelissen, F., Lauwers, W., and Van Cutsem, J. (1980). *In vitro* and *in vivo* effects of the antimycotic drug ketoconazole on sterol synthesis. *Antimicrobial Agents and Chemotherapy*, **17**, 922–8.

Vanden Bossche, H., Lauwers, W., Willemsens, G., and Cools, W. (1985a). The cytochrome P-450 dependent C17,20-lyase in subcellular fractions of the rat testis: differences in sensitivity to ketoconazole and itraconazole. In *Microsomes and drug oxidations* (ed. A. R. Boobis, J. Caldwell, F. de Matteis, and C. R. Elcombe), pp. 63–73. Taylor and Francis, London.

Vanden Bossche, H., Lauwers, W., Willemsens, G., and Cools, W. (1985b). Ketoconazole an inhibitor of the cytochrome P-450 dependent testosterone biosynthesis. In *EORTC genitourinary group monograph 2. Part A: Therapeutic principles in metastatic prostatic cancer* (ed. F. H. Schroeder and B. Richards), pp. 187–96. Liss, New York.

Vanden Bossche, H., De Coster, R., and Amery, W. (1987). Pharmacological and clinical uses of ketoconazole. In *Pharmacology and clinical uses of inhibitors of hormone secretion and action*. (ed. B. J. A. Furr and A. E. Wakeling), pp. 288–307. Baillière Tindall, London.

Vanden Bossche, H., Marichal, P., Gorrens, J., Coene, M. C., Willemsens, G., Bellens, D., *et al.* (1989). Biochemical approaches to selective antifungal activity. Focus on azole antifungals. *Mycoses*, **32** (Suppl. 1), 35–52.

Vanden Bossche, H., Marichal, P., Gorrens, J., Bellens, D., Coene, M-C., Lauwers, W., *et al.* (1990a). Mode of action of antifungals of use in immunocompromised patients. Focus on *Candida glabrata* and *Histoplasma capsulatum*. In *Mycoses in AIDS patients* (ed. H. Vanden Bossche, D. W. R. Mackenzie, G. Cauwenbergh, J. Van Cutsem, E. Drouhet, and B. Dupont), pp. 223–43. Plenum Press, New York.

Vanden Bossche, H., Willemsens, G., Bellens, D., Roels, I., and Janssen, P. A. J. (1990b). From 14α-demethylase inhibitors in fungal cells to androgen and oestrogen biosynthesis inhibitors in mammalian cells. *Biochemical Society Transactions*, **18**, 10–13.

Vanden Bossche, H., Moereels, H., and Janssen, P. A. J. (1991). Role of cytochrome P-450 in the anabolism and catabolism of endobiotics. In *Molecular Aspects of Monooxygenases and Bioactivation of Toxic Compounds* (ed. E. Arinç, J. B. Schenkman, and E. Hodgson), pp. 305–30. Plenum Press, New York.

Van Ginckel, R., De Coster, R., Wouters, W., Vanherck, W., van der Veer, R., Goeminne, N., *et al.* (1990) *Prostate* 16, 313–23.

Van Wauwe, J. P., Coene, M.-C., Goossens, J., Van Nijen, G., Cools, W., and Janssen, P. A. J. (1988). Ketoconazole inhibits the *in vitro* and *in vivo* metabolism of all-*trans*-retinoic acid. *Journal of Pharmacology and Experimental Therapeutics*, 245, 718–22.

Van Wauwe, J. P., Coene, M.-C., Goossens, J., Cools, W., and Monbaliu, J. (1990). Effects of cytochrome P-450 inhibitors on the *in vivo* metabolism of all-*trans*-retinoic acid in rats. *Journal of Pharmacology and Experimental Therapeutics*, 252, 365–9.

Voutilainen, R. and Miller, W. L. (1986). Development expression of genes for the steroidogenic enzymes P450scc (20,22-desmolase), P450c17 (17a-hydroxylase/17,20-lyase), and P450c21 (21-hydroxylase) in the human fetus. *Journal of Clinical Endocrinology and Metabolism*, 63, 1145–50.

Voutilainen, R., Tapanainen, J., Chung, B-C., Matteson, K. J., and Miller, W. L. (1986). Hormonal regulation of P450scc (20,22-desmolase) and P450c17 (17a-hydroxylase/17,20-lyase) in cultured human granulosa cells. *Journal of Clinical Endocrinology and Metabolism*, 63, 202–7.

Weber, M. M., Will, A., Adelmann, B., and Engelhardt, D. (1991). Effect of ketoconazole on human ovarian C17,20-desmolase and aromatase. *Journal of Steroid Biochemistry and Molecular Biology*, 38, 213–18.

White. P. C., New, M. I., and Dupont, B. (1986). Structure of human steroid 21-hydroxylase genes. *Proceedings of the National Academy of Sciences of the United States of America*, 83, 5111–15.

Williams, J. B. and Napoli, J. L. (1985). Metabolism of retinoic acid and retinol during differentiation of F9 embryonal carcinoma cells. *Proceedings of the National Academy of Sciences of the United States of America*, 82, 4658–62.

Williams, J. B. and Napoli, J. L. (1987). Inhibition of retinoic acid metabolism by imidazole antimycotics in F9 embryonal carcinoma cells. *Biochemical Pharmacology*, 36, 1386–8.

Yanagibashi, K. and Hall, P. F. (1986). Role of electron transport in the regulation of the lyase activity of C_{21} side-chain cleavage P-450 from porcine adrenal and testicular microsomes. *Journal of Biological Chemistry*, 261, 8429–33.

Yanase, T., Sanders, D., Shibata, A., Matsui, N., Simpson, E. R., and Waterman, M. R. (1990). Combined 17a-hydroxylase/17,20-lyase deficiency due to a 7-basepair duplication in the N-terminal region of the cytochrome $P450_{17a}$ (*CYP17*) gene. *Journal of Clinical Endocrinology and Metabolism*, 70, 1325–9.

Yanase, T., Simpson, E. R., and Waterman, M. R. (1991). 17a-Hydroxylase/17,20-lyase deficiency: from clinical investigation to molecular definition. *Endocrine Reviews*, 12, 91–108.

Zuber, M. X., Simpson, E. R., and Waterman, M. R. (1986a). Expression of bovine 17a-hydroxylase cytochrome P-450 cDNA in nonsteroidogenic (COS 1) cells. *Science*, 234, 1258–61.

Zuber, M. X., John, M. E., Okamura, T., Simpson, E. R., and Waterman, M. R. (1986b). Bovine adrenocortical cytochrome $P450_{17a}$. Regulation of gene expression by ACTH and elucidation of primary sequence. *Journal of Biological Chemistry*, 261, 2475–82.

Section 9D

Inhibitors of hydroxysteroid dehydrogenases: 17β-hydroxysteroid dehydrogenase

Trevor M. Penning

9D.1   Introduction

Hydroxysteroid dehydrogenases (HSDs) are a group of pyridine-nucleotide-dependent oxidoreductases that catalyse the interconversion of ketones to secondary alcohols in a positional and stereospecific manner on the steroid nucleus or side-chain (Talalay 1963) (Fig. 9D.1). 17β-Hydroxysteroid dehydrogenase (17β-HSD) belongs to this group and catalyses the final step in androgen biosynthesis by converting androstenedione to testosterone.

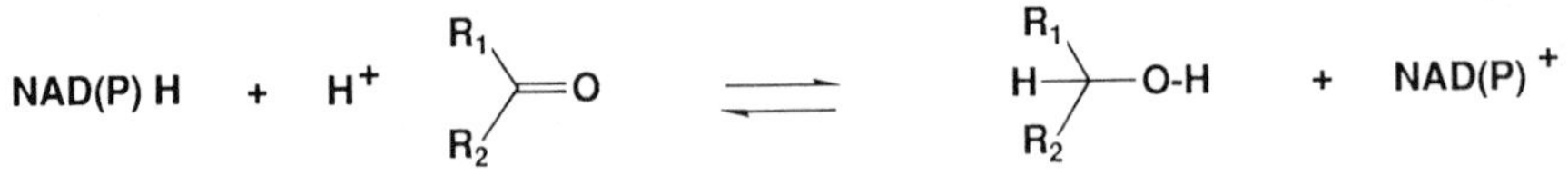

$$NAD(P)H \quad + \quad H^+ \quad {R_1 \atop R_2}{>}{=}O \quad \rightleftharpoons \quad {R_1 \atop R_2}{>}H{-}O{-}H \quad + \quad NAD(P)^+$$

Fig. 9D.1 Generalized reaction catalysed by HSDs. R_1 and R_2 are components of either the steroid nucleus or the side-chain. (Reproduced with permission from Penning and Ricigliano 1991.)

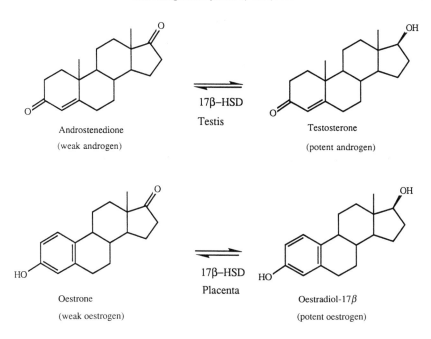

Fig. 9D.2 Specific reactions catalysed by 17β-HSD.

The enzyme will also convert oestrone to 17β-oestradiol (Fig. 9D.2). A feature of both reactions is that a biologically less potent steroid is converted to a highly potent steroid hormone. By virtue of these reactions, 17β-HSD can regulate androgen and oestrogen biosynthesis.

The reactions described are freely reversible *in vitro* and the reaction direction can be driven by the concentration of steroid substrate, the pyridine nucleotide cofactor, and pH. In the Leydig or interstitial cells of the testis, the reduction of androstenedione to testosterone is highly favoured. Deficiencies in testicular 17β-HSD have been associated with pseudo-hermaphroditism (Gross *et al.* 1986; Wilson *et al.* 1987, 1988), implicating the importance of this enzyme in testosterone production. It follows that inhibition of this enzyme could block androgen biosynthesis and androgen action. On this basis, selective inhibitors of testicular 17β-HSD could have the potential to prevent the growth of androgen-dependent tumours, for example benign hypertrophy and cancer of the prostate. Moreover, effective inhibitors could be used as adjuvants to enhance the efficacy of androgen receptor antagonists.

In human placenta, oestradiol-17β dehydrogenase catalyses the irreversible reduction of 16α-hydroxyoestrone to form the major oestrogen of pregnancy, oestriol (Engel and Inano 1978). Multiple forms of 17β-HSD exist in human breast tissue, and they vary in their capacity to catalyse the reduction and oxidation of oestrogens (Tait *et al*. 1989). Since the reduced products (oestriol and 17β-oestradiol) are more potent oestrogens than their oxidized substrates (16α-hydroxyoestrone and oestrone), these enzymes clearly control the production of potent oestrogens. Inhibitors of tumour-specific isoforms of 17β-HSD, which preferentially form oestradiol-17β, have the potential to attenuate the growth of oestrogen-dependent cancers, such as cancer of the breast. Therefore effective inhibitors of 17β-HSD could block the synthesis of potent oestrogens and might be useful as adjuvants to enhance the efficacy of oestrogen receptor antagonists.

9D.2   17β-Hydroxysteroid dehydrogenase isoforms

17β-HSD activity has been described in many rodent and human tissues. It has been purified from the liver of mouse (Bolcsak and Nerland 1983; Sawada *et al*. 1988), rabbit (Antoun *et al*. 1985; Hara *et al*. 1986), and guinea-pig (Kobayashi and Kochakian 1978; Hara *et al*. 1985). The enzyme has also been purified from the testis of rat (Bogovich and Payne 1980) and pig (Inano and Tamaoki 1986). In rat testis it coexists with 17-keto-reductase (Bogovich and Payne 1980). 17β-HSD as been described in the following human tissues: placenta (Jarabak *et al*. 1962), erythrocytes (Mulder *et al*. 1972), and breast and adipose tissue (Tait *et al*. 1989). Although the foregoing list is not comprehensive, it is important to realize that the most thoroughly characterized forms of this enzyme are the homogeneous preparations obtained from porcine testis microsomes (Inano and Tamaoki 1986) and human placental cytosol (Jarabak *et al*. 1962). Both enzymes copurify to homogeneity with additional 20α-HSD activity, and it has been shown that the 17β- and 20α-HSD activities are catalysed at the same active site of these proteins (Strickler *et al*. 1981; Tobias *et al*. 1982; Inano and Tamaoki 1986). In rodent liver the 17β-HSDs may exist as multiple isozymes (Bolcsak and Nerland 1983; Sawada *et al*. 1988). These isozymes can copurify with aldehyde reductase(s) and dihydrodiol dehydrogenases (Sawada *et al*. 1988); these activities are important in the detoxication of drugs, xenobiotics, and carcinogens. The demonstration that homogeneous enzyme may have dual HSD activity, which may play an important role in detoxication in some tissues, may have important consequences in targeting these enzymes for inhibition. When designing inhibitors, failure to consider the distribution of these isozymes and associated activities of a target HSD could result in inappropriate specificity or inadvertent loss of secondary (dual) enzyme activity.

The porcine testis enzyme exists as a monomer (M_r = 36 kDa) and can exhibit charge heterogeneity giving rise to subunits which have pI values equal to 5.5 and 4.8 (Inano and Tamaoki 1986). In contrast, the human placental enzyme has a similar monomeric molecular mass (35 kDa), but evidence exists that at least three different monomers may exist which combine to give a series of heterodimers with a molecular mass of 68 kDa (Engel and Inano 1978).

In considering inhibitors of 17β-HSD, it is also important to discuss 3(17)β-hydroxysteroid dehydrogenase from *Pseudomonas testosteroni*. This prokaryotic enzyme was first described some years ago and, because of its general availability, it has been used by many investigators to evaluate potential inhibitors for 3β- and 17β-HSDs.

9D.3   Cloning of 17β-hydroxysteroid dehydrogenases

A full-length cDNA clone for 17β-HSD has been isolated by immuno-screening a λgt-11 expression library constructed against human placental poly(A)$^+$-RNA (Peltoketo *et al.* 1988; Luu-The *et al.* 1989a). The cDNA sequenced by the two separaté groups is identical. The human placental enzyme displays no peptide homology with other HSDs that have recently been cloned and sequenced, including rat liver 3α-HSD (Pawlowski *et al.* 1991), human placental 3β-HSD/ketosteroid isomerase (Luu-The *et al.* 1989b), and rat liver 11β-HSD (Agarwal *et al.* 1989). The identity of the human placental 17β-HSD cDNA has been confirmed by locating the sequence of known peptides, within the clone, including the active site peptide sequenced by Murdock *et al.* (1986). Despite the heterogeneity observed in monomers of the placental 17β-HSD, cDNA probes show the existence of two mRNA species in human placental poly(A$^+$)-RNA which differ only in the length of their 5′-untranslated regions (Luu-The *et al.* 1989a). To date, the successful overexpression of the 17β-HSD cDNA has not been described.

9D.4   Reaction mechanism

In designing inhibitors for 17β-HSD it is important to consider the catalytic and kinetic mechanisms that drive this reaction.

9D.4.1   Catalytic mechanism

HSDs catalyse the direct transfer of a hydride ion from the C4 position of a reduced nicotinamide cofactor to the acceptor carbonyl of the steroid substrate (Fisher *et al.* 1953; Loweus *et al.* 1953). Moreover, the hydride ion is transferred with a high degree of stereospecificity from either the A or the B face of the pyridine ring, resulting in the transfer of the pro(*R*)-hydrogen or the pro(*S*)-hydrogen respectively. The stereochemistry of hydride transfer has been determined for both the porcine testis (Inano and Tamaoki 1975) and human placental 17β-HSDs (Jarabak and Talalay 1960), and in each case it is the pro(*S*)-hydrogen that is transferred. This

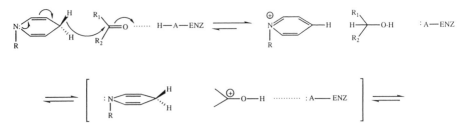

Fig. 9D.3 Catalytic mechanism for hydroxysteroid dehydrogenases: ENZ, enzyme; A–H, general acid at the enzyme active site; R_1 and R_2, components of either the steroid nucleus or the side-chain. The polarization of the acceptor carbonyl with the formation of a formal carbonium ion is shown in parenthesis. (Reproduced with permission from Bloxham *et al.* 1975.)

is in agreement with the general rule that the hydrogen atom transferred to the α face of steroids originates from the pro(S) side of the cofactor. A transition state for the reduction of androstenedione by NADPH, catalysed by 17β-HSD, has been proposed by Inano and Tamaoki (1986).

To facilitate the hydride transfer there is polarization of the acceptor carbonyl at the active site. This polarization may lead to the generation of a partial or full carbonium ion (Bloxham *et al.* 1975) (Fig. 9D.3). In alcohol dehydrogenase, the group that is responsible for the polarization of the acceptor carbonyl is atomic zinc. Investigators have examined homogeneous preparations of human placental 17β-HSD (Murdock *et al.* 1991) and 3(17)β-HSD (Levy *et al.* 1987) for the presence of zinc by atomic absorption spectrometry and have found no evidence for its participation in the catalytic mechanism. Evidence exists for both enzymes, based on either affinity-labelling or chemical modification studies (Murdock *et al.* 1986; Levy *et al.* 1987), that the general acid involved in polarizing the acceptor carbonyl may be the imidazole ring of a histidine residue. It is conceivable that the same histidine residue functions as both a general acid and a base in the reduction and oxidation directions.

9D.4.2   Kinetic mechanism

As a consequence of the direct hydride transfer between pyridine nucleotide and steroid substrate, all HSDs have sequential bisubstrate kinetic mechanisms. These mechanisms can be random, in which case either substrate can bind first to form a binary complex, or they can be compulsory ordered mechanisms in which the pyridine nucleotide binds first and leaves last (Fig. 9D.4).

The kinetic mechanisms of many HSDs have been determined. In nearly every instance the mechanism appears to be ordered. The exception to this

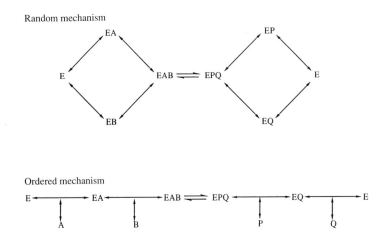

Fig. 9D.4 Kinetic mechanisms for hydroxysteroid dehydrogenases E, enzyme; A, $NAD(P)^+$; B, steroid substrate; P, steroid product; Q, NAD(P)(H). (Reproduced with permission from Penning and Ricigliano 1991.)

rule is seen with human placental (Betz 1971) and porcine testis (Inano and Tamaoki 1986) 17β-HSDs, where a random Bi-Bi mechanism appears to operate. In contrast, 3(17)β-HSD from *Pseudomonas testosteroni* displays an ordered kinetic mechanism (Levy *et al.* 1987). The kinetic mechanism of other mammalian 17β-HSDs is yet to be determined.

Understanding the kinetic mechanism for 17β-HSDs offers important insights into inhibitor design. For eukaryotic 17β-HSDs, which display random mechanisms, the species subjected to inhibition or inactivation by a steroid analogue could be either E or E·NAD(P)(H). The resultant binary and ternary complexes may differ in their dissociation constants for an inhibitor and may have variable susceptibility to alkylation by an enzyme inactivator.

The kinetic mechanism is also important in considering the design of transition state or intermediate-state analogues for 17β-HSDs. If these compounds are based on bisubstrate analogues, their ability to form tight-binding complexes with 17β-HSDs which display random mechanisms may be diminished by the prevailing concentrations of either steroid substrate or cofactor.

9D.5 Inhibitors of 17β-hydroxysteroid dehydrogenases

Compounds which inhibit 17β-HSD have the potential to regulate the production of androgens and oestrogens, and fall into one of several classes:

(1) selective reversible inhibitors;

(2) tight-binding inhibitors;

(3) affinity alkylators;

(4) enzyme-generated inhibitors;

(5) epoxide-based inhibitors.

9D.5.1   Reversible inhibitors

Reversible inhibitors rely on binding affinity for selectivity. These agents exclude substrate access to the catalytic site by direct competition. Such compounds are effective as therapeutic agents as long as appropriate concentrations can be maintained. In general, they would be short-acting drugs. Jarabak and Sack (1969) were among the first to show that non-steroidal oestrogens (diethylstilbestrol, hexestrol) and anti-oestrogens (*cis-* and *trans-*clomiphene) are potent competitive inhibitors of human placental 17β-HSD. This work was extended by Blomquist *et al.* (1984), and these findings might be anticipated since the enzyme has an oestrogen binding site. Because these non-steroids display an even higher affinity for the oestrogen receptor, it is unlikely that they can act as selective inhibitors of 17β-HSD. However, it is conceivable that, at high concentrations, non-steroidal anti-oestrogens can be used to block oestrogen action by both acting as oestrogen receptor antagonists and inhibiting oestrogen biosynthesis at the level of 17β-HSD. Moreover, non-steroidal anti-oestrogens may provide important leads to the development of selective inhibitors of 17β-HSD with no affinity for the oestrogen receptor.

9D.5.2   Tight-binding inhibitors

Tight-binding inhibitors include transition state and intermediate state analogues. For a compound to belong to this group, its structure must mimic that intermediate on the reaction pathway and must display nanomolar affinity for the target enzyme. Unlike inactivators which covalently modify their target enzyme, these compounds can produce stoichiometric pseudo-irreversible inhibition owing to their slow rate of dissociation and will predominantly affect V_{max} (Fig. 9D.5, eqn (1)).

The concept that steroid pyrazoles may display high affinity for HSDs has been developed recently by Levy *et al.* (1987) based on the classical work of Theorell (Theorell and Yonetani 1963; Theorell *et al.* 1969), which demonstrated that liver alcohol dehydrogenase is potently inhibited by the zinc chelator pyrazole. Crystallographic studies indicate that the basis of this inhibition is the formation of a coordinate complex in which one pyrazole ring nitrogen is coordinated to zinc while the other pyrazole nitrogen is coordinated with the C4 position of the nicotinamide ring. Although

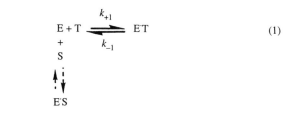

$$E + T \underset{k_{-1}}{\overset{k_{+1}}{\rightleftharpoons}} E{\cdot}T \qquad (1)$$

$$E + I \underset{k_{-1}}{\overset{k_{+1}}{\rightleftharpoons}} E{\cdot}I \overset{k_{+2}}{\longrightarrow} E{\cdot}Inact \qquad (2)$$

$$E + pI \underset{k_{-1}}{\overset{k_{+1}}{\rightleftharpoons}} E{\cdot}pI \underset{k_{-2}}{\overset{k_{+2}}{\rightleftharpoons}} E{\cdot}I^* \overset{k_{+3}}{\longrightarrow} E{\cdot}Inact \qquad (3)$$

Fig. 9D.5 Simple kinetic schemes which depict modes of hydroxysteroid dehydrogenase inhibition or inactivation: (1) inhibition by a tight binding inhibitor T where S is a substrate; (2) inactivation by an affinity alkylator; (3) inactivation by a suicide substrate where pI is a proinhibitor and I is an enzyme-generated inhibitor.

human placental 17β-HSD and $3(17)\beta$-HSD from *P. testosteroni* do not contain essential metal ions at their active sites, they do employ a general acid to facilitate the polarization of the acceptor carbonyl, suggesting that pyrazole inhibition of HSDs might be possible. Levy *et al.* (1987) have developed this concept by synthesizing a series of 2,3- and 3,4-fused ring steroidal pyrazoles (Fig. 9D.6, **1–4**). These compounds were effective inhibitors of *Pseudomonas* $3(17)\beta$-HSD, yielding K_i values as low as 20 nM.

In the case of $3(17\beta)$-HSD these steroid pyrazoles bind to the $E{\cdot}NAD^+$ complex which effectively prevents the pyrazole ring from acting as a pyridine ring substitute. Chemical modification studies with diethylpyrrocarbonate have provided evidence for the involvement of an essential histidine at the enzyme's active site which may act as the general acid in catalysis. Based on these observations, Levy *et al.* (1987) have proposed a model in which $E{\cdot}NAD^+$, the active-site histidine, and the steroid pyrazole form an activated ternate. In this model the pyrazole ring is oriented to

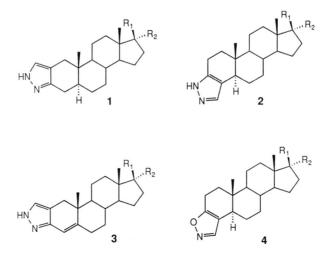

Fig. 9D.6 2,3- and 3,4-Fused steroid pyrazoles examined as inhibitors of 3(17)β-HSD.

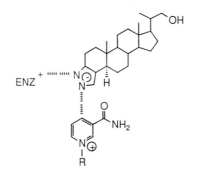

Fig. 9D.7 An activated ternate formed with a 3,4-fused pyrazole during the inhibition of 3(17)β-HSD. (Reproduced with permission from Levy *et al.* 1987.)

share the hydrogen of one of its ring nitrogens, with a lone pair provided by the enzyme histidine, while the lone pair of the remaining nitrogen on the pyrazole ring coordinates with C4 of the nicotinamide ring (Fig. 9D.7). The obligatory requirement for the steroid pyrazoles to bind to an E·NAD$^+$ complex is substantiated by monitoring the inhibition of the NADH dependent reduction of androstenedione. In this reverse direction, a hundred times more steroid pyrazole is required for enzyme inhibition. This implies that the pyridinium ion on the oxidized cofactor is essential for the formation of the ternate.

It is of interest that placental 17β-HSD is believed to contain an active-site histidine (Murdock *et al.* 1986), yet fused ring steroidal pyrazoles have not been examined as inhibitors of this enzyme. It could be argued that, since the original pyrazoles are 2,3- and 3,4-fused ring derivatives, these molecules have the wrong structure to act as tight-binding inhibitors of mammalian 17β-HSD. What may be required is the synthesis of D-ring fused pyrazoles, i.e. (15,16- and 16,17-fused ring derivatives).

9D.5.3 Affinity alkylators

Affinity alkylators are compounds which contain an affinity-labeling moiety attached to either an analogue of a steroid substrate or a steroid inhibitor. The selectivity built into these agents relies on their affinity for the active site. Archetypal HSD affinity alkylators are the bromoacetoxysteroids (Sweet *et al.* 1972; Arias *et al.* 1973; Strickler *et al.* 1975). The interaction of an affinity alkylator with its target enzyme is shown in Fig. 9D.5, eqn (2). This simplified scheme does not account for the complications introduced by kinetic mechanism. One advantage of affinity alkylators is a potentially long duration of action, since *de novo* protein synthesis is presumably required for the restoration of enzyme activity. However, because affinity alkylators are introduced as reactive molecules, they can interact with low molecular mass nucleophiles or cellular macromolecules prior to reaching their target, and therefore have diminished specificity. While such compounds have been highly effective for active-site mapping, their high reactivity with extraneous nucleophiles renders them ineffective as therapeutic agents.

9D.5.4 Enzyme-generated inhibitors

Enzyme-generated inhibitors include the suicide substrates and enzyme-generated affinity-alkylating agents. Suicide substrates are those compounds which bind in a latent form to the target enzyme, and are then turned over by the enzyme to form a reactive species which covalently modifies it at the active site prior to dissociation (Rando 1974a,b; Walsh 1982; Silverman 1986). By definition, these compounds have a partition ratio of 1.0. Here the partition ratio k_{cat}/k_{inact} is defined as the number of molecules of latent inhibitor that have to be turned over before one molecule of enzyme is inactivated, i.e. the k_{-4} term is insignificant (see Fig. 9D.5, eqn (3)). In contrast, enzyme-generated affinity-alkylating agents are compounds that behave in the same manner as suicide substrates except that their partition ratio is much greater than 1.0, i.e. the k_{-4} term is significant (see Fig. 9D.5, eqn (3)). In this instance, the reactive species generated by the enzyme preferentially dissociates from the enzyme and at a later time re-associates to form covalently inactivated enzyme. The selectivity inherent in the design of the inhibitor may be lost, since the reactive species may either be scavenged by extraneous nucleophiles or modify the target enzyme at a site other than the active site.

Enzyme-generated inhibitors have several advantages. First, since the inactivators are introduced in an innocuous form, they are more likely to alkylate their target enzyme rather than other macromolecules. Second, the requirement for activation by the target enzyme provides them with an increased specificity over reversible inhibitors and affinity-labelling agents. Third, like affinity alkylators these compounds covalently modify their target enzyme and should have a long duration of action which can only be overcome by *de novo* protein synthesis.

The inactivation of yeast alcohol dehydrogenase by allyl alcohol in the presence of NAD^+ (Rando 1974b) has had a significant impact on work in this area and has led to the concept that steroid allylic alcohols may effectively inactivate an HSD (Fig. 9D.8). This, in turn, led to the concept that one method of exploiting the catalytic mechanism of 17β-HSD would be to introduce an *a,β*-unsaturated alcohol (latent Michael acceptor) into either the D ring of the steroid or the 17β-side-chain. Upon enzymatic oxidation, this group would be converted to an *a,β*-unsaturated ketone (a Michael acceptor) which could ultimately lead to suicide inactivation.

Covey and his coworkers (Covey 1979; Strickler *et al.* 1980) were the first to develop unsubstituted steroidal latent Michael acceptors as potential suicide substrates for human placental 17β-HSD. The first compounds evaluated contained either a propynyl alcohol on the side-chain (e.g. 17β-(1[*R*]-1-hydroxy-2-propynyl)-androst-4-en-3-one (**5**), a latent Michael acceptor) or a propynyl ketone on the side-chain (e.g. 17β-(1-oxo-2-propynyl-androst-4-en-3-one (**8**), an active Michael acceptor) (Table 9D.1). The structures of these molecules predict that they would inactivate 17β-HSD

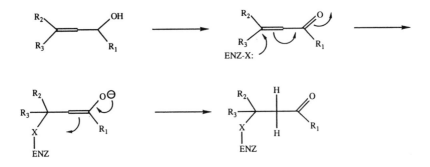

Fig. 9D.8 Enzyme generation of active Michael acceptors: ENZ-X, enzyme nucleophile; R_1–R_3, components of the steroid nucleus and/or the side-chain (Reproduced with permission from Penning and Ricigliano 1991.)

Table 9D.1 Comparison of steroid latent and active Michael acceptors as inactivators of 17β-HSD

Latent or active Michael acceptor	Enzyme	Oxidation			Inactivation		
		Turnover (%)	K_m (μM)	V_{max} (μmol min^{-1} mg^{-1})	K_i (μM)	k_{inact} (S^{-1})	$t_{1/2}$ (min)
	5 17β,20α-HSD* Human placenta	0.03[†]	435	0.04	—	ND	500 at 50 μM
	6 17β,20α-HSD‡ Human placenta	108[†]	8	2.8	—	ND	60 at 100 μM§
	7 17β,20α-HSD¶ Human placenta	0.02[†]	79	0.008	—	ND	45 at 50 μM
	8 17β,20α-HSD* Human placenta	—	—	—	190	9.4×10^{-2}	
	9 17β,20α-HSD‡ Human placenta	—	—	—	261	—	7.2 at 25 μM
	10 17β,20α-HSD¶ Human placenta	—	—	—	2	—	12 (limiting)

ND, — not determined. *Values taken from Tobias et al. (1982). [†]Values are given as a percentage of the utilization ration V_{max}/K_m observed with the normal substrate. ‡Values taken from Thomas et al. (1983). §Inactivation rates observed at pH 9.2. ¶Values taken from Auchus and Covey (1986).

only if it shared dual activity with 20α-HSD. Indeed, these compounds have been used to corroborate the finding that 17β- and 20α-HSD activities are catalysed at the same active site (Tobias *et al.* 1982). The propynyl alcohols caused time-dependent inactivation of the human placental 17β-HSD in a concentration-dependent manner, and this inactivation had an obligatory requirement for a pyridine nucleotide, indicating that turnover was essential. Unfortunately, the alcohol **5** displayed a high K_m and low V_{max} for 17β-HSD, indicating that it was a poor substrate; as a result of this poor turnover, the enzyme was inactivated with a half-life $t_{1/2}$ of 500 minutes at 50 μM. The corresponding ketone (the enzyme-generated product) rapidly inactivated the enzyme with $k_{+3} = 9.4 \times 10^{-2}$ s^{-1} which translated to a $t_{1/2}$ at saturation of 8 seconds or less (Table 9D.1). The problem associated with this pair of latent and active Michael acceptors appears to be poor turnover.

In an attempt to exploit the oxidation of the 17β-hydroxy group directly, 16-methylene-17β-oestradiol (**6**) was synthesized as a potential suicide substrate for the human placental 17β-HSD (Thomas *et al.* 1983). This compound was an excellent substrate for the enzyme, yielding a K_m of 8.0 μM and a V_{max} of 2.8 μmol min^{-1} mg^{-1}. However, inactivation by the parent alcohol was still unimpressive, yielding a half-life for the enzyme at saturation of 60 minutes. Examination of the inactivation of the enzyme with 16-methylene-estrone (**9**) (the active Michael acceptor) showed that this compound produced inactivation with a limiting half-life of 7.2 minutes at a concentration of 25 μM. These data indicate that, for this pair of latent and active Michael acceptors, the problem is one of low reactivity of the enzyme-generated Michael acceptor.

It should be emphasized that none of the attempts to make effective suicide substrates for 17β-HSD have the desirable property of a low partition ratio. In every instance these enzyme-generated inactivators inactivate 17β-HSD by a release and return mechanism. Therefore these compounds fit more closely the definition of enzyme-generated affinity alkylators.

In an attempt to optimize both turnover and reactivity, Auchus and Covey (1986) elected to synthesize seco-oestrogens in which portions of the D ring were removed. However, compounds such as 14,15-seco-oestra-1,3,5(10)-trien-15-yne-3,17β-diol (**7**) were found to be poor substrates and the corresponding ketone (**10**) produced a limiting half-life of 12 minutes. However, compounds of this type have been useful in identifying amino acid residues modified at the active site of 17β-HSD. By using natural abundance ^{13}C-NMR, resonances that correspond to a lysyl-enaminone adduct were detected in a pronase digest of the inactivated enzyme (Auchus and Covey 1987). These findings have been corroborated using solid state NMR (Auchus *et al.* 1988).

Interpretation of these data implies that, although unsubstituted latent and active Michael acceptors provide interesting leads to suicide substrates for 17β-HSD, they do not have the desirable properties sought in ideal compounds. Either they are poorly oxidized by the target enzyme or the enzyme-generated electrophile is not reactive enough to permit rapid Michael addition which would prevent dissociation from the active site. This leads to the question of how the turnover and reactivity of these compounds can be improved. One possible method is to substitute these compounds with electron-donating and electron-withdrawing groups which may, in turn, influence the reactivity.

A priori it might be predicted that introduction of an electron-withdrawing group to the unsaturated bond of a latent Michael acceptor would lead to an increase in their reactivity of the resultant enzyme-generated α,β-unsaturated ketone. In contrast, introduction of an electron-withdrawing group geminal to the hydroxyl group of a latent Michael acceptor would promote turnover by facilitating the deprotonation event that occurs during oxidation; it would also increase the reactivity of the enzyme-generated Michael acceptor. Moreover, electron-withdrawing groups introduced adjacent to the hydroxyl group leave the electrophilic carbon sterically unhindered and more accessible to nucleophilic attack. Although these arguments are duly noted, it is clear that it is difficult to take advantage of these features because of the steric hindrance associated with C17 and its position in the D ring of the steroid. Here, the synthesis of seco-oestrogens described by Auchus and Covey (1986) may provide a means that will permit the introduction of appropriate electron-withdrawing and electron-donating groups into the latent Michael acceptor. Using this approach it was found that substitution of a triple bond of a seco-oestrogen with a trifluoromethyl group (**11**) (Fig. 9D.9) resulted in the formation of a potent affinity alkylator for human placental 17β-HSD and that this compound did not require oxidation of the alcohol for enzyme inactivation (Lawate and Covey 1990). These findings may not have been surprising, based on the known electron-withdrawing capabilities of the trifluoromethyl-group. Unfortunately, substitution of latent Michael acceptors at C17 or the equivalent position of a secosteroid with appropriate electron-withdrawing and electron-donating groups has not been systematically explored.

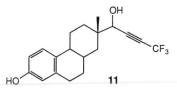

Fig. 9D.9 Trifluoromethylacetylenic seco-oestradiol inhibitor of placental 17β-HSD.

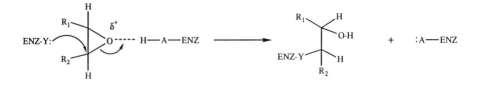

Fig. 9D.10 Inactivation of HSDs by steroid epoxides: ENZ-Y, enzyme nucleophile; R_1 and R_2, components of either the steroid nucleus or the side-chain; H-A-ENZ, general acid at the active site of an HSD. (Reproduced with permission from Penning and Ricigliano 1991.)

9D.5.5   Epoxide-based inhibitors

The presumptive catalytic mechanism for HSDs involves compulsory polarization of the acceptor carbonyl to facilitate hydride transfer. This portion of the enzyme mechanism could be exploited by replacing the acceptor carbonyl with either an epoxide or cyclopropyl ring to form an enzyme-activated inactivator. Protonation of the oxiranyl oxygen or bridge-head carbon at the active site would increase ring strain and facilitate nucleophilic attack at a ring carbon (Fig. 9D.10). Work by Bloxham *et al.* (1975) with epoxide inhibitors of two aliphatic alcohol dehydrogenases (lactate and β-hydroxybutyrate dehydrogenase) demonstrates the formation of such protonated species without subsequent enzyme inactivation.

A number of steroid epoxides have been synthesized and tested as inactivators of 3α-, 3β- and 20α-HSDs in the presence and absence of pyridine nucleotide (Penning *et al.* 1991). In general, no binding to the target HSD was observed. A number of 17β-spiro-epoxides, including some based on equine oestrogens, have been synthesized and evaluated as inhibitors of Δ^5-3-ketosteroid isomeras (Bevins *et al.* 1980; Kayser *et al.* 1983); however, none have been examined as potential inhibitors or inactivators of 17β-HSDs.

9D.6   Studies *in vivo* with 17β-hydroxysteroid dehydrogenase inactivators

It has been argued that the administration of selective 17β-HSD inhibitors or inactivators *in vivo* would result in the attenuation of androgen and oestrogen action. The only study performed *in vivo* examined the effect of administering 16-methylene oestradiol (**6**) to immature rats (McDonald *et al.* 1988). In those studies it was found that inactivation of 17β-HSD led to an enhancement in oestradiol potency, as judged by an increase in the weight of the immature rat uterus. However, no other studies have been conducted to verify this effect in other species. Moreover, these data may be difficult to interpret if a separate 17-ketoreductase and 17β-HSD exists in all rat tissues. It will be recalled that Bogovich and Payne (1980) found that these two enzymes coexist in rat testis.

9D.7 Summary

In designing 17β-HSD inhibitors, attempts have been made to exploit its catalytic mechanism by testing compounds that give rise to activated ternates (steroid pyrazoles) and enzyme-generated affinity alkylators (latent steroid Michael acceptors). This field is still ripe for development; no attempt has been made to synthesize transition state analogues based on bisubstrate analogues, and appropriate D-ring fused pyrazoles have not been synthesized as potential activated ternates. The effect of electron-withdrawing and electron-donating effects on the turnover and reactivity of steroid latent and active Michael acceptors has not been systematically explored. Even though it has been documented that 17β-HSD will bind non-steroidal oestrogens and anti-oestrogens as competitive inhibitors, no attempts have been made to exploit this finding by using these compounds as leads for the synthesis of either more potent reversible inhibitors or non-steroidal suicide substrates for 17β-HSD. Studies in this laboratory have shown that it is feasible to synthesize effective non-steroidal suicide substrates for 3α-HSD (Ricigliano and Penning 1989, 1990; Penning *et al.* 1991). The advantage of such compounds is their ease of synthesis and the flexibility that they permit for the introduction of different enzyme-activatable functionalities.

Acknowledgements

TMP is grateful to the National Institutes of Health for support during the writing of this review through GM 33464 and CA 35904. He is also a recipient of a Research Career and Development Award from the National Cancer Institute, CA01335.

References

Agarwal, A. K., Monder, C., Eckstein, B., and White, P. C. (1989). Cloning and expression of rat cDNA encoding corticosteroid 11β-dehydrogenase. *Journal of Biological Chemistry*, **264**, 18939–43.

Antoun, G. R., Brglez, I., and Williamson, D. G. (1985). A 17β-hydroxysteroid dehydrogenase of female rabbit liver cytosol. Purification and characterization of multiple forms of the enzyme. *Biochemical Journal*, **225**, 383–90.

Arias, F., Sweet, F., and Warren, J. C. (1973). Affinity labeling of steroid binding sites: study of the active site of 20β-hydroxysteroid dehydrogenase with 6β- and 11α-bromoacetoxyprogesterone. *Journal of Biological Chemistry*, **248**, 5641–7.

Auchus, R. J. and Covey, D. F. (1986). Mechanism-based inactivation of 17β,20α-hydroxysteroid dehydrogenase by an acetylenic secoestradiol. *Biochemistry*, **25**, 7295–300.

Auchus, R. J. and Covey, D. F. (1987). Dehydrogenase inactivation by an enzyme generated acetylenic ketone; identification of a lysyl enaminone by ^{13}C-NMR. *Journal of the American Chemical Society*, **109**, 280–2.

Auchus, R. J., Covey, D. F., Bork, V., and Schaefer, J. (1988). Solid-state NMR observation of cysteine and lysine Michael adducts of inactivated oestradiol-17β dehydrogenase. *Journal of Biological Chemistry*, **263**, 11640–5.

Betz, G. (1971). Reaction mechanism of 17β-estradiol dehydrogenase determined by equilibrium rate exchange. *Journal of Biological Chemistry*, **246**, 2063–8.

Bevins, C. I., Kayser, R. H., Pollack, R. M., Ekiko, D. B., and Sadoff, S. (1980). Irreversible active-site directed inhibition of Δ^5-3-ketosteroid isomerase by steroidal 17β-oxiranes. Evidence for two modes of binding in steroid-enzyme complexes. *Biochemical and Biophysical Research Communications*, **95**, 1131–7.

Blomquist, C. H., Lindemann, N. J., and Hakanson, E. Y. (1984). Inhibition of 17β-HSD activities of human placenta by steroids and nonsteroidal hormone agonists and antagonists. *Steroids*, **44**, 571–86.

Bloxham, D. P., Giles, I. G., Wilton, D. C., and Akhtar, M. (1975). The mechanism of the bond forming events in pyridine nucleotide oxidoreductases. Studies with epoxide inhibitors of lactate dehydrogenase and β-hydroxybutyrate dehydrogenase. *Biochemistry*, **14**, 2235–41.

Bogovich, K. and Payne, A. H. (1980). Purification of rat testicular microsomal 17-ketosteroid reductase. Evidence that 17-ketosteroid reductase and 17β-HSD are distinct enzymes. *Journal of Biological Chemistry*, **255**, 5552–9.

Bolcsak, L. E. and Nerland, D. E. (1983). Purification of mouse liver benzene-dihydrodiol dehydrogenases. *Journal of Biological Chemistry*, **258**, 7252–5.

Covey, D. F. (1979). Synthesis of 17β-[(1S)-1-hydroxy-2-propynyl]- and 17β-[(1R)-1-hydroxy-2-propynyl]androst-4-en-3-one. Potential suicide substrates of 20α- and 20β-hydroxysteroid dehydrogenases. *Steroids*, **34**, 199–206.

Engel, L. L. and Inano, H. (1978). Some kinetic properties of human placental estradiol-17β dehydrogenase. Patterns of inhibition by adenine dinucleotides. *Advances in Enzyme Regulation*, **17**, 363–71.

Fisher, H. F., Conn, E. E., Vennesland, B., and Westheimer, F. H. (1953). The enzymatic transfer of hydrogen I. The reaction catalyzed by alcohol dehydrogenase. *Journal of Biological Chemistry*, **202**, 687–97.

Gross, D. J., Landau, H., Kohn, G., Farkas, A., Elrayyes, E., El-Shawwa, R., et al. (1986). Male pseudohermaphroditism due to 17β-HSD deficiency: gender reassessment in early pregnancy. *Acta Endocrinologica*, **112**, 238–46.

Hara, A., Hayashibara, M., Nakayama, T., Hasebe, K., Usui, S., and Sawada, H. (1985). Guinea-pig liver testosterone 17β-hydroxysteroid dehydrogenase (NADP$^+$) and aldehyde reductase exhibit benzenedihydrodiol dehydrogenase activity. *Biochemical Journal*, **225**, 177–81.

Hara, A., Kariya, K., Nakamura, M., Nakayama, T., and Sawada, H. (1986). Isolation of multiple forms of indanol dehydrogenase associated with 17β-hydroxysteroid dehydrogenase activity from male rabbit liver. *Archives of Biochemistry and Biophysics*, **249**, 225–36.

Inano, H. and Tamaoki, B.-I. (1975). Relationship between steroids and pyridine nucleotides in the oxido-reduction catalyzed by the 17β-hydroxysteroid dehydrogenase purified from the porcine testicular fraction. *European Journal of Biochemistry*, **53**, 319–26.

Inano H. and Tamaoki, B.-I. (1986). Testicular 17β-hydroxysteroid dehydrogenase: Molecular properties and reaction mechanism. *Steroids*, **48**, 1–26.

Jarabak, J. and Talalay, P. (1960). Stereospecificity of hydrogen transfer by pyridine nucleotide linked hydroxysteroid dehydrogenases. *Journal of Biological Chemistry*, **235**, 2147–54.

Jarabak, J. and Sack, G. H. (1969). Soluble 17β-hydroxysteroid dehydrogenase from human placenta. The binding of pyridine nucleotides and steroids. *Biochemistry*, **8**, 2203–11.

Jarabak, J., Adams, J. A., Williams-Ashman, H. G., and Talalay, P. (1962). Purification of a 17β-hydroxysteroid dehydrogenase of human placenta and studies on its transhydrogenation function. *Journal of Biological Chemistry*, **257**, 345–57.

Kayser, R. H., Bounds, P. L., Bevins, C. L., and Pollack, R. M. (1983). Affinity-alkylation of bacterial Δ^5-3-ketosteroid isomerase. Identification of the amino acid modified by steroidal 17β-oxiranes. *Journal of Biological Chemistry*, **258**, 909–15.

Kobayashi, K. and Kochakian, C. D. (1978). 17β-Hydroxy-C$_{19}$-steroid dehydrogenases from male guinea-pig liver. Purification and characterization. *Journal of Biological Chemistry*, **253**, 3635–42.

Lawate, S. S. and Covey, D. F. (1990). Trifluoromethylacetylenic alcohols as affinity labels. Inactivation of oestradiol dehydrogenase by a trifluoromethyl-acetylenic secoestradiol. *Journal of Medicinal Chemistry*, **33**, 2319–21.

Levy, M. A., Holt, D. A., Brandt, M., and Metcalf, B. W. (1987). Inhibition of 3(17)β-hydroxysteroid dehydrogenase from *Pseudomonas testosteroni* by steroidal A ring fused pyrazoles. *Biochemistry*, **26**, 2270–9.

Loweus, F. A., Olfner, P., Fisher, H. F., Westheimer, F. H., and Vennesland, B. (1953). The enzymatic transfer of hydrogen II. The reaction catalyzed by lactate dehydrogenase. *Journal of Biological Chemistry*, **202**, 699–704.

Luu-The, V., Labrie, C., Zhao, H. F., Couet, J., Lachance, Y., Simard, J., *et al.* (1989a). Characterization of cDNA's for human estradiol-17β dehydrogenase and assignment of the gene to chromosome 17: Evidence of two mRNA species with distinct 5′ termini in human placenta. *Molecular Endocrinology*, **3**, 1301–9.

Luu-The, V., Lachance, Y., Labrie, C., Leblanc, G., Thomas, J. L., Strickler, R. C., and Labrie, F. (1989b). Full length cDNA structure and deduced amino acid sequence of human 3β-hydroxy-5-ene steroid dehydrogenase. *Molecular Endocrinology*, **3**, 1310–12.

McDonald, Z. A., Slikker, W., Fu, P. P., Bailey, J. R., Lipe, G. W., and Unruh, L. E. (1988). Enhancement of estradiol potency by the 17β-hydroxysteroid dehydrogenase inhibitor, 16-methylene-estradiol *in vivo*. *Journal of Pharmacology and Experimental Therapeutics*, **214**, 428–31.

Mulder, E., Lamers-Stahlhofen, G. J. M., and van der Molen, H.-J. (1972). Isolation and characterization of 17β-hydroxysteroid dehydrogenase from human erythrocytes. *Biochemical Journal*, **127**, 649–59.

Murdock, G. L., Chang-Chen, C., and Warren, J. C. (1986). Human placental estradiol 17β-dehydrogenase: sequence of a histidine-bearing peptide in the catalytic region. *Biochemistry*, **25**, 641–6.

Murdock, G. L., Pineda, J., Nagorsky, N., Lawrence, S. S., Heritage, R., and

Warren, J. C. (1991). Estradiol 17β-dehydrogenase: full enzymatic activity in the absence of zinc. *Biochimica et Biophysica Acta*, **1076**, 197–202.

Pawlowski, J. E., Huizinga, M., and Penning, T. M. (1991). Cloning and sequencing of the cDNA for rat liver 3α-hydroxysteroid/dihydrodiol dehydrogenase. *Journal of Biological Chemistry*, **266**, 8820–5.

Peltoketo, H., Isomaa, V., Maentausta, O., and Vihko, R. (1988). Complete amino acid sequence of human placental 17β-HSD deduced from cDNA. *Federation of European Biochemical Societies Letters* **239**, 73–7.

Penning, T. M. and Ricigliano, J. W. (1991). Mechanism-based inhibition of hydroxy steroid dehydrogenase. *Journal of Enzyme Inhibition*, **5**, 165–98.

Penning, T. M., Thornton, R., and Ricigliano, J. W. (1991). Clues to the development of mechanism-based inactivators of 3α-hydroxysteroid dehydrogenases: comparison of steroidal and nonsteroidal Michael acceptors and epoxides. *Steroids*, **56**, 420–7.

Rando, R. R. (1974a). Chemistry and enzymology of k_{cat} inhibitors. *Science*, **185**, 320–4.

Rando, R. R. (1974b). Allyl alcohol-induced irreversible inhibition of yeast alcohol dehydrogenase. *Biochemical Pharmacology*, **23**, 2328–31.

Ricigliano, J. W. and Penning, T. M. (1989). Synthesis and evaluation of nonsteroidal mechanism based inactivators of 3α-hydroxysteroid dehydrogenase. *Biochemical Journal*, **262**, 139–49.

Ricigliano, J. W. and Penning, T. M. (1990). Evidence that enzyme-generated aromatic Michael acceptors covalently modify the nucleotide binding site of 3α-hydroxysteroid dehydrogenase. *Biochemical Journal*, **269**, 749–55.

Sawada, H., Hara, A., Nakayama, T., Nakagawa, M., Inoue, Y., Hasebe, K., and Zhang, Y.-P. (1988). Mouse liver dihydrodiol dehydrogenases: identity of the predominant and a minor form with 17β-hydroxysteroid dehydrogenase and aldehyde reductase. *Biochemical Pharmacology*, **37**, 453–8.

Silverman, R. B. (1986). In *Mechanism-based enzyme inactivation: chemistry and enzymology* Vol. 1, pp. 3–27. CRC Press, Boca Raton, Fl.

Strickler, R. C., Sweet, F., and Warren, J. C. (1975). Affinity labeling of steroid binding sites. Study of the active site of 20β-hydroxysteroid dehydrogenase with 2α-bromoacetoxyprogesterone and 11α-bromoacetoxyprogesterone. *Journal of Biological Chemistry*, **250**, 7656–62.

Strickler, R. C., Covey, D. F., and Tobias, B. (1980). Study of 3α,20β-hydroxysteroid dehydrogenase with an enzyme-generated affinity alkylator: dual enzyme activities at a single active site. *Biochemistry*, **19**, 4950–4.

Strickler, R. C., Tobias, B., and Covey, D. F. (1981). Human placental 17β-estradiol dehydrogenase and 20α-hydroxysteroid dehydrogenase. Two activities at a single enzyme active site. *Journal of Biological Chemistry*, **256**, 316–21.

Sweet, F., Arias, F., and Warren, J. C. (1972). Affinity-labeling of steroid binding sites. Synthesis of 16α-bromoacetoxyprogesterone and its use for affinity-labeling 20β-hydroxysteroid dehydrogenase. *Journal of Biological Chemistry*, **247**, 3424–33.

Tait, G. H., Newton, C. J., Reed, M. J., and James, V. H. T. (1989). Multiple forms of 17β-hydroxysteroid oxidoreductase in human breast tissue. *Journal of Molecular Endocrinology*, **2**, 71–80.

Talalay, P. (1963). Hydroxysteroid dehydrogenases, In *The enzymes* (2nd edn), Vol. 7, pp. 177–202. Academic Press, New York.

Theorell, H. and Yonetani, T. (1963). Liver alcohol dehydrogenase-DPN-pyrazole complex: a model of a ternary intermediate in the enzyme reaction. *Biochemische Zeitschrift*, **338**, 537–53.

Theorell, H., Yonetani, T., and Sjoberg, B. (1969). On the effects of some heterocyclic compounds on the enzyme activity of liver alcohol dehydrogenase. *Acta Chemica Scandinavica*, **23**, 255–60.

Thomas, J. L., LaRochelle, M. C., Covey, D. F., and Strickler, R. C. (1983). Inactivation of human placental 17β,20α-hydroxysteroid dehydrogenase by 16-methylene estrone an affinity alkylator enzymatically generated from 16-methylene estradiol-17β. *Journal of Biological Chemistry*, **258**, 11500–4.

Tobias, B., Covey, D. F., and Strickler, R. C. (1982). Inactivation of human placental 17β-estradiol dehydrogenase and 20α-hydroxysteroid dehydrogenase with active site directed 17β-propynyl-substituted progestin analogs. *Journal of Biological Chemistry*, **257**, 2783–86.

Walsh, C. T. (1982). Suicide substrates, mechanism-based enzyme inactivators: recent developments. *Annual Review of Biochemistry*, **53**, 493–535.

Wilson, S. C., Hodgins, M. B., and Scott, J. S. (1987). Incomplete masculinization due to a deficiency of 17β-hydroxysteroid dehydrogenase: comparison of prepubertal and peripubertal siblings. *Clinical Endocrinology*, **26**, 459–69.

Wilson, S. C., Oakey, R. E., and Scott, J. S. (1988). Steroid metabolism in testes of patients with incomplete masculinization due to androgen insensitivity or 17β-hydroxysteroid dehydrogenase deficiency and normally differentiated males. *Journal of Steroid Biochemistry*, **29**, 649–55.

Section 9E

Inhibition of steroid sulphatases

M. J. Reed and A. Purohit

9E.1 Introduction

Tumours that develop in steroid responsive tissues such as breast, endometrium or prostate are hormone dependent (James and Reed 1980). Such tumours can respond to surgical ablative procedures performed to remove the source(s) of steroid production. However, the mortality and morbidity associated with surgery led to a search for alternative means of inhibiting steroid production, and the development of specific inhibitors of steroid synthesis has been a major advance in the treatment of patients with hormone-dependent tumours. So far attention has been directed mainly at the development of aromatase and 5 a-reductase inhibitors for use in the treatment of breast and prostatic cancer respectively. While the synthesis of such inhibitors is a logical step in the production of steroidogenic enzyme inhibitors, there is now considerable interest in the development of steroid sulphatase inhibitors. In this chapter we examine the requirement for steroid sulphatase inhibitors and review the somewhat limited attempts made so far to develop such inhibitors.

9E.2   Steroid sulphates and sulphatases

For many years sulphate conjugates of steroids were believed to represent the end-products of steroid metabolism, but it is now generally accepted that steroid sulphates are important intermediates in the synthesis, transport, and action of steroid hormones (Purdy *et al.* 1961; Rosenthal *et al.* 1975; Vignon *et al.* 1980). While many steroids exist in the body in a sulphated form, the potential role that steroid sulphates may have in supporting tumour growth has mainly concentrated on two steroid sulphates, oestrone sulphate (E1S) and dehydroepiandrosterone sulphate (DHA-S). Concentrations of E1S and DHA-S in plasma (1 nmol l^{-1} and 1 μmol l^{-1}) are much higher than those of the unconjugated forms of these steroids (Reed *et al.* 1983; Vermeulen *et al.* 1986). The half-lives of steroid sulphates in blood of about 7.5 hours are much longer than those of unconjugated steroids (30 minutes), thus making steroid sulphates a potential circulating reservoir for the formation of active steroid hormones (Ruder *et al.* 1972; Hawkins *et al.* 1985).

Significant concentrations of DHA-S and E1S have also been detected in breast tumours (Vermeulen *et al.* 1986; Pasqualini *et al.* 1989; Thijssen and Blankenstein 1989). However, concentrations of E1S detected in breast tumours vary from 16−207 pg g^{-1} of tissue (Vermeulen *et al.* 1986, Thijssen and Blankenstein 1989) to the much higher levels of 2120 ± 974 pg g^{-1} reported by Pasqualini *et al.* (1989). In addition, extremely high concentrations of steroid sulphates are present in breast cyst fluid collected from women with gross cystic breast disease, a condition which may be associated with an increased risk for the development of breast cancer (Bradlow *et al.* 1981).

The enzymes involved in the sulphation (sulphotransferase) and hydrolysis of steroid sulphates (sulphatase) are widely distributed throughout the body, including normal and malignant breast tissues, endometrium, prostate, gonads, adrenal cortex, and liver. Measurement of oestrone sulphatase and oestrone sulphotransferase activities in breast tissues and breast cancer cells indicates that sulphatase activity is much higher than sulphotransferase activity, thus favouring the formation of the unconjugated steroid moiety (Tseng *et al.* 1983; Pasqualini *et al.* 1989).

Although hydrolysis of DHA-S and E1S involves the removal of a sulphate group, it is still not clear whether the hydrolysis of DHA-S and E1S is mediated by the same or different sulphatases. In the original study to investigate the ability of breast tumours to hydrolyse E1S and DHA-S, Dao *et al.* (1974) noted that a greater proportion of tumours could hydrolyse E1S than DHA-S, suggesting the presence of distinct sulphatases. The ability of pregnenolone sulphate to inhibit DHA sulphatase and E1 sulphatase activities in a placental preparation led Townsley *et al.* (1970) to question the existence of distinct sulphatases. Using an endometrial preparation, however, Prost and Addessi (1983) showed that E1 sulphatase and DHA sulphatase have different pH requirements, that DHA sulphatase is more sensitive to thermal inactivation, and that magnesium chloride enhances E1 sulphatase but not DHA sulphatase activity. They also demonstrated that DHA-S inhibits E1 sulphatase and E1S inhibits DHA sulphatase in a non-competitive manner, suggesting the presence of different sulphatase enzymes with different binding sites. MacIndoe *et al.* (1988) have recently carried out a similar study using an MCF-7 breast cancer microsomal preparation and again obtained evidence to support the existence of different sulphatases for the hydrolysis of DHA-S and E1S. Recent investigations employing purified placental sulphatase preparations support the presence of only one sulphatase which is capable of hydrolysing E1S and DHA-S (Burns 1983; Dibbelt and Kuss 1986; Kawano *et al.* 1989).

A steroid sulphatase has now been purified from human placenta, cloned, and sequenced (Yen *et al.* 1987). Results indicate that the mature steroid sulphatase is a 492 amino acid hydrophobic glycoprotein derived following the removal of a 22 amino acid signal peptide. Its molecular mass is in the region of 120 kDa with subunits of 60–62 kDa, suggesting that the active enzyme is most likely to be a homodimer. Expression studies with cDNA should reveal whether the same or different sulphatases are involved in the hydrolysis of E1S and DHA-S.

9E.3   Tissue availability of steroid sulphates

Two important questions remain to be resolved with regard to the potential role of steroid sulphates as substrates for the formation of biologically active steroids.

1. Are polar steroid conjugates, as such, able to cross cell membranes and be taken up by tissues?

2. What is the cellular location of the steroid sulphatase complex?

In an original investigation, Vignon *et al.* (1980) injected ^{3}H oestradiol into CH3 mice with mammary tumours and found that 50–70 per cent of the radioactivity was present as polar metabolites with chromatographic properties similar to those of oestrogen sulphates. While this was taken as evidence to suggest that oestrogen sulphates are taken up by tumour tissues, most tumours also possess oestrogen sulphotransferase activity. It is therefore possible that, after injection of ^{3}H oestradiol, unconjugated oestradiol enters the tumour where it is subsequently sulphated.

Holinka and Gurpide (1980), using a double-isotope technique, showed that, while E1S was taken up by the liver in the rabbit, there was no evidence for the entry of E1S into the endometrium. This finding is supported by our own results in which we have examined the uptake of [3]H E1S or E1-^{35}S by normal and malignant breast tissues but have so far found no evidence to support the uptake of E1S, as such, by these tissues (Reed *et al.* 1989; Purohit *et al.* 1990).

Steroid sulphatases are membrane-bound enzymes and both E1 sulphatase and DHA sulphatase activities have been found to reside in the cytoplasmic particulate fraction (MacIndoe *et al.* 1988). This finding led MacIndoe and colleagues to conclude that, as steroid sulphatases appear to be localized to cell microsomes, transmembrane transport of polar steroid sulphates would be a prerequisite for steroid hydrolysis. Schwenk and Del Pino (1980) obtained evidence to support the active up-take of E1S by rat liver cells. Influx of E1S was similar to the uptake of the polar bile acid taurocholate, being a saturable energy and pH-dependent process. As no evidence of oestrone sulphatase activity was detected in isolated liver cell membranes, they concluded that the influx of E1S requires the involvement of an energy-dependent carrier. However, evidence for oestrone sulphatase activity has been found in breast tissue cell membranes (approximately 5 per cent of the total cell sulphatase activity), suggesting that hydrolysis may occur at the cell membrane, allowing the liberated steroid to enter the cell (Tseng *et al.* 1983).

While further studies are required to examine the mechanisms by which steroid sulphates are made available to cells and tissues, the high circulating levels of steroid sulphates and the potential for hydrolysis within the liver and/or other peripheral tissues makes these conjugates an important circulating reservoir for the formation of biologically active steroids.

9E.4 The role of oestrone sulphate in oestrogen synthesis in breast tumours

Recent interest in the development of steroid sulphatase inhibitors has arisen as a result of a number of studies carried out to examine the biological activity of oestrogen sulphates and the origin of oestrogens in breast tumours. In post-menopausal women, breast tumour concentrations of oestrogens are much higher than oestrogen concentrations in plasma (Bonney *et al.* 1983; Van Landeghem *et al.* 1985; Vermeulen *et al.* 1986). While retention of oestrogens in breast tumours by high affinity binding proteins will contribute to the level of oestrogens in breast tumours, oestrogen concentrations are similar in receptor-positive and receptor-negative tumours (Fishman *et al.* 1977). Therefore it is likely that local formation of oestrogens from oestrogen precursors will also make an important contribution to the oestrogen content of breast tumours.

In post-menopausal women, when ovarian production of oestrogens has ceased, oestrogens are formed almost exclusively from the peripheral conversion of androstenedione to oestrone (Siiteri and MacDonald 1973; Reed *et al.* 1979). The presence of the enzymes required for oestrogen synthesis in breast tumours has been confirmed by a number of research groups (Miller and Forrest 1976; Tilson-Mallett *et al.* 1983; James *et al.* 1987). An outline of potential pathways for oestrogen synthesis in breast tumours, together with plasma precursor concentrations, is shown in Fig. 9E.1. While all oestrogens are formed by the action of the aromatase enzyme complex, aromatase activity in breast tumours is considerably lower than E1 sulphatase activity (James *et al.* 1987). As plasma concentrations of E1S are much higher than those of unconjugated E1, the potential role of E1S as a substrate for oestrogen synthesis or a mediator of oestrogen action has been examined in breast cancer cells and breast-tumour tissues.

Using MCF-7 breast cancer cells, which possess oestrone sulphatase activity, Vignon *et al.* (1980) demonstrated that E1S stimulates the synthesis of well-characterized oestrogen induced proteins. In view of this finding and the high circulating concentrations of E1S, Santner *et al.* (1984) examined the relative contribution that the aromatase and E1 sulphatase enzyme complexes make to the synthesis of oestrone in breast tumours. Under the conditions of limited substrate availability used, 10 times more

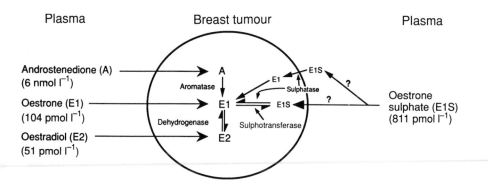

Fig. 9E.1 The origin of oestrogens in breast tumours.

oestrone was found to originate from E1S than from androstenedione, suggesting that the oestrone sulphatase pathway may be the primary mechanism for the local production of oestrogens in breast tumours.

Further evidence to support the role of E1S in regulating breast tumour growth was recently obtained by Santner *et al.* (1990) using the nitro-somethylurea(NSMU)-induced breast carcinoma model in rats. This tumour possesses E1 sulphatase activity, but not aromatase activity, and the majority of tumours regress after castration. Administration of E1S resulted in a dose-dependent stimulation of the NSMU-induced tumour, suggesting that E1S is biologically active *in vivo*. Pasqualini *et al.* (1982) had previously shown that E1S increases uterine weights in fetal guinea pigs. However, such investigations do not allow a distinction to be drawn between hydrolysis *in situ* and hydrolysis in peripheral tissues with subsequent transport to endocrine-sensitive tissues. As conversion of E1S to oestradiol can occur in NSMU-induced tumour cells, it is possible that a combination of both *in situ* and peripheral conversion occurs.

A further stimulus to the development of steroid sulphatase inhibition has arisen from recent studies in which women with breast cancer have been treated with specific inhibitors of aromatase activity. A number of aromatase inhibitors are currently being developed, but one of the most promising compounds tested so far is 4-hydroxyandrostenedione (4-OHA) Dowsett *et al.* 1987). Our investigations have revealed that treatment with 4-OHA effectively abolishes the peripheral conversion of androstenedione to oestrone, yet significant concentrations of E1 are still detectable in plasma and normal and malignant breast tissues (Reed *et al.* 1990, 1991). A possible explanation for the continued presence of E1 in plasma and tissues of women after treatment with 4-OHA is that E1 continues to be formed from the large slowly turning over pool of E1S which is present in blood and other tissues. In order to improve the response rate in women with breast cancer, it may be necessary to inhibit both the aromatase and sulphatase pathways of oestrogen synthesis.

The potential role of oestrone sulphate in regulating the growth of hormone-dependent breast tumours has led to the development of inhibitors of steroid sulphatase activity but, in contrast with the development of aromatase inhibitors, this area of research is still at a very early stage.

9E.5   Inhibitors of steroid sulphatase activity

The regulation of steroid sulphatase activity has been investigated using enzyme preparations derived from placental (Townsley *et al.* 1970), prostatic (Farnsworth 1973), and testicular (Notation and Ungar 1969) tissues. These early investigations revealed that, while a number of unconjugated steroids can inhibit steroid sulphatase activity in general, a greater degree of inhibition is achieved using steroid sulphates. Kinetic data for E1 sulphatase and DHA sulphatase, together with K_i values for some steroid inhibitors, are shown in Table 9E.1.

While these initial studies suggested the potential importance of steroid sulphatases as key regulatory enzymes in the balance between the formation of inactive and active steroids, it is only recently that the development of steroid sulphatase inhibitors has been seriously pursued. So far the most widely studied inhibitor of steroid sulphatase activity is the synthetic steroid danazol, an isoxazole derivative of 17α-ethinyltestosterone (Fig. 9E.2(a)). Although danazol had been shown to inhibit the growth of an endometrial carcinoma cell line (Terakawa *et al.* 1987) and to inhibit DMBA-induced mammary carcinogenesis in the rat (Peters *et al.* 1977), Carlstrom *et al.* (1984a) initially suggested that this compound inhibited steroid sulphatase activity. Treatment of women with endometriosis by the administration of danazol was found to result in an increase in circulating levels of DHA-S with a corresponding decrease in DHA concentrations, suggesting inhibition of steroid sulphatase activity. Carlstrom *et al.* (1984b) subsequently demonstrated that danazol inhibits steroid sulphatase activity in human liver cells and breast tumour tissue *in vitro*. Our own studies have also shown that danazol (10 μM) significantly inhibits E1 sulphatase activity in MCF-7 and MDA-MB-231 breast cancer cells and also inhibits

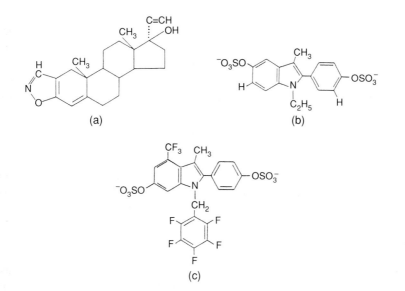

(a)

(b)

(c)

Fig. 9E.2 Steroid sulphatase inhibitors: (a) danazol (2,4,17α-pregnadien-20-yno[2,3-d] isoxazol-17-ol); (b) ethyl-3-methyl-5-sulphooxy-2(4-sulphooxy-phenyl)-indole, disodium salt; (c) 3-methyl-1-pentafluorphenylmethyl-6-sulphooxy-2-(4-sulphooxy-phenyl)-4-trifluormethylindole, disodium salt.

Table 9E.1 Inhibitors of steroid sulphatase activity

	Substrate	K_m (μM)	Enzyme system	Species
1	E1S	6.83	Placenta microsomal	Human
	E1S	8.91	Breast carcinoma microsomal	Human
2	E1S	–	Breast carcinoma	Human
		–	NSMU- mammary tumour	Rat
3	DHAS	33.00	Placenta post- mitochondrial Supernatant	Human
4	E1S	20.80	Liver microsomal	Rat
5	DHAS	2.04	Testes microsomal	Rat
	5-Androstene-3β,17β-diol-3-S	0.93		
6	Pregnenolone Sulphate	0.73	Testes microsomal	Human
	DHAS	3.85		
	5-Androstene-3β,17β-diol-3-S	3.13		
7	E1S	–	Uterus 1000 $\times$g Supernatant	Calf

the growth of MCF-7 cells (Purohit and Reed 1991). We have also examined the effect of Danazol (800 mg daily for 2 weeks) on the conversion of E1S to E1 and the plasma concentration of E1 in women with advanced breast cancer (Reed *et al.* 1989). In two out of three women examined so far, treatment with danazol resulted in a 40 per cent decrease in the peripheral conversion of E1S to E1 and the plasma oestrone concentration decreased from 100 ± 39 pmol l^{-1} to 69 ± 17 pmol l^{-1}. E1 sulphatase activity in normal breast tissue also decreased after treatment. While the

Inhibitor	K_i (μM)	Type of inhibition	Reference
Danazol	–		
5-Androstene-3β,17β-diol-3-S	2.0	Competitive	Evans *et al*. 1991
			Santner and Santen 1991
Tamoxifen	1000.0	Non-competitive	
4-Hydroxytamoxifen	300.0	Non-competitive	
ICI 164384	10.0	Non-competitive	
Oestradiol	7.0	Competitive	
DHA	32.5	–	Townsley 1973
Androstenedione	37.5	–	
Oestradiol	11.5	–	
Progesterone	17.0	–	
Pregnenolone-Sulphate	0.6	–	
E1S	0.5	–	
Oestrone	19.1	Competitive	Dolly *et al*. 1972
Oestradiol	3.2	Competitive	
Oestriol	–		
Stilboestrol			
5α-Androstane-3β,17β-diol	1.7	Competitive	Payne *et al*. 1969
5α-Androstane-3α,17β-diol	3.6	Competitive	
Testosterone	11.8	–	
5-Pregnen-3β,21-diol-20-one	–	–	Payne 1972
5-Pregnene-3β,20α-diol	15.0	–	
5α-Androstane-3β,17β-diol	40.0	–	
2-Phenylindols			Birnbock and Von Angerer 1990
Structure **2b**	4000.0 [*]	–	
Structure **2c**	80.0 [*]	–	

[*] IC$_{50}$ (μM).

results from this preliminary study suggest that danazol does act as a steroid sulphatase inhibitor *in vivo*, inhibition of sulphatase activity is much less than the inhibition of aromatase activity (> 90 per cent) achieved with 4-OHA (Reed *et al*. 1990) and indicates the need for more potent inhibitors of steroid sulphatase activity.

The search for more potent sulphatase inhibitors is proceeding by two routes: the development of non-steroidal and steroidal compounds with potential inhibitory properties. Birnbock and Von Angerer (1990) have developed a series of steroid sulphatase inhibitors based on a new class of mammary tumour inhibitory compounds, the 2-(hydroxyphenyl) indoles. One of the most potent inhibitors of mammary tumour growth, 5-acetoxy-2-(4-acetoxyphenyl)-1-ethyl-3-methylindole, was shown to be metabolized to a sulphoconjugate *in vivo* (Fig. 9E.2(b)). Therefore the ability of the sulphated derivative to inhibit E1 sulphatase activity was examined using a calf uterine preparation. In this system the IC_{50} values for oestradiol sulphate and DHA-S were 35 μM and 80 μM respectively. Sulphate groups were also introduced at other suitable positions of this compound and a number of sulphated derivatives were found to be active, with mono-sulphates exhibiting stronger enzyme-inhibiting properties than disulphates. The most potent inhibitor tested ($IC_{50} = 80$ μM) had a large substituent at the indole nitrogen (Fig. 9E.2(c)). Incubation of one of the derivatives with the enzyme preparation revealed that the sulphated derivative was converted to the free hydroxy compound, raising doubts about whether such compounds will be active *in vivo*.

A number of other research groups are currently designing and synthesizing steroid sulphatase inhibitors, although details of some of the compounds under development have still to emerge (Li and Pillai 1991). Evans *et al*. (1991) have compared the ability of a number of natural and synthetic steroids to inhibit E1 sulphatase activity using a placental enzyme preparation. In this system danazol (50 μM) produced a 20 per cent inhibition of E1 sulphatase activity. Tamoxifen, *cis*-tamoxifen, 4-OHA, and stilboestrol also inhibited E1 sulphatase activity but to a lesser extent than that obtained with danazol. For natural steroids, the possession of a sulphate group at position C3 of the steroid nucleus was found to be the major factor in determining the degree of inhibitory activity. In this series the most potent inhibitor found so far was 5-androstene-$3\beta,17\beta$-diol-3 sulphate, resulting in 70 per cent inhibition of E1 sulphatase activity.

The ability of anti-oestrogens to inhibit E1 sulphatase activity has also been examined in cultured breast cancer cells (Pasqualini and Gelly 1988; Pasqualini and Nguyen 1991) and breast tumour preparations (Santner and Santen 1991). In a series of experiments, Pasqualini and his colleagues have demonstrated that the anti-oestrogen tamoxifen and ICI 164,384, a newly developed anti-oestrogen, reduce the concentrations of oestradiol in MCF-7 breast cancer cells after exposure to E1S. So far, however, it is not clear whether the anti-oestrogens are inhibiting the uptake of E1S into the cells or inhibiting E1 sulphatase activity. However, Santner and Santen (1991) have shown that tamoxifen, 4-OH tamoxifen, and ICI 164,384 all inhibit E1 sulphatase activity in a breast tumour preparation, acting as mixed or non-competitive inhibitors (Table 9E.1). The findings suggest that the effects of anti-oestrogen on the uptake of E1S and/or inhibition of E1 sulphatase activity may contribute to the ability of anti-oestrogens to inhibit breast tumour growth.

While it is apparent that the development of potent steroid sulphatase inhibitors is still at an early stage, there is an urgent need for such inhibitors to determine the role that steroid sulphates have in regulating breast tumour growth and also to examine their potential therapeutic applications. Results from a number of the investigations reviewed have indicated that the addition of a sulphate group to potential non-steroidal and steroidal inhibitors enhances sulphatase inhibitory activity. However, the ubiquitous distribution of the family of steroid sulphatases throughout the body suggests that such compounds may have little effect *in vivo*, being rapidly metabolized by the liver. Even so, using such compounds as models, it should be possible to design stable inhibitors with similar molecular configurations to steroid sulphates, which should retain their inhibitory activity *in vivo*.

So far, interest in the potential therapeutic use of sulphate inhibitors has been directed towards their possible employment in the treatment of breast cancer. The presence of steroid sulphates in the endometrium and prostate suggest that such compounds may also have a wider role for the treatment of other endocrine-dependent tumours.

References

Birnbock, H. and Von Angerer, E. (1990). Sulfate derivatives of 2-phenylindols as novel steroid sulfatase inhibitors. *Biochemical Pharmacology*, **39**, 1709–13.

Bonney, R. C., Reed, M. J., Davidson, K., Beranek, P. A., and James, V. H. T. (1983). The relationship between 17β-hydroxysteroid dehydrogenase activity and oestrogen concentrations in human breast tumours and in normal breast tissue. *Clinical Endocrinology*, **19**, 727–39.

Bradlow, H. L., Rosenfeld, R. S., Kream, J., Fleisher, M., O'Connor, J., and Schwartz, M. K. (1981). Steroid hormone accumulation in human breast cyst fluid. *Cancer Research*, **41**, 105–7.

Burns, G. R. J. (1983). Purification and partial characterization of acylsulphatase C from human placental microsomes. *Biochemica et Biophysica Acta*, **759**, 199–204.

Carlstrom, K., Doberl, A., Gershagen, S., and Rannevik, G. (1984a). Peripheral levels of dehydroepiandrosterone sulfate, dehydroepiandrosterone, androstenedione, and testosterone following different doses of Danazol. *Acta Obstetrica et Gynecologica Scandinavica*, Suppl. 123, 125–9.

Carlstrom, K., Doberl, A., Pousette, A., Rannevik, G., and Wilking, N. (1984b). Inhibition of steroid sulfatase activity by Danazol. *Acta Obstetrica et Gynecologica Scandinavica*, Suppl. 123, 107–11.

Dao, T. L., Hayes, C., and Libby, P. R. (1974). Steroid sulfatase activities in human breast tumours. *Proceedings of the Society for Experimental Biology and Medicine*, **146**, 381–4.

Dibbelt, L. and Kuss, E. (1986). Human placental steryl-sulfatase. *Biological Chemistry Hoppe Seyler*, **367**, 1223–9.

Dolly, J. O., Dodgson, K. S., and Rose, F. A. (1972). Studies on the oestrogen sulphatase and arylsulphatase C activities of rat liver. *Biochemical Journal*, **128**, 337–45.

Dowsett, M., Goss, P. E., Powles, T. J., Hutchinson, G., Brodie, A. M. H., Jeffcoate, S. L., and Coombes, R. C. (1987). Use of aromatase inhibitor 4-hydroxy-androstenedione in postmenopausal breast cancer: optimization of therapeutic dose and route. *Cancer Research*, **47**, 1957–61.

Evans, J., Rowlands, M., Jarman, M., and Coombes, R. C. (1991). Inhibition of oestrone sulphatase enzyme in human placenta and human breast carcinoma. *Journal of Steroid Biochemistry and Molecular Biology*, **39**, 493–9.

Farnsworth, W. E. (1973). Human prostatic dehydroepiandrosterone sulfate sulfatase. *Steroids*, **21**, 647–64.

Fishman, J., Nisselbaum, J. S., Menendez-Botet, C. J., and Schwartz, M. K. (1977). Estrone and estradiol content in human breast tumours: relationship to estradiol receptors. *Journal of Steroid Biochemistry*, **8**, 893–6.

Hawkins, R. A., Thomson, M. L., and Killen, E. (1985). Oestrone sulphate, adipose tissue and breast cancer. *Breast Cancer Research and Treatment*, **6**, 75–87.

Holinka, C. F. and Gurpide, E. (1980). *In vivo* uptake of estrone sulfate by rabbit uterus. *Endocrinology*, **106**, 1193–7.

James, V. H. T. and Reed, M. J. (1980). Steroid hormones and human cancer. *Progress in Cancer Research and Therapy*, **14**, 471–87.

James, V. H. T., McNeill, J. M., Lai, L. C., Newton, C. J., Ghilchik, M. W., and Reed, M. J. (1987). Aromatase activity in normal breast and breast tumour tissue: *in vivo* and *in vitro* studies. *Steroids*, **50**, 269–79.

Kawano, J.-I., Kotani, T., Ohtaki, S., Minamino, N., Matsuo, H., Oinuma, T., and Aikawa, E. (1989). Characterization of rat and human steroid sulfatases. *Biochimica et Biophysica Acta*, **997**, 199–205.

Li, P. K. and Pillai, R. (1991). Biochemical studies and synthesis of estrone sulfatase inhibitors as antitumour agents for estrogen dependent breast cancer. In *Endocrine Society, Program Abstracts*, p. 176, Abstr. 580.

MacIndoe, J. H., Woods, G., Jeffries, L., and Hinkhouse, M. (1988). The hydrolysis of estrone sulfate and dehydroepiandrosterone sulfate by MCF-7 human breast cancer cells. *Endocrinology*, **123**, 1281–7.

Miller, W. R. and Forrest, A. P. M. (1976). Oestradiol synthesis from C19 steroids by human breast cancers. *British Journal of Cancer*, **33**, 116–18.

Notation, A. D. and Ungar, F. (1969). Rat testis sulfatase: 2.Kinetic study. *Steroids*, **14**, 151–9.

Pasqualini, J. R. and Gelly, C. (1988). Effect of tamoxifen and tamoxifen derivatives on the conversion of estrone sulfate to estradiol in the MCF-7 mammary cell line. *Cancer Letters*, **40**, 115–21.

Pasqualini, J. R. and Nguyen, B.-L. (1991). Estrone sulphatase activity and effects of antioestrogens on transformation of oestrone sulphate in hormone-dependent vs. independent human breast cancer cells. *Breast Cancer Research and Treatment*, **18**, 93–8.

Pasqualini, J. R., Lanzone, A., Tahri-Joutei, A., and Nguyen, B.-L. (1982). Effects of seven different oestrogen sulphates on uterine growth and on progesterone receptor in the foetal uterus of guinea pig after administration to the mother. *Acta Endocrinologica*, **101**, 630–5.

Pasqualini, J. R., Gelly, C., Nguyen, B.-L., and Vella, C. (1989). Importance of estrogen sulfates in breast cancer. *Journal of Steroid Biochemistry*, **34**, 155–63.

Payne, A. H. (1972). Gonadal steroid sulfates and sulfatase. V. Human testicular steroid sulfatase: partial characterization and possible regulation by free steroids. *Biochimica et Biophysica Acta*, **258**, 473–83.

Payne, A. H., Mason, M., and Jaffe, R. B. (1969). Testicular steroid sulfatase. Substrate specificity and inhibition. *Steroids*, **14**, 685–704.

Peters, T. G., Lewis, J. D., Wilkinson, E. J., and Fuhrman, T. M. (1977). Danazol therapy in hormone-sensitive mammary carcinoma. *Cancer*, **40**, 2797–800.

Prost, O. and Adessi, G. L. (1983). Estrone and dehydroepiandrosterone sulfatase activities in normal and pathological human endometrium biopsies. *Journal of Clinical Endocrinology and Metabolism*, **56**, 653–61.

Purdy, R. H., Engel, L. L., and Oncley, J. L. (1961). The characterization of estrone sulfate from human plasma. *Journal of Biological Chemistry*, **236**, 1043–50.

Purohit, A. and Reed, M. J. (1991). Oestrogen sulphatase activity in hormone-dependent and hormone independent breast cancer cells: modulation by steroidal and non-steroidal therapeutic agents. *International Journal of Cancer*, **50**, 901–5.

Purohit, A., Ross, M. S., Lai, L. C., Ghilchik, M. W., Shotria, S., James, V. H. T., and Reed, M. J. (1990). Inability of normal and malignant breast tissues to take up oestrone-^{35}S-sulphate. *Journal of Endocrinology*, **127**, (Suppl.), Abstr. 69.

Reed, M. J., Hutton, J. D., Baxendale, P. M., James, V. H. T., Jacobs, H. S., and Fisher, R. P. (1979). The conversion of androstenedione to oestrone and production of oestrone in women with endometrial cancer. *Journal of Steroid Biochemistry*, **11**, 905–11.

Reed, M. J., Cheng, R. W., Noel, C. T., Dudley, H. A. F., and James, V. H. T. (1983). Plasma levels of estrone, estrone sulfate, and estradiol and the percentage of unbound estradiol in postmenopausal women with or without breast disease. *Cancer Research*, **43**, 3940–3.

Reed, M. J., Ross, M. S., Lai, L. C., Ghilchik, M. W., and James, V. H. T. (1989). *In vivo* uptake and metabolism of ^{3}H oestrone sulphate by normal breast and breast tumour tissues: effect of treatment with Danazol. *Journal of Endocrinology*, **123** (Suppl.), Abstr. 146.

Reed, M. J., Lai, L. C., Owen, A. M., Singh, A., Coldham, N. G., Purohit, A., *et al.* (1990). Effect of treatment with 4-hydroxyandrostenedione on the peripheral conversion of androstenedione to oestrone and *in vitro* tumour aromatase activity in postmenopausal women with breast cancer. *Cancer Research*, **50**, 193–6.

Reed, M. J., Aherne, G. W., Ghilchik, M. W., Patel, S., and Chakraborty, J. (1991). Concentrations of oestrone and 4-hydroxyandrostenedione in malignant and normal breast tissues. *International Journal of cancer*, **49**, 562–5.

Rosenthal, H. E., Ludwig, G. A., Pietrzak, E., and Sandberg, A. A. (1975). Binding of the sulfates of estradiol-17β to human serum albumin and plasma. *Journal of Clinical Endocrinology and Metabolism*, **41**, 1144–54.

Ruder, H. J., Lorraux, D. L., and Lipsett, M. B. (1972). Estrone sulfate: production rate and metabolism in man. *Journal of Clinical Investigation*, **51**, 1020–33.

Santner, S. J. and Santen, R. J. (1991). Inhibition of estrone sulfatase by anti-estrogens and estradiol. In *Endocrine Society, Program Abstracts*, p. 175, Abstr. 578.

Santner, S. J., Feil, P. D., and Santen, R. J. (1984). *In situ* estrogen production via estrone sulfatase pathway in breast tumours: relative importance versus the aromatase pathway. *Journal of Clinical Endocrinology and Metabolism*, **59**, 29–33.

Santner, S. J., Levin, M. C., and Santen, R. J. (1990). Estrone sulfate stimulates growth of nitrosomethylurea-induced breast carcinoma *in vivo* in the rat. *International Journal of Cancer*, **46**, 73–8.

Schwenk, M. and Del Pino, V. (1980). Uptake of estrone sulphate by isolated rat liver cells. *Journal of Steroid Biochemistry*, **13**, 669–73.

Siiteri, P. K. and MacDonald, P. C. (1973). Role of extraglandular estrogen in human endocrinology. In *Handbook of Physiology, Endocrinology* (ed. G. D. Astwood and R. O. Greep), Section 7, pp. 615–29. American Physiological Society, Washington, DC.

Terakawa, N., Ikegami, H., Shimizu, I., Aono, T., Tanizawa, O., and Matsumoto, K. (1987). Growth inhibition by danazol in a human endometrial cancer cell line with estrogen-independent progesterone receptors. *Journal of Steroid Biochemistry*, **28**, 571–4.

Thijssen, J. H. H. and Blankenstein, M. A. (1989). Endogenous oestrogens and androgens in normal and malignant endometrial and mammary tissues. *European Journal of Cancer and Clinical Oncology*, **25**, 1953–9.

Tilson-Mallett, N., Santner, S. J., Feil, P. D., and Santen, R. J. (1983). Biological significance of aromatase activity in human breast tumours. *Journal of Clinical Endocrinology and Metabolism*, **57**, 1125–8.

Townsley, J. D. (1973). Further studies on the regulation of human placental steroid 3-sulfatase activity. *Endocrinology*, **93**, 172–81.

Townsley, J. D., Schul, D. A., and Rubin, E. J. (1970). Inhibition of steroid 3-sulfates by endogenous steroids. A possible mechanism controlling placental estrogen synthesis from conjugated precursors. *Journal of Clinical Endocrinology and Metabolism*, **31**, 670–8.

Tseng, L., Mazella, J., Lee, L. Y., and Stone, M. L. (1983). Estrogen sulfatase and estrogen sulfo-transferase in human primary mammary carcinoma. *Journal of Steroid Biochemistry*, **19**, 1413–17.

Van Landeghem, A. A. J., Poortman, J., Nabuurs, M., and Thijssen, J. H. H. (1985). Endogenous concentration and sub-cellular distribution of estrogens in normal and malignant breast tissue. *Cancer Research*, **45**, 2900–6.

Vermeulen, A., Deslypere, J. P., Pavidaens, R., Leclercq, G., Roy, F., and Henson, J. C. (1986). Aromatase, 17β-hydroxysteroid dehydrogenase and intra-tissular sex hormone concentrations in cancerous and normal breast tissue in postmenopausal women. *European Journal of Cancer and Clinical Oncology*, **26**, 515–25.

Vignon, F., Terqui, M., Westley, B., Derocq, D., and Rochefort, H. (1980). Effect of plasma estrogen sulfates in mammary cancer cells. *Endocrinology*, **106**, 1079–86.

Yen, P. H., Allen, E., Marsh, B., Mohandas, T., Wang, N., Taggart, R. T., and Shapiro, L. J. (1987). Cloning and expression of steroid sulfatase cDNA and the frequent occurrence of deletions in STS deficiency: implications for x-y interchange. *Cell*, **49**, 443–54.

9F.1　Introduction

In 1963 Farnsworth and Brown (1963) reported that 5α-dihydrotestosterone (DHT) is the major metabolite produced when testosterone is incubated with rat or human prostate preparations. Bruchovsky and Wilson (1968) later administered radiolabelled testosterone intravenously to rats and observed that the radioactivity recovered from prostatic nuclei is present almost exclusively in the DHT fraction. These findings led to the hypothesis that testosterone is a prohormone in the prostate and that locally produced DHT is the androgen actually utilized by the organ (Anderson and Liao 1968; Baulieu *et al*. 1968). In fact, Dorfman and Kincl (1963) had previously shown that DHT is more active than testosterone for promoting prostate growth in castrated rats.

Very little *de novo* synthesis of DHT occurs in the testes or adrenals, and most or all of that found in the circulation is provided through the peripheral conversion of testosterone into DHT (Wilson and Gloyna 1970). For this transformation to occur, testosterone must undergo 5α-reduction. Early studies by Shimazaki *et al*. (1966), demonstrated the presence of a 5α-reductase capable of catalysing this process in the prostate. Certain other tissues including the liver (McGuire and Tomkins 1959), areas of the central nervous system (CNS) (Martini 1982; Celotti *et al*. 1992), and areas of the skin (Wilson and Walker 1969; Bingham and Shaw 1973; Stewart *et al*. 1977; Takayasu *et al*. 1980) convert testosterone to DHT, but there is evidence, cited later, which indicates that more than one 5α-reductase may be mediating such conversions.

The consequences of a 5α-reductase deficiency in males have been clearly outlined (Imperato-McGinley *et al*. 1974; Walsh *et al*. 1974). Among other phenomena, the levels of circulating DHT in affected individuals were much reduced, although testosterone levels were not significantly different from those seen in normal males. The prostate was grossly under-developed in both children and adults. Post-pubertal development of these individuals resulted in normal male physique and libido directed toward females, indicating that testosterone was sufficient for the initiation and maintenance of these male characteristics.

These observations strongly indicated that DHT is the primary androgen necessary for prostate growth and provided an impetus to discover inhibitors of 5α-reductase for treatment of benign prostatic hyperplasia (BPH) and carcinoma of the prostate. It was anticipated that if a potent inhibitor of prostatic 5α-reductase could be found which did not bind to the androgen receptor, then the formation of DHT could be selectively prevented without compromising the action of testosterone in those areas, such as skeletal muscle development, where it plays an important role.

BPH is androgen dependent since it does not develop in men castrated before puberty (Wendel *et al.* 1972), and some positive responses have been noted with the use of anti-androgens (agents which block androgen action at the receptor level) including flutamide (Caine *et al.* 1975), cyproterone acetate (Scott and Wade 1969), and medrogestone (Rangno *et al.* 1971). Prostatic hyperplasia is common in older men (over 50 years) and is characterized by bladder obstruction in the periurethral and bladder neck regions.

Transurethral prostatic resection (TURP) to remove tissue impinging upon the urethra is the most common treatment for BPH and usually affords symptomatic relief, but some degree of morbidity is often associated with the operation (Milroy and Chapple 1988; Roos *et al.* 1989). Impotence, retrograde ejaculation, and even death may occur as a consequence of TURP. Further, in a significant number of patients a second TURP is needed in a few years. Therefore it would seem desirable to avoid the necessity of surgery by treatment with a safe effective drug which would prevent or reverse the prostatic growth which leads to symptomatic BPH.

The growing medical significance of 5α-reductase in hormone action has led to increased investigation of the enzyme(s) ranging from molecular biology to the clinical use of inhibitors in the treatment of prostatic disease. Some progress in these areas has been reviewed elsewhere (Rasmusson 1987; Metcalf *et al.* 1989b; Smith 1989; Tenover 1991).

9F.2   *In vitro* studies of 5α-reductase

Steroid 5α-reductase (EC 1.3.99.5) catalyses the NADPH-dependent 5α-reduction of Δ^4-3-ketosteroids. This enzyme is found in all tissues where DHT is the physiologically important androgen. These tissues include prostate, epididymis, seminal vesicles, and skin (Wilson and Gloyna 1970). The enzyme is membrane bound in all species and tissues, although its subcellular localization varies. The best characterized of the reductases are those from rat liver and human prostate. In rat liver, enzyme activity is localized to the microsomal fraction whereas, in the human prostate, the reductase is found mainly in the nuclear membrane (Wilson and Gloyna 1970; Houston *et al*. 1985a). Many groups have been successful with the solubilization of both rat liver and human prostate reductase (Golf and Graff 1978; Scheer and Robaire 1983; Houston *et al*. 1985b; Ichihara and Tanaka 1987; Watkins *et al*. 1988; Enderle-Schmitt *et al*. 1989; Sargent and Habib 1991) but to date no one has reported its purification.

As described above, 5a-reductase deficiency is characterized by normal to slightly elevated plasma levels of testosterone and low, but detectable, levels of DHT. There is also a decrease in all urinary 5a-reduced metabolites of the C19 and C21 steroids (Imperato-McGinley and Gautier 1986). Thus it appears that 5a-reductase is an enzyme with broad substrate specificity. Steroid 5a-reductase is capable of utilizing a variety of Δ^4-3-ketosteroid substrates. Progesterone, 20a-hydroxypregn-4-ene-3-one, epitestosterone, and 17a-hydroxyprogesterone are all good substrates for the rat prostate reductase with apparent K_m values of 0.2–0.4 μM compared with 0.8 μM for testosterone (Frederiksen and Wilson 1971). Deoxycorticosterone, cortexolone, and androstenedione are similar to testosterone in affinity for the enzyme. Androstenediol is a poorer substrate than testosterone, while cortisol, corticosterone, and cortisone are inactive as substrates. With regard to cofactor specificity, there is an absolute requirement for NADPH. No activity is observed when NADPH is replaced by NADH (McGuire and Tomkins 1960; Frederiksen and Wilson 1971).

Thus far, the limiting amounts of enzyme activity, together with the membrane nature of the enzyme, has restricted its characterization to kinetic studies. Early on, it was demonstrated that the C5 hydrogen of DHT originates from the 4S position of NADPH (Bjorkhem 1969; Abul-Hajj 1972). These data are consistent with a mechanism for reduction of the substrate which involves direct hydride transfer from the 4S position of NADPH to the 5a-position of the steroid, leading to an enolate at C3,C4. Presumably, the enolate is stabilized by a group at the active site of the enzyme. Tautomerization then leads to the 5a-reduced product. The kinetic mechanism of 5a-reductase has been studied extensively (Campbell *et al*. 1986; Houston *et al*. 1987; Campbell and Karavolas 1989; Levy *et al*. 1990a). With solubilized rat liver enzyme, Levy *et al*. (1990a) found that there is ordered addition of substrates, with NADPH binding occurring first followed by Δ^4-3-ketosteroid. Furthermore, the competitive inhibition of NADP$^+$ versus NADPH is consistent with a mechanism where the two nicotinamides (NADPH and NADP$^+$) bind to the same form of the enzyme. The non-competitive inhibition of NADP$^+$ versus Δ^4-3-ketosteroid suggests that these species bind to different enzyme–substrate complexes. These data are in agreement with the ordered release of products where

5α-reduced steroid leaves first followed by $NADP^+$. Similar results were found with the rat anterior pituitary (Campbell *et al.* 1986), rat hypothalamic (Campbell and Karavolas 1989), and human prostate and human liver 5α-reductases (Houston *et al.* 1987).

Despite the indication from the genetic deficiency state that a single 5α-reductase exists (Imperato-McGinley *et al.* 1986), there have been many reports regarding the presence of isozymes in both rats and humans (McGuire and Tomkins 1960; Moore and Wilson 1976; Martini *et al.* 1986; Hudson 1987; Bruchovsky *et al.* 1988). Martini *et al.* (1986) proposed that, in rat ventral prostate, one isozyme is responsible for the reduction of testosterone and the other is responsible for the reduction of androstenedione. Similarly, Zoppi *et al.* (1992) demonstrated the selective inhibition of rat epididymal 5α-reductase by 17β-methoxy-17α-methyl-(5α)-$1H'$-androstane-[3,2c]pyrazole. No inhibition of rat prostate reductase by this compound was observed. In human prostate, Hudson (1987) and Bruchovsky *et al.* (1988) found different 5α-reductase activities in the stromal and epithelial fractions. Additionally, Moore and Wilson (1976) described two distinct human reductases with peaks of activities at either pH 5.5 or pH 7–9. The pH 5.5 form was similar to the enzyme found in prostate and was found only in fibroblasts from genital skin, whereas the pH 7–9 form was present in all fibroblasts assayed. Similarly, Itami *et al.* (1991) showed that there are two forms of 5α-reductase in dermal papilla cells from human scalp and beard hair. The enzyme in the beard dermal papilla cells has an optimum of pH 5.5, whereas the reductase in scalp dermal papilla cells has an optimum of pH 6.0–9.0. Taken altogether these findings are consistent with the existence of isozymes of 5α-reductase.

Recently, cDNAs encoding the rat and human 5α-reductases have been isolated. Farkash *et al.* (1988) first demonstrated that *Xenopus* oocytes could synthesize catalytically active steroid 5α-reductase when microinjected with rat liver and prostate RNA. Similar methodology was utilized by Andersson *et al.* (1989) to identify a mRNA of 2.4 kb that encodes the steroid 5α-reductase (reductase type 1) in both rat prostate and rat liver. The relative abundance of this mRNA in female rat liver, male rat liver, and prostate parallels enzyme activity in these tissues with the level of 5α-reductase activity decreasing in the order female rat liver > male rat liver > rat prostate (Moore and Wilson 1973; Liang *et al.* 1985a). This mRNA encodes a hydrophobic protein of 255 amino acids with a predicted molecular mass of 29 kDa. Over 50 per cent of the amino acids in this sequence are hydrophobic, consistent with the membrane nature of this protein. The properties of this enzyme expressed in COS cells (Andersson and Russell 1990), *Saccharomyces cerevisiae* (Ordman *et al.* 1991), and *Escherichia coli* (Harris and Azzolina 1990) are identical to the native enzyme. These findings support the proposal that a single mRNA is sufficient to encode a functional 5α-reductase.

The transcriptional regulation of this mRNA in rats was examined in castrated animals treated with testosterone (Andersson *et al.* 1989). These studies revealed that there is differential regulation of the mRNA by androgens. Castration had no effect on the level of the 5α-reductase mRNA in the prostate, while subsequent testosterone administration increased the level of this mRNA. In contrast, castration increased the 5α-reductase mRNA in liver but there was no further change following testosterone administration. These changes in mRNA levels in the two tissues are in agreement with the changes in enzyme activity described previously (Moore and Wilson 1973). These data indicate that this mRNA is transcriptionally regulated differently in prostate and liver.

A second cDNA encoding a rat 5α-reductase (reductase type 2, based on order of identification) has also been identified (Normington and Russell 1992). This isozyme is found in most male reproductive organs and probably represents the reductase activity in rat epididymis studied by Zoppi *et al.* (1992). This enzyme is unique among the known 5α-reductases in having a K_m for steroid substrates in the nanomolar range rather than micromolar range as found with other reductases. On the basis of the different affinities for substrates, Normington and Russell (1992) propose that the type 1 reductase plays a catabolic role in the metabolism of androgens whereas the type 2 enzyme plays an anabolic role.

In humans there also appear to be two genes encoding 5α-reductase (Andersson *et al.* 1989, 1991). Two cDNAs encoding 5α-reductase (designated 5α-reductase 1 and 5α-reductase 2 based on the order of their identification) were isolated from human prostate. Both proteins encoded by these genes are hydrophobic, with a molecular mass of 29 kDa, similar to that found for the cloned rat reductase. Expression studies in 293 cells showed that 5α-reductases 1 and 2 have similar substrate specificities for steroid hormones. However, these enzymes vary in their pH profile and sensitivity to inhibition by 4-azasteroids. Steroid 5α-reductase 1 has a pH optimum centred around pH 7.0 and is poorly inhibited by the 4-azasteroid, MK906 (**6**) (Andersson *et al.* 1989). In contrast, reductase 2 is most active at pH 5.0–5.5 and is inhibited by **6** (Andersson *et al.* 1991). Reductase 1 may represent the neutral pH form of the enzyme as described by Moore and Wilson (1976) in fibroblasts, while reductase 2 most closely resembles the enzyme found in human prostatic homogenates. As expected, mutations in reductase 2 cDNA give rise to 5α-reductase deficiency (Andersson *et al.* 1991).

9F.3 Development of 5α-reductase inhibitors

9F.3.1 Development of 4-azasteroids

Shortly after DHT was demonstrated as the primary androgen in prostatic tissue and it was realized that it is the agent interacting in the nucleus of sensitive cells, a new approach to control of androgen action became apparent—inhibition of 5α-reductase and formation of DHT. For a short period after the discovery of DHT action, it was not clear if all androgen responses in the body were mediated by DHT and whether blocking its synthesis would lead to the side-effects (feminization and feedback effects) noted with the androgen antagonists studied earlier. However, since DHT is generally produced at its site of action and there is a potential for the enzyme to be tissue specific, there was some hope that a selective action could be attained which might avoid the problems of androgen antagonists.

Initial efforts in the Merck laboratories focused on the skin as a target organ and, to minimize the potential of sexual side-effects, the aim was to develop a topically active agent. This interest was largely fuelled by the early studies of Voigt et al. (1970) and Voigt and Hsia (1973) who demonstrated that human skin 5α-reductase could be inhibited by non-hormonal steroidal compounds and that, upon topical application, one of these inhibitors, 17βC (**1a**), could block the local effects of applied testosterone, but not applied DHT, in an animal model (hamster flank organ) for androgenic acne. Studies in the Merck laboratories led to the diethyl amide of 17βC (**1b**) which showed higher, more consistent, and equally selective activity in this model (Johnston and Arth 1980).

Reports of pseudohermaphroditism due to 5α-reductase deficiency appeared during these studies (Imperato-McGinley et al. 1974; Walsh et al. 1974). The fact that affected males, although undergoing normal testosterone stimulated masculine development at puberty, failed to show prostatic growth provided support for the premise that a 5α-reductase inhibitor would be an effective treatment for BPH. Because of the difficulty of developing and proving a topical agent completely free of systemic effects and the attendant fears of treating adolescents with agents which modify hormone action, the acne target was abandoned and a new direction was taken to develop an orally active inhibitor for BPH treatment.

Substrate type 5α-reductase inhibitors such as **1a** and **1b** appeared desirable for topical treatment, since they were virtually inactive upon systemic administration. Presumably the reductases of the liver and other tissues convert these Δ^4-3-oxosteroids to inactive dihydroderivatives before they can affect internal DHT-sensitive organs. It was thus necessary to develop an approach to metabolically stable inhibitors.

A lead was derived from the discovery in the topical programme of the high in vitro activity of the 4-cyano derivative, **1c** (Rasmusson et al. 1983, 1986). The activity of **1c** was presumed to be a result of the formation on the enzyme of the intermediate **2**. This Δ^3-enol would be stabilized by the 4-cyano group and, as a result, would be less prone to tautomerize to the ketone, as would normal intermediates on the enzyme. Such 'transition state' mimicry would be expected to block turnover on the enzyme and provide a mechanism for inhibition. However, compound **1c** showed no observable 5α-reductase inhibitory activity when administered systemically to animals. Again, reductive metabolism must have quickly deactivated this unsaturated ketone.

More metabolically stable analogues were provided by 3-oxo-4-aza-5α-steroids. The conformation and atom positions of the A ring of these compounds very closely approximate those of the transition state 3-enol formed on the enzyme in the course of reduction of the steroidal enone to the saturated ketone. The azasteroids turned out to be potent competitive inhibitors of rat 5α-reductase.

Optimal *in vitro* activity resided in 4-methyl derivatives and attention quickly centred on the 17-diethylcarbamoyl derivative **3** which was to become known as 4-MA (sometimes called DMAA) (Brooks *et al*. 1981; Liang and Heiss 1981; Rasmusson *et al*. 1984). This compound inhibited rat and human prostatic 5α-reductases with apparent K_i = 5nM and 8nM, respectively (Liang *et al*. 1985a). In general, other modifications on the A or B rings of the steroid led to lower *in vitro* activity, while a variety of semipolar groups attached to the 17β-position retained high activity (Rasmusson *et al*. 1984, 1986). The relative potency of various analogues against 5α-reductase from different tissues in the rat (Liang *et al*. 1983) or from different disease states of the human prostate (Liang *et al*. 1985a) remained the same. However, enzyme from prostate of different species showed quite different responses to various analogues. When given orally or subcutaneously to male rats or dogs, many of these analogues selectively lowered DHT levels in the prostate gland (Brooks *et al*. 1986a,b). In castrate rats, a number of the azasteroids reduced the growth-promoting effect of administered testosterone, but not that of added DHT, on the prostate (Brooks *et al*. 1986a). In intact and testosterone-maintained castrate dogs, **3** lowered circulating DHT levels and caused regression of the prostate (Brooks *et al*. 1982; Wenderoth *et al*. 1983).

Although **3** proved unsuitable for development as a treatment for BPH in humans (see below), it has provided the basic researcher with a tool for the investigation of androgen action. Studies with different forms and substrates of 5α-reductase have shown **3**, in general, to be a potent inhibitor. It provided a means of studying hormone oxidative metabolism in liver cell culture without complicating reductive metabolism (Sonderfan and Parkinson 1988; Swinney 1990). It reverses or slows the progression of several animal models (Dunning, Noble, PC-82) of androgen-sensitive prostatic carcinoma (Kadohama *et al*. 1985; Andriole *et al*. 1987; Geldof *et al*. 1990). Animal models of 5α-reductase deficiency have been developed using 4-MA (Imperato-McGinley *et al*. 1985; Connolly and Resko 1989). Prolonged topical treatment of a primate model of androgenic alopecia with **3** prevented hair loss without significantly changing circulating testosterone levels (Rittmaster *et al*. 1987). In castrated monkeys, 4-MA blockage of DHT formation had no effect on HDL-cholesterol suppression by

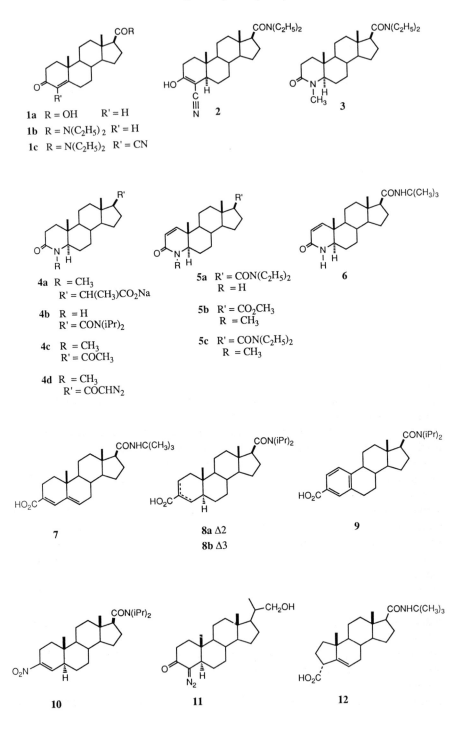

1a R = OH   R' = H
1b R = N(C₂H₅)₂ R' = H
1c R = N(C₂H₅)₂ R' = CN

2

3

4a R = CH₃
    R' = CH(CH₃)CO₂Na

4b R = H
    R' = CON(iPr)₂

4c R = CH₃
    R' = COCH₃

4d R = CH₃
    R' = COCHN₂

5a R' = CON(C₂H₅)₂
    R = H

5b R' = CO₂CH₃
    R = CH₃

5c R' = CON(C₂H₅)₂
    R = CH₃

6

7

8a Δ2
8b Δ3

9

10

11

12

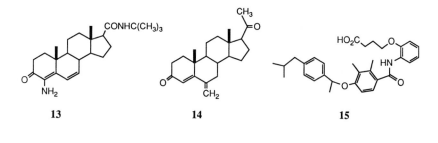

13　　　　　　　14　　　　　　　15

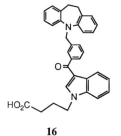

16

administered testosterone (Greger *et al*. 1990). In the hamster, **3** showed high 5*a*-reductase inhibitory activity but failed to suppress sebaceous gland growth, indicating that DHT is not necessary for stimulation of this androgen-dependent structure (Schroeder *et al*. 1989).

Several analogues developed at about the same time as **3** have also been used to study the enzyme and androgen action in various systems. The water-soluble carboxylate **4a** (4-MAPC), a potent 5*a*-reductase inhibitor in the rat, shows reduced androgen receptor binding and 3β-hydroxy-Δ^5-steroid dehydrogenase/3-keto-Δ^5-steroid isomerase (3β-ol DH) inhibitory activities relative to **3**. This material has been used to study testosterone metabolism in rat testis (Verhoeven and Cailleau 1983; Murono and Washburn 1989) and prostate tumour tissue *in vitro* (Kadohama *et al*. 1985). In the rat, **4a** blocked androgen-related prostatic tumour growth (Kadohama *et al*. 1984) and provided models of pre- and post-natal 5*a*-reductase deficiency in this species (Imperato-McGinley *et al*. 1985; Ngyuen *et al*. 1991). Detailed studies in prostate size reduction with **4a** showed that 5*a*-reductase inhibition causes a decrease in cell synthetic activity, secretory cell atrophy, and a reduction of cell number (Ghusn *et al*. 1991). The 4-unsubstituted diisopropyl amide **4b** is also very active against the rat prostatic enzyme and has no ability to bind to the androgen receptor. In studies on cell type morphogenesis **4b** was used to show that, in the mouse, development of the seminal vesicle, but not the epididymis, requires a fully active 5α-reductase (Shima *et al*. 1990; Tsuji *et al*. 1991). In the fetal and post-natal development of the male rat, **4b** was used to demonstrate the necessity of DHT for development of external genitalia as well as for nipple regression (Imperato-McGinley *et al*. 1986). Along with 4-MA, **4b** has been used to show that conversion of testosterone to DHT is not necessary for the *in vitro* suppression of gonadotropin release stimulated by luteinizing-hormone-releasing hormone (LH-RH) (Liang *et al*. 1984b; Kamel and Krey 1991). The azapregnane analogue **4c** (AMPD) has been shown to inhibit progesterone 5α-reductase of rat hypothalamus and pituitary selectively (Bertics *et al*. 1984a,b). A photoreactive analogue **4d** (diazo-MAPD) has been used to label rat liver 5α-reductase (Liang *et al*. 1985b). The Δ^1-azasteroid **5a**, a good *in vivo* inhibitor of rat 5α-reductase, was used to demonstrate that 7α-methyl-19-norandrogens act directly, without metabolic amplification, in the prostate. Testosterone and 7α-methyl-19-norandrogens, in the presence of **5a**, were not altered in their anabolic or gonadotropin action (Kumar *et al*. 1992). The azasteroidal ester **5b**, a modest rat enzyme inhibitor but good androgen receptor binder *in vitro*, showed good topical activity in reversing androgen-stimulated hamster flank organ development and sebaceous gland growth (Brooks *et al*. 1991b).

Safety studies in the rat found **3** to be well tolerated without significant side-effects, but high doses (≥ 40mg kg^{-1}) in the dog caused a reversible elevation of liver transaminases. Drug-related testicular hypertrophy was observed in the dog and gynaecomastia occurred in juvenile monkeys. These later two observations are thought to be the combined manifestations of the modest anti-androgenic activity of the compound (IC$_{50}$ = 2.8 μM vs. the rat androgen receptor) (Liang and Heiss 1981) and its ability to inhibit 3β-ol DH, the enzyme which forms the 3-oxo-Δ^4 system of T and other steroid hormones (Chan *et al*. 1987; Takahashi *et al*. 1990; Brandt and Levy 1989).

For optimal activity in the dog, **3** was most effective when given twice daily. Metabolism of the side-chain of **3** was found to occur rapidly in the dog to give, in relatively rapid order, the corresponding mono- and bis-deethylated amides. The unsubstituted amide has greatly reduced 5α-reductase activity relative to **3**.

Development of a clinical candidate from the 4-MA lead thus required a compound with an improvement in selectivity for 5α-reductase inhibition over androgen receptor interaction and 3β-ol DH inhibition. A compound which had good pharmacodynamics and which was free of potential liver toxicity in the dog was also required for further development. Of these requirements, liver toxicity appeared most critical, as it was not clear whether blockage of 5α-reductase, prevalent in the liver, might be directly related to the liver changes that had been observed in the dog.

An observation that the Δ^1-analogue of 4-MA, **5c**, and certain other azasteroids containing this unsaturation possess more *in vivo* 5α-reductase activity (as measured by DHT levels in the prostate) in the rat than would have been predicted from *in vitro* results led to a study of the selectivity and safety aspects of this series of compounds (Brooks *et al.* 1986a). With some relief, it was found that none of these agents when tested at high levels in the dog elevated liver transaminases to serious levels. Removal of the 4-methyl group actually increased the *in vitro* activity of these analogues and retained the high *in vivo* activity seen with the methyl derivatives. This change also had the added benefit of considerably reducing androgen receptor binding (Liang *et al.* 1984a) and 3β-ol DH inhibiting activities. To alter the metabolic disposition seen with **3**, a *t*-butyl carbox-amide was prepared at the 17-position to block the α-oxidation process which probably led to the dealkylations observed.

The result of these modifications was *N*-(1,1-dimethylethyl)-3-oxo-4-aza-5α-androst-1-ene-17β-carboxamide **6**, MK-906, finasteride, PROSCAR®. Finasteride was highly active both *in vitro* and *in vivo* as a 5α-reductase inhibitor (Brooks *et al.* 1986a), caused prostate regression in mature male dogs (Brooks *et al.* 1986b; Cohen *et al.* 1991), and was remarkably free of toxicity in safety assessment studies. Because of its lack of inherent activities other than 5α-reductase inhibitory potency, it was used in several studies which further elucidated certain biological phenomena. For example, George *et al.* (1989) treated male rats with finasteride from birth to the onset of puberty and confirmed that, while DHT is needed for normal post-natal growth of the prostate, seminal vesicles, epididymis, and penis, it has no major role in spermatogenesis or muscle development. Wise *et al.* (1991) observed that, while finasteride caused decreased fertility in male rats treated for prolonged periods (up to 32 weeks), the infertility was due to finasteride-induced inhibition of accessory gland secretions and not to any observable gross or histological changes in the testis itself. Diani *et al.* (1992) noted that an oral dose of 0.5 mg of finasteride daily given for 20 weeks increased hair weight in balding male adult stumptailed macaques. The results were very similar to those obtained by topical administration of the hair growth drug minoxidil. A combination of finasteride and minoxidil produced an additive effect on hair growth, indicating that the two drugs reverse the balding process by different modes of action.

In the clinic, Geller (1990) found that a 1 week regimen of 50 or 100 mg of finasteride daily caused a significant reduction in prostatic tissue DHT (0.302 ng g^{-1} versus 4.5 ng g^{-1} in controls). In addition, Stoner (1990), McConnell *et al.* (1992), and Rittmaster *et al.* (1992) have all reported that the compound markedly suppresses serum DHT levels in man without lowering testosterone levels. This latter result is of great importance since it indicates that those tissues and processes in which testosterone itself is utilized, such as skeletal muscle and libido, will not be affected by the presence of finasteride. Rittmaster *et al.* (1992) observed that chronic suppression of endogenous DHT in men receiving 5 mg of finasteride daily did not appear to influence serum gonadotropin levels, thus implying that physiological levels of circulating DHT do not modulate luteinizing hormone (LH) and follicle-stimulating hormone (FSH) secretion. Finally, a multicentre, double-blind placebo-controlled phase III clinical study was carried out to determine the efficacy of finasteride for treating men suffering from BPH (Stoner 1990; GROUP 1991). Daily oral doses of 1 or 5 mg of the compound were given over a 12 month period. A significant drug-related effect was obtained on each of the efficacy parameters. These included serum DHT level, prostate volume, maximum urinary flow, and symptomatic improvement score. It was concluded that finasteride is safe and effective for the treatment of BPH

In terms of the potential for 5α-reductase inhibitors as agents against prostatic carcinoma (PCA), the picture is not at all clear. Several investigators (Petrow et al. 1984; Gormley 1991) have expressed the opinion that reducing the amount of DHT, or available testosterone in an androgen-responsive prostatic tumour might attenuate its growth. Indeed, as mentioned above, Kadohama et al. (1985) reported that in the Noble rat model of prostatic adenocarcinoma two different 4-methyl-4-aza steroidal inhibitors of 5α-reductase, 4-MA and 4-MAPC, each significantly increased tumour volume doubling time, i.e. retarded tumour growth rate. Similarly, Andriole et al. (1987) showed that 4-MA slowed growth of the human androgen-responsive cancers PC 82 and R198 grown in athymic male mice. Geldof et al. (1992) used male rats bearing the androgen-responsive rat PCA R 3327H to demonstrate that daily injections of 4-MA decreased tumour growth rate in a dose-dependent manner.

In contrast with the report cited above, two recent studies failed to show that finasteride has any effect on the progression of the R-3327 tumour in rats (Pode et al. 1990; Brooks et al. 1991a). It is of interest that Brooks et al. 1991a) found that, although tumour concentrations of DHT were greatly reduced in treated animals (0.76 ng g^{-1} of tumour tissue versus 5.18 mg g^{-1} in controls), tumour growth rate was not altered. Presti et al. (1992) found that men afflicted with stage D PCA who received 10 mg of finasteride daily over periods of 6–24 weeks showed significant decreases in serum DHT and prostatic specific antigen (PSA) but no change in prostatic acid phosphatase (PAP), serum testosterone, prostatic volume, or appearance of bone scans from pretreatment baselines.

Some explanation for the seemingly contradictory findings from these various laboratories may have been provided by Lamb et al. (1992). They demonstrated that the growth of rat and human tumour lines characterized by low or undetectable levels of tissue 5α-reductase (R-3327G and PC82 respectively) was inhibited by the 5α-reductase inhibitor episteride (7, SK&F 105657) whereas growth of R-3327H, a subline with a much higher tissue level of 5α-reductase, was not. Further, tumour DHT content was reduced by **7** in both the R-3327G and PC82 tumours but not in the R-3327H carcinoma. On the basis of these results, they postulated that antitumour effects can be produced by a 5α-reductase inhibitor if it can bring about a depletion in tumour DHT below that level which maintains tumour growth. An alternative possibility suggested by Brooks *et al.* (1991a) was that, unlike BPH tissue, androgen-responsive PCA cells in the R-3327H type of tumour may proliferate under the stimulus of either testosterone or DHT. Therefore, both androgens would have to be blocked if any decrease in tumour growth rate was to be expected. A pure 5α-reductase inhibitor such as finasteride, which does not affect the availability of testosterone to the PCA, might be unlikely to alter the course of the disease. This latter explanation might account for the ineffectiveness of finasteride in the studies by Pode *et al.* (1990), Brooks *et al.* (1991a), and Presti *et al.* (1992).

9F.3.2   Development of other 5α-reductase inhibitors

A series of novel 5α-reductase inhibitors has been unveiled in the laboratories of Smith Kline Beecham. The most detailed reports have centred on the 3-carboxy-3,5-dienic steroid (**7**). This compound is one of the more potent ($K_i \approx 30$nM for rat or human prostatic enzyme) of a group of 3-carboxy-A-ring-unsaturated steroidal 5α-reductase inhibitors (Metcalf *et al.* 1989a; Holt *et al.* 1990b). Similar to the azasteroid **4a**, compound **7** in rats was able to reduce secretion, inhibit glandular cell proliferation, and decrease cell number in the prostate (Lamb *et al.* 1992). As mentioned above, against prostatic tumours in rodents, **7** was effective in suppressing tumour growth in two cases where 5α-reductase activity was low in the tumour (rat Dunning R-3327G and mouse PC-82), but not where intra-tumour levels of the enzyme are relatively high (rat Dunning R-3327H) (Lamb *et al.* 1992). When **7** was administered to pregnant rats over days 7–21 of gestation, the external genitalia, coagulating gland, and prostate of the male fetuses did not develop normally, as would be expected from selective 5α-reductase inhibition. The affected offspring without hypospadias were subsequently able to mate and fertilize females (Wier *et al.* 1990).

Epristeride has been submitted for clinical trials for the treatment of BPH. Phase I data indicate the drug was well tolerated at oral doses up to 160 mg daily. Upon multiple dosing, a twofold accumulation of **7** in plasma was found and correlations were made between the drug's plasma levels and DHT serum concentrations (Chalpelsky *et al.* 1992).

Analogues of epristeride have been prepared which have high 5α-reductase inhibitory activity. The arrangement and number of double bonds can be changed in these types of inhibitors without seriously interfering with activity against the human enzyme, as long as the 3-position of the steroid remains trigonal and the A-B ring framework is kept planar. Thus, Δ^2- and Δ^3-5α mono-unsaturated 3-carboxy analogues (i.e. **8a**, **8b**) have good activity (Holt *et al*. 1990b). A-ring aromatic analogues such as **9** also show good activity, with and without additional unsaturation elsewhere in the molecule (Holt *et al*. 1990a). The 3-carboxyl group can be replaced by phosphinic, phosphonic, or sulphonic acid moieties with retention of inhibitory activity (Holt *et al*. 1991b; Levy *et al*. 1991). For optimal activity against the human prostatic enzyme, the 17-position of the steroid has been substituted with alkyl carbamoyl groups. Fluorine substitution at positions 4 or 6, methylation at 4, or oxygenation (oxo or β-hydroxy) at 7 are permissive changes for retained activity (Metcalf *et al*. 1991).

The mechanism of enzyme inhibition by this class of compound has been carefully studied in a rat liver preparation (Levy *et al*. 1990b). Whereas the azasteroids competitively block this enzyme (Liang *et al*. 1983), these acidic steroids inhibit the enzyme in an uncompetitive manner with respect to the substrate testosterone. The kinetics indicate that the inhibition is occurring at that stage in the ordered process where freshly reduced steroid dissociates from the enzyme leaving the enzyme: $NADP^+$ complex. At this point, the inhibitor in its anionic form effectively binds in a transition-state-like configuration, resulting in an inactive enzyme, with the association supposedly enhanced through a charge interaction with the oxidized cofactor.

Interestingly, the 3-nitrocompound **10**, which is isosteric with an active 3-carboxysteroid, does not show similar inhibition kinetics to the anionic carboxylates but displays standard competitive kinetics versus the substrate testosterone (Holt *et al*. 1991a). The nitro compound, when given orally to monkeys, lowered plasma DHT levels by 50 per cent, which was equivalent to that seen with a potent 3-carboxy analogue.

Studies of inhibitors of 5α-reductase have continued at Merrell-Dow Research Laboratories over a period of time. Early efforts focused on substrate analogues (Benson and Blohm 1978), but later studies resulted in more significant activity with the 4-diazo-5α-steroid **11** (RMI 18,341). This material shows time-dependent inhibition of the rat enzyme, which is believed to be due to an activated intermediate which reacts to block the enzyme covalently (Blohm *et al*. 1980). This material was orally active in the castrate rat maintained on testosterone and showed no indication of interaction with the androgen receptor or with testosterone-mediated events (Blohm *et al*. 1986). Recent patent applications from these laboratories claim A-nor analogues (i.e. **12**) related to the SK&F series and 4-aminodienones (i.e. **13**) as effective 5α-reductase inhibitors (Flynn *et al*. 1991; Weintraub *et al*. 1992).

The k_{cat} inhibitor 6-methyleneprogesterone (**14**, LY207320) has been investigated in several *in vivo* systems. In the Dunning R3327 prostatic carcinoma model, this compound was able to reduce tumour growth without changing plasma testosterone levels (Damber *et al.* 1992). Male mice exposed prenatally to **14** had shortened anogenital distances with some hypospadias and feminization of the nipples. Development of the prostate, coagulating gland, and bulbourethral gland were suppressed. These effects were temporary, however, as maturation to adults was accompanied by regrowth of the sensitive tissues to normal (Iguchi *et al.* 1991). In an *in vivo* study of the conversion of radioactive testosterone to DHT in the rat prostate, **14** was much less effective than 4-MA (**3**) in preventing DHT formation (Toomey *et al.* 1991). In this study, **14** appeared to block uptake of testosterone into the prostate. This compound, which is not orally active, in addition to acting by 5*a*-reductase inhibition apparently restricts androgen action by other means (Neubauer *et al.* 1988).

A number of non-steroidal 5*a*-reductase inhibitors have been described in the patent literature. Compounds with potent activity have been reported by the Japanese research laboratories of Ono and Fujisawa Pharmaceuticals (Nakai *et al.* 1988; Okada *et al.* 1991). These compounds are distinguished by a terminal butyric acid chain attached to a bent polyaromatic nitrogen-containing residue. Examples of these structures are **15** and **16** (from Ono and Fujisawa Pharmaceuticals respectively). A recent observation has shown that certain *cis* unsaturated fatty acids are uncompetitive 5*a*-reductase inhibitors, and it has been suggested that such compounds may play a role in the regulation of the enzyme in target cells (Liang and Liao 1992).

9F.4   Conclusion

Progress in the development of 5*a*-reductase inhibitors has reached the point where the clinical effects of DHT reduction can be observed. Two agents studied in man, finasteride and episteride, appear to be well tolerated and cause circulating levels of DHT to decrease rapidly. In both, the target of treatment appears to be BPH. In clinical studies, the response of the prostate to finasteride has been slow, but positive with regard to alleviation of symptoms and gland size change. Questions about the effects of these agents on prostatic cancer in humans remain to be answered, as a brief human trial with finasteride and tests of these agents in animal models have given inconclusive responses. Other possible uses, such as the treatment of acne, hirsutism, and androgenic alopecia, will also have to await more definitive studies before possible development in humans.

In basic science, the utilization of molecular biological methods has resulted in the discovery of new isozymes of 5*a*-reductase in rats and humans. The new enzymes appear quite different from each other and give rise to the questions: Why are additional enzymes necessary? What are their substrates? What are their functions? The development of inhibitors specific for these enzymes and the use of the inhibitors in defining the contribution of each enzyme should be fertile areas for future research. It is to be hoped that new areas of therapeutic treatment will eventually evolve from such studies.

References

Abul-Hajj, Y. J. (1972). Stereospecificity of hydrogen transfer from NADPH by steroid Δ^4-5α and Δ^4-5β-reductase. *Steroids*, **20**, 215–22.

Anderson, K. M. and Liao, S. (1968). Selective retention of dihydrotestosterone by prostatic nuclei. *Nature, London*, **219**, 277–9.

Andersson, S. and Russell, D. W. (1990). Structural and biochemical properties of cloned and expressed human and rat steroid 5α-reductases. *Proceedings of the National Academy of Sciences of the United States of America*, **87**, 3640–4.

Andersson, S., Bishop, R. W., and Russell, D. W. (1989). Expression cloning and regulation of steroid 5α-reductase, an enzyme essential for male sexual differentiation. *Journal of Biological Chemistry*, **264**, 16249–55.

Andersson, S., Berman, D. M., Jenkins, E. P., and Russell, D. W. (1991). Deletion of steroid 5α-reductase 2 gene in male pseudohermaphroditism. *Nature, London*, **354**, 159–61.

Andriole, G. L., Rittmaster, R. S., Loriaux, D. L., Kish, M. L., and Linehan, W. M. (1987). The effect of 4MA, a potent inhibitor of 5 alpha-reductase, on the growth of androgen-responsive human genitourinary tumors grown in athymic nude mice. *Prostate*, **10**, 189–97.

Baulieu, E. E., Lasnitzki, I., and Robel, P. (1968). Metabolism of testosterone and action of metabolites on prostate glands grown in organ culture. *Nature, London*, **219**, 1155–6.

Benson, H. D. and Blohm, T. R. (1978). Testosterone 5α-reductase inhibitors US Patent 4,088,760 to Richardson Merrill Pharmaceutical Co.

Bertics, P. J., Edman, C. F., and Karavolas, H. J. (1984a). A high affinity inhibitor of pituitary progesterone 5α-reductase. *Endocrinology*, **114**, 63–9.

Bertics, P. J., Edman, C. F., and Karavolas, H. J. (1984b). Potent inhibition of the hypothalamic progesterone 5α-reductase by a 5α-dihydroprogesterone analog. *Journal of Biological Chemistry*, **259**, 107–11.

Bingham, K. D. and Shaw, D. A. (1973). The metabolism of testosterone by human male scalp skin. *Journal of Endocrinology*, **57**, 111–21.

Bjorkhem I. (1969). Mechanism and stereochemistry of the enzymic conversion of a Δ^4-3-oxosteroid into a 3-oxo-5α-steroid. *European Journal of Biochemistry*, **8**, 345–51.

Blohm, T. R., Laughlin, M. E., Benson, H. D., Johnston, J. O., Wright, C. L., Schatzman, G. L., and Weintraub, P. M. (1986). Pharmacological induction of 5α-reductase deficiency in the rat: separation of testosterone-mediated and 5α-dihydrotestosterone-mediated effects. *Endocrinology*, **119**, 959–66.

Blohm, T. R., Metcalf, B. W., Laughlin, M. E., Sjoerdsma, A., and Schatzman, G. L. (1980). Inhibition of testosterone 5α-reductase by a proposed enzyme-activated, active site-directed inhibitor. *Biochemical and Biophysical Research Communications*, **95**, 273–80.

Brandt, M., and Levy, M. A. (1989). 3β-Hydroxy-Δ^5-steroid dehydrogenase/3-

keto-Δ^5-steroid isomerase from bovine adrenal: mechanism of inhibition by 3-oxo-4-aza steroids and kinetic mechanism of the dehydrogenase. *Biochemistry*, **28**, 140–8.

Brooks, J. R., Baptista, E. M., Berman, C., Ham, E. A., Hichens, M., Johnston, D. B. R., *et al.* (1981). Response of rat ventral prostate to a new and novel 5α-reductase inhibitor. *Endocrinology*, **109**, 830–6.

Brooks, J. R., Berman, D., Glitzer, M. S., Gordon, L. R., Primka, R. L., Reynolds, G. F., and Rasmusson, G. R. (1982). Effect of a new 5α-reductase inhibitor on size, histologic characteristics, and androgen concentrations of the canine prostate. *Prostate*, **3**, 35–44.

Brooks, J. R., Berman, C., Primka, R. L., Reynolds, G. F., and Rasmusson, G. H. (1986a). 5α-Reductase inhibitory and anti-androgenic activities of some 4-aza-steroids in the rat. *Steroids*, **47**, 1–19.

Brooks, J. R., Berman, C., Garnes, D., Giltinan, D., Gordon, L. R., Malatesta, P. F., *et al.* (1986b). Prostatic effects induced in dogs by chronic or acute oral administration of 5α-reductase inhibitors. *Prostate*, **9**, 65–75.

Brooks, J. R., Berman, C., Nguyen, H., Prahalada, S., Primka, R. L., Rasmusson, G. H., and Slater, E. E. (1991a). Effect of castration, DES, flutamide, and the 5α-reductase inhibitor, MK-906, on the growth of the Dunning rat prostatic carcinoma, R-3327. *Prostate*, **18**, 215–27.

Brooks, J. R., Primka, R. L., Berman, C., Krupa, D. A., Reynolds, G. F., and Rasmusson, G. H. (1991b). Topical anti-androgenicity of a new 4-azasteroid in the hamster. *Steroids*, **56**, 428–33.

Bruchovsky, N. and Wilson, J. D. (1968). The conversion of testosterone to 5α-androstan-17β-ol-3-one by rat prostate *in vivo* and *in vitro*. *Journal of Biological Chemistry*, **243**, 2012–21.

Bruchovsky, N., Rennie, P. S., Batzold, F. H., Goldenberg, S. L., Fletcher, T., and McLoughlin, M. G. (1988). Kinetic parameters of 5α-reductase activity in stroma and epithelium of normal, hyperplastic, and carcinomatous human prostates. *Journal of Clinical Endocrinology and Metabolism*, **67**, 806–816.

Caine, M., Perlberg, S., and Gordon, R. (1975). The treatment of benign prostatic hypertrophy with flutamide (SCH: 13521): a placebo-controlled study. *Journal of Urology*, **114**, 564–8.

Campbell, J. S. and Karavolas, H. J. (1989). The kinetic mechanism of the hypo-thalamic progesterone 5α-reductase. *Journal of Steroid Biochemistry*, **32**, 283–9.

Campbell, J. S., Bertics, P. J., and Karavolas, H. J. (1986). The kinetic mechanism of the anterior pituitary progesterone 5α-reductase. *Journal of Steroid Biochemistry*, **24**, 801–6.

Celotti, F., Melcangi, R. C., and Martini, L. (1992). The 5α-reductase in brain: Molecular aspects and relation to brain function. *Frontiers in Neuroendocrinology*, **13**, 163–215.

Chalpelsky, M. C., Nichols, A. L., Jorkasky, D. K., Pue, M. A., Lundberg, D. E., Knox, S. H., and Audet, P. R. (1992). Pharmacokinetics and pharmaco-dynamics of SK&F 105657 in healthy elderly male subjects. *Clinical Pharmacology and Therapeutics*, **51**, 154.

Chan, W. K., Fong, C. Y., Tiong, H. H., and Tan, C. H. (1987). The inhibition of 3βHSD activity in porcine granulosa cells by 4-MA, a potent 5α-reductase inhibitor. *Biochemical and Biophysical Research Communications*, **144**, 166–71.

Cohen, S. M., Taber, K. H., Malatesta, P. F., Shpungin, J., Berman, C., Carlin,

J. R., Werrmann, J. G., Prahalada, S., Bryan, R. N., and Cordes, E. H. (1991). Magnetic resonance imaging of the efficacy of specific inhibition of 5α-reductase in canine spontaneous benign prostatic hyperplasia. *Magnetic Resonance in Medicine*, **21**, 55–70.

Connolly, P. B., and Resko, J. A. (1989). Role of steroid 5α-reductase activity in sexual differentiation of the guinea pig. *Neuroendocrinology*, **49**, 324–30.

Damber, J., Bergh, A., Daehlin, L., Petrow, V., and Landstrom, M. (1992). Effects of 6-methylene progesterone on growth, morphology, and blood flow of the Dunning R3327 prostatic adenocarcinoma. *Prostate*, **20**, 187–97.

Diani, A. R., Mulholland, M. J., Shull, K. L., Kubicek, M. F., Johnson, G. A., Schostarez, H. J., *et al.* (1992). Hair growth effects of oral administration of finasteride, a steroid 5α-reductase inhibitor, alone and in combination with topical minoxidil in the balding stumptail macaque. *Journal of Clinical Endocrinology and Metabolism*, **74**, 345–50.

Dorfman, R. I., and Kincl, F. A. (1963). Relative potency of various steroids in an anabolic-androgenic assay using the castrated rat. *Endocrinology*, **72**, 259–66.

Enderle-Schmitt, U., Neuhaus, C., and Aumuller, G. (1989). Solubilization of nuclear steroid 5α-reductase from rat ventral prostate. *Biochimica et Biophysica Acta*, **987**, 21–8.

Farkash, Y., Soreq, H., and Orly, J. (1988). Biosynthesis of catalytically active rat testosterone 5α-reductase in microinjected *Xenopus* oocytes: Evidence for tissue-specific differences in translatable mRNA. *Proceedings of the National Academy of Sciences of the United States of America*, **85**, 5824–8.

Farnsworth, W. E. and Brown, J. R. (1963). Metabolism of testosterone by the human prostate. *Journal of the American Medical Association*, **183**, 436–9.

Flynn, G. A., Bey, P., and Blohm, T. R. (1991). Novel A-nor-steroid-3-carboxylic acid derivatives, European Patent 0435321 to Merrell Dow Pharmaceutical Inc.

Frederiksen, D. W. and Wilson, J. D. (1971). Partial characterization of the nuclear reduced nicotinamide adenine dinucleotide phosphate: Δ^4-3-ketosteroid 5α-oxidoreductase of rat prostate. *Journal of Biological Chemistry*, **246**, 2584–603.

Geldof, A. A., de Voogt, H. J., and Rao, B. R. (1990). Enzyme inhibitors in hormone dependent prostate cancer treatment. *European Journal of Cancer*, **26**, 188.

Geldof, A. A., Meulenbroek, M. F. A., Dijkstra, I., Bohlken, S., and Rao, B. R. (1992). Consideration of the use of 17β-*N*,*N*-diethylcarbamoyl-4-methyl-4-aza-5α-androstan-3-one (4MA), a 5α-reductase inhibitor, in prostate cancer therapy. *Journal of Cancer Research and Clinical Oncology*, **118**, 50–5.

Geller, J. (1990). Effect of finasteride, a 5α-reductase inhibitor on prostate tissue androgens and prostate-specific antigen. *Journal of Clinical Endocrinology and Metabolism*, **71**, 1552–5.

George, F. W., Johnson, L., and Wilson, J. D. (1989). The effect of a 5α-reductase inhibitor on androgen physiology in the immature male rat. *Endocrinology*, **125**, 2434–8.

Ghusn, H. F., Shao, T. C., Klima, M., and Cunningham, G. R. (1991). 4-MAPC, a 5α-reductase inhibitor, reduces rat ventral prostate weight, DNA, and prostatein concentrations. *Journal of Andrology*, **12**, 315–22.

Golf, S. W. and Graff, V. (1978). Reconstitution of NADPH: 4-ene-3-oxosteroid-5α-oxidoreductase from solubilized components of rat liver microsomes. *Journal of Steroid Biochemistry*, **9**, 1087–92.

Gormley, G. (1991). Role of 5α-reductase inhibitors in the treatment of advanced prostatic carcinoma. *Urologic Clinics of North America*, **18**, 93–8.

Greger, N. G., Insull, W., Jr, Probstfield, J. L., and Keenan, B. S. (1990). High-density lipoprotein response to 5α-dihydrotesterone and testosterone in *Macaca fascicularis*: a hormone-responsive primate model for the study of atherosclerosis. *Metabolism*, **39**, 919–24.

GROUP, MK906. Study. (1991). One-year experience in the treatment of benign prostatic hyperplasia with finasteride. *Journal of Andrology*, **12**, 372–5.

Harris, G. and Azzolina, B. (1990). 5α-Reductase, a mammalian membrane-bound protein: cloning and expression in *Escherichia coli*. *FASEB Journal*, **4**, 2127a.

Holt, D. A., Levy, M. A., Ladd, D. L., Oh, H.-J., Erb, J. M., Heaslip, J. I., *et al.* (1990a). Steroidal A ring aryl carboxylic acids: a new class of steroid 5α-reductase inhibitors. *Journal of Medicinal Chemistry*, **33**, 937–42.

Holt, D. A., Levy, M. A., Oh, H.-J., Erb, J. M., Heaslip, J. I., Brandt, M., *et al.* (1990b). Inhibition of steroid 5α-reductase by unsaturated 3-carboxysteroids. *Journal of Medicinal Chemistry*, **33**, 943–50.

Holt, D. A., Levy, M. A., Yen, H.-K., Oh, H.-J., and Metcalf, B. (1991a). Inhibition of steroid 5α-reductase by 3-nitrosteroids: synthesis, mechanism of inhibition, and *in vivo* activity. *Bioorganic and Medicinal Chemistry Letters*, **1**, 27–32.

Holt, D. A., Oh, H.-J., Levy, M. A., and Metcalf, B. (1991b). Synthesis of a steroidal A ring aromatic sulfonic acid as an inhibitor of steroid 5α-reductase. *Steroids*, **56**, 4–7.

Houston, B., Chisholm, G. D., and Habib, F. K. (1985a). Evidence that human prostatic 5α-reductase is located exclusively in the nucleus. *Federation of European Biochemical Societies Letters*, **185**, 231–5.

Houston, B., Chisholm, G. D., and Habib, F. K. (1985b). Solubilization of human prostatic 5α-reductase. *Journal of Steroid Biochemistry*, **22**, 461–7.

Houston, B., Chisholm, G., and Habib, F. (1987). A kinetic analysis of the 5α-reductases from human prostate and liver. *Steroids*, **49**, 355–69.

Hudson, R. W. (1987). Comparison of nuclear 5α-reductase activities in the stromal and epithelial fractions of human prostatic tissue. *Journal of Steroid Biochemistry*, **26**, 349–53.

Ichihara, K. and Tanaka, C. (1987). Some properties of progesterone 5α-reductase solubilized from rat liver microsomes. *Biochemistry International*, **15**, 1005–11.

Iguchi, T., Uesugi, Y., Takasugi, N., and Petrow, V. (1991). Quantitative analysis of the development of genital organs from the urogenital sinus of the fetal male mouse treated prenatally with a 5α-reductase inhibitor. *Journal of Endocrinology*, **128**, 395–401.

Imperato-McGinley, J., Guerrero, T., Gautier, T., and Peterson, R. E. (1974). Steroid 5α-reductase deficiency in man: an inherited form of male pseudo-hermaphroditism. *Science*, **186**, 1213–15.

Imperato-McGinley, J. and Gautier, T. (1986). Inherited 5α-reductase deficiency in man. *Trends in Genetics*, **2**, 130–3.

Imperato-McGinley, J., Binienda, Z., Arthur, A., Mininberg, D. T., Vaughan, E. D., Jr., and Quimby, F. W. (1985). The development of a male psdeudo-hermaphroditic rat using an inhibitor of the enzyme 5α-reductase. *Endocrinology*, **116**, 807–12.

Imperato-McGinley, J., Binienda, Z., Gedney, J., and Vaughan, E. D., Jr. (1986).

Nipple differentiation in fetal male rats treated with an inhibitor of the enzyme 5α-reductase: definition of a selective role for dihydrotestosterone. *Endocrinology*, **118**, 132–7.

Itami, S., Kurata, S., Sonada, T., and Takayasu, S. (1991). Characterization of 5α-reductase in cultured human dermal papilla cells from beard and occipital scalp hair. *Journal of Investigative Dermatology*, **96**, 57–60.

Johnston, D. B. R. and Arth, G. E. (1980). N-Substituted 17β-carbamoylandrost-4-en-3-one 5α-reductase inhibitors. US Patent 4,191,759 to Merck & Co.

Kadohama, N., Karr, J. P., Murphy, G. P., and Sandberg, A. A. (1984). Selective inhibition of prostatic tumor 5α-reductase by a 4-methyl-4-aza-steroid. *Cancer Research*, **44**, 4947–54.

Kadohama, N., Wakisaka, M., Kim, U., Karr, J. P., Murphy, G. P., and Sandberg, A. A. (1985). Retardation of prostate tumor progression in the Noble rat by 4-methyl-4-aza-steroidal inhibitors of 5α-reductase. *Journal of National Cancer Institute*, **74**, 475–86.

Kamel, F. and Krey, L. C. (1991). Testosterone processing by pituitary cells in culture: an examination of the role of 5α-reduction in androgen action on the gonadotroph. *Steroids*, **56**, 22–9.

Kumar, N., Didolkar, A. K., Monder, C., Bardin, C. W., and Sundaram, K. (1992). The biological activity of 7α-methyl-19-nortestosterone is not amplified in male reproductive tract as is that of testosterone. *Endocrinology*, **130**, 3677–83.

Lamb, J. C., Levy, M. A., Johnson, R. K., and Isaacs, J. T. (1992). Response of rat and human prostatic cancers to the novel 5α-reductase inhibitor, SK&F 105657. *Prostate*, **21**, 15–34.

Levy, M. A., Brandt, J., and Greway, A. T. (1990a). Mechanistic studies with solubilized rat liver steroid 5α-reductase: elucidation of the kinetic mechanism. *Biochemistry*, **29**, 2808–15.

Levy, M. A., Brandt, M., Heys, R., Holt, D. A., and Metcalf, B. W. (1990b). Inhibition of rat liver steroid 5α-reductase by 3-androstene-3-carboxylic acids: mechanism of enzyme inhibitor interaction. *Biochemistry*, **29**, 2815–24.

Levy, M. A., Metcalf, B. W., Brandt, M., Erb, J. M., Oh, H.-J., Heaslip, J. I., *et al.* (1991). 3-Phosphinic acid and 3-phosphonic acid steroids as inhibitors of steroid 5α-reductase: species comparison and mechanistic studies. *Bioorganic Chemistry*, **19**, 245–60.

Liang, T., and Heiss, C. E. (1981). Inhibition of 5α-reductase, receptor binding, and nuclear uptake of androgens in the prostate by a 4-methyl-4-aza-steroid. *Journal of Biological Chemistry*, **256**, 7998–8005.

Liang, T. and Liao, S. (1992). Inhibition of steroid 5α-reductase by specific aliphatic unsaturated fatty acids. *Biochemical Journal*, **285**, 557–62.

Liang, T., Heiss, C. E., Ostrove, S., Rasmusson, G. H., and Cheung, A. (1983). Binding of a 4-methyl-4-aza-steroid to 5α-reductase of rat liver and prostate, microsomes. *Endocrinology*, **112**, 1460–8.

Liang, T., Heiss, C. E., Cheung, A. H., Reynolds, G. F., and Rasmusson, G. H. (1984a). 4-Azasteroidal 5α-reductase inhibitors without affinity for the androgen receptor. *Journal of Biological Chemistry*, **259**, 734–9.

Liang, T., Brady, E. J., Cheung, A., and Saperstein, R. (1984b). Inhibition of luteinizing hormone (LH)-releasing hormone-induced secretion of LH in rat anterior pituitary cell culture by testosterone without conversion to 5α-dihydrotestosterone. *Endocrinology*, **115**, 2311–17.

Liang, T., Cascieri, M. A., Cheung, A. H., Reynolds, G. F., and Rasmusson, G. H. (1985a). Species differences in prostatic steroid 5a-reductases of rat, dog, and human. *Endocrinology*, **117**, 571–9.

Liang, T., Cheung, A. H., Reynolds, G. F., and Rasmusson, G. H. (1985b). Photoaffinity labeling of steroid 5a-reductase of rat liver and prostate microsomes. *Biological Chemistry*, **260**, 4890–5.

McConnell, J. D., Wilson, J. D., George, F. W., Geller, J., Pappas, F., and Stoner, E. (1992). Finasteride, an inhibitor of 5a-reductase, suppresses prostatic dihydrotestosterone in men with benign prostatic hyperplasia. *Journal of Clinical Endocrinology and Metabolism*, **74**, 505–8.

McGuire, J. S., Jr and Tomkins, G. M. (1959). The effects of thyroxin administration on the enzymic reduction of Δ^4-3-ketosteroids. *Journal of Biological Chemistry*, **234**, 791–4.

McGuire, J. S., Jr. and Tomkins, G. M. (1960). The heterogeneity of Δ^4-3-ketosteroid reductases. *Journal of Biological Chemistry*, **235**, 1634–8.

Martini, L. (1982). The 5a-reduction of testosterone in the neuroendocrine structures: biochemical and physiological implications. *Endocrine Reviews*, **3**, 1–25.

Martini, L., Zoppi, S., and Motta, M. (1986). Studies on the possible existence of two 5a-reductases in the rat prostate. *Journal of Steroid Biochemistry*, **24**, 177–82.

Metcalf, B. W., Holt, D. A., Levy, M. A., Erb, J. M., Heaslip, J. I., Brandt, M., and Oh, H.-J. (1989a). Potent inhibition of human steroid 5a-reductase (EC 1.3.1.30) by 3-androstene-3-carboxylic acids. *Bioorganic Chemistry*, **17**, 372–6.

Metcalf, B. W., Levy, M. A., and Holt, D. A. (1989b). Inhibitors of steroid 5a-reductase in benign prostatic hyperplasia, male pattern baldness and acne. *Trends in Pharmacological Sciences*, **10**, 491–5.

Metcalf, B. W., Holt, D. A., and Levy, M. A. (1991). 7-Keto or hydroxy-3,5-diene steroids as inhibitors of steroid 5a-reductase. US Patent 5,032,586 to Smith Kline French Corporation.

Milroy, E. and Chapple, C. (1988). The aetiology and treatment of benign prostatic obstruction. *Practitioner*, **232**, 1141–2.

Moore, R. J. and Wilson, J. D. (1973). The effect of androgenic hormones on the reduced nicotinamide adenine dinucleotide phosphate: Δ^4-3-ketosteroid 5a-oxidoreductase of rat ventral prostate. *Endocrinology*, **93**, 581–92.

Moore, R. J. and Wilson, J. D. (1976). Steroid 5a-reductase in cultured human fibroblasts: biochemical and genetic evidence for two distinct enzyme activities. *Journal of Biological Chemistry*, **251**, 5895–900.

Murono, E. P. and Washburn, A. L. (1989). 5a-reductase activity regulates testosterone accumulation in two bands of immature cultured Leydig cells isolated on Percoll density gradients. *Acta Endocrinologica*, **121**, 538–44.

Nakai, H., Terashima, H., and Arai, Y. (1988). Benzoylaminophenoxybutanoic acid derivatives. Patent applications 291245, 291247, 294035, 294937 to Ono Pharmaceutical Co.

Neubauer, B. L., Best, K. L., Clemens, J. A., Fuller, R. W., Goode, R. L., Petrow, V., *et al.* (1988). Regressive effects of the 5a-reductase inhibitor, LY207320 (6-methylene-4-pregnene-3,20-dione) on accessory sex organs of the male rat. *Program of the 70th Annual Meeting of the Endocrine Society*, **89**, no. 276.

Ngyuen, M. M., Lemmi, C. A. E., and Rajfer, J. (1991). Effect of 5-alpha-reductase inhibitor, 4-MAPC, on testicular descent in male rat. *Journal of Urology*, **145**, 1096–8.

Normington, K. and Russell, D. W. (1992). Tissue distribution and kinetic characteristics of rat steroid 5α-reductase isozymes. *Journal of Biological Chemistry*, **267**, 19548–54.

Okada, S., Sawada, K., Kayakiri, N., Saitoh, Y., Tanaka, H., and Hashimoto, M. (1991). Indole derivatives. European Patent Application EP 458,207 to Fujisawa Pharmaceutical Co.

Ordman, A. B., Farley, D., Meyhack, B., and Nick, H. (1991). Expression of rat 5α-reductase in *Saccharomyces cerevisiae*. *Journal of Steroid Biochemistry and Molecular Biology*, **39**, 487.

Petrow, V., Padilla, G. M., Mukherji, S., and Marts, S. A. (1984). Endocrine dependence of prostatic cancer upon dihydrotestosterone and not upon testosterone. *Journal of Pharmacy and Pharmacology*, **36**, 352–3.

Pode, D., Heston, W. D. W., Hun, K. R., and Fair, W. R. (1990). Effect of 5α-reductase inhibitors on the rat prostate and rat prostatic carcinoma. In *Proceedings of the Congress of the European Association of Urology, Amsterdam*.

Presti, J. C., Fair, W. R., Andriole, G., Sogani, P. C., Seidmon, E. J., Ferguson, D., *et al.* (1992). Multicenter, randomized, double-blind, placebo controlled study to investigate the effect of finasteride (MK906) on stage D prostate cancer. *Journal of Urology*, **148**, 1201–4.

Rangno, R. E., McLeod, P. J., Ruedy, J., and Ogilvie, R. I. (1971). Treatment of benign prostatic hypertrophy with medrogestone. *Clinical Pharmacology and Therapeutics*, **12**, 658–65.

Rasmusson, G. H. (1987). Biochemistry and pharmacology of 5α-reductase inhibitors. In *Pharmacology and clinical uses of inhibitors of hormone secretion and action* (ed. B. J. A. Furr and A. E. Wakeling), pp. 308–25. Baillière Tindall, London.

Rasmusson, G. H., Liang, T., and Brooks, J. R. (1983). A new class of 5α-reductase inhibitors. In *Gene regulation by steroid hormones II* (ed. A. K. Roy and J. H. Clark), pp. 311–34. Springer-Verlag, New York.

Rasmusson, G. H., Reynolds, G. F., Utne, T., Jobson, R. B., Primka, R. L., Berman, C., and Brooks, J. R. (1984). Azasteroids as inhibitors of rat prostatic 5α-reductase. *Journal of Medicinal Chemistry*, **27**, 1690–1701.

Rasmusson, G. H., Reynolds, G. F., Steinberg, N. G., Walton, E., Patel, G. F., Liang, T., *et al.* (1986). Azasteroids: Structure–activity relationships for inhibition of 5α-reductase and of androgen receptor binding. *Journal of Medicinal Chemistry*, **29**, 2298–315.

Rittmaster, R. S., Uno, H., Provar, M. L., Mellin, T. N., and Loriaux, D. L. (1987). The effects of N,N-diethyl-4-methyl-3-oxo-4-aza-5α-androstane-17β-carboxamide, a 5α-reductase inhibitor and antiandrogen, on the development of baldness in the stumptail macaque. *Journal of Clinical Endocrinology and Metabolism*, **65**, 188–93.

Rittmaster, R. S., Lemay, A., Zwicker, H., Capizzi, T. P., Winch, S., Moore, E., and Gormley, G. J. (1992). Effect of finasteride, a 5α-reductase inhibitor, on serum gonadotropins in normal men. *Journal of Clinical Endocrinology and Metabolism*, **75**, 484–8.

Roos, N. P., Wennberg, J. E., Malenka, D. J., Fisher, E. S., McPherson, K., Andersen, T. F., *et al.* (1989). Mortality and reoperation after open and transurethral resection of the prostate for benign prostatic hyperplasia. *New England Journal of Medicine*, **320**, 1120–4.

Sargent, N. S. E., and Habib, F. K. (1991). Partial purification of human prostatic 5α-reductase (3-oxo-5α-steroid:NADP$^+$ 4-ene-oxido-reductase: EC 1.3.1.22) in a stable and active form. *Journal of Steroid Biochemistry and Molecular Biology*, **38**, 73–7.

Scheer, H., and Robaire, B. (1983). Solubilization and partial characterization of rat epididymal Δ^4-steroid 5α-reductase (cholestenone 5α-reductase). *Biochemistry Journal*, **211**, 65–74.

Schroeder, H. G., Ziegler, M., Nickisch, K., Kaufmann, J., and El Etreby, M. F. (1989). Effects of topically applied antiandrogenic compounds on sebaceous glands of hamster ears and flank organs. *Journal of Investigative Dermatology*, **92**, 769–73.

Scott, W. W. and Wade, J. C. (1969). Medical treatment of benign nodular prostatic hyperplasia with cyproterone acetate. *Journal of Urology*, **101**, 81–5.

Shima, H., Tsuji, M., Young, P., and Cunha, G. R. (1990). Postnatal growth of mouse seminal vesicle is dependent on 5α-dihydrotestosterone. *Endocrinology*, **127**, 3222–33.

Shimazaki, J., Kurihara, H., Ito, Y., and Shida, K. (1966). Testosterone metabolism in prostate; formation of androstan-17β-ol-3-one and androst-3-ene-3, 17-dione, and inhibitory effect of natural and synthetic estrogens. *Gunma Journal of Medical Science*, **14**, 313–25.

Smith, H. J. (1989). 5α-reductase inhibitors. In *Design of Enzyme Inhibitors as Drugs* (ed. M. Sandler and H. J. Smith), pp. 777–90. Oxford University Press.

Sonderfan, A. and Parkinson, A. (1988). Inhibition of steroid 5α-reductase and its effects on testosterone hydroxylation by rat liver microsomal cytochrome P-450. *Archives of Biochemistry and Biophysics*, **265**, 208–18.

Stewart, M. E., Pochi, P. E., Wotiz, H. H., and Clark, S. J. (1977). *In vitro* metabolism of [^{3}H]testosterone by scalp and back skin: Conversion of testosterone into 5α-androstane-3β-diol. *Journal of Endocrinology*, **72**, 385–90.

Stoner, E. (1990). The clinical development of a 5α-reductase inhibitor, finasteride. *Journal of Steroid Biochemistry and Molecular Biology*, **37**, 375–8.

Swinney, D. C. (1990). Progesterone metabolism in hepatic microsomes. Effect of the cytochrome P-450 inhibitor, ketoconazole, and the NADPH 5α-reductase inhibitor, 4-MA, upon the metabolic profile in human, monkey, dog, and rat. *Drug Metabolism and Disposition*, **18**, 859–65.

Takahashi, M., Luu-The, V., and Labrie, F. (1990). Inhibitory effect of synthetic progestins, 4-MA and cyanoketone on human placental 3β-hydroxysteroid de-hydrogenase/5,4-ene-isomerase activity. *Journal of Steroid Biochemistry and Molecular Biology*, **37**, 231–6.

Takayasu, S., Wakimoto, H., Itami, S., and Sano, S. (1980). Activity of testosterone 5α-reductase in various tissues of human skin. *Journal of Investigative Dermatology*, **74**, 187–91.

Tenover, J. S. (1991). Prostates, pates and pimples: the potential medical uses of 5α-reductase inhibitors. In *Steroid hormones: synthesis, metabolism and action in health and disease* (ed. J. F. Strauss III), pp. 893–909. W. B. Saunders, Philadelphia, PA.

Toomey, R. E., Goode, R. L., Petrow, V., and Neubauer, B. L. (1991). *In vivo* assay for conversion of testosterone to dihydrotestosterone by rat prostatic steroid 5α-reductase and comparison of two inhibitors. *Prostate*, **19**, 63–72.

Tsuji, M., Shima, H., and Cunha, G. R. (1991). *In vitro* androgen-induced growth and morphogenesis of the Wolffian duct within urogenital ridge. *Endocrinology*, **128**, 1805–11.

Verhoeven, G. and Cailleau, J. (1983). Inhibition by a 4-methyl-4-aza-steroid of NADPH: Δ^4-oxosteroid-5a-oxido-reductase activity in interstitial cells derived from immature rat testis. *Journal of Steroid Biochemistry*, **18**, 365–7.

Voigt, W. and Hsia, S. L. (1973). The antiandrogenic action of 4-androsten-3-one-17β-carboxylic acid and its methyl ester on hamster flank organ. *Endocrinology*, **92**, 1216–22.

Voigt, W., Fernandez, E. P., and Hsia, S. L. (1970). Transformation of testosterone into 17β-hydroxy-5a-androstan-3-one by microsomal preparation of human skin. *Journal of Biological Chemistry*, **245**, 5594–9.

Walsh, P. C., Madden, J. D., Herrod, M. J., Goldstein, J. L., MacDonald, P. C., and Wilson, J. D. (1974). Familial incomplete male pseudohermaphroditism type 2: Decreased dihydrotestosterone formation in pseudovaginal perineoscrotal hypospadias. *New England Journal of Medicine*, **291**, 944–9.

Watkins, W. J., Goldring, C. E. P., and Gower, D. B. (1988). Properties of 4-ene-5a-reductase and studies on its solubilization from porcine testicular microsomes. *Journal of Steroid Biochemistry*, **29**, 325–31.

Weintraub, P. M., Burkhart, J. P., and Blohm, T. R. (1992). New 4-amino-Δ^4-steroids as 5a-reductase inhibitors for treating DHT-mediated disease e.g. benign prostatic hypertrophy, acne vulgaris, androgenic alopecia, seborrhea and female hirsutism. European Patent Application 469,548, Merrill Dow Pharmaceutical Co.

Wendel, E. F., Brannen, G. E., Putong, P. B., and Grayhack, J. T. (1972). The effect of orchiectomy and estrogens on benign prostatic hyperplasia. *Journal of Urology*, **108**, 116–19.

Wenderoth, U. K., George, F. W., and Wilson, J. D. (1983). The effect of a 5a-reductase inhibitor on androgen-mediated growth of the dog prostate. *Endocrinology*, **113**, 569–73.

Wier, P. J., Connor, M., and Johnson, C. M. (1990). Abnormal development of male urogenital sinus derivatives produced by a 5a-reductase inhibitor. *Teratology*, **41**, 599.

Wilson, J. D., and Gloyna, R. E. (1970). The intranuclear metabolism of testosterone in the accessory organs of reproduction. *Recent Progress in Hormone Research*, **26**, 309–36.

Wilson, J. D. and Walker, J. D. (1969). The conversion of testosterone to 5a-androstan-17β-ol-3-one (dihydrotestosterone) by skin slices of man. *Journal of Clinical Investigation*, **48**, 371–9.

Wise, L. D., Minsker, D. H., Cukierski, M. A., Clark, R. L., Prahalada, S., Antonello, J. M., *et al.* (1991). Reversible decreases of fertility in male Sprague-Dawley rats treated orally with finasteride, a 5a-reductase inhibitor. *Reproductive Toxicology*, **5**, 337–46.

Zoppi, S., Lechuga, M., and Motta, M. (1992). Selective inhibition of the 5a-reductase of the rat epididymis. *Journal of Steroid Biochemistry and Molecular Biology*, **42**, 509–14.

10

HMG-CoA reductase inhibitors

M.J. Ashton and G. Fenton

10.1   Introduction

Numerous clinical studies evaluating the effects of diet and/or cholesterol-lowering drugs on reducing morbidity and mortality from coronary heart disease (CHD) have been performed in the previous decades. The outcome of many of these trials has been reviewed by Havel (1988). These results, combined with studies of experimentally induced atherosclerosis in animals and observations from patients genetically predisposed to CHD, has led to a wide acceptance that elevated plasma cholesterol, associated with raised concentrations of low density lipoprotein (LDL), is linked to an increased risk of morbidity in CHD but not conclusively to mortality.

Dietary control of hyperlipidaemia is occasionally successful but, for many patients, pharmacological intervention is required. Prior to the introduction of 3-hydroxy-3-methylglutaryl-coenzyme A reductase (HMG-CoA) inhibitors the main drugs available to the physician were the bile acid sequestrants (cholestyramine, colestipol), fibric acids (bezafibrate, fenofibrate, gemfibrozil), probucol, and nicotinic acid (Hoeg *et al.* 1986). Patient compliance, adverse effects, and in some cases lack of efficacy limited the widespread use of these agents. The bile acid sequestrants reduce plasma levels of LDL-cholesterol as a result of an increase in the hepatic conversion of cholesterol to bile acids stimulated by their removal from the enterohepatic circulation by irreversible binding to the sequestrant and subsequent elimination in the faeces. However, there is a compensating increase in cholesterol biosynthesis which may diminish their overall effectiveness in lowering plasma LDL-cholesterol.

Clearly, there was a requirement for a safe effective agent which could be used in single therapy or in combination with some of the established agents. Cholesterol biosynthesis can be inhibited at several steps in the biosynthetic pathway from acetate to cholesterol. Work in the 1960s uncovered several agents, of which triparanol was the most noteworthy, but these agents acted at the later stages of biosynthesis and caused an accumulation of desmosterol which had serious side-effects in man. This earlier work has been surveyed by Kritchevsky (1987). Attention then turned towards inhibition of earlier events in the cascade, in particular the inhibition of HMG-CoA reductase, the rate-determining step in cholesterol biosynthesis, and this review will focus on this topic.

10.2 HMG-CoA reductase

10.2.1 Enzyme structure

In man, most plasma-derived cholesterol is synthesized in the liver, although many other human cell types are capable of sterol biosynthesis (Sabine 1983). The biosynthetic pathway from acetyl-CoA to cholesterol is shown in Fig. 10.1. HMG-CoA reductase (EC 1.1.1.34) in mammalian cells catalyses the conversion of 3-hydroxy-3-methylglutaryl-coenzyme A to mevalonate, mediated by NADPH, and is the rate-determining step in this biosynthetic sequence (Fig. 10.2). Therefore inhibition of this enzyme became a principal target in the search for effective hypocholesterolaemic agents.

Although the enzyme has not been isolated in a pure form from a mammalian source, much information has accrued from studies with isolated

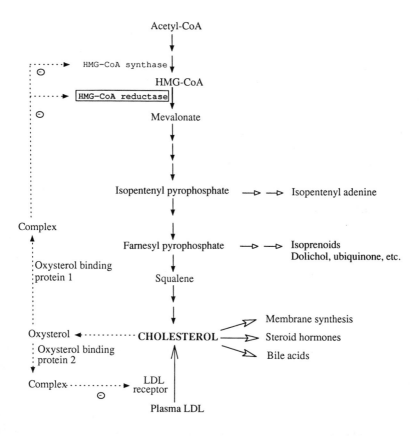

Fig. 10.1 Biosynthetic pathway for cholesterol biosynthesis (—►) from acetyl-CoA and internalization of exogenous cholesterol (—▷) via LDL receptor. The regulatory feedback pathways for HMG-CoA reductase, HMG-CoA synthase, and the LDL receptor (---►) are also shown. (Adapted from Goldstein and Brown 1990.)

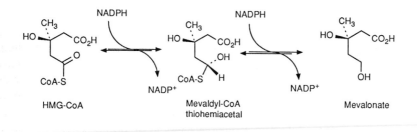

Fig. 10.2 The two-step reduction of HMG-CoA to mevalonate showing the enzyme-bound thiohemiacetal intermediate. The stereochemistry at the β centre is as shown and is retained.

microsomes. The enzyme is a 97 kDa transmembrane glycoprotein, residing in the endoplasmic reticulum of mammalian cells. The complete amino acid sequence was determined by Chin *et al*. (1984). A model of the secondary structure (Liscum *et al*. 1985) predicts that the protein consists of seven helical membrane-spanning regions which anchor the amino terminus and a 62 kDa fragment bearing the carboxy terminus which is exposed to the cytosol. The 62 kDa fragment can be further proteolysed to give a 53 kDa unit which contains the active site. The membrane-spanning and catalytic domains are highly conserved between rodents, humans, and also a cytosolic yeast-derived enzyme (Luskey and Stevens 1985; Basson *et al*. 1986). The linking region joining together these two domains is less well conserved between species. Thus both rodent and yeast-derived HMG-CoA reductases have been employed for the study of enzyme inhibitors.

Prior to this sequencing, the nature of the catalytic site was examined by Qureshi *et al*. (1976) using a yeast-derived enzyme. They attempted to elucidate the kinetics of the reaction and a model for the double reduction was proposed (Fig. 10.2). This was further developed to provide a chemically based mechanism of action (Veloso *et al*. 1981), whereby a cationic centre, probably a histidine residue, and a carboxyl group (glutamic or aspartic acid) assist in the formation of the putative enzyme-bound mevaldate thiohemiacetal. These, and related studies, have been summarized by Rogers *et al*. (1983). Evidence for the active-site histidine has been provided by Dugan and Katiyar (1986) using chemical probes. The nature of the active-site carboxyl group has been examined by Wang *et al*. (1990) who compared the catalytic domains of 11 eukaryotic HMG-CoA reductases with that from *Pseudomonas mevalonii* and found that only three acidic residues were conserved, one aspartate and two glutamate residues. Glu[83] was found to be the catalytically involved acid residue from a site-directed mutagenesis study using the *P. mevalonii* HMG-CoA reductase, and by extension the conserved motif (Pro-Met-AIa-Thr-Thr-Glu-Gly-Cys-Leu-Val-Ala) present in eukaryotic HMG-CoA reductases contains the glutamate residue active in catalysis.

Kinetic studies indicate that the enzyme can bind each of its substrates independently, which suggests that the catalytic site consists of two non-overlapping domains, an NADP(H) domain and a HMG-CoA domain (Qureshi et at. 1976). Furthermore the work of Nakamura and Abeles (1985) suggests that the HMG-CoA domain can be subdivided into an HMG binding site and a CoA site. The enzyme is known to require reduction by thiols in order to bind HMG-CoA and to be inhibited by agents which alkylate or oxidize sulphydryl groups (Rogers *et al*. 1983). Cysteine residues have been thought to participate in catalysis by HMG-CoA reductase (Dugan and Katiyar 1986), and recent studies using an enzyme from rat liver microsomes suggest a role for the binding of the CoA moiety to the catalytic site (Roitelman and Shechter 1989). Alternative findings by Jordan-Starck and Rodwell (1989a,b) using the NADH-dependent *P. mevalonii* HMG-CoA reductase indicate that a cysteine residue is not required for substrate binding or catalysis but may play a role in maintaining the enzyme structure. A full analysis of the substrate-binding domain and catalytic mechanism awaits determination of the three-dimensional structure.

10.2.2 Physiological regulation

A wider analysis of the involvement of HMG-CoA reductase in the maintenance of cholesterol homeostasis reveals its more complex relationship with plasma LDL-cholesterol levels. Intracellular cholesterol levels are regulated by a combination of biosynthesis and recruitment of plasma LDL-cholesterol. The plasma LDL-cholesterol enters the cell via receptor-mediated endocytosis with subsequent release of the cholesterol by lysosomal hydrolysis, as shown by the seminal work of Brown and Goldstein (1986) and reviewed by Bilheimer (1988).

In the absence of LDL-cholesterol cultured cells maintain high levels of HMG-CoA reductase and hence cholesterol biosynthesis, whereas in the presence of LDL-cholesterol HMG-CoA reductase activity is substantially reduced, although enough mevalonate is still produced to satisfy the cellular requirement for mevalonate-dependent isoprenoid biosynthesis (dolichol, ubiquinone, etc.) (Fig. 10.1). HMG-CoA reductase activity is not fully suppressed until the need for these isoprenoids, which are essential for cell growth, are satisfied (Brown and Goldstein 1980). In conditions of low mevalonate production the high affinity enzymes of the non-sterol pathway shunt a higher proportion of available mevalonate into isoprenoid biosynthesis. Thus LDL-cholesterol effects a feedback regulation of HMG-CoA reductase and the latter is further controlled by feedback regulation from the isoprenoid pathway (cumulative feedback regulation). As the cellular requirement for cholesterol becomes satisfied, the expression of cell surface LDL receptors is down-regulated.

The feedback regulatory mechanism(s) following internalization of LDL-cholesterol could be expected to be mediated by either the cholesterol itself or a metabolite, probably an oxysterol. The term oxysterol is used to describe derivatives of cholesterol possessing one or more additional oxygenation sites. Cholesterol has been shown not to be the mediator, as high levels of pure cholesterol fail to suppress HMG-CoA reductase activity, provided that autooxidation is prevented, whereas oxysterols (e.g. 25-hydroxycholesterol) effectively down-regulate HMG-CoA reductase activity. The isolation of a cytosolic oxysterol binding protein (OSBP) (Taylor and Kandutsch 1985) and the correlation between the binding affinity of a large variety of oxysterols with OSBP and their ability to repress HMG-CoA reductase activity provided further evidence for the role of oxysterols

(Taylor *et al.* 1984). In addition, the down-regulation of HMG-CoA reductase is prevented by inhibitors of cytochrome P450 enzymes, such as
ketoconazole, thus decreasing the oxidation of cholesterol to oxysterols.

Although the physiological role of the OSBP–oxysterol complex is
uncertain, it is believed to play a regulatory role whereby it interacts with
DNA either directly or, more likely, via transcription factors to repress
the transcription of genes encoding for HMG-CoA reductase, HMG-CoA
synthase, and the gene for the LDL receptor. More detailed aspects of the
regulatory elements of gene transcription have been reviewed by Goldstein
and Brown (1990), and the structure and role of the LDL receptor have
recently been reviewed by Innerarity (1991).

The existence of OSBP subtypes, whereby endogenous cholesterol synthesis and cholesterol uptake may be differentially controlled at the level
of gene transcription, has not been demonstrated. Furthermore, the structure
of the physiological oxysterol mediator(s) has yet to be elucidated. These
pathways may well provide suitable sites for pharmacological intervention
in the control of HMG-CoA reductase and cholesterol homeostasis.

10.3   Natural products and semisynthetic derivatives

10.3.1   Isolation and microbiological modification

The discovery of three inhibitors of HMG-CoA reductase—ML-236A, ML-
236B, and ML-236C—from the culture broth of the fungus *Penicillium
citrinum* (Endo *et al.* 1976) and the isolation of ML-236B from *Penicillium
brevicompactum* as an antifungal agent (known as compactin, later given
the generic name mevastatin) (Brown *et al.* 1976) initiated the search for
potent HMG-CoA reductase inhibitors from microbial sources. Later, a
potent inhibitor was isolated, independently by two groups, from *Monascus
ruber* (Endo 1979) and *Aspergillus terreus* (Alberts *et al.* 1980) (mevinolin,
generic name lovastatin) (Fig. 10.3).

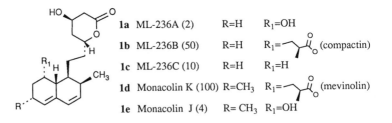

Fig. 10.3 The structure of compactin and related compounds from microbial
sources. The numbers in parentheses represent their relative potencies in inhibiting
HMG-CoA reductase. (From Endo 1985a.)

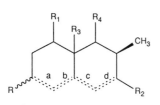

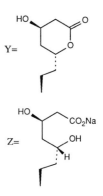

2 a-h

	Source	R	R₁	R₂	R₃	R₄	a	b	c	d	Reference
2a	B	α-CH₃		H	β-H	Y	sb	sb	sb	db	Albers-Schönberg *et al.* 1981
2b	MC	H		α-OH	β-H	Y	db	sb	db	sb	Serizawa *et al.* 1983a
2c	B	α-CH₃	H	H	β-H	Y	sb	sb	sb	db	Endo and Hasumi 1985
2d	B	α-CH₃		H	β-H	Y	sb	db	sb	db	Endo and Hasumi 1985
2e	MC	H		H	α-OH	Y	sb	db	sb	db	Yamashita *et al.* 1985
2f	MC	α-CH₃		H	α-OH	Y	sb	db	sb	db	Yamashita *et al.* 1985
2g	MC	β-OH		H	β-H	Z	sb	db	sb	db	Serizawa *et al.* 1983b
2h	MC	H		α-OH	β-H	Z	db	sb	db	sb	Serizawa *et al.* 1983c

Fig. 10.4 Compounds 2a–2h are related to mevinolin or compactin and were isolated from microbial sources (B) or derived by microbiological transformation of mevinolin or compactin (MC). Bonds a,b,c, and d are either single (sb) or double (db).

The therapeutic potential of compactin and mevinolin prompted the examination of many fungal broths for other active metabolites. Microbial hydroxylation of compactin and mevinolin was examined after the finding that the urine of compactin-treated dogs produced a metabolite which was as potent as compactin (Haruyama *et al.* 1986). Figure 10.4 shows the metabolite 3β-hydroxycompactin (**2g**, CS-514, generic name pravastatin) in addition to some of the derivatives of compactin and mevinolin which were isolated during these studies (Endo 1985b). Pravastatin is now produced by microbial hydroxylation of compactin using *Nocardia autotrophica* (Tsujita *et al.* 1986). Both lovastatin and pravastatin are now marketed as hypolipidaemic agents, whereas the development of compactin was discontinued.

10.3.2   Semisynthetic compounds

The compactin-like molecules can be divided into four groups for consideration of structure–activity relationships: side-chain ester, lactone, hexahydronaphthalene system, and the link between the hexahydronaphthalene system and the lactone.

10.3.2.1   Side-chain ester

Compounds **1a** and **1e**, (Fig. 10.3), which lack the 2(S)-methylbutyryl side-chain ester, have about 25 times less inhibitory potency than compactin and mevinolin respectively. Since this side-chain appears to be important for potency, the nature of this moiety has been investigated extensively in the mevinolin series of compounds. Chemical modification of mevinolin to introduce a range of side-chain esters (Hoffman *et al.* 1986a) and ethers (Lee *et al.* 1991) has been examined. In general, ether groups were much less potent than the corresponding ester analogues, indicating that the carbonyl of the ester function is important for potent inhibitory activity. An exception to this was the 4-fluorobenzyl ether **3a** (Fig. 10.5), which had an activity comparable with compactin. The role of 4-fluoroaryl substituents will be described later in the section on synthetic inhibitors. In contrast, modifications to the ester chain revealed that the stereochemistry of the carbon α to the carbonyl group was not crucial, since the enantiomeric 2(R)-methylbutyryl residue **3b** was equiactive with the natural product and an additional methyl group at this centre gave a 2.5-fold increase in potency over mevinolin. This latter compound, **3c** (synvinolin, generic name simvastatin), is the first semisynthetic agent to be marketed. Increasing the length of the side-chain led to a reduction in potency in this series.

10.3.2.2   The lactone

The lactone is considered to be the inactive prodrug form of the physiologically active 3,5-dihydroxypentanoic acid (pravastatin (Fig. 10.4, **2g**) is

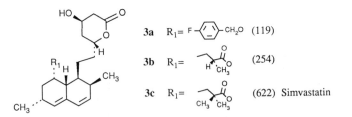

Fig. 10.5 The structures of ether and ester side-chains. The numbers in parentheses are the inhibitory potencies relative to compactin which was assigned a value of 100. Mevinolin had a relative inhibitory potency of 254. (Data from Lee *et al.* (1991) and Hoffman *et al.* (1986a).)

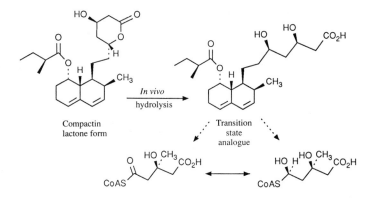

Fig. 10.6 Potential of the dihydroxy acid form to act as a transition state mimic of the first reduction of the natural substrate.

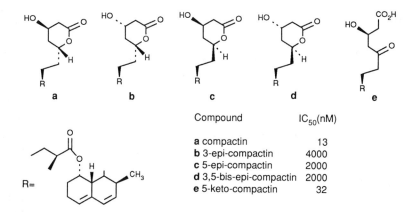

Compound	IC$_{50}$(nM)
a compactin	13
b 3-epi-compactin	4000
c 5-epi-compactin	2000
d 3,5-bis-epi-compactin	2000
e 5-keto-compactin	32

Fig. 10.7 Structure and inhibitory activities of the lactone isomers and the 5-keto form of compactin. (After Heathcock *et al.* 1987.)

isolated in this form as a sodium salt), which is generated by hydrolysis *in vivo*. The dihydroxy acid can be regarded as a transition state mimic of the natural substrate, or its half-reduced form mevaldate SCoA thiohemiacetal (Fig. 10.6), and probably occupies the same binding region.

Modification of the dihydroxy acid/lactone section of the natural products has had limited success. The introduction of a methyl group on to the hydroxy-bearing carbon of mevinolin lactone to give a direct analogue of the natural substrate (3-hydroxy-3-methylglutaryl CoA) with the same stereochemistry was a logical step (Lee *et al.* 1982). Surprisingly, this compound was much less active than mevinolin. In addition, Endo and Hasumi (1989) reported that esterification of the hydroxy groups of the dihydroxy acid or conversion of the carboxy group to an amide abolishes activity. Activity was also lost when the dihydroxy acid form of mevinolin was homologized to a 4,6-dihydroxy acid. Heathcock *et al.* (1987) have examined the 3-*epi*, 5-*epi*, and 3,5-bis-*epi* lactone isomers of compactin and found them to be less potent than compactin by a factor of about 200, whereas oxidation of the 5-hydroxy group to a ketone (5-keto-compactin) resulted in almost the same potency as the natural product (Fig. 10.7). It is possible that the 5-keto derivative binds to the enzyme and is then reduced to give the natural product.

10.3.2.3   *The hexahydronaphthalene system*

Chemical reduction of the hexahydronaphthalene system has been employed to give various di- and tetrahydro derivatives, most of which, with a *trans* ring junction, had comparable potency with the parent compounds (DeCamp *et al.* 1989). However, Duggan *et al.* (1991) reported the synthesis of 5-oxygenated derivatives of synvinolin and found some derivatives (Fig. 10.8) with enhanced activity.

Most modifications to the hexahydronaphthalene section of the natural products have concentrated on replacing this system with totally synthetic and diverse structures. This has served two purposes. (a) to find agents with superior pharmacological, metabolic, and toxicological profiles; (b) to move to synthetically less complex structures even though several excellent total syntheses of the natural products have been published.

10.3.2.4   *The linker group*

Variations of the linking group and the totally synthetic agents are covered in a later section.

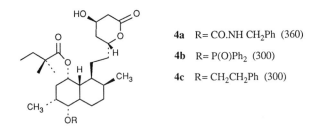

4a   R= CO.NH CH₂Ph (360)

4b   R= P(O)Ph₂ (300)

4c   R= CH₂CH₂Ph (300)

Fig. 10.8 Chemical modification of synvinolin to introduce 5-oxygenation. The numbers in parentheses are the relative potencies compared with compactin which is assigned a value of 100. In the same study synvinolin had a relative potency of 235.

10.3.3 Mechanism of HMG-CoA reductase inhibition by natural and semisynthetic compounds

Compactin, mevinolin, synvinolin, and pravastatin in their dihydroxy acid forms are potent reversible inhibitors of HMG-CoA reductase with inhibitor dissociation constants K_i in the low nanomolar range, whereas the K_m value for the natural substrate HMG-CoA is 4×10^{-6} M, i.e. the enzyme having ca. 10^4 times higher affinity for these inhibitors than for the natural substrate. This affinity is surprising since the inhibitors only partially resemble the natural substrate (Fig. 10.9). The basis for this strong binding affinity has been studied by Nakamura and Abeles (1985), using compactin and yeast HMG-CoA reductase, and they showed that compactin binding is competitive with respect to HMG-CoA and CoASH, and noncompetitive with respect to NADPH. In addition, DL-3,5-dihydroxyvaleric acid, which resembles the dihydroxy acid moiety of compactin, is a weak inhibitor and competitive with HMG-CoA, and compounds **5a** and **5b** (Fig. 10.9), which are related to the hexahydronaphthalene system, are inactive. Thus Nakamura and Abeles proposed that compactin binds to two sites in the enzyme, the hydroxymethylglutaryl domain and an adjacent hydrophobic pocket via its hexahydronaphthalene moiety, and that this moiety also overlaps the CoASH domain even though this may not be a strong interaction. The strong binding of compactin (and presumably related

(a)

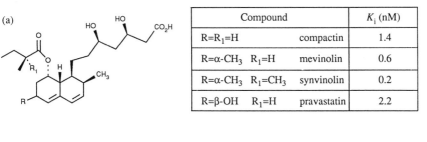

Compound			K_i (nM)
$R=R_1=H$		compactin	1.4
$R=\alpha\text{-}CH_3$ $R_1=H$		mevinolin	0.6
$R=\alpha\text{-}CH_3$ $R_1=CH_3$		synvinolin	0.2
$R=\beta\text{-}OH$ $R_1=H$		pravastatin	2.2

(b)

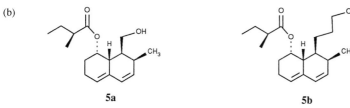

5a   5b

Fig. 10.9 (a) The K_i values for the natural and semisynthetic inhibitors displayed as their dihydroxy acid forms (Slater and MacDonald 1988); (b) compounds representing the hexahydronaphthalene portion of compactin used to determine binding domains.

structures) is believed to be derived from its simultaneous interaction at the two separate sites, the hydroxymethylglutaryl domain and the hydrophobic pocket.

10.3.4 Evaluation of the efficacy and side-effects of natural and semisynthetic inhibitors

These classes of compounds represented by mevinolin (lovastatin), synvinolin (simvastatin), and pravastatin are the only HMG-CoA reductase inhibitors currently available to the clinician and therefore are the only ones to have undergone extensive clinical evaluation. They are effective in inhibiting hepatic cholesterol synthesis in animal models and man. Lovastatin and simvastatin treatment resulted in an increase in receptor-dependent hepatic LDL uptake with a concomitant reduction in plasma LDL-cholesterol levels in animal models; in man all three agents reduce total plasma cholesterol by 20–30 per cent and plasma LDL-cholesterol by 30–40 per cent. Furthermore, lovastatin in combination with a bile acid sequestrant has reduced plasma LDL-cholesterol concentration by 50 per cent or more. Clinical efficacy, tolerance, and safety profiles have been thoroughly reviewed (Henwood and Heel 1988; Slater and MacDonald 1988; Todd and Goa 1990; Illingworth 1991; Tobert 1991).

The subject of tissue selectivity, where liver to peripheral tissue drug concentration should be as high as possible so as to target the drug to the principal site of cholesterol production and minimize its impact on extrahepatic cells, has been examined. Tsujita *et al.* (1986) administered pravastatin, compactin, or mevinolin orally to rats at a dose of 25 mg kg^{-1}. After 2 hours the animals were sacrificed and *in vitro* sterol biosynthesis was measured in slices taken from various organs. The results indicated that all three agents had potent inhibitory effects in the liver and ileum but in other tissues (kidney, lung, spleen, cerebrum, prostate, testis, adrenal, muscle, and skin) pravastatin had weak or no inhibitory effects. In the case of mevinolin and compactin, significant inhibition was observed in adrenal, lung, spleen, prostate, and testis in particular. These results indicated that pravastatin is tissue selective relative to mevinolin and compactin, and this was attributed to the slower transfer of the hydrophilic pravastatin across the peripheral tissue membranes. In contrast, however, Germershausen *et al.* (1989) described *in vivo* studies which determined the tissue distribution of mevinolin, sinvinolin, and pravastatin and total exposure to these agents over a 24 hour period following oral administration of 25 mg kg^{-1} to rats. At each time point the hepatic concentrations of mevinolin and sinvinolin were higher than those of pravastatin, and in the other tissues examined (kidney, spleen, testis, stomach, and adrenal) the levels of pravastatin were higher than or equal to those of mevinolin or sinvinolin. Germershausen *et al.* concluded that mevinolin and sinvinolin were more tissue selective than pravastatin; this may reflect the efficient hepatic uptake of lactones compared with dihydroxy acids.

The two different approaches taken by these two groups, tissue bio-synthetic activity versus total exposure to drug substance, have not resolved the problem of tissue selectivity. These results have been appraised by Sirtori (1990) and Tobert (1991) who also considered other factors, including the extent of plasma protein binding and the role of metabolites.

Resolution of this issue might indicate the preference for developing agents in lactone (prodrug) form or as dihydroxy acids (active form). As an adjunct to this, the physiological disposition of HMG-CoA reductase inhibitors has been reviewed by Duggan and Vickers (1990).

10.4   Totally synthetic HMG-CoA reductase inhibitors

10.4.1   Keynote studies

Early rational design involved the synthesis of arylalkyl hydrogen suc-cinates and glutarates (Boots *et al.* 1973; Guyer *et al.* 1976) as substrate mimics, with the aryl and alkyl moieties being varied to maximize lipophilic binding. The more active compounds are shown in Fig. 10.10. Compound **6b** was examined further, and the inhibition was found to be reversible and non-competitive with respect to HMG-CoA and NADPH. Furthermore, kinetic data indicated that the enzyme must bind three molecules of **6b** before inhibition occurs; presumably, the compound is acting allosterically.

Compactin and mevinolin were discovered shortly after the publication of these reports and, armed with the knowledge of these natural com-pounds, many of the major pharmaceutical companies initiated programmes to develop totally synthetic inhibitors. Their success is reflected in the patent literature (more than 300 patents reported in the last 8 years) although none has yet reached the market.

Merck researchers published keynote studies on the synthetic inhibi-tors. They were wide ranging, encompassing modifications to the lactone, the bridging group, and the lipophilic anchor (the moiety to replace the hexahydronaphthalene ring of the natural products). The initial series (Stokker *et al.* 1985) (Fig. 10.11), although only moderately active *in vitro*,

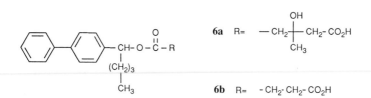

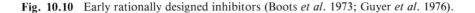

Fig. 10.10   Early rationally designed inhibitors (Boots *et al.* 1973; Guyer *et al.* 1976).

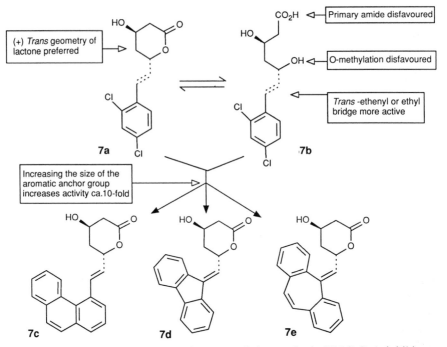

Fig. 10.11 The key structural requirements of the synthetic HMG-CoA inhibitors. The IC$_{50}$ values for **7b** (ethenyl bridge) and for **7c**, **7d**, and **7e**, evaluated as their sodium salts, were 22 μM, 1.9 μM, 0.89 μM, and 1.6 μM respectively.

delineated several key features which have held true for many subsequent series of HMG-CoA reductase inhibitor.

1. This study confirmed that the dihydroxy acid form was the active species and that the stereochemical requirements of the lactone 'prodrug' form were crucial for maximal activity, with the (+)*trans*-substituted lactone being the most active isomer. Thus the stereochemistry is identical with that of compactin and mevinolin.

2. Introduction of a 4-methyl group into the lactone, thus forming a closer analogue of the natural substrate, provided no enhancement of potency, and oxidation of the 4-hydroxy function to a keto/enol system substantially reduced activity. In the dihydroxy acid form, amide formation and methylation of the 5-hydroxy group abolished potency. An extension of amide formation is the preparation of δ-lactams. This was reported by Ashton *et al.* (1989) for a related series, and these compounds were found to be inactive, possibly because of the stability of the lactam towards proteolysis or the adverse effects of a 5-amino group following ring opening.

3. The bridging group is preferentially a *trans*-ethenyl or ethyl group with the *cis*-ethenyl, ethynyl, and oxymethylene links being far less active. Lengthening or removing the bridge also reduces activity.

4. The lipophilic anchor can be a simple aryl or cycloalkyl group and larger aromatic residues afford increased potency (Fig. 10.11, compounds **7c–7e**). The sensitivity of the size and shape of the anchor group towards inhibitor binding highlighted it as a key structural feature for modification in order to obtain increased inhibitory potency and, possibly, tissue selectivity.

A second publication (Hoffman *et al.* 1986b) described the effects of different substitution patterns around the aryl ring of compound **7a** using a limited set of substituent types — chloro, methyl, phenyl, aryl, and substituted methyl ethers. The structure–activity relationship (SAR) showed that a 2,4,6-trisubstituted aryl ring was preferred and, in particular, that a bulky benzyl ether substituent should be located *ortho* to the bridging link to maximize potency (Fig. 10.12, compound **8a**). As discussed above, inhibitory potency was enhanced by the introduction of a large lipophilic anchor group. In addition, substitution of a methyl group in place of a chloro group produced little change in potency, but a *p*-fluoro substituent in the *o*-benzyloxy group increased potency. Furthermore, within this series, compounds with an ethyl bridge were two to four times more potent than those with a *trans*-ethenyl bridge, leading to compound **8b** which has about 50 per cent of the inhibitory potency of compactin. The interaction

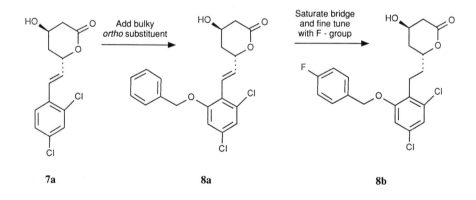

Fig. 10.12 Addition of bulky *ortho* substituent to improve inhibitory activity (Hoffman *et al.* 1986b). The IC$_{50}$ values for **7a**, **8a**, and **8b** as sodium salts are 22 μM, 0.43 μM, and 0.076 μM respectively, and the relative potencies are 0.08, 3.5 and 38 compared with compactin which is assigned a value of 100.

between the flexible benzyloxy substituent and the spatial orientation of
the lactone and bridging group were not discussed.

The third series based on a less flexible biphenyl anchor group, was
found to give more potent inhibitors (Stokker *et al.* 1986a). These were
derived from **8a**, when the benzyloxy group was replaced by a phenyl
group giving a moderately active compound (Fig. 10.13, **9a**). Using this as
a starting point, systematic modifications revealed that the 3,5-dichloro
substituents could be replaced by methyl groups with retention of activity
(compare **9b** with **9c**, and the four compounds **9d**–**9g**). Moreover the
type and position of substitution on the phenyl ring, *ortho* to the alkenyl
bridging group, proved to have a greater influence on intrinsic potency,
with a 4′-fluoro substituent being beneficial and a 4′-fluoro-3′-methyl
substitution pattern giving high inhibitory potency. Compounds possessing
a *trans*-ethenyl bridging link in this series, where the *o*-aryl ring is conformationally restricted (X-ray data for **9b** indicated that the dihedral
angle subtended by the planes of the two aryl rings is 54.7 ° and that of

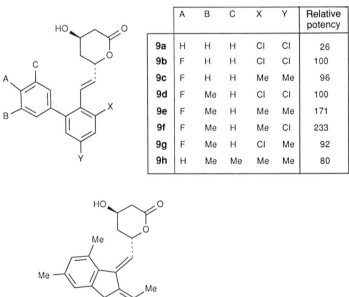

	A	B	C	X	Y	Relative potency
9a	H	H	H	Cl	Cl	26
9b	F	H	H	Cl	Cl	100
9c	F	H	H	Me	Me	96
9d	F	Me	H	Cl	Cl	100
9e	F	Me	H	Me	Me	171
9f	F	Me	H	Me	Cl	233
9g	F	Me	H	Cl	Me	92
9h	H	Me	Me	Me	Me	80

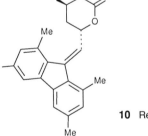

10 Relative potency=1.7

Fig. 10.13 Racemic compounds based on biphenylyl and fluorenylidene anchor
groups. The potency is expressed relative to compactin which is assigned a value
of 100. (After Stokker *et al.* 1986a,b.)

the aryl ring and the ethenyl bridge is 57.5 °), were the most potent inhibitors. The fluorenylidene **7d** can be considered as a rigid analogue of **9a–9h**, holding the two phenyl rings coplanar. Stokker *et al.* (1986b) prepared substituted analogues in the fluorenylidene series to evaluate these constraints; for example, comparison of the relative activities of compounds **10** and **9h** shows that forcing the aryl rings to be coplanar leads to a large reduction in activity. Hence a non-coplanar biphenyl anchor group is desirable for greater inhibitory potency. The relative potency of the biphenyl series compared with that of the *o*-benzyloxy substituted series, which is more conformationally mobile, reveals the former to be far more potent. Compounds **9b–9g** (Fig. 10.13 shows the relative potencies of racemates) have demonstrated that synthetic analogues can be as potent as, or more potent than, the natural product compactin. Resolution to give the (+)*trans* forms further increases potency. Furthermore, the nature of the lipophilic anchor group has been partially defined to show some of the constraints required for high potency, in particular an aryl ring attached *ortho* to the bridging link and a chloro or methyl group occupying the other *ortho* position.

10.4.2 Replacement of aryl anchor groups by heterocycles

Studies with the biphenyl series served as a starting point for many structure–activity investigations. Studies of five- and six-membered alicyclic and heterocyclic rings as lipophilic anchor groups Z (Fig. 10.14) have been made such that the indicated substitution pattern could be accommodated. Many publications describe compounds which fit this general structure, but only those describing a design element will be discussed here.

Roth *et al.* (1990) noted that the key feature of these compounds was a large lipophilic group held in a particular spatial arrangement with respect to the 4-hydroxypyranone and prepared a series of pyrrole analogues with

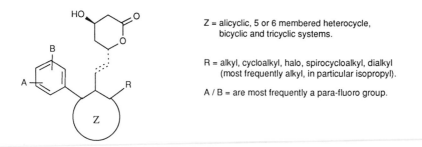

Z = alicyclic, 5 or 6 membered heterocycle, bicyclic and tricyclic systems.

R = alkyl, cycloalkyl, halo, spirocycloalkyl, dialkyl (most frequently alkyl, in particular isopropyl).

A / B = are most frequently a para-fluoro group.

Fig. 10.14 A general model: Z, acyclic five- or six-membered heterocycle, bicyclic, and tricyclic systems; R, alkyl, cycloalkyl, halo, spirocycloalkyl, dialkyl (most frequently alkyl, in particular isopropyl); A/B, most frequently a *p*-fluoro group.

the bridging group attached to the ring nitrogen. Structure–activity relationships showed that an ethyl bridge (an ethenyl bridge was not examined, possibly because of stability problems), a 4-fluorophenyl moiety, and a C5 isopropyl group were required for optimal potency (Fig. 10.15, **11a**). High potency was also seen with a trifluoromethyl substituent (Fig. 10.15, **11b**), and the activity was attributed to stabilization of the pyrrole ring by its electron-withdrawing effect.

Molecular modelling of the compactin and biphenyl series was performed to help identify size constraints of the substituted pyrrole anchor, favourable torsional conformations of the ethyl bridge/lactone, and electronic characteristics of the phenyl substituent. This revealed the size constraints shown in Fig. 10.16, accommodating the more potent inhibitor **11a** which also has a significant dipole in the same region of space as does the butyryl ester of compactin, possibly accounting for additional potency exhibited by the 4-fluorophenyl substituent. Furthermore, minimum

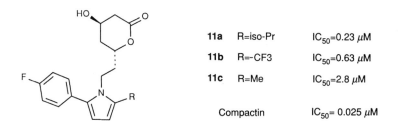

11a	R=iso-Pr	IC$_{50}$=0.23 μM
11b	R=-CF3	IC$_{50}$=0.63 μM
11c	R=Me	IC$_{50}$=2.8 μM
	Compactin	IC$_{50}$= 0.025 μM

Fig. 10.15 Pyrrole series (Roth *et al.* 1990).

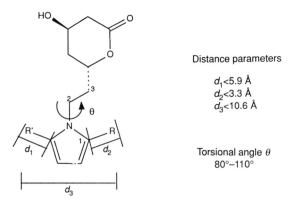

Distance parameters

d_1<5.9 Å
d_2<3.3 Å
d_3<10.6 Å

Torsional angle θ
80°–110°

Fig. 10.16 Distance constraints and range of preferred torsional angle θ (Roth *et al.* 1990). The torsional angle θ is defined by the angle C1, N, C2, C3.

energy calculations indicate that, whilst maintaining the flanking aryl group orthogonal to the plane of the pyrrole ring, the ethyl bridge/lactone is twisted out of plane ($\theta = 80°-110°$) in the more potent analogues, similar to the calculated minimum energy conformation of compactin. Thus this simplified model indicates that the flanking alkyl group plays an important role in influencing the population of active conformations of the bridge/lactone system (compare **11a** and **11c**) and, although the Merck group often used a flanking chloro substituent, the majority of studies show a preference for an alkyl group, particularly isopropyl.

Later, Roth *et al.* (1991a) found that substitution of the 3- and 4-positions of the pyrrole with a combination of electron-withdrawing and lipophilic groups further enhanced *in vitro* potency (Fig. 10.17). The data indicated a trend towards increasing bulk and lipophilicity (**12a** and **12c–12f** compared with **11a**) at these positions and that electron-withdrawing effects had a rather ambiguous role (**12b** versus **11a** and **12a** versus **12d**). Moreover the regiochemistry of the substituents appears to be important (compare **12c** and **12d**), but whether lipophilicity or tolerance of an electron-withdrawing group governs this remains unclear. Replacement of the iso-propyl group of **12f** with a trifluoromethyl group also affords a potent inhibitor, as was found with compound **11b**.

Several other groups have examined substituted pyrroles bearing an additional lipophilic residue and found compounds with potent *in vitro* activity, comparable with or better than mevinolin and compactin. These potent compounds, in which the bridging group was connected via N1, C2, or C3 indicated that the heteroatom position had much less effect on

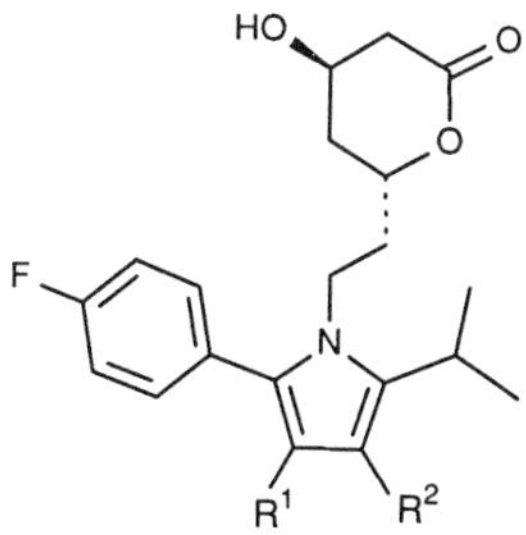

	R¹	R²	Relative potency
12a	H	Ph	36.3
12b	CO₂Et	CO₂Et	2.8
12c	Ph	CO₂Et	35.5
12d	CO₂Et	Ph	100
12e	2-pyridyl	H	76
12f	Ph	CONHPh	81.4
12g*	Ph	CONHPh	500

*(+)*trans* lactone from resolution of **12f**.

Fig. 10.17 Pyrroles substituted at the 3- and 4-positions (Roth *et al.* 1991a). Data for (±)trans-lactones unless otherwise indicated. The potency is expressed relative to compactin which is assigned a value of 100. The relative potency of compound **11a** ($R^1 = R^2 = H$) is 10.9.

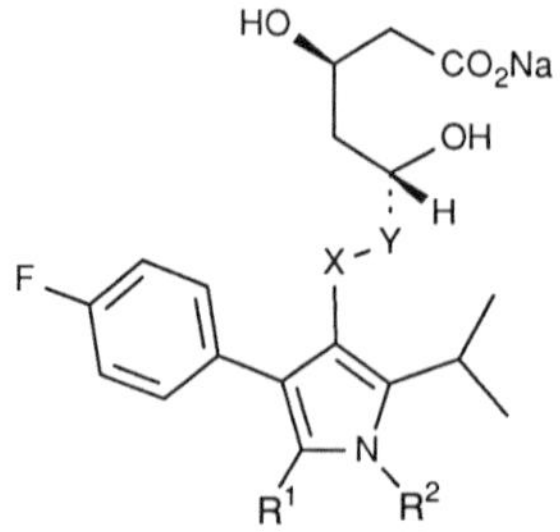

	R^1	R^2	A-B	Relative potency
13a	H	Ph	CH=CH	110
13b	H	Ph	CH$_2$CH$_2$	128
13c*	H	Ph	CH$_2$CH$_2$	257
13d	H	iPr	CH=CH	6
13e	H	iPr	CH$_2$CH$_2$	42
13f	H	Cyclohexyl	CH$_2$CH$_2$	92

*3R,5R-enantiomer.

Fig. 10.18 Substituted pyrroles (after Jendralla *et al.* 1990) prepared as erythro-dihydroxycarboxylic acid sodium salts. The *in vitro* potency is expressed relative to mevinolin which is assigned a value of 100.

potency than the nature and position of the substituents. Jendralla *et al.* (1990) reported on pyrroles with the bridge attached to C3 (Fig. 10.18, **13a–13d**). Flanking 4-fluorophenyl and isopropyl groups were preferred within this series, and increasing the lipophilicity of the anchor group by additional bulky phenyl and cyclohexyl substituents led to an increase in potency (compare **13b** and **13f** with **13e**). An additional methyl group at R^1 increased or decreased potency, depending on other substituents. Generally, in this series, a *trans*-ethenyl bridge and an ethyl bridge had similar potencies *in vitro* but, with the electron-rich pyrrole system, the former were susceptible to acid catalysed decomposition and this may result in decreased *in vivo* activity. The 3R,5R-enantiomer **13c** was shown to be the active isomer.

In a whole-cell assay (HEP G2 cells) measuring acetate incorporation into cholesterol, the racemic compounds **13a**, **13b**, and **13e** were respectively three, five, and 25 times more potent than mevinolin. In normal fed rabbits racemic **13b** decreased total plasma cholesterol by 34 per cent (dosed at 20 mg kg^{-1} orally for 10 days) compared with mevinolin (dosed at 10 mg kg^{-1} orally for 10 days) which gave a 25 per cent reduction. Compound **13a** was inactive, and this was suggested to be a result of acid-catalysed decomposition of the compound in the stomach. Further studies in the dog revealed that **13b** (20 mg kg^{-1} orally for 14 days) reduced LDL-cholesterol levels by 48 per cent compared with an 18 per cent reduction effected by mevinolin (10 mg kg^{-1} orally for 19 days).

Thus the investigation of a pyrrole-based series of compounds resulted in the discovery of totally synthetic inhibitors of HMG-CoA reductase, with comparable or greater potency than the natural products both *in vitro* and *in vivo*.

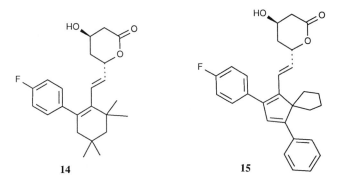

Fig. 10.19 Alicyclic replacements of the pyrrole nucleus: **14**, $IC_{50} = 0.15$ μM; **15**, $IC_{50} = 0.0034$ μM. (From WO Patent 89/05639, 29 June 1989, and US Patent 4,904,691, 27 February 1990, to Rorer Pharmaceutical Corporation.)

A survey of six-membered heterocycles and other five-membered heterocycles as alternatives to the pyrrole ring reveals similar structure–activity relationships. Table 10.1 shows examples of these systems and their *in vitro* activities. Compounds with an isoxazole anchor group (entry 4) cannot accommodate a further lipophilic substituent and are less potent inhibitors compared with entries 1,2, and 3, which bear an additional group. The pyridine-based compound (entry 2) has a cholesterol-lowering effect in a normolipidaemic rabbit model, reducing total serum and LDL-cholesterol levels by 35 per cent and 53 per cent respectively when administered orally at 10 mg kg^{-1} for 19 days. Mevinolin for the same dose and duration caused 17% and 30 % reductions in total serum and LDL-cholesterol respectively.

Since the position of the heteroatom in the lipophilic anchor appears to have little effect on activity, some groups have examined partially saturated alicyclic systems such as compounds **14** and **15** (Fig. 10.19). One of the flanking groups in these compounds now has geminal dimethyl substitution or a spirocyclopentyl group replacing the usual isopropyl moiety in order to confer the necessary conformational modulation of the lactone–bridge system. These compounds have *in vitro* activities of the same order as mevinolin.

10.4.3   Compounds possessing bicyclic lipophilic anchor groups

Several groups have explored bi- and tricyclic -systems, and these have been derived from two converging studies.

1. Direct replacement of the hexahydronaphthalene unit of compactin with naphthalene (Fig. 10.20) (Prugh *et al.* 1990); these compounds are

Table 10.1 Alternative monocyclic heterocycles used as anchor groups

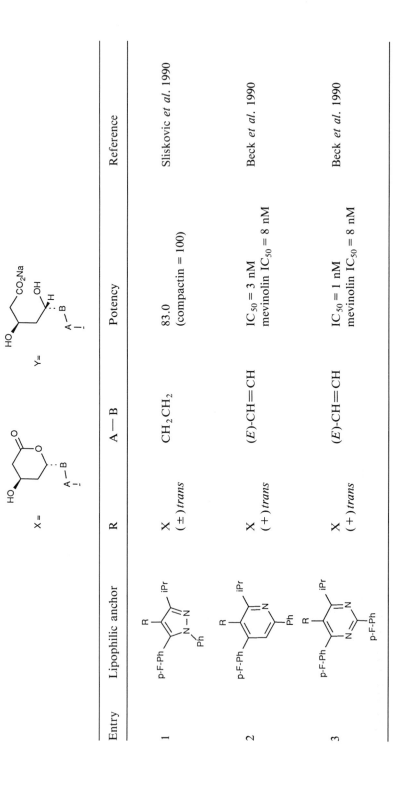

Entry	Lipophilic anchor	R	A — B	Potency	Reference
1	p-F-Ph, iPr, R, N—N, Ph (pyrazole)	X (±) *trans*	CH₂CH₂	83.0 (compactin = 100)	Sliskovic *et al.* 1990
2	p-F-Ph, iPr, R, N, Ph (pyridine)	X (+) *trans*	(E)-CH=CH	IC₅₀ = 3 nM mevinolin IC₅₀ = 8 nM	Beck *et al.* 1990
3	p-F-Ph, iPr, R, N, N, p-F-Ph (pyrimidine)	X (+) *trans*	(E)-CH=CH	IC₅₀ = 1 nM mevinolin IC₅₀ = 8 nM	Beck *et al.* 1990

Table 10.1 (*continued*)

Entry	Lipophilic anchor	R	A—B	Potency	Reference
4		X (+) *trans*	(*E*)-CH=CH	$IC_{50} = 0.91\ \mu M$ mevinolin $IC_{50} = 0.2\ \mu M$	Ashton 1991
5		Y mainly erythro	(*E*)-CH=CH	$ED_{50} = 0.076\ mg\ kg^{-1}$ mevinolin $ED_{50} =$ $0.41\ mg\ kg^{-1}$	WO Patent 87/02662, 7 May 1987, to Sandoz
6		Y erythro	(*E*)-CH=CH	$IC_{50} = 2.6\ nM$ mevinolin $IC_{50} =$ $0.14\ \mu M$	US Patent 4,755,606, 5 July 1988, to Sandoz

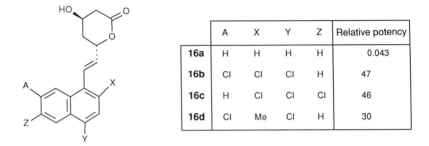

	A	X	Y	Z	Relative potency
16a	H	H	H	H	0.043
16b	Cl	Cl	Cl	H	47
16c	H	Cl	Cl	Cl	46
16d	Cl	Me	Cl	H	30

Fig. 10.20 Substituted naphthalenes to replace the bicyclic system of compactin (Prugh *et al.* 1990). *In vitro* potency is expressed relative to compactin which is assigned a value of 100.

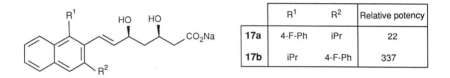

	R^1	R^2	Relative potency
17a	4-F-Ph	iPr	22
17b	iPr	4-F-Ph	337

Fig. 10.21 Modified naphthalenes to introduce two *ortho* flanking groups (Kathawala 1991). *In vitro* potency is expressed relative to compactin which is assigned a value of 100.

racemates and, allowing for this, the more potent compounds **16b−16d** with *ortho* substitution at C2, were of similar potency to compactin. Although substitution of chlorine or methyl groups in the 2-position of the naphthyl ring led to an increase in potency over the unsubstituted compound, no investigation of 2,8-disubstituted compounds was undertaken. These may have shown increased potency. However, moving the bridge−lactone system to C2 allows simple functionalization of positions 1 and 3 to give compounds **17a** and **17b** (Fig. 10.21) (Kathawala 1991) and there is a surprising difference in activity between the two regio-isomers.

2. The addition of fused rings to the previously discussed monocyclic systems in order to increase the steric bulk and lipophilicity of the anchor group (Fig. 10.22).

The indoles **18a−18c** were investigated by workers at Sandoz, followed by the indenes **19**, and the quinolines **20a** and **20b**. Kathawala (1991) has reviewed the SAR of the indole and indene series and surveyed many of

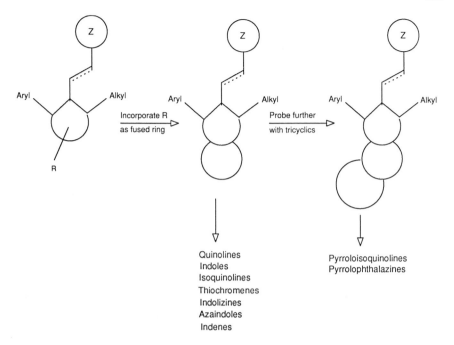

Quinolines
Indoles
Isoquinolines
Thiochromenes
Indolizines
Azaindoles
Indenes

Pyrroloisoquinolines
Pyrrolophthalazines

Fig. 10.22 Fusion onto the monocyclic system to produce bi- and tricyclic anchor groups: R, aryl, cycloalkyl, or bulky alkyl; Z, lactone or dihydroxy acid.

the patented aza and polyaza bicyclic compounds, and Sliskovic *et al.* (1991) reported the evaluation of the quinolines with **20a** and **20b** as the most potent compounds (Fig. 10.23). The marked difference in potency between the regio-isomers **18a** and **18b** and the high potency of 6-substituted indole **18c** suggests that the enzyme can tolerate larger anchor groups. This is borne out when considering the tricyclic structures **21a** and **21b** whose activity *in vitro* surpasses that of mevinolin.

The indole **18a** (generic name fluvastatin) is reported to be in phase III clinical trials. The compound lowers LDL + VLDL-cholesterol by 47 per cent at an oral dose of 2 mg kg^{-1} daily in the dog and by 30 per cent at 30 mg kg^{-1} daily in the rhesus monkey. Furthermore, in man dose-dependent reductions in LDL-cholesterol of 15–28 per cent were achieved at doses ranging from 5 to 40 mg four times daily.

Compounds with electron-rich heterocyclic lipophilic anchor groups like **17a**, **21a**, and **21b**, which also possess an ethenyl bridge, are susceptible to acid-catalysed decomposition to give trienes and trienoic acids. This could account for the apparent loss of *in vivo* potency compared with their intrinsic *in vitro* potency. Moreover acid catalysis can cause epimerization of the lactones at the C6 position or the C5 hydroxy group of the di-hydroxy acid form, which would lead to production of an inactive isomer.

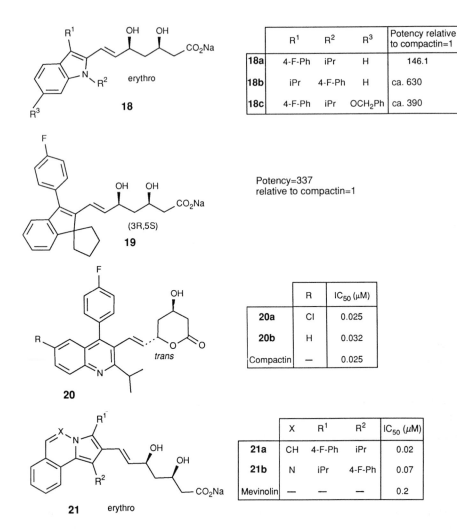

	R¹	R²	R³	Potency relative to compactin=1
18a	4-F-Ph	iPr	H	146.1
18b	iPr	4-F-Ph	H	ca. 630
18c	4-F-Ph	iPr	OCH₂Ph	ca. 390

Potency=337
relative to compactin=1

	R	IC₅₀ (µM)
20a	Cl	0.025
20b	H	0.032
Compactin	—	0.025

	X	R¹	R²	IC₅₀ (µM)
21a	CH	4-F-Ph	iPr	0.02
21b	N	iPr	4-F-Ph	0.07
Mevinolin	—	—	—	0.2

Fig. 10.23 Examples of bicyclic anchor groups (after Kathawala 1991; Sliskovic *et al.* 1991) and tricyclic systems (after Patents EP303446, 15 February 1989, and EP319330, 7 June 1989, to May & Baker).

Ideally, only the single active enantiomer of these inhibitors should be assessed clinically. To meet this criterion and achieve acid stability a further design feature was incorporated (Ashton 1991). This involved incorporation of an 'electron sink' into the anchor which not only permits formation of the *trans* ethenyl bridge but also allows the formation of one enantiomer of the lactone, which is stable. Compounds **22a** and **22b** (Fig. 10. 24) were

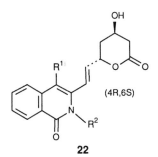

	R¹	R²	IC_{50} (μM)
22a	4-F-Ph	iPr	0.4
22b	iPr	4-F-Ph	0.2
Mevinolin	—	—	0.2

22

(4R,6S)

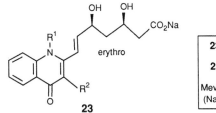

	R¹	R²	IC_{50} (μM)
23a	4-F-Ph	iPr	0.049
23b	iPr	4-F-Ph	3.75
Mevinolin	—	—	0.35
(Na salt)	—	—	0.068

erythro

23

Fig. 10.24 Stabilized anchor groups permitting the facile formation of enantio-merically pure lactones (after Patent EP326386, 8 June 1989, to May & Baker) and quinolone (after Coppola 1989).

developed on this basis and shown to be as active as mevinolin *in vitro*. Similarly, the quinolones **23a** and **23b** reported by Coppola (1989) can be expected to be stable to acid-catalysed decomposition.

10.4.4 Further modifications of the bridging group and lactone/dihydroxy acid functions

The general guidelines invoking the use of ethyl or *trans*-ethenyl bridges to the exclusion of ethynyl or oxymethylene groups have been reinvesti-gated in compounds where the lipophilic anchor groups have greater affinity for the active site. Jendralla *et al.* (1991) reported the activity of compounds bearing an ethynyl link with IC_{50} values less than 10 nM and went on to describe inhibitors having oxymethylene links with *in vitro* potencies close to that of mevinolin. Figure 10.25 shows the more potent *in vitro* inhibitors **24a** and **24c** in which the *o*-isopropyl and 4-fluorophenyl groups are retained but the nature of the Z substituent appears to diverge from that in foregoing series (compare the loss of activity in exchanging iPr for alternative bulky substituents 4-F-Ph or tBu (**24a** compared with **24b** or **24d**)). This was reflected *in vivo* in a rat model. Activity in a rabbit model did not completely parallel the *in vitro* results, as **24a** and **24c** were

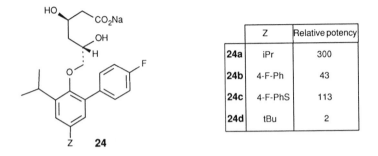

	Z	Relative potency
24a	iPr	300
24b	4-F-Ph	43
24c	4-F-PhS	113
24d	tBu	2

Fig. 10.25 Active oxymethylene-bridged compounds in optically pure form (after Jendralla *et al.* 1991). *In vitro* potency is expressed relative to mevinolin which is assigned a value of 100.

more active than mevinolin and **24b** (lactone form) was also as active as mevinolin. Surprisingly, this activity was not evident in the dog and this was attributed to metabolic deactivation by oxidative cleavage of the oxymethylene link. Although potent *in vitro* activity can be achieved with this alternative bridging group, metabolic degradation leads to loss of activity *in vivo*.

Variation of the bridge unit, accompanied by a major change to the dihydroxy acid system, was reported by workers from Bristol-Myers Squibb. Their hypothesis was based on the mechanism of action of HMG-CoA reductase, where the enzyme acts as an acid–base catalyst for the transfer of hydride ion between NADPH and the natural substrate. Karanewsky *et al.* (1990) designed hydroxyphosphinyl-containing inhibitors which are proposed to interact with the catalytic unit so as to bind by forming ion pairs between the corresponding phosphinate anion and the protonated catalytic moiety. Initially, using the well-defined biphenyl anchor group, the phosphinic acid was shown to be more potent than the corresponding methyl esters, possibly indicating that the proposed binding was occurring. Different types of bridge were examined (Fig. 10.26, **25**, R = Me) and it was found that a two-atom link, in particular a *trans*-ethenyl link, was most potent. However, on replacing **25** (R = methyl for R = isopropyl) there was a dramatic enhancement in potency for the acetylenic and oxymethylene-linked compounds. Compounds **26d** and **26f** were orally active in rabbit and dog and the former has been selected for studies in man. The use of phosphinic acid residues can also be considered as an alternative method for providing stabilized bridge–lactone systems for electron-rich anchor groups.

A second report from the same group concentrated on a series of pyridyl-based compounds (Fig. 10.27) optimizing the ring substituents with respect

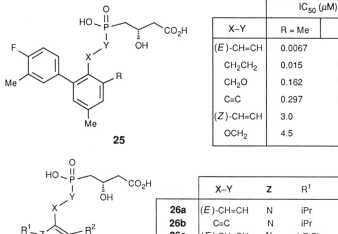

	IC_{50} (μM)	
X–Y	R = Me	R = iPr
(E)-CH=CH	0.0067	—
CH_2CH_2	0.015	0.0038
CH_2O	0.162	0.0012
C≡C	0.297	0.0085
(Z)-CH=CH	3.0	—
OCH_2	4.5	—

25

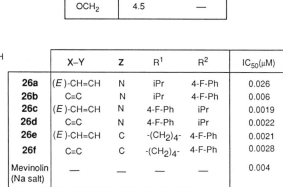

	X–Y	Z	R^1	R^2	IC_{50}(μM)
26a	(E)-CH=CH	N	iPr	4-F-Ph	0.026
26b	C≡C	N	iPr	4-F-Ph	0.006
26c	(E)-CH=CH	N	4-F-Ph	iPr	0.0019
26d	C≡C	N	4-F-Ph	iPr	0.0022
26e	(E)-CH=CH	C	-$(CH_2)_4$-	4-F-Ph	0.0021
26f	C≡C	C	-$(CH_2)_4$-	4-F-Ph	0.0028
Mevinolin (Na salt)	—		—	—	0.004

Fig. 10.26 *In vitro* activity of phosphinic and phosphonic acid analogues of the dihydroxy acid and the various bridging links examined for this modification. (After Karanewsky *et al.* 1990.)

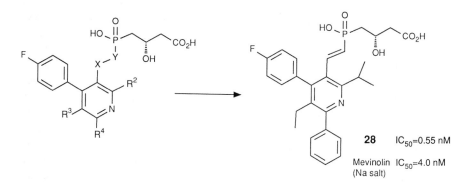

Fig. 10.27 Variation of bridge X — Y and R^2 — R^4 gives the potent pyridyl analogue of the phosphinic acid series 28. (After Robl *et al.* 1991.)

to the type of bridge. The *trans*-ethenyl link was generally superior, the group R^2 had to be tailored to suit the individual bridge links, and substitution at R^3 and R^4 was preferred, in particular R^3 = methyl or ethyl and R^4 = phenyl, culminating in the very potent analogue **28** (Robl *et al.* 1991).

Phosphinic acid analogues have also been disclosed by Dreyer *et al.* (1991) and shown to be potent inhibitors of recombinant human HMG-CoA reductase. However, the potency was very much reduced in tests in whole cells (HEP G2 cells) which was attributed to the poor membrane permeability of these doubly charged species.

Further modifications to the dihydroxy acid have been reported by workers from Merck who patented a series of 5-thiaheptanoic acids, exemplified by **29**, and the 5-keto-3-hydroxy acids **30**, (Fig. 10.28). No activities were given for these compounds, although Bone *et al.* (1992) and Heathcock *et al.* (1987) have reported that the 5-keto-3-hydroxy acid derivatives of 4,4a-dihydromevinolin and compactin have similar *in vitro* activities to the parent compounds. The geminally fluoro-substituted 5-keto-3-hydroxy acids **31a** and **31b** were prepared for their potential ability to bind to the enzyme in a similar manner to the 3,5-dihydroxy acids, since a-fluoro-ketones are potent inhibitors of other enzyme classes by virtue of

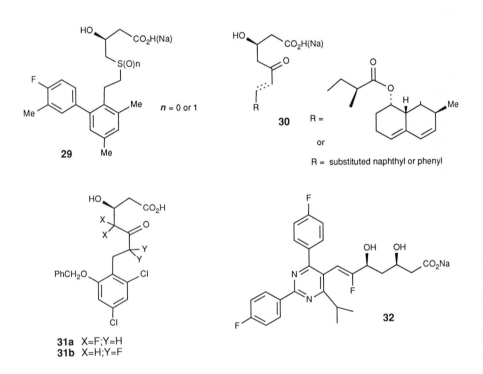

Fig. 10.28 Other modifications to the dihydroxy acid−bridge system. Compounds **29** and **30** after Patents EP127848, 12 December 1984, and EP142146, 22 May 1985, to Merck.

their propensity to form stable hydrates and adducts with active-site nucleophiles. These compounds were reported to be effective inhibitors of HMG-CoA reductase *in vitro* (no data given) (Dreyer and Metcalf 1988). Nevertheless the use of 5-keto-3-hydroxy acids has not been widely adopted by other groups.

Structure **32**, which is fluorinated in the bridge, is based on the premise that fluorination in other classes of compound afforded agents with more desirable characteristics. This compound was active *in vitro* (IC_{50} = 2.9 nM compared with IC_{50} = 8.0 nM for mevinolin sodium salt) but no other comparative data were given (Baader *et al*. 1989).

10.4.5 Diverse changes to the anchor group

Balasubramanian *et al*. (1989) and Sit *et al*. (1990) disclosed a series of inhibitors based on a 6,8-nonadienoic acid system (Fig. 10.29). This change leads to a diversity in the substitution pattern of the C8 position of the dienoic acid, and molecular modelling studies were used to examine the active conformations of the molecules with respect to other potent inhibitors, for example **18a**, so as to define a unified model. The calculated bioactive conformation of **33a** involved adoption of a non-planar conformation by the butadiene and the tetrazole ring twisted out of planarity with respect to the C8–C9 double bond. The lost delocalization energy of the non-planar diene should easily be compensated by the resulting improved interaction with the enzyme binding site. A further feature of this system is that the tetrazole ring is hydrophilic, yet it appears to be binding in the same region as the hydrophobic isopropyl group of other inhibitors.

Thus binding to this site could be dependent on steric factors, and a volume map of the site has been generated with the substituents at C9 held constant. From this, it was proposed that (1) inactive compounds arise

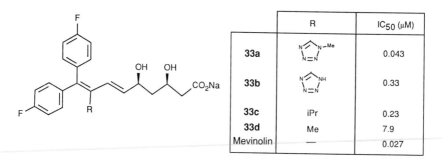

	R	IC_{50} (µM)
33a	N‑N‑N=N‑Me (methyltetrazole)	0.043
33b	N‑NH tetrazole	0.33
33c	iPr	0.23
33d	Me	7.9
Mevinolin	—	0.027

Fig. 10.29 The 6,8-nonadienoic acid series tested *in vitro* as racemates. (After Sit *et al*. 1990.)

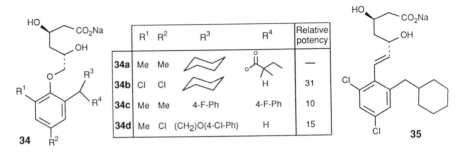

Fig. 10.30 Variations in the type of *ortho* substituent (after Jendralla *et al.* 1991). Potency is expressed relative to mevinolin which is assigned a value of 100.

because the substituent needs to occupy space outside this volume, resulting in steric repulsions and a weak inhibitor–enzyme complex, (2) moderate activity is a result of insufficient occupancy of the site and a low net stabilization of the complex, for example **33d**, and (3) high potency was achieved when 50 per cent or more of the defined volume was occupied, for example **33a** where the 1-methyltetrazole had 65 per cent occupancy and **33c** where the isopropyl had 58 per cent occupancy. A fuller account of this work has been published by Motoc *et al.* (1991).

Further deviations from the accepted substitution pattern around the anchor group were compounds **34a**, which encompassed the synvinolin side-chain ester, and **34b–34d**, which have bulky or flexible side-chains, (Fig. 10.30) (Jendralla *et al.* 1991). Although the intrinsic *in vitro* potencies were much less than in mevinolin, compounds **34b** and **34d** are nearly as potent as mevinolin *in vivo* (rat model). The poor metabolic stability of the oxymethylene bridge, discussed earlier, has been eliminated by returning to the *trans*-ethenyl bridge culminating in compound **35** which was still less potent than mevinolin *in vitro* but was twice as active on inhibition of cholesterol biosynthesis in whole cells. Thus **35** was reported to be undergoing further evaluation. An explanation for the lack of correlation between the *in vitro* and *in vivo* activities of these compounds was not given.

10.4.6 Rationalization and definition of the pharmacophore of HMG-CoA reductase inhibitors

The main structural features of the inhibitors described are as follows:

(1) a *trans* stereochemistry of the lactone substituents with the 4-hydroxy group having the (*R*)-configuration;

(2) a large lipophilic anchor group, a hexahydronaphthalene in the natural substrates, and mono-, bi-, or tricyclic aryl or heteroaryl ring systems for the synthetic inhibitors;

(3) the lactone is connected to the anchor group by a two-atom unit, preferably a two-carbon unit and in particular a *trans*-ethenyl group;

(4) the presence of two bulky substituents *ortho* to the bridge;

(5) a polar group (most frequently a fluoro substituent) located ca. 6 Å from the anchor group.

Using these criteria, Cosentino *et al.* (1992) carried out a principal component analysis (PCA) on representative examples from several series, including **1b**, **9b**, **11b**, **18a**, **33c**, and the additional structures **36a**, **36b**, and **37–40** (Fig. 10.31). Compounds **36b**, **39**, and **40** were inactive, compounds **11b**, **37**, and **38** were moderately active, and the remainder had good to excellent activity.

Minimum energy conformations were obtained for each compound (lactone form), retaining those within 6 kcal mol^{-1} of the global minimum, and a set of common interatomic distances were determined for each structure. PCA revealed that three interatomic distances were critical in defining active conformations, and mapping of electrostatic potentials provided a further discriminator showing the need for a zone of negative potential associated with the polar fluoro group and a second zone of positive potential, common to the active compounds, around group L of Fig. 10.32.

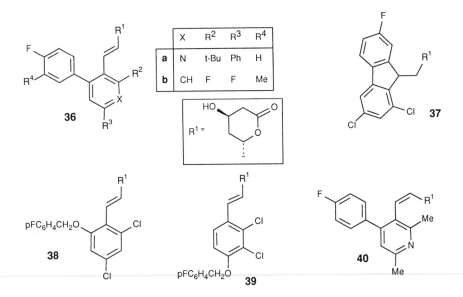

Fig. 10.31 Additional compounds used by Cosentino *et al.* (1992) for PCA to determine a unified model of an HMG-CoA reductase pharmacophore.

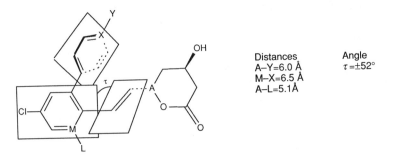

Fig. 10.32 The key distances and torsional angle τ for the proposed HMG-CoA pharmacophore using a biphenyl analogue to illustrate the model (Cosentino *et al.* 1992).

Similar findings have been presented by Ashton (1991). The key distances are shown in Fig. 10.32 for the biphenyl analogue, together with the average torsional angle τ thus generated.

In addition the determination of quantitative structure–activity relationships for substituted derivatives of the biphenyl series reinforced the need for a polar substituent in the *para* position and showed that increasing polar and decreasing resonance contributions will lead to greater activity (Prabhakar *et al.* 1989).

It is anticipated that this unifying model might be used as a tool in the assessment and design of new inhibitors.

10.5 Tissue selectivity and synthetic inhibitors

The inhibition of extrahepatic cholesterol biosynthesis probably contributes little to plasma cholesterol lowering and may lead to undesirable side-effects. Workers from Bristol Myers (Balasubramanian *et al.* 1989; Sit *et al.* 1990) compared the relative inhibitory potency of BMY21950 (**33a**) and XU-62320 (**18a**) with that of mevinolin in cell cultures isolated from several rat tissue types. The data indicated that BMY21950 was more selective for hepatocytes than extrahepatic tissues compared with the other two agents. An *in vivo* rat study, comparing BMY21950 and its corresponding lactone form (BMY22089) with mevinolin (dihydroxy acid form) and mevinolin respectively, showed that the two synthetic compounds had less inhibitory effect on sterol synthesis in ileal tissue than in hepatic tissue. Furthermore, mevinolin (dihydroxy acid form) had more marked effects than its lactone moiety in ileal tissue, which is consistent with the lower hepatic extraction and higher plasma levels of this dihydroxy acid form. In contrast, BMY21950 and the corresponding lactone form had similar activity in ileal tissue (Parker *et al.* 1990).

Karanewsky *et al.* (1990) and Robl *et al.* (1991) have compared the relative potency of the phosphinic acid analogues **26d** and **26f** with mevinolin and pravastatin in human skin fibroblasts and rat hepatocytes. Both phosphinic acid analogues were weaker inhibitors of cholesterol synthesis in fibroblasts than in hepatocytes, as was pravastatin. Conversely, mevinolin was a weaker inhibitor in hepatocytes than in fibroblasts.

Roth *et al.* (1991b) have examined the relationship between tissue selectivity and lipophilicity for a diverse range of inhibitors. Lipophilicity has been proposed as an influential factor affecting selectivity, with the more hydrophilic agents exhibiting higher hepatoselectivity. Compounds were tested as their sodium salts for their ability to inhibit the incorporation of $[^{14}C]$-acetate into sterols in tissue cubes from rat liver spleen and testis. The calculated octanol–water partition coefficients ($C \log P$) values for the selected inhibitors covered a range of nearly 5 logarithmic units, and so any trends could be detected. Generally, the results of a quantitative structure activity analysis indicated that compounds with $C \log P < 2$ were more selective for hepatic tissue and those with a $C \log P > 2$ were more selective for spleen and testis. Moreover the analysis revealed that peripheral tissue discriminated more on the basis of $C \log P$ with a parabolic dependence and an optimum around 2.5–3.0, whereas liver tissue was relatively insensitive to lower values of $C \log P$. Thus these studies suggest that liver selectivity is based on differential membrane selectivity, with compounds having a low $C \log P$ value being more selective for the liver.

Permeability in hepatic versus extrahepatic cells may account for these apparent selectivities. Furthermore, bioavailability, metabolism, and protein binding will almost certainly complicate the picture *in vivo*.

The concept of tissue selectivity has been addressed more recently (Menear *et al.* 1992). The affinity of bile acids for the enterohepatic circulation has been used to design agents targeted to the liver (Fig. 10.33). The requirements for bile acid transport depend on the topology of the molecule (the presence of a C17 side-chain terminating in an acid function and a chain length no greater than eight atoms) and on the presence of C3, C7 and C12 hydroxy groups. Thus the hybrid structure **41a** with the necessary structure of a bile acid and incorporating the 3,5-dihydroxy acid of most HMG-CoA reductase inhibitors has been evolved. The acylated derivative **41b** was prepared to introduce a side-chain ester proximate to the dihydroxy acid function, as in mevinolin. The *in vitro* activity of unresolved **41a** and **41b** was weak (IC$_{50}$ values of 39.2 μM and 12.3 μM respectively) compared with mevinolin (IC$_{50}$ = 3.69 nM). Compound **41b** was shown to be transported non-specifically, indicating that the predominant mode of transport does not involve bile acid binding protein and so might not be expected to exhibit tissue selectivity by passage through the enterohepatic circulation.

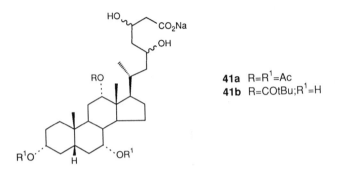

41a R=R^1=Ac
41b R=COtBu;R^1=H

Fig. 10.33 Inhibitors based on bile acids with potential to target agents to the liver (Menear *et al.* 1992).

10.6   Approaches based on other models

10.6.1   Inhibitors based on the natural substrate

Compounds designed to mimic the hemithioacetal intermediate reduction product of the natural substrate (HMG-CoA), but which cannot be reduced further to liberate mevalonic acid, have been reported by Fischer *et al.* (1985) and Turakhia *et al.* (1986). These agents bear a pantetheine-type residue rather than the complete coenzyme A-type chain (since mevaldic acid pantetheine hemithioacetal is a substrate for the second reduction) and have the natural labile C—S bond replaced by either a C—C or a C—N bond to give the ketones and alcohols **42a–42d** and the amide **42e** (Fig. 10.34). The ketones and alcohols are already in reduced form compared with the natural substrate, and none of the compounds has a good leaving group like the CoASH moiety. These compounds were only weak inhibitors of HMG-CoA reductase *in vitro*.

A similar approach has been outlined by Gordon *et al.* (1991a,b) who prepared compounds **42f–42h** with an extra methylene inserted between the pantetheinyl and glutaryl moieties, the amide analogues **42i** and **42j**, and the amine **42k**. These compounds also lacked significant inhibitory potency.

3-Hydroxy-3-methylglutaric acid (HMG) is known to be active as an inhibitor, and researchers at Searle have examined the effect of replacing the 3-methyl group with longer alkyl chains (Baran *et al.* 1985). The potency depends on the chain length, with C13–C17 being more potent (IC$_{50}$ = 50–100 μM, cf. compactin IC$_{50}$ = 1 μM) and exhibiting competitive inhibition. Ester derivatives, conversion of the diacid to a lactone, and removal of the 3-hydroxy function resulted in loss of activity. *In vivo*, the

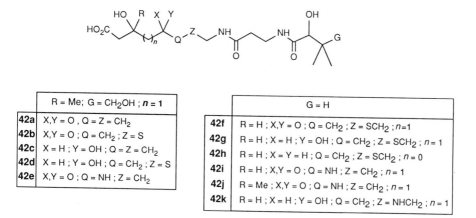

R = Me; G = CH₂OH ; n = 1	
42a	X,Y = O , Q = Z = CH$_2$
42b	X,Y = O ; Q = CH$_2$; Z = S
42c	X = H ; Y = OH ; Q = Z = CH$_2$
42d	X = H ; Y = OH ; Q = CH$_2$; Z = S
42e	X,Y = O ; Q = NH ; Z = CH$_2$

G = H	
42f	R = H ; X,Y = O ; Q = CH$_2$; Z = SCH$_2$; n=1
42g	R = H ; X = H ; Y = OH ; Q = CH$_2$; Z = SCH$_2$; n = 1
42h	R = H ; X = Y = H ; Q = CH$_2$; Z = SCH$_2$; n = 0
42i	R = H ; X,Y = O ; Q = NH ; Z = CH$_2$; n = 1
42j	R = Me ; X,Y = O ; Q = NH ; Z = CH$_2$; n = 1
42k	R = H ; X = H ; Y = OH ; Q = CH$_2$; Z = NHCH$_2$; n = 1

Fig. 10.34 Irreducible analogues of mevaldic acid coenzyme A thiohemiacetal.

pentadecyl derivative lowered serum cholesterol in triton-treated rats and prevented a rise in HMG-CoA reductase activity in rats pretreated with diazasterol, albeit at doses higher than for a comparable effect with compactin. The space-filling effect of the alkyl chain was likened to the pantetheine residue of coenzyme A and considered to play a significant role in binding to the enzyme.

10.6.2 Steroid-based modulators of cholesterogenesis

Oxygenated sterols play a role in the regulation of the expression of HMG-CoA reductase as described earlier, and there have been several reports of steroidal compounds which suppress cholesterol biosynthesis in this manner. Most notable are the cholestenes **43a** and **43b** described by Shroepfer's group (Swaminathan *et al.* 1992 and references cited therein) and the investigation of the metabolism and oxidative products of **43a** (Herz *et al.* 1992) affording another active compound **44** (Fig. 10.35). Compounds **43a** and **43b** reduce HMG-CoA reductase activity in CHO-K1 cells, with a 50 per cent reduction occurring at concentrations in the range 0.1–1.0 μM; compound **44** shows slightly weaker activity.

Workers at Du Pont have also patented a wide range of steroid derivatives, exemplified by **45**, which are capable of suppressing HMG-CoA reductase activity in Chinese hamster ovary (CHO) cells and inhibiting lanosterol-14α-demethylase from a rat microsomal preparation. These effects should be synergistic in inhibiting cholesterol biosynthesis. This was demonstrated for **45** by determining [^{14}C]-acetate incorporation into cholesterol in CHO cells where, at a concentration of 1 μM, cholesterol synthesis was reduced to 1 per cent of that of controls.

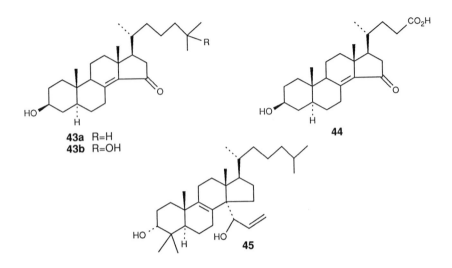

Fig. 10.35 Steroid-based modulators of HMG-CoA reductase: 43a, 43b, and 44 after Swaminathan *et al.* (1992); **45** after US Patent 5,041,432, 20 August 1991, to Du Pont.

This area of modulating HMG-CoA reductase activity is relatively un-explored and the search for agents which control the feedback mechanisms of cholesterol biosynthesis continues.

10.7 Conclusions

The discovery of HMG-CoA reductase inhibitors represented a major milestone in the treatment of hyperlipidaemia. Apart from providing an effective class of compounds for the treatment of elevated plasma choles-terol concentrations, they have played an important role in our under-standing of cholesterol homeostasis in man. The serendipitous discovery of the natural product compactin, and Endo's foresight in recognizing its value, resulted in the first potent HMG-CoA reductase which has served as a tool for mechanistic studies and a benchmark for medicinal chemists. The area has been further enhanced by the elegant work of Brown and Goldstein who forged the crucial link between inhibition of HMG-CoA reductase and reduction of plasma cholesterol levels via up-regulation of LDL receptors.

These factors have catalysed much effort to discover new inhibitors derived from microbial sources, to modify natural products, and to de-velop totally synthetic agents, with the first two categories providing the commercially available agents mevinolin (lovastatin, Mevacor®), eptastatin (pravastatin, Pravachol®), and synvinolin (simvastatin, Zocor®). In the case of the synthetic agents, many potent compounds have been discovered and the 'rules' for the design of compounds of this type are reasonably well defined. A number of these synthetic compounds are undergoing clinical evaluation but none have yet reached the market. Particularly notable are compounds **18a** (fluvastatin, Sandoz) and **14** (dalvastatin, Rhône Poulenc Rorer) which are currently in phase II–III of development. It remains to be seen whether these agents find a place in the treatment of hyperlipidaemia.

References

Albers-Schönberg, G., Joshua, H., Lopez, M. B., Hensens, O. D., Springer, J. P., Chen, J., *et al*. (1981). Dihydromevinolin, a potent hypocholesterolaemic metabolite produced by Aspergillus terreus. *Journal of Antibiotics*, **34**, 507–12.

Alberts, A. W., Chen, J., Kuron, G., Hunt, V., Huff, J., Hoffman, C., *et al*. (1980). Mevinolin, a highly potent competitive inhibitor of HMG-CoA reductase and cholesterol lowering agent. *Proceedings of the National Academy of Sciences of the United States of America*, **77**, 3957–61.

Ashton, M. J. (1991). HMG-CoA reductase inhibitors—recent developments. Drugs for the Treatment of Hyperlipidaemia, SCI Meeting, London, May 1991.

Ashton, M. J., Hills, S. J., Newton, C. G., Taylor, J. B., and Tondu, S. C. D. (1989). Synthesis of 6-aryl-4-hydroxypiperidin-2-ones and a possible application to the synthesis of a novel HMG-CoA reductase inhibitor. *Heterocycles*, **28**, 1015–31.

Baader, E., Bartmann, W., Beck, G., Below, P., Bergmann, A., Jendralla, H., *et al*. (1989). Enantioselective synthesis of a new fluoro-substituted HMG-CoA reductase inhibitor. *Tetrahedron Letters*, **30**, 5115–8.

Balasubramanian N., Brown, P. J., Catt, J. D., Han, W. T., Parker, R. A., Sit, S. Y., and Wright, J. J. (1989). A potent tissue-selective, synthetic inhibitor of HMG-CoA reductase. *Journal of Medicinal Chemistry*, **32**, 2038–41.

Baran, J. S., Laos, I., Langford, D. D., Miller, J. E., Jett, C., Taite, B., Rohrbacher, E. (1985). 3-Alkyl-3-hydroxyglutaric acids: a new class of hypocholesterolemic HMG-CoA reductase inhibitors. 1. *Journal of Medicinal Chemistry*, **28**, 597–601.

Basson, M. E., Thorsness, M., and Rine, J. (1986). Saccharomyces cerevisiae contains two functional genes encoding 3-hydroxy-3-methylglutaryl co-enzyme A reductase. *Proceedings of the National Academy of Sciences of the United States of America*, **83**, 5563–7.

Beck, G., Kesseler, K., Baader, E., Bartmann, W., Bergmann, A., Granzer, E., *et al*. (1990). Synthesis and biological activity of new HMG-CoA reductase inhibitors. 1. Lactones of pyridine- and pyrimidine-substituted 3,5-dihydroxy-6-heptenoic (-heptanoic) acids. *Journal of Medicinal Chemistry*, **33**, 52–60.

Bilheimer, B. W. (1988). The lipoprotein receptor concept. *Drugs*, **36** (Suppl. 3), 55–62.

Bone, E. A., Cunningham, E. M., Davidson, A. H., Galloway, W. A., Lewis, C. N., Morrice, C. M., *et al*. (1992). The design and biological evaluation of a series of 3-hydroxy-3-methylglutaryl co-enzyme A (HMG-CoA) inhibitors related to dihydromevinolin. *Bioorganic and Medicinal Chemistry Letters*, **2**, 223–8.

Boots, M. R., Boots, S. G., Noble, C. M., and Guyer, K. E. (1973). Hypercholesterolaemic agents II: Inhibition of β-hydroxy-β-methylglutaryl coenzyme A reductase by arylalkyl hydrogen succinates and glutarates. *Journal of Pharmaceutical Sciences*, **62**, 952–7.

Brown, M. S. and Goldstein, J. L. (1980). Multivalent feedback regulation of HMG CoA reductase, a control mechanism coordinating isoprenoid synthesis and cell growth. *Journal of Lipid Research*, **21**, 505–17.

Brown, M. S. and Goldstein, J. L. (1986). A receptor-mediated pathway for cholesterol homeostasis. *Angewandte Chemie International Edition*, **25**, 583–602.

Brown, A. G., Smale, T. C., King, T. J., Hasenkamp, R., and Thompson, R. H. (1976). Crystal and molecular structure of Compactin, a new antifungal metabolite from *Penicillium brevicompactum*. *Journal of the Chemical Society, Perkin Transactions I, Part I*, 1165–70.

Chin, J. C., Gil, G., Russell, G. W., Liscum, L., Luskey, K. L., Basu, S. K., *et al.* (1984). Nucleotide sequence of 3-hydroxy-3-methylglutaryl coenzyme A reductase, a glycoprotein of endoplasmic reticulum. *Nature, London*, **308**, 613–17.

Coppola, G. M. (1989). Design and synthesis of 4-oxoquinolin-2-yl-6-heptenoic acid derivatives as HMG-CoA reductase inhibitors. *Heterocycles*, **29**, 1497–1516.

Cosentino, U., Moro, G., Pitea, D., Scolastico, S., Todeschini, R., and Scolastico, C. (1992). Pharmacophore identification by molecular modeling and chemometrics: The case of HMG-CoA reductase inhibitors. *Journal of Computer-Aided Molecular Design*, **6**, 47–60.

DeCamp, A. E., Verhoeven, T. R., and Shinkai, I. (1989). Synthesis of (+)-dihydromevinolin by selective reduction of mevinolin. *Journal of Organic Chemistry*, **54**, 3207–8.

Dreyer, G. R. and Metcalf, B. W. (1988). *a,a*-Difluoroketone inhibitors of HMG-CoA reductase. *Tetrahedron Letters*, **29**, 6885–8.

Dreyer, G. B., Garvie, C. T., Metcalf, B. W., Meek, T. D., and Mayer, R. J. (1991). Phosphinic acid inhibitors of 3-hydroxy-3-methylglutaryl-coenzyme A reductase. *Bioorganic and Medicinal Chemistry Letters*, **1**, 151–4.

Dugan, R. E. and Katiyar, S. S. (1986). Evidence for catalytic site cysteine and histidine by chemical modification of β-hydroxy-β-methylglutaryl coenzyme A reductase. *Biochemical and Biophysical Research Communications*, **141**, 278–84.

Duggan, D. E. and Vickers, S. (1990). Physiological disposition of HMG-CoA reductase inhibitors. *Drug Metabolism Reviews*, **22**, 333–62.

Duggan, M. E., Alberts, A. W., Bostedor, R., Chao, Y., Germerhausen, J. I., Gilfillan, J. L., *et al.* (1991). 3-Hydroxy-3-methylglutaryl coenzyme A reductase inhibitors. 7. Modification of the hexahydronaphthalene moiety of simvastatin: 5-oxygenated and 5-oxa derivatives. *Journal of Medicinal Chemistry*, **34**, 2489–95.

Endo, A. (1979). Monacolin K, a new hypocholesterolaemic agent produced by a Monascus species. *Journal of Antibiotics*, **32**, 852–4.

Endo, A. (1985a). Compactin (ML-236B) and related compounds as potential cholesterol-lowering agents that inhibit HMG-CoA reductase. *Journal of Medicinal Chemistry*, **28**, 401–5.

Endo, A. (1985b). Drugs inhibiting HMG-CoA reductase. *Pharmacology and Therapeutics*, **31**, 257–67.

Endo, A. and Hasumi, K. (1985). Dihydromonacolin L and monacolin X, new metabolites those inhibit cholesterol biosynthesis. *Journal of Antibiotics*, **38**, 321–32.

Endo, A. and Hasumi, K. (1989). Biochemical aspect of HMG-CoA reductase inhibitors. *Advances in Enzyme Regulation*, **28**, 53–64.

Endo, A., Kuroda, M., and Tsujita, Y. (1976). ML-236A, ML-236B and ML-236C, new inhibitors of cholesterogenesis produced by *Penicillium citrinum*. *Journal of Antibiotics*, **29**, 1346–8.

Fischer, G. C., Turakhia, R. H., and Morrow, C. J. (1985). Irreducible analogues of mevaldic acid coenzyme A hemithioacetal as potential inhibitors of HMG-CoA reductase. Synthesis of a carbon-sulphur interchanged analogue of mevaldic acid pantetheine hemithioacetal. *Journal of Organic Chemistry*, **50**, 2011–19.

Germershausen, J. I., Hunt, V. M., Bostedor, R. G., Bailey, P. J., Karkas, J. D., and Alberts, A. W. (1989). Tissue selectivity of the cholesterol-lowering agents lovastatin, simvastatin and pravastatin in rats *in vivo*. *Biochemical and Biophysical Research Communications*, **158**, 667–75.

Goldstein, J. L. and Brown, M. S. (1990). Regulation of the mevalonate pathway. *Nature, London*, **343**, 425–30.

Gordon, E. M., Pluscec, J., and Ciosek, Jr., C. P. (1991a). Synthesis of substrate-based inhibitors of HMG-CoA reductase. *Bioorganic and Medicinal Chemistry Letters*, **1**, 61–4.

Gordon, E. M., Pluscec, J., and Ciosek, Jr., C. P. (1991b). Synthesis of substrate-based inhibitors of HMG-CoA reductase (II). *Bioorganic and Medicinal Chemistry Letters*, **1**, 161–4.

Guyer, K. E., Boots, S. G., Marecki, P. E., and Boots, M. R. (1976). Hyper-cholesterolaemic agents III: Inhibition of β-hydroxy-β-methylglutaryl coenzyme A reductase by half acid esters of 1-(4-biphenylyl)pentanol. *Journal of Pharmaceutical Sciences*, **65**, 548–52.

Haruyama, H., Kuwamo, H., Kinoshita, T., Terahara, A., Nishigaki, T., and Tamura, C. (1986). Structure elucidation of the bioactive metabolites of ML-236B (mevastatin) isolated from dog urine. *Chemical and Pharmaceutical Bulletin of Japan*, **34**, 1459–67.

Havel, R. J. (1988). Lowering cholesterol, rationale, mechanisms, and means. *Journal of Clinical Investigation*, **81**, 1653–60.

Heathcock, C. H., Hadley, C. R., Rosen, T., Theisen, P. D., and Hecker, S. J. (1987). Total synthesis and biological evaluation of structural analogues of compactin and dihydromevinolin. *Journal of Medicinal Chemistry*, **30**, 1858–73.

Henwood, J. M. and Heel, R. C. (1988). Lovastatin: A preliminary review of its pharmacodynamic properties and therapeutic use in hyperlipidaemia. *Drugs*, **36**, 429–54.

Herz, J. E., Swaminathan, S., Pinkerton, F. D., Wilson, W. K., and Schroepfer, Jr, G. J. (1992). Inhibitors of sterol synthesis. A highly efficient and specific side-chain oxidation of 3β-acetoxy-5α-cholest-8(14)-en-15-one for construction of metabolites and analogs of the 15-ketosterol. *Journal of Lipid Research*, **33**, 579–98.

Hoeg, J. M., Gregg, R. E., and Brewer, H. B., Jr. (1986). An approach to the management of hyperlipidaemia. *Journal of the American Medical Association*, **255**, 512–21.

Hoffman, W. F., Alberts, A. W., Anderson, P. S., Chen, J. S., Smith, R. L., and Willard, A. K. (1986a). 3-Hydroxy-3-methylglutaryl coenzyme A reductase inhibitors. 4. Side chain ester derivatives of mevinolin. *Journal of Medicinal Chemistry*, **29**, 849–52.

Hoffman, W. F., Alberts, A. W., Cragoe, E. J., Deana, A. A., Evans, B. E., Gilfillan, J. L., *et al.* (1986b). 3-Hydroxy-3-methylglutaryl-coenzyme A reductase inhibitors. 2. Structural modification of 7-(substituted aryl)-3,5-dihydroxy-6-heptenoic acids and their lactone derivatives. *Journal of Medicinal Chemistry*, **29**, 160–9.

Illingworth, D. R. (1991). Clinical implications of new drugs for lowering plasma cholesterol concentrations. *Drugs*, **41**, 151–60.

Innerarity, T. L. (1991). The low-density lipoprotein receptor. *Current Opinion in Lipidology*, **2**, 156–61.

Jendralla, H., Baader, E., Bartmann, W., Beck, G., Bergmann, A., Granzer, E., *et al.* (1990). Synthesis and biological activity of new HMG-CoA reductase inhibitors 2. Derivatives of 7-(1H-pyrrol-3-yl)-substituted-3,5-dihydroxyhept-6(*E*)-enoic (-heptanoic) acids. *Journal of Medicinal Chemistry*, **33**, 61–70.

Jendralla, H., Granzer, E., von. Kerekjarto, B., Krause, R., Schacht, U., Baader, E., *et al.* (1991). Synthesis and biological activity of new HMG-CoA reductase inhibitors. 3. Lactones of 6-phenoxy-3,5-dihydroxyhexanoic acids. *Journal of Medicinal Chemistry*, **34**, 2962–83.

Jordan-Starck, T. C. and Rodwell, V. W. (1989a). *Pseudomonas mevalonii* 3-hydroxy-3-methylglutaryl coenzyme A reductase: characterisation and chemical modification. *Journal of Biological Chemistry*, **264**, 17913–18.

Jordan-Starck, T. C. and Rodwell, V. W. (1989b). Role of cysteine residues in *Pseudomonas mevalonii* 3-hydroxy-3-methylglutaryl coenzyme A reductase. *Journal of Biological Chemistry*, **264**, 17919–23.

Karanewsky, D. S., Badia, M. C., Ciosek, Jr. C. P., Robl, J. A., Sofia, M. J., Simpkins, L. M., *et al.* (1990). Phosphorus-containing inhibitors of HMG-CoA reductase. 1. 4-[(2-Arylethyl)hydroxyphosphinyl]-3-hydroxybutanoic acids: a new class of cell-sensitive inhibitors of cholesterol biosynthesis. *Journal of Medicinal Chemistry*, **33**, 2952–6.

Kathawala, F. G. (1991). HMG-CoA reductase inhibitors: an exciting development in the treatment of hyperlipoproteinaemia. *Medicinal Research Reviews*, **11**, 121–46.

Kritchevsky, D. (1987). Inhibition of cholesterol synthesis. *Journal of Nutrition*, **117**, 1330–4.

Lee, T.-J., Holtz, W. J., and Smith, R. L. (1982). Structural modification of mevinolin. *Journal of Organic Chemistry*, **47**, 4750–7.

Lee, T.-J., Holtz, W. J., Smith, R. L., Alberts, A. W., and Gilfillan, J. L. (1991). 3-Hydroxy-3-methylglutaryl coenzyme A reductase inhibitors. 8. Side chain ether analogues of lovastatin. *Journal of Medicinal Chemistry*, **34**, 2474–7.

Liscum, L., Finer-Moore, J., Stroud, R. M., Luskey, K. L., Brown, M. S., and Goldstein, J. L. (1985). Domain structure of 3-hydroxy-3-methylglutaryl coenzyme A reductase, a glycoprotein of the endoplasmic reticulum. *Journal of Biological Chemistry*, **260**, 522–30.

Luskey, K. L. and Stevens, B. (1985). Human 3-hydroxy-3-methylglutaryl co-enzyme A reductase; conserved domains responsible for catalytic activity and sterol-regulated degradation. *Journal of Biological Chemistry*, **260**, 10271–7.

Menear, K. A., Patel, D., Clay, V., Howes, C., and Taylor, P. (1992). A novel approach to the site specific delivery of potential HMG-CoA reductase inhibitors. *Bioorganic and Medicinal Chemistry Letters*, **2**, 285–90.

Motoc, I., Sit, S. Y., Harte, W. E., Balasubramanian, N., and Wright, J. J. (1991). 3-Hydroxy-3-methylglutaryl-coenzyme A reductase: molecular modelling, three dimensional structure–activity relationships, inhibitor design. *Quantitative Structure–activity Relationships*, **10**, 30–5.

Nakamura, C. E. and Abeles, R. H. (1985). Mode of interaction of β-hydroxy-β-methylglutaryl coenzyme A reductase with strong binding inhibitors: Compactin and related compounds *Biochemistry*, **24**, 1364–76.

Parker, R. A., Clark, R. W., Sit, S. Y., Lanier, T. L., Grosso, R. A., and Wright, J. J. K. (1990). Selective inhibition of cholesterol synthesis in liver versus extrahepatic tissues by HMG-CoA reductase inhibitors. *Journal of Lipid Research*, **31**, 1271–82.

Prabhakar, Y. S., Saxena, A. K., and Doss, M. J. (1989). QSAR study of the role of hydrophobicity in the activity of HMGR inhibitors. *Drug Design and Delivery*, **4**, 97–108.

Prugh, J. D., Alberts, A. W., Deana, A. A., Gilfillian, J. L., Huff, J. W., Smith, R. L., and Wiggins, J. M. (1990). 3-Hydroxy-3-methylglutaryl-coenzyme A reductase inhibitors. 6. *Trans*-6-[2-(substituted -1-naphthyl)ethyl(or ethenyl)]-3,4,-5,6-tetrahydro-4-hydroxy-2*H*-pyran-2-ones. *Journal of Medicinal Chemistry*, **33**, 758–65.

Qureshi, N., Dugan, R. E., Cleland, W. W., and Porter, J. W. (1976). Kinetic analysis of the individual reductive steps catalysed by β-hydroxy-β-methylglutaryl coenzyme A reductase obtained from yeast. *Biochemistry*, **15**, 4191–7.

Robl, J. A., Duncan, L. A., Plusec, J., Karanewsky, D. S., Gordon, E. M., Ciosek, C. P., Jr, *et al*. (1991). Phosphorus-containing inhibitors of HMG-CoA reductase. 2. Synthesis and biological activities of a series of substituted pyridines containing a hydroxyphosphinyl moiety. *Journal of Medicinal Chemistry*, **34**, 2804–15.

Rogers, D. H., Panini, S. R., and Rudney, H. (1983). Properties of HMG-CoA reductase and its mechanism of action. In *3-Hydroxy-3-methylglutaryl co-enzyme A reductase* (ed. J. R. Sabine), pp. 57–75. CRC Press, Boca Raton, FL.

Roitelman, J. and Shechter, I. (1989). Studies on the catalytic site of rat liver HMG-CoA reductase: interaction with CoA-thioesters and inactivation by iodo-acetamide. *Journal of Lipid Research*, **30**, 97–107.

Roth, B. D., Ortwine, D. F., Hoefle, M. L., Stratton, C. D., Sliskovic, D. R., Wilson, M. W., and Newton, R. S. (1990). Inhibitors of cholesterol biosynthesis. 1. *Trans*-6-(2-pyrrol-1-ylethyl)-4-hydroxypyran-2-ones, a novel series of HMG-CoA reductase inhibitors. 1. Effects of structural modifications at the 2- and 5-positions of the pyrrole nucleus. *Journal of Medicinal Chemistry*, **33**, 21–31.

Roth, B. D., Blankley, C. J., Chucholowski, A. W., Ferguson, E., Hoefle, M. L., Ortwine, D. F., *et al*. (1991a). Inhibitors of cholesterol biosynthesis. 3. Tetra-hydro-4-hydroxy-6-[2-(1H-pyrrol-1-yl)ethyl]-2H-pyran-2-one inhibitors of HMG-CoA reductase. 2. Effects of introducing substituents at positions three and four of the pyrrole nucleus. *Journal of Medicinal Chemistry*, **34**, 357–66.

Roth, B. D., Bocan, T. M. A., Blankley, C. J., Chucholowski, A. W., Creger, P. L., Creswell, M. W., *et al*. (1991b). Relationship between tissue selectivity and lipophilicity for inhibitors of HMG-CoA reductase. *Journal of Medicinal Chemistry*, **34**, 463–6.

Sabine, J. R. (1983). General distribution and importance of HMG-CoA reductase.

In *3-Hydroxy-3-methylglutaryl coenzyme A reductase* (ed. J. R. Sabine), pp. 3–10. CRC Press, Boca Raton, FL.

Serizawa, N., Nakagawa, K., Tsujita, Y., Terahara, A., Kuwano, H., and Tanaka, M. (1983a). 6α-Hydroxy -iso-ML-236B (6α-hydroxy -iso-compactin) and ML-236A, microbial transformation products of ML-236B. *Journal of Antibiotics*, **36**, 918–20.

Serizawa, N., Serizawa, S., Nakagawa, K., Furuya, K., Okazaki, T., and Terahara, A. (1983b). Microbial hydroxylation of ML-236B (compactin) studies on organisms capable of 3β-hydroxylation of ML-236B. *Journal of Antibiotics*, **36**, 887–91.

Serizawa, N., Nakagawa, K., Hamano, K., Tsujita, Y., Terahara, A., and Kuwano, H. (1983c). Microbial hydroxylation of ML-236B (compactin) and monacolin K (MB-530B). *Journal of Antibiotics*, **36**, 604–7.

Sirtori, C. R. (1990). Pharmacology and mechanism of action of the new HMG-CoA reductase inhibitors. *Pharmacological Research*, **22**, 555–63.

Sit, S. Y., Parker, R. A., Motoc, I., Han, W., Balasubramanian, N., Catt, J. D., *et al.* (1990). Synthesis, biological profile, and quantitative structure–activity relationship of a series of novel 3-hydroxy-3-methylglutaryl coenzyme A reductase inhibitors. *Journal of Medicinal Chemistry*, **33**, 2982–99.

Slater, E. E. and MacDonald, J. S. (1988). Mechanism of action and biological profile of HMG-CoA reductase inhibitors. A new therapeutic alternative. *Drugs*, **36** (Suppl. 3), 72–82.

Sliskovic, D. R., Roth, B. D., Wilson, M. W., Hoefle, M. L., and Newton, R. S. (1990). Inhibitors of cholesterol biosynthesis. 2. 1,3,5-Trisubstituted [2-(tetrahydro-4-hydroxy-2-oxopyran-6-yl)ethyl]pyrazoles. *Journal of Medicinal Chemistry*, **33**, 31–8.

Sliskovic, D. R., Picard, J. A., Roark, W. H., Roth, B. D., Ferguson, E., Krause, B. R., *et al.* (1991). Inhibitors of cholesterol biosynthesis. 4. *Trans*-6-[2-(substituted-quinolinyl)ethenyl/ethyl]tetrahydro-4-hydroxy-2*H*-pyran-2-ones, a novel series of HMG-CoA reductase inhibitors. *Journal of Medicinal Chemistry*, **34**, 367–73.

Stokker, G. E., Hoffman, W. F., Alberts, A. W., Cragoe, E. J., Deana, A. A., Gilfillan, J. L., *et al.* (1985). 3-Hydroxy-3-methylglutaryl-coenzyme A reductase inhibitors. 1. Structural modification of 5-substituted 3,5-dihydroxypentanoic acids and their lactone derivatives. *Journal of Medicinal Chemistry*, **28**, 347–58.

Stokker, G. E., Alberts, A. W., Anderson, P. S., Cragoe, E. J., Deana, A. A., Gilfillan, J. L., *et al.* (1986a). 3-Hydroxy-3-methylglutaryl-coenzyme A reductase inhibitors 3. 7-(3,5-Disubstituted[1,1′-biphenyl]-2-yl)-3,5-dihydroxy-6-heptenoic acids and their lactone derivatives. *Journal of Medicinal Chemistry*, **29**, 170–81.

Stokker, G. E., Alberts, A. W., Gilfillan, J. L., Huff, J. W., and Smith, R. L. (1986b). 3-Hydroxy-3-methylglutaryl-coenzyme A reductase inhibitors. 5. 6-(Fluoren-9-yl)- and 6-(fluoren-9-ylidenyl)-3,5-dihydroxyhexanoic acids and their lactone derivatives. *Journal of Medicinal Chemistry*, **29**, 852–5.

Swaminathan, S., Pinkerton, F. D., and Schroepfer, Jr., G. J. (1992). Inhibitors of sterol synthesis. 3β,25-Dihydroxy-5α-cholest-8(14)-en-15-one, an active metabolite of 3β-hydroxy-5α-cholest-8(14)-en-15-one. *Journal of Medicinal Chemistry*, **35**, 793–5.

Taylor, F. R. and Kandutsch, A. A. (1985). Oxysterol binding protein. *Chemistry and Physics of Lipids*, **38**, 187–94.

Taylor, F. R., Saucier, S. E., Shown, E. P., Parish, E. J., and Kandutsch, A.

(1984). Correlation between oxysterol binding to a cytosolic binding protein and potency in the repression of hydroxymethylglutaryl coenzyme A reductase. *Journal of Biological Chemistry*, **259**, 12382–7.

Tobert, J. A. (1991). The HMG-CoA reductase inhibitors: similarities and differences. *Current Drugs: Antiatherosclerotic Agents*, B21–9.

Todd, P. A. and Goa, K. L. (1990). Simvastatin: A review of its pharmacological properties and therapeutic potential in hypercholesterolaemia. *Drugs*, **40**, 583–607.

Tsujita, Y., Kuroda, M., Shimada, Y., Tanzawa, K., Arai, M., Kaneko, I., *et al.* (1986). CS-514, a competitive inhibitor of 3-hydroxy-3-methylglutaryl coenzyme A reductase: tissue selective inhibition of sterol synthesis and hypolipidaemic effect on various animal species. *Biochimica et Biophysica Acta,* **877**, 50–60.

Turakhia, R. H., Fischer, G. C., Morrow, C. J., Maschhoff, B. L., Toubbeh, M. I., and Zbur-Wilson, J. I. (1986). Irreducible analogues of mevaldic acid coenzyme A hemithioacetal as potential inhibitors of HMG-CoA reductase. Synthesis of a secondary alcohol analogue of mevaldic acid pantetheine hemithioacetal and an amide analogue of 3-hydroxy-3-methylglutaryl-S-pantetheine. *Journal of Organic Chemistry*, **51**, 1955–60.

Veloso, D., Cleland, W. W., and Porter, J. W. (1981). pH properties and chemical mechanism of action of 3-hydroxy-3-methylglutaryl coenzyme A reductase. *Biochemistry*, **20**, 887–94.

Wang, Y., Darnay, B. G., and Rodwell, V. W. (1990). Identification of the principal catalytically important acidic residue of 3-hydroxy-3-methylglutaryl coenzyme A reductase. *Journal of Biological Chemistry*, **265**, 21634–41.

Yamashita, H., Tsubokawa, S., and Endo, A. (1985). Microbial hydroxylation of compactin (ML-236B) and monacolin K. *Journal of Antibiotics*, **38**, 605–9.

11

DNA topoisomerases

Jennifer Fostel and Linus L. Shen

11.1   Topoisomerase function and characteristics

11.1.1   Catalytic functions

DNA topoisomerases are a class of enzymes that modulate the topological structure of DNA. Since the discovery of the first topoisomerase 20 years ago (Wang 1971), many of the properties of this class of enzymes have been elucidated and this progress has been the subject of many reviews (Cozzarelli 1980; Gellert 1981; Liu 1983; Drlica 1984; Wang 1985, 1987b; Maxwell and Gellert 1986; Yanagida and Wang 1987; Osheroff 1989a; Austin and Fisher 1990, Champoux 1990; Hsieh 1990; Osheroff et al. 1991). In purified systems, topoisomerases relax supercoiled DNA, and can tie and untie DNA knots, and link and unlink catenated DNA circles. In eukaryotic cells, type I topoisomerases are associated with elongating transcription and replication forks, while type II topoisomerases are essential for segregating daughter chromosomes after DNA replication is complete (Yanagida and Wang 1987). Topoisomerases are also the target of a number of antineoplastic and antibacterial agents whose cytotoxic effects appear to arise from the stabilization of a complex between the topoisomerase and DNA (Ross 1985; Glisson and Ross 1987; Drlica and Franco 1988; Liu 1989; Smith 1990).

11.1.1.1 *DNA topology*

Topoisomerases are enzymes which change the topological structure of DNA, therefore it is necessary to give some definitions relating to DNA topology itself before summarizing the characteristics of these enzymes (Crick 1976; Wang 1980). The number of times that the two strands of DNA are interwound in a covalently closed molecule is defined as the linking number of that molecule. Since the average helical pitch of unconstrained DNA is 10.4 base pairs per turn (Wang 1979), a relaxed covalently closed DNA circle will have a linking number equal to an integral value near $N/10.4$, where N is the length of the DNA in base pairs. Underwound, or negatively supercoiled, DNA circles will have linking numbers smaller than this value, while overwound, or positively supercoiled, circles have linking numbers greater than this value. The linking number of a DNA circle cannot be altered unless at least one of the DNA strands is transiently broken to allow the interwinding of the two strands to be changed.

DNA molecules that are otherwise identical and differ only in their linking number are referred to as topological isomers, or topoisomers, and can easily be resolved by agarose gel electrophoresis (Keller 1975). Some topoisomerases can supertwist DNA and some relax positively or negatively supercoiled DNA circles to generate a population of relaxed topoisomers. In addition, circular DNA molecules can form other topological isomers, for instance knotted structures, which can be isolated from bacteriophage P4 capsids (Liu *et al.* 1981), and catenated rings, which are often the initial product of the replication of DNA circles (Hudson *et al.* 1968; Yang *et al.* 1987). These DNA species can also serve as substrates for topoisomerases, which are able to introduce and remove knots, under different reaction conditions, and also reversibly catenate and decatenate DNA circles (Fig. 11.1). Not all topoisomerases can carry out all of these reactions, and topoisomerases are classified as either type I or type II enzymes on the basis of this mechanistic difference.

11.1.1.2 *Reaction mechanism distinguishes type I and type II topoisomerases*

The action of a topoisomerase must include the formation of a transient break in the DNA backbone, since the linking number of DNA cannot change without such a break, and topoisomerases are classified as either type I or type II on the basis of this break. Type I topoisomerases introduce a transient break in one strand of DNA at a time, whereas type II topoisomerases introduce concerted breaks in both DNA strands to produce a double-strand break in the DNA. This difference in mechanism allows type II topoisomerases to catenate and decatenate covalently closed double-stranded DNA rings (Hsieh and Brutlag 1980; Kreuzer and Cozzarelli 1980),

I Knotting – unknotting

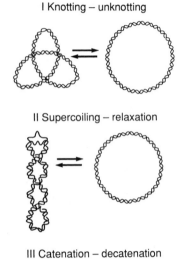

II Supercoiling – relaxation

III Catenation – decatenation

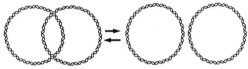

Fig. 11.1 Schematic representation of the interconversion of circular double-stranded DNA topoisomers catalysed by DNA topoisomerases.

and also to knot and unknot covalently closed double-stranded circles (Liu *et al.* 1980; Hsieh 1983). The type I topoisomerases, however, cannot catenate or decatenate double-stranded DNA unless a nick or gap is present in one of the circles (Tse and Wang 1980; Brown and Cozzarelli 1981).

The bacterial type II topoisomerase can utilize the energy of ATP hydrolysis to introduce negative supercoils into DNA and for this reason is referred to as a DNA 'gyrase' (Gellert *et al.* 1976a). Only the bacterial topoisomerase II can perform this reaction; the purified eukaryotic type II topoisomerases can only relax DNA. The mechanistic basis for this difference appears to lie in the interactions of these enzymes with DNA. The eukaryotic topoisomerase II interacts with a stretch of only 25 nucleotides (Lee *et al.* 1989), whereas during the gyrase reaction a DNA segment of approximately 150 nucleotides is wrapped around gyrase with a positive superhelical sense (Liu and Wang 1978a; Kirkegaard and Wang 1981, Morrison and Cozzarelli 1981; Kirchhausen *et al.* 1985) and this imparts directionality to the strand passage reaction.

11.1.1.3   *Strand passage model of topoisomerase mechanism*

The mechanism of the type II topoisomerase is believed to involve the passage of a DNA segment through this transient double-strand break (Brown and Cozzarelli 1979; by Hsieh 1990; Osheroff *et al*. 1991), and the type II topoisomerases alter the linking number of the DNA in steps of two which is consistent with this mechanistic model (Brown and Cozzarelli 1979; Hsieh and Brutlag 1980; Liu *et al*. 1980). ATP is hydrolysed during the topoisomerase II reaction. This step is likely to occur after strand passage and prior to reinitiation of catalysis, since the type II eukaryotic topoisomerases that have been studied display limited strand-passing activity in the presence of non-hydrolysable ATP analogues (Hsieh 1990; Osheroff *et al*. 1991). Two models of the type I topoisomerase mechanism have been proposed (Champoux 1990). Experimental evidence reveals that the type I topoisomerase binds DNA and introduces a nick in one strand. The enzyme could then pass the unbroken strand through this nick in a mechanism similar to the type II topoisomerases, or the type I topoisomerase could swivel the nicked strand around the unbroken strand which would have the same net topological effect. The type I topoisomerase would then reseal the nick and dissociate or reinitiate a new round of catalysis.

11.1.2   Structure and characteristics of topoisomerase enzymes

11.1.2.1   *Prokaryotic type I topoisomerases*

The first topoisomerase identified was the type I topoisomerase from *Escherichia coli* (Wang 1971). This enzyme has a molecular weight of 97.4 kDa, and acts as a monomer (Depew *et al*. 1978; Tse-Dinh and Wang 1986). The prokaryotic type I topoisomerase can only relax negatively supercoiled DNA under normal conditions, although it can relax positively supercoiled DNA if a single-stranded loop has been introduced into one strand of the DNA substrate to provide a binding site for the enzyme (Kirkegaard and Wang 1985). The bacterial topoisomerase I requires exogenous magnesium for activity (Wang 1971; Kung and Wang 1977). These last two properties distinguish the prokaryotic topoisomerase I from the eukaryotic topoisomerase I, which can relax both positively and negatively supercoiled DNA and is active in the presence of EDTA (Champoux and Dulbecco 1972).

In addition to topoisomerase I, a second type I topoisomerase, termed topoisomerase III, has been isolated from *E. coli*. Topoisomerase III has a molecular weight of 75 kDa, which is distinct from that of *E. coli* topoisomerase I. The two topoisomerases also show different spectra of cleavage sites (Dean *et al*. 1982; Srivenugopol *et al*. 1984). Topoisomerase III shows a greater ability *in vitro* to decatenate nicked DNA than to relax supercoiled DNA (DiGate and Marians 1988), in contrast with topoi-somerase I which displays a higher level of DNA relaxation activity. Since topoisomerases I and III appear to have different properties in terms of both activity and structure, it is possible that each of these enzymes will serve as a target for novel antibacterial agents.

11.1.2.2 Eukaryotic type I topoisomerases

Type I topoisomerases with apparent molecular weights of 100 kDa have been isolated from a variety of eukaryotic sources, including HeLa cells (Liu and Miller 1981), human placenta (Holden et al. 1990), mouse FM3A cells (Ishii et al. 1983), chicken erythrocytes (Tricoli and Kowalski 1983), Saccharomyces cerevisiae (Goto et al. 1984), and wheat germ (Dynan et al. 1981). These enzymes act as monomers (Liu and Miller 1981; Ishii et al. 1983; Tricoli and Kowalski 1983). The eukaryotic topoisomerase I appears to contain structures in addition to its catalytic domain, since proteolysed forms of the enzyme retain activity in vitro (Martin et al. 1983). Genetic truncations of the type I topoisomerase structure reveal that the N-terminal portion can be removed without loss of activity (Bjornsti and Wang 1987; D'Arpa et al. 1988), suggesting that this region is not necessary for catalysis.

In addition to type I topoisomerases with molecular weights of approxi-mately 100 kDa, type I enzymes with higher apparent molecular weights have been isolated from Xenopus laevis oocytes and from Drosophila melanogaster embryos. These enzymes have apparent molecular weights of 165 kDa and 135 kDa respectively (Javaherian et al. 1982; Richard and Bogenhagen 1989). In X. laevis, the 165 kDa topoisomerase I is found in ovaries, while a 100 kDa topoisomerase I is isolated from somatic tissue. These two forms are immunologically distinct, and thus the 100 kDa somatic topoisomerase I is not likely to be a proteolytic fragment of the 165 kDa species. The 165 kDa topoisomerase is lost as the oocyte matures (Richard and Bogenhagen 1991). Therefore it appears that X. laevis oocytes contain a specific topoisomerase I which has a substantially larger apparent molecular weight than the topoisomerase isolated from somatic tissue.

11.1.2.3 Sequence homology among type I topoisomerases

The DNA sequences encoding the type I topoisomerase from human (D'Arpa et al. 1988), Schizosaccharomyces pombe (Uemura et al. 1987), S. cerevisiae (Goto and Wang 1985; Thrash et al. 1985), and the eukaryotic virus vaccinia (Shuman and Moss 1987) have been determined, as have the sequence of the two E. coli type I topoisomerases (Tse-Dinh and Wang 1986; DiGate and Marians 1989). The two genes encoding the bacterial type I topoisomerases (E. coli topoisomerases I and III) show homology in the central portion of the coding region; however, there are structural differences outside this region. Most notably, the putative zinc-finger domain motifs found in topoisomerase I (Tse-Dinh and Beran-Steed 1988) are not detected in the gene encoding topoisomerase III (DiGate and Marians 1989).

There appears to be very little sequence conservation between the *E. coli* topoisomerase I and eukaryotic type I topoisomerases, although it is possible to pick out a short stretch of conserved amino acids near the amino terminus of the protein (Tse *et al*. 1980). The lack of common sequence structure is perhaps not surprising in the light of the different catalytic characteristics and requirements displayed by these two classes of topoisomerases.

The sequences encoding the type I topoisomerases from human and *S. pombe* and *S. cerevisiae* show conservation over the major portion of the gene, encompassing all but the N-terminal 25 per cent. With conservative substitutions, the degree of homology between human and fission and budding yeast topoisomerase sequences is approximately 50 per cent (Thrash *et al*. 1985; Uemura *et al*. 1987; D'Arpa *et al*. 1988; Lynn *et al*. 1989). A conserved 70 amino acid domain has been identified near the C-terminal of eukaryotic type I topoisomerases which appears to contain the active site of the enzyme (Lynn *et al*. 1989). The amino acid in topoisomerase I which becomes linked to DNA has been identified by physical means, and found to be tyrosine-727 in *S. cerevisiae* (Eng *et al*. 1989; Lynn *et al*. 1989) and the homologous tyrosine-771 in *S. pombe* (Eng *et al*. 1989). When the tyrosine residue at position 727 of the *S. cerevisiae* topoisomerase I is replaced by a phenylalanine residue, the resulting protein is inactive (Eng *et al*. 1989), suggesting that this tyrosine is necessary for catalytic activity.

Recently, two additional genes from *S. cerevisiae* have been identified which appear to encode proteins with homology to known type I topoisomerases. These are the *HPR*1 gene which has a domain homologous to the yeast topoisomerase I (Aguilera and Klein 1990), and the *TOP*3 gene which is homologous to the *E. coli* topoisomerase I (Wallis *et al*. 1989). The protein products encoded by these genes are still being characterized, although it appears that the *TOP*3 gene product has topoisomerase activity (Drlica 1990). The *TOP*3 gene was identified by the hyper-recombination phenotype displayed by cells deficient in this locus, and the *HPR*1 gene was identified through a defect in extra-ribosomal DNA recombination; and thus it is likely that the *TOP*3 and *HPR*1 gene products are involved in recombination of genes outside the nucleolus (Wallis *et al*. 1989; Aguilera and Klein 1990).

11.1.2.4 *Type II topoisomerases*

Type II topoisomerases have been isolated from a number of eukaryotic sources, including human (Miller *et al*. 1981), calf thymus (Halligan *et al*. 1985), *D. melanogaster* (Hsieh and Brutlag 1980), and *S. cerevisiae* (Goto and Wang 1982) cells. The eukaryotic type II topoisomerases are homo-dimers consisting of two identical subunits with apparent molecular weight ranging from 155 to 170 kDa, resulting in a holoenzyme of apparent molecular weight 310–340 kDa (Miller *et al.* 1981; Goto and Wang 1982; Sander and Hsieh 1983). Recently, an additional form of topoisomerase II has been isolated from human cells (Drake *et al.* 1989). This enzyme has an apparent subunit molecular weight of 180 kDa, and appears to be encoded in a different genetic locus from the locus encoding the topoisomerase with 170 kDa subunits (Chung *et al.* 1989; Tan *et al.* 1992).

Type II topoisomerases isolated from prokaryotic cells (DNA gyrase) have a tetrameric A_2B_2 structure (Higgins *et al.* 1978; Liu and Wang 1978b; Mizuuchi *et al.* 1978). The *E. coli* gyrase enzyme consists of two A subunits and two B subunits, which are ca. 105 kDa and ca. 95 kDa respectively. An additional type II topoisomerase is found in *E. coli* cells infected by the bacteriophage T4. This T4-encoded enzyme is a complex of at least two copies of each of three subunits of 58 kDa, 50 kDa, and 18 kDa respectively (Liu *et al.* 1979; Stetler *et al.* 1979; Kreuzer and Jongeneel 1983). The T4 topoisomerase is interesting in that it appears to share several properties with eukaryotic type II topoisomerases. For instance, the T4 topoisomerase can relax supercoiled DNA but is unable to introduce superhelical turns into relaxed DNA. Additionally, the T4 topoisomerase is sensitive to a number of compounds that target eukaryotic type II topoisomerases, and is relatively insensitive to nalidixic acid and oxolinic acid which target the bacterial gyrases (Huff *et al.* 1989; Huff and Kreuzer 1990).

The function of the gyrase subunits has been dissected by physical and genetic techniques. Mutations conferring resistance to novobiocin, a competitive inhibitor of ATP binding, have been mapped to the *gyrB* gene (Drlica 1984), and affinity labelling of the ATP binding site has localized this domain to amino acid residues 93–131 in the *gyrB* subunit (Tamura and Gellert 1990). Most mutations conferring resistance to nalidixic acid and other new quinolones that stimulate gyrase-mediated DNA cleavage occur in the *gyrA* locus (Drlica 1984), and are frequently found in a region spanning residues 67–106 (Yamagishi *et al.* 1981; Yoshida *et al.* 1988; Sreedharan *et al.* 1990). The gyrase A subunit is the portion of gyrase that interacts with DNA (Sugino *et al.* 1980; Tse *et al.* 1980), and Tyr-122 of this subunit is found linked to DNA after the reaction is interrupted (Horowitz and Wang 1987). The gyrase A subunit can be dissected into two functional domains, with the N-terminal 64 kDa domain responsible for DNA breaking and rejoining (Reece and Maxwell 1991b) while the C-terminal 33 kDa domain has DNA-binding activity (Reece and Maxwell 1991a).

11.1.2.5 *Sequence homology among type II topoisomerases*
The sequences encoding several eukaryotic type II topoisomerases have been determined, including the human (Tsai-Pflugfelder *et al.* 1988),

D. melanogaster (Wyckoff *et al*. 1989), *S. pombe* (Uemura *et al*. 1986), and *S. cerevisiae* (Giaever *et al*. 1986) enzymes. A striking homology is revealed when the predicted amino acid sequences of the *D. melanogaster*, *S. cerevisiae* and *S. pombe* type II topoisomerases are aligned (Wyckoff *et al*. 1989). The sequence of the N-terminal 1200 amino acids is highly conserved among these different species, while the C-terminal third diverges. In this N-terminal portion, 46 per cent of the residues are identical between *D. melanogaster*, *S. cerevisiae*, and *S. pombe* (Wyckoff *et al*. 1989). The sequences of the genes encoding the DNA gyrases from *E. coli* (Yamagishi *et al*. 1981; Adachi *et al*. 1987; Swanberg and Wang 1987) and *Bacillus subtilis* (Moriya *et al*. 1985) also contain many of these conserved residues. The gyrase B subunit is homologous to the first third of the eukaryotic type II topoisomerase, and the N-terminal domain of the gyrase A subunit is homologous to the middle third (Wyckoff *et al*. 1989). This conserved protein structure is also seen in the sequence of the T4-encoded topoisomerase II (Huang 1986a,b; Huang *et al*. 1988).

Recently, the sequences of two *E. coli* genes, *parC* and *parE*, have been determined. These genes appear to encode protein products that share homology with the *E. coli* gyrase A and B subunits (Kato *et al*. 1990). The *parC* gene product is essential for DNA partitioning after cell division. Lysates of cells that overexpress *parC* and *parE* contain elevated levels of DNA relaxation activity, and for this reason the authors proposed the name topoisomerase IV for the *parC/parE* gene products (Kato *et al*. 1990). The question of whether eukaryotes possess a gene homologous to the *E. coli parC/parE* locus remains to be answered. In this context it is interesting to note that two genes, encoding different type II topoisomerases, have been identified in human cells (Tsai-Pflugfelder *et al*. 1988; Tan *et al*. 1992).

11.1.3 Physiological role of DNA topoisomerases

11.1.3.1 *Eukaryotic topoisomerases*

Topoisomerase I molecules have been physically localized to regions of transcriptional activity in eukaryotic cells by a variety of methods, including physical fractionation of the cell (Higashinakagawa *et al*. 1977), immunological staining (Fleischmann *et al*. 1984; Muller *et al*. 1985), and UV-induced cross-linking (Gilmour *et al*. 1986). In addition, when antibodies to topoisomerase I are injected into isolated salivary glands of *Chironomus tentans*, the synthesis of large transcripts is decreased markedly. The injection of exogenous topoisomerase I isolated from rat cells can overcome this effect; thus the decrease in transcription arises from insufficient topoisomerase I rather than blockage of transcription forks by the antibody–enzyme complex (Egyhazi and Durban 1987). The movement of the transcription machinery along DNA requires the relative rotation of large molecules. Consideration of the physical forces involved led to the suggestion that this rotation occurs in the DNA (Liu and Wang 1987). In eukaryotic cells this is most likely to occur through the action of topoisomerase I.

Genetic studies using *S. cerevisiae* and *S. pombe* have demonstrated that, while the presence of a topoisomerase I gene is not essential for viability in cells containing normal levels of topoisomerase II (Thrash *et al.* 1984; Goto and Wang 1985; Uemura *et al.* 1987), the lack of a functional type I topoisomerase leads to reduced rate of growth and a decrease in large RNA transcripts (Brill *et al.* 1987), much as is observed when topoisomerase I activity is reduced by the injection of antibodies to the enzyme. Topoisomerase II, however, is an essential enzyme (Yanagida and Wang 1987). Yeast cells without functional topoisomerase II die when they attempt to segregate of daughter chromosomes during cell division (DiNardo *et al.* 1984; Holm *et al.* 1985); thus it is likely that topoisomerase II plays a major role in this process. The segregation of daughter chromosomes is topologically equivalent to the decatenation of linked DNA circles, a reaction carried out by topoisomerase II *in vitro*.

Yeast cells containing deletions in the gene encoding topoisomerase I and a temperature-sensitive mutation in the topoisomerase II gene demonstrate alterations in the genetic organization of their ribosomal RNA genes. Cells with low levels of topoisomerase show 100-fold increases in the level of recombination in the rDNA (Christman *et al.* 1988) and excise their rDNA in the form of extrachromosomal circles, which reintegrate once the level of topoisomerase in the cell is increased (Kim and Wang 1989). Both these observations correlate increased levels of recombination in the ribosomal genes with decreased levels of topoisomerase. An interpretation of this observation is that diminished topoisomerase I activity leads to an increase in torsional strain, particularly in the heavily transcribed rDNA genes. This, in turn, may lead to increased interactions between different DNA segments, thereby facilitating recombination. However, since the newly identified *S. cerevisiae* genes, whose products share sequence homology with topoisomerases, are also associated with recombination, and since these gene products do not show major topoisomerase activity within the cell (Wang *et al.* 1990), the role of topoisomerase I in recombination may be more fundamental than simply controlling the torsional strain of DNA.

11.1.3.2 *Role of topoisomerases in prokaryotic cells*

As is the case for eukaryotic topoisomerase II, gyrase is required for DNA segregation after cell division (Steck and Drlica 1984). However, the gene encoding the *E. coli* topoisomerase I cannot be deleted without a compensatory genetic change, often affecting gyrase activity (DiNardo *et al.* 1982; Pruss *et al.* 1982). The reason for this difference may lie in the observation that the topoisomerases found in prokaryotic cells carry out different reactions from those performed by their eukaryotic counterparts. Eukaryotic topoisomerase I and topoisomerase II can both relax positively and negatively supercoiled DNA. In contrast, the prokaryotic gyrase introduces negative supercoils into relaxed DNA, thus unwinding the DNA strands, while the prokaryotic topoisomerase I is capable of relaxing negatively supercoiled DNA but under normal conditions is unable to relax positively supercoiled DNA.

A model has been put forward by Liu and Wang (1987) based on the observation that, during transcription, the nascent transcript must rotate relative to the DNA strand. An analysis of the physical forces involved and the rate of transcription led to the hypothesis that the DNA, rather than the transcription complex, is rotating and that this rotation is performed by topoisomerases. As the transcription complex moves along the DNA, positive supercoils build up in front of the moving complex while negative supercoils are found behind it. Thus the transcription complex partitions the transcribed DNA into twin domains with opposite senses of supercoiling handedness. The bacterial topoisomerase I acts on negative supercoils and so relaxes the domain behind the transcription complex, while the gyrase is able to act ahead of the complex, introducing negative supercoils to relax the overwound strands. Extensive evidence has been gathered to support this hypothesis, both in purified systems (Yang *et al*. 1987; Wu *et al*. 1988; Tsao *et al*. 1989; Ostrander *et al*. 1990) and in cells (Figueroa and Bossi 1988; Giaever *et al*. 1988; Giaever and Wang 1988).

11.2 Interactions of different therapeutic drugs with DNA topoisomerases

11.2.1 Mechanism and specificity of topoisomerase poisons

11.2.1.1 *Cleavable complex formation and interactions with drugs* in vitro

As part of their interaction with DNA, both type I and type II topoisomerases reversibly form a complex with DNA (Champoux 1977; Gellert *et al*. 1977; Sugino *et al*. 1977; Depew *et al*. 1978; Sander and Hsieh 1983). This has been termed the cleavable complex (Liu *et al*. 1983; Chen and Liu 1986) since, although the form of DNA in the complex is unknown, the addition of protein denaturants leads to DNA nicking, in the case of a type I topoisomerase, or DNA breakage, in the case of a type II topoisomerase. The denatured topoisomerase is covalently linked to one of the newly formed DNA ends through a phosphodiester linkage with a tyrosine residue. The eukaryotic type I topoisomerase is attached to the 3′ end of the nick (Champoux 1978), while the subunits of the eukaryotic type II topoisomerase (Liu *et al*. 1983; Sander and Hsieh 1983), the prokaryotic type I topoisomerase (Depew *et al.* 1978; Tse *et al.* 1980), and the gyrase A subunit of the prokaryotic type II topoisomerase (Sugino *et al.* 1980; Tse *et al.* 1980) are linked to the new 5′ end of the DNA. The mechanistic significance of this polarity difference is unknown.

This cleavable complex can be stabilized by the addition of a number of compounds to the reaction mixture using purified topoisomerase (Ross 1985; Glisson and Ross 1987; Drlica and Franco 1988; Liu 1989; Smith 1990). The antitumour drug camptothecin and its derivatives (see §11.2.4.1) target the eukaryotic type I topoisomerase (Hsiang *et al.* 1985). A number of different drugs target the eukaryotic type II topoisomerase, including intercalators such as adriamycin (Tewey *et al.* 1984) (see §11.2.3.2), amsacrine (Nelson *et al.* 1984), and ellipticine (Ross *et al.* 1984; Tewey *et al.* 1984) (see §11.2.3.5), and the epipodophyllotoxins, which do not intercalate into DNA (Chen *et al.* 1984) (see §11.2.3.3). DNA gyrase is the target of the quinolone family of antibacterial agents (Gellert *et al.* 1977; Sugino *et al.* 1977) (see §11.2.2). More details of studies relating to these interactions are presented later in this chapter.

11.2.1.2   *Topoisomerase poisons target the topoisomerase in the cell*
It is likely that topoisomerases are the target of these drugs in the cell as well as *in vitro*, as demonstrated by genetic experiments. The topoisomerase I gene can be disrupted in *S. cerevisiae* using genetic techniques, leading to a yeast strain that does not contain a functional topoisomerase I. When this is done in strains of yeast that are normally sensitive to camptothecin, the disruption of topoisomerase I is correlated with the acquisition of a camptothecin-resistant phenotype. When topoisomerase I is reintroduced into the cell, the cell regains its sensitivity to camptothecin (Eng *et al.* 1988; Nitiss and Wang 1988). When the gene encoding the human topoisomerase I is introduced into the topoisomerase-I-deficient yeast strains, the cells regain camptothecin sensitivity, demonstrating that the human topoisomerase I is also the target of camptothecin in these cells (Bjornsti *et al.* 1989).

It is difficult to perform similar experiments in mammalian cells; however, it is likely that the mammalian topoisomerase I is the target of camptothecin in these cells as is the case in yeast. Two mammalian cell lines, which were selected on the basis of resistance to camptothecin, have been found to contain an altered form of topoisomerase I which is itself resistant to camptothecin *in vitro* (Gupta *et al.* 1988; Kjeldsen *et al.* 1988). Thus mammalian cells containing a camptothecin-resistant form of topoisomerase I are themselves more resistant than wild-type cells to the cytotoxic effects of camptothecin.

Similar experiments, in which the topoisomerase II is genetically removed, cannot be performed since topoisomerase II is essential for cell growth. However, the recent reports of drug-resistant topoisomerase II enzymes isolated from cells resistant to etoposide (Sullivan *et al.* 1989) or amsacrine (Hinds *et al.* 1991) suggest that topoisomerase II is the intracellular target of these drugs in mammalian cells. In addition, the isolation and characterization of the protein linked to DNA following exposure to topoisomerase II poisons has revealed that this protein is topoisomerase II (Minford *et al.* 1986).

The formation of the topoisomerase–DNA complex in the cell can be monitored by lysing the cell with sodium dodecylsulphate (SDS) which traps the topoisomerase–DNA complex and leads to protein-linked DNA damage. A correlation between the level of protein-linked DNA damage and cell cytotoxicity in the presence of different topoisomerase poisons has been observed in several studies (Zwelling *et al.* 1981; Wozniak and Ross 1983; Rowe *et al.* 1985; Hsiang *et al.* 1989c), and thus it is likely that the formation of the topoisomerase–DNA complex in the cell triggers cell death (D'Arpa and Liu 1989; Liu 1989). In this sense, the drug converts the topoisomerase into a cellular poison. Therefore these drugs are fundamentally different from classical enzyme inhibitors. In the case of enzyme inhibitors, increasing the amount of target enzyme can overcome the effects of the inhibitors. The opposite is true in the case of topoisomerases, where the presence of more enzyme molecules leads to a higher level of stabilized topoisomerase–DNA complexes, thus making the cell more sensitive to the drug.

11.2.1.3 *Basis of cytotoxicity of type I topoisomerase poison*

Exposure of cells to camptothecin leads to inhibition of DNA and RNA synthesis, blocking of the cell-cycle progression into mitosis, reversible DNA fragmentation, and cell death (Li *et al.* 1972; Horwitz and Horwitz 1973). The presence of camptothecin blocks transcription in purified systems containing eukaryotic topoisomerase I (Bendixen *et al.* 1990). Interestingly, cells undergoing DNA replication are much more sensitive to the cytotoxic effects of topoisomerase poisons than are cells in other stages of the cell cycle. Cells exposed to camptothecin during different stages of the cell cycle show up to 1000-fold more sensitivity when it is administered while the cells are undergoing DNA replication (Li *et al.* 1972; Drewinko *et al.* 1974). When aphidicolin, a DNA synthesis inhibitor which stops the progression of DNA replication forks, is administered concurrently with camptothecin, the cells are protected from camptothecin cytotoxicity (Holm *et al.* 1989; Hsiang *et al.* 1989b). Thus if the replication fork is halted, the stabilization of the topoisomerase–DNA complex does not result in cytotoxicity.

Interestingly, the level of cleavable complex formed in the cell after exposure to camptothecin does not necessarily correlate with cytotoxocity. When aphidicolin is added to cells cultured in camptothecin, the level of camptothecin-stabilized topoisomerase I cleavable complexes is unchanged relative to a control culture without aphidicolin; however, the cells with

aphidicolin are completely protected from the cytotoxic effects of camptothecin (Holm *et al.* 1989). These observations have led to a model
of cell killing that involves an interaction between the topoisomerase–
DNA complex and the moving replication fork (Holm *et al.* 1989; Hsiang
et al. 1989b; Liu 1989). The fork may become stalled at the topoisomerase–
DNA complex and trigger a G2 arrest similar to that induced in yeast
by different DNA-damaging agents (Weinert and Hartwell 1988). If the
topoisomerase I complex occurred on the leading strand template, then
disruption of the topoisomerase–DNA complex by collision with the fork
could lead to an irreparable double—strand break.

11.2.1.4 *Cytotoxicity of mammalian type II topoisomerase poisons*

Exposure of mammalian cells to topoisomerase II poisons leads to inhibition of DNA and RNA synthesis, an increase in sister chromatid exchanges
and chromosomal aberrations, and reversible DNA fragmentation (Loike
and Horwitz 1976; Deaven *et al.* 1978; Ross *et al.* 1978). The cytotoxic
effects of topoisomerase II poisons shows some cell-cycle dependence,
increasing in toxicity from 2- to 15-fold in the S phase (Bhuyan *et al.*
1972; Chow and Ross 1987; Estey *et al.* 1987); however in contrast with
the experimental results obtained with camptothecin, aphidicolin does not
protect cells from the cytotoxic effects of topoisomerase II poisons (Holm
et al. 1989). Intracellular topoisomerase II protein levels rise during the
cell cycle to a peak level which occurs in the late M phase (Chow and
Ross 1987; Heck *et al.* 1988) or early G1 (Hsiang *et al.* 1988). It is
possible that this increase in the intracellular concentration of topoisomerase II leads to increased sensitivity to topoisomerase poisons during
the S phase, and that the cytotoxic effect of topoisomerase poisons arises
from a collision of transcription or replication forks with the trapped
complex, leading to irreparable DNA strand breaks (Liu 1989).

Cell-cycle-dependent variations in the level of topoisomerase-II-mediated
DNA cleavage also occur, with a maximum in the late G2 or M phase (Chow
and Ross 1987; Estey *et al.* 1987). This may reflect the peak in topoisomerase levels that is observed at this point in the cell cycle. In addition,
the peak in DNA cleavage is temporally correlated with chromosome segregation, an essential function of topoisomerase II which, if interrupted,
could lead to tearing of entangled chromosomes as the mitotic spindles
move apart.

Another result of drug stabilization of the topoisomerase II–DNA
complex may be the facilitation of illegitimate recombination. There is
evidence linking topoisomerase II with illegitimate recombination *in vitro*
(Ikeda *et al.* 1982; Ikeda 1986; Bae *et al.* 1988; Sperry *et al.* 1989). It has
been proposed that topoisomerase II holoenzymes in close proximity in the
cell could undergo subunit exchange, leading to illegitimate recombination

and sister chromatid exchanges, and these effects could be lethal (Drlica 1984; Pommier *et al.* 1985; Long and Stringfellow 1988).

11.2.1.5 *Specificity of topoisomerase poisons for enzymes from different species*

Topoisomerases from prokaryotes display sensitivity to a different spectrum of drugs than eukaryotic topoisomerases (Drlica and Franco 1988). There are no drugs known that target the bacterial topoisomerase I (Wang 1987a; Drlica and Franco 1988). The bacterial topoisomerase II (DNA gyrase) is very sensitive to novobiocin and other coumarins, which appear to interact with the gyrase B subunit, the ATP-binding domain of this enzyme (Gellert *et al.* 1976b). The quinolone family of compounds were developed from the bacterial poison nalidixic acid and primarily target DNA gyrase, although a few quinolone derivatives have recently been shown to target the eukaryotic topoisomerase II (Oomori *et al.* 1988; Gootz *et al.* 1990; Akahane *et al.* 1991; Robinson *et al.* 1991). Most of the antitumour agents that target the eukaryotic type II topoisomerase appear to be specific for this enzyme and do not poison the bacteria-specific DNA gyrase (Drlica and Franco 1988).

The specificity of different chemical agents for the different topoisomerases is due to the difference in the gross protein structures of these enzymes. The bacterial and eukaryotic topoisomerase I share very little sequence homology, and there are differences in the reaction mechanisms of the purified enzymes; thus it may be anticipated that these enzymes will exhibit different drug sensitivities. The bacterial and eukaryotic type II topoisomerases share more points of sequence homology but appear to interact with DNA in fundamentally different ways, since it appears that a segment of DNA is wrapped around the bacterial gyrase during its catalytic cycle whereas the eukaryotic topoisomerase II only binds a small segment of DNA. Thus it is likely that the DNA binding sites of these two classes of enzymes are structurally distinct. However, the site of drug interaction with the enzyme and/or DNA is not fully established.

The specificity shown by eukaryotic and prokaryotic enzymes has allowed the quinolones to be developed into a highly effective series of therapeutic agents which specifically target the bacterial topoisomerase, while the eukaryotic topoisomerase II is essentially insensitive to this class of drug. A similar specificity may also hold for the topoisomerases from other organisms. The type II topoisomerases isolated from *S. cerevisiae* and human cells show differential sensitivity to inhibition of catalysis by a number of etoposide derivatives (Figgitt *et al.* 1989). In addition, the type II topoisomerase from the pathogenic fungus *Candida albicans* shows sensitivity to a different spectrum of compounds than the topoisomerase II isolated from human cells (Shen *et al.* 1991). It is possible that this differential sensitivity can be exploited to develop a novel class of antifungal agents which targets the fungal topoisomerase but does not interact strongly with the host topoisomerase.

11.2.1.6 *Specificity of topoisomerase poisons for neoplastic cells*

Intracellular levels of topoisomerase II are controlled during the cell cycle. The level of topoisomerase II in the cell decreases sharply after mitosis in early G1 phase, and then rises during the subsequent cell cycle (Heck *et al.* 1988). Additionally, quiescent cells have low levels of topoisomerase II activity (Taudou *et al.* 1984; Tricoli *et al.* 1985; Sullivan *et al.* 1986) and protein (Heck and Earnshaw 1986; Nelson *et al.* 1987) compared with dividing cells. When the growth of normal cells is interrupted through serum depletion or cell–cell contact inhibition, their topoisomerase II levels drop and then increase again when normal growth is allowed to resume (Hsiang *et al.* 1988). Topoisomerase II levels also drop as cells become differentiated and stop dividing; thus the level of topoisomerase II in cells can be used as a marker of cell proliferation (Heck and Earnshaw 1986).

Tumour cells have a higher proliferative rate than normal cells and as expected, have higher intercellular levels of topoisomerase II than non-proliferating normal cells (Nelson *et al.* 1987; Hsiang *et al.* 1988; Potmesil *et al.* 1988). Additionally, the regulation of intercellular topoisomerase II levels appears to be altered in tumour cells since they do not fall after growth in culture is arrested by cell contact inhibition or serum starvation, nor do they drop after mitosis as is observed in normal cells (Hsiang *et al.* 1988). Since the level of topoisomerase II in the cell has been observed to correlate with the sensitivity of the cell to topoisomerase II poisons, these observations explain why tumour cells are more sensitive to topoisomerase II poisons than quiescent normal cells, and this is supported by clinical observations.

Levels of topoisomerase I protein do not change during the cell cycle (Heck *et al.* 1988; Hsiang *et al.* 1988), or in lymphoblasts stimulated by phytohaemagglutinin (PHA) (Hwang *et al.* 1989). However, an increase in mRNA encoding topoisomerase I has been reported in cells infected with adenovirus or stimulated to divide by the presence of PHA (Hwong *et al.* 1989; Romig and Richter 1990). In contrast with protein levels, topoisomerase I activity has been reported to increase in cells stimulated to divide by the presence of mitogens such as phorbol diester (Gorsky *et al.* 1989) or other stimuli (Tricoli *et al.* 1985), or in cells infected with adenovirus (Chow and Pearson 1985). This suggests that the specific activity of topoisomerase I may change in response to a stimulation of cell growth. The heightened sensitivity of tumour cells to camptothecin is probably based on the increased rate of proliferation, since it has been observed that DNA replication plays a key part in determining the sensitivity of a cell to camptothecin and the molar abundance of topoisomerase protein does not appear to change in growing cells.

11.2.2 Bacterial topoisomerase II poisons—the quinolones

DNA gyrase, a bacterial type II topoisomerase, is specifically inhibited by two types of antibacterial agents: the coumarins (Drlica and Coughlin 1989) and the quinolones which target the gyrase A and gyrase B units respectively. In this section, we focus on the gyrase-A-targeted quinolones only, as this class of inhibitors has demonstrated an overwhelming success in clinical applications.

11.2.2.1 *History of discovery*

The first member of the quinolone antibacterial family, nalidixic acid, was discovered in 1962 as a by-product of the synthesis of chloroquine (Lesher *et al.* 1962). Nalidixic acid has an antibacterial spectrum limited essentially to certain Gram-negative microorganisms and, clinically, was used primarily to treat urinary tract infections. Other first-generation quinolones include oxolinic acid, pipemidic acid, piromidic acid, cinoxacin, and flume-quine (Fig. 11.2) (Albrecht 1977). The discovery of DNA gyrase in 1976 (Gellert *et al.* 1976) and the subsequent studies showing that the enzyme is the target of nalidixic acid action have triggered the development of new quinolones, including the fluoroquinolones. Norfloxacin was the first fluorinated quinolone to be used in clinics, and it has a much broader antibacterial spectrum in that many Gram-positive organisms are now susceptible to clinically achievable doses. Other significant members of the second-generation quinolone family include pefloxacin, ciprofloxacin, ofloxacin, lomefloxacin, fleroxacin, sparfloxacin, temafloxacin, and tosuflox-acin (Fig. 11.2).

11.2.2.2 *Structure–activity relationships of quinolones*

The structure–activity relationships (SARs) of quinolones have been extensively reviewed (Chu and Fernandes 1989; Mitscher *et al.* 1989, 1990; Rosen 1990; Wentland 1990). The current SARs of quinolones are summarized in Fig. 11.3 and are discussed below.

1. N1 requires a hydrophobic and comparatively small substituent, and the substitution can be aromatic, can contain heteroatoms, and can be cyclopropyl or even tert-butyl. Bridging an N1 substituent to C2 or C8 usually gives good potency.

2. Few substitutions at the C2 position have been made. The CH group can be replaced by N, but the replacement of H by OH, OMe, or other such groups results in poor potency unless the group is bridged to N1 or C3.

3. The carboxyl group at C3 is required, with the single exception of an isothiazolone group bridging from C2 to C3. The series of compounds

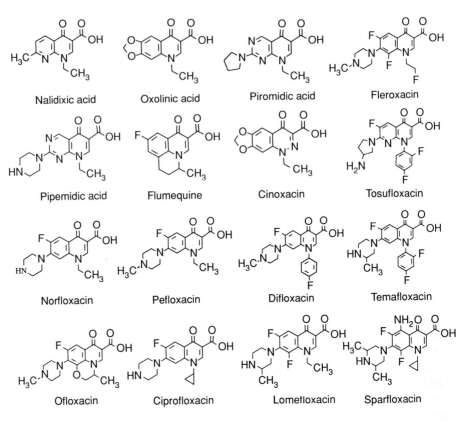

Fig. 11.2 Chemical structures of some first- and second-generation quinolones.

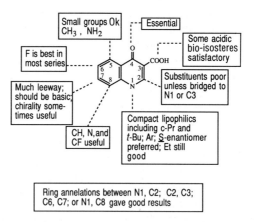

Fig. 11.3 Current SARs of quinolone antibacterial agents.

with such a modification to the carboxyl group have greatly enhanced *in vitro* activity, but are without *in vivo* value.

4. The C4 keto group is an absolute requirement for activity.

5. Groups at C5 must be small. Those with a methyl group or an amino moiety appear to be active.

6. C6 has been optimized with $C-F$.

7. A variety of substitutions at C7 are allowed. In most series, a piper-azinyl or a 3-ethylaminomethylpyrrolidinyl moiety gives good results. This position also allows: substitutions with a wide variety of five- and six-membered cycloaliphatic amines and bicycloderivatives.

8. Substitutions at C8 are generally limited to small groups such as $C-H$, N, or $C-F$. Bridging to N1 is acceptable. Bridging to C7 results in decreased potency.

11.2.2.3 *Model of action of quinolones*

Early progress in the development of quinolone antibacterial agents was made mainly through use of semi-empirical synthetic approaches. However, the discovery of DNA gyrase (Gellert *et al*. 1976a) stimulated and accele-rated the research and development of this class of antibacterial agents. Subsequent extensive studies on the mechanism of the gyrase-catalysed DNA supercoiling process and on the genetic analysis of quinolone-resistant bacterial mutants led to the conclusion that the primary functional target of quinolone drugs is the A subunit of the enzyme (reviewed in Cozzarelli 1980; Gellert 1981), and this laid the ground work for systematic drug develop-ment. However, the conclusion that the gyrase A subunit is the exclusive target of quinolones has been complicated by the finding that, while the majority of mutations leading to high-level drug resistance are in *gyrA* (Higgins *et al*. 1978; Yamagishi *et al*. 1981, 1986), mutations leading to quinolone resistance have also been found in *gyrB* (Yamagishi *et al*. 1981, 1986).

In 1985, Shen and coworkers, using a radioligand binding technique, found that ^{3}H-norfloxacin does not bind to DNA gyrase but instead binds to pure DNA (Shen and Pernet 1985). Further studies on the DNA binding specificity revealed that the drug binds preferentially to single-stranded DNA rather than to double-stranded DNA. A preference in binding can be demonstrated only if the strands are separated: the drug prefers guanine to the other three bases. The binding of the drug to double-stranded DNA is determined by the topological state of the DNA, i.e. the drug binds at inhibitory concentrations only to the underwound (supercoiled) form rather than to the linear or the relaxed form. Presumably, the drug preferentially binds to a partially denatured DNA pocket found in supercoiled DNA and binding occurs in a cooperative manner. However, it was subsequently found that the binding of the drug to relaxed forms of DNA may be induced by the action of DNA gyrase. The amount of the drug binding under these conditions is far more than the total amount of the binding to the DNA or to the enzyme separately. The increased drug binding was not due to the conversion of the substrate DNA to the supercoiled form since only a non-hydrolysable triphosphate nucleotide was used in the binding mixture so that such conversion was restricted (Shen *et al*. 1989c). The binding of the drug to the gyrase–DNA complex strongly resembles that of the binding to supercoiled DNA in terms of binding affinity, maximum molar binding ratio at saturation, and binding cooperativity (Shen *et al*. 1989a). These results suggest that the binding of DNA gyrase to the DNA substrate creates a site that allows the drug to bind in a cooperative manner.

On the basis of all the experimental observations described above, a quinolone–DNA cooperative binding model for the inhibition of DNA gyrase has been proposed (Shen *et al*. 1989d). All lines of experimental evidence favour the notion that the bound enzyme induces the formation of a drug binding site on the relaxed DNA substrate. It was proposed that the binding site is formed during the gate-opening step which requires the binding of ATP. The separated short single DNA strands between the four base-pair staggered cuts form a simulated denatured DNA bubble that is an ideal binding site for the drug (Fig. 11.4). Drug molecules

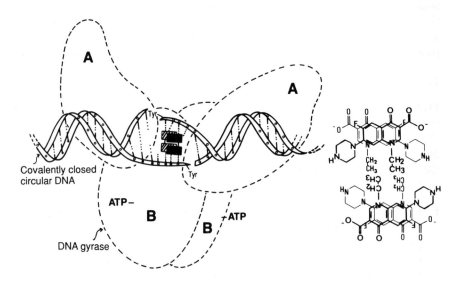

Fig. 11.4 Model of the proposed ternary complex among quinolone molecules, DNA gyrase, and duplex DNA substrate (■ and ▨ refer to stacked quinolone molecules shown in the inset). (From Shen *et al*. 1989d)

acquire high binding affinity through a cooperative binding mechanism achieved via self-association of the drug molecules inside the binding pocket. Two types of interactions, supported by observations in the structure of nalidixic acid crystal, are feasible: π-π stacking between the quinolone rings and tail-to-tail hydrophobic interactions between the N1 substitution groups (Fig, 11.4, inset). Such interactions result in the formation of a supermolecular complex with multiple sets of hydrogen bond acceptors in a consolidated unit, so that the assembled drug molecules can act together to occupy a site on DNA with binding groups distributed in a three-dimensional space.

This working model has two main features: (i) the appearance of a drug binding site induced on DNA by the action of DNA gyrase, and (ii) the unique ability of the drug molecules to occupy such a site via a self-assembly process. Both aspects are equally important in determining drug binding affinity and specificity. It is evident that the DNA binding specificity at the enzyme inhibition level is controlled by the binding of the enzyme that creates a favourable DNA site for the drug. This can be viewed as a third level of drug binding specificity.

This binding model offers an answer to questions concerning quinolone-resistance mutants. The model predicts that any mutations, either in *gyrA* or in *gyrB*, which alter the configuration of the drug binding pocket on DNA could lead to drug resistance. Such a mutation may be more likely to occur in *gyrA* since the gyrase A subunit is directly involved in creating such a binding site and in stabilizing the drug bound to DNA. However, the gyrase B subunit, the energy-transduction machinery which provides a conformational change to assist the DNA gate opening and strand passing, is obviously also important in the formation of such a site.

11.2.2.4 *Implications of the model for drug design*

11.2.2.4.1 *The model is consistent with quinolone structure−activity relationships* The proposed model suggests three functional domains on the quinolone molecule: the DNA binding domain, the drug self-association domain, and the drug−enzyme interaction domain (Fig. 11.5). Accordingly, the implications in drug design relative to the model can be summarized as follows, and these features are consistent with the SAR of quinolones.

1. Hydrophobic substitutions at the N1 position are essential for activity. The requirement that the N1 substituent be relatively small and lipophilic is consistent with its role as the central self-assembly part of the molecule. If the groups are the wrong size, then they will not fit into the space made available by the enzyme. If they are too polar, then they will not self-associate in the interior. Although the strength of these interactions is not expected to be the sole determinant for maximum activity, a minimum level of interaction between these hydrophobic

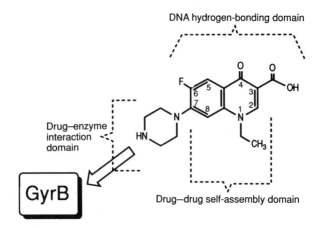

Fig. 11.5 Current concept of the functional domains of a quinolone antibacterial agent. The norfloxacin molecule is used as an example. The C7 substitutions may interact with the hypothetical 'quinolone pocket' on the gyrase B subunit (Yoshida *et al.* 1991).

groups is necessary for optimal potency. It is evident from Fig. 11.2 that substituents at the N1 positions of these active drug molecules, namely ethyl, cyclopropyl, and phenyl groups, are indeed hydrophobic.

2. Since drug self-association at the binding pocket is important for co-operative binding, it can be predicted that highly potent compounds may be very insoluble, and this is generally true (Shen *et al.* 1989d). An appropriate pharmaceutical formulation method or a prodrug approach is recommended for increasing the solubility of the final product.

3. The C4 keto group is absolutely essential for activity. The model assigns specific functional roles to the C4 keto moiety. This group, together with the C3 carboxyl group in the coplanar position, constitute the portions of the molecule proposed to be in contact with DNA through strong hydrogen-bonding interactions with the DNA bases in the short regions of duplex DNA made single-stranded by DNA gyrase. This vital role is consistent with the empirical observation that this part of the quinolone molecule is indispensable. The polar nature of these functional groups requires them to face outwards towards polar environmental factors (solvent in solution, DNA bases in the active site).

4. Substitutions at C5 with hydrogen-bond donors or acceptors are allowed, since it is within the DNA-binding domain. This is consistent with the good potency shown by sparfloxacin (Fig. 11.2). The requirement that groups attached to C5 and C6 be small is understandable as they

cannot be allowed to prevent interaction between the DNA bases and the upper portion of the molecule.

5. Extensive substitutions at C7 are allowed. The wide structural latitude available at C7 is understandable as this part of the molecule is distant from the pharmacophore or the self-assembly region. It is possible that these groups find auxiliary binding sites on the protein. This would rationalize the finding that there are volume limits for the C7 substituent which, while permissive, may not be exceeded. However, the function of this domain is less well defined by the proposed model and deserves more exploration. It may be speculated that this is the area responsible for the drug–enzyme interaction. In a recent publication (Yoshida et al. 1991) it is suggested that the C7 substitutions may indeed interact with the 'quinolone pocket' in the gyrase B subunit, judged from the differential response of quinolones with charged and non-charged substitutions at the C7 position to two different mutations that have altered charge property at the hypothetical quinolone pocket.

6. The requirement that C8 be small is also consistent with the idea that this side of the molecule must be capable of close approach to another quinolone molecule. The helpful influence of bridging is also seen as a consequence of the need for the adjacent molecules to approach each other closely and to form a compact virtual supermolecule. Bridging reduces the net volume requirements of the substituents.

The strong influence of chirality at N1 as compared with C7 is also understandable, since N1 is the site of closest approach between quinolone molecules; this region of the molecule dictates the nature of the stacking interaction and must be complimentary in absolute stereochemistry to the pocket opened in the DNA by the action of the enzyme. This feature is discussed in greater detail in the next section. The relatively lesser effect of optical asymmetry at C7 follows from its distance from either the pharmacophore or the self-assembly region.

However, there are some molecules whose SARs, in accord with the model, remain puzzling. The N-t-butyl analogues are very bulky and, of necessity, at least one of the methyl groups must lie below the plane of the molecule when associated in the way proposed. However, these agents are more active against Gram-positive bacteria than against Gram-negative bacteria where enzyme studies have shown there to be a smaller binding pocket (Shen et al. 1989d).

11.2.2.4.2 *Interpretation of the large activity difference of ofloxacin enantiomers* As suggested in the previous section, the groups attached to N1 and C8 represent areas of close contact between adjacent quinolone monomers in the model. As the binding pocket opened in DNA by DNA gyrase is likely to be chiral, a compatible chirality effect must be present in those drugs which possess chirality.

Ofloxacin (synthesized at Daiichi Seiyaku Co.) has an antibacterial potency against *E. coli* roughly equal to that of norfloxacin (Une *et al.* 1988) and has a supercoiling inhibition activity slightly less than that of norfloxacin (Shen *et al.* 1989d). The compound has a unique tricyclic structure with a methyl group attached to the asymmetric C3 on the oxazine ring. Studies with selected laboratory bacterial strains revealed that the [*S*-(−)-ofloxacin] isomer is approximately 8–128 times more potent than the [*R*-(+)-ofloxacin] (Hayakawa *et al.* 1986). Evidently, the stereochemical effect is on the enzyme rather than on other factors such as the drug transport mechanism, since the *S*-isomer has also shown about 30 times and 3 times more potency than the *R*-isomer for inhibiting DNA gyrases isolated from *E. coli* and from *Micrococcus luteus* respectively.

Molecular modelling (Shen *et al.* 1990) shows that there are two different ways in which *S*-ofloxacin can stack—methyls outside and methyls inside —and each puckers such that the methyls are either equatorial or axial. When the methyls are outside, in the *endo* form of *S*-ofloxacin or in the *exo* form of *R*-ofloxacin, the stack is compact in the lateral dimension, i.e. the distance between the two rings is shortest as shown by the (A) and (d) conformers in Fig. 11.6. Therefore the methyl groups strongly affect the closeness of approach of molecules in the virtual supermolecule that is intrinsically chiral. This means, in particular, that the pharmacophoric regions (hydrogen bond acceptors) have a reverse screw sense when the stacked *R*- and *S*-monomers are compared with each other. In the more active *S*-analogue the hydrogen-bond acceptors on the two quinolone rings are oriented 'northwest–southeast' whereas in the *R*-analogue they are oriented 'northeast–southwest'. Thus the models predicts a particular complementary chirality to the enzyme-induced single-stranded DNA pocket. It is not possible at present to verify or choose between these possibilities as the detailed structure of the ternary complex is unknown except by inference. None the less, this provides an important and ultimately testable consequence of the model. The substituent at C7 does not affect the closeness of approach nor the chirality of the stack, but this area is proposed to be the enzyme–drug interaction domain. Chirality may also be important from this point of view.

11.2.2.5 *Clinical utility and potential problems*

The clinical applications and potential problems of quinolone antibacterial agents have been extensively reviewed (Wolfson and Hooper 1989b; Neu 1990; Hooper and Wolfson 1991; Talley 1991). The new quinolones are highly potent against many *Enterobacteriaceae* and have reasonably good activity against *Pseudomonas aeruginosa* and *Staphylococci*. *Streptococci* and anaerobes are less susceptible. The drugs are well absorbed orally and

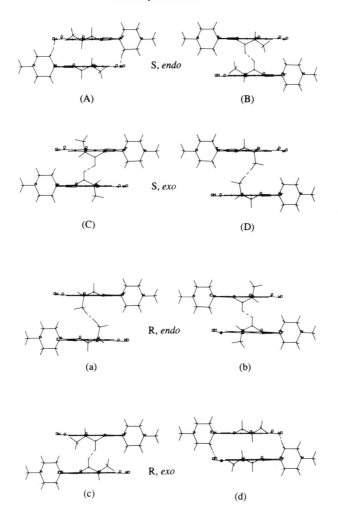

Fig. 11.6 Eight possible stacking conformations of ofloxacin enantiomers as seen with quinolone rings perpendicular to the plane of the paper. A and B represent *S, endo* methyls equatorial; they differ in the pucker conformation of the aliphatic ring bridging N1–C8. C and D represent *S, exo* methyls axial; they also differ in the pucker conformation of the aliphatic ring. Molecular pairs a – d represent the same conformers in the *R* series. The most compact orientations are A and d in which both the methyls and the ring pucker are away from adjacent stacked molecules. (From Shen *et al.* 1990.)

can usually achieve high serum levels with long half-life, thus twice daily dosing is normally allowed. Quinolones are orally effective antibacterial agents. They are highly effective for the treatment of the following infectious diseases: urinary tract infections such as cystitis and pyelonephritis, gastrointestinal infections such as bacterial gastroenteritis and diarrhoeal diseases, and some sexually transmitted diseases such as gonorrhoea and chancroid. They are also effective, but less uniformly, for the treatment of infections such as prostatitis, respiratory infections, Gram-negative osteomyelitis, and skin and soft-tissue infections. According to the current trend in the development, it may be predictable that the new quinolone antibacterials agents will be widely used as cost-effective and clinically effective alternatives for the treatment of various infectious diseases.

Common side-effects, including gastrointestinal effects, central nervous system effects, and allergic reactions, have been observed during clinical usage. However, these adverse effects are mild. The frequency of adverse experience was not greater than that for comparative agents such as ampicillin, pivampicillin, doxycycline, and cefotaxime.

Quinolones can be classified as DNA-targeted chemotherapeutic agents. However, the binding to DNA is weak and reversible, and in mammalian cells may be further decreased by the presence of histones and other chromosomal proteins (Shen et al. 1989b). They have fused heterocyclic structures, and extensive modifications of the ring structure could result in DNA unwinding and intercalation (Shen et al. 1990), imposing a potential carcinogenic effect. Surveillance for the DNA-unwinding effect during quinolone development should not be ignored.

A potentially serious problem that may limit the future clinical application of quinolone antibacterial agents is the development of resistant bacterial strains. The mechanism of bacterial resistance to quinolones has been the focus of intensive research efforts, and has been the subject of several reviews (Wolfson and Hooper 1989a; Fernandes and Shen 1989; Hooper and Wolfson 1990). The resistance can be divided into two categories: (1) mutations in DNA gyrase and (2) outer-membrane mutations affecting the drug transport process.

Mutations in DNA gyrase have been mapped either in gyrA or, usually with a lower degree of resistance, in gyrB. Most of the known mutations resulting in quinolone resistance are caused by a point mutation within a narrow region of amino acids 67–106 in the A subunit termed the quinolone-resistance-determining region (Yamagishi et al. 1981, 1986). In the gyrB gene, two quinolone-resistance sites have been identified at amino acids 426 and 447 (Yoshida et al. 1988, 1990). Molecular cloning and site-directed mutagenesis studies suggested that mutations of serine-83 to alanine or to tryptophan in the E. coli gyrase A subunit (Cullen et al. 1989; Hallett and Maxwell 1991) are responsible for high level resistance to new quinolones. Corresponding mutation of serine-84 to leucine or serine-85 to proline in the Staphylococcus aureus gyrase A subunit (Sreedharan et al. 1990) brings about similar high level resistance.

Resistance related to the mutation, other than those in the gyrase gene, appears to be involved only with the drug permeation process. Such E. coli mutants resistant to the newer fluoroquinolones, norfloxacin and cipro-floxacin have been selected in laboratories and several resistance loci have been identified: *nfxB*, *cfxB*, *norB*, and *norC* (Hirai *et al.* 1986; Hooper *et al.* 1986; 1987). All these mutants have common phenotypes, including low level resistance (about fourfold) to other fluoroquinolones and cross-resistance with other structure-unrelated agents such as tetracycline, chloram-phenicol, and some β-lactams. They also exhibited substantial reduction of the *OmpF* porin outer-membrane protein which constitutes the diffusion channel for small molecules through the barrier. The reduction in drug accumulation, at least in the cells of *nfxB* and *cfxB* mutants, is believed to involve an energy-dependent carrier-mediated efflux system present at the bacterial inner membrane, since norfloxacin accumulation in these mutants increases to the normal level after treatment with energy inhibitors (Hooper *et al.* 1989).

More recently, the development of high level resistance to new quino-lones among methicillin-resistance *S. aureus* (MRSA) strains has been identified (Harnett *et al.* 1991), suggesting a re-evaluation of the efficacy of the use of quinolones in the treatment of these important nosocomial pathogens. While the mechanism of quinolone resistance to Staphylococci still remains unclear, recent results indicate that the *norA* gene may be involved in such a resistance process (Ubukata *et al.* 1989). The *NorA* polypeptide may play a role in the membrane-associated active efflux pump of quinolones (Yoshida *et al.* 1990).

11.2.3   Eukaryotic topoisomerase II poisons

11.2.3.1   *Introduction*

Topoisomerase II is the target of a number of therapeutically important compounds (Liu 1989; Smith 1990). These include intercalating agents such as the aminoacridine amsacrine (Nelson *et al.* 1984), anthracyclines such as doxorubicin (also called adriamycin) (Tewey *et al.* 1984b), ellipticine and its derivatives (Tewey *et al.* 1984a), and compounds which do not strongly intercalate, such as the epipodophyllotoxins etoposide and teni-poside (Chen *et al.* 1984; Ross *et al.* 1984). In all cases, these drugs stabilize a complex between purified topoisomerase II and DNA which leads to cell death. In this section we focus on doxorubicin and etoposide, re-presentatives of two distinct classes of topoisomerase II poisons which are widely used clinically.

11.2.3.2   *Doxorubicin*

Adriamycin, or doxorubicin, consists of an adriamycinone chromophore attached to a daunosamine sugar moiety (Fig. 11.7). It is closely related, both structurally and biologically, to daunorubicin which is also shown in Fig. 11.7. Both doxorubicin and daunorubicin have been intensively

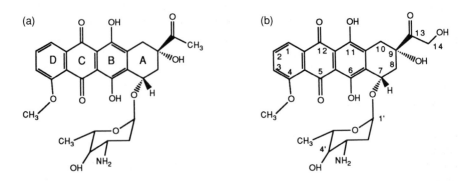

Fig. 11.7 (a) Daunomycin and (b) doxorubicin (adriamycin).

studied for several decades (Di Marco 1967; Carter 1975, Arcamone 1981; Zunino and Capranico 1990), and so only a few of the documented properties of this class of drug will be summarized here.

11.2.3.2.1 *History of doxorubicin* Daunomycin was first isolated from a culture of *Streptomyces peucetius* in the early 1960s (Grein *et al.* 1963; Di Marco 1967; Arcamone 1981). The biological properties of daunomycin were studied, and the drug was found to be very effective when tested in animals (Di Marco 1967). One early study found that 60 per cent of patients with childhood leukaemia responded to a single dose of daunomycin (Tan *et al.* 1967). Unfortunately, the narrow therapeutic index of daunomycin has limited its therapeutic usefulness (Carter 1975).

Doxorubicin, also known as adriamycin, was similarly isolated from cultures of *S. peucetius* (Arcamone *et al.* 1969; Arcamone 1981). Doxorubicin differs from daunorubicin only by the presence of a hydroxyl group at C14 (Fig. 11.7), yet doxorubicin has proven to be highly effective in clinical use. Doxorubicin is effective against a number of malignancies, and is used alone or in combination therapy in 60–65 per cent of chemotherapeutic courses (Scrip 1989).

11.2.3.2.2 *Structure–activity studies with derivatives of doxorubicin* A vast amount of effort has been devoted to understanding and improving the biological activity of doxorubicin and daunorubicin. Most derivatives have lower activity than the parent compound, for example derivatives in which the A ring is opened or in which the hydroxyl groups at carbons 6, 9, or 11 are altered have decreased activity (Arcamone 1981). 5-Imino-daunorubicin has similar activity to the parent compound, but its decreased toxicity makes it potentially useful. A study of six derivatives of doxorubicin, modified at positions 4, 5, 6, 11, and 14 of the chromophore, found a good correlation between strength of intercalation into DNA and stimulation of topoisomerase-II-mediated cleavage using purified enzyme, and also a direct correlation between cytotoxicity and potency in stabilizing the complex between purified topoisomerase II and DNA (Capranico *et al.* 1990b). In this study, C4-demethoxy daunorubicin was found to be more potent than doxorubicin, in terms of both stabilizing the topoisomerase II cleavable complex and the cytotoxicity.

The two chiral centres of adriamycin, C7 and C9 in the chromophore, have been the focus of many studies, as has position C14, particularly since a substitution at C14 transforms the relatively toxic daunorubicin into the highly effective doxorubicin. No derivatives with properties much improved over doxorubicin have been produced (Arcamone 1981). Substitutions at position C14 interfere with the ability of these compounds to stabilize the topoisomerase II–DNA complex (Bodley *et al.* 1989).

The C7 position is the site of attachment of the daunosamine moiety, a sugar which appears to be unique to this class of compounds. For this reason, the effect that replacing daunosamine with different sugars has on the activity of doxorubicin has also been the focus of much attention (Arcamone 1981). Aglycone derivatives are inactive, possible because of the decreased solubility of these compounds. 4'-*epi*-isomers have similar activity but appear to act against a different spectrum of tumours than the parent compound, making these of potential clinical utility. Both doxorubicin and 4'-*epi*-doxorubicin are equally effective in stabilizing the topoisomerase II cleavable complex (Capranico *et al.* 1990b).

A study of 3'-*N*-substituted anthracyclines reported that many of these compounds show decreased binding to DNA compared with the parent drug, and are almost ineffective in stabilizing the topoisomerase II–DNA complex in a purified system (Bodley *et al.* 1989). Substitutions at position C14 in the chromophore also interfere with the ability of these compounds to stabilize the topoisomerase II–DNA complex (Bodley *et al.* 1989). Thus doxorubicin appears to interact with topoisomerase II at two sites, the C14 position of the chromophore and the 3'-N of the daunosamine moiety. Analysis of crystals formed with daunomycin and DNA oligomers has revealed that the chromophore binds to DNA by intercalating into the DNA helix, while the A ring and sugar bind to the minor groove (Wang *et al.* 1987). This mode of binding would leave the C14 position of the chromophore, and the 3'-N of the daunosamine moiety accessible to interact with the topoisomerase as it contacts the DNA, in agreement with the SAR studies. Comparison of the structure of cocrystals of daunomycin with DNA and doxorubicin with DNA reveals a difference in solvation at the C14 position, which appears to confer on daunomycin a preference for an A–T pair outside the intercalation site (Frederick *et al.* 1990). The effect that this difference may have on the topoisomerase II cleavable complex is unclear.

11.2.3.2.3 *Mechanism of action of doxorubicin*   Both daunorubicin and doxorubicin bind to DNA, and these drugs have an unusual activity profile with a bell-shaped dose–response curve. At low drug concentrations these drugs stabilize the topoisomerase II cleavable complex, while at high concentrations of drug the topoisomerase II complex is diminished. This has been attributed to suppression of topoisomerase II binding to DNA by the excessive DNA unwinding effect imposed by these intercalative drugs (Tewey *et al.* 1984b; Zunino and Capranico 1990). This property makes it difficult to measure the extent of DNA damage accurately, particularly when comparing different compounds with different DNA binding affinities. For example, it is possible to see an increase in drug-dependent DNA damage after the drug has been removed from the media, as the intracellular drug concentration drops to a point where the drug no longer inhibits the formation of topoisomerase II cleavable complex but in fact stabilizes it (Zunino and Capranico 1990). With this caveat, the conclusion of recent studies is that DNA binding, stabilization of topoisomerase II cleavable complex, and cytotoxicity can be correlated for many derivatives of doxorubicin (Bodley *et al.* 1989; Capranico *et al.* 1990a; Zunino and Capranico 1990).

The mechanism of stabilization of the topoisomerase cleavable complex by doxorubicin has not been established; however, a model for stabilization by this class of DNA intercalative drugs has been suggested (D'Arpa and Liu 1989; Capranico *et al.* 1990a). In this model, the drug would bind to the DNA held in the topoisomerase II DNA binding pocket in the cleavable complex. The DNA in the pocket is known to be topologically constrained, since free rotation of the DNA does not occur until the topoisomerase is denatured. Thus the intercalation of a single drug molecule into the DNA helix after it has been cleaved by the topoisomerase would introduce localized twist into the DNA, forcing the DNA ends out of alignment and making the resealing of the two ends energetically costly. Analysis of the nucleotide sequences found at cleavage sites in the presence of doxorubicin (or amsacrine) has revealed a drug-dependent sequence preference, for an A at the 3′ terminus of the cleavage site of doxorubicin-stabilized sites and an A at the 5′ terminus of amsacrine-stabilized sites (Capranico *et al.* 1990; Pommier *et al.* 1991). These nucleotide positions are between the two cutting sites of topoisomerase II and thus would fall into the region of DNA constrained topologically by topoisomerase II. These data support a model of drug stabilization of the cleavable complex deriving from the untwisting of the DNA held by the topoisomerase.

Although adriamycin and its derivatives have been used to treat patients for a number of years, the mechanism of action of this family of drugs has not been fully resolved. As mentioned above, studies with purified topoisomerase II have shown that the topoisomerase II–DNA complex is stabilized by adriamycin, and this could lead to cell death, as is thought to be the case for other topoisomerase II poisons such as amsacrine or epipodophyllotoxins (Liu 1989). This hypothesis is supported by observations of direct correlations between potency in stabilizing the topoisomerase II–DNA complex and biological activity. However, a series of derivatives at the 3'-N position of doxorubicin have recently been synthesized, and these appear to have retained biological activity while showing little or no stabilization of the topoisomerase II–DNA complex (Bodley et al. 1989). This suggests that adriamycin has two distinct mechanisms of action, and that these can be chemically separated. It has been suggested that adriamycin damages DNA through a mechanism involving the production of free radicals (Lown et al. 1977; Bachur et al. 1978). Thus it is possible that adriamycin has two distinct cytotoxic effects, one targeting topoisomerase II and one independent of the enzyme.

11.2.3.3 *Epipodophyllotoxins*

The epipodophyllotoxins were originally synthesized as part of an attempt to improve the efficacy of podophyllotoxin. Podophyllotoxin is extracted from the roots and rhizomes of the American mandrake or may apple. While podophyllotoxin itself has antitumour activity, clinical trials were terminated owing to high toxicity (Kelly and Hartwell 1954; Jardine 1980). Podophyllotoxin binds to tubulin and is inactive against topoisomerase II, while its congeners etoposide and teniposide are very potent against topoisomerase II but do not bind to tubulin. The structure of these compounds is shown in Fig. 11.8. Interestingly, the effect of podophyllotoxin on cells is to block the formation of the mitotic spindle, so that the cells accumulate with condensed chromosomes and eventually die. However,

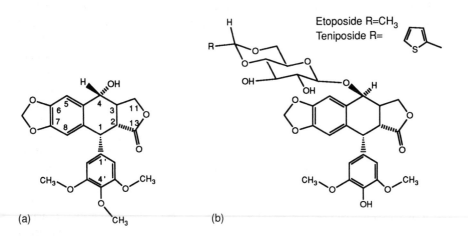

Fig. 11.8 (a) Podophyllotoxin and (b) the epipodophyllotoxin derivatives etoposide and teniposide.

etoposide and teniposide cause cells to arrest in the S-phase, prior to mitosis. Thus the terminal phenotype of cells killed by podophyllotoxin and epipodophyllotoxins is different, as is their mechanism of action.

11.2.3.3.1 *History of epipodophyllotoxins* Etoposide and teniposide are two of a number of semisynthetic derivatives of podophyllotoxin that were synthesized in the 1960s (Keller-Juslen *et al.* 1971; Stahelin and von Wartburg 1989, 1991). These derivatives were not antimicrotubule agents, but since they were found to have biological activity, the determination of their mechanism of action became the focus of research effort. Loike and Horwitz (1976) reported that exposure to these compounds resulted in intracellular DNA damage which led to observations of a correlation between drug-dependent DNA breakage and cytotoxicity (Wozniak *et al.* 1984; Sullivan *et al.* 1986; Markovits *et al.* 1987). Exposure of purified DNA to these drugs did not result in breakage of the DNA; thus there was another component in the cell that was responsible for the DNA damage following exposure to the epipodophyllotoxins. Studies in isolated nuclei demonstrated that DNA breakage did not require the intact cell (Filipski and Kohn 1982; Glisson *et al.* 1984; Pommier *et al.* 1984; Long *et al.* 1986), thus suggesting a component of the nucleus as the missing link. The identification of topoisomerase II as the key to drug-dependent DNA damage followed quickly (Chen *et al.* 1984; Minocha and Long 1984; Ross *et al.* 1984; Yang *et al.* 1985), and a number of corroborative studies have supported this hypothesis (van Maanen *et al.* 1988).

Teniposide and etoposide entered clinical trials in 1970 (Stahelin and von Wartburg 1989, 1991), and while teniposide was more active in pre-clinical tests, etoposide was more active in animal studies (Rozencweig *et al.* 1977; O'Dwyer *et al.* 1984; Stahelin and von Wartburg 1989, 1991). At present, etoposide is currently used either alone or as part of a combination therapy programme to treat patients with small-cell lung cancer, germ cell tumours, and lymphomas (Aisner and Lee 1991; Slevin 1991). One study reports that etoposide is responsible for complete remissions in approximately 20 per cent of previously treated patients with acute non-lymphocytic leukaemia (Bishop 1991). Additional studies with altered dosing schedules and delivery modes have opened the door to the possibility of using etoposide to treat a wider variety of malignancies (Aisner and Lee 1991; Johnson *et al.* 1991).

11.2.3.3.2 *Structure–activity relationships among derivatives of epipodo-phyllotoxins* Once it was determined that epipodophyllotoxins act by means of a different mechanism than podophyllotoxin, the structural features that are necessary to convert the tubulin-binding podophyllotoxin into the topoisomerase targeting etoposide were identified. The conclusions of this work are that four changes to podophyllotoxin are crucial (Long *et al.*

1984): (1) demethylation at the 4' position, (2) epimerization at position 4, (3) addition of a glucose moiety at position 4, and (4) aldehyde condensation with the glucose moiety.

Etoposide is metabolized to *o*-dihydroxy and *o*-quinone derivatives which are both less cytotoxic than the parent etoposide and also less potent in stabilizing the topoisomerase II–DNA complex (Sinha *et al.* 1990). Another study of epipodophyllotoxin structure focused on C4 derivatives in which the glycosidic moiety was replaced by different arylamino substitutions. These authors reported a correlation between intracellular DNA breaks, inhibition of topoisomerase II catalytic activity, and stabilization of the topoisomerase II–DNA complex for the six derivatives studied (Chang *et al.* 1991).

11.2.3.3.3 *Mechanism of action of epipodophyllotoxins* The epipodophyllotoxins appear to bind to DNA in a manner reminiscent of the way in which quinolones bind to DNA (Chow *et al.* 1988; Shen *et al.* 1989a,d). Unlike doxorubicin and amsacrine, which appear to bind DNA by intercalation, the epipodophyllotoxins have limited binding sites on DNA. Etoposide binds to single-stranded DNA preferentially and this binding is stimulated by the presence of magnesium in the buffer (Chow *et al.* 1988). Interestingly, competition studies show that both teniposide and etoposide compete equally well with the binding of radiolabelled etoposide to DNA, although teniposide is more potent in stabilizing the topoisomerase II–DNA complex (Chow *et al.* 1988). This observation suggests that additional interactions between epipodophyllotoxins and topoisomerase II are important for stabilization of the cleavable complex.

Similar to the case of intercalating topoisomerase poisons, a sequence preference for C at the 3' terminus of the cleavage site in teniposide-stimulated topoisomerase II cleavage has been observed (Pommier *et al.* 1991). This suggests that teniposide interacts with the DNA that is constrained in the topoisomerase–DNA complex and, by analogy with the model for intercalating topoisomerase poisons, the binding of teniposide to the DNA in the complex may introduce sufficient localized twist to interfere with resealing of the DNA ends. This model is supported by reports that the presence of etoposide interferes with the religation step of the topoisomerase II reaction (Osheroff 1989b).

Recently, the sequence of the topoisomerase II from two human leukaemia cell lines selected for resistance to teniposide has been determined (Bugg *et al.* 1991). The topoisomerase II activity in nuclear extracts from these cells has previously been reported to have an altered ATP requirement, and this prompted the authors to determine the sequence of the region corresponding to a consensus ATP binding site of the topoisomerase II. The enzyme of both mutant cell lines contains the same sequence change from the wild-type sequence in this region: the change of arginine-449 to glutamine. The position is distinct from the region of the eukaryotic type II topoisomerase homologous to amino acid residues 93–131 of gyrase B subunit, which have been shown by physical methods to be the ATP binding region (Tamura and Gellert 1990).

11.2.3.4 *Concerns about the therapeutic use of topoisomerase II poisons*

Exposure of cells to some topoisomerase II poisons leads to sister chromatid exchanges and other chromosomal damage (Pommier *et al.* 1985; Dillehay *et al.* 1987). The stabilization of topoisomerase II complexes with DNA *in vitro* has been linked to increased levels of illegitimate recombination, presumably occurring through subunit exchange between neighbouring topoisomerase molecules (Ikeda *et al.* 1982; Ikeda 1986; Bae *et al.* 1988; Sperry *et al.* 1989). In addition to causing chromosomal rearrangement, these compounds are mutagenic (Singh and Gupta 1983), leading to increases in frame-shift mutations in bacteria treated with intercalating topoisomerase poisons (Masurekar *et al.* 1991).

There are many examples of cell lines selected for resistance to topoisomerase II poisons, as well as resistant cell lines derived from naturally occurring tumours. The mechanistic basis for this elevated resistance has been the focus of much study. Cells can acquire resistance through both alterations in the topoisomerase target and another mechanism termed multipdrug resistance (MDR).

The MDR phenotype is correlated with the overexpression or amplification of the gp170 drug transporter which contributes to the efflux of particular compounds from the cell (Endicott and Ling 1989). The gp 170 protein transports several natural products including topoisomerase II poisons as well as other drugs such as vinblastine or methotrexate. Cells which acquire the MDR phenotype display elevated resistance to most drugs in this class, including topoisomerase II poisons, hence the name multidrug resistance.

Cells also acquire resistance to topoisomerase II poisons through alterations to topoisomerase II. Two different phenotypes of this class of resistant cells have been described. Cell lines with resistant forms of topoisomerase II have been isolated and characterized (Sullivan *et al.* 1989; Hinds *et al.* 1991). Additionally, cell lines with reduced topoisomerase II levels, which are less sensitive to topoisomerase II poisons, have also been isolated (Deffie *et al.* 1989). The phenotype of cell lines with reduced levels of topoisomerase II has been termed atypical MDR, since these cell lines are frequently cross-resistant to the spectrum of topoisomerase II poisons but not to the family of compounds included in the 'classical' MDR phenotype (Danks *et al.* 1987).

11.2.3.5 *Perspective for the use of topoisomerase II poisons*

The improvement of topoisomerase II targeted therapy is being followed along three paths. First, analogues of known topoisomerase II poisons are

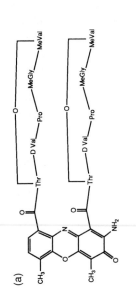

(a)

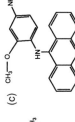

(b)

(c)

(d)

(e)

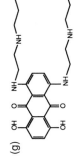

(f)

(g)

(h)

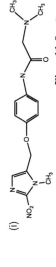

(i)

(j)

(k)

(l)

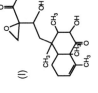

(b)

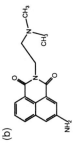

Fig. 11.9 Compounds which target type II topoisomerases: (a) actinomycin D (Tewey et al. 1984); (b) amonafide (Hsiang et al. 1989a); (c) amsacrine (Nelson et al. 1984); (d) BE 10988 (Suda et al. 1991); (e) flavone (Yamashita et al. 1990b); (f) ellipticine (Ross et al. 1984; Tewey et al. 1984b); (g) mitoxantrone (Tewey et al. 1984b); (h) MST-16 (Tanabe et al. 1991); (i) Ro-15-0216 (Sorensen et al. 1990); (j) saitopin (Yamashita et al. 1990c); (k) streptonigrin (Yamashita et al. 1990a); (l) terpentecin (Kawada et al. 1991).

being synthesized and characterized. This builds on a library of such studies, which so far, with the exception of etoposide, have not resulted in the production of new therapeutic compounds. Second, combination therapies are being tested in which the effects of treating patients simultaneously or sequentially with several therapeutic compounds are being determined. These results are promising, but are not directly related to the action of topoisomerase II within the cell and so will not be considered further here. Finally, there are ongoing screening projects to discover novel topoisomerase II poisons.

A number of new compounds which stabilize the cleavable complex formed between mammalian topoisomerase II and DNA have recently been described. The structure of some representative compounds is given in Fig. 11.9. The structures presented in this figure reveal the wide range of chemical structures which are able to interact with the topoisomerase II–DNA complex. This information, combined with structural information about the eukaryotic topoisomerase II, will facilitate the design of novel topoisomerase II poisons in the not too distant future.

11.2.4　Camptothecin and other drugs that target the eukaryotic topoisomerase I

11.2.4.1　*Introduction*

Camptothecin is a naturally derived compound which is capable of stabilizing the complex formed between the purified eukaryotic topoisomerase I and DNA (Hsiang *et al.* 1985). The stabilization by camptothecin of the topoisomerase I/DNA complexes in the cell is thought to be the basis of the cytotoxic and antitumour activity of this class of compounds (reviewed by Liu 1989). The structures of camptothecin and several of its analogues are shown in Fig. 11.10.

Camptothecin was first isolated from the bark of the Chinese tree *Camptotheca acuminata* (Wall *et al.* 1966). After its antitumour activity was demonstrated in L1210 cells, camptothecin became the target for extensive chemical synthesis and a number of analogues have been synthesized (Schultz 1973; Wall and Wani 1980). Both camptothecin and the sodium salt of the acid form of camptothecin demonstrated antitumour activity in animal models, although camptothecin acid, while more water soluble, was approximately 10-fold less potent than camptothecin lactone. Because of promising results in animal studies and favourable solubility, the sodium salt of camptothecin acid was chosen for clinical evaluation (Gottlieb *et al.* 1970; Gottlieb and Luce 1972; Moertel *et al.* 1972; Muggia *et al.* 1972). Unfortunately, despite reports of possible activity against leukaemia and gastrointestinal tumours, clinical studies with sodium camptothecin were discontinued because of severe toxic side-effects.

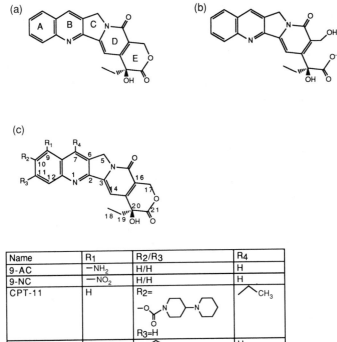

Fig. 11.10 Camptothecin and its derivatives: (a) lactone form of camptothecin; (b) sodium salt of camptothecin; (c) camptothecin derivatives.

Recently, derivatives of camptothecin which are more water soluble have been synthesized (Wall *et al.* 1986; Wani *et al.* 1986, 1987; Hsiang *et al.* 1989c; Kingsbury *et al.* 1991) and tested in cell culture and animal models (Giovanella *et al.* 1989, 1991; Kaufmann 1991b). One study, performed with xenografts of human cancers in nude mice, found that camptothecin was more effective than other clinically available drugs tested and, in addition, three synthetic derivatives (9-nitrocamptothecin (9-NC), 9-aminocamptothecin (9-AC) and 10,11 -methylenedioxycamptothecin (10,11-MDC)) were even more effective than camptothecin in this system (Giovanella *et al.* 1991). A phase I study of 7-ethyl-10-[4-(1-piperidino)-1-piperidino]carbonyloxycamptothecin (CPT-11) reported a response rate of 18 per cent in 17 patients with advanced non-small-cell lung cancer. In addition, however, this study noted substantial interpatient variation in toxicity due to CPT-11 (Negoro *et al.* 1991). *In vivo*, CPT-11 appears to be metabolized to 7-ethyl-10-hydroxycamptothecin (SN-38) which is more active than the parent compound. Phase I studies of another camptothecin derivative, 9-dimethylaminomethyl-10-hydroxycamptothecin (topotecan), are underway (Kaufmann 1991a).

11.2.4.2   *Structure–activity relationships of camptothecin derivatives*

A number of derivatives of camptothecin have been synthesized and their properties determined (Wall and Wani 1980; Wani *et al.* 1980; Wall *et al.* 1986; Wani *et al.* 1986, 1987; Jaxel *et al.* 1989; Hertzberg *et al.* 1989a,b; Hsiang *et al.* 1989c). These studies have reported that compounds which fail to stabilize the topoisomerase I–DNA complex do not show cytotoxic or antitumour activity. Moreover, in some cases there is a quantitative correlation between effect on topoisomerase I and antitumour potency (Jaxel *et al.* 1989), in good agreement with the hypothesis that topoisomerase I is the intracellular target of camptothecin and its derivatives.

A major conclusion of these studies is that an intact *a*-hydroxy lactone in ring E is essential for both antitumour activity and stabilization of the topoisomerase I–DNA complex (Schultz 1973; Wall and Wani 1980). The sodium salt of camptothecin acid, which has a carboxyl group rather than the lactone ring found in camptothecin, has a lower potency than camptothecin in animal models. It is probable that the activity of sodium camptothecin *in vivo* results from a low level of recyclization to form camptothecin in the plasma. The planar configuration of rings A–D is also an important factor in the activity of the camptothecin analogue (Wall and Wani 1980). Additionally, substitutions at positions 9 and/or 10 of the A ring of camptothecin are well tolerated, whereas only non-bulky substitutions at position 11 result in a compound able to stabilize the topoisomerase I–DNA complex (Wall and Wani 1980; Wall *et al.* 1986; Wani *et al.* 1986, 1987; Kingsbury *et al.* 1991).

In a study of substitutions in the E ring it has been concluded that the stereochemistry of camptothecin is important for activity (Jaxel *et al.* 1989). Whereas natural camptothecin has an *R* conformation at position 20, a synthetic analogue with the *S* configuration at this position has greatly reduced activity (Jaxel *et al.* 1989). This suggests that camptothecin interacts with an asymmetric site on its target. Additional substitutions at positions 20 and 21 of the E ring decrease activity further, as do bulky substitutions at position 12 in the A ring which would be expected to hinder an interaction with camptothecin at position 20.

The chemical structure of the E ring is fundamental to camptothecin activity. The natural camptothecin structure is 20-hydroxy-21-lactone, which allows facile ring opening and reclosing under physiological conditions. Modifications to this ring, which tend to inhibit this opening and closing, have a diminished potency in terms of both cytotoxicity and the stabilization of the topoisomerase I–DNA complex (Wall and Wani 1980;

Hertzberg *et al.* 1989b). This has been interpreted as suggesting that the interaction of camptothecin with topoisomerase I may involve a covalent intermediate in which camptothecin binds to topoisomerase I through an ester exchange reaction, and that this reaction may be facilitated by a hydrogen-bonding interaction of the hydroxyl group at position 20 with a chiral site on the topoisomerase (Hetzberg *et al.* 1989b; Jaxel *et al.* 1989).

11.2.4.3 *Mechanism of action of camptothecin and other compounds that target topoisomerase I*

Under catalytic conditions, topoisomerase I forms a complex with DNA and the addition of camptothecin to the reaction stabilizes this complex. Camptothecin does not unwind DNA, since the linking number of DNA topoisomers relaxed in the presence and absence of camptothecin is similar (Hsiang *et al.* 1985; Jaxel *et al.* 1989). Equilibrium dialysis studies have demonstrated that camptothecin reversibly binds to the topoisomerase I DNA complex, but not to either the topoisomerase or the the DNA in the absence of the other (Hertzberg *et al.* 1989a).

Genetic experiments with *S. cerevisiae* have demonstrated that topoisomerase I is the intracellular target of camptothecin (Eng *et al.* 1988; Nitiss and Wang 1988). Topoisomerase I is also likely to be the target of camptothecin in mammalian cells, and this hypothesis is supported by the observation that the stabilization of the topoisomerase I–DNA complex is quantitatively correlated with antitumour potency (Jaxel *et al.* 1989), and that the protein linked to DNA breaks after treatment with camptothecin is recognized by antibodies raised to topoisomerase I (Hsiang and Liu 1988). This conclusion is further supported by the isolation of a resistant topoisomerase I from mammalian cells selected for resistance to the cytotoxic effects of camptothecin (Gupta *et al.* 1988; Kjeldsen *et al.* 1988).

The topoisomerase I isolated from a camptothecin-resistant Chinese hamster cell line is resistant to both the inhibition of catalysis by camptothecin and the stabilization of the cleavable complex by camptothecin (Gupta *et al.* 1988). The topoisomerase I isolated from a human camptothecin-resistant cell line is also less sensitive to the effects of camptothecin (Kjeldsen *et al.* 1988). In the absence of camptothecin, the resistant human topoisomerase I cleaves DNA more efficiently than the wild-type topoisomerase I, and the kinetic stability of the cleavable complex formed by the mutant topoisomerase I with DNA is higher than that of the wild-type cleavable complex. In the presence of camptothecin, however, the kinetic stability of the cleavable complex formed by the wild-type topoisomerase I is substantially increased, whereas the kinetic stability of the complex formed by the mutant enzyme and DNA is only slightly enhanced (Kjeldsen *et al.* 1988). The mechanistic basis of this behaviour is not known.

An analysis of the gene encoding the resistant topoisomerase I revealed two points of difference between the sensitive wild-type topoisomerase I and the resistant mutant: asparagine to glycine at amino acid position 533 and asparagine to glycine at position 583 (Tamura *et al.* 1991). These are both found in evolutionarily conserved regions, and further studies of topoisomerase I with a single amino acid mutation are required to determine whether one or both of the two changes confers resistance to camptothecin. The tyrosine residue implicated in binding to DNA is at position 773 of the human topoisomerase I (Lynn *et al.* 1989); thus the site of interaction with camptothecin may be distinct from the DNA binding domain of the enzyme. This question cannot be conclusively answered until the three-dimensional structure of the DNA binding domain is determined.

A model of the interaction between camptothecin and topoisomerase I has been proposed in which camptothecin acts to stabilize a topoisomerase–DNA complex that accumulates after catalysis is complete (Hertzberg *et al.* 1989a). However, the complex formed by the topoisomerase I and DNA may occur as part of the catalytic cycle of the enzyme (Wang 1971). If this is the case, then stabilization of this complex would be expected to interfere with catalysis. Interestingly, much higher concentrations of camptothecin are required to interfere with catalysis than to have a detectable effect on topoisomerase II–DNA complex stability (Hsiang *et al.* 1985). This may arise from differential sensitivity of the two assays or from a twofold effect of camptothecin on topoisomerase I.

Compounds other than camptothecin and its derivatives also interfere with the topoisomerase I catalytic cycle (Fig. 11.11). These include intercalators such as ethidium and a number of aminoacridine analogues (Pommier *et al.* 1987) and DNA binding drugs such as distamycin (Mortensen *et al.* 1990). These drugs appear to interfere with catalysis by disturbing the binding of topoisomerase I to DNA rather than by stabilizing the topoisomerase I–DNA complex. In contrast, actinomycin D appears to stabilize the topoisomerase I–DNA complex but does not affect the strand-passing activity (Trask and Muller 1988).

11.2.4.4   *Concerns about the therapeutic use of camptothecin*

The therapeutic use of camptothecin and its derivatives has been hindered by unacceptably high toxicity. This could arise from poor solubility of the parent compound, in which case the more hydrophilic new derivatives would be expected to surmount this problem. If toxicity is due to lack of specificity between topoisomerase I in tumour and in normal cells, it is possible that altered delivery schemes could bypass this and allow effective camptothecin therapy.

Camptothecin has been shown to produce an increased frequency of sister chromatid exchanges and other chromosomal aberrations in human lymphocytes (Degrassi *et al.* 1989). If camptothecin is present during the

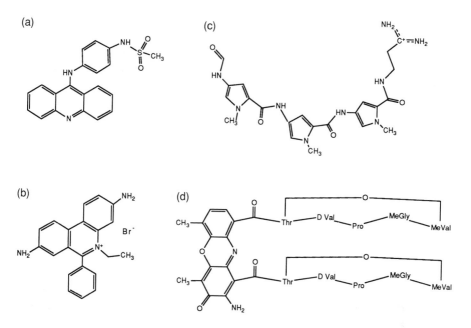

Fig. 11.11 Compounds which inhibit the catalytic activity of topoisomerase I: (a) amsacrine; (b) ethidium bromide; (c) distamycin; (d) actinomycin D.

S phase, then the damage involves both chromatids, whereas removal of camptothecin from the medium before the cells enter the S phase results in chromatid damage, probably reflecting events on only one DNA strand. This study suggests that cytotoxic damage could occur in patients treated with camptothecin.

11.2.4.5   *Future prospects for camptothecin and its derivatives*
Camptothecin is specifically toxic to cells in the S phase (Li *et al.* 1972; Drewinko *et al.* 1974; Del Bino *et al.* 1991), and thus it might be expected that rapidly dividing cells would be particularly sensitive to it. For this reason, the combination of camptothecin with other drugs which themselves interfere with cell division might be expected to diminish its efficacy. This is supported by studies demonstrating that concomitant treatment with aphidicolin and camptothecin appears to protect cells from the cytotoxic effects of camptothecin, presumably since traversal of the replication complex through the site of the topoisomerase I complex is a key determinant of camptothecin cytotoxicity (Holm *et al.* 1989; Hsiang *et al.* 1989b). It has been proposed that the synchronization of tumour cells by treatment with aphidicolin prior to camptothecin therapy may heighten the sensitivity of these cells to camptothecin by arresting cells in the S phase (Del Bino

et al. 1991), and it is probable that sequential treatment of cells with poisons of topoisomerases I and ll will have a synergistic effect on cyto-toxicity (Oguro 1990).

Two cell lines resistant to camptothecin have been selected and found to contain a camptothecin-resistant topoisomerase I. Other modes of camptothecin resistance are possible; for example, camptothecin-resistant cell lines have been described in which camptothecin resistance is correlated with reduced levels of topoisomerase I (Eng *et al.* 1990). The reduction in target enzyme capable of forming a toxic complex with DNA would be expected to decrease the sensitivity of the cell to the effects of camptothecin. In two cell lines which have developed camptothecin resistance correlating with reduced levels of topoisomerase I, a concomitant increase in topoisomerase II levels is seen (Sugimoto *et al.* 1990). This may render these cells more sensitive to topoisomerase II poisons, as is the case for the Chinese hamster cell line selected for resistance to camptothecin which has a two- to threefold increased sensitivity towards topoisomerase II poisons (Gupta *et al.* 1988). Unfortunately, an antagonism between camptothecin and topoisomerase II poisons has been observed in studies using cultured cells (Kaufmann 1991b), so that therapy with both camptothecin and topoisomerase II poisons may require sequential rather than simultaneous administration for optimal effect.

11.3 Summary

Topoisomerases play important catalytic roles in prokaryotic and eukaryotic cells. The activity of these enzymes has been implicated in many aspects of DNA metabolism, including DNA replication, recombination, transcription, and chromosomal segregation. In addition to the well-characterized topoisomerases, new enzymes of this family have recently been identified, with at present unidentified physiological functions.

Topoisomerases are the targets of a number of therapeutically important drugs, for example the quinolone class of antibacterial agents. These drugs stabilize a complex between topoisomerase and DNA *in vitro*, and it appears that the stabilization of this complex within the cell can trigger a cascade of events leading to cell death. The specificity shown by these agents for different topoisomerases has allowed the development of highly effective antibacterial agents. This process is continuing, with the topoisomerases of additional pathogenic organisms now becoming the targets of novel drug discovery programmes.

Topoisomerases are also the targets of several anticancer drugs, such as doxorubicin and etoposide, which appear to target actively proliferating cells. This area of research is following two paths: new derivatives of known topoisomerase poisons are being developed and tested clinically, and novel compounds are being also discovered and developed.

The mechanisms by which cells become resistant to topoisomerase drugs include alterations in uptake or efflux of the drug from the cell, a decrease in the intracellular level of topoisomerase, and also alterations in the structure of the topoisomerase enzyme, making it less sensitive to the cytotoxic effects of topoisomerase poisons. The study of these alterations, in combination with structural information derived from ongoing physical characterization of these enzymes, will allow the drug-sensitive domains of topoisomerases to be identified. In turn, this will allow novel compounds which specifically target the topoisomerase to be designed.

References

Adachi, T., Mizuuchi, M., Robinson, E. A., Appella, E., O'Dea, M. H., Gellert, M., and Mizuuchi, K. (1987). DNA sequence of the *E. coli gyr*B gene: Application of a new sequencing strategy. *Nucleic Acids Research*, **15**, 771–84.

Aguilera, A. and Klein, H. L. (1990). HPR1, a novel yeast gene that prevents intrachromosomal excision recombination, shows carboxy-terminal homology to the *Saccharomyces cerevisiae* TOP1 gene. *Molecular and Cell Biology*, **10**, 1439–51.

Aisner, J. and Lee, E. J. (1991). Etoposide. Current and future status. *Cancer*, **67**, 215–19.

Akahane, K., Hoshino, K., Sato, K., Kimura, Y., Une, T., and Osada, Y. (1991). Inhibitory effects of quinolones on murine hematopoetic progenitor cells and eukaryotic topoisomerase II. *Chemotherapy*, **37**, 224–6.

Albrecht, R. (1977). Development of antibacterial agents of the nalidixic acid type. *Progress in Drug Research*, **21**, 9–104.

Arcamone, F. (1981). *Doxorubicin. Anticancer antibiotics.* New York, Academic Press.

Arcamone, F., Cassinelli, G., Fantini, G., Grein, A., Orezzi, P., Pol, C., and Spalla, C. (1969). Adriamycin, 14-hydroxydaunomycin, a new antitumor antibiotic from *S. peucetius var. caesius*. *Biotechnology and Bioengineering*, **11**, 1101–10.

Austin, C. A. and Fisher, L. M. (1990). DNA topoisomerases: enzymes that change the shape of DNA. *Science Progress*, **74**, 147–62.

Bachur, N. R., Gordon, S. L., and Gee, M. V. (1978). A general mechanism for microsomal activation of quinolone anticancer agents to free radicals. *Cancer Research*, **38**, 1745–50.

Bae, Y.-S., Kawasaki, I., Ikeda, H., and Liu, L. F. (1988). Illegitimate recombination mediated by calf thymus DNA topoisomerase II *in vitro*. *Proceedings of the National Academy of Sciences of the United States of America*, **85**, 2076–80.

Bendixen, C., Thomsen, B., Alsner, J., and Westergaard, O. (1990). Camptothecin-stabilized topoisomerase I-DNA adducts cause premature termination of transcription. *Biochemistry*, **29**, 5613–19.

Bhuyan, B. K., Fraser, T. J., and Li, L. H. (1972). Cell cycle phase specificity and biochemical effects of ellipticine on mammalian cells. *Cancer Research*, **32**, 2538–44.

Bishop, J. F. (1991). Etoposide in the management of leukemia: a review. *Seminars in Oncology*, **18**, 62–9.

Bjornsti, M.-A. and Wang, J. C. (1987). Expression of yeast DNA topoisomerase I can complement a conditional-lethal DNA topoisomerase I mutation in *Escherichia coli. Proceedings of the National Academy of Sciences of the United States of America*, **84**, 9871–5.

Bjornsti, M.-A., Benedetti, P., Viglianti, G. A., and Wang, J. C. (1989). Expression of human DNA topoisomerase I in yeast cells lacking yeast DNA topoisomerase I: restoration of sensitivity of the cells to the antitumor drug camptothecin. *Cancer Research*, **49**, 6318–23.

Bodley, A., Liu, L. F., Israel, M., Seshadri, R., Koseki, Y., Giuliani, F. C., *et al.* (1989). DNA topoisomerase II-mediated interaction of doxorubicin and daunomycin congeners with DNA. *Cancer Research*, **49**, 5969–78.

Brill, S. J., DiNardo, S., Voelkel-Meiman, K., and Sternglanz, R. (1987). Need for DNA topoisomerase activity as a swivel for DNA replication and for transcription of ribosomal RNA. *Nature, London*, **326**, 414–16.

Brown, P. O. and Cozzarelli, N. R. (1979). A sign inversion mechanism for enzymatic supercoiling of DNA. *Science*, **206**, 1081–3.

Brown, P. O. and Cozzarelli, N. R. (1981). Catenation and knotting of duplex DNA by type 1 topoisomerases: A mechanical parallel with type 2 topoisomerases. *Proceedings of the National Academy of Sciences of the United States of America*, **78**, 843–7.

Bugg, B. Y., Danks, M. K., Beck, W. T., and Suttle, D. P. (1991). Expression of a mutant DNA topoisomerase II in CCRF-CEM human leukemic cells selected for resistance to teniposide. *Proceedings of the National Academy of Sciences of the United States of America*, **88**, 7654–8.

Capranico, G., Kohn, K. W., and Pommier, Y. (1990a). Local sequence requirements for DNA cleavage by mammalian topoisomerase II in the presence of doxorubicin. *Nucleic Acids Research*, **18**, 6611–19.

Capranico, G., Zunino, F., Kohn, K. W., and Pommier, Y. (1990b). Sequence-selective topoisomerase II inhibition by anthracycline derivatives in SV40 DNA: Relationship with DNA binding affinity and cytotoxicity. *Biochemistry*, **29**, 562–9.

Carter, S. K. (1975). Adriamycin—a review. *Journal of National Cancer Institute*, **55**, 1265–74.

Champoux, J. J. (1977). Strand breakage by the DNA untwisting enzyme results in covalent attachment of the enzyme to DNA. *Proceedings of the National Academy of Sciences of the United States of America*, **74**, 3800–4.

Champoux, J. J. (1978). Mechanism of the reaction catalzed by the untwisting enzyme: Attachment of the enzyme to the 3′ terminus of the nicked DNA. *Journal of Molecular Biology*, **118**, 441–6.

Champoux, J. J. (1990). Mechanistic aspects of type-I topoisomerases. In *DNA topology and its biological effects* (ed. N. R. Cozzarelli and J. C. Wang), pp. 217–42. Cold Spring Harbor Laboratory Press, New York.

Champoux, J. J. and Dulbecco, R. (1972). An activity from mammalian cells that untwists superhelical DNA—a possible swivel for DNA replication. *Proceedings of the National Academy of Sciences of the United States of America*, **69**, 143–6.

Chang, J.-Y., Han, F.-S., Liu, S.-Y., Wang, Z.-Q., Lee, K.-H., and Cheng, Y.-C. (1991). Effect of 4β-arylamino derivatives of 4′-O-demethylepipodophyllotoxin on human DNA topoisomerase II, tubulin polymerization, KB cells, and their resistant variants. *Cancer Research*, **51**, 1755–9.

Chen, G. L. and Liu, L. F. (1986). DNA topoisomerases as therapeutic targets in cancer chemotherapy. *Annual Reports of Medicinal Chemistry*, **21**, 257–62.

Chen, G. L., Yang, L., Rowe, T. C., Halligan, B. D., Tewey, K. M., and Liu, L. F. (1984). Nonintercalative antitumor drugs interfere with the breakage–reunion reaction of mammalian DNA topoisomerase II. *Journal of Biological Chemistry*, **259**, 13560–6.

Chow, K. C. and Pearson, G. D. (1985). Adenovirus infection elevates levels of cellular topoisomerase I. *Proceedings of the National Academy of Sciences of the United States of America*, **82**, 2247–51.

Chow, K.-C. and Ross, W. E. (1987). Topoisomerase-specific drug sensitivity in relation to cell cycle progression. *Molecular and Cell Biology*, **7**, 3119–23.

Chow, K.-C., MacDonald, T. L., and Ross, W. E. (1988). DNA binding by epipodophyllotoxins and *N*-acyl anthracyclines: Implications for mechanism of topoisomerase II inhibition. *Molecular Pharmacology*, **34**, 467–73.

Christman, M. F., Dietrich, F. S., and Fink, G. S. (1988). Mitotic recombination in the rDNA of *S. cerevisiae* is suppressed by the combined action of DNA topoisomerases I and II. *Cell*, **55**, 413–25.

Chu, D. T. and Fernandes, P. B. (1989). Structure-activity relationships of the fluoroquinolones. *Antimicrobial Agents and Chemotherapy*, **33**, 131–5.

Chung, T. D. Y., Drake, F. H., Tan, K. B., Per, S. R., Crooke, S. T., and Mirabelli, C. K. (1989). Characterization and immunological identification of cDNA clones encoding two human topoisomerase isozymes. *Proceedings of the National Academy of Sciences of the United States of America*, **86**, 9331–5.

Cozzarelli, N. R. (1980). DNA gyrase and the supercoiling of DNA. *Science*, **207**, 953–60.

Crick, F. H. C. (1976). Linking numbers and nucleosomes. *Proceedings of the National Academy of Sciences of the United States of America*, **73**, 2639–43.

Cullen, M. E., Wyke, A. W., Kuroda, R., and Fisher, L. M. (1989). Cloning and characterization of a DNA gyrase A gene from *Escherichia coli* that confers clinical resistance to 4-quinolones. *Antimicrobial Agents and Chemotherapy*, **33**, 886–94.

Danks, M. K., Yalowich, J. C., and Beck, W. T. (1987). Atypical multiple drug resistance in a human leukemic cell line selected for resistance to teniposide (VM-26). *Cancer Research*, **47**, 1297–1301.

D'Arpa, P. and Liu, L. F. (1989). Topoisomerase-targeting antitumor drugs. *Biochimica et Biophysica Acta*, **989**, 163–77.

D'Arpa, P., Machlin, P. S., Ratrie, H., III, Rothfield, N. F., Cleveland, D. W., and Earnshaw, W. C. (1988). c-DNA cloning of human DNA topoisomerase I: catalytic activity of a 67.7-kDA carboxyl-terminal fragment. *Proceedings of the National Academy of Sciences of the United States of America*, **85**, 2543–7.

Dean, F., Krasnow, M. A., Otter, R., Matzuk, M. M., Spengler, S. J., and Cozzarelli, N. R. (1982). *Escherichia coli* type-I topoisomerases: identification, mechanism, and role in recombination. *Cold Spring Harbor Symposia on Quantitative Biology*, **47**, 769–77.

Deaven, L. L., Oka, M. S., and Tobey, R. A. (1978). Cell cycle-specific chromosome damage following treatment of cultured Chinese hamster cells with 4'-[(9-acridinyl)amino]methanesulphon-*m*-aniside-HCl. *Journal of National Cancer Institute*, **60**, 1155–61.

Deffie, A. M., Bosman, D. J., and Goldenberg, G. J. (1989). Evidence for a mutant allele of the gene for DNA topoisomerase II in adriamycin-resistant P388 murine leukemia cells. *Cancer Research*, **49**, 6879–82.

Degrassi, F., De Salva, R., Tanzarella, C., and Palitti, F. (1989). Induction of chromosomal aberrations and SCE by camptothecin, an inhibitor of mammalian topoisomerase I. *Mutation Research*, **211**, 125–30.

Del Bino, G., Lassota, P., and Darzynkiewicz, Z. (1991). The S-phase cytotoxicity of camptothecin. *Experimental Cell Research*, **193**, 27–35.

Depew, R. E., Liu, L. F., and Wang, J. C. (1978). Interaction between DNA and *Escherichia coli* protein ω. Formation of a complex between single-stranded DNA and ω protein. *Journal of Biological Chemistry*, **253**, 511–18.

DiGate, R. J. and Marians, K. J. (1988). Identification of a potent decatenating enzyme from *Escherichia coli*. *Journal of Biological Chemistry*, **263**, 13366–73.

DiGate, R. J. and Marians, K. J. (1989). Molecular cloning and DNA sequence analysis of *Escherichia coli* topB, the gene encoding topoisomerase III. *Journal of Biological Chemistry*, **264**, 17924–30.

Dillehay, L. E., Denstman, S. C., and Williams, J. R. (1987). Cell cycle dependence of sister chromatid exchange induction by DNA topoisomerase II inhibitors in Chinese hamster V79 cells. *Cancer Research*, **47**, 206–9.

Di Marco, A. (1967). Daunomycin and related antibiotics. In *Antibiotics* (ed. D. Gottleib and P. D. Shaw), pp. 190–210. Springer-Verlag, New York.

DiNardo, S., Voelkel, K. A., Sternglanz, R., Reynolds, A. E., and Wright, A. (1982). *Escherichia coli* DNA topoisomerase I mutants have compensatory mutations in DNA gyrase genes. *Cell*, **31**, 43–51.

DiNardo, S., Voelkel, K. A., Sternglanz, R. (1984). DNA topoisomerase II mutant of *Saccharomyces cerevisiae*: Topoisomerase II is required for segregation of daughter molecules at the termination of DNA replication. *Proceedings of the National Academy of Sciences of the United States of America*, **81**, 2616–20.

Drake, F. H., Hofmann, G. A., Bartus, H. F., Mattern, M. F., Crooke, S. T., and Mirabelli, C. K. (1989). Biochemical and pharmacological properties of p170 and p180 forms of topoisomerase II. *Biochemistry*, **28**, 8154–60.

Drewinko, B., Freireich, E. J., and Gottleib, J. A. (1974). Lethal activity of camptothecin sodium on human lymphoma cells. *Cancer Research*, **34**, 747–50.

Drlica, K. (1984). Biology of bacterial deoxyribonucleic acid topoisomerases. *Micobiological Reviews*, **48**, 273–89.

Drlica, K. (1990). Bacterial topoisomerases and the control of DNA supercoiling. *Trends in Genetics*, **6**, 433–7.

Drlica, K. and Coughlin, S. (1989). Inhibitors of DNA gyrase. *Pharmacology and Therapeutics*, **44**, 107–22.

Drlica, K. and Franco, R. J. (1988). Inhibitors of DNA topoisomerases. *Biochemistry*, **27**, 2253–9.

Dynan, W. S., Jendrisak, J. J., Hager, D. A., and Burgess, R. R. (1981). Purification and characterization of wheat germ DNA topoisomerase I (nicking-closing enzyme). *Journal of Biological Chemistry*, **256**, 5860–5.

Egyhazi, E. and Durban, E. (1987). Microinjection of anti-topoisomerase I immunoglobulin G into nuclei of *Chironomus tentans* salivary gland cells leads to blockage of transcription elongation. *Molecular and Cell Biology*, **7**, 4308–16.

Endicott, J. A. and Ling, V. (1989). The biochemistry of P-glycoprotein-mediated multidrug resistance. *Annual Review of Biochemistry*, **58**, 137–71.

Eng, W.-K., Faucette, L., Johnson, R. K., and Sternglanz, R. (1988). Evidence that DNA topoisomerase I is necessary for the cytotoxic effects of camptothecin. *Molecular Pharmacology*, **34**, 755–60.

Eng, W.-K., Pundit, S. D., and Sternglanz, R. (1989). Mapping of the active site tyrosine of eukaryotic DNA topoisomerase I. *Journal of Biological Chemistry*, **264**, 13373–6.

Eng, W. K., McCabe, F. L., Tan, K. B., Mattern, M. R., Hofmann, G. A., Woessner, R. D., *et al.* (1990). Development of a stable camptothecin-resistant subline of P388 leukemia with reduced topoisomerase I content. *Molecular Pharmacology*, **38**, 471–80.

Estey, E., Adlakha, R. C., Hittelman, W. N., and Zwelling, L. A. (1987). Cell cycle stage dependent variations in drug-induced topoisomerase II mediated DNA cleavage and cytotoxicity. *Biochemistry*, **26**, 4338–44.

Fernandes, P. B. and Shen, L. L. (1989). Quinolones: mode of action and mechanism of resistance. In *Clinical implications of antimicrobial resistance: mechanism, testing problems and epidemiology* (ed. P. Actor, G. Shockman, E. Hinks, and L. R. Walsh), pp. 40–56. Eastern Pennsylvania Branch, American Society of Microbiology, Philadelphia, PA.

Figgitt, D. P., Denyer, S. P., Dewick, P. M., Jackson, D. E., and Williams, P. (1989). Topoisomerase II: a potential target for novel antifungal agents. *Biochemical and Biophysical Research Communications*, **160**, 257–62.

Figueroa, N. and Bossi, L. (1988). Transcription induces gyration of the DNA template in *Escherichia coli*. *Proceedings of the National Academy of Sciences of the United States of America*, **85**, 9416–20.

Filipski, J. and Kohn, K. W. (1982). Ellipticine-induced protein-associated DNA breaks in isolated L1210 nuclei. *Biochimica et Biophysica Acta*, **698**, 280–6.

Fleischmann, G., Pflugfelder, G., Steiner, E. K., Javaherian, K., Howard, G. C., Wang, J. C., and Elgin, S. C. R. (1984). *Drosophila* DNA topoisomerase I is associated with transcriptionally active regions of the genome. *Proceedings of the National Academy of Sciences of the United States of America*, **81**, 6958–62.

Frederick, C. A., Williams, L. D., Ughetto, G., van der Marel, G. A., van Boom, J. H., Rich, A., and Wang, A. H.-J. (1990). Structural comparison of anticancer drug-DNA complexes: adriamycin and daunomycin. *Biochemistry*, **29**, 2538–49.

Gellert, M. (1981). DNA topoisomerases. *Annual Review of Biochemistry*, **50**, 879–910.

Gellert, M., Mizuuchi, K., O'Dea, M. H., Itoh, T., and Tomizawa, J.-I. (1976a). DNA gyrase: an enzyme that introduces superhelical turns into DNA. *Proceedings of the National Academy of Sciences of the United States of America*, **73**, 3872–6.

Gellert, M., O'Dea, M. H., Itoh, T., and Tomizawa, J. (1976b). Novobiocin and coumermycin inhibit DNA supercoiling catalzed by DNA gyrase. *Proceedings of the National Academy of Sciences of the United States of America*, **73**, 4474–8.

Gellert, M., Mizuuchi, K., O'Dea, M. H., Itoh, T., and Tomizawa, J-I. (1977). Nalidixic acid resistance: a second genetic character involved in DNA gyrase activity. *Proceedings of the National Academy of Sciences of the United States of America*, **74**, 4772–6.

Giaever, G. N. and Wang, J. C. (1988). Supercoiling of intracellular DNA can occur in eukaryotic cells. *Cell*, **55**, 849–56.

Giaever, F., Lynn, R., Goto, T., and Wang, J. C. (1986). The complete nucleotide sequence of the structural gene TOP2 of yeast DNA topoisomerase II. *Journal of Biological Chemistry*, **261**, 12448–54.

Giaever, G. N., Snyder, L., and Wang, J. C. (1988). DNA supercoiling *in vivo*. *Biological Chemistry*, **29**, 7–15.

Gilmour, D. S., Pflugfelder, G., Wang, J. C., and Lis, J. T. (1986). Topoisomerase I interacts with transcribed regions in *Drosophila* cells. *Cell*, **44**, 401–7.

Giovanella, B. C., Stehlin, J. S., Wall, M. E., Wani, M. C., Nicholas, A. W., Liu, L. F., *et al.* (1989). DNA topoisomerase I-targeted chemotherapy of human colon cancer in xenografts. *Science*, **246**, 1046–8.

Giovanella, B. C., Hinz, H. R., Kozielski, A. J., Stehlin, J. S., Jr, Silber, R., and Potmesil, M. (1991). Complete growth inhibition of human cancer xenografts in nude mice by treatment with 20-(S)-camptothecin. *Cancer Research*, **51**, 3052–5.

Glisson, B. S. and Ross, W. E. (1987). DNA topoisomerase II: A primer on the enzyme and its unique role as a multidrug target in cancer chemotherapy. *Pharmacology and Therapeutics*, **32**, 89–106.

Glisson, B. S., Smallwood, S. E., and Ross, W. E. (1984). Characterization of VP-16-induced DNA damage in isolated nuclei from L1210 cells. *Biochimica et Biophysica Acta*, **783**, 74–9.

Gootz, T. D., Barrett, J. F., Holden, H. E., Ray, V. A., and McGuirk, P. R. (1990). Selective toxicity: the activities of 4-quinolones against eukaryotic DNA topoisomerases. In *The 4-quinolones: antibacterial agents in vitro* (ed. C. Crumplin), pp. 159–72. London: Springer-Verlag.

Gorsky, L. D., Cross, S. M., and Morin, M. J. (1989). Rapid increase in the activity of DNA topoisomerase I, but not topoisomerase II, in HL-60 promyelocytic leukemia cells treated with a phorbol diester. *Cancer Communications*, **1**, 83–92.

Goto, T. and Wang, J. C. (1982). Yeast DNA topoisomerase II: an ATP-dependent type II topoisomerase that catalzes the catenation, decatenation, unknotting and relaxation of double-stranded DNA rings. *Journal of Biological Chemistry*, **257**, 5866–72.

Goto, T. and Wang, J. C. (1985). Cloning of yeast TOP1, the gene encoding DNA topoisomerase I, and construction of mutants defective in both DNA topoisomerase I and DNA topoisomerase II. *Proceedings of the National Academy of Sciences of the United States of America*, **82**, 7178–82.

Goto, T., Laipis, P., and Wang, J. C. (1984). The purification and characterization of DNA topoisomerases I and II of the yeast *Saccharomyces cerevisiae*. *Journal of Biological Chemistry*, **259**, 10422–9.

Gottlieb, J. A. and Luce, J. K. (1972). Treatment of malignant melanoma with camptothecin (NSC-100880). *Cancer Chemotherapy Reports, Part I*, **56**, 103–5.

Gottlieb, J. A., Guarino, A. M., Call, J. B., Oliverio, V. T., and Black, J. B. (1970). Preliminary pharmacologic and clinical evaluation of camptothecin sodium (NSC-100880). *Cancer Chemotherapy Reports, Part I*, **54**, 461–70.

Grein, A., Spalla, C., Di Marco, A., and Canevazzi, G. (1963). Descrizione e classificazione di un attinomicete (*Streptomyces peucetius sp. nova*) produttore di una sostanza ad attivita antitumorale: la daunomicina. *Giornale microbiologia*, **11**, 109–18.

Gupta, R. S., Gupta, R., Eng, B., Lock, R. B., Ross, W. E., Hertberg, R. P., *et al.* (1988). Camptothecin-resistant mutants of Chinese hamster ovary cells containing a resistant form of topoisomerase I. *Cancer Research*, **48**, 6404–10.

Hallett, P. and Maxwell, A. (1991). Novel quinolone resistance mutations of the *Escherichia coli* DNA gyrase A protein: enzymatic analysis of the mutant proteins. *Antimicrobial Agents and Chemotherapy*, **35**, 335–40.

Halligan, B. D., Edwards, K. A., and Liu, L. F. (1985). Purification and characterization of a type II DNA topoisomerase from bovine calf thymus. *Journal of Biological Chemistry*, **260**, 2475–82.

Harnett, N., Brown, S., and Krishnan, C. (1991). Emergence of quinolone resistance among clinical isolates of methicillin-resistant *Staphylococcus aureus* in Ontario, Canada. *Antimicrobial Agents and Chemotherapy*, **35**, 1911–13.

Hayakawa, I., Atarashi, S., Yokohama, S., Imamura, M., Sakano, K.-I., and Furukawa, M. (1986). Synthesis and antibacterial activities of optically active ofloxacin. *Antimicrobial Agents and Chemotherapy*, **29**, 163–4.

Heck, M. M. S. and Earnshaw, W. C. (1986). Topoisomerase II: a specific marker for cell proliferation. *Journal of Cell Biology*, **103**, 2569–81.

Heck, M. M. S., Hittelman, W. N., and Earnshaw, W. C. (1988). Differential expression of DNA topoisomerases I and II during the eukaryotic cell cycle. *Proceedings of the National Academy of Sciences of the United States of America*, **85**, 1086–90.

Hertzberg, R. P., Caranfa, M. J., and Hecht, S. M. (1989a). On the mechanism of topoisomerase I inhibition by camptothecin: evidence for binding to an enzyme-DNA complex. *Biochemistry*, **28**, 4629–38.

Hertzberg, R. P., Caranfa, M. J., Holden, K. G., Jakas, D. R., Gallagher, G., Mattern, M. R., *et al.* (1989b). Modification of the hydroxy lactone ring of camptothecin: inhibition of mammalian topoisomerase I and biological activity. *Journal of Medicinal Chemistry*, **32**, 715–20.

Higashinakagawa, T., Wahn, H., and Reeder, R. H. (1977). Isolation of ribosomal gene chromatin. *Developmental Biology*, **55**, 375–86.

Higgins, N. P., Peebles, C. L., Sugino, A., and Cozzarelli, N. R. (1978). Purification of subunits of *Escherichia coli* DNA gyrase and reconstitution of enzymatic activity *Proceedings of the National Academy of Sciences of the United States of America*, **75**, 1773–7.

Hinds, M., Deisseroth, K., Mayes, J., Altschuler, E., Jansen, R., Ledley, F. D., and Zwelling, L. A. (1991). Identification of a point mutation in the topoisomerase II gene from a human leukemia cell line containing an amsacrine-resistant form of topoisomerase II. *Cancer Research*, **51**, 4729–31.

Hirai, K., Aoyama, H., Suzue, S., Irikura, T., Iyobe, S., and Mitsuhashi, S. (1986). Isolation and characterization of norfloxacin-resistant mutants in *Escherichia coli* K12. *Antimicrobial Agents and Chemotherapy*, **30**, 248–53.

Holden, J. A., Rolfson, D. H., and Low, R. L. (1990). DNA topoisomerase I from human placenta. *Biochimica et Biophysica Acta*, **1049**, 303–10.

Holm, C., Goto, T., Wang, J. C., and Botstein, D. (1985). DNA topoisomerase II is required at the time of mitosis in yeast. *Cell*, **41**, 553–63.

Holm, C., Covey, J. M., Kerrigan, D., and Pommier, Y. (1989). Differential requirements of DNA replication of cytotoxicity of DNA topoisomerase I and II inhibitors in Chinese hamster DC3F cells. *Cancer Research*, **49**, 6365–8.

Hooper, D. C. and Wolfson, J. S. (1990). Mechanisms of resistance to 4-quinolones. In *The 4-quinolones: antibacterial agents in vitro* pp. 201–14. Springer-Verlag, New York.

Hooper, D. C. and Wolfson, J. S. (1991). Fluoroquinolone antimicrobial agents. *New England Journal of Medicine*, **324**, 384–95.

Hooper, D. C., Wolfson, J. S., Ng, E. Y., and Swartz, M. N. (1987). Mechanisms of action and resistance to ciprofloxacin. *American Journal of Medicine*, **82** (Suppl. 4A), 12–20.

Hooper, D. C., Wolfson, J. S., Souza, K. S., Tung, C., McHugh, G. L., and Swartz, M. N. (1986). Genetic and biochemical characterization of norfloxacin resistance in *Escherichia coli*. *Antimicrobial Agents and Chemotherapy*, **29**, 639–44.

Hooper, D. C., Wolfson, J. S., Souza, K. S., Ng, E. Y., McHugh, G. L., and Swartz, M. N. (1989). Mechanisms of quinolone resistance in *Escherichia coli*: Characterization of *nfxB* and *cfxB*, two mutant resistance loci decreasing norfloxacin accumulation. *Antimicrobial Agents and Chemotherapy*, **33**, 283–90.

Horowitz, D. S. and Wang, J. C. (1987). Mapping the active site tyrosine of *Escherichia coli* DNA gyrase. *Journal of Biological Chemistry*, **262**, 5339–44.

Horowitz, S. B. and Horowitz, M. S. (1973). Effects of camptothecin on the breakage and repair of DNA during the cell cycle. *Cancer Research*, **33**, 2834–36.

Hsiang, Y.-H. and Liu, L. F. (1988). Identification of mammalian DNA topoisomerase I as an intracellular target of the anticancer drug camptothecin. *Cancer Research*, **48**, 1722–6.

Hsiang, Y.-H., Hertzberg, R., Hecht, S., and Liu, L. F. (1985). Camptothecin induces protein-linked DNA breaks via mammalian DNA topoisomerase I. *Journal of Biological Chemistry*, **260**, 14873–8.

Hsiang, Y.-H., Wu, H. Y., and Liu, L. F. (1988). Proliferation-dependent regulation of DNA topoisomerase II in cultured human cells. *Cancer Research*, **48**, 3230–5.

Hsiang, Y.-H., Jiang, J. B., and Liu, J. F. (1989a). Topoisomerase II-mediated DNA cleavage by amonafide and its structural analogs. *Molecular Pharmacology*, **36**, 371–6.

Hsiang, Y.-H., Lihou, M. G., and Liu, L. F. (1989b). Arrest of replication forks by drug-stabilized topoisomerase I-DNA cleavable complexes as a mechanism of cell killing by camptothecin. *Cancer Research*, **49**, 5077–82.

Hsiang, Y.-H., Liu, L. F., Wall, M. E., Wani, M. C., Nicholas, A. W., Manikumar, G., *et al.* (1989c). DNA topoisomerase I-mediated DNA cleavage and cytotoxicity of camptothecin analogues. *Cancer Research*, **49**, 4385–9.

Hsieh, T.-S. (1983). Knotting of circular duplex DNA by type II DNA topoisomerase from *Drosophila melanogaster*. *Journal of Biological Chemistry*, **258**, 8413–20.

Hsieh, T.-S. (1990). Mechanistic aspects of type-II topoisomerases. In *DNA topology and its biological effects* (ed. N. R. Cozzarelli and J. C. Wang), pp. 243–63. Cold Spring Harbor Laboratory Press, New York.

Hsieh, T.-S. and Brutlag, D. (1980). ATP-dependent DNA topoisomerase from *D. melanogaster* reversibly catenates duplex DNA rings. *Cell*, **21**, 115–25.

Huang, W. M. (1986a). Nucleotide sequence of a type II DNA topoisomerase gene. Bacteriophage T4 gene 52. *Nucleic Acids Research*, **14**, 7379–90.

Huang, W. M. (1986b). Nucleotide sequence of a type II DNA topoisomerase gene. Bacteriophage T4 gene 39. *Nucleic Acids Research*, **14**, 7751–65.

Huang, W. M., Ao, S.-H., Casjens, S., Orlandi, R., Zeikus, R., Weiss, R., *et al.* (1988). A persistent untranslated sequence within bacteriophage T4 DNA topoisomerase gene 60. *Science*, **239**, 1005–12.

Hudson, B., Clayton, D. A., and Vinograd, J. (1968). Complex mitochondrial DNA. *Cold Spring Harbor Symposia on Quantitative Biology*, **30**, 435–42.

Huff, A. C. and Kreuzer, K. N. (1990). Evidence for a common mechanism of action for antitumor and antibacterial agents that inhibit type II DNA topoisomerases. *Journal of Biological Chemistry*, **265**, 20496–505.

Huff, A. C., Leatherwood, J. K., and Kreuzer, K. N. (1989). Bacteriophage T4 DNA topoisomerase is the target of antitumor agent 4′-(9-acridinylamino)-

methanesulfon-*m*-aniside (*m*-AMSA) in T4-infected *Escherichia coli*. *Proceedings of the National Academy of Sciences of the United States of America*, **86**, 1307–11.

Hwang, J., Shyy, S., Chen, A. Y., Juan, C.-C., and Whang-Peng, J. (1989). Studies of topoisomerase-specific antitumor drugs in human lymphocytes using rabbit antisera against recombinant human topoisomerase II polypeptide. *Cancer Research*, **49**, 958–62.

Hwong, C.-L., Chen, M.-S., and Hwang, J. (1989). Phorbol ester transiently increases topoisomerase I mRNA levels in human skin fibroblasts. *Journal of Biological Chemistry*, **264**, 14923–6.

Ikeda, H. (1986). Bacteriophage T4 DNA topoisomerase mediates illegitimate recombination *in vitro*. *Proceedings of the National Academy of Sciences of the United States of America*, **83**, 922–6.

Ikeda, H., Aoki, K., and Naito, A. (1982). Illegitimate recombination mediated *in vitro* by DNA gyrase of *Escherichia coli*: Structure of recombinant DNA molecules. *Proceedings of the National Academy of Sciences of the United States of America*, **79**, 3724–8.

Ishii, K., Hasegawa, T., Fujisawa, K., and Andon, T. (1983). Rapid purification and characterization of DNA topoisomerase I from cultured mouse mammary carcinoma FM3A cells. *Journal of Biological Chemistry*, **258**, 12728–32.

Jardine, I. (1980). Podophyllotoxins. In *Anticancer agents based on natural product models* (ed. J. M. Cassidy and J. D. Douros), pp. 319–51. Academic Press, New York.

Javaherian, K., Tse, Y.-C., and Vega, J. (1982). *Drosophila* topoisomerase I: Isolation, purification and characterization. *Nucleic Acids Research*, **10**, 6945–55.

Jaxel, C. J., Kohn, K. W., Wani, M. C., Watt, M. E., and Pommier, Y. (1989). Structure-activity study of the actions of camptothecin derivatives on mammalian topoisomerase I: evidence for a specific receptor site and a relation to antitumor activity. *Cancer Research*, **49**, 1465–9.

Johnson, D. H., Hainsworth, J. D., Hande, K. R., and Greco, F. A. (1991). Current status of etoposide in the management of small cell lung cancer. *Cancer*, **67**, 231–44.

Kato, J.-I., Nishimura, Y., Imamura, R., Niki, H., Hiraga, S., and Suzuki, H. (1990). New topoisomerase essential for chromosome segregation in *E. coli*. *Cell*, **63**, 393–404.

Kaufmann, S. (1991a). DNA topoisomerases in chemotherapy. *Cancer Cells*, **3**, 24–7.

Kaufmann, S. H. (1991b). Antagonism between camptothecin and topoisomerase II-directed chemotherapeutic agents in a human leukemia cell line. *Cancer Research*, **51**, 1129–36.

Kawada, S.-Z., Yamashita, Y., Fujii, N., and Nakano, H. (1991). Induction of a heat-stable topoisomerase II-DNA cleavable complex by nonintercalative terpenoides, terpentecin and clerocidin. *Cancer Research*, **51**, 2922–5.

Keller, W. (1975). Characterization of purified DNA-relaxing enzyme from human tissue culture cells. *Proceedings of the National Academy of Sciences of the United States of America*, **72**, 2550–4.

Keller-Juslen, C., Kuhn, M., von Wartburg, A., and Stahelin, H. (1971). Synthesis and antimitotic activity of glycosidic lignan derivatives related to podophyllotoxin. *Journal of Medicinal Chemistry*, **14**, 936–40.

Kelly, M. G. and Hartwell, J. L. (1954). The biological effects and the chemical composition of podophyllotoxin. A review. *Journal of National Cancer Institute*, **14**, 967–1010.

Kim, R. A. and Wang, J. C. (1989). A subthreshold level of DNA topoisomerases leads to the excision of yeast rDNA as extrachromosomal rings. *Cell*, **57**, 975–85.

Kingsbury, W. D., Boehm, J. C., Jakas, D. R., Holden, K. G., Hecht, S. M., Gallagher, G., *et al.* (1991). Synthesis of water-soluble (aminoalkyl)camptothecin analogues: inhibition of topoisomerase I and antitumor activity. *Journal of Medicinal Chemistry*, **34**, 98–107.

Kirchhausen, T., Wang, J. C., and Harrison, S. C. (1985). DNA gyrase and its complexes with DNA: Direct observation by electron microscopy. *Cell*, **41**, 933–43.

Kirkegaard, K. and Wang, J. C. (1981). Mapping the topography of DNA wrapped around gyrase by nucleolytic and chemical probing of complexes of unique DNA sequences. *Cell*, **23**, 721–9.

Kirkegaard, K. and Wang, J. C. (1985). Bacterial DNA topoisomerase I can relax positively supercoiled DNA containing a single-stranded loop. *Journal of Molecular Biology*, **185**, 625–37.

Kjeldsen, E., Bonven, J. B., Andoh, T., Ishii, K., Okada, K., Bolund, L., and Westergaard, O. (1988). Characterization of a camptothecin-resistant human DNA topoisomerase I. *Journal of Biological Chemistry*, **263**, 3912–16.

Kreuzer, K. N. and Cozzarell, N. R. (1980). Formation and resolution of DNA catenanes by DNA gyrase. *Cell*, **20**, 245–54.

Kreuzer, K. N. and Jongeneel, C. V. (1983). *Escherichia coli* phage T4 topoisomerase. *Methods in Enzymology*, **100**, 144–60.

Kung, V. T. and Wang, J. C. (1977). Purification and characterization of an omega protein from *Micrococcus luteus*. *Journal of Biological Chemistry*, **252**, 5398–402.

Lee, M. P., Sander, M., and Hsieh, T.-S. (1989). Nuclease protection by *Drosophila* DNA topoisomerase II. Enzyme/DNA contacts at the strong topoisomerase II cleavage site. *Journal of Biological Chemistry*, **264**, 21779–87.

Lesher, G. Y., Froelich, E. J., Gruett, M. D., Bailey, J. H., and Brundage, R. P. (1962). 1,8-Naphthyridine derivatives. A new class of chemotherapeutic agents. *Journal of Medicinal Chemistry*, **5**, 1063–5.

Li, L. H., Fraser, T. J., Olin, E. J., and Bhuyab, B. K. (1972). Action of camptothecin on mammalian cells in culture. *Cancer Research*, **32**, 2550–63.

Liu, L. F. (1983). DNA topoisomerases—enzymes that catalyze the breaking and rejoining of DNA. *CRC Critical Review of Biochemistry*, **15**, 1–24.

Liu, L. F. (1989). DNA topoisomerase poisons as antitumor drugs. *Annual Review of Biochemistry*, **58**, 351–75.

Liu, L. F. and Miller, K. G. (1981). Eukaryotic DNA topoisomerases: two forms of type I DNA topoisomerases from HeLa cell nuclei. *Proceedings of the National Academy of Sciences of the United States of America*, **78**, 3487–91.

Liu, L. F. and Wang, J. C. (1978a). DNA–DNA gyrase complex: the wrapping of the DNA duplex outside the enzyme. *Cell*, **15**, 979–84.

Liu, L. F. and Wang, J. C. (1978b). *Micrococcus luteus* DNA gyrase: active components and a model for its supercoiling of DNA. *Proceedings of the National Academy of Sciences of the United States of America*, **75**, 2098–102.

Liu, L. F. and Wang, J. C. (1987). Supercoiling of the DNA template during transcription. *Proceedings of the National Academy of Sciences of the United States of America*, **84**, 7024–7.

Liu, L. F., Liu, C. C., and Alberts, B. M. (1979). T4 DNA topoisomerase: A new ATP-dependent enzyme essential for initiation of T4 DNA replication. *Nature, London*, **281**, 456–61.

Liu, L. F., Liu, C. C., and Alberts, B. M. (1980). Type II DNA topoisomerases: enzymes that can unknot a topologically knotted DNA molecule via a reversible double-strand break. *Cell*, **19**, 697–707.

Liu, L. F., Davis, J. L., and Calendar, R. (1981). Novel topologically knotted DNA from bacteriophage P4 capsids: Studies with DNA topoisomerase. *Nucleic Acids Research*, **9**, 3979–89.

Liu, L. F., Rowe, T. C., Yang, L., Tewey, K. M., and Chen, G. L. (1983). Cleavage of DNA by mammalian DNA topoisomerase II. *Journal of Biological Chemistry*, **258**, 15365–70.

Loike, J. D. and Horwitz, S. B. (1976). Effect of VP-16–213 on the intracellular degradation of DNA in HeLa cells. *Biochemistry*, **15**, 5443–8.

Long, B. H. and Stringfellow, D. A. (1988). Inhibitors of topoisomerase II: Structure-activity relationships and mechanism of action of podophyllotoxin congeners. *Advances in Enzyme Regulation*, **27**, 223–56.

Long, B. H., Musial, S. T., and Brattain, M. G. (1984). Comparison of cytotoxicity and DNA breakage activity of congeners of podophyllotoxin including VP 16–213 and VM26: a quantitative structure–activity relationship. *Biochemistry*, **23**, 1183–8.

Long, B. H., Musial, S. F., and Brattain, M. G. (1986). DNA breakage in human lung carcinoma cells and nuclei that are naturally sensitive or resistant to etoposide and teniposide. *Cancer Research*, **46**, 3809–16.

Lown, J. W., Sim, S.-K., Makumdar, K. C., and Chang, R. K. (1977). Strand scission of DNA by bound adriamycin and daunorubicin in the presence of reducing agents. *Biochemical and Biophysical Research Communications*, **76**, 705–10.

Lynn, R. M., Bjornsti, M.-A., Caron, P. R., and Wang, J. C. (1989). Peptide sequencing and site-directed mutagenesis identify tyrosine-727 as the active site tyrosine of *Saccharomyces cerevisiae* DNA topoisomerase I. *Proceedings of the National Academy of Sciences of the United States of America*, **86**, 3559–63.

Markovits, J., Pommier, Y., Kerrigan, D., Covey, J. M., Tilchen, E. J., and Kohn, K. W. (1987). Topoisomerase II-mediated DNA breaks and cytotoxicity in relation to cell proliferation and the cell cycle in NIH 3T3 fibroblasts and L1210 leukemia cells. *Cancer Research*, **47**, 2050–5.

Martin, S. R., McCoubrey, W. K., Jr, McConaughy, B. L., Young, L. S., Been, M. D., Brewer, B. J., and Champoux, J. J. (1983). Multiple forms of rat liver type I topoisomerase. *Methods in Enzymology*, **100**, 137–44.

Masurekar, M., Kreuzer, K. N., and Ripley, L. S. (1991). The specificity of topoisomerase-mediated DNA cleavage defines acridine-induced frameshift specificity within a hotspot in bacteriophage T4. *Genetics*, **127**, 453–62.

Maxwell, A. and Gellert, M. (1986). Mechanistic aspects of DNA topoisomerases. *Advances in Protein Chemistry*, **38**, 69–107.

Miller, K. G., Liu, L. F., and Englund, P. T. (1981). A homogeneous type II DNA topoisomerase from HeLa cell nuclei. *Journal of Biological Chemistry*, **256**, 9334–9.

Minford, J., Pommier, Y., Filipski, J., Kohn, K. W., Kerrigan, D., Mattern, M., *et al.* (1986). Isolation of intercalator-dependent protein-linked DNA strand cleavage activity and identification as topoisomerase II. *Biochemistry*, **25**, 9–16.

Minocha, A. and Long, B. H. (1984). Inhibition of the DNA catenation activity of type II topoisomerase by VP16–213 and VM26. *Biochemical and Biophysical Research Communications*, **122**, 165–70.

Mitscher, L. A., Zavod, R. M., and Sharma, P. N. (1989). Structure-activity relationships of the newer quinolone antibacterial agents. In *International Telesymposium on Quinolones* (ed. P. Fernandes), pp. 3–22. J. R. Prous, Barcelona.

Mitscher, L. A., Devasthale, P. V., and Zavod, R. M. (1990). Structure-activity relationships of fluoro-4-quinolones. In *The 4-quinolones: antibacterial agents in vitro* (ed. C. Crumplin), pp. 115–46. Springer-Verlag, New York.

Mizuuchi, K., O'Dea, M. H., and Gellert, M. (1978). DNA gyrase: Subunit structure and ATPase activity of the purified enzyme. *Proceedings of the National Academy of Sciences of the United States of America*, **75**, 5960–3.

Moertel, C. G., Schutt, A. J., Reitmeier, R. J., and Hahn, R. G. (1972). Phase II study of camptothecin (NSC-100880) in treatment of advanced gastrointestinal cancer. *Cancer Chemotherapy Reports, Part I*, **56**, 95–101.

Moriya, S., Ogasawara, N., and Yoshikawa, H. (1985). Structure and function of the region of the replication origin of the *Bacillus subtilis* chromosome. III. Nucleotide sequence of some 10,000 base pairs in the origin region. *Nucleic Acids Research*, **13**, 2251–65.

Morrison, A. and Cozzarelli, N. R. (1981). Contacts between DNA gyrase and its binding site on DNA: features of symmetry and asymmetry revealed by protection from nucleases. *Proceedings of the National Academy of Sciences of the United States of America*, **78**, 1416–20.

Mortensen, U. H., Stevnsner, T., Krogh, S., Olesen, K., Westergaard, O., and Bonven, B. J. (1990). Distamycin inhibition of topoisomerase I-DNA interaction: a mechanistic analysis. *Nucleic Acids Research*, **18**, 1983–9.

Muggia, F. M., Craven, P. J., Hansen, H. H., Cohen, M. H., and Selawry, O. S. (1972). Phase I clinical trial of weekly and daily treatment with camptothecin (NSC-100880): Correlation with preclinical studies. *Cancer Chemotherapy Reports, Part I*, **56**, 515–21.

Muller, M. T., Pfund, W. P., Mehta, V. B., and Trask, D. K. (1985). Eukaryotic type I topoisomerase is enriched in the nucleolus and catalytically active on ribosomal DNA. *EMBO Journal*, **4**, 1237–43.

Negoro, S., Fukuoka, M., Masuda, N., Tadaka, M., Kusunoki, Y., Matsui, K., *et al.* (1991). Phase I study of weekly intravenous infusions of CPT-11, a new derivative of camptothecin, in the treatment of advanced non-small-cell lung cancer. *Journal of National Cancer Institute*, **83**, 1164–9.

Nelson, E. M., Tewey, K. M., and Liu, L. F. (1984). Mechanism of antitumor drug action: Poisoning of mammalian DNA topoisomerase II on DNA by 4'-(9-acridinylamino)-methanesulfon-*m*-anisidide. *Proceedings of the National Academy of Sciences of the United States of America*, **81**, 1361–5.

Nelson, W. G., Cho, K. R., Hsiang, Y.-H., Liu, L. F., and Coffey, D. S. (1987). Growth-related elevations of DNA topoisomerase II levels found in Dunning R3327 rat prostatic adenocarcinomas. *Cancer Research*, **47**, 3246–50.

Neu, H. C. (1990). Quinolones in perspective. *Journal of Antimicrobial Chemotherapy*, **26**, 1–6.

Nitiss, J. and Wang, J. C. (1988). DNA topoisomerase-targeting antitumor drugs can be studied in yeast. *Proceedings of the National Academy of Sciences of the United States of America*, **85**, 7501–5.

O'Dwyer, P. J., Alonso, M. T., Leyland-Jones, B., and Marsoni, S. (1984). Teniposide: a review of 12 years of experience. *Cancer Treatment Reports*, **678**, 1455–66.

Oguro, M. (1990). A topoisomerase I inhibitor, CPT-11: its enigmatic anti-tumor activity in combination with other agents *in vitro*. *Abstracts of 3rd Conf. on DNA Topoisomerases in Cancer Chemotherapy, New York*, Abstr. 54.

Oomori, Y., Yasue, T., Aoyama, H., Hirai, K., Suzue, S., and Yokota, T. (1988). Effects of fleroxacin on HeLa cell functions and topoisomerase II. *Journal of Antimicrobial Chemotherapy*, **22**, 91–7.

Osheroff, N. (1989a). Biochemical basis for the interactions of type I and type II topoisomerases with DNA. *Pharmacology and Therapeutics*, **41**, 223–41.

Osheroff, N. (1989b). Effect of antineoplastic agents on the DNA cleavage/relegation reaction of eukaryotic topoisomerase II: Inhibition of DNA religation by etoposide. *Biochemistry*, **28**, 6157–60.

Osheroff, N., Zechiedrich, E. L., and Gale, K. C. (1991). Catalytic function of DNA topoisomerase II. *BioEssays*, **13**, 269–74.

Ostrander, E. A., Benedetti, P., and Wang, J. C. (1990). Template supercoiling by a chimera of yeast GAL4 protein and phage T4 RNA polymerase. *Science*, **249**, 1261–5.

Pommier, Y., Schwartz, R. E., Kohn, K. W., and Zwelling, L. A. (1984). Formation and rejoining of deoxyribonucleic acid double-strand breaks induced in isolated cell nuclei by antineoplastic intercalating agents. *Biochemistry*, **23**, 3194–201.

Pommier, Y., Zwelling, L. A., Kao-Shan, C.-S., Whang-Peng, J., and Bradley, M. O. (1985). Correlations between intercalator-induced DNA strand breaks and sister chromatid exchanges, mutations, and cytotoxicity in Chinese hamster cells. *Cancer Research*, **45**, 3143–49.

Pommier, Y., Covey, J. M., Kerrigan, D., Markovits, J., and Pham, R. (1987). DNA unwinding and inhibition of mouse leukemia L1210 DNA topoisomerase I by intercalation. *Nucleic Acids Research*, **15**, 6713–31.

Pommier, Y., Capranico, G., Orr, A., and Kohn, K. W. (1991). Local base sequence preferences for DNA cleavage by mammalian topoisomerase II in the presence of amsacrine or teniposide. *Nucleic Acids Research*, **19**, 5973–80.

Potmesil, M., Hsiang, Y.-H., Liu, L. F., Bank, B., Grossberg, H., Kirschenbaum, S., *et al.* (1988). Resistance of human leukemic and normal lymphocytes to drug-induced DNA cleavage and low levels of DNA topoisomerase II. *Cancer Research*, **48**, 3537–43.

Pruss, G. J., Manes, S. H., and Drlica, K. (1982). *Escherichia coli* DNA topoisomerase I mutants: Increased supercoiling is corrected by mutations near gyrase genes. *Cell*, **31**, 35–42.

Reece, R. J. and Maxwell, A. (1991a). The C-terminal domain of the *Escherichia coli* DNA gyrase A subunit is a DNA-binding protein. *Nucleic Acids Research*, **19**, 1399–1405.

Reece, R. J. and Maxwell, A. (1991b). Probing the limits of the DNA gyrase breakage-reunion domain of the *Escherichia coli* DNA gyrase A protein. *Journal of Biological Chemistry*, **266**, 3540–6.

Richard, R. E. and Bogenhagen, D. F. (1989). A high molecular weight topoisomerase I from *Xenopus laevis* ovaries. *Journal of Biological Chemistry*, **264**, 4704–9.

Richard, R. E. and Bogenhagen, D. F. (1991). The 165-kDa DNA topoisomerase from *Xenopus laevis* oocytes is a tissue-specific variant. *Developmental Biology*, **146**, 4–11.

Robinson, M. J., Martin, B. A., Gootz, T. D., McGuirk, P. R., Moynihan, M., Sutcliffe, J. A., and Osheroff, N. (1991). Effects of quinolone derivatives on eukaryotic topoisomerase II. A novel mechanism for enhancement of enzyme-mediated DNA cleavage. *Journal of Biological Chemistry*, **266**, 14585–92.

Romig, H. and Richter, A. (1990). Expression of the type I DNA topoisomerase gene in adenovirus-5 infected human cells. *Nucleic Acids Research*, **18**, 801–8.

Rosen, T. (1990). The fluoroquinolone antibacterial agents. *Progress in Medicinal Chemistry*, **27**, 235–95.

Ross, W. E. (1985). DNA topoisomerases as target for cancer therapy. *Biochemical Pharmacology*, **34**, 4191–5.

Ross, W. E., Glaubiger, D. L., and Kohn, K. W. (1978). Protein associated DNA breaks in cells treated with adriamycin or ellipticine. *Biochimica et Biophysica Acta*, **519**, 23–30.

Ross, W., Rowe, T., Yang, L., Glisson, B., Yalowich, J., and Liu, L. F. (1984). Role of topoisomerase II in mediating epipodophyllotoxin-induced DNA cleavage. *Cancer Research*, **44**, 5857–60.

Rowe, T., Kupfer, G., and Ross, W. (1985). Inhibition of epipodophyllotoxin cytotoxicity by interference with topoisomerase-mediated DNA cleavage. *Biochemical Pharmacology*, **34**, 2483–7.

Rozencweig, M., Von Hoff, D. D., Henney, J. E., and Muggia, F. M. (1977). VM 26 and VP 16–213: a comparative analysis. *Cancer*, **40**, 334–2.

Sander, M. and Hsieh, T.-S. (1983). Double-strand DNA cleavage by type II DNA topoisomerase from *Drosophila melanogaster*. *Journal of Biological Chemistry*, **258**, 8421–8.

Schultz, A. G. (1973). Camptothecin. *Chemical Reviews*, **73**, 385–405.

Scrip (1989). *Cancer chemotherapy report*. Scrip, Richmond.

Shen, L. L. and Pernet, A. G. (1985). Mechanism of inhibition of DNA gyrase by analogues of nalidixic acid: the target of the drugs is DNA. *Proceedings of the National Academy of Sciences of the United States of America*, **82**, 307–11.

Shen, L. L., Baronowski, J., and Pernet, A. G. (1989a). Mechanism of inhibition of DNA gyrase by quinolone antibacterials: Specificity and cooperativity of drug binding to DNA. *Biochemistry*, **28**, 3879–85.

Shen, L. L., Baranowski, J., Wai, T., Chu, D. T. W., and Pernet, A. G. (1989b). The binding of quinolones to DNA: should we worry about it?. In *International Telesymposium on Quinolones* (ed. P. Fernandes), pp. 159–70. J. R., Prous, Barcelona.

Shen, L. L., Kohlbrenner, W. E., Weigl, D., and Baranowski, J. (1989c). Mechanism of quinolone inhibition of DNA gyrase. Appearance of unique norfloxacin binding sites in enzyme–DNA complexes. *Journal of Biological Chemistry*, **264**, 2973–8.

Shen, L. L., Mitscher, L. A., Sharma, P. N., O'Donnell, T. J., Chu, D. W. T., Cooper, C. S., *et al.* (1989d). Mechanism of inhibition of DNA gyrase by quinolone antibacterials. A cooperative drug-DNA binding model. *Biochemistry*, **28**, 2886–94.

Shen, L. L., Bures, M. G., Chu, D. T. W., and Plattner, J. J. (1990). Quinolone–DNA interaction: how a small drug molecule acquires high DNA binding affinity and specificity. In *Molecular Basis of Specificity in Nucleic Acid-Drug Interaction* (ed. B. Pullman and J. Jortner), pp. 495–512. Kluwer, Dordrecht.

Shen, L. L., Baranowski, J., Fostel, J., and Lartey, P. A. (1991). DNA topoisomerases from pathogenic fungi: targets of anti-fungal drug discovery. *Proc. Int. Symp. on DNA Topoisomerases in Chemotherapy*, Nagoya, p. 99, Abstr. P-33.

Shuman, S. and Moss, B. (1987). Identification of a vaccinia virus gene encoding a type I DNA topoisomerase. *Proceedings of the National Academy of Sciences of the United States of America*, **84**, 7478–82.

Singh, B. and Gupta, R. S. (1983). Mutagenic responses of thirteen anticancer drugs on mutation induction at multiple genetic loci and on sister chromatid exchanges in Chinese hamster ovary cells. *Cancer Research*, **43**, 577–84.

Sinha, B. K., Politi, P. M., Eliot, H. M., Kerrigan, D., and Pommier, Y. (1990). Structure–activity relations, cytotoxicity and topoisomerase II dependent cleavage induced by pendulum ring analogs of etoposide. *European Journal of Cancer*, **26**, 590–3.

Slevin, M. L. (1991). The clinical pharmacology of etoposide. *Cancer*, **67**, 319–29.

Smith, P. J. (1990). DNA topoisomerase dysfunction: a new goal for antitumor chemotherapy. *BioEssays*, **12**, 167–72.

Sorensen, B. S., Jensen, P. S., Andersen, A. H., Christiansen, K., Alsner, J., Thomsen, B., and Westergaard, O. (1990). Stimulation of topoisomerase II mediated DNA cleavage at specific sequence elements by the 2-nitroimidazole Ro 15–0216. *Biochemistry*, **29**, 9507–15.

Sperry, A. O., Blasquez, V. C., and Gerrard, W. T. (1989). Dysfunction of chromosomal loop attachment sites: illegitimate recombination linked to matrix association regions and topoisomerase II. *Proceedings of the National Academy of Sciences of the United States of America*, **86**, 5497–501.

Sreedharan, S., Oram, M., Jensen, B., Peterson, L. R., and Fisher, L. M. (1990). DNA gyrase *gyrA* mutations in ciprofloxacin-resistant strains of *Staphylococcus aureus*: close similarity with quinolone resistance mutations in *Escherichia coli*. *Journal of Bacteriology*, **172**, 7260–2.

Srivenugopal, K. S., Lockson, D., and Morris, D. R. (1984). *Escherichia coli* DNA topoisomerase III: purification and characterization of a new type I enzyme. *Biochemistry*, **23**, 1899–1906.

Stahelin, H. and von Wartburg, A. (1989). From podophyllotoxin glucoside to etoposide. *Progress in Drug Research*, **33**, 171–266.

Stahelin, H. F. and von Wartburg, A. (1991). The chemical and biological route from podophyllotoxin glucoside to etoposide: Ninth Cain Memorial Award lecture. *Cancer Research*, **51**, 5–15.

Steck, T. R. and Drlica, K. (1984). Bacterial chromosome segregation: evidence for DNA gyrase involvement in decatenation. *Cell*, **36**, 1081–8.

Stetler, G. L., King, G. J., and Huang, W. M. (1979). T4 DNA-delay proteins required for specific DNA replication form a complex that has ATP-dependent DNA topoisomerase activity. *Proceedings of the National Academy of Sciences of the United States of America*, **76**, 3737–41.

Suda, H., Matsunga, K., Yamamura, S., and Shizuri, Y. (1991). Structure of a new topoisomerase II inhibitor BE 10988. *Tetrahedron Letters*, **32**, 2791–2f.

Sugimoto, Y., Tsukahara, S., Oh-hara, T., Liu, L. F., and Tsuruo, T. (1990).

Elevated expression of DNA topoisomerase II in camptothecin-resistant human tumor cell lines. *Cancer Research*, **50**, 7962–5.

Sugino, A., Peebles, C. L., Cozzarelli, N. R., and Kreuzer, K. N. (1977). Mechanism of action of nalidixic acid: Purification of *E. coli nalA* gene product and its relationship to DNA gyrase and a novel nicking-closing enzyme. *Proceedings of the National Academy of Sciences of the United States of America*, **74**, 4767–71.

Sugino, A., Higgins, N. P., and Cozzarelli, N. R. (1980). DNA gyrase subunit stoichiometry and the covalent attachment of subunit A to DNA during DNA cleavage. *Nucleic Acids Research*, **8**, 3865–74.

Sullivan, D. M., Glisson, B. S., Hodges, P. K., Smallwood-Kentro, S., and Ross, W. E. (1986). Proliferation dependence of topoisomerase II mediated drug action. *Biochemistry*, **25**, 2248–56.

Sullivan, D. M., Latham, M. D., Rowe, T. C., and Ross, W. E. (1989). Purification and characterization of an altered topoisomerase II from a drug-resistant Chinese hamster ovary cell line. *Biochemistry*, **28**, 5680–7.

Swanberg, S. L. and Wang, J. C. (1987). Cloning and sequencing of the *Escherichia coli gyrA* gene coding for the A subunit of DNA gyrase. *Journal of Molecular Biology*, **197**, 729–36.

Talley, J. H. (1991). Fluoroquinolones: new miracle drugs? *Postgraduate Medicine*, **89**, 101–13.

Tamura, J. K. and Gellert, M. (1990). Characterization of the ATP binding site on *Escherichia coli* DNA gyrase. Affinity labeling of lys-103 and lys-110 of the B subunit by pyridoxal 5′-diphospho-5′-adenosine. *Journal of Biological Chemistry*, **265**, 21342–9.

Tamura, H.-O., Kohchi, C., Yamada, R., Ikeda, T., Koiwai, O., Patterson, E., *et al.* (1991). Molecular cloning of a cDNA of a camptothecin-resistant human DNA topoisomerase I and identification of mutation sites. *Nucleic Acids Research*, **19**, 69–75.

Tan, C., Tasaka, H., Yu, K.-P., Murphy, M. L., and Karnofsky, D. A. (1967). Daunomycin, an antitumor antibiotic, in the treatment of neoplastic disease. Clinical evaluation with special reference to childhood leukemia. *Cancer*, **20**, 333–53.

Tan, K. B., Dorman, T. E., Falls, K. M., Chung, T. D. Y., Mirabelli, C. K., Crooke, S. T., and Mao, J.-I. (1992). Topoisomerase IIa and topoisomerase IIb genes: Characterization and mapping to human chromosomes 17 and 3, respectively. *Cancer Research*, **52**, 321–34.

Tanabe, K., Ikegami, Y., Ishida, R., and Andoh, T. (1991). Inhibition of topoisomerase II by antitumor agents bis(2,6-dioxopiperazine) derivatives. *Cancer Research*, **51**, 4903–8.

Taudou, G., Mirambeau, G., Lavenot, C., der Garabedian, A., Vermeersch, J., and Duguet, M. (1984). DNA topoisomerase activities in concanavalin A-stimulated lymphocytes. *Federation of European Biochemical Societies Letters*, **176**, 431–5.

Tewey, K. M., Chen, G. L., Nelson, E. M., and Liu, L. F. (1984a). Intercalative antitumor drugs interfere with the breakage-reunion reaction of mammalian DNA topoisomerase II. *Journal of Biological Chemistry*, **259**, 9182–7.

Tewey, K. M., Rowe, T. C., Yang, L., Halligan, B. D., and Liu, L. F. (1984b). Adriamycin-induced DNA damage mediated by mammalian DNA topoisomerase II. *Science*, **226**, 466–8.

Thrash, C., Voekel, K., DiNardo, S., and Sternglanz, R. (1984). Identification of *Saccharomyces cerevisiae* mutants deficient in DNA topoisomerase I activity. *Journal of Biological Chemistry*, **259**, 1375–7.

Thrash, C., Bankier, A. T., Barrell, B. G., and Sternglanz, R. (1985). Cloning, characterization, and sequence of the yeast DNA topoisomerase I gene. *Proceedings of the National Academy of Sciences of the United States of America*, **82**, 4374–8.

Trask, D. K. and Muller, M. T. (1988). Stabilization of type I topoisomerase-DNA covalent complexes by actinomycin D. *Proceedings of the National Academy of Sciences of the United States of America*, **85**, 1417–21.

Tricoli, J. V. and Kowalski, D. (1983). Topoisomerase I from chicken erythrocytes: purification, characterization, and detection by a deoxyribonucleic acid binding assay. *Biochemistry*, **22**, 2025–31.

Tricoli, J. V., Sahai, B. M., McCormick, P. J., Jarlinski, S. J., Bertram, J. S., and Kowalski, D. (1985). DNA topoisomerase I and II activities during cell proliferation and the cell cycle in cultured mouse embryo fibroblast (C3H 10T1/2) cells. *Experimental Cell Research*, **158**, 1–14.

Tsai-Pflugfelder, M., Liu, L. F., Liu, A. A., Tewey, K. M., Whang-Peng, J., Knutsen, T., *et al.* (1988). Cloning and sequencing of cDNA encoding human DNA topoisomerase II and localization of the gene to chromosome region 17q21–22. *Proceedings of the National Academy of Sciences of the United States of America*, **85**, 7177–81.

Tsao, Y.-P., Wu, H.-Y., and Liu, L. F. (1989). Transcription-driven supercoiling of DNA: direct biochemical evidence from *in vitro* studies. *Cell*, **56**, 111–18.

Tse, Y.-C. and Wang, J. C. (1980). *E. coli* and *M. luteus* DNA topoisomerase I can catalze catenation or decatenation of double-stranded DNA rings. *Cell*, **22**, 269–76.

Tse, Y.-C., Kirkegaard, K., and Wang, J. C. (1980). Covalent bonds between protein and DNA. Formation of phosphotyrosine linkage between certain DNA topoisomerases and DNA. *Journal of Biological Chemistry*, **255**, 5560–5.

Tse-Dinh, Y.-C. and Beran-Steed, R. K. (1988). *Escherichia coli* DNA topoisomerase I is a zinc metalloprotein with three repetitive zinc-binding domains. *Journal of Biological Chemistry*, **263**, 15857–9.

Tse-Dinh, Y.-C. and Wang, J. C. (1986). Complete nucleotide sequence of the *topA* gene encoding *Escherichia coli* DNA topoisomerase I. *Journal of Molecular Biology*, **191**, 321–31.

Ubukata, K., Itoh, N.-Y., and Konno, M. (1989). Cloning and expression of the norA gene for fluoroquinolone resistance in *Staphylococcus aureus*. *Antimicrobial Agents and Chemotherapy*, **33**, 1535–9.

Uemura, T., Morikawa, K., and Yanagida, M. (1986). The nucleotide sequence of the fission yeast DNA topoisomerase II gene: structural and functional relationships to other DNA topoisomerases. *EMBO Journal*, **5**, 2355–61.

Uemura, T., Morino, K., Uzawa, S., Shiozaki, K., and Yanagida, M. (1987). Cloning and sequencing of *Schizosaccharomyces pombe* DNA topoisomerase I gene, and effect of gene disruption. *Nucleic Acids Research*, **15**, 9727–39.

Une, T., Fujimoto, T., Sato, K., and Osada, Y. (1988). *In vitro* activity of DR-3355, an optically active ofloxacin. *Antimicrobial Agents and Chemotherapy*, **32**, 1336–40.

van Maanen, J. M. S., Retel, J., de Vries, J., and Pinendo, H. M. (1988).

Mechanism of action of antitumor drug etoposide: a review. *Journal of National Cancer Institute*, **80**, 1526–33.

Wall, M. E. and Wani, M. C. (1980). Camptothecin. In *Anticancer agents based on natural product models* (ed. J. M. Cassidy and J. D. Douros), pp. 417–36. Academic Press, New York.

Wall, M. E., Wani, M. C., Cook, C. E., Palmer, K. H., McPhail, A. T., and Sim, G. A. (1966). Plant antitumor agents. I. The isolation and structure of camptothecin, a novel alkaloidal leukemia and tumor inhibitor from *Camptotheca acuminata*. *Journal of the American Chemical Society*, **88**, 3888–90.

Wall, M. E., Wani, M. C., Natschke, S. M., and Nicholas, A. W. (1986). Plant antitumor agents 22. Isolation of 11-hydroxycamptothecin from *Camptotheca acuminata Decne*: Total synthesis and biological activity. *Journal of Medicinal Chemistry*, **29**, 1553–55.

Wallis, J. W., Chrebet, G., Brodsky, G., Rolfe, M., and Rothstein, R. (1989). A hyperrecombination mutation in *S. cerevisiae* identifies a novel eukaryotic topoisomerase. *Cell*, **58**, 409–19.

Wang, A. H.-J., Ughetto, G., Quigley, G. J., and Rich, A. (1987). Interactions between an anthracycline antibiotic and DNA: molecular structure of daunomycin complexed to d(CpGpTpApCpG) at 1.2-Å resolution. *Biochemistry*, **26**, 1152–63.

Wang, J. C. (1971). Interaction between DNA and *E. coli* protein ω. *Journal of Molecular Biology*, **55**, 523–33.

Wang, J. C. (1979). Helical repeat of DNA in solution. *Proceedings of the National Academy of Sciences of the United States of America*, **76**, 200–3.

Wang, J. C. (1980). Superhelical DNA. *Trends in Biological Sciences*, **5**, 219–21.

Wang, J. C. (1985). DNA topoisomerases. *Annual Review of Biochemistry*, **54**, 665–97.

Wang, J. C. (1987a). Recent studies of DNA topoisomerases. *Biochimica et Biophysica Acta*, **909**, 1–9.

Wang, J. C. (1987b). DNA topoisomerases: nature's solution to the topological ramifications of the double-helix structure of DNA. *Harvey Lectures*, **81**, 93–110.

Wang, J. C., Caron, P. R., and Kim, R. A. (1990). The role of DNA topoisomerases in recombination and genome stability: a double-edged sword? *Cell*, **62**, 403–6.

Wani, M. C., Ronman, P. E., Lindley, J. T., and Wall, M. E. (1980). Plant antitumor agents. 18. Synthesis and biological activity of camptothecin analogues. *Journal of Medicinal Chemistry*, **23**, 554–60.

Wani, M. C., Nicholas, A. W., and Wall, M. E. (1986). Plant antitumor agents. 23. Synthesis and antileukemic activity of camptothecin analogs. *Journal of Medicinal Chemistry*, **29**, 2358–63.

Wani, M. C., Nicholas, A. W., Manikumar, G., and Wall, M. E. (1987). Plant antitumor agents. 25. Total synthesis and antileukemic activity of ring A substituted camptothecin analogs. Structure-activity correlation. *Journal of Medicinal Chemistry*, **30**, 1774–9.

Weinert, T. A. and Hartwell, L. H. (1988). The RAD9 gene controls the cell cycle response to DNA damage in *Saccharomyces cerevisiae*. *Science*, **241**, 317–22.

Wentland, M. P. (1990). Structure-activity relationships of fluoroquinolones. In *The new generation of quinolones* (ed. S. Siporin, C. L. Heifetz, and J. M. Dimagala), pp. 1–43. Marcel Dekker, New York.

Wolfson, J. S. and Hooper, D. C. (1989a). Bacterial resistance to quinolones: mechanism and clinical importance. *Review of Infectious Diseases*, **11**, S960–8.

Wolfson, J. S. and Hooper, D. C. (1989b). Fluoroquinolone antimicrobial agents. *Clinical Microbiology Reviews*, **2**, 378–424.

Wozniak, A. J. and Ross, W. E. (1983). DNA damage as a basis for 4′-demethyl-epipodophyllotoxin-9-(4,6-*O*-ethylidene-b-D-glucopyranoside) (etoposide) cytotoxicity. *Cancer Research*, **43**, 120–4.

Wozniak, A. J., Glisson, B. S., Hande, K. R., and Ross, W. E. (1984). Inhibition of etoposide-induced DNA damage and cytotoxicity in L1210 cells by dehydrogenase inhibitors and other agents. *Cancer Research*, **44**, 626–32.

Wu, H. Y., Shyy, S., Wang, J. C., and Liu, L. F. (1988). Transcription generates positively and negatively supercoiled domains in the template. *Cell*, **53**, 433–40.

Wyckoff, E., Natalie, D., Nolan, J. M., Lee, M., and Hsieh, T.-S. (1989). Structure of the *Drosophila* DNA topoisomerase II gene: nucleotide sequence and homology among topoisomerase II. *Journal of Molecular Biology*, **251**, 1–14.

Yamagishi, J., Furutani, Y., Inoue, S., Ohue, T., Nakamura, S., and Shimizu, M. (1981). New nalidixic acid resistance mutations related to deoxyribonucleic acid gyrase activity. *Journal of Bacteriology*, **148**, 450–8.

Yamagishi, J., Yoshida, H., Yamayoshi, M., and Nakamura, S. (1986). Nalidixic acid-resistant-mutations of the *gyrB* gene of *Escherichia coli*. *Molecular and General Genetics*, **204**, 367–73.

Yamashita, Y., Kawada, S.-Z., Fujii, N., and Nakano, H. (1990a). Induction of mammalian DNA topoisomerase II dependent DNA cleavage by antitumor antibiotic streptonigrin. *Cancer Research*, **50**, 5841–4.

Yamashita, Y., Kawada, S.-Z., and Nakano, H. (1990b). Induction of mammalian topoisomerase II dependent DNA cleavage by nonintercalative flavonoids, genistein and orobol. *Biochemical Pharmacology*, **39**, 737–44.

Yamashita, Y., Siatoh, Y., Ando, K., Takahashi, K., Ohno, H., and Nakano, H. (1990c). Saintopin, a new antitumor antibiotic with topoisomerase II dependent DNA cleavage activity, from *Paecilomyces*. *Journal of Antibiotics*, **43**, 1344–6.

Yanagida, M. and Wang, J. C. (1987). Yeast DNA topoisomerases and their structural genes. In *Nucleic acids and molecular biology* (ed. F. Eckstein and D. M. J. Lilley), pp. 196–209. Springer-Verlag, Berlin.

Yang, L., Rowe, T. C., and Liu, L. F. (1985). Identification of DNA topoisomerase II as an intracellular target of antitumor epipodophyllotoxins in simian virus 40-infected monkey cells. *Cancer Research*, **45**, 5872–6.

Yang, L., Wold, M. S., Li, J. J., Kelly, T. J., and Liu, L. F. (1987). Roles of DNA topoisomerases in simian virus 40 DNA replication *in vitro*. *Proceedings of the National Academy of Sciences of the United States of America*, **84**, 950–4.

Yoshida, H., Kojima, T., Yamagishi, J., and Nakamura, S. (1988). Quinolone-resistant mutations of the *gyrA* gene of *Escherichia coli*. *Molecular and General Genetics*, **211**, 1–7.

Yoshida, H., Bogaki, M., Nakamura, S., Ubukata, K., and Konno, M. (1990). Nucleotide sequence and characterization of the *Staphylococcus aureus norA* gene, which confers resistance to quinolones. *Journal of Bacteriology*, **172**, 6942–9.

Yoshida, H., Bogaki, M., Nakamura, M., Yamanaka, L. M., and Nakamura, S. (1991). Quinolone resistance-determining region in the DNA gyrase *gyrB* gene of *Escherichia coli*. *Antimicrobial Agents and Chemotherapy*, **35**, 1647–50.

Zunino, F. and Capranico, G. (1990). DNA topoisomerase II as the primary target of anti-tumor anthracyclines. *Anti-Cancer Drug Design*, **5**, 307–17.

Zwelling, L. A., Michaels, S., Erikson, L. C., Ungerleider, R. S., Nichols, M., and Kohn, K. W. (1981). Protein-associated deoxyribonucleic acid strand breaks in L1210 cells treated with DNA intercalating agents 4'-(9-acridinylamino)-methanesulfon-*m*-anisidide and adriamycin. *Biochemistry*, **20**, 6553−63.

12

Catechol O-methyltransferase (COMT) and COMT inhibitors

P.T. Männistö, I. Ulmanen, J. Taskinen, and S. Kaakkola

12.1 Introduction

Catechol O-methyltransferase (COMT, EC 2.1.1.6) is a ubiquitous enzyme in nature, occurring in various plants, microorganisms (e.g. bacteria and yeasts), invertebrates, and vertebrates, including elasmobranchs (e.g. sharks), amphibians (e.g. frogs), birds, and mammals (Guldberg and

Marsden 1975; Sariaslani and Rosazza 1983). It is unlikely that all of them share the same COMT protein(s).

COMT is distributed throughout the various organs. In mammals, the highest activities are in liver and kidney. COMT also occurs in heart, lung, smooth and skeletal muscle, intestinal tract, reproductive organs, various glands, adipose tissue, skin, blood cells, and neural tissues, including both neurones and glial cells (Guldberg and Marsden 1975)

COMT is a cellular enzyme: little or no activity is present in extra-cellular fluids such as plasma or cerebrospinal fluid. In vertebrates most of the COMT protein appears in soluble form (S-COMT) and a small fraction is associated with membranes (membrane-bound or MB-COMT) (Guldberg and Marsden 1975). MB-COMT is found as microsomal protein, but the actual membrane association is not known. In *Candida tropicalis*, however, COMT is located solely in cell wall and plasma membrane (Veser *et al.* 1981).

COMT catalyses transfer of the methyl group of S-adenosyl-L-methionine (AdoMet) to the phenolic group of a substrate which must have a cate-chol structure (Axelrod and Tomchick 1958; Axelrod *et al.* 1958). Physio-logical substrates of COMT include dopa, catecholamines (dopamine, noradrenaline, adrenaline), their hydroxylated metabolites, catechol oestro-gens, and ascorbic acid. Several dietary and medicinal products are also good substrates, for example 3,4-dihydroxycinnamic acid, 3,4-dihydroxy-benzoic acid, triphenols and substituted catechols, dobutamide, isopre-naline, rimiterol, α-methyldopa, benserazide and carbidopa. The general function of COMT is the elimination of biologically active or toxic cate-chols and some other hydroxylated metabolites (see also p. 640).

12.2   COMT gene(s) and proteins

The two types of COMT protein from various mammalian tissues have already been partially characterized using conventional protein purification methods. The molecular mass of cytoplasmic S-COMT is about 23 kDa and that of the integral membrane protein MB-COMT is about 26 kDa (Borchardt *et al.* 1974; Jeffery and Roth 1985).

Recent progress in molecular biological methods has made cloning of COMT possible. This is necessary to resolve the molecular basis and interrelationship of S-COMT and MB-COMT proteins. It also enables the regulation of the COMT gene to be studied and the three-dimensional structure of COMT to be determined after production of sufficient amounts of recombinant enzyme.

12.2.1   Cloning of COMT

Salminen *et al.* (1990) cloned cDNA and the gene of rat liver COMT, and Lundström *et al.* (1991b) cloned human placental COMT cDNAs. Both rat and human sequences contain an open reading frame of 663 nucleotides, apparently coding for the S-COMT polypeptide. In two out of four placental clones, the open reading frame starts from another AUG codon located upstream. This sequence could code for a 50 amino acid extension to S-COMT. Because the amino-terminal end of the sequence resembles eukaryotic signal sequences of membrane proteins, it may code for the human MB-COMT (Lundström *et al*. 1991b).

Recently, Bertocci *et al*. (1991) have isolated a cDNA clone from the human hepatoma cell line G2. This sequence is virtually identical with that published by Lundström *et al*. (1991b). However, the hepatoma cDNA is longer in the 5′ end and is shorter in the 3′ end than the placental clones. It is unclear whether the differences in cDNA sequences are real or due to cloning artefacts.

12.2.2 COMT gene localization and transcription

The genomic organizations of COMT in rat, man, monkey, and canine DNA have been analysed using cDNA clones (Salminen *et al*. 1990; Lundström *et al*. 1991b). The results suggest that there is only one COMT gene in these mammals. This agrees with the genetic data derived from segregation analysis of human erythrocyte COMT (Weinshilboum and Raymond 1977; Goldin 1985; Weinshilboum 1988). Applying the *in situ* hybridization and cell hybrid techniques, Winqvist *et al*. (1992) localized the human COMT gene in the band q11.2 on chromosome 22, confirming the biochemical mapping employing somatic cell hybrids (Brahe *et al*. 1986). They also detected a relatively frequent two-allele COMT gene restriction fragment length polymorphism (RFLP) in human DNAs digested with BglI. Rat liver contains a 1.8 kb COMT specific transcript (Salminen *et al*. 1990). The human COMT transcript is slightly smaller at 1.4–1.5 kb (Bertocci *et al*. 1991; Lundström *et al*. 1991b). It is not known how the two COMT forms are produced from a single gene.

12.2.3 Primary structure of COMT

The open reading frame of 663 nucleotides of the rat and human clones (Salminen *et al*. 1990; Bertocci *et al*. 1991; Lundström *et al*. 1991b) codes for S-COMT containing 221 amino acids. This is proved by analysing amino acid sequences of tryptic peptides of rat liver and human placental S-COMT (Tilgmann and Kalkkinen 1990, 1991). The predicted molecular masses of rat and human S-COMT are 24.7 kDa and 24.4 kDa respectively. There are neither hydrophobic domains nor *N*-glycosylation sites. Rat S-COMT is a unique protein and does not have any direct homology with any other protein. Rat and human S-COMT amino acid sequences have 80 per cent similarity (Fig. 12.1). Four conserved cysteine residues are

```
   MB-COMT →
R - MP------LAAVSLGLLLLA-LLLLLRHLGWGLVTIFWFEYVLQPVHNLI  -43
    .:.      :::: :::.::   :::::::: ::::   : : :..:::.:::.
H - MPEAPPLLLAAVLLGLVLLVVLLLLLRHWGWGLCLIGWNEFILQPIHNLL   -50


   S-COMT →
R - MGDTKEQRILRYVQQNAKPGDPQSVLEAIDTYCTQKEWAMNVGDAKGQIM   -93
    .::::::::::  : : :  ::   :::::::::::::: :::::::::::: :: :.
H - MGDTKEQRILNHVLQHAEPGNAQSVLEAIDTYCEQKEWAMNVGDKKGKIV  -100
                                      :: :: :: ::: ::
P -                               KERAMHVGRKKGQIV   -15



R - DAVIREYSPSLVLELGAYCGYSAVRMARLLQPGARLLTMEMNPDYAAITQ  -143
    :::: : :  ::..:::::::::::::::::  :::::.:.:.::: :::::
H - DAVIQEHQPSVLLELGAYCGYSAVRMARLLSPGARLITIEINPDCAAITQ  -150
    :.:.:: :::::::::::::::::::::::: : :::.:::.::: :::.:
P - DTVVQEQRPSVLLELGAYCGYSAVRMARLLLPSARLLTIELNPDNAAIAQ   -65



R - QMLNFAGLQDKVTILNGASQDLIPQLKKKYDVDTLDMVFLDHWKDRYLPD  -193
    :. :::. :::::.. :::::.::::::::::::::::::::::::::::::
H - RMVDFAGVKDKVTLVVGASQDIIPQLKKKYDVDTLDMVFLDHWKDRYLPD  -200
    .:::::. :.::.:::::::::::::::::::::::::::::::::::::::
P - QVVDFAGLQDRVTVVVGASQDIIPQLKKKYDVDTLDMVFLDHWKDRYLPD  -115



R - TLLLEKCGLLRKGTVLLADNVIVPGTPDFLAYVRGSSSFECTHYSSYLEY  -243
    :::::  ::::::::::::::::: ::.:::::  ::::: :::::: :.:::
H - TLLLEECGLLRKGTVLLADNVICPGAPDFLAHVRGSSCFECTHYQSFLEY  -250
    :::::::::::::::::::::::::::::::::   :::::. :.::::
P - TLLLEECGLLRKGTVLLADNVICPGAPDFLAHVRGCGRFECTHFSSYLEY  -165



R - MKVVDGLEKAIYQGPSSPDKS   -264
    :::::::::::: :: :
H - REVVDGLEKAIYKGPGSEAGP   -271
    .::::::::.:::::: : :
P - SQMVDGLEKAVYKGPGSPAQP   -186
```

Fig. 12.1 The alignment of rat (R), human (H), and porcine (P) COMT amino acid sequences derived from cloned DNA (Salminen *et al.* 1990; Bertocci *et al.* 1991; Lundström *et al.* 1991b). The putative signal peptides of the MB-COMT amino termini are underlined. The initiation methionines for the MB-COMT and S-COMT are enclosed in boxes. Identical amino acids are shown by two dots and similar amino acids by one dot.

found in both rat and human sequences. The 165 amino acids in the porcine clone (Bertocci *et al.* 1991) have 82 per cent similarity with the human sequence, and three of the conserved cysteine residues are found in the porcine clone (Fig. 12.1). The amino-terminal elongation of the putative MB-COMT adds 43 and 50 amino acids to the S-COMT polypeptide in rat and man respectively (Bertocci *et al.* 1991; Lundström *et al.* 1991b). The amino end of this sequence carries 17 and 24 hydrophobic residues in rat and man respectively (Fig. 12.1). This sequence may form an *a*-helical transmembrane domain, responsible for the membrane association of MB-COMT. The hydrophobic sequence is flanked in its carboxyl terminus by arginine and histidine. This structure suggests that MB-COMT may be oriented towards the cytoplasmic side of the membrane (von Hejne and Gavel 1988; Singer 1990), thus representing the class Ib type of membrane proteins. In fact we have recently obtained evidence, by expressing the MB-COMT clones in cell-free lysates, that its amino end indeed functions as a signal-anchor sequence with the predicted topology (Ulmanen and Lundström 1991). The amino terminal sequence of MB-COMT and the sequence organizations of mitochondrial signals are different (Pfanner and Neupert 1990). Therefore MB-COMT is unlikely to be a component of the outer mitochondrial membrane, as suggested by Grossman *et al.* (1985). The subcellular localization of MB-COMT must be re-evaluated.

12.2.4   Expression of recombinant COMT

The recombinant clones of S-COMT (Lundström *et al.* 1991b) and MB-COMT (Bertocci *et al.* 1991) have been expressed in transfected mammalian cells. In both cases, increases of COMT activity were found after transfection and immunoreactive polypeptides of the predicted sizes could be seen. MB-COMT is transiently expressed in transfected human embryonic kidney 293 cells. It is associated with the membrane fraction, whereas S-COMT is in the soluble fraction (Bertocci *et al.* 1991). *In vitro* transcription and translation experiments show that the MB-COMT associates cotranslationally with the microsomal membranes (Ulmanen and Lundström 1991). No processing of the signal peptide is detected. Neither is any indication obtained that S-COMT would cleave proteolytically from MB-COMT *in vitro*. In fact, S-COMT is synthesized *in vitro* from the MB-COMT mRNA by initiation from the second internal AUG of the transcript. The expression of the coding sequence of rat S-COMT in *Escherichia coli* produces high amounts of active COMT enzyme. Bacterial COMT has similar mobilities in SDS PAGE as the rat liver and human placental polypeptides. Recently, recombinant S-COMT has been purified to homogeneity and crystallized (Lundström *et al.* 1992; Vidgren *et al.* 1991). Lundström *et al.* (1991a) also reported preliminary data on site-directed mutagenesis of rat enzyme produced in the bacterial system. The successful expression of active recombinant COMT polypeptides will soon be used to reveal the structure–function relationships of S-COMT and MB-COMT.

12.3   Reaction mechanisms and kinetics of COMT

COMT catalyses transfer of the methyl group of AdoMet to one of the hydroxyl groups of the catechol substrate in the presence of Mg^{2+}. The mechanism and kinetics of the reaction have been studied using partially purified enzyme preparations from various sources, mostly from rat liver and rat or human brain.

Early kinetic studies gave conflicting results. Both a rapid equilibrium random-order mechanism (Flohe and Schwabe 1970; Coward et al. 1973) and a ping-pong mechanism (Borchardt 1973) are suggested. However, studies of the stereochemical course of the reaction show evidence that the methyl transfer proceeds through a direct nucleophilic attack by one of the hydroxyl groups of the catechol substrate on the methyl carbon of AdoMet in a tight S_N2-like transition state (Woodard et al. 1980). Product inhibition studies by Rivett and Roth (1982) and Tunnicliff and Ngo (1983) have established a sequential ordered mechanism. AdoMet is the first substrate to bind and S-adenosyl-homocysteine (AdoHcy) the last product to dissociate from the enzyme. Subsequently, Jeffery and Roth (1987) showed that Mg^{2+} ions bind to the free enzyme in a rapid equilibrium reaction. The picture of the kinetic mechanism emerging from these studies is shown in Fig. 12.2.

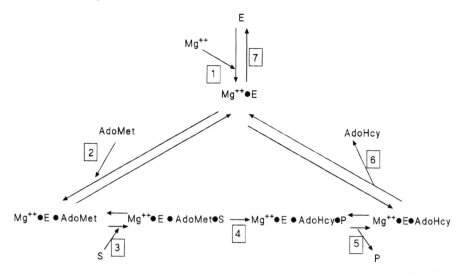

Fig. 12.2 Kinetic mechanism of COMT: E, COMT enzyme; S, catechol substrate; P, O-methylated product; AdoMet, S-adenosyl-L-methionine; AdoHcy, S-adenosyl-L-homocysteine. The order of the reactions is shown by numbers enclosed in boxes.

S-COMT and MB-COMT react via a similar mechanism. The main difference observed is the higher affinity of MB-COMT for the catechol substrate. Rivett and Roth (1982) reported K_m values of 3.3 μM (MB-COMT) and 280 μM (S-COMT) for dopamine. K_m values for AdoMet were 3.9 μM and 9.0 μM for MB-COMT and S-COMT respectively. Other kinetic constants of S-COMT or MB-COMT are not well characterized. The V_{max} values reported seem to refer to enzyme activities in various tissues rather than to basic constants of the enzyme reaction.

In addition to Mg^{2+}, some other divalent cations (e.g. Cd^{2+} promote methylation (Axelrod and Tomchick 1958), while others (e.g. Ca^{2+}) non-competitively inhibit the reaction even in the presence of saturating concentrations of Mg^{2+} (Weinshilboum and Raymond 1976).

Which of the hydroxyl groups of the catechol substrate is preferentially methylated depends on the substitution pattern and the nature of the substituents on the catechol ring. Substituents can change the relative nucleophilicity of the hydroxyls. They may also have direct stereo-electronic interactions with the enzyme affecting the orientation of the substrate on the active site. Normal catecholamine substrates (e.g. dopamine and noradrenaline) are methylated *in vivo* almost exclusively on the *m*-hydroxyl (cf. Guldberg and Marsden 1975). *p-O*-methylation accounts for 10–25 per cent of methylations *in vitro*. Similar *meta*-to-*para* ratios occur with dihydroxybenzoic acid as the substrate (Nissinen 1984). However, 40–45 per cent of 3,4-dihydroxybenzylalcohol is *p*-methylated. It seems that an ionized substituent, negative or positive, guides the orientation of the substrate, perhaps to avoid unfavourable interaction with a hydrophobic region in the active site. The importance of the relative nucleophilicity of the hydroxyl groups, which can be reversed by substituent effects, has been shown using ring-fluorinated catecholamines (Kirk and Creveling 1984; Thakker *et al.* 1986). For instance, *p-O*-methylation accounts for 70–88 per cent of the methylated products of 5-fluoronoradrenaline. There is some evidence that the ratio of *m*-methylated to *p*-methylated products is greater for MB-COMT than for S-COMT (Nissinen 1984).

12.4 Importance of S-COMT and MB-COMT

Although the basic kinetic mechanisms of S-COMT and MB-COMT may be the same (Ca^{2+} inhibition, Mg^{2+} requirement, pH optimum, similar K_m for AdoMet, and recognition by S-COMT antiserum), they are certainly different enzymes as shown above. High salt concentrations or alkali do not release MB-COMT from the membranes and strong detergent treatment is needed. The observed increase in K_m is apparently caused by competitive inhibition of MB-COMT by Triton X-100 (Jeffery and Roth 1984).

As mentioned above, S-COMT has a low affinity for catecholamine substrates but very high capacity (V_{max} from 50 pmol min^{-1} (mg protein)$^{-1}$

in skeletal muscle to as high as 14690 pmol min^{-1} (mg protein)$^{-1}$ in the liver). MB-COMT has much higher affinity but low capacity (2–40 pmol min^{-1} (mg protein)$^{-1}$; cf. Guldberg and Marsden (1975)). At present, nothing is known about possible differences in the substrate selectivity of the two enzyme forms. Physiological substrate concentrations are crucial when the relative importance of either enzyme subtype is considered. Striatal and hypothalamic dopamine levels in brain homogenates are about 65 μM and 3 μM respectively, and striatal and hypothalamic noradrenaline concentrations are 0.8 μM and 12 μM respectively. However, there is no method available at present to measure amine levels inside the cells, in the milieu where COMT enzymes exists, or to measure the activity and concentrations of COMT at these sites. All data obtained are from various homogenates. With these serious reservations, it seems that the natural concentrations of catecholamines may well be in the optimum range for MB-COMT. Roth and coworkers (Rivett and Roth 1982; Rivett *et al.* 1982; Jeffery and Roth 1984; Roth 1992) have thoroughly discussed and modelled this point. Their conclusion is that MB-COMT is the predominant enzyme at dopamine concentrations below 10 μM and at noradrenaline concentrations below 300 μM. They also state that the opposite view held by others are based on the use of excessive substrate concentrations that favour S-COMT.

12.5　Localization of COMT

12.5.1　Peripheral COMT

Both neuronal and extra-neuronal locations of MB-COMT are indicated. Denervation decreases COMT activity (Marsden *et al.* 1972; Jarrott 197B; Broch 1974). However, it also decreases the degree of differentiation of the smooth muscle cells, which are under the trophic influence of adrenergic nerves. Transformed cells lose extraneuronal uptake and/or extraneuronal COMT (Branco *et al.* 1984). Hence, the evidence for the existence of COMT in the peripheral autonomic nervous system is weak.

12.5.2　Brain COMT

Lesion experiments in rat brain have shown that destruction of the substantia nigra by 6-hydroxydopamine does not affect striatal COMT activity (Kaakkola *et al.* 1987). However, kainic acid injections into the striatum decrease MB-COMT by 20 per cent and nearly double S-COMT (Rivett *et al.* 1983). In another study (Kaakkola *et al.* 1987), S-COMT was only slightly increased without any significant change in MB-COMT. Since local toxin infusions destroy neuronal cells only at the site of injection, these results do not support a presynaptic localization of MB-COMT; however, a partial postsynaptic localization in the striatum remains possible. This would be an optimum site for the regulation of newly released dopamine. There has been some discussion of the orientation of the MB-COMT in the cell membrane. Preliminary data from molecular biological studies suggest that MB-COMT might be facing into the cytoplasm (see above). Basic biochemical concepts also support the cytoplasmic orientation of MB-COMT: Ca^{2+} concentrations in the extracellular fluid are high enough to inhibit COMT activity (Head *et al.* 1985); the IC_{50} of Ca^{2+} as a COMT inhibitor is 8 mM in the presence of Mg^{2+} (Weinshilboum and Raymond 1976). In contrast, concentrations of AdoMet are too low (cf. Baldessarini 1987) for the optimum activity of COMT. Intracellular, but not extracellular, Mg^{2+} concentration is also optimum for COMT (Jeffery and Roth 1987; Schultz and Nissinen 1989). The low affinity uptake system of COMT substrates works, at least in glial membranes, making an intracellular orientation physiologically relevant (Trendelenburg 1989).

Immunohistochemical studies using antibodies to S-COMT (Kaplan *et al.* 1979) and other studies (Rivett *et al.* 1983) have localized the soluble enzyme to glial cells. Thus the present view is that most of the brain S-COMT is located outside the neurons.

12.6   COMT inhibitors

12.6.1   First-generation COMT inhibitors

Guldberg and Marsden (1975) comprehensively reviewed early COMT inhibitors that are not dealt with in detail here. It is surprising that no real progress in developing COMT inhibitor was made until 1988 when a new generation emerged. The K_i values for the early compounds were in the micromolar range or higher (Guldberg and Marsden 1975). Several of these compounds may still be practical *in vitro* tools (e.g. tropolone, U-0521). However, their efficacy *in vivo* is low and transient, usually because of pharmacokinetic factors. Moreover, most of them lack selectivity and are quite toxic (Guldberg and Marsden 1975; Törnwall and Männistö 1991).

Until recently, clinical experience in Parkinson's disease with the COMT inhibitors available (e.g. gallates, tropolone, ascorbic acid, U-0521, 3′,4′-dihydroxy-2-methyl-propiophenone) has been disappointing owing to the lack of potent and specific compounds (cf. Männistö and Kaakkola 1989, 1990).

12.6.2   Second-generation COMT inhibitors

Three groups (Bäckström *et al.* 1989; Borgulya *et al.* 1989; Waldmeier *et al.* 1990a) have independently developed very potent, highly selective, and orally active COMT inhibitors. Apart from CGP 28014, nitrocatechol is

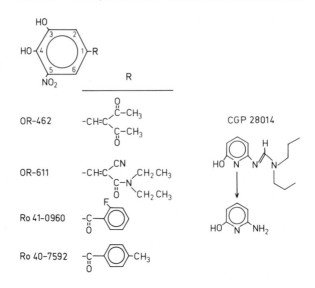

Fig. 12.3 Chemical structures of 5-nitrocatechols [(OR-462 (nitecapone), OR-611 (entacapone), Ro 41–0960, and Ro 40–7592 (tolcapone)] and of CGP 28014 and one of its metabolites.

the key structure for most of these molecules (Fig. 12.3). The properties of the new compounds are discussed below.

12.6.3   Structure–activity relationships of catechol-type inhibitors

In the search for new COMT inhibitors, extensive random screening of catechols, systematic synthetic modification, and quantitative structure–activity relationship (SAR) studies have been undertaken (Bäckström *et al.* 1989; Borgulya *et al.* 1989; Taskinen *et al.* 1989; Lotta *et al.* 1992). These studies have revealed several structural features determining the inhibitory activity of catechol-type compounds. Substitution of the aromatic ring, particularly in the 1- and 5-positions (see Fig. 12.3), with strongly electron-withdrawing substituents increases affinity of the inhibitors for COMT. This substitution raises the acidity of the catechol, with 4-OH being the first ionizing hydroxyl. However, this is not the only effect of the substituents. Studies of the ring-fluorinated catecholamines as substrates (Kirk and Creveling 1984) have shown that substitution in position 5 also resulted in a 10–20-fold increase in methylation rate. This is probably an unfortunate side effect of the electron-withdrawing acyl substituent at position 1 of U-0521.

The nitro group seems to be the optimal substituent at position 5. As well as effectively lowering the pK_a of the phenolic hydroxyls, it may have additional attractive interactions with the binding site. It also seems to convert the catechol to a very poor substrate for COMT. Larger electron-withdrawing substituents are not tolerated at this position, probably because of steric hindrance. At position 1, however, the binding site can accommodate fairly large substituents. Quantitative SAR studies imply that the size and hydrophobicity of the substituent at this site increase activity, while ionic groups decrease activity.

12.6.4 Individual compounds

Nitecapone (OR-462, 3-(3,4-dihydroxy-5-nitro-benzylidene)-2,4-pentanedione) and entacapone (OR-611, N,N-diethyl-2-cyano-3-(3,4-dihydroxy-5-nitro-phenyl) acrylamide) are highly effective inhibitors of rat soluble COMT (IC$_{50}$, 3−35 nM). They are also selective, since their *in vitro* IC$_{50}$ values for tyrosine hydroxylase, dopamine-β-hydroxylase, dopa decarboxylase, and monoamine oxidases A and B are in the micromolar range (Männistö *et al.* 1988; Nissinen *et al.* 1988).

In rats, oral nitecapone (3−30 mg kg^{-1}), in combination with levodopa and carbidopa, is effective in reducing 3-O-methyldopa (3-OMD) formation and in elevating serum and brain dopa, dopamine, 3,4-dihydroxyphenyl-acetic acid (DOPAC), and homovanillic acid (HVA) levels (Lindén *et al.* 1988; Nissinen *et al.* 1988). Similar findings have been reported in cyno-molgus monkeys with no difference between the intravenous efficacy of nitecapone and entacapone (Cedarbaum *et al.* 1991). Evidently, part of the dopa saved from COMT is metabolized through alternative pathways since the increase in serum dopa is smaller than the decrease in 3-OMD. Increases in striatal dopamine levels correlate with behavioural changes. Nitecapone potentiates dose dependently the action of carbidopa and levodopa on the motility of reserpine-treated mice and on the turning movements of rats with unilateral nigral lesions (Lindén *et al.* 1988; Männistö *et al.* 1988). OR-611 resembles nitecapone in potentiating the turning behaviour in-duced by levodopa and carbidopa in rats with unilateral nigral lesions (Etemadzadeh *et al.* 1989). At the doses studied, the action of nitecapone can be judged to be peripheral since, in *in vivo* studies in rats, oral nitecapone (up to 30 mg kg^{-1}) mainly inhibits duodenal COMT but does not affect striatal COMT (Nissinen *et al.* 1988; Zürcher *et al.* 1990b).

Comparative studies (Männistö *et al.* 1990, 1992; Männistö and Tuo-mainen 1991) have shown that inhibition of COMT outside the brain (as with nitecapone and OR-611) made an equal to brain dopamine levels as the inhibition that also occurred in the brain (as with Ro 41−0960, see below). These studies also revealed upper limits of brain dopamine levels after single doses of levodopa and carbidopa (both 100 mg kg^{-1}), of sixfold greater in the striatum and 45-fold greater in the hypothalamus than those in saline-treated control rats (Männistö and Tuomainen 1991).

Ro 41−0960 (2′-fluoro-3,4-dihydroxy-5-nitrobenzophenone) has IC_{50} values of 16 nM and 42 nM for rat brain and liver soluble COMT respectively. Oral ED_{50} values have varied from 1.3 mg kg^{-1} (rat liver) to 36 mg kg^{-1} (rat brain) measured as *ex vivo* inhibition of COMT at 4 hours (Da Prada *et al.* 1988). In another report, the oral ED_{50} value at 1 hour was 1.2 mg kg^{-1} (rat liver) (Zürcher *et al.* 1990b). Ro 41−0960 is 10 times more effective than nitecapone as a COMT inhibitor in the liver. Ro 41−0960 lacks activity on amine-synthesizing and other metabolizing enzymes, including several methyltransferases (Borgulya *et al.* 1989; Zürcher *et al.* 1990b).

Ro 41−0960 differs from nitecapone in having central effects. It effectively inhibits the formation of 3-*O*-methylated metabolites (i.e. 3-methoxytyramine (3-MT), HVA, and 4-hydroxy 3-methoxy-phenylethyleneglycol (HMPG)) in the brain.

Ro 40−7592 (tolcapone) resembles Ro 41−0960 both chemically and biologically. Its IC_{50} values in rat liver preparations are 30−36 nmol l^{-1} and its K_i value is 30 nmol l^{-1} (Zürcher *et al.* 1990a,b). After oral administration, ED_{50} values according to *ex vivo* experiments are 1−3 mg kg^{-1} in rat liver and kidney. Ro 40−7592 does not affect monoamine oxidase (MAO), hydroxyindole-*O*-methyl transferase, histamine-*N*-methyl transferase, or phenyl-*N*-methyl transferase activities or adrenergic (a, β), serotonergic, or cholinergic receptors (Zürcher *et al.* 1990a,b).

After oral administration of 30 mg kg^{-1} of Ro 40−7592 together with 10 mg kg^{-1} of levodopa and 15 mg kg^{-1} of benserazide, plasma and whole-brain dopa increases fourfold and 3-OMD decreases to very low levels. Dopamine formation in the whole brain increased, at least for 6 hours (Zürcher *et al.* 1990a,b).

Maj *et al.* (1990) reported further neurochemical and behavioural effects of Ro 40−7592. Oral Ro 40−7592 itself does not modify dopamine levels in the striatum, nucleus accumbens, or frontal cortex. However, DOPAC was increased dose dependently, and HVA and 3-MT were decreased by 10 mg kg^{-1} and 30 mg kg^{-1} of Ro 40−7592 at 1 hour. Surprisingly, 5 mg kg^{-1} of Ro 40−7592 elevates HVA levels in the striatum and nucleus accumbens. Ro 40−7592 increases exploratory activity of the rats at 10 and 30 mg kg^{-1} orally. Amphetamine- and nomifensine-induced hyperactivity and stereotypy are potentiated by Ro 40−7592. Ro 40−7592 slightly antagonises fluphenazine-induced catalepsy but does not relieve pimozide or haloperidol catalepsy. When given together with levodopa and benserazide, Ro 40−7592 potentiates motor activity, antihypothermic effects, and anticataleptic activity of levodopa or levodopa plus pargyline (Maj *et al.* 1990).

12.6.5   Toxicity of nitrocatechols

The acute toxicity of nitrocatechols is generally low (Borgulya *et al.* 1989). The intraperitoneal LD_{50} of Ro 41−0960 in mice (about 100 mg/kg) is

5 times higher than that of nitecapone and OR-611 (Borgulya *et al.* 1989; Törnwall and Männistö 1991). Levodopa and carbidopa treatments do not significantly enhance their acute toxicity (Törnwall and Männistö 1991). Oral LD_{50} values in mice and rats are greater than 2 g/kg (Borgulya *et al.* 1989). Since their effective doses are in the range of 3–30 mg/kg, the therapeutic ratio in the oral treatment of rodents is > 50.

12.6.6   Mechanism and kinetics of inhibition of nitrocatechols

An inhibition kinetic study is available only on nitecapone, whose effect on S-COMT from rat liver and duodenum has been studied (Schultz and Nissinen 1989). Nitecapone is a reversible competitive inhibitor with respect to catechol substrate and an uncompetitive inhibitor with respect to AdoMet. Nitecapone seems to bind to the Mg^{2+}-AdoMet—enzyme complex in the same manner as the substrate. The K_i value is lower if the inhibitor is preincubated with COMT in the presence of Mg^{2+} and AdoMet. After preincubation for 1 hour, $K_i \approx 1$ nM. These results imply that binding may involve rapid formation of an initial collision complex followed by slow isomerization to a tight complex. Consequently, nitecapone may be classified as a slow tight-binding inhibitor (Morrison and Walsh 1988). In view of the structural similarity of OR-611, Ro 41–0960, and Ro 40–7592 to nitecapone, they can also be expected to be competitive inhibitors with respect to catechol substrates. A K_i value of 30 nM has been reported for Ro 40–7592 (Zürcher *et al.* 1990a).

The IC_{50} values for all these inhibitors of S-COMT are in the low nanomolar range. It is important to point out that if some inhibitors show slow binding kinetics, IC_{50} measurements could give a poor indication of their relative potencies. Nitrocatechols inhibit both S-COMT and MB-COMT, but not much is known about their selectivity (Roth 1992; E. Schultz, personal communication).

12.6.7   Conclusion

The new COMT inhibitors (nitrocatechols) alter dopa metabolism and potentiate the action of levodopa plus a dopa decarboxylase inhibitor much more effectively than the early COMT inhibitors (e.g. gallates, tropolone, U-0521). Some of the new compounds (e.g. nitecapone, entacapone) scarcely penetrate the blood—brain barrier but increase striatal dopamine levels to a similar extent as the brain-penetrating compounds (i.e. Ro 41–0960, tolcapone).

12.7   CGP 28014—a pyridine derivative

CGP 28014, first described by Waldmeier *et al.* (1990 a, b), mimics the effects of COMT inhibitor although it is not a COMT inhibitor *in vitro*.

Its ED_{50} values are $2-8$ mg kg^{-1} orally when the end-points are the decrease of striatal HVA, the decrease of striatal 3-MT after clorgyline treatment (both without exogenous levodopa), or the formation of 3-OMD from exogenous levodopa (without dopa decarboxylase inhibitor). It is also long acting when given at high doses of 100 mg kg^{-1} (more than 12 hours) or 300 mg kg^{-1} (more than 24 hours but less than 36 hours). CGP 28014 increases striatal AdoMet levels. It is quite selective, since it does not have any affinity for nearly 20 receptors for the common neurotransmitters and other endogenous substances studied (less than 15 per cent displacement at 10^{-5} mol l^{-1}). It does not modify noradrenaline uptake into the heart, 5-hydroxytryptamine (5-HT) or noradrenaline release by electrical stimulation from the cortical slices, H75/12-induced depletion of 5-HT from the whole brain. However, it increases striatal 5-hydroxyindoleacetic acid and tryptophan dose dependently in a dose range of $1-10$ mg kg^{-1}.

We have found that CGP 28014 appears to be a poor COMT inhibitor in the periphery, or at least its inhibitory effect on 3-OMD formation is slow, becoming significant only after 3 hours. However, it behaves as an efficient COMT-inhibitor-like compound in the brain, preventing the formation of both HVA and 3-MT (Männistö *et al.* 1991). This kind of brain selectivity is an extraordinary feature of CGP 28014, and has not been described previously for COMT inhibitors. In fact, in earlier studies, CGP 28014 inhibited both 3-OMD and HVA levels in the brain to an equal extent after both oral and intraperitoneal administration (Waldmeier *et al.* 1990a,b). However, it is noteworthy that the earlier studies were either performed without levodopa or levodopa was given without a peripheral dopa decarboxylase inhibitor. Hence only moderate amounts of 3-OMD were produced in the periphery since most of the dopa was decarboxylated to dopamine.

The mechanism of action of CGP 28014 is not known. It is not a COMT inhibitor *in vitro* except in millimolar concentrations, and its major metabolite 2-amino-6-hydroxypyridine is not active. In our studies (Männistö *et al.* 1992), dopa, dopamine, and DOPAC levels in the striatum or hypothalamus are not much elevated by CGP 28014. It may just inhibit the transfer of COMT substrates to the enzyme, i.e. it might inhibit uptake$_2$. Since peripheral uptake is not identical with brain uptake$_2$ (Trendelenburg 1989), it may be argued that CGP 28014 preferentially inhibits central type uptake$_2$.

12.8   Experiences with new COMT inhibitors in man

The pharmacokinetics of OR-462 and OR-611 have been studied in healthy volunteers (Pentikäinen *et al.* 1989; Keränen *et al.* 1991). Bioavailability of orally administered OR-462 is $38-59$ per cent. Hepatic first-pass metabolism may occur. The distribution volume is $6-8$ l. The total clearance of nitecapone is 340 ml min^{-1} and that of OR-611 are 750 ml min^{-1}. Both have a similar elimination half-life of 30–40 minutes. Nitecapone is mainly excreted as glucuronide conjugates of the intact drug or its reduced metabolites (Taskinen *et al.* 1991).

Nitecapone (100 mg orally to healthy volunteers) has no influence on resting or exercise heart rate, blood pressure, systolic time intervals, or plasma dopamine, noradrenaline, and adrenaline levels. It increases 3,4-dihydroxyphenylethyleneglycol levels significantly and decreases HMPG levels in human plasma (Sundberg *et al.* 1990). It does not affect the tyramine pressor response (Sundberg and Gordin 1991).

Both nitecapone (10–100 mg orally) and OR-611 (50–400 mg orally) inhibit, S-COMT activity in erythrocytes dose dependently, decrease plasma levels of 3-OMD, and increase slightly the bioavailability of levodopa when given to human volunteers concomitantly with levodopa (100 mg) and carbidopa (25 mg) (Kaakkola *et al.* 1990; Keränen *et al.* 1991). Nitecapone also increases plasma levels of DOPAC and decreases plasma and urine HVA levels (Kaakkola *et al.* 1990). At 400 mg of Ro 40–7592, maximum COMT inhibition in erythrocytes (over 90 per cent) takes place 30 minutes after dosing and complete recovery occurs within 24 hours. Up to 800 mg of Ro 40–7952 orally was well tolerated (Zürcher *et al.* 1990a).

OR-462 (100 mg thrice daily) causes significant COMT inhibition in erythrocytes and decreases 3-OMD levels in plasma of parkinsonian patients. Compared with levodopa and dopa decarboxylase inhibitor therapy alone, this triple treatment significantly decreased disability when studied in seven parkinsonian patients (Teräväinen *et al.* 1990).

Studies in human volunteers and pilot studies in parkinsonian patients indicate that nitecapone, OR-611, and Ro 40–7592 are well tolerated. Urine discoloration is the only significant adverse effect. No human data for Ro 41–0960 are available at present.

CGP 28014 (20–600 mg orally) reduces plasma concentrations of 3-OMD (by 67 per cent) and HVA (by 17 per cent), and increases that of DOPAC (by 36 per cent), when given to human volunteers concomitantly with levodopa (250 mg, without a dopa decarboxylase inhibitor). 3-OMD reduction is not dose dependent (Bieck *et al.* 1990).

12.9   Clinical potential of the new COMT inhibitors

The main clinical application of COMT inhibitors would be as an adjuvant in the drug therapy of Parkinson's disease (Männistö and Kaakkola 1989, 1990). The standard therapy for Parkinson's disease is oral levodopa given with a dopa decarboxylase inhibitor (e.g. carbidopa or benserazide) which does not normally enter the brain. When dopa decarboxylase is inhibited, 3-OMD becomes the major plasma metabolite and its concentration is usually many times that of dopa. Since the half-life of 3-OMD is about 15 hours compared to about 1 hour for dopa, the concentration of 3-OMD remains particularly high during chronic therapy, particularly if new slow release levodopa preparations are used (Da Prada *et al.* 1984).

COMT inhibitors should improve the brain entry of dopa by decreasing metabolism to 3-OMD and increasing the bioavailability of levodopa. Hence, the dose of levodopa could be decreased compared with the present combination dosage, with a reduction in dopamine effects in the peripheral tissues. The dosing interval for levodopa could probably be prolonged. Finally, COMT inhibitors should decrease fluctuations in the subsequent formation of dopamine.

Problems may arise in the use of COMT inhibitors. When benserazide, an inhibitor of dopa decarboxylase, is coadministered with Ro 40–7592 (10 mg kg^{-1}) to Rhesus monkeys, a dose-dependent decrease in brain dopamine formation takes place with an apparent ED$_{50}$ of 3 mg kg^{-1}. No such effect occurs when 3.5 mg kg^{-1} of carbidopa (claimed to be equipotent with 10 mg kg^{-1} of benserazide) is given (Tedroff *et al.* 1991). Both benserazide and carbidopa are COMT substrates and weak COMT inhibitors. The affinity of carbidopa to COMT is much weaker than that of benserazide (Hagan *et al.* 1980). COMT inhibition is therefore likely to cause an increase in plasma levels in particular and subsequent brain penetration of benserazide.

COMT activity (Amin *et al.* 1983) and oestrogen concentrations are high in breast cancer tissue. Oestrogens are easily hydroxylated to catecholoestrogens, which serve as COMT substrates. Oestrogens stimulate tumour growth while catecholoestrogens inhibit it (Vandewalle and Lefebvre 1989). Thus COMT inhibition should inhibit cancer growth. However, an opposite phenomenon has also been reported. Oestrogen loading induces renal carcinoma in hamsters, which have low COMT activity, but not in rats, which have high COMT activity. Accumulation of catecholoestrogens occurs only in the former animals where COMT activity is inadequate (Li *et al.* 1989). The consequences of using COMT inhibitors to prevent the metabolism of catecholoestrogens need further study.

Oestrogen-induced ovum implantation may be mediated through formation of catecholoestrogens which stimulate the synthesis or release of prostaglandins (Paria *et al.* 1990). The time course of the development of COMT activity in the conceptus also favours the view that catecholoestrogens have a role in conceptus–maternal signalling during the establishment of pregnancy (Chakraborty *et al.* 1990). Interference in this delicate system by COMT inhibitors would be worth studying as a novel contraceptive mechanism.

However, it should be noted that that during the first trimester COMT is likely to have another role: protecting the placenta and the developing embryo from activated hydroxylated compounds formed from aryl hydrocarbon and oestrogen hydroxylases (Barnea and Avigdor 1990).

Noradrenaline deficiency characterizes some forms of depression. Enhancement of this deficit by tricyclic uptake inhibitors and MAO inhibitors has become an established therapy for depression. By analogy, the COMT inhibitors reaching the brain should decrease the metabolism of noradrenaline and dopamine and be beneficial in this type of depression, probably in combination with other drugs.

12.10   Use of COMT inhibitors in positron emission tomography

One of the many problems of positron emission tomography (PET) using 6-[^{18}F]-fluoro-L-dopa (6-FD) to visualize brain dopamine metabolism, is the peripheral formation of 3-O-methyl-6-[^{18}F]-fluoro-L-dopa (3-OMFD) by COMT. 3-OMFD contaminates brain radioactivity analysis since, like 3-OMD, it is easily transported to the brain. Mathematical modelling must be used to correct the results. Selective COMT inhibition would reduce the formation of 3-OMFD and remove some of the sources of error in PET analysis.

Despite the incomplete COMT inhibition achieved by U-0521 (Cumming *et al.* 1987), a significant reduction of 3-OMFD was found with enhancement of striatal 6-fluoro-dopamine and 6-fluoro-DOPAC content. Preliminary reports using nitecapone and OR-611 have given even better results in monkeys (Léger *et al.* 1990; Guttman *et al.* 1993). This finding was recently confirmed, using nitecapone, in man (Laihinen *et al.* 1992). A decrease in the isotope dose used would be one of the major advantages of using COMT inhibitors as adjuncts for PET research.

Acknowledgements

The authors' work described in this review has been partially financed by grants from the Sigrid Juselius Foundation and Orion Pharmaceutica.

References

Amin, A. M., Creveling, C. R., and Lowe, M. C. (1983). Immunohistochemical localization of catechol methyltransferase in normal and cancerous breast tissues of mice and rats. *Journal of National Cancer Institute*, **70**, 337–42.

Axelrod, J. and Tomchick, R. (1958). Enzymatic O-methylation of epinephrine and other catechols. *Journal of Biological Chemistry*, **233**, 702–5.

Axelrod, J., Senoh, S., and Witkop, B. (1958). O-Methylation of catechol amines *in vivo*. *Journal of Biological Chemistry*, **233**, 697–701.

Bäckström, R., Honkanen, E., Pippuri, A., Kairisalo, P., Pystynen, J., Heinola, K., *et al.* (1989). Synthesis of some novel potent and selective catechol-O-methyltransferase inhibitors. *Journal of Medicinal Chemistry*, **32**, 841–6.

Baldessarini, R. J. (1987). Neuropharmacology of S-adenosyl-L-methionine. *American Journal of Medicine*, **83**, 95–103.

Barnea, E. R. and Avigdor, S. (1990). Coordinated induction of estroger hydroxy-lase and catechol-O-methyl transferase by xenobiotics in 1st trimester human placental explants. *Journal of Steroid Biochemistry*, **35**, 327–31.

Bertocci, B., Miggiano, V., Da Prada, M., Dembic, Z., Lahm, H. W., and Malherbe, P. (1991). Human catechol-O-methyltransferase—cloning and expres-sion of the membrane-associated form. *Proceedings of the National Academy of Sciences of the United States of America*, **88**, 1416–20.

Rieck, P. R., Nilsson, E., and Antonin, K. H. (1990). Effect of the new selective COMT inhibitor CGP 28014a on the formation of 3-O-methyldopa (3OMD) in plasma of healthy subjects. *Journal of Neural Transmission*, **32** (Suppl.), 387–91.

Borchardt, R. T. (1973). Catechol-O-methyltransferase.1. Kinetics of tropolone inhibition. *Journal of Medicinal Chemistry*, **16**, 377–82.

Borchardt, R. T., Cheng, C., Cooke, P., and Creveling, C. (1974). The puri-fication and kinetic properties of liver microsomal catechol-O-methyltransferase. *Life Sciences*, **14**, 1089–100.

Borgulya, J., Bruderer, H., Bernauer, K., Zürcher, G., and Da Prada, M. (1989). Catechol-O-methyltransferase-inhibiting pyro-catechol derivatives—synthesis and structure–activity studies. *Helvetica Chimica Acta*, **72**, 952–68.

Brahe, C., Banetta, P., Meera Khan, P., Arwert, F., and Serra, A. (1986). Assignment of the catechol-O-methyltransferase gene to human chromosome 22 in somatic cell hybrids. *Human Genetics*, **74**, 230–4.

Branco, D., Teixeira, A., Azevedo, I., and Osswald, W. (1984). Structural and functional alterations caused at the extraneuronal level by sympathetic denerva-tion of blood vessels. *Naunyn-Schmiedebergs Archives of Pharmacology*, **326**, 302–12.

Broch, O. J. (1974). Effect of reserpine on catechol-O-methyl transferase in rat submaxillary gland. *Journal of Pharmacy and Pharmacology*, **26**, 375–7.

Cedarbaum, J. M., Léger, G., and Guttman, M. (1991). Reduction of circulating 3-O-methyldopa by inhibition of catechol-O-methyl-transferase with OR-611 and OR-462 in cynomolgus monkeys: implications for the treatment of Parkinson's disease. *Clinical Neuropharmacology*, **14**, 330–42.

Chakraborty, C., Davis, D. L., and Dey, S. K. (1990). The O-methylation of catechol oestrogens by pig conceptuses and endometrium during the peri-implantation period. *Journal of Endocrinology*, **127**, 77–84.

Coward, J. K., Slisz, E. P., and Wu, F. Y. (1973). Kinetic studies on catechol-O-methyltransferase. Product inhibition and the nature of the catechol binding site. *Biochemistry*, **12**, 2291–6.

Cumming, P., Boyes, B. E., Martin, W. R. W., Adam, M. J., Ruth, T. J., and McGeer, E. G. (1987). Altered metabolism of [18F]-6-fluorodopa in the hooded rat following inhibition of catechol-O-methyl-transferase with U-0521. *Biochemical Pharmacology*, **36**, 2527–31.

Da Prada, M., Keller, H. H., Pieri, L., Kettler, R., and Haefely, W. E. (1984). The pharmacology of Parkinson's disease: basic aspects and recent advances. *Experientia*, **40**, 1165–72.

Da Prada, M., Kettler, R., Zürcher, G., and Keller, H. H. (1988). Hemmer der MAO-B und COMT: Möglichkeiten ihrer Anwendung bei der Parkinson-Thera-pie aus heutiger Sicht. In *Modifizierende Faktoren bei der Parkinson-Therapie* (ed. P.-A. Fischer), pp. 309–22. Editiones Roche, Basel.

Etemadzadeh, E., Koskinen, L., and Kaakkola, S. (1989). Computerized rotometer apparatus for recording circling behavior. *Methods and Findings in Experimental and Clinical Pharmacology*, **11**, 399–407.

Flohe, L. and Schabe, K. (1970). Kinetics of purified catechol-*O*-methyltransferase. *Biochimica et Biophysica Acta*, **220**, 469–76.

Goldin, L. R. (1985). Segregation analysis of dopamine-beta-hydroxylase (DBH) and catechol-*O*-methyltransferase (COMT): identification of major locus and polygenic components. *Genetic Epidemiology*, **2**, 317–25.

Grossman, M., Creveling, C. R., Rybczynski, R., Braverman, M., Isersky, C., and Breakefield, X. (1985). Soluble and particulate forms of rat catechol-*O*-methyltransferase distinguished by gel electrophoresis and immune fixation. *Journal of Neurochemistry*, **44**, 421–32.

Guldberg, H. C. and Marsden, C. A. (1975). Catechol-*O*-methyl transferase: pharmacological aspects and physiological role. *Pharmacological Reviews*, **27**, 135–206.

Guttman, M., Léger, G., Reches, A., Evans, A., Diksic, M., Cedarbaum, J. M., and Gjedde, A. (1993). Administration of the new COMT inhibitor OR-611 increases striatal uptake of fluorodopa. *Movement Disorders*, **8**, 298–304.

Hagan, R. M., Raxworthy, M. J., and Gulliver, P. A. (1980). Benserazide and carbidopa as substrates of catechol-*O*-methyl-transferase: a new mechanism of action in Parkinson's disease. *Biochemical Pharmacology*, **29**, 3123–6.

Head, R. J., Irvice, R. J., Barone, S., Stitzel, R. E., and de la Lande, I. S. (1985). Nonintracellular, cell-associated *O*-methylation of isoproterenol in the isolated rabbit thoracic aorta. *Journal of Pharmacology and Experimental Therapeutics*, **234**, 184–9.

Jarrott, B. (1973). The cellular localization and physiological role of catechol-*O*-methyltransferase in the body. In *Frontiers in catecholamine research* (ed. E. Usdin and S. H. Snyder), pp. 113–15. Pergamon Press, New York.

Jeffery, D. and Roth, J. A. (1984). Characterization of membrane-bound and soluble catechol-*O*-methyltransferase from human frontal cortex. *Journal of Neurochemistry*, **42**, 826–32.

Jeffery, D. and Roth, J. A. (1985). Purification and kinetic mechanism of human brain soluble catechol-*O*-methyltransferase. *Journal of Neurochemistry*, **44**, 881–5.

Jeffery, D. and Roth, J. A. (1987). Kinetic reaction mechanism for magnesium binding to membrane-bound and soluble catechol-*O*-methyltransferase. *Biochemistry*, **26**, 2955–8.

Kaakkola, S., Männistö, P. T., and Nissinen, E. (1987). Striatal membrane-bound and soluble catechol-*O*-methyltransferase after selective neural lesions in the rat. *Journal of Neural Transmission*, **69**, 221–8.

Kaakkola, S., Gordin, A., Järvinen, M., Wikberg, T., Schultz, E., Nissinen, E., *et al.* (1990). Effect of a novel catechol-*O*-methyltransferase inhibitor, nitecapone, on the metabolism of L-DOPA in healthy volunteers. *Clinical Neuropharmacology*, **13**, 436–47.

Kaplan, G., Hartman, B., and Creveling, C. (1979). Immunohistochemical demonstration of catechol-*O*-methyltransferase in mammalian brain. *Brain Research*, **167**, 241–50.

Keränen, T., Gordin, A., Karlsson, M., Korpela, K., Pentikäinen, P. J., Schultz, E., *et al.* (1991). Effect of the novel catechol-*O*-methyltransferase inhibitor OR-611 in healthy volunteers. *Neurology*, **41**, 213.

Kirk, K. L. and Creveling, C. R. (1984). The chemistry and biology of ring-fluorinated biogenic amines. *Medical Research Reviews*, **4**, 189–220.

Laihinen, A., Rinne, J. O., Rinne, U. K., Haaparanta, M., Ruotsalainen, U., Bergman, J., and Solin, O. (1992). [^{18}F]-6-fluorodopa PET scanning in Parkinson's disease after selective COMT inhibition with nitecapone (OR-462). *Neurology*, **42**, 199–203.

Léger, G., Reches, A., Cedarbaum, J. M., Guttman, M., Leblanc, C., and Gjedde, A. (1990). Inhibition of 3-O-methylfluorodopa formation with OR-462: attempts to simplify the fluorodopa model for PET analysis. *Neurology*, **20**, 156.

Li, S. A., Purdy, R. H., and Li, J. J. (1989). Variations in catechol O-methyltransferase activity in rodent tissues: possible role in estrogen carcinogenicity. *Carcinogenesis*, **10**, 63–7.

Linden, I. B., Nissinen, E., Etemadzadeh, E., Kaakkola, S., Männistö, P. T., and Pohto, P. (1988). Favorable effect of catechol-O-methyltransferase inhibition by OR-462 in experimental models of Parkinson's disease. *Journal of Pharmacology and Experimental Therapeutics*, **247**, 289–93.

Lotta, T., Taskinen, J., Bäckström, R., and Nissinen, E. (1992). PLS modelling of structure–activity relationship of catechol-O-methyltransferase inhibitors. *Journal of Computer-Aided Molecular Design*, **6**, 253–72.

Lundström, K., Ahti, H., and Ulmanen, I. (1991a). *In vitro* mutagenesis of rat catechol-O-methyltransferase. In *Site-directed mutagenesis and protein engineering* (ed. M. R. El-Gewely), pp. 119–22. Elsevier, New York.

Lundström, K., Salminen, M., Jalanko, A., Savolainen, R., and Ulmanen, I. (1991b). Cloning and characterization of human placental catechol-O-methyltransferase cDNA. *DNA and Cell Biology*, **10**, 181–9.

Lundström, K., Tilgmann, C., Peränen, J., Kalkkinen, N., and Ulmanen, I. (1992). Expression of enzymatically active rat liver and human placental catechol-O-methyltransferase in *E. coli*: purification and partial characterization. *Biochimica et Biophysica Acta*, **1129**, 149–54.

Maj, J., Rogóz, Z., Skuza, G., Sowinska, H., and Superata, J. (1990). Behavioural and neurochemical effects of Ro 40–7592, a new COMT inhibitor with a potential therapeutic activity in Parkinson's disease. *Journal of Neural Transmission—Parkinson's Disease and Dementia Section*, **2**, 101–12.

Männistö, P. T. and Kaakkola, S. (1989). New selective COMT inhibitors: useful adjuncts for Parkinson's disease? *Trends in Pharmacological Sciences*, **10**, 54–6.

Männistö, P. T. and Kaakkola, S. (1990). Rationale for selective COMT inhibitors as adjuncts in the drug treatment of Parkinson's disease. *Pharmacology and Toxicology*, **66**, 31–23.

Männistö, P. T. and Tuomainen, P. (1991). Effect of high single doses of levodopa and carbidopa on brain dopamine and its metabolites: modulation by selective inhibitors of monoamine oxidase and/or catechol-O-methyltransferase in the male rat. *Naunyn-Schmiedebergs Archives of Pharmacology*, **344**, 412–18.

Männistö, P. T., Kaakkola, S., Nissinen, E., Lindén, I.-B., and Pohto, P. (1988). Properties of novel effective and highly selective inhibitors of catechol-O-methyltransferase. *Life Sciences*, **43**, 1465–71.

Männistö, P. T., Tuomainen, P., Toivonen, M., Törnwall, M., and Kaakkola, S. (1990). Effect of acute levodopa on brain catecholamines after selective MAO and COMT inhibition in male rats. *Journal of Neural Transmission—Parkinson's Disease and Dementia Section*, **2**, 31–43.

Männistö, P. T., Tuomainen, P., and Tuominen, R. K. (1991). Different *in vivo* properties of three new inhibitors of catechol-O-methyltransferase in the rat. *British Journal of Pharmacology*, **105**, 569–74.

Marsden, C., Broch, O., and Guldberg, H. (1972). Effect of nigral and raphe lesions on the catechol-O-methyltransferase and monoamine oxidase activities in the rat striatum. *European Journal of Pharmacology*, **19**, 35–42.

Morrison, J. F. and Walsh, C. T. (1988). The behavior and significance of slow-binding enzyme inhibitors. *Advances in Enzymology*, **61**, 201–301.

Nissinen, E. (1984). The site of O-methylation by membrane-bound catechol-O-methyltransferase. *Biochemical Pharmacology*, **33**, 3105–8.

Nissinen, E., Lindén, I.-B., Schultz, E., Kaakkola, S., Männistö, P. T., and Pohto, P. (1988). Inhibition of catechol-O-methyl-transferase activity by two novel disubstituted catechols in the rat. *European Journal of Pharmacology*, **153**, 263–9.

Paria, B. C., Chakraborty, C., and Dey, S. K. (1990). Catechol estrogen formation in the mouse uterus and its role in implantation. *Molecular and Cellular Endocrinology*, **69**, 25–32.

Pentikäinen, P. J., Vuorela, A., Järvinen, M., Wikberg, T., and Gordin, A. (1989). Human pharmacokinetics of OR-462, a new catechol-O-methyltransferase inhibitor. *European Journal of Clinical Pharmacology*, **36**, A110.

Pfanner, N. and Neupert, W. (1990). The mitochondrial protein import apparatus. *Annual Review of Biochemistry*, **59**, 331–53.

Rivett, A. and Roth, J. A. (1982). Kinetic studies on the O-methylation of dopamine by human brain membrane-bound catechol-O-methyltransferase. *Biochemistry*, **21**, 1740–2.

Rivett, A., Eddy, B., and Roth, J. A. (1982). Contribution of sulfate conjugation, deamination and O-methylation of dopamine and norepinephrine in human brain. *Journal of Neurochemistry*, **39**, 1009–16.

Rivett, A., Francis, A., and Roth, J. A. (1983). Distinct cellular localization of membrane-bound and soluble forms of catechol-O-methyltransferase in brain. *Journal of Neurochemistry*, **40**, 215–19.

Roth, J. A. (1992). Membrane-bound catechol-O-methyltransferase: a re-evaluation of its role in the O-methylation of the catecholamine neurotransmitters. *Physiology, Biochemistry and Pharmacology*, **120**, 1–29.

Salminen, M., Lundström, K., Tilgmann, C., Savolainen, R., Kalkkinen, N., and Ulmanen, I. (1990). Molecular cloning and characterization of rat liver catechol-O-methyltransferase. *Gene*, **93**, 241–7.

Sariaslani, S. F. and Rosazza, J. P. (1983). Novel biotransformations of 7-ethoxycoumarin by *Streptomyces griseus*. *Applied and Environmental Microbiology*, **46**, 468–74.

Schultz, E. and Nissinen, E. (1989). Inhibition of rat liver and duodenum soluble catechol-O-methyltransferase by a tight-binding inhibitor OR-462. *Biochemical Pharmacology*, **38**, 3953–6.

Singer, S. J. (1990). The structure and insertion of integral proteins in membranes. *Annual Review of Cell Biology*, **6**, 247–96.

Sundberg, S. and Gordin, A. (1991). COMT inhibition with nitecapone does not affect the tyramine pressor response. *Clinical Pharmacology*, **32**, 130–2.

Sundberg, S., Scheinin, M., Ojala-Karlsson, P., Kaakkola, S., Akkila, J., and Gordin, A. (1990). Exercise hemodynamics and catecholamine metabolism after catechol-O-methyltransferase inhibition with nitecapone. *Clinical Pharmacology and Therapeutics*, **48**, 356–64.

Taskinen, J., Vidgren, J., Ovaska, M., Bäckström, R., Pippuri, A., and Nissinen, E. (1989). QSAR and binding model for inhibition of rat liver catechol-O-methyltransferase by 1,5-substituted-3,4-dihydroxybenzenes. *Quantitative Structure-Activity Relationships*, **8**, 210–13.

Taskinen, J., Wikberg, T., Ottoila, P., Kanner, L., Lotta, T., Pippuri, A., and Bäckström, R. (1991). Identification of major metabolites of the catechol-O-methyltransferase-inhibitor nitecapone in human urine. *Drug Metabolism and Disposition*, **19**, 178–83.

Tedroff, J., Hartvig, P., Bjurling, P., Andersson, Y., Antoni, G., and Långström, B. (1991). Central actions of benserazide after COMT inhibition demonstrated *in vivo* by PET. *Journal of Neural Transmission-General Section*, **85**, 11–17.

Teräväinen, H., Kaakkola, S., Järvinen, M., and Gordin, A. (1990). Selective COMT inhibitor, nitecapone, in Parkinson's disease. *Neurology*, **40**, 271.

Thakker, D. R., Boelert, C., Kirk, K. L., Anthowiak, R., and Creveling, C. R. (1986). Regioselectivity of catechol-O-methyltransferase. The effect of pH on the site of O-methylation of fluorinated norepinephrine. *Journal of Biological Chemistry*, **261**, 178–84.

Tilgmann, C. and Kalkkinen, N. (1990). Purification and partial characterization of rat liver soluble catechol-O-methyltransferase. *Federation of European Biochemical Societies Letters*, **264**, 95–9.

Tilgmann, C. and Kalkkinen, N. (1991). Purification and partial sequence analysis of the soluble catechol-O-methyltransferase from human placenta—comparison to the rat liver enzyme. *Biochemical and Biophysical Research Communications*, **174**, 995–1002.

Törnwall, M. and Männistö, P. T. (1991). Acute toxicity of three new selective COMT inhibitors in mice with a special emphasis on interactions with drugs increasing catecholaminergic neurotransmission. *Pharmacology and Toxicology*, **69**, 64–70.

Trendelenburg, U. (1989). The uptake and metabolism of ^{3}H-catecholamines in rat cerebral cortex slices. *Naunyn-Schmiedebergs Archives of Pharmacology*, **339**, 293–7.

Tunnicliff, G. and Ngo, T. T. (1983). Kinetics of rat brain soluble catechol-O-methyltransferase and its inhibition by substrate analogues. *International Journal of Biochemistry*, **15**, 733–8.

Ulmanen, I. and Lundström, K. (1991). Cell-free synthesis of rat and human catechol-O-methyltransferase: insertion of the membrane bound form into microsomal membranes *in vitro*. *European Journal of Biochemistry*, **202**, 1013–20.

Vandewalle, B. and Lefebvre, J. (1989). Opposite effects of estrogen and catecholestrogen on hormone-sensitive breast cancer cell growth and differentiation. *Molecular and Cellular Endocrinology*, **61**, 2391–46.

Veser, J., Martin, R., and Thomas, H. (1981). Immunocytochemical demonstration of catechol-O-methyltransferase in *Candida tropicalis*. *Journal of General Microbiology*, **126**, 97–101.

Vidgren, J., Tilgmann, C., Lundström, K., and Liljas, A. (1991). Crystallization and preliminary X-ray investigation of a recombinant form of rat catechol-O-methyltransferase. *Proteins: Structure, Function and Genetics*, **11**, 233–6.

von Hejne, G. and Gavel, Y. (1988). Topogenic signals in integral membrane proteins. *European Journal of Biochemistry*, **174**, 671–8.

Waldmeier, P. C., Baumann, P. A., Feldtrauer, J. J., Hauser, K., Bittiger, H., Bischoff, S., and Von Sprecher, G. (1990a). CGP 28014, a new inhibitor of cerebral catechol-O-methylation with a non-catechol structure. *Naunyn-Schmiedebergs Archives of Pharmacology*, **342**, 305–11.

Waldmeier, P. C., De Herdt, P., and Maitre, L. (1990b). Effects of the COMT inhibitor, CGP 28014, on plasma homovanillic acid and O-methylation of exogenous L-DOPA in the rat. *Journal of Neural Transmission* **32** (Suppl.), 381–6.

Weinshilboum, R. (1988). Pharmacogenetics of methylation: relationship to drug metabolism. *Clinical Biochemistry*, **21**, 201–10.

Weinshilboum, R. and Raymond, F. A. (1976). Calcium inhibition of rat liver catechol-O-methyltransferase. *Biochemical Pharmacology*, **25**, 573–9.

Weinshilboum, R. and Raymond, F. A. (1977). Inheritance of low erythrocyte catechol-O-methyltransferase activity in man. *American Journal of Medical Genetics*, **29**, 125–35.

Winqvist, R., Lundström, K., Salminen, M., Laatikainen, M., and Ulmanen, I. (1991). The human catechol-O-methyltransferase gene maps to band q11.2 of chromosome 22 and shows a frequent RFLP with BglI. *Cytogenetics and Cell Genetics*, **59**, 253–7.

Woodard, R. W., Tsai, M.-D., Floss, H. G., Crooks, P. A., and Coward, J. K. (1980). Stereochemical course of the transmethylation catalzed by catechol-O-methyltransferase. *Journal of Biological Chemistry*, **255**, 9124–7.

Zürcher, G., Colzi, A., and Da Prada, M. (1990a). Ro 40–7592—inhibition of COMT in rat brain and extracerebral tissues. *Journal of Neural Transmission* **32** (Suppl.), 375–80.

Zürcher, G., Keller, H. H., Kettler, R., Borgulya, J., Bonetti, E. P., Eigenmann, R., and Da Prada, M. (1990b). Ro 40–7592, a novel, very potent, and orally active inhibitor of catechol-O-methyl-transferase—a pharmacological study in rats. *Advances in Neurology*, **53**, 497–503.

Inhibitors of phospholipase A_2

Dominick Mobilio and Guy A. Schiehser

13.1 Introduction

As the first rate-limiting enzyme in the arachidonic acid cascade, phospholipase A_2 (PLA_2) has long held promise as a strategic target for therapeutic intervention. In hydrolysing arachidonyl esters from the *sn*-2 position of membrane phospholipids, this enzyme class initiates the generation of a host of humoral mediators including the leucotrienes, prostaglandins, thromboxanes, and lipoxins. When utilizing 1-*O*-alkyl phosphatidylcholines as substrates, PLA_2s liberate lyso-platelet-activating factor (lyso-PAF), the progenitor of the potent lipid mediator platelet-activating factor (PAF). This 'remodelling pathway' is the primary biosynthetic route for the generation of PAF following cellular activation. In addition to its pivotal role in mediator biosynthesis, the direct effects of PLA_2s on phospholipid catabolism and the preferential hydrolysis of oxidized substrates suggest a role in membrane remodelling and homeostasis. As a consequence of its multiple physiological effects, unregulated PLA_2 activity is suspected of major involvement in inflammatory pathologies. Despite intense efforts to identify modulators of these enzymes, selective inhibitors and clinically useful agents have proved to be frustratingly elusive.

Since the constraints of this chapter do not permit a comprehensive treatment of PLA_2 research, the reader is referred to a number of specialized reviews (Verheij *et al.* 1981; Chang *et al.* 1987; Dennis 1987; Waite 1987; Mobilio and Marshall 1989; Bereziat *et al.* 1990; Langton 1990; Van Den Bosch *et al.* 1990; Wilkerson 1990; Pruzanski and Vadas 1991). In this chapter we shall focus on recent research that may have relevance to inhibitor design and testing or to potential therapeutic applications and we shall provide a selective review of PLA$_2$ inhibitors.

13.2 Sources and primary structure

PLA$_2$s, which are widely distributed phylogenetically, were historically categorized into secreted forms present in large quantities in snake venom, and mammalian pancreatic juices, and low abundance cell-associated enzymes that are found in virtually all cell types examined. To date, over 60 enzymes from a variety of organisms and cellular sources have been sequenced and, with few exceptions, all possess a high degree of sequence homology and are now known to be secretable upon appropriate stimulation (Dennis *et al.* 1991).

Low molecular weight (LMW) PLA$_2$s (14–18 kDa) found in snake venom and pancreatic secretions provided early researchers with an abundance of enzyme for structural studies. Based upon amino acid sequences, two broad classifications were proposed (Heinrikson *et al.* 1977). Type I enzymes include those from pancreatic, cobra (*Elapidae*) and sea snake (*Hydrophidae*) sources, and are characterized by a Cys-11–Cys-77 disulphide bridge and a 57–66 'elapid loop'. The type II enzymes from vipers (*Viperidae*), pit vipers (*Crotalidae*), and non-pancreatic eucaryotic cells possess a carboxy-terminal extension terminating in a Cys-133–Cys-50 disulphide bridge and a deletion between amino acids 57 and 66. The honey-bee (*Apis mellifera*) venom PLA$_2$, a glycoprotein containing an asparagine-linked oligosaccharide (Shipolini *et al.* 1974), has historically been viewed as a distinct class. Recently, examination of the revised amino acid sequence deduced from the corresponding cDNA has revealed conspicuous homology to the type I enzymes (Kuchler *et al.* 1989).

Isolation and characterization of clinically relevant 'pro-inflammatory' PLA$_2$s and identification of their cellular sources in humans remains an area of intense interest and controversy. The first human sequence published was of pancreatic PLA$_2$, an enzyme whose primary function is digestive (Verheij *et al.* 1983). Presumed to be of pathological significance because of their presence at inflammatory sites, non-pancreatic PLA$_2$s were isolated from human platelets and synovial fluids of rheumatoid arthritis patients (Kramer *et al.* 1989). Partial sequencing revealed both enzymes to have identical amino-terminal (19 amino acids) sequences. Screening of a cDNA library with oligonucleotide probes produced a sequence encoding a 124 amino acid sequence characteristic of type II enzymes (Kramer *et al.* 1989; Seilhamer *et al.* 1989b). Additional PLA$_2$s isolated from human placenta

(Lai and Wada 1988) and spleen (Kanda *et al.* 1989) also proved to be identical to the platelet enzyme. Despite identical primary structures, these LMW human PLA$_2$s may yet reveal differential physiological effects through cell-selective activation and regulatory mechanisms.

A number of reports have appeared describing cytosolic high molecular weight (HMW) (56−110 kDa) PLA$_2$s from non-human (Channon and Leslie 1990; Gronich *et al.* 1990; Krause *et al.* 1991; Leslie 1991) and human (Clark *et al.* 1990; Diez and Mong 1990; Rehfeldt *et al.* 1991; Takayama *et al.* 1991) sources. The range of molecular weights should be accepted with caution as the 56−60 kDa proteins may be proteolytic artefacts (Leslie 1991) or unrelated impurities (Gronich *et al.* 1990). Recently, the HMW cytosolic PLA$_2$ isolated from U937 cells was tryptically cleaved and complementary oligonucleotide probes were prepared (Clark *et al.* 1990). The cloned cDNA encoded a 85.2 kDa PLA$_2$ which migrates on SDS-PAGE gel with an apparent molecular weight of 110 kDa (Clark *et al.* 1991). The 749 amino acid sequence bears no apparent homology to any known PLA$_2$; however, the 140 amino acid amino-terminal fragment does exhibit homology to phospholipase C (PLC) and the C2 region (calcium binding translocation domain) of protein kinase C (PKC). This sequence similarity may provide a structural correlate for the membrane-directed calcium-dependent translocation commonly observed in the HMW species. The resemblance to other translocated enzymes such as 5-lipoxygenase (5-LO) (Miller *et al.* 1990) may reflect an analogous regulatory and activation mechanism for PLA$_2$. Notably, the substrate specificity for arachidonate-containing phospholipids strongly implicates HMW PLA$_2$s in eicosanoid generation. This direct link of HMW PLA$_2$s to arachidonate mobilization offers hope that selective inhibition of mediator release is achievable and provides an alternative to the LMW variants for *in vitro* assays to guide drug design.

13.3   Structure and catalytic mechanism

The molecular mechanism by which PLA$_2$ hydrolyses phospholipids is essential to understanding substrate specificity, enzyme−substrate interactions at lipid−water interfaces, and ultimately, through design of inhibitor probes, the physiological and clinical significance of this enzyme class. On the basis of chemical, spectroscopic, and structural information, early investigations of bovine, equine, and porcine PLA$_2$s led to a proposed catalytic site architecture and a hydrolytic mechanism (Fig. 13.1) (Verheij *et al.* 1980). X-ray crystallography data revealed an apparent active site containing a histidine residue (His-48) and the obligate calcium ion ligated by the carbonyl oxygens of Tyr-28, Gly-30, and Gly-32 (calcium binding domain), Asp-49, and two water molecules (Dijkstra *et al.* 1981a). Mechanistically, the calcium, acting as a Lewis acid, would activate the *sn*-2 ester carbonyl of the bound phospholipid to nucleophilic attack by a water

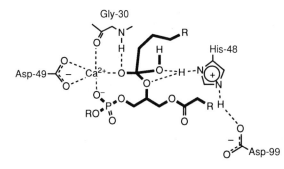

Fig. 13.1 Proposed transition state in the hydrolysis of phospholipids by PLA₂.

molecule. Hydrolysis would be facilitated by removal of a proton from the water by the imidazole of His-48 and the resulting charge would be delocalized through the carboxylate of Asp-99 (Scott *et al.* 1990b). Stabilization of the postulated oxyanionic tetrahedral intermediate was accommodated in the model by coordination to the calcium and the NH group of Gly-30. In addition, calcium coordination to the phosphate group and the scissile ester carbonyl was invoked to account for the observed stereochemical preference for L-phospholipids.

X-ray structures for bovine pancreatic PLA₂ (Dijkstra *et al.* 1981b), porcine pancreatic PLA₂ (Dijkstra *et al.* 1983), and *Crotalus atrox* PLA₂ (Brunie *et al.* 1985) have been described and the coordinates deposited in the Brookhaven Crystallographic Database. Recent PLA₂–inhibitor complexes which have yielded X-ray structures include bovine pancreatic PLA₂–*p*-bromophenacylbromide (Renetseder *et al.* 1988), *Naja naja atra* and honey-bee venom PLA₂ complexed with a phosphonate transition state analogue (Scott *et al.* 1990a; White *et al.* 1990), and porcine pancreatic PLA₂ mutant–substrate analogue (Thunnissen *et al.* 1990). As well as providing substantial confirmation of the original catalytic mechanism (Verheij *et al.* 1980), new insights regarding the nature of the hydrophobic channel, the interfacial binding phenomenon the hydrolytic acceleration with aggregated substrates have become apparent (Scott *et al.* 1990b). The specific inhibitors used for these crystal structures are discussed in § 13.5.5.

13.4   Clinical indications

Although the clinical utility of a 'pure' PLA₂ inhibitor has yet to be demonstrated, a number of potential applications have been suggested based on the known involvement of lipid mediators in disease states, pathogenic manifestations upon exogenous administration of PLA₂ and existing therapeutic agents (non-steroidal anti-inflammatory drugs (NSAIDs), 5-LO inhibitors, and PAF antagonists). Elevated levels of PLA_2s also support therapeutic indications in pancreatitis (Schmidt and Creutzfeld 1969), rheumatoid arthritis and osteoarthritis (Stefanski et al. 1986), malaria and psoriasis (Nevalainen et al. 1985), and septic shock (Seeger 1987).

Given its abundance, it is not surprising that the first recognized pathogenic role for PLA_2 was in pancreatitis (Zieve and Vogel 1961). Acute pancreatitis is an autodigestive disease wherein the resulting catabolic products, including fatty acids and lysolecithin, contribute to secondary complications such as shock and circulatory collapse. Increases in immunoreactive PLA_2 titres and catalytic activity have been measured in acute pancreatitis (Nevalainen et al. 1983), and serum PLA_2 activity has been correlated with disease severity and clinical outcome (Schroder et al. 1980).

Increased levels of PLA_2 activity have been reported in synovial fluids of patients with rheumatoid and osteoarthritis (Pruzanski et al. 1985). Two isoforms of LMW PLA_2 (peaks A and B) were isolated from synovial fluids of arthritic patients (Seilhamer et al. 1989a). In osteoarthritis, peak B is the predominant form while peak A occurs in greater abundance in rheumatoid joints.

Peripheral monocytes (Bomalaski et al. 1986), polymorphonuclear leucocytes (PMNs) (Bomalaski et al. 1985), and epidermis (Taylor et al. 1991) also exhibit markedly enhanced PLA_2 activities in rheumatoid arthritis. Correlations of serum PLA_2 activity with clinical markers of disease severity have been demonstrated (Silverman et al. 1987; Pruzanski et al. 1988). Intra-articular injection of the isolated PLA_2 generates an inflammatory response (Vadas et al. 1986) mediated in part by the release of superoxide and lysosomal enzymes from human PMNs and monocytes (Pruzanski et al. 1991b). Investigations of the source of the synovial fluid PLA_2 revealed significantly higher levels of enzymatic activity in both superficial and deep layers of cartilage compared with the synovium in both rheumatoid and osteoarthritic joints (Pruzanski et al. 1991a). By implication, articular cartilage may be a significant source of PLA_2 in arthritic joints, although its contribution to the chronic inflammatory reaction is unknown.

Septic shock, which is clinically associated with a 40–60 per cent mortality rate (Rackow and Astiz 1991), is characterized by high levels of tumour necrosis factor (TNF), interleukin-1 (IL-1), and endogenous mediators from the arachidonic acid cascade (Dammas et al. 1989). Serum PLA_2 activity is increased up to 200-fold in patients presenting with septic shock, and the enzymatic activity correlates with the degree and time course of circulatory collapse (Vadas et al. 1988), adult respiratory distress syndrome (ARDS), and acute renal failure (Baur et al. 1989). Consistent with increased PLA_2 activity and its role in eicosanoid generation, clinical studies (Haupt et al. 1991) with ibuprofen and animal studies with the 5-LO inhibitor SKF104353 (Eckardt and Weston 1988) have shown significant effects in outcome in septic shock.

Several additional therapeutic targets have been proposed for which PLA$_2$ involvement has experimental support. A recent study of reperfusion following myocardial ischaemia in rats using anti-PLA$_2$ antibody suggests that the enzyme is involved in the degradation of cardiac phospholipids with resultant cellular damage and decreases in contractility and coronary blood flow (Prasad *et al.* 1991). Although the aetiology of inflammatory bowel disease is not known, recent interest has focused on the role of leucotrienes. In addition to evidence from animal models, clinical studies of leucotriene antagonists and lipoxygenase/translocation inhibitors should establish the viability of this mechanistic approach. If these drugs prove successful, PLA$_2$ inhibitors would, in principle, offer similar therapeutic potential. Psoriasis is a chronic hyperproliferative inflammatory condition characterized in part by abnormal arachidonate metabolism. Increased levels of 12-HETE, LTB$_4$, and PAF, as well as PLA$_2$, have been noted. NSAIDs, which are believed to shunt arachidonic acid metabolism to the lipoxygenase pathway, exacerbate psoriatic lesions when given orally or topically. PLA$_2$ inhibition may provide the broad reduction in mediators necessary to modulate this disease. In asthma, the clinical data generated on leucotriene modulating agents will also provide impetus for the use of PLA$_2$ inhibitors.

13.5 Inhibitors

Abundant enzymes, a defined catalytic mechanism, X-ray crystal structures, and a point of intervention upstream of the therapeutically successful NSAIDs make PLA$_2$ an attractive target for the medicinal chemist. Inhibitor design has followed a predictable evolution from substrate analogues and natural products to transition state analogues and suicide inhibitors, with ever-increasing assistance from X-ray crystallography and molecular modelling. Unfortunately, marked differences in inhibitory activity depending on enzyme source, substrate structure, and lipid architecture often render *in vitro* assay results equivocal. In view of the apparent promiscuity of enzymatic assays, few of the numerous micromolar inhibitors of PLA$_2$ known to date have proved of mechanistic or pharmacological significance. Increased reliance on cellular assays may provide a more predictable and fertile source of pharmacological agents. Although it has been assumed that PLA$_2$ inhibitors, by virtue of their reduction of lipid mediator generation, should exhibit activity in classical anti-inflammatory assays, the limited *in vivo* activity demonstrated to date remains problematic and emphasizes the need for alternative animal models.

A search of the patent literature reveals numerous claims of PLA$_2$ inhibitory activity which are beyond the scope of the following discussion. Thus, only those compounds which have appeared in the open literature will be described with specific emphasis on recent disclosures.

13.5.1 Substrate analogues

In a study that used molecular modelling to explore the relationship between phospholipid analogues and natural phospholipids, various conformations (keto–enol tautomers and *cis–trans* isomers) of a constrained analogue (±)1, were overlapped with the best enzyme-docked conformation of di-lauryl-phosphatidylcholine (Campbell *et al.* 1988, 1989). While the keto form with the (3S,4R) configuration had the best fit, only racemic 1 was tested and shown to inhibit rat neutrophil cell-free PLA$_2$ (IC$_{50}$ = 64 μM) and rat macrophage PLA$_2$ (IC$_{50}$ = 44 μM).

Replacement of the ester at the *sn*-2 position of a phospholipid with an amide has resulted in potent and reversible inhibitors of PLA$_2$. In the first study, a single compound, 1-stearyl-2-stearoylaminodeoxy phosphatidyl-choline, was found to inhibit *N. naja naja* PLA$_2$ (N-PLA$_2$) in the Triton X-100–phospholipid mixed micelle system with an IC$_{50}$ value of 38 μM (Davidson *et al.* 1986).

A second study, which included detailed kinetic parameters, examined amide replacements at both the *sn*-1 and *sn*-2 positions of phospholipids (de Haas *et al.* 1990a). Both enantiomers of the amides were examined. The conclusions were that replacement of either ester with an amide results in inhibitors of porcine pancreatic PLA$_2$, but potent inhibitors had the amide at the *sn*-2 position with the naturally occurring R phospholipid stereochemistry. The unnatural enantiomers were only weakly active.

The study was then extended and inhibitor activities in different assay systems were examined (de Haas *et al.* 1990b). The results emphasize the caution that must be taken when evaluating potential PLA$_2$ inhibitors. The water-soluble acylamino analogues exhibit inhibitory activity only when incorporated into an organized substrate–water interface (micelle). When the assays were run on molecularly dispersed substrate solutions, the compounds lost their inhibitory activity.

It has long been known that the activity of PLA$_2$ is greatly enhanced when the substrate is above its critical micelle concentration (CMC). Two groups have reported the synthesis and potentials for hydrolysis of constrained phospholipid analogues 2 to see whether this activation results from a change in the substrate conformation (substrate theory of activation) in the micelle (Barlow *et al.* 1988a,b; Gialih *et al.* 1988; Lister and Hancock 1988). The (−)enantiomer of 2 (R = C$_5$H$_{11}$) was a substrate and was hydrolysed at the same rate whether above or below its CMC. This supported the theory, because it was believed that the compound would be unable to undergo a conformational change at the CMC because of its constrained nature. If the rate increase above the CMC for natural sub-strates resulted instead from a conformational change in the enzyme, then one would have expected to see a rate change at the CMC for the constrained compounds.

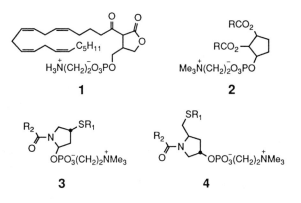

Similar conformationally restricted compounds **3** and **4** were prepared by another group and tested against porcine pancreatic PLA$_2$ (Magolda and Galbraith 1989). Direct comparisons of three corresponding pairs (R$_2$ = PhCh$_2$O, R$_1$ = C$_{12}$H$_{25}$, C$_{16}$H$_{25}$, and C$_{18}$H$_{25}$) showed that isomers **4** were two to five times more potent than isomers **3** (IC$_{50}$ values from 4.7 to 40 μM). Computer modelling of these inhibitors and either bovine or porcine pancreatic PLA$_2$ indicated that the difference in activity was because of the degree to which the enzyme could accommodate both side-chains.

Attempts to prepare fluorinated phospholipid transition state analogues resulted in the production of inhibitors **5** and **6** and their corresponding alcohol reduction products. The compounds were tested against N-PLA$_2$ in mixed micelles (Gelb 1986; Yuan *et al.* 1987). The single-chain compounds were the most potent inhibitors and were partially hydrated in the micelle as evidenced by ^{19}F NMR (IC$_{50}$ values of 0.7 mM, 1.6 mM, and 0.07 mM for **5a**, **5b**, and **5c** respectively). This was not the case with compound **6**. Reduction of **5a** to the alcohol resulted in a loss of activity.

Use of the transition state analogue approach also resulted in phosphonate-containing phospholipid analogues **7** (R = H, O-alkyl) (Yuan and Gelb 1988). Although the monoesters (X = NH$_3^+$, R = CH$_2$OC$_{16}$H$_{33}$, IC$_{50}$ = 5 μM) showed significant activity, this was greatly reduced upon conversion to the methyl phosphonates. A later report extended this work to include detailed kinetic and inhibition studies on phosphonates **7** as well as thiophosphonates **8** and thioesters **9** (Yuan *et al.* 1990).

Arachidonic acid analogues **10** (R = alkenyl or alkynyl) have been reported as inhibitors of N-PLA$_2$ (Foster *et al.* 1987). The most potent compound (**10**, R = C≡C—C$_{11}$H$_{23}$) had an IC$_{50}$ value of 0.7 μM against N-PLA$_2$ and was active as an inhibitor of slow reacting substance of anaphylaxis (SRS-A) release in an *in vivo* rat passive peritoneal model of anaphylaxis (51 per cent inhibition at 200 μM). The same study also

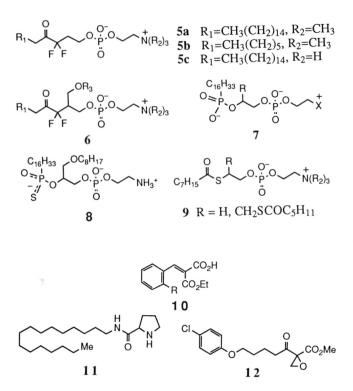

5a R$_1$=CH$_3$(CH$_2$)$_{14}$, R$_2$=CH$_3$
5b R$_1$=CH$_3$(CH$_2$)$_5$, R$_2$=CH$_3$
5c R$_1$=CH$_3$(CH$_2$)$_{14}$, R$_2$=H

6

7

8

9 R = H, CH$_2$SCOC$_5$H$_{11}$

10

11

12

reported the PLA$_2$ inhibitory activity of 5,8,11,14-eicosatetraynoic acid (ETYA, IC$_{50}$ = 20 μM versus N-PLA$_2$). ETYA was a weak and inconsistent inhibitor of SRS-A release. Others also found ETYA to be an inhibitor of PLA$_2$ from rabbit peritoneal neutrophil sonicates and acid extracts (Lanni and Becker 1985). IC$_{50}$ values were 12 and 22 μM, respectively.

Two series of compounds, typified by **11** and **12**, were designed as transition state inhibitors and have been studied both *in vitro* and *in vivo* (Marshall and Chang 1990). *In vitro* activity was assessed against human platelet and human synovial fluid PLA$_2$, and both compounds proved to be inhibitors (IC$_{50}$ values of: 16.1 μM and 120 μM respectively for **11**, and of 18.4 μM and 36.3 μM respectively for **12**). Given the expectation that a PLA$_2$ inhibitor should be active in classical *in vivo* models of inflammation involving arachidonic acid metabolites, the compounds were examined in the rat carrageenan paw oedema and 12-*O*-tetradecanoate phorbol-13-acetate (TPA) induced mouse ear oedema models. Both compounds reduced carrageenan paw oedema when administered orally at 50 or 100 mg kg^{-1}. Ear oedema was reduced upon oral administration of **11** (ED$_{50}$ = 69 mg kg^{-1}) but only upon topical administration of **12** (ED$_{50}$ $\approx$ 1 mg per ear).

13.5.2 Suicide inhibitors

The design and synthesis of the first suicide inhibitors of PLA$_2$ based upon the enzyme's mechanism has recently been reported and is illustrated in eqn (13.1) (Washburn and Dennis 1990a,b; 1991). The inhibitors **13**, which are termed suicide inhibitory bifunctionally linked substrates (SIBLINKS), are dibasic acids linking the glycerol backbone of a phospholipid at the *sn*-2 position to a *p*-nitrophenol chromophore. The actual inhibitor **16** is formed at the active site by PLA$_2$ hydrolysis of **13**, liberating **14**. Compound **14** then cyclizes to the reactive anhydride **16** that acylates the PLA$_2$. The SIBLINKS examined had R$_1$ = R$_2$ = H (n = 0, 1), R$_1$ = H, R$_2$ = Me (n = 0, 1) or R$_1$ = Me, R$_2$ = H (n = 1). Except for the unsubstituted glutarate (R$_1$ = R$_2$ = H, n = 1), cyclization of **14** to **16** occurs at the active site. The anhydride then acylates PLA$_2$ rather than reacting with the bulk solution. However, the unsubstituted glutarate cyclizes more slowly and diffuses from the active site. The resulting anhydride then reacts with water and does not have any suicide inhibitory effect.

The size of R was varied from 8 to 18 carbon atoms and, while not influencing the rate of hydrolysis, it had the effect of modulating the ratio of the number of moles of SIBLINK hydrolysed per number of moles of enzyme inactivated. In the case of **13** (R$_1$ = H, R$_2$ = Me, n = 1), the

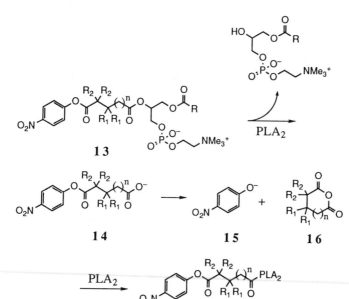

(13.1)

trend is to increase this ratio from 19:1 to 58:1 (thereby decreasing the efficiency of acylation by **16**) as the size of R increases from 10 to 18 carbons. However, the generality of this trend is in doubt since similar ratios are produced when R is eight carbons (52:1) as when it is 18 carbons (58:1).

13.5.3   Natural products

Sesterterpene (**18**) was isolated from the marine sponge *Halichondriidae* (Kernan and Faulker 1988). The compound produced 100 per cent inhibition of bee venom PLA_2 at 16 μg ml^{-1} and was also active in the mouse TPA ear oedema assay.

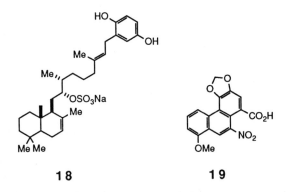

1 8   **1 9**

Aristolochic acid (**19**), an inhibitor of *Vipera russelli* venom PLA_2 ($IC_{50} = 50$ μM, $K_i = 9.9 \times 10^{-4}$ M) (Vishwanath and Gowda 1987) was the subject of a circular dichroism binding study (Vishwanath *et al.* 1987b). It was found to bind to the venom PLA_2 with an association constant of 5.0×10^3 M^{-1} ($\Delta G° = -5.1$ kcal mol^{-1}) in the absence of substrate. Kinetics showed the inhibition to be non-competitive. However, competitive inhibition ($IC_{50} = 25$ μM, $K_i = 3.9 \times 10^{-7}$ M) was observed against the basic *Trimeresurus flavoviridis* venom PLA_2. *In vivo* activity was demonstrated by the compounds ability to inhibit the edema caused by both *V. russelli* and *T. flavoviridis* venom PLA_2 upon injection into mice paws (Vishwanath *et al.* 1987a).

Retinoids have been shown to possess anti-inflammatory activity in animals and humans. Recent studies have shown that this might be because of the compound's ability to inhibit PLA_2 (Hope *et al.* 1990). A series of naturally occurring retinoids and analogues were tested for their ability to inhibit human synovial fluid (HSF) PLA_2 and N-PLA_2 (Fiedler-Nagy

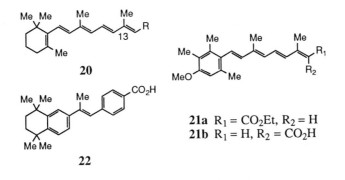

20

21a R$_1$ = CO$_2$Et, R$_2$ = H
21b R$_1$ = H, R$_2$ = CO$_2$H

22

et al. 1987). The most active naturally occurring retinoids (**20**) were retinal, all-*trans*-retinoic acid and 13-*cis*-retinoic acid (IC$_{50}$ values against HSF PLA$_2$/N-PLA$_2$ of 6/25 μM, 10/37 μM and 15/45 μM respectively). Synthetic analogues **21** and **22** were also found to inhibit N-PLA$_2$ (IC$_{50}$ values from 37 to 83 μM), while **22** was also active against HSF-PLA$_2$ (IC$_{50}$ = 12 μM). In addition, **21b** was shown to be an inhibitor of 5-LO and cyclooxygenase.

Two related sesterterpenes, luffariellolide (**23**) (Albizati *et al.* 1987) and manoalide **24** (Jacobs *et al.* 1985; Mayer *et al.* 1988), have been isolated from marine sources. Both inhibit bee venom PLA$_2$ (IC$_{50}$ values of 230 nM and 50–120 nM for **23** and **24** respectively), but the inhibition by **24** is irreversible while that by **23** is partially reversible. Compound **23** demonstrated *in vivo* activity in the TPA-induced mouse ear inflammation assay at a dose of 50 μg per ear. Compound **24** has entered phase I clinical trials as an anti-inflammatory agent and is the only reported PLA$_2$ inhibitor to have been studied in man thus far (Hutton 1991).

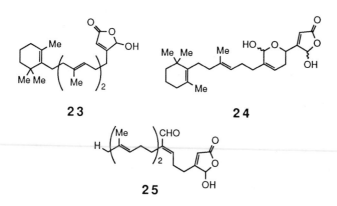

23

24

25

The wide range of reported IC$_{50}$ values for **24** demonstrate the care that must be taken when comparing activities among inhibitors (0.05–0.12 μM, bee venom PLA$_2$ (Mayer *et al*. 1988); 0.7 μM, rattlesnake venom PLA$_2$ (Bennett *et al*. 1987); 30 μM, cobra venom PLA$_2$ (Lombardo and Dennis 1985; Bennett *et al*. 1987; Deems *et al*. 1987); 30 μM, porcine pancreatic PLA$_2$ (Bennett *et al*. 1987); 0.2 and 0.02 μM for HSF-PLA$_2$ with dipalmitoylphosphatidylcholine and *Escherichia coli* respectively as substrates (Jacobson *et al*. 1990)). Knowledge of the enzyme, substrate, and assay conditions is crucial for making comparisons.

A series of manoalide analogues, typified by 'manoalogue' (**25**), have been prepared as inhibitors of PLA$_2$ (Deems *et al*. 1987; Mihelich *et al*. 1988; Reynolds *et al*. 1988). The aim was to identify the specific structural features of **24** responsible for its irreversible inhibition. Comparisons of the various analogues led to the conclusion that both an α,β-unsaturated aldehyde (hemiacetal in **24**) and an open γ-lactone ring are necessary for irreversible inhibition. Compound **25** is undergoing preclinical evaluation (Hutton 1991).

A curious collection of anti-oxidant natural products have shown PLA$_2$ inhibitory activity. Gossypol (**26**), a male contraceptive, completely inhibits the ability of human spermatozoa to hydrolyse monolayers of phosphatidylglycerol at 100 μM (Vainio *et al*. 1985). Quercetin (**27**) inhibits the PLA$_2$ activity of neutrophil sonicates and acid extracts (IC$_{50}$ values of 57 μM and 100 μM respectively) (Lanni and Becker 1985). The inhibitory activity of nordihydroguaiaretic acid (**28**) against neutrophil sonicates and extracts is shown in the same paper. IC$_{50}$ values were about 10 μM in both assays. Finally, vitamin E (**29**) was shown to inhibit rat platelet PLA$_2$ by 20–50 per cent at 116 μM (Douglas *et al*. 1986). It is unknown whether the anti-oxidant potential for these compounds is related to their PLA$_2$

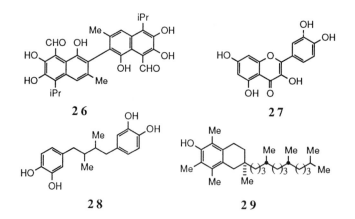

inhibitory activity. A redox system has not been proposed as part of the hydrolytic mechanism of PLA$_2$, and the anti-oxidant activity of these compounds may be irrelevant to their inhibitory mechanism.

Finally, searches for naturally occurring PLA$_2$ inhibitors do not always produce small organic molecules. One such quest produced two peptidic inhibitors of human PMN and synovial fluid PLA$_2$ (Fredenhagen *et al.* 1990). The *Streptoverticillium* strain R2075 and the *Streptomyces griseoluteus* strain R2107 yielded the lanthionine-containing peptides duramycin B (**30**) and duramycin C (**31**) respectively. Inhibitory IC$_{50}$ values for **30** and **31** were 1.5 μM and 1.0 μM respectively against human PMN PLA$_2$, and 0.8 μM and 1.0 μM respectively against HSF-PLA$_2$. The compounds possess weak antibacterial activity against *Bacillus subtilis* only and are inactive against other strains.

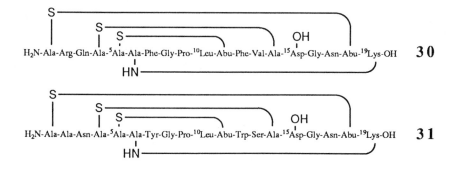

13.5.4 Computer-aided design

The X-ray structure of bovine pancreatic PLA$_2$ was examined with the aim of designing compounds that fit both sterically and electronically into the active site. This led to the identification of a series of acenaphthenes typified by **32**, the most potent compound (IC$_{50}$ = 0.2 μM) (Ripka *et al.* 1987). It is believed that the naphthalene ring might mimic the double bonds in the arachidonyl chain and fit in the slot between Leu-2 and Tyr-69. The benzyl group takes advantage of the hydrophobic residues in the active site. The compounds are active in the croton oil ear oedema and contact sensitivity ear assays (Wilkerson 1990).

Another modelling study of the same X-ray structure led to a series of long-chain alkylamine inhibitors of porcine pancreatic PLA$_2$ (Davis *et al.* 1988). The compounds, typified by **33** (IC$_{50}$ = 10 μM, both enantiomers), were designed to interact with His-48 and Asp-49, the only two accessible polar residues at the active site, and with Tyr-69. The first two residues

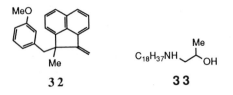

32   33

are highly conserved among different PLA$_2$s and are involved in the hydrolysis.

13.5.5 Inhibitor-enzyme crystal structures

Four crystal structures of inhibitor-PLA$_2$ complexes have been reported. The first of these was the 2.5 Å resolution crystal structure of the co-valently bound complex of *p*-bromophenacyl bromide (BPB) with bovine pancreatic PLA$_2$ (Renetseder *et al.* 1988). The substrate was covalently bound to active-site residue His-48, and its presence produced no change in the conformations of the remaining active-site residues when compared with the native enzyme. However, there were some large differences in other regions of the enzyme. Hydrophobic interactions between Phe-5 and Cys-45 with BPB are present, and this may explain why the inhibitor is rather specific for PLA$_2$.

Next to appear was the 2.4 Å crystal structure of **34** bound to a porcine PLA$_2$ mutant (Thunnissen *et al.* 1990). The mutant, which was obtained by site-directed mutagenesis, was used because of its crystalliza-tion properties. As in the case of the BPB structure (Renetseder *et al.* 1988), the conformations of the active-site residues were unchanged by the bound inhibitor. However, two water molecules near His-48 had been displaced.

Crystal structures of inhibitor **35** bound to PLA$_2$ from *Naja naja atra* venom (White *et al.* 1990) and bee venom (Scott *et al.* 1990a, 1991) have also been reported. Compound **35** was designed as a transition-state ana-logue with the tetrahedral phosphorus mimicking the intermediate in the hydrolysis of natural substrates. In the snake PLA$_2$–inhibitor complex, the *sn*-1 chain is less tightly bound than the *sn*-2 chain while the methylene

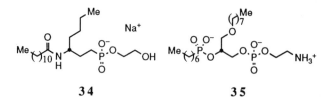

34   35

units and methyl groups furthest from the glycerol have the least order. The two chains lie almost parallel in a 14 Å hydrophobic channel. A similar 9 Å channel contains the two chains of **35** in the bee venom structure. The interactions in both complexes, including the coordination of the calcium cofactors, are essentially identical. Detailed inhibition studies with **35** have been reported (Yuan *et al.* 1990).

13.5.6 Miscellaneous

A series of 3-(4-alkyl)benzoylacrylic acids (**36**) has been reported to inhibit *V. russelli* PLA$_2$ (Kohler *et al.* 1991). The IC$_{50}$ values were strongly dependent on the length of R and varied from more than 500 μM (R = Et) to 0.07 μM (R = octadecyl). After 5 hours of dialysis no PLA$_2$ activity was recovered, supporting a mechanism of irreversible inhibition. Kinetic data agreed with a Michaelis–Menten model of inhibition. A dissociable enzyme–inhibitor complex was formed which then went on to the irreversibly bound complex. Toxicity issues relating to the acrylic acid structure have to be addressed before the usefulness of these compounds can be established.

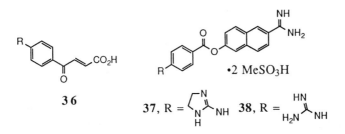

In a study against 17 enzymes, serine protease inhibitors FUT-187 (**37**) and FUT-175 (**38**) were reported to inhibit PLA$_2$ with the same IC$_{50}$ value of 20 μM (Oda *et al.* 1990). The compounds were not specific for PLA$_2$ as IC$_{50}$ values against nine proteases were either comparable with or much lower (23 μM to 2.1 nM) than that against PLA$_2$. The conclusion was that **37** is a potent and selective inhibitor of the trypsin-like serine proteases and should be a useful therapeutic agent for various inflammatory diseases involving overactivity of the complement system. Its PLA$_2$ activity is irrelevant.

13.6 Conclusion

The intense scientific interest in PLA$_2$ is evidenced by the numerous patent and literature compounds with reported enzyme inhibitory activity. Progress in basic research continues to enhance our understanding of the interaction of diverse PLA$_2$s with lipid substrates and the biological implications of those interactions. Efforts to define the contributions of PLA$_2$s from various cellular and compartmental sources to physiological and patho-physiological events has expanded the potential therapeutic applications for future PLA$_2$ inhibitors. The recent characterization of HMW cytosolic species is a significant step in identifying a specific source of arachidonic acid release and mediator generation.

Attempts to correlate inhibitory activity in enzyme assays with *in vivo* models have encountered difficulties. Drug design and evaluation would thus appear to profit from increased emphasis on cellular models which more closely approximate physiological substrates and environments. Progress continues to be hindered by the lack of a 'pure' PLA$_2$ inhibitor; however, the commercial availability of monoclonal antibodies should provide a powerful tool for elucidating the biochemical and clinical involvement of PLA$_2$. As understanding of molecular mechanisms of the enzyme grows, selective inhibitors of PLA$_2$s will emerge to illuminate the pharmacological and pathogenic roles of this significant enzymatic target.

References

Albizati, K. F., Holman, T., Faulkner, D. J., Glaser, K. B., and Jacobs, R. S. (1987). Luffariellolide, an anti-inflammatory sesterterpene from the marine sponge *Luffariella* sp. *Experientia*, **43**, 949–50.

Barlow, P. N., Lister. M. D., Sigler, P. B., and Dennis, E. A. (1988a). Probing the role of substrate conformation in phospholipase A$_2$ action on aggregated phospholipids using constrained phosphatidylcholine analogues. *Journal of Biological Chemistry*, **263**, 12954–58.

Barlow, P. N., Vidal, J.-C., Lister, M. D., Hancock, A. J., and Sigler, P. B. (1988b). Synthesis and some properties of constrained short-chain phosphatidylcholine analogues: (+)- and (−)- (1,3/2)-1-*O*-(phosphocholine)-2,3-*O*-dihexanoylcyclopentane-1,2,3-triol. *Chemistry and Physics of Lipids*, **46**, 157–64.

Baur, M., Schmid, T.-O., and Landauer, B. (1989). Role of phospholipase A in multiorgan failure with special reference to ARDS and acute renal failure (ARF). In *Phospholipase A: Recent developments in methodology, pathophysiology and clinical application* (ed. M. Buchler and H. G. Beger), pp. 196–202. Springer-Verlag, Berlin.

Bennett, C. F., Mong, S., Clark, M. A., Kruse, L. I., and Crooke, S. T. (1987). Differential effects of manoalide on secreted and intracellular phospholipases. *Biochemical Pharmacology*, **36**, 733–40.

Bereziat, G., Etienne, J., Kokkinidis, M., Olivier, J. L., and Pernas, P. (1990). New trends in mammalian non-pancreatic phospholipase-A$_2$ research. *Journal of Lipid Mediators*, **2**, 159–72.

Bomalaski, J. S., Clarke, M. A., Douglas, S. D., and Zurier, R. B. (1985). Enhanced phospholipase A$_2$ and C activities of peripheral blood polymorphonuclear leukocytes from patients with rheumatoid arthritis. *Journal of Leukocyte Biology*, **38**, 649–54.

Bomalaski, J. S., Clarke, M. A., and Zurier, R. B. (1986). Enhanced phospholipase activity in peripheral blood monocytes from patients with rheumatoid arthritis. *Arthritis and Rheumatism*, **29**, 312–18.

Brunie, S., Bolin, J., Gewirth, D., and Sigler, P. B. (1985). The refined crystal structure of dimeric phospholipase A_2 at 2.5 Å. *Journal of Biological Chemistry*, **260**, 9742–9.

Campbell, M. M., Long-Fox, J., Osguthorpe, D., Sainsbury, M., and Sessions, R. B. (1988). Inhibition of phospholipase A_2; a molecular recognition study. *Journal of the Chemical Society, Chemical Communications*, 1560–62.

Campbell, M. M., Fox, J. L., Sainsbury, M., and Liu, Y. (1989). Synthesis of structural variants of phospholipids: inhibition of phospholipase A_2. *Tetrahedron*, **45**, 4551–6.

Chang, J., Musser, J. H., and McGregor, H. (1987). Phospholipase A_2: function and pharmacological regulation. *Biochemical Pharmacology*, **13**, 2429–36.

Channon, J. Y. and Leslie, C. C. (1990). A calcium-dependent mechanism for associating a soluble arachidonoyl-hydrolyzing phospholipase A_2 with membrane in the macrophage cell line RAW 264.7. *Journal of Biological Chemistry*, **265**, 5409–13.

Clark, J. D., Milona, N., and Knopf, J. L. (1990). Purification of a 110-kilodalton cytoplasmic phospholipase A_2 from the human monocytic cell line U937. *Proceedings of the National Academy of Sciences of the United States of America*, **87**, 7708–12.

Clark, J. D., Lin, L.-L., Kriz, R. W., Ramesha, C. S., Sultzman, L. A., Lin, A. Y., *et al.* (1991). A novel arachidonic acid-selective cytosolic PLA_2 contains a Ca^{2+}-dependent translocation domain with homology to PKC and GAP. *Cell*, **65**, 1043–51.

Dammas, P., Reuter, A., Gysen, P., Demonty, J., Lainy, M., and Franchimonst, P. (1989). Tumor necrosis factor and interleukin-1 serum levels during severe sepsis. *Critical Care Medicine*, **17**, 975–8.

Davidson, F. F., Hajdu, J., and Dennis, E. A. (1986). 1-Stearyl, 2-stearoylamino-deoxy phosphatidylcholine, a potent reversible inhibitor of phospholipase A_2. *Biochemical and Biophysical Research Communications*, **137**, 587–92.

Davis, P. D., Nixon, J. S., Wilkinson, S. E., and Russell, M. G. N. (1988). Inhibition of phospholipase A_2 by some long chain alkylamines. *Biochemical Society Transactions*, **16**, 816–17.

Deems, R. A., Lombardo, D., Morgan, B. P., Mihelich, E. D., and Dennis, E. A. (1987). The inhibition of phospholipase A_2 by manoalide and manoalide analogues. *Biochimica et Biophysica Acta*, **917**, 258–68.

de Haas, G. H., Dijkman, R., van Oortt, M. G., and Verger, R. (1990a). Competitive inhibition of lipolytic enzymes. III. Some acylamino analogues of phospholipids are potent competitive inhibitors of porcine pancreatic phospholipase A_2 *Biochimica et Biophysica Acta*, **1043**, 75–82.

de Haas, G. H., Dijkman, R., Ransac, S., and Verger, R. (1990b). Competitive inhibition of lipolytic enzymes. IV. Structural details of acylamino phospholipid analogues important for the potent inhibitory effects on pancreatic phospholipase A_2. *Biochimica et Biophysica Acta*, **1046**, 249–57.

Dennis, E. A. (1987). Phospholipase A_2 mechanism inhibition and role in arachidonic acid release. *Drug Development Research*, **10**, 205–20.

Dennis, E. A., Rhee, S. G., Billah, M. M., and Hannun, Y. A. (1991). Role of phospholipases in generating lipid 2nd messengers in signal transduction. *FASEB Journal*, **5**, 2068–77.

Diez, E. and Mong, S. (1990). Purification of a phospholipase A$_2$ from human monocytic leukemic U937 cells. *Journal of Biological Chemistry*, **265**, 14654–61.

Dijkstra, B. W., Drenth, J., and Kalk, K. H. (1981a). Active site and catalytic mechanism of phospholipase A$_2$. *Nature, London*, **289**, 604–6.

Dijkstra, B. W., Kalk, K. H., Hol, W. G. J., and Drenth, J. (1981b). Structure of bovine pancreatic phospholipase A$_2$ at 1.7 Å resolution. *Journal of Molecular Biology*, **147**, 97–123.

Dijkstra, B. W., Renetseder, R., Kalk, K. H., Hol, W. G. J., and Drenth, J. (1983). Structure of porcine pancreatic phospholipase A$_2$ at 2.6 Å and comparison with bovine phospholipase A$_2$. *Journal of Molecular Biology*, **168**, 163–79.

Douglas, C. E., Chan, A. C., and Choy, P. C. (1986). Vitamin E inhibits platelet phospholipase A$_2$. *Biochimica et Biophysica Acta*, **876**, 639–45.

Eckardt, R. O. and Weston, J. F. (1988). Beneficial effects of the peptidoleukotriene receptor antagonist SK&F104353 on the responses to experimental endotoxemia in the conscious rat. *Circulatory Shock*, **25**, 21–31.

Fiedler-Nagy, C., Wiltreich, B. H., Georgiadis, A., Hope, W. C., Welton, A. F., and Coffey, J. W. (1987). Comparative study of natural and synthetic retinoids as inhibitors of arachidonic acid release and metabolism in rat peritoneal macrophages. *Dermatologica*, **175** (Suppl. 1), 81–92.

Foster, K. A., Buckle, D. R., Crescenzi, K. L., Fenwick, A. E., and Taylor, J. E. (1987). Arachidonic acid analogues as inhibitors of phospholipase A$_2$ activity. *Biochemical Society Transactions*, **15**, 418–19.

Fredenhagen, A., Fendrich, G., Marki, F., Marki, W., Gruner, J., Raschdorf, F., and Peter, H. H. (1990). Duramycin-B and duramycin-C, two new lanthionine containing antibiotics as inhibitors of phospholipase A$_2$-structural revision of duramycin and cinnamycin. *Journal of Antibiotics*, **43**, 1403–12.

Gelb, M. H. (1986). Fluoro ketone phospholipid analogues: new inhibitors of phospholipase A$_2$. *Journal of the American Chemical Society*, **108**, 3146–7.

Gialih, L., Noel, J., Loffredo, W., Stable, H. Z., and Tsai, M.-D. (1988). Use of short-chain cyclopentano-phosphatidylcholines to probe the mode of activation of phospholipase A$_2$ from bovine pancreas and bee venom. *Journal of Biological Chemistry*, **263**, 13208–14.

Gronich, J. H., Bonventre, J. V., and Nemenoff, R. A. (1990). Purification of a high-molecular-mass form of phospholipase A$_2$ from rat kidney activated at physiological calcium concentrations. *Biochemical Journal*, **271**, 37–43.

Haupt, M. T., Jastremski, M. S., Clemmer, T. P., Metz, C. A., Brown, B., and Goris, G. B. (1991). Effect of ibuprofen in patients with severe sepsis: a randomized, double-blind, multicenter study. *Critical Care Medicine*, **19**, 1339–47.

Heinrikson, R. L., Krueger, E. T., and Keim, P. S. (1977). Amino acid sequence of phospholipase A$_2$ from the venom of *Crotalus adamanteus*. A new classification of phospholipase A$_2$ based upon structural determinants. *Journal of Biological Chemistry*, **252**, 4913–21.

Hope, W. C., Patel, B. J., Fiedler-Nagy, C., and Wittreieh, B. H. (1990). Retinoids inhibit phospholipase A$_2$ in human synovial fluid and arachidonic acid release from rat peritoneal macrophages. *Inflammation*, **14**, 543–59.

Hutton, I. (1991). Pharmaprojects, Therapeutic Categories Main Volume, Vol. 12, p. a1239. PJB Publications Ltd. Richmond, Surrey.

Jacobs, R. S., Culver, P., Langdon, R., O'Brien, T., and White, S. (1985). Some pharmacological observations on marine natural products. *Tetrahedron*, **41**, 981–4.

Jacobson, P. B., Marshall, L. A., Sung, A., and Jacobs, R. S. (1990). Inactivation of human synovial fluid phospholipase A$_2$ by the marine natural product, manoalide. *Biochemical Pharmacology*, **39**, 1557–64.

Kanda, A., Ono, T., Yoshida, N., Tojo, H., and Okamoto, M. (1989). The primary structure of a membrane-associated phospholipase A$_2$ from human spleen. *Biochemical and Biophysical Research Communications*, **183**, 42–8.

Kernan, M. R. and Faulker, D. J. (1988). Sesterterpene sulfates from a sponge of the family *Halichondriidae*. *Journal of Organic Chemistry*, **53**, 4574–8.

Kohler, T., Friedrich, G., and Nuhn, P. (1991). Phospholipase-A$_2$ inhibition by alkylbenzoylacrylic acids. *Agents and Actions*, **32**, 70–2.

Kramer, R. M., Hession, C., Johansen, B., Hayes, G., McGray, P., Chow, E. P., *et al.* (1989). Structure and properties of a human non-pancreatic phospholipase A$_2$. *Journal of Biological Chemistry*, **264**, 5768–75.

Krause, H., Dieter, P., Schulze-Specking, A., Ballhorn, A., and Decker, K. (1991). Ca^{2+}-induced reversible translocation of phospholipase A$_2$ between the cytosol and the membrane fraction of rat liver macrophages. *European Journal of Biochemistry*, **199**, 355–9.

Kuchler, K., Gmachl, M., Sippl, M. J., and Kreil, G. (1989). Analysis of the cDNA for phospholipase A$_2$ from honeybee venom glands. *European Journal of Biochemistry*, **184**, 249–54.

Lai, C.-Y. and Wada, K. (1988). Phospholipase A$_2$ from human synovial fluid: purification and structural homology to the placental enzyme. *Biochemical and Biophysical Research Communications*, **157**, 488–93.

Langton, S. R. (1990). Phospholipase A$_2$: its measurement and implications in disease. *Australian Journal of Medical Laboratory Science*, **11**, 78–86.

Lanni, C. and Becker, E. L. (1985). Inhibition of neutrophil phospholipase A$_2$ by *p*-bromophenacyl bromide, nordihydroguaiaretic acid, 5,8,11,14-eicosatetrayenoic acid and quercetin. *International Archives of Allergy and Applied Immunology*, **76**, 214–17.

Leslie, C. C. (1991). Kinetic properties of a high molecular mass arachidonoyl-hydrolyzing phospholipase-A$_2$ that exhibits lysophospholipase activity. *Journal of Biological Chemistry*, **266**, 11366–71.

Lister, M. D. and Hancock, A. J. (1988). Cyclopentanoid analogs of phosphatidylcholine: susceptibility to phospholipase A$_2$. *Journal of Lipid Research*, **29**, 1297–1308.

Lombardo, D. and Dennis, E. A. (1985). Cobra venom phospholipase A$_2$ inhibition by manoalide. *Journal of Biological Chemistry*, **260**, 7234–40.

Magolda, R. L. and Galbraith, W. (1989). Design and synthesis of conformationally restricted phospholipids as phospholipase A$_2$ inhibitors. *Journal of Cellular Biochemistry*, **40**, 371–86.

Marshall, L. A. and Chang, J. Y. (1990). Pharmacological control of phospholipase A$_2$ activity *in vitro* and *in vivo*. In *Phospholipase A$_2$* (ed. P. Y.-K. Wong), pp. 169–82. Plenum Press, New York.

Mayer, A. M. S., Glaser, K. B., and Jacobs, R. S. (1988). Regulation of eicosanoid biosynthesis *in vitro* and *in vivo* by the marine natural product manoalide:

a potent inactivator of venom phospholipases. *Journal of Pharmacology and Experimental Therapeutics*, **244**, 871–8.

Mihelich, E. D., Morgan, B. P., Ho, P. P. K., Walters, C. P., and Bertsch, B. A. (1988). Inhibition of 5-lipoxygenase and phospholipase A$_2$ by manoalide analogues. *Annals of the New York Academy of Sciences*, **524**, 445–7.

Miller, D. K., Gillard, J. W., Vickers, P. J., Sadowski, S., Leveille, C., Mancini, J. A., *et al.* (1990). Identification and isolation of a membrane protein necessary for leukotriene production. *Nature, London*, **343**, 278–81.

Mobilio, D. and Marshall, L. A. (1989). Inhibitors of phospholipase A$_2$ and their assessment *in vitro*. In *Annual reports in medicinal chemistry*, Vol. 24 (ed. R. C. Allen), pp. 157–66. Academic Press, San Diego, CA.

Nevalainen, T. J., Aho, A. J., Eskola, J. U., and Suonpaa, A. K. (1983). Immuno-histochemical localization of phospholipase A$_2$ in human pancreas in acute and chronic pancreatitis. *Acta Pathologica et Microbiologica Scandinavica A*, **91**, 97–102.

Nevalainen, T. J., Eskola, J. U., Aho, A. J., Havia, V. T., Lovgren, T. N.-E., and Nanto, V. (1985). Immunoreactive phospholipase A$_2$ in serum in acute pancreatitis and pancreatic cancer. *Clinical Chemistry*, **31**, 1116–20.

Oda, M., Ino, Y., Nakamura, K., Kuramoto, S., Shimamura, K., Iwaki, M., and Fujii, S. (1990). Pharmacological studies on 6-amidino-2-naphthy[4-(4,5-dihydro-1*H*-imidazoyl-2-yl)amino] benzoate dimethane sulfonate (FUT-187). I: Inhibitory activities on various kinds of enzymes *in vitro* and anticomplement activity *in vivo*. *Japanese Journal of Pharmacology*, **52**, 23–4.

Prasad, M. R., Popescu, L. N., Moraru, I. I., Liu, X., Maity, S., Engelman, R. M., and Das, D. K. (1991). Role of phospholipases-A$_2$ and phospholipase-C in myocardial ischemic reperfusion injury. *American Journal of Physiology*, **260**, H877–83.

Pruzanski, W. and Vadas, P. (1991). Phospholipase-A$_2$—a mediator between proximal and distal effectors of inflammation. *Immunology Today*, **12**, 143–6.

Pruzanski, W., Vadas, P., Stefanski, E., and Urowitz, M. B. (1985). Phospholipase A$_2$ activity in sera and synovial fluids in rheumatoid arthritis and osteoarthritis. Its possible role as a proinflammatory enzyme. *Journal of Rheumatology*, **12**, 211–16.

Pruzanski, W., Keystone, E. C., Sternby, B., Bombardier, C., Snow, K. M., and Vadas, P. (1988). Serum phospholipase A$_2$ correlates with disease activity in rheumatoid arthritis. *Journal of Rheumatology*, **15**, 1351–5.

Pruzanski, W., Bogoch, E., Stefanski, E., Wloch, M., and Vadas, P. (1991a). Enzymatic activity and distribution of phospholipase-A$_2$ in human cartilage. *Life Sciences*, **48**, 2457–62.

Pruzanski, W., Saito, S., Stefanski, E., and Vadas, P. (1991b). Comparison of group-I and group-II soluble phospholipases-A$_2$ activities on phagocytic functions of human polymorphonuclear and mononuclear phagocytes. *Inflammation*, **15**, 127–35.

Rackow, E. C. and Astiz, M. E. (1991). Pathophysiology and treatment of septic shock. *Journal of the American Medical Association*, **266**, 548–54.

Rehfeldt, W., Hass, R., and Goppeltstruebe, M. (1991). Characterization of phospholipase-A$_2$ in monocytic cell lines—functional and biochemical aspects of membrane association. *Biochemical Journal*, **276**, 631–6.

Renetseder, R., Dijkstra, B. W., Huizinga, K., Kalk, K. H., and Drenth, J.

(1988). Crystal structure of bovine pancreatic phospholipase A_2 covalently inhibited by p-bromophenacylbromide. *Journal of Molecular Biology*, **200**, 181–8.

Reynolds, L. J., Morgan, B. P., Hite, G. A., Mihelich, E. D., and Dennis, E. A. (1988). Phospholipase A_2 inhibition and modification by manoalogue. *Journal of the American Chemical Society*, **110**, 5172–7.

Ripka, W. C., Sipio, W. J., and Blaney, J. M. (1987). Molecular modeling and drug design: strategies in the design and synthesis of phospholipase A_2 inhibitors. *Lectures in Heterocyclic Chemistry*, **9**, 95–104.

Schmidt, H. and Creutzfeld, W. (1969). The possible role of phospholipase A in the pathogenesis of acute pancreatitis. *Scandinavian Journal of Gastroenterology*, **4**, 39–48.

Schroder, T., Kivilaakso, E., Kinnunen, P. K. J., and Lempinen, M. (1980). Serum phospholipase A_2 in human acute pancreatitis. *Scandinavian Journal of Gastroenterology*, **15**, 633–6.

Scott, D. L., Otwinowski, M. H., Gelb, M. H., and Sigler, P. B. (1990a). Crystal structure of bee-venom phospholipase-A_2 in a complex with a transition-state analogue. *Science*, **250**, 1563–6.

Scott, D. L., White, S. P., Otwinowski, Z., Yuan, W., Gelb, M. H., and Sigler, P. B. (1990b). Interfacial catalysis: the mechanism of phospholipase A_2. *Science*, **250**, 1541–6.

Scott, D. L., Otwinowski, Z., Gelb, M. H., and Sigler, P. B. (1991). Crystal structure of bee-venom phospholipase A_2 correction. *Science*, **252**, 764.

Seeger, W. (1987). Clinical features and pathophysiology of lung failure in shock. *Journal of Clinical Chemistry and Clinical Biochemistry*, **25**, 209–11.

Seilhamer, J. J., Plant, S., Pruzanski, W., Schilling, J., Stefanski, E., Vadas, P., and Johnson, L. K. (1989a). Multiple forms of phospholipase A_2 in arthritic synovial fluid. *Journal of Biochemistry*, **106**, 38–42.

Seilhamer, J. J., Pruzanski, W., Vadas, P., Plant, S., Miller, J. A., Kloss, J., and Johnson, L. K. (1989b). Cloning and recombinant expression of phospholipase A_2 present in rheumatoid arthritic synovial fluid. *Journal of Biological Chemistry*, **264**, 5335–8.

Shipolini, K. A., Callewaert, G. L., Cottrell, R. C., and Vernon, C. A. (1974). The amino acid sequence and carbohydrate content of phospholipase A_2 from bee venom. *European Journal of Biochemistry*, **48**, 465–76.

Silverman, E., Pruzanski, W., Laxer, R., Albin-Cook, K., Stepanovic, E., and Vadas, P. (1987). Correlation of phospholipase A_2 level and disease activity in juvenile rheumatoid arthritis. *Arthritis and Rheumatism*, **30**, S127.

Stefanski, E., Pruzanski, W., Sternby, B., and Vadas, P. (1986). Purification of a soluble phospholipase A_2 from synovial fluid in rheumatoid arthritis. *Journal of Biochemistry*, **100**, 1297–1303.

Takayama, K., Kudo, I., Kim, D. K., Nagata, K., Nozawa, Y., and Inoue, K. (1991). Purification and characterization of human platelet phospholipase-A_2 which preferentially hydrolyzes an arachidonoyl residue. *Federation of European Biochemical Societies Letters*, **282**, 326–30.

Taylor, H. G., Dawes, P. T., Ilchyshyn, A., Shadforth, M. F., Ilderton, E., and Yardley, H. J. (1991). Raised epidermal phospholipase A_2 activity in rheumatoid arthritis. *Clinical and Experimental Rheumatology*, **9**, 275–7.

Thunnissen, M. M. G. M., Eiso, A. B., Kalk, K. H., Drenth, J., Dijkstra, B. W.,

Kuipers, O. P., *et al.* (1990). X-ray structure of phospholipase A$_2$ complexed with a substrate-derived inhibitor. *Nature, London*, **347**, 689–91.

Vadas, P., Pruzanski, W., Kim, J., and Fornasier, V. (1986). The proinflammatory effect of intra-articular injection of soluble human and venom phospholipase A$_2$. *American Journal of Pathology*, **134**, 807–11.

Vadas, P., Pruzanski, W., Stefanski, E., Sternby, B., Mustard, R., Bohnen, J., *et al.* (1988). Pathogenesis of hypotension in septic shock: correlation of circulating phospholipase A$_2$ levels with circulatory shock. *Critical Care Medicine*, **16**, 1–7.

Vainio, P., Thuren, T., Wichman, K., Luukkainen, T., and Kinnunen, P. K. J. (1985). Hydrolysis of phospholipid monolayers by human spermatozoa. Inhibition by male contraceptive gossypol. *Biochimica et Biophysica Acta*, **814**, 405–8.

Van Den Bosch, H., Aarsman, A. J., Van Schaik, R. H. N., Schalkwijk, C. G., Neijs, F. W., and Sturk, A. (1990). Structural and enzymological properties of cellular phospholipases A$_2$. *Biochemical Society Transactions*, **18**, 781–5.

Verheij, H. M., Volwerk, J. J., Jansen, E. H. J. M., Puyk, W. C., Dijkstra, B. W., Drenth, J., and de Haas, G. H. (1980). Methylation of histidine-48 in pancreatic phospholipase A$_2$. Role of histidine and calcium ion in the catalytic mechanism. *Biochemistry*, **19**, 743–50.

Verheij, H. M., Slotboom, A. J., and de Haas, G. H. (1981). Structure and function of phospholipase A$_2$. *Reviews of Physiology and Biochemical Pharmacology*, **91**, 92–203.

Verheij, H. M., Westerman, J., Sternby, B., and de Haas, G. H. (1983). The complete primary structure of phospholipase A$_2$ from human pancreas. *Biochimica et Biophysica Acta*, **747**, 93–9.

Vishwanath, B. S. and Gowda, T. V. (1987). Interaction of aristolochic acid with *Vipera russelli* phospholipase A$_2$: its effect on enzymatic and pathological activities. *Toxicon*, **25**, 929–37.

Vishwanath, B. S., Kini, R. M., and Gowda, T. V. (1987a). Characterization of three edema-inducing phospholipase A$_2$ enzymes from Habu (*Trimeresurus flavoviridis*) venom and their interaction with the alkaloid aristolochic acid. *Toxicon*, **25**, 501–15.

Vishwanath, B. S., Rao, A. G. A., and Gowda, T. V. (1987b). Interaction of phospholipase A$_2$ from *Vipera russelli* venom with aristolochic acid: a circular dichroism study. *Toxicon*, **25**, 939–46.

Waite, M. (1987). *The phospolipases: handbook of lipid research*, Vol. 5. (ed. D. J. Hanahan), Plenum Press, New York.

Washburn, W. and Dennis, E. (1990a). Novel general approach for the assay and inhibition of hydrolytic enzymes utilizing suicide-inhibitory bifunctionally linked substrates (SIBLINKS)—exemplified by a phospholipase A-2 assay. *Journal of the American Chemical Society*, **112**, 2040–1.

Washburn, W. and Dennis, E. (1990b). Suicide-inhibitory bifunctionally linked substrates (SIBLINKS) as phospholipase A$_2$ inhibitors. **112**, 2042–3.

Washburn, W. N. and Dennis, E. A. (1991). Suicide-inhibitory bifunctionally linked substrates (SIBLINKS) as phospholipase-A$_2$ inhibitors—mechanistic implications. *Journal of Biological Chemistry*, **266**, 5042–8.

White, S. P., Scott, D. L., Otwinowski, Z., Gelb, M. H., and Sigler, P. B. (1990). Crystal structure of cobra-venom phospholipase-A$_2$ in a complex with a transition-state analogue. *Science*, **250**, 1560–3.

Wilkerson, W. W. (1990). Anti-inflammatory phospholipase A_2 inhibitors. *Drugs of the Future*, **15**, 139–48.

Yuan, W., Berman, R. J., and Gelb, M. H. (1987). Synthesis and evaluation of phospholipid analogues as inhibitors of cobra venom phospholipase A_2. *Journal of the American Chemical Society*, **109**, 8071–81.

Yuan, W. and Gelb, M. H. (1988). Phosphonate-containing phospholipid analogues as tight-binding inhibitors of phospholipase A_2. *Journal of the American Chemical Society*, **110**, 2665–6.

Yuan, W., Quinn, D. M., Sigler, P. B., and Gelb, M. H. (1990). Kinetic and inhibition studies of phospholipase A_2 with short-chain substrates and inhibitors. *Biochemistry*, **29**, 6082–94.

Zieve, L. and Vogel, W. C. (1961). Measurement of lecithinase A in serum and other fluids. *Journal of Laboratory and Clinical Medicine*, **57**, 586–99.

14

Inhibitors of gastric H$^+$,K$^+$-ATPase

Björn Wallmark, David Keeling, and Per Lindberg

14.1 Rationale for the use of H$^+$,K$^+$-ATPase inhibitors

Acid-related diseases include reflux oesophagitis, duodenal ulcer, gastric ulcer, and the Zollinger–Ellison syndrome. These disorders are treated by a reduction of gastric acid secretion which can be achieved by surgery, antacids, or pharmacological agents. Several classes of antisecretory agent have been developed and introduced into clinical use. These include anticholinergic compounds, such as pirenzipine, and the histamine H$_2$-receptor antagonists (H$_2$RAs), such as cimetidine (Black *et al.* 1972). The introduction of cimetidine was followed later by other H$_2$RAs, such as ranitidine and famotidine. In addition, stable prostaglandin analogues with antisecretory properties have been developed. However, these agents have been found to possess relatively weak ulcer healing properties (Nicholson 1985).

Recently, inhibitors of gastric H$^+$,K$^+$-ATPase, the 'acid pump' of the stomach, have been introduced in therapy. The most documented compound of this class is omeprazole, which has been investigated in the acid-related disorders mentioned above. The accumulated clinical data show that omeprazole exhibits superior healing rates and better symptom relief in all these disorders compared with previously available therapy (McTavish *et al.* 1991).

Thus H^+,K^+-ATPase is an important target enzyme for antisecretory drugs. This survey will focus on the chemistry, mechanism of action, and pharmacology of drugs which inhibit this enzyme.

14.2 Gastric H^+,K^+-ATPase

Secretion of gastric acid is physiologically stimulated by food. Three agents are fundamentally important in this process: histamine which is locally released in the gastric mucosa, acetylcholine which is released from the cholinergic nerve fibres innervating the gastric epithelium, and gastrin which is released into the blood from the lower part of the stomach, the antrum (Fig. 14.1).

H^+,K^+-ATPase, the 'acid pump', is located in the parietal cells of the stomach. As a result of its activity, the pH of the stomach falls

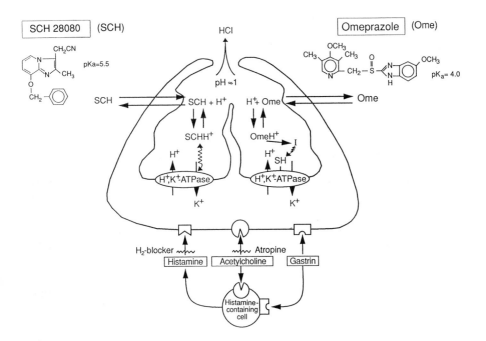

Fig. 14.1 The acid-secreting parietal cell. The pathways for receptor-mediated stimulation of acid secretion are shown together with the way in which covalent (omeprazole) and non-covalent (SCH 28080) inhibitors of acid secretion interact with H^+,K^+-ATPase in the acid-secreting membrane.

below 1, which means that the enzyme is capable of generating a proton gradient in excess of a millionfold. It is found predominantly in parietal cells (Smolka *et al.* 1983; Canfield *et al.* 1990), although some reports indicate that related enzymes may occur in the kidney and in the colon (Takeguchi *et al.* 1990; Wingo *et al.* 1990).

Gastric H$^+$, K$^+$-ATPase was first discovered in bullfrog gastric mucosa (Ganser and Forte 1973) and was later demonstrated in several species, including man (Saccomani *et al.* 1979). Its H$^+$ transport ability was demonstrated in membrane vesicles isolated from gastric mucosa and was shown to depend upon the presence of ATP and K$^+$ ions (Lee *et al.* 1974). A direct correlation was established between gastric H$^+$, K$^+$-ATPase activity and acid secretion in the whole animal, confirming the role of this enzyme as the gastric 'acid pump' (Wallmark *et al.* 1985).

The H$^+$, K$^+$-ATPase belongs to a family called P-type ATPases. This class includes Na$^+$, K$^+$-ATPase and Ca^{2+}-ATPase. These cation transport enzymes are all transmembrane proteins that utilize ATP as substrate and form an acid stable phosphorylenzyme intermediate during the catalytic cycle (Pedersen and Carafoli 1987). Like the closely related Na$^+$, K$^+$-ATPase, H$^+$, K$^+$-ATPase consists of a catalytic α-subunit and a smaller glycosylated β-subunit of unknown function (Shull and Lingrel 1986; Canfield *et al.* 1990). Despite the general similarities between enzymes of this class, they all differ in their specificities towards transported ions.

H$^+$, K$^+$-ATPase catalyses the electroneutral counter-transport of H$^+$ and K$^+$ ions (Sachs *et al.* 1976). The stoichiometry for transport of H$^+$ ions has been reported to be either one or two per ATP molecule (Rabon *et al.* 1982; Skrabanja *et al.* 1987; Norberg and Mårdh 1990). However, under physiological conditions, the H$^+$, K$^+$-ATPase cannot transport more than one H$^+$ ion per ATP molecule hydrolysed when working against the large H$^+$ gradient observed in the stomach.

Gastric H$^+$, K$^+$-ATPase offers a unique target for antisecretory drugs for the following reasons:

(1) it is primarily located in the parietal cell, a fact which permits a selective pharmacological action;

(2) it generates a very low extracellular pH, which can be used for drug targeting (see below);

(3) it is the final step in the physiological process leading to formation of gastric acid, and thus blockade of the enzyme will inhibit acid secretion irrespective of the stimulus.

14.3   Covalent inhibitors of H$^+$, K$^+$-ATPase

The development of covalent inhibitors of H$^+$, K$^+$-ATPase began as early as 1972 (Sjöstrand *et al.* 1978; Brändström *et al.* 1985; Lindberg *et al.*

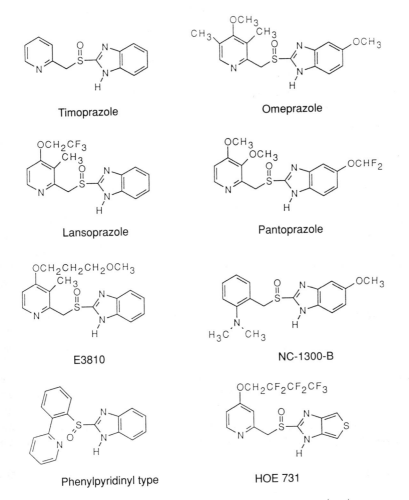

Fig. 14.2 The structures of selected covalent inhibitors of H^+, K^+-ATPase.

1986, 1990). The lead structure for this series of compounds was pyridinylthioacetamide (CMN 131) which had antiviral properties but, as a side-effect was observed to inhibit acid secretion. This screening work led to the discovery of compound H83/69, timoprazole, which was the parent compound of the group of pyridinmethylsulphinylbenzimidazoles (Fig. 14.2). In 1977, picoprazole was prepared and was found effectively to counteract acid secretion in animals and in man. At this stage, it also became clear that picoprazole acted by inhibiting H^+, K^+-ATPase (Fellenius *et al.* 1981, 1982; Wallmark *et al.* 1983b). In 1979, omeprazole was synthesized and was found to be about 10 times more potent than picoprazole

(Larsson *et al.* 1983; Lind *et al.* 1983; Wallmark *et al.* 1983a; Konturek *et al.* 1984). Omeprazole is now approved for use in acid-related disorders in most countries.

The covalent H^+,K^+-ATPase inhibitors have attracted much attention and several related drugs are now in various stages of development, most notably lansoprazole and pantoprazole (Fig. 14.2). However, since the best documented and most advanced drug in this class is omeprazole, in the remainder of this section we shall focus principally on this compound.

14.3.1   Mechanism of action

It is now well established that omeprazole and related compounds inhibit acid secretion by blockade of H^+,K^+-ATPase. An early series of experiments involving autoradiography with ^{3}H-omeprazole (Helander *et al.* 1985) showed that animal parietal cell membranes containing H^+,K^+-ATPase were selectively labelled by administration of ^{3}H-omeprazole. It was concluded from these studies that the drug selectively labels parietal cell membranes but not that H^+,K^+-ATPase is the target. This was subsequently shown in a study in rabbits where labelled H^+,K^+-ATPase was purified from animals treated with ^{3}H-omeprazole. No other protein in the secretory portion of the stomach was found to be labelled (Fryklund *et al.* 1988a). The linkage between acid secretion and activity of H^+,K^+-ATPase has also been studied (Im *et al.* 1985a; Wallmark *et al.* 1985). A linear correlation was found between inhibition of maximally stimulated acid secretion and H^+,K^+-ATPase activity, demonstrating directly that the degree of inhibition of H^+,K^+-ATPase is related to the rate of acid secretion under *in vivo* conditions.

Omeprazole acts as a prodrug for an active compound which is generated by acid-catalysed conversion of omeprazole, and the active compound (the sulphenamide derivative) reacts with extracellular cysteine residues on H^+,K^+-ATPase. *In vivo*, it was found that inhibition of acid secretion by other means prior to administration of omeprazole markedly reduces its capacity to inhibit H^+,K^+-ATPase (Im *et al.* 1985b; de Graef and Woussen-Colle 1986b; Fryklund *et al.* 1988b). In isolated gastric glands, it was shown that reduction of intraglandular acid prevents the chemical conversion of omeprazole (Wallmark *et al.* 1984). In vesicles containing H^+,K^+-ATPase it was demonstrated that the inhibitory effect depends on intravesicular acid (Keeling *et al.* 1987; Lorentzon *et al.* 1987). All these studies in different biological preparations clearly indicated that omeprazole is converted in acid to an active compound.

The stoichiometry for binding of inhibitor to H^+,K^+-ATPase has been investigated. In order to do this, the number of functional H^+,K^+-ATPase units present has been assessed by measuring the steady state level of the phosphoenzyme intermediate of H^+,K^+-ATPase. Since the rate of phosphorylation is much faster than the rate of dephosphorylation (Wallmark *et al.* 1980) it is assumed that this steady state level represents the true number of phosphorylation sites and hence the number of functional α-subunits present. Binding studies involving either *in vivo* or *in vitro* inhibited H⁺,K⁺-ATPase revealed that 2 moles of inhibitor are bound per mole of functional phosphorylation site (Keeling *et al.* 1987; Lorentzon *et al.* 1987; Fryklund *et al.* 1988a). The covalent enzyme–inhibitor complex is stable and is eliminated at a slow rate.

14.3.2   Chemical reactions in acid leading to inhibition

Several studies of the acid degradation of omeprazole have been performed in order to obtain mechanistic information at a molecular level (Im *et al.* 1985b; Rackur *et al.* 1985; Figala *et al.* 1986; Lindberg *et al.* 1986, 1990; Senn-Bilfinger *et al.* 1987; Sturm *et al.* 1987; Brändström *et al.* 1989). Investigation of the acid decomposition of omeprazole (**1**) has resulted in the isolation of an intermediate, the sulphenamide (**2**), which effectively inhibits the H⁺,K⁺-ATPase preparation *in vitro* and reacts rapidly with mercaptans, e.g. β-mercaptoethanol, to form the disulphide (**3**) (Fig. 14.3). This reaction with mercaptans suggests that a similar process could occur on H⁺,K⁺-ATPase, leading to a reaction with cysteine residues as outlined above. Thus in the acidic canaliculus of the parietal cell omeprazole (**1**) is converted ($t_{1/2} = 2$ min) into the sulphenamide **2** by an acid-catalysed Smiles-type rearrangement. This compound, which is the active inhibitor, reacts rapidly with luminally accessible cysteines of H⁺,K⁺-ATPase to form disulphide inhibitor complex **4**.

In neutral conditions omeprazole, which is a lipid-permeable weak base ($pK_a = 4$), exists predominantly in its neutral base form in which it is able to cross cell membranes freely. However, because of the low pH (< 1) of the canaliculus of the parietal cell, it becomes protonated and

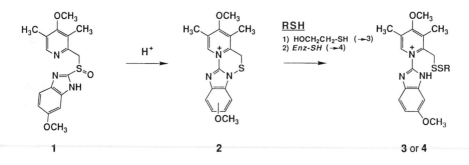

Fig. 14.3 The chemical reactions of omeprazole leading to inhibition of H⁺,K⁺-ATPase.

concentrated in these compartments. Furthermore, the active sulphen-amide formed is a permanent cation and therefore cannot penetrate back through the secretory membrane. Consistent with this, the isolated sul-phenamide can immediately inhibit purified H$^+$,K$^+$-ATPase (Wallmark *et al.* 1984), but is inactive when tested in the gastric gland model (Lindberg *et al.* 1990) probably because of the difficulty that this permanent cation encounters in crossing the cell membrane (or decomposing in the medium).

The disulphide enzyme–inhibitor complex is stable unless mercaptan is present. This stable complex is believed to be the reason for the long duration of the antisecretory action of omeprazole. Regeneration of active enzyme following exposure to β-mercaptoethanol has been demonstrated *in vitro* (Wallmark *et al.* 1984; Lorentzon *et al.* 1987; Fryklund *et al.* 1988a). *In vivo*, the recovery of acid secretion after inhibition could be due to chemical displacement by endogenous mercaptans or to resynthesis of H$^+$,K$^+$-ATPase subunits. Studies in the rat have favoured the latter alternative (Im *et al.* 1985a), whereas studies with other agents of the pyridinmethylsulphinylbenzimidazole class have indicated that endogenous mercaptans may play an important role in the recovery of acid secretion (Fujisaki *et al.* 1991). Since omeprazole and its analogues are acid acti-vated, it is possible that these compounds are also activated in other weakly acidic compartments in the body. Lysosomes are acidic com-partments, although they are not as strongly acid (pH 4.5) as the parietal cell canaliculus (pH < 1). However, omeprazole and pantoprazole have been shown to act selectively on H$^+$,K$^+$-ATPase of the parietal cell (Simon *et al.* 1990).

14.3.3   Structure–activity relationships

Since the sulphenamide (the active principle) formed is very reactive towards SH groups on H$^+$,K$^+$-ATPase, the degree of inhibition depends only on the amount of sulphenamide formed in the acid compartment of the parietal cell. Furthermore, the substituents on the sulphenamide, once formed, are of little importance. This means that once the sulphoxide has been taken up into the parietal cell canaculiculus, the substitution pattern is only important for the rate of conversion to the sulphenamide. Strong support for this view has been provided by *in vitro* testing of various omeprazole analogues in the isolated gastric gland model (Lindberg *et al.* 1987). In the *in vivo* situation, factors like absorption, distribution, and metabolism will also influence the potency of the compound.

The structural framework of omeprazole consists of three elements (the timoprazole template), the pyridine ring, the benzimidazole ring, and the chain between these two rings (Fig. 14.2). During the development of omeprazole, substitution of a variety of heterocyclic rings for the pyridine ring or the benzimidazole ring resulted in compounds with no antisecretory effect. However, a few compounds with ring systems closely related to benzimidazole showed weak activity. The only ring-connecting chains that gave *in vivo* biological effect were $-CH_2S-$, $-CH_2SO-$ and $-CH(CH_3)SO$. Moreover, the attachment points of the connecting chain were critical. Thus, CH_2SO must be attached by the CH_2 carbon in the 2-position of the pyridine ring and by the sulphur atom in the 2-position of the benzimidazole ring (Lindberg *et al.* 1987, 1990).

Substituents in the pyridine ring are of great importance for the biological effect. Thus the effect is enhanced with increasing pK_a of the pyridine ring. The 3,5-dimethyl-4-methoxy-substituted pyridine of omeprazole, with $pK_a = 4$, gives the most potent compound *in vivo* (when tested in the dog). The effect of substituents in the benzimidazole ring is less dramatic. Thus most of the compounds synthesized with various substituents in the benzimidazole ring, but with the same 3,5-dimethyl-4-methoxy-pyridine ring, have been found to be active (Brändström *et al.* 1985).

14.3.4 Pharmacology

The effects of omeprazole have been investigated in rat, dog, and man. In man, omeprazole was found to counteract basal and stimulated acid secretion with equal potency (Lind *et al.* 1983, 1986). The drug has also been shown to block 24 hour intragastric acidity more effectively than the histamine H_2RA ranitidine, the predominant difference being a more pronounced inhibition of daytime acidity (Lanzon-Miller *et al.* 1987). During continous treatment, either in animals or man, no escape from inhibition has been observed (Carlsson *et al.* 1986). In addition, in patients with excessive hypersecretion, i.e. in Zollinger–Ellison syndrome, secretion has been found to be controlled by a once daily dose regimen without the need for dose adjustment (Lloyd-Davies *et al.* 1988). Long duration of antisecretory effect is characteristic of the covalent H^+, K^+-ATPase blockers. The antisecretory effect of omeprazole and of related compounds persists after the decline in its plasma levels. In fact, there is no correlation between the plasma level of omeprazole and its inhibitory effect at a given time point. However, the inhibitory effect of a given dose is closely related to the area under the plasma concentration curve (AUC), i.e. to the amount of omeprazole that is available for inhibition of the H^+, K^+-ATPase (Larsson *et al.* 1983; Lind *et al.* 1983). In man and dog acid secretion returns to normal 4–5 days after cessation of treatment, whereas in rat the duration of the antisecretory effect is somewhat shorter. Following long-term treatment, the same duration of antisecretory effect has been found as for single dose administration (Carlsson *et al.* 1986).

14.3.5 Toxicology

One hurdle in the development of omeprazole emerged from long-term carcinogenic studies, where gastric carcinoids developed in the rat. These carcinoids consisted of enterochromaffin-like (ECL) cells, located exclusively in the corpus region of the stomach, and were observed in the late phase of the life-span of the rats involved (Ekman *et al.* 1985; Havu 1986). In a large series of studies, the occurrence of ECL cell carcinoids was shown not to be caused by omeprazole itself, but by the hypergastrinaemia associated with a pronounced suppression of gastric acid secretion during lifelong treatment. Evidence for this conclusion emerged from studies in which ECL cell carcinoids also developed after gastric acid secretion was reduced either surgically or by histamine H_2RAs (ranitidine, loxtidine, SKF 93479) (Poynter *et al.* 1985; Betton *et al.* 1988; Havu *et al.* 1990; Mattson *et al.* 1991). The mechanism for the development of ECL cell carcinoids in rat has been established.

The induced suppression of gastric acid results in secretion of the hormone gastrin, which is trophic for the corpus region of the stomach in general and for ECL cells in particular. When the hypergastrinaemia is maintained chronically, this leads to a proliferation of ECL cells and, after lifelong treatment, to ECL cell tumours in the rat. During continuous long-term treatment with omeprazole in man, using moderate to high doses for up to 5 years, there has been no development of dysplasia or neoplasia of endocrine cells. The only change observed was some increase in hyperplasia of endocrine cells (Creutzfeldt and Lambert 1991). However, this was correlated with an increase in the degree of gastritis in the corpus region of the stomach. A similar increase in gastritis and a corresponding and similar increase in hyperplasia of endocrine cells has been observed in patients with peptic ulcer disease who had never received any treatment with antisecretory drugs (Havu *et al.* 1991).

14.3.6   Classes of covalent inhibitors

About 40 pharmaceutical companies have now patented compounds in this area. Most of these have described sulphoxides which contain the timoprazole template. However, few compounds have reached the clinic. As well as omeprazole, other pyridinylmethylsulphinylbenzimidazoles known to be in development include lansoprazole (Nagaya *et al.* 1989), pantoprazole (Simon *et al.* 1990), and E-3810 (Morii *et al.* 1990) (Fig. 14.2). In addition to the pyridinmethylsulphinylbenzimidazoles, three other classes of inhibitor have been described—the aniline type, the thienimidazole type, and the phenylpyridyl type (Fig. 14.2).

In the aniline-type compounds, the pyridine ring of omeprazole has been substituted for an aniline, usually an alkylated aniline, as in NC 1 300-B (Okabe *et al.* 1988). In the thienoimidazole-type compounds, the benzimidazole part of omeprazole has been substituted, as in S 1924 (Herling *et al.* 1988b) and HOE-731 (Herling *et al.* 1988a). In phenylpyridyl-type compounds (Suschitzky and Wells 1990), a phenyl group has been inserted in the linking chain of omeprazole. These compounds appear to possess potent antisecretory properties, similar to those of omeprazole.

14.4 Non-covalent inhibitors of H^+,K^+-ATPase

The development of covalent long-acting inhibitors of gastric H^+,K^+-ATPase has made it possible to inhibit acid secretion for extended periods of time. As discussed above, the pharmacological effect of these compounds persists after they have been cleared from plasma and other body compartments. Although not yet available clinically, non-covalent inhibitors of this ion pump have also been identified which inhibit acid secretion as effectively as omeprazole, but for shorter periods of time. The rate of recovery of acid secretion in this case is most likely to be determined by the rate of clearance of the compound from plasma. Whilst H^+,K^+-ATPase inhibitors have been described from many sources, the discussion here will be restricted to those that have been shown to be non-covalent and reversible in nature. Many such compounds share common structural features, in that they are all heterocycles that are either protonatable or already exist in a cationic form. The imidazopyridines, e.g. SCH 28080 (Kaminski *et al.* 1985), the guanidinothiazoles (LaMattina *et al.* 1990), and analogues of 4-(arylamino)-quinolines, e.g. SKF 96067 (Munson and Reevis 1982; Brown *et al.* 1990), can be included in this group (Fig. 14.4). Similar compounds include aminopyridines (Hioki *et al.* 1990) and a number of organic amines such as nolinium bromide (Nandi *et al.* 1983, 1990; Im *et al.* 1984). By far the most studied of these compounds to date is the imidazopyridine SCH 28080. Much of the following discussion will centre on this compound.

14.4.1 Mechanism of action

In contrast with inhibitors of acid secretion that block receptors on the basolateral membrane of the parietal cell, inhibitors of H^+,K^+-ATPase are effective even when secretion is stimulated distal to the receptor. Thus SCH 28080 has been shown to inhibit acidification in intact rabbit gastric glands equipotently, whether stimulated by histamine or dibutyryl cAMP (Wallmark *et al.* 1987). A common property of this group of short-acting H^+,K^+-ATPase inhibitors is that inhibition is competitive with respect to the activating cation K^+ (Nandi *et al.* 1983; Beil *et al.* 1986; Brown *et al.* 1990; LaMattina *et al.* 1990). This has stimulated speculation that they interact at the extracytosolic, high affinity site for K^+. At present there is evidence both for and against this idea. In favour, most of these compounds have been shown to interact with the extracytosolic face of the enzyme (Nandi *et al.* 1983; Briving *et al.* 1988; Keeling *et al.* 1988; Brown *et al.* 1990). In addition, SCH 28080 has been shown to bind only

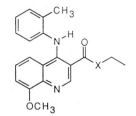

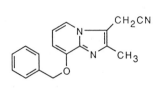

SCH 28080

Prototype quinoline (X=O)
SK&F 96067 (X=CH$_2$)

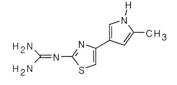

Guanidinothiazole

Fig. 14.4 The structures of selected non-covalent inhibitors of H$^+$, K$^+$-ATPase.

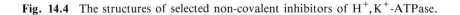

to the E$_2$ form of the enzyme, i.e. the form in which the K$^+$ ion binds with high affinity to the extracytosolic site of the pump (Keeling *et al.* 1989b; Mendlein and Sachs 1990). Accordingly, both SCH 28080 and the 4-(arylamino)quinoline SK&F 96067 appear to be predominantly active in their positively charged protonated forms (Keeling *et al.* 1988, 1991). Against the idea that the inhibitor binding site and the K$^+$-translocating site are one and the same is the finding that SK&F 96067 becomes a mixed type inhibitor relative to K$^+$ at high pH (Keeling *et al.* 1991). This implies that, under these conditions, inhibitor and K$^+$ can bind simultaneously to the enzyme and therefore that the binding sites cannot be the same.

SCH 28080 is a potent inhibitor of H$^+$, K$^+$-ATPase, with K_i in the range 20–50 nM at neutral pH (Beil *et al.* 1986; Keeling *et al.* 1988). The thermodynamics of binding have been studied using radiolabelled compound and indicate a slow rate of association between enzyme and inhibitor (Keeling *et al.* 1989b). Thus there is a significant energy barrier that must be overcome before binding can occur. The half-life for binding (at K_i concentrations) was approximately 30 seconds at room temperature and significantly longer on ice. This slow binding is unlikely to affect the action of the compound *in vivo*, but it could have implications for the design experiments *in vitro* (Keeling *et al.* 1988).

The stoichiometry of binding of imidazopyridines to H$^+$,K$^+$-ATPase has also been investigated. Direct binding studies have suggested a stoichiometry of two molecules of SCH 28080 per phosphorylation site (Keeling *et al.* 1989b). This has also been found for a photoaffinity analogue (mATIP) based upon SCH 28080 (Keeling *et al.* 1989a), and is in agreement with that found for the binding of omeprazole to H$^+$,K$^+$-ATPase. A further study using the fluorescent 4-aminopyridine analogue MDPQ gave a stoichiometry of 1.4 moles per phosphorylation site (Rabon *et al.* 1991). The reason for these differences in stoichiometry unclear at present.

Since the covalent inhibitor omeprazole also reacts with the extra-cytosolic face of H$^+$,K$^+$-ATPase, the relationship between the binding sites of these two classes of inhibitor is of interest. Covalent inhibition by omeprazole was reduced in the presence of SCH 28080, suggesting an interaction between these sites (Hersey *et al.* 1988). This effect could not be explained by SCH 28080 blocking acid formation, thereby preventing the activation of omeprazole.

H$^+$,K$^+$-ATPase is one of a family of cation pumps, of which the most closely related is Na$^+$,K$^+$-ATPase with a 62 per cent amino acid homology (Shull and Lingrel 1986). This enzyme also transports K$^+$ at a high affinity extracytosolic site. Nevertheless, SCH 28080 is a very weak inhibitor of Na$^+$,K$^+$-ATPase (Beil *et al.* 1986) and SK&F 96067 is more than 30-fold less potent on this enzyme (Keeling *et al.* 1991). There are significant differences in the amino acid sequences of the predicted first extracytosolic domains of these two ion pumps (Shull and Lingrel 1986) which may account for this selectivity of action.

14.4.2 Pharmacology

Like the covalent H$^+$,K$^+$-ATPase inhibitors such as omeprazole, SCH 28080 has been shown to inhibit gastric acid secretion irrespective of the stimulus used (Chiu *et al.* 1983; Long *et al.* 1983; Mårdh *et al.* 1988). Complete inhibition of acid output was achieved 1 hour after oral dosing of SCH 28080 (8 mg kg^{-1}) to dogs, although acid secretion recovered to 80 per cent of control after a further 3 hours (Long *et al.* 1983), demonstrating the reversible short-acting nature of this inhibitor.

In a clinical study in human volunteers, SCH 28080 inhibited both basal and pentagastrin-stimulated acid output in a dose-related manner. An 86 per cent reduction in acid output was observed 2–3 hours after an intragastric dose of 200 mg. Mean gastric pH during this time was pH 6.1 (Ene *et al.* 1982). Subsequent clinical development of this compound was suspended as a result of liver toxicity (Kaminski *et al.* 1987).

14.4.3   Structure–activity relationships

The K^+-competitive inhibitors of H^+, K^+-ATPase arise from a number of different heterocyclic systems (Fig. 14.4). To date, no single structure–activity relationship can account for all these systems. Whilst it is known, for example, that the imidazopyridine SCH 28080 and the 4-(arylamino)-quinoline SK&F 96067 cannot bind to the enzyme at the same time (Keeling *et al.* 1991), this does not necessarily mean that their binding sites are exactly superimposable and that they should have an equivalent structure–activity profile. However, certain characteristics do appear to be important for activity. In both heterocycles, methylation of the protonatable nitrogen atom to form a permanent cation does not destroy potency against H^+, K^+-ATPase when assayed in permeable vesicles. In contrast, activity is greatly reduced in ion-tight gastric vesicles, indicating that the neutral (unprotonated) form of these compounds is needed to cross the membrane and gain access to the extracytosolic face of the enzyme (Briving *et al.* 1988; Keeling *et al.* 1988; Brown *et al.* 1990). However, for optimal activity, protonation must occur. This has been demonstrated both by pH studies on the isolated enzyme, where the potencies of SCH 28080 (Keeling *et al.* 1988) and SK&F 96067 (Keeling *et al.* 1991) correlated with their degrees of protonation, and by the inactivity of an isosteric analogue of SCH 28080 whose low pK_a precluded significant protonation (Briving *et al.* 1988). Low pK_a has also been suggested as a reason for reduced potency of selected analogues of the 4-(arylamino)-quinolines (Brown *et al.* 1990).

In the imidazopyridine series, the substituents in the five-membered ring, particularly that in the 3-position have a very pronounced influence on the pharmacological effect of the compound (Kaminski *et al.* 1985). Thus, of at least 30 different 3-substituents tested, very few gave compounds with potency comparable with SCH 28080, which has a $3-CH_2CN$ substituent. Among the acceptable 3-substituents for high activity are CH_3 (but not C_2H_5) and CH_2OH. Strong electron-withdrawing groups, like CN and carbonyl-containing groups, or bulky groups like $C(CH_3)_2CN$ gave totally inactive compounds. The very detrimental effect of electron-withdrawing groups in the five-membered ring may come from their influence on the pK_a. An aromatic ring connected to the pyridine ring (preferentially in the 8-position) via a spacer arm is also of crucial importance for effect.

Structural modifications of 4-(arylamino)quinoline-3-carboxylic esters (Munson and Reevis 1982) have resulted in a large number of very active H^+, K^+-ATPase inhibitors, some of which have been reported in the literature (Brown *et al.* 1990). Exchanging the 3-carboxylic ester group of the prototype quinoline structure for a 3-butyryl group led to SK&F 96067, which was selected for further studies (Keeling *et al.* 1991).

An extensive structure–activity relationship investigation of 4-substituted guanidinothiazoles showed that (**1**) replacement of the thiazole unit is very detrimental for activity (2) pyrrolyl, phenyl, and indolyl groups can be used as the C4 substituent, (3) substituents on these rings gave no consistent trends, and (4) monoalkylation of the guanidine or alkylation of the thiazole at C5 often gave improved *in vitro* activity which, however, was not additive. Despite a hundredfold increase in *in vitro* activity over the initial lead compound, only a threefold increase in *in vivo* potency was observed (LaMattina *et al.* 1990).

14.5   Other inhibitors

The depside salvianolic acid has been reported to be an inhibitor of H^+, K^+-ATPase (Murakami *et al.* 1990). In contrast with the K^+-competitive inhibitors described above, this compound inhibits H^+, K^+-ATPase activity competitively with respect to ATP and non-competitively with respect to potassium. This compound is also effective *in vivo* as an inhibitor of gastric acid output in the pylorus-ligated rat.

14.6   Conclusion

The introduction of histamine H_2RAs made possible the pharmacological control of acid secretion, which has had a large impact on treatment of acid-related disorders. More recently, the discovery of selective inhibitors of gastric H^+, K^+-ATPase has led to the development of new therapeutic principles for acid-related disease. Thus blockade of this enzyme by omeprazole has led to more effective control of acid secretion compared with that obtained with histamine H_2RAs. This is also manifested in better therapeutic results.

In addition, research has provided mechanistically different inhibitors of H^+, K^+-ATPase, both covalent and reversible. The future role in therapy of the latter group of compounds awaits clinical investigation, whereas the covalent blockers, such as omeprazole, have already established their role in acid-related disorders.

References

Beil, W., Hackbarth, I., and Sewing, K.-Fr. (1986). Mechanism of gastric antisecretory effect of SCH 28080. *British Journal of Pharmacology*, **88**, 19–23.

Betton, G. R., Dormer, C. S., Wells, T., Pert, P., Price, C. A., and Buckley, P. (1988). Gastric ECL-cell hyperplasia and carcinoids in rodents following chronic administration of H2-antagonists SK&F 93479 and oxmetidine and omeprazole. *Toxicologic Pathology*, **16**, 288–98.

Black, J. W., Duncan, W. A. M., Durant, C. J., Ganellin, C. R., and Parsons, E. M. (1972). Definition and antagonism of histamine H2-receptors. *Nature, London*, **236**, 385–90.

Brändstrom, A., Lindberg, P., and Junggren, U. (1985). Structure activity relationships of substituted benzimidazoles. *Scandinavian Journal of Gastroenterology*, **108** (Suppl.), 15–22.

Brändström, A., Lindberg, P., Bergman, N.-A., Alminger, T., Ankner, K., Junggren, U., *et al.* (1989). Chemical reactions of omeprazole analogues I-VI (six articles). *Acta Chemica Scandinavica*, **43**, 536–611.

Briving, C., Andersson, B.-M., Nordberg, P., and Wallmark, B. (1988). Inhibition of gastric H⁺/K⁺-ATPase by substituted imidazol[1,2-a]pyridines. *Biochimica et Biophysica Acta*, **946**, 185–92.

Brown, T. H., Ife, J. R., Keeling, D. J., Laing, S. M., Leach, C. A., Parsons, M. E., *et al.* (1990). Reversible inhibitors of the gastric (H⁺/K⁺)-ATPase. 1. 1-aryl-4-methylpyrrolo[3,2-c]quinolines as conformationally restrained analogues of 4-(arylamino)quinolines. *Journal of Medicinal Chemistry*, **33**, 527–33.

Canfield, V. A., Okamoto, C. T., Chow, D., Dorfman, J., Gros, P., Forte, J. G., and Levenson, R. (1990). Cloning of the H⁺, K⁺-ATPase β subunit. *Journal of Biological Chemistry*, **265**, 19878–84.

Carlsson, E., Larsson, H., Mattsson, H., Ryberg, B., and Sundell, G. (1986). Pharmacology and toxicology of omeprazole with special reference to the effects on the gastric mucosa. *Scandinavian Journal of Gastroenterology*, **118**, (Suppl.), 31–8.

Chiu, P. J. S., Casciano, C., Tetzloff, G., Long, J. F., and Barnett, A. (1983). Studies on the mechanisms of the antisecretory and cytoprotective actions of SCH 28080. *Journal of Pharmacology and Experimental Therapeutics*, **226**, 121–5.

Creutzfeldt, W. and Lamberts, R. (1991). Is hypergastrinaemia dangerous to man? *Scandinavian Journal of Gastroenterology*, **26** (suppl. 180), 179–91.

de Graef, J. and Woussen-Colle, M.-C. (1986). Influence of the stimulation state of the parietal cells on the inhibitory effect of omeprazole on gastric acid secretion in dogs. *Gastroenterology*, **91**, 333–7.

Ekman, L., Hansson, E., Havu, N., Carlsson, E., and Lundberg, C. (1985). Toxicological studies on omeprazole. *Scandinavian Journal of Gastroenterology*, **108** (Suppl.), 53–69.

Ene, M. D., Khan-Daneshmend, T., and Roberts, G. J. C. (1982). A study of the inhibitory effects of SCH 28080 on gastric secretion in man. *British Journal of Pharmacology*, **76**, 389–91.

Fellenius, E., Berglindh, G., Sachs, G., Olbe, L., Elander, B., Sjöstrand, S.-E., and Wallmark, B. (1981). Substituted benzimidazoles inhibit gastric acid secretion by blocking H⁺, K⁺-ATPase. *Nature, London*, **290**, 159–61.

Fellenius, E., Elander, B., Wallmark, B., Helander, H. F., and Berglindh, T. (1982). Inhibition of acid secretion in isolated gastric glands by substituted benzimidazoles. *American Journal of Physiology*, **243**, G505–10.

Figala, V., Klemm, K., Kohl, B., Krüger, U., Rainer, G., Schaefer, H., *et al.* (1986). Acid activation of H⁺, K⁺-ATPase inhibiting 2-(2-pyridylmethylsulfinyl)-benzimidazoles: isolation and characterization of the thiophilic 'active principle' and its reactions. *Journal of the Chemical Society Chemical Communications*, 125–7.

Fryklund, J., Gedda, K., and Wallmark, B. (1988a). Specific labelling of gastric H⁺, K⁺-ATPase by omeprazole. *Biochemical Pharmacology*, **37**, 2543–9.

Fryklund, J., Helander, H. F., Elander, B., and Wallmark, B. (1988b). Function and structure of parietal cells after H^+,K^+-ATPase blockade. *American Journal of Physiology*, **254**, G399–407.

Fujisaki, H., Shibata, H., Oketani, K., Murakami, M., Fujimoto, M., Wakabayashi, T., *et al.* (1991). Inhibitions of acid secretion by E3810 and omeprazole, and their reversal by glutathione. *Biochemical Pharmacology*, **42**, 321–8.

Ganser, A. L. and Forte, J. G. (1973). K^+-stimulated ATPase in purified microsomes of bullfrog oxyntic cells. *Biochimica et Biophysica Acta*, **307**, 169–80.

Havu, N. (1986). Enterochromaffin-like cell carcinoids of gastric mucosa in rats after life-long inhibition of gastric secretion. *Digestion*, **35** (Suppl. 1), 42–55.

Havu, N., Mattsson, H., Ekman, L., and Carlsson, E. (1990), Enterochromaffin-like cell carcinoids in the rat gastric mucosa following long-term administration of raniditine. *Digestion*, **45**, 189–95.

Havu N., Maaroos, H.-I., and Sipponen, P. (1991). Argyrophil cell hyperplasia associated with chronic corpus gastritis in gastric ulcer disease. *Scandinavian Journal of Gastroenterology*, **26**, (Suppl. 186), 90–4.

Helander, H. F., Ramsay, C.-H., and Regårdh, C.-G. (1985). Localisation of omeprazole and metabolites in the mouse. *Scandinavian Journal of Gastroenterology*, **20** (Suppl 108), 95–104.

Herling, A. W., Bickel, M., Lang, H.-J., Scheunemann, K., and Metzger, H. (1988a). HOE 731 a novel H^+,K^+-ATPase inhibitor with a different biological profile compared to omeprazole. *International Conference on Gastroenteric Biology*, Oxnard, CA, 25–28 October 1988, Abstract P27.

Herling, A. W., Bickel, M., Lang, H.-J., and Weidmann, A. (1988b). Substituted thieno[3.4-d]imidazole versus substituted benzimidazoles as H^+,K^+-ATPase inhibitors. *Pharmacology*, **36**, 289–7.

Hersey, S. J., Steiner, L., Mendlein, J., Rabon, E., and Sachs, G. (1988). SCH 28080 prevents omeprazole inhibition of the gastric H^+/K^+-ATPase. *Biochimica et Biophysica Acta*, **956**, 49–57.

Hioki, Y., Takada, J., Hidaka Y., Takeshita, H., Hosoi, M., and Yano, M. (1990). A newly synthesized pyridine derivative, (Z)-5-methyl-2-[2-(1-naphthyl-(ethenyl]-4-piperidinopyridine hydrochloride (AU-1421), as a reversible gastric proton pump inhibitor. *Archives Internationales de Pharmacodynamie et de Therapie.* **305**, 32–44.

Im, W. B., Blakeman, D. P., Mendlein, J., and Sachs, G. (1984). Inhibition of $(H^+ + K^+)$-ATPase and H^+ accumulation in hog gastric membranes by trifluoperazine, verapamil and 8-(N,N-diethylamino)octyl-3,4,5-trimethoxybenzoate. *Biochimica et Biophysica Acta*, **770**, 65–72.

Im, W. B., Blakeman, D. P., and Davis, J. P. (1985a). Irreversible inactivation of rat gastric $(H^+ - K^+)$-ATPase *in vivo* by omeprazole. *Biochemical and Biophysical Research Communications*, **126**, 78–82.

Im, W. B., Sih, J. C., Blakeman, D. P., and McGrath, J. P. (1985b). Omeprazole, a specific inhibitor of gastric $(H^+ - K^+)$-ATPase is a H^+-activated oxidizing agent of sulfhydryl groups. *Journal of Biological Chemistry*, **260**, 4591–7.

Kaminski, J. J., Bristol, J. A., Puchalski, C., Lovey, R. G., Elliott, A. J., Guzik, H., *et al.* (1985). Antiulcer agents. 1. Gastric antisecretory and cytoprotective properties of substituted imidazo[1,2-a]pyridines. *Journal of Medicinal Chemistry*, **28**, 876–92.

Kaminski, J. J., Perkins, D. G., Frantz, J. D., Solomon, D. M., Elliott, A. J., Chiu, P. J. S., and Long, J. F. (1987). Antiulcer agents. 3. Structure-activity-toxicity relationships of substituted imidazo[1,2-a]pyridines and a related imidazo-[1,2-a]pyrazine. *Journal of Medicinal Chemistry*, **30**, 2047–51.

Keeling, D. J., Fallowfield, C., and Underwood, A. H. (1987). The specificity of omeprazole as an (H⁺,K⁺)-ATPase inhibitor depends upon the means of its activation. *Biochemical Pharmacology*, **36**, 339–44.

Keeling, D. J., Laing, S. M., and Senn-Bilfinger, J. (1988). SCH 28080 is a lumenally acting, K⁺-site inhibitor of the gastric (H⁺ + K⁺)-ATPase. *Biochemical Pharmacology*, **37**, 2231–6.

Keeling, D. J., Fallowfield, C., Lawrie, K. M. W., Saunders, D., Richardson, S., and Ife, R. J. (1989a). Photoaffinity labeling of the luminal K⁺-site of the gastric (H⁺,K⁺)-ATPase. *Journal of Biological Chemistry*, **264**, 5552–8.

Keeling, D. J., Taylor, A. G., and Schudt, C. (1989b). The binding of a K⁺ competitive ligand, 2-methyl,8-(phenylmethoxy)imidazol(1,2-a)pyridine 3-acetonitrile, to the gastric (H⁺,K⁺)-ATPase. *Journal of Biological Chemistry*, **264**, 5545–51.

Keeling, D. J., Malcolm, R. C., Laing, S. M., Ife, R. J., and Leach, C. A. (1991). SK&F 96067 is a reversible, luminally acting inhibitor of the gastric (H⁺ + K⁺)-ATPase. *Biochemical Pharmacology*, **42**, 123–30.

Konturek, S. J., Cieszkowski, M., Kwiecien, N., Konturek, J., Tasler, J., and Bilski, J. (1984). Effects of omeprazole, a substituted benzimidazole, on gastrointestinal secretions, serum gastrin, and gastric mucosal blood flow in dogs. *Gastroenterology*, **86**, 71–7.

LaMattina, J. L., McCarthy, P. A., Reiter, L. A., Hoit, W. F., and Yeh. L-A. (1990). Antiulcer agents. 4-substituted 2-guanidinothiazoles: reversible, competitive, and selective inhibitors of gastric H⁺,K⁺-ATPase. *Journal of Medicinal Chemistry*, **33**, 543–52.

Lanzon-Miller, S., Pounder, R. E., Hamilton, M. R., Ball, S., Chronos, N. A. F., Raymond, F., *et al.* (1987). Twenty-four-hour intragastric acidity and plasma gastrin concentration before and during treatment with either ranitidine or omeprazole. *Alimentary Pharmacology and Therapeutics*, **1**, 239–51.

Larsson, H., Carlsson, E., and Junggren, U. (1983). Inhibition of gastric acid secretion by omeprazole in the dog and cat. *Gastroenterology*, **85**, 900–7.

Lee, J., Simpson, G., and Scholes, P. (1974). ATPase from dog gastric mucosa. Changes of outer pH in suspensions of membrane vesicles. *Biochemical and Biophysical Research Communications*, **60**, 825–32.

Lind, T., Cederberg, C., Ekenved, G., Haglund, U., and Olbe L. (1983). Effect of omeprazole—a gastric proton pump inhibitor—on pentagastrin stimulated acid secretion in man. *Gut*, **24**, 270–6.

Lind, T., Cederberg, C., Ekenved, G., and Olbe, L. (1986). Inhibition of basal and betazole—and sham-feeding-induced acid secretion by omeprazole in man. *Scandinavian Journal of Gastroenterology*, **21**, 1004–10.

Lindberg, P., Nordberg, P., Alminger, T., Brändström, A., and Wallmark, B. (1986). The mechanism of action of the gastric acid secretion inhibitor omeprazole. *Journal of Medicinal Chemistry*, **29**, 1327–9.

Lindberg, P., Brändström, A., and Wallmark, B. (1987). Structure–activity relationships of omeprazole analogues and their mechanism of action. *Trends in Pharmacological Sciences*, **8**, 399–402.

Lindberg, P., Brändström, A., Wallmark, B., Mattsson, H., Rikner, L., and Hoffman, K-J. (1990). Omeprazole: the first proton pump inhibitor. *Medicinal Research Reviews*, **10**, 1–54.

Lloyd-Davies, K. A., Rutgersson, K., and Sölvell L. (1988). Omeprazole in the treatment of Zollinger–Ellison syndrome: a 4-year international study. *Alimentary Pharmacology and Therapeutics*, **2**, 13–32.

Long, J. F., Chiu, P. J. S., Derelanko, M. J., and Steinberg, M. (1983). Gastric antisecretory and cytoprotective activities of SCH 28080. *Journal of Pharmacology and Experimental Therapeutics*, **226**, 114–20.

Lorentzon, P., Jackson, R., Wallmark B., and Sachs, G. (1987). Inhibition of (H$^+$, + K$^+$)-ATPase by omeprazole in isolated gastric vesicles requires proton transport. *Biochimica et Biophysica Acta*, **897**, 41–51.

McTavish, D., Buckley, M.-T., and Heel, R. C. (1991). Omeprazole—an updated review of its pharmacology and therapeutic use in acid-related disorders. *Drugs*, **42**, 138–70.

Mårdh, S., Song, Y.-H., and Wallmark, B. (1988). Effects of some antisecretory drugs on acid production, intracellular free Ca^{2+} and cyclic AMP production in isolated pig parietal cells. *Scandinavian Journal of Gastroenterology*, **23**, 977–82.

Mattsson, H., Havu, N., Bräutigam, J., Carlsson, K., Lundell, L., and Carlsson, E. (1991). Partial gastric corpectomy results in hypergastrinemia and development of gastric enterochromaffinlike cell carcinoids in the rat. *Gastroenterology*, **100**, 311–9.

Mendlein, J. and Sachs, G. (1990). Interaction of a K$^+$-competitive inhibitor, a substituted imidazo[1,2a]pyridine, with the phospho- and dephosphoenzyme forms of H$^+$,K$^+$-ATPase. *Journal of Biological Chemistry*, **265**, 5030–6.

Morii, M., Takata, H., Fujisaki, H., and Takeguchi, N. (1990). The potency of substituted benzimidazoles such as E3810, omeprazole, Ro 18–5364 to inhibit gastric H$^+$,K$^+$-ATPase is correlated with the rate of acid-activation of the inhibitor. *Biochemical Pharmacology*, **39**, 661–7.

Munson, H. R., Jr and Reevis, S. A. (1982). *US Patent 4, 343, 804*.

Murakami, S., Kijima, H., Isobe, Y., Muramatsu, M., Aihara, H., Otomo, S., *et al.* (1990). Effect of salvianolic acid A, a depside from roots of Salvia miltiorrhiza, on gastric H$^+$,K$^+$-ATPase. *Planta Medica*, **56**, 360–3.

Nagaya, H., Satoh, H., Kubo, K., and Maki, Y. (1989). Possible mechanism for the inhibition of gastric (H$^+$ + K$^+$)-adenosine triphosphatase by the proton pump inhibitor AG-1749. *Journal of Pharmacology and Experimental Therapeutics*, **248**, 799–805.

Nandi, J., Wright, M. V., and Ray, T. K. (1983). Mechanism of gastric anti-secretory effects of nolinium bromide. *Gastroenterology*, **85**, 938–45.

Nandi, J., King, R. L., Kaplan, D. S., and Levine, R. A. (1990). Mechanisms of gastric proton pump inhibition by calcium channel antagonists. *Journal of Pharmacology and Experimental Therapeutics*, **252**, 1102–7.

Nicholson, P. A. (1985). A multicenter international controlled comparison of two dosage regimes of misoprostol and cimetidine in the treatment of duodenal ulcer in out-patients. *Digestive Diseases and Sciences*, **30**, 171S-7S.

Norberg, L. and Mårdh, S. (1990). A continuous-flow technique for analysis of stoichiometry and transport kinetics of gastric H$^+$,K$^+$-ATPase. *Acta Physiologica Scandinavica*, **140**, 567–73.

Okabe, S., Akimoto, Y., Yamasaki, S., and Nagai, H. (1988). Effects of NC-1300-B, a new benzimidazole derivative, on hog gastric H$^+$,K$^+$-ATPase, gastric acid secretion and HCl ethanol-induced gastric lesions in rats. *Digestive Diseases and Sciences*, **33**, 1425–34.

Pedersen, P. L. and Carafoli, E. (1987). Ion motive ATPases. I. Ubiquity, properties, and significance to cell function. *Trends in Biochemical Sciences*, **12**, 146–50.

Poynter, D., Pick, C. R., Harcourt, R. A., Selway, S. A. M., Ainge, G., Harman, I. W., *et al.* (1985). Association of long lasting unsurmountable histamine H2 blockade and gastric carcinoid tumours in the rat. *Gut*, **26**, 1284–95.

Rabon, E., McFall, T. L., and Sachs, G. (1982). The gastric H$^+$,K$^+$-ATPase H$^+$/ATP stochiometry. *Journal of Biological Chemistry*, **257**, 6296–9.

Rabon, E., Sachs, G., Bassilian, S., Leach, C., and Keeling, D. (1991). A K$^+$-competitive fluorescent inhibitor of the H$^+$,K$^+$-ATPase. *Journal of Biological Chemistry*, **266**, 12395–401.

Rackur, G., Bickel, M., Fehlhaber, H.-W., Herling, A., Hitzel, V., Lang, H. J., *et al.* (1985). 2-((2-pyridylmethyl)sulfinyl)benzimidazoles: acid sensitive suicide inhibitors of the proton transport system in the parietal cell. *Biochemical and Biophysical Research Communications*, **128**, 477–84.

Saccomani, G., Chang, H. H., Mihas, A. A., Crago, S., and Sachs, G. (1979). An acid transporting enzyme in human gastric mucosa. *Journal of Clinical Investigation*, **64**, 627–35.

Sachs, G., Chang, H. H., Rabon, E., Schachmann, R., Lewin, H., and Saccomani, G. (1976). A non electrogenic H$^+$ pump in plasma membrane of hog stomach. *Journal of Biological Chemistry*, **251**, 7690–8.

Senn-Bilfinger, J., Krüger, U., Sturm, E., Figala, V., Klemm, K., Kohl, B., *et al.* (1987). H$^+$,K$^+$-ATPase inhibiting 2-[(2-pyridylmethyl)sulfinyl]benzimidazoles. 2. The reaction cascade induced by treatment with acids. Formation of 5H-pyrido-[1′,2′:4,5][1,2,4]thiadiazino[2,3-a]benzimidazol-13-ium salts and their reactions with thiols. *Journal of Organic Chemistry*, **52**, 4573–81.

Shull, G. E. and Lingrel, J. B. (1986). Molecular cloning of the rat stomach (H$^+$ + K$^+$)-ATPase. *Journal of Biological Chemistry*, **261**, 16788–91.

Simon, W. A., Keeling, D. J., Laing, S. M., Fallowfield, C., and Taylor A. G. (1990). BY 1023/SK&F 96022: Biochemistry of a novel (H$^+$ + K$^+$)-ATPase inhibitor. *Biochemical Pharmacology*, **39**, 1799–1806.

Sjöstrand, S-E., Ryberg, B., and Olbe, L. (1978). Stimulation and inhibition of acid secretion in the isolated guinea pig gastric mucosa. *Acta Physiologica Scandinavica. Special Supplement*, 181–5.

Skrabanja, A. T. P., van der Hijden, H. T. W. M., and de Pont, J. J. H. H. M. (1987). Transport ratios of reconstituted H$^+$,K$^+$-ATPase. *Biochimica et Biophysica Acta*, **903**, 434–40.

Smolka, A., Helander, H. F., and Sachs, G. (1983). Monoclonal antibodies against gastric H$^+$,K$^+$-ATPase. *American Journal of Physiology*, **245**, G589–96.

Sturm, E., Krüger, U., Senn-Bilfinqer, J., Figala, V., Klemm, K., Kohl, B., *et al.* (1987). (H$^+$ + K$^+$)-ATPase inhibiting 2-[(2-pyridylmethyl)sulfinyl]benzimidazoles. 1. Their reaction with thiols under acidic condions. Disulfide containing 2-pyridinobenzimidazolides as mimics for the inhibited enzyme. *Journal of Organic Chemistry*, **52**, 4573–81.

Suschitzky, J. L. and Wells, E. (1990). Agents acting on active ion transport. In *Comprehensive medicinal chemistry*, Vol. 2, (ed. P. G. Sammes), pp. 193–212. Pergamon Press, New York.

Takeguchi, M., Asano, S., Tabuchi, Y., and Takeguchi, N. (1990). The presence of H$^+$,K$^+$-ATPase in the crypt of rabbit distal colon demonstrated with monoclonal antibodies against gastric H$^+$,K$^+$-ATPase. *Gastroenterology*, **99**, 1339–46.

Wallmark, B., Stewart, H. B., Rabon, E., Saccomani, G., and Sachs, G. (1980). The catalytic cycle of gastric $(H^+ + K^+)$-ATPase. *Journal of Biological Chemistry*, **255**, 5313–19.

Wallmark, B., Jaresten, B.-M., Larsson, H., Ryberg, B., Brändström, A., and Fellenius, E. (1983a). Differentiation among inhibitory actions of omeprazole, cimetidine and SCN^- on gastric acid secretion. *American Journal of Physiology*, **245**, G64–71.

Wallmark, B., Sachs, G., Mårdh, S., and Felienius, E. (1983b). Inhibition of gastric (H^+, K^+)-ATPase by the substituted benzimidazole, picoprazole. *Biochimica et Biophysica Acta*, **728**, 31–8.

Wallmark, B., Brändström, A., and Larsson, H. (1984). Evidence for acid-induced transformation of omeprazole into an active inhibitor of proton-potassium ATPase within the parietal cell. *Biochimica et Biophysica Acta*, **778**, 549–58.

Wallmark, B., Larsson, H., and Humble, L. (1985). The relationship between gastric acid secretion and gastric H⁺,K⁺-ATPase activity. *Journal of Biological Chemistry*, **260**, 13681–4.

Wallmark, B., Briving, C., Fryklund, J., Munson, K., Jackson, R., Mendlein J., et al. (1987). Inhibition of gastric H⁺,K⁺-ATPase and acid secretion by SCH 28080, a substituted pyridyl(1,2a)imidazole. *Journal of Biological Chemistry*, **262**, 2077–84.

Wingo, C. S., Madsen, K. M., Smolka, A., and Tisher, C. C. (1990). H⁺,K⁺-ATPase immunoreactivity in cortical and outer medullary collecting duct. *Kidney International*, **38**, 985–90.

15

Inhibitors of mammalian collagenases

W.H. Johnson, K.M.K. Bottomley,
M.J. Broadhurst, P.A. Brown, and J.S. Nixon

15.1 Introduction

The matrix metalloproteinase (MMP) family of enzymes contains at least 11 members, subdivided into three groups, gelatinases, stromelysins, and collagenases. They are zinc metalloenzymes, which have a requirement for calcium, operate optimally at neutral pH, and are secreted as latent proforms requiring activation. Sequence homology between family members is 55 per cent between human fibroblast collagenase and stromelysin, and 57 per cent between human fibroblast and neutrophil collagenases. The zinc-binding motif and three cysteine residues are totally conserved. All MMPs are inhibited by tissue inhibitors of metalloproteinases (TIMP 1–4) (Docherty *et al.* 1985; Williamson *et al.* 1990) and by a_2-macroglobulin, although a physiological role for this inhibitor is questionable.

Under normal circumstances, the MMPs are probably involved in the remodelling of the extracellular matrix of connective tissue. This is required to facilitate cell migration, morphogenesis, and growth. In various pathological conditions such as arthritis, tumour metastasis, and periontal disease, they are implicated in abnormal remodelling and tissue degradation (Krane *et al.* 1988; Liotta *et al.* 1991). Amongst these enzymes, two mammalian collagenases, one derived from neutrophils (58 kDa and 75 kDa forms (MMP8)) and the other from synovial fibroblasts, chondrocytes, and keratinocytes (55 kDa (MMP1)), are unique in their ability to cleave triple helical collagen (types I, II, and III). At physiological temperature this single cleavage causes spontaneous denaturation of the collagen fragments, which are then subject to further degradation by other MMPs and less specific proteinases. Therefore inhibition of the collagenases should have a marked effect on the increased turnover and degradation of tissue observed in a number of pathological conditions.

15.2   Properties of collagenases

15.2.1   Purification

Medium from fibroblasts cultured with the cytokine interleukin 1 (IL-1), or from neutrophils stimulated with phorbol esters, is the usual starting point for MMP purification (Mainardi *et al.* 1988; Murphy 1990). Procollagenase may be activated before or after purification. The former permits optimal activation by contaminating stromelysin during isolation, while the latter allows storage of purified proenzyme at high concentrations for long periods since the activated enzyme is subject to degradation by autocatalysis. Strategies used to separate collagenases from other MMPs include the following: selective removal of progelatinase by chromatography on gelatin/agarose (Murphy *et al.* 1989), separation of collagenase from stromelysin by heparin/sepharose chromatography (Galloway *et al.* 1983), and selective binding of collagenase to an affinity matrix bearing synthetic peptide inhibitors (Moore and Spilburg 1986a). Recombinant collagenase has been expressed in both bacterial and mammalian cell lines (Brinckerhoff *et al.* 1990; O'Hare *et al.* 1991). Milligram quantities of recombinant enzyme requiring little purification and free from contaminating MMPs have been produced.

15.2.2   Structure and activation

Human fibroblast (HFC) and human neutrophil procollagenase (HNC) are very similar in both size and domain organization. The protein sequences (c. 450 residues) (Goldberg *et al.* 1986; Hasty *et al.* 1990) are arranged into three functional domains. The N-terminal propeptide (80 residues) contains a highly conserved sequence around Cys-73 (RCGVPDV). This residue may bind to the active-site zinc in the latent enzyme preventing substrate binding. Propeptide removal results in disruption of this $Cys-Zn^{2+}$ interaction and triggers enzyme activation (Springman *et al.* 1990). The second domain contains the zinc-binding motif (HELGH) identified in other zinc metalloproteases. In the bacterial metalloproteinase thermolysin, both histidines bind to the zinc with the third ligand (Glu-166) lying outside the HELGH motif. The glutamic acid between the two histidines is a key residue in the catalytic mechanism for thermolysin (Matthews 1988). The confirmation of a similar mechanism for collagenase and the identification of the third zinc ligand will require a crystal structure determination. The C-terminal domain confers substrate specificity on collagenase. Loss of this domain, which occurs during enzyme autolysis, yields an enzyme able to cleave casein and gelatin but not collagen (Clark and Cawston 1989). Point mutation or deletion of bases encoding either of the conserved cysteine residues in this domain (Cys-259, Cys-447) also gives an active enzyme which cannot cleave type I collagen (Windsor *et al.* 1991).

Activation of collagenase requires a conformational change in domain 1 to expose the active site. *In vitro*, this may be achieved by treatment with organomercurials (Stricklin *et al.* 1983), which allows removal of the propeptide by autocatalysis. Alternatively, direct cleavage of the proenzyme to active collagenase may be achieved by treatment with a range of proteases (trypsin, kallikrein). Physiological activation may be initiated by plasmin, a serine protease generated from plasminogen by plasminogen activator (Gavrilovic and Murphy 1989). However, optimal activation of collagenase probably requires further processing by the related MMP stromelysin (Suzuki *et al.* 1990).

5.2.3 Substrate specificity

Although collagenase cleaves only one bond in collagen (Gly-775 — Ile/ Leu-776), it is known to cleave a variety of other peptides and proteins. Systematic investigation of the differences between HNC and HFC, using oligopeptide substrates covering P_4-P_5' residues (nomenclature of Schechter and Berger (1967)), suggest that both enzymes prefer alanine in P_1 and tryptophan or phenylalanine in P_2' but HNC accommodates aromatic residues in subsite P_1' more readily than HFC (Netzel-Arnett *et al.* 1991a). These studies do not explain the failure of collagenases to hydrolyse other potential sites in the native substrate and support the concept that additional elements in the triple helix of collagen determine the cleavage site. HFC and HNC have different affinities towards types I, II, and III collagens (HFC, III > II > I; HNC, I > II > III) (Netzel-Arnett *et al.* 1991a). For HFC the preferred sequences adjacent to the scissile bond (775 — 776) in these collagens are

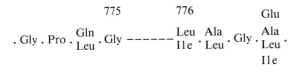

15.2.4 Assay methods

Collagenase assays using the physiological substrate rely on the production of soluble fragments from insoluble prelabelled collagen or on the
separation by sodium dodecyl sulphate (SDS) polyacrylamide gel electrophoresis of the 1/4–3/4 products from the digestion of soluble collagen
(Cawston and Barrett 1979; Johnson-Wint 1980; Gadher *et al.* 1988).
These methods allow assay of collagenase in the presence of other MMPs,
since only collagenase will cleave native collagen. However, interpretation
of kinetic data, used to determine the binding mode of inhibitors, is
complicated by the use of an insoluble substrate.

The use of synthetic peptides simplifies analysis of kinetic data. However,
these peptides are also cleaved by other MMPs, and so pure collagenase
is required. A number of strategies have been devised to simplify detection
of the products of collagenase action. When an N-protected peptide is
used (e.g. acetyl.Pro.Gln.Gly––Leu.Leu.Gly.OEt), collagenase produces
a tripeptide with a free amino group which is derivatized by reaction
with picrylsulphonic acid to generate a chromophore which can be detected
spectrophotometrically (Johnson *et al.* 1987). Dinitrophenylpeptides, such
as DNP.Pro.Leu.Gly.Ile.Ala.Gly.Arg.NH$_2$, have been used as substrates,
but these entail time-consuming extraction of the DNP fragments (Masui
et al. 1977). These peptide substrates do not allow continuous monitoring
of enzyme activity, but this has been achieved with fluorogenic substrates
such as DNP.Pro.Leu.Gly.Leu.Trp.Ala.D.Arg.NH$_2$ (Stack and Gray
1989). In these peptides, the quenching of tryptophan fluorescence in the
intact substrate is diminished on hydrolysis and this results in. an increase
in tryptophan fluorescence which can be continuously recorded. Sequence
optimization for different MMPs has resulted in DNP.Pro.Leu.Ala.Leu.-
Trp.Ala.Arg.OH as the best substrate for HFC, and DNP.Pro.Leu.Ala.-
Tyr.Trp.Ala.Arg.OH for HNC (Netzel-Arnett *et al.* 1991b).

15.2.5 Physiological control of collagenase

Physiological control of collagenase activity is exerted at several levels,
with the signal transduction pathways mediating collagenase expression,
activation of collagenase, and its inhibition by natural inhibitors (TIMPs).
Collagenase is expressed by connective tissue cells (fibroblasts and chondrocytes) in response to IL-1, tumour necrosis factor *a*, basic fibroblast

growth factor, and transforming growth factor β (Murphy and Docherty 1988). Early events in the signal transduction pathway mediating the effects of these cytokines are unclear. Increased concentration of IL-1 in plasma (Eastgate *et al.* 1988) and the presence of collagenase in involved tissue have been demonstrated in some connective tissue pathologies, notably in synovial explants from rheumatoid arthritis patients where the most probable source of MMPs is synovial type B fibroblasts (Krane *et al.* 1988). The transcriptional events involved in collagenase expression have been investigated using phorbol esters which, as direct and specific activators of protein kinase C, will induce expression of collagenase in fibroblasts. The precise molecular mechanism is unclear, but it is known to involve prior induction of a transcription factor (AP-1) which binds to a phorbol ester-responsive element (TRE) present in the collagenase gene promoter (Angel *et al.* 1987a,b; Auble and Brinckerhoff 1991). In contrast with fibroblasts, which do not store preformed MMPs, collagenase and gelatinase are packaged in specific granules in neutrophils and are secreted in response to various stimuli (phorbol esters, Ca^{2+} ionophore, formyl.Met.Leu.Phe.OH) (Mainardi *et al.* 1988).

The last level of control of MMPs is by inhibition with protein inhibitors. TIMPs are the most important interstitial inhibitors of collagenase in fibroblasts and chondrocytes, and are frequently coexpressed with MMPs. They form stable complexes with the active enzyme with 1:1 stoichiometry. In the case of rabbit bone TIMP and purified rabbit collagenase, the K_D value of 1.4×10^{-10} M indicates tight binding (Cawston *et al.* 1983).

15.3   Design of active-site-directed inhibitors

The strategy used to prepare inhibitors of angiotensin-converting enzyme (ACE), first described by Ondetti *et al.* (1977), has provided the basis for the rational design of collagenase inhibitors. Similar approaches have been reported for the inhibition of other zinc metalloproteases, carboxypeptides A and B (Ondetti *et al.* 1979), and enkephalinase (Schwartz 1989). Conceptually, a zinc ligand is placed at the position of the cleaved amide bond and parts of the adjacent substrate sequence are incorporated to give improved binding and specificity for the target enzyme. The mammalian collagenases have been shown to cleave protected octapeptides (Nagai *et al.* 1976; Masui *et al.* 1977) and hexapeptides (Weingarten *et al.* 1985) related to the conserved cleavage site in the natural substrate. With the hexapeptide substrate Ac.Pro.Leu.Gly.Leu.Leu.Gly.OEt (1), the collagenases cleave the central amide bond to yield two tripeptide derivatives, Ac.Pro.Leu.Gly.OH and H.Leu.Leu.Gly.OEt. For the design of inhibitors, the zinc ligand can be placed in the N-terminal triplet (Ac.Pro.Leu.Gly.ligand), in the C-terminal triplet (ligand.Leu.Leu.Gly.OEt),

or at the centre of the full hexapeptide substrate (Ac.Pro.Leu.Gly.ligand.-
Leu.Leu.Gly.OEt).

15.3.1   Thiols

The first inhibitors of vertebrate collagenase with modest activity (IC_{50}
in the submillimolar range) were reported by Gray et al. (1981). By replacing the amino group in the cleaved product of a synthetic octapeptide
with a thiol, they produced a 2-mercapto-4-methylpentanoyl tetrapeptide
amide (P_1'-P_5') which had an IC_{50} of 10 μM against tadpole backskin
collagenase. Sundeen and Dejneka (1981) incorporated a methylene spacer
group between the ligand and the P_1' side-chain by using derivatives of
2-mercaptomethyl-4-methylpentanoic acid. No biological data were reported
for these compounds, however, the same ligand and spacer gave compound
(2), with activities below 10 μM against the pig synovial enzyme (Gray
et al. 1986). A surprising feature of these compounds was the lack of
stereospecificity at the P_1' position.

Substitution of the methylene spacer with alkyl groups gave the first
thiols with activities below 1 μM (Donald et al. 1986). Substituents containing carbonyl groups (e.g. $R \cdot CO \cdot CH_2$—, $R \cdot O \cdot CO \cdot CH_2$—, and
$R \cdot NHCO \cdot CH_2$—) form the basis of a number of patent applications
(Markwell et al. 1988, 1989). Activities of the best diastereoisomers (3)
are 4–14 nM against rabbit bone collagenase. It is not known whether the
improvement in potency with these compounds is due to the conformational
restraint in the area of the ligand and the P_1' side-chain or whether the
additional group interacts with the enzyme.

With their natural substrates, the collagenases show high specificity for
the side-chain groups in the S_1' to S_3' subsites. In the inhibitors reported
the S_1' subsite has shown a strong preference for leucine type side-chains.
Replacement of the isobutyl group by methyl or benzyl results in significant loss of activity (Gray et al. 1986). Schwartz et al. (1991) have
shown that, for potent compounds, the difference between the S and R
stereoisomers is about one order of magnitude and that the R configuration
which corresponds to the unnatural D-amino acid, is the most potent.
(4). This is an unexpected finding and is the opposite result to that obtained
with other zinc ligands. The S_2' site binds aromatic groups, tyrosine
derivatives (Donald et al. 1986), phenylalanine, tryptophan, and a larger
aromatic group β-naphthaloylalanine (Nal) (Darlak et al. 1990). The P_3'
residue can be glycine derivatives with esters and amides in P_4' (Johnson
et al. 1987; Darlak et al. 1990), alanine derivatives with the natural
stereochemistry (Darlak et al. 1990), and simple amides (Donald et al.
1986). Occupancy of binding sites above $S_3'S_4'$ has little effect on inhibitor binding. The compound $HSCH_2CH(^{i}Bu)CO.Nal.Ala.NH_2$ (5) (isomer

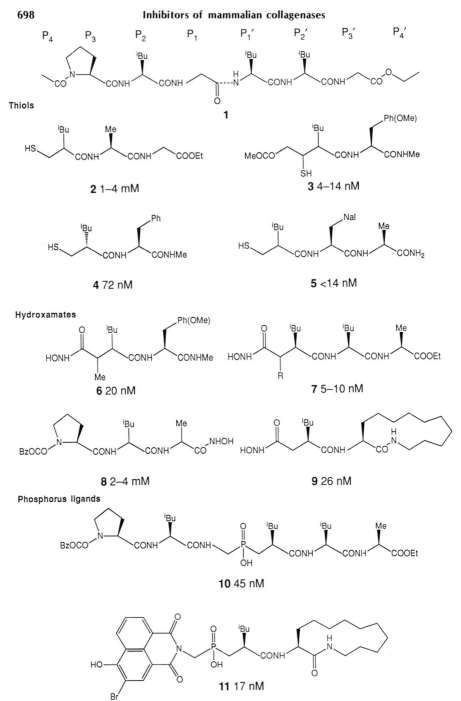

Fig. 15.1 Synthetic substrate for collagenase (**1**) and representative inhibitors containing different zinc ligands.

A, Darlak *et al*. 1990) has an IC_{50} of 14 nM or better against porcine collagenase using soluble type I collagen as substrate.

The P_2' phenylalanine analogue, $HSCH_2CH(^iBu)CO.Phe.Ala.NH_2$ has been reported by two groups. There is good agreement with respect to potency: IC_{50} is 40nM against porcine collagenase (Darlak *et al*. 1990), 42 nM against human neutrophil enzyme, and 56 nM against human fibroblast collagenase (Schwartz *et al*. 1991). However, there is a discrepancy with regard to stability. Darlak *et al*. (1990) state that the compound has a half-life of approximately 30 min. When assayed against rabbit corneal collagenase, the IC_{50} was $1-3$ μM when assayed for 3 hours with collagen type I as substrate but 10 nM when assayed rapidly against a synthetic substrate (Burns *et al*. 1989). Schwartz *et al*. (1991) found a decrease of less than 20 per cent in inhibitor potency after incubation with enzyme for 4 hours. Thus the inhibitor potency and rate of oxidative dimerization appear to depend on the assay conditions. This could be a serious disadvantage of thiol-containing inhibitors when they are progressed to *in vivo* studies.

Thiol-containing inhibitors related to the N-terminal portion of the substrate (P_3-P_1), for example acetyl.Pro.Leu.$NHCH_2CH_2SH$, show very poor activity (100 μM) against the human synovial enzyme (Johnson *et al*. 1987).

15.3.2   Hydroxamic acids

Dickens *et al*. (1986) claimed in a patent the first sub-100 nM inhibitors of human fibroblast collagenase. The compounds contained hydroxamate as the ligand and a one-carbon spacer group, which could be substituted with alkyl groups, between the ligand and the specificity side-chain. Isobutyl was used as the P_1' residue, *O*-methyltyrosine in P_2', and methylamide in P_3'. These compounds are the direct analogues of the thiols (Donald *et al*. 1986), where the $HS \cdot CH(R)$ group has been replaced by $HONHCO \cdot CH(R) -$. The most active compounds (R = H, R = Me (6)) had IC_{50} values of 20 nM, which is an order of magnitude more active than the corresponding thiols. In a systematic study aimed at identifying the subsite requirements of the enzyme, identifying the contribution of the different side-chains and amide bonds, and testing a range of ligands, Johnson *et al*. (1987) showed that hydroxamic acids with a one-carbon spacer group were the most potent inhibitors of human synovial collagenase. For good activity, changes in the critical P_1' subsite are limited to alkyl groups related to leucine/isoleucine and there is an absolute requirement for the P_1' group to have stereochemistry equivalent to the natural amino acid. The requirements for the P_2' position were identified using a series of peptide ethylamides, $HONHCOCH_2CH(^iBu)$-$CO.AA.Gly.NHEt$. All L-amino acids, except proline, were more active

(IC_{50} = 0.2 μM) than alanine (IC_{50} = 1.3 μM), the most frequently oc-curring amino acid in the natural substrates. No upper size limitation was found at this position; even N^{ε}-protected lysine derivatives are accom-modated, indicating that most of this side-chain points away from the enzyme and towards the solvent. There were two major surprises when changes were made in the P_3' and P_4' positions. First L-alanine was preferred to the natural residue glycine in P_3', and second replacement of the amide in the P_4' subsite by ketone, ether, carboxylate, and ester groups gave improvement in activity ($-NHCH_2CH_3$, IC_{50} = 0.2 μM; $-OCH_2CH_3$, IC_{50} = 26 nM). The amino acid residue in P_3' may be replaced with a simple amide (e.g. methylamide) without significant loss of activity. The amide bonds between $P_1'-P_2'$ and $P_2'-P_3'$ could not be replaced by ester bonds, and methylation ($-CONMe-$) of amide $P_2'-P_3'$ gave a loss of activity, similar to proline in the P_3' site. The size of the group in P_4' has little effect on activity and probably does not interact with the enzyme. The changes in each position are independent of each other, and when the optimal groups are incorporated into one molecule, $HONHCOCH_2CH(^{i}Bu)CO.Leu.Ala.OEt$ (7), the potency increases (IC_{50} = 8.5 nM; K_i = 5.0 nM). A further improvement in activity was found by stereospecific substitution of the methylene spacer group. A methyl group gave a slight improvement and larger groups ($-(CH_2)_4.N.Pth$) resulted in a significantly more active compound (IC_{50} = 5.0 nM). This increase in activity is probably due to conformational restraint, fixing the ligand with respect to the specificity side-chain. For the methyl com-pound, this has been demonstrated by NMR which shows only one con-formation in solution (Johnson *et al.* 1987).

Anticollagenase activity was detected in the supernatant of an *Actino-mycete* strain (Faucher *et al.* 1987). Isolation and structural studies iden-tified the compound as the known pseudopeptide antibiotic actinonin $HONHCOCH_2CH(nC_5H_9)CO.Val.Prolinol$ (K_i = 1.4 μM against porcine synovial enzyme). Replacement of the *n*-pentyl group failed to increase activity as did replacement of prolinol by morpholino functions (Lelievre *et al.* 1989).

Hydroxamic-acid-containing inhibitors based on the P_1-P_4 residues of the acylated hexapeptide substrate have been reported (Moore and Spilburg 1986b; Johnson *et al.* 1987; Odake *et al.* 1990). Compounds containing glycine (P_1), leucine (P_2), and acetyl (P_3) have poor activity; however, incorporation of proline (P_3) and acetyl (P_4) gives a compound active at 10 μM (Johnson *et al.* 1987). Odake *et al.* (1990) have shown that P_1 may be alanine and that leucine (P_2) must have the natural stereochemistry, but if both residues are D then the compound is fully active (2–4 μM) (8). These data indicate that it is the residues in P_3 and P_4 or the amide (P_3-P_2) which interact with the enzyme.

15.3.3   Phosphorus-containing ligands

In a systematic investigation (Broadhurst *et al.* unpublished study) of collagenase inhibitors based on the P'_1–P'_3 sequence of the substrate, it was found that activity depends markedly on the spacer between the phosphorus atom and the P'_1 side-chain and also on the nature of the groups coordinating phosphorus. Compounds with a phosphonic acid ligand $[PO(OH)_2]$ directly attached to the P'_1 residue had little activity; however, incorporation of a methylene spacer resulted in modest activity (IC_{50} = 1–3 μM) for one of the isomers at the P'_1 position. A considerable loss of potency was observed when the methylene spacer was replaced by either sulphur or oxygen. Compounds with two methylene groups as the spacer showed relatively poor activity which was improved (IC_{50} = 6 μM) when the carbon adjacent to the P'_1 position was replaced by nitrogen. Further small improvements could be obtained by introducing small non-polar alkyl groups next to phosphorus ($(HO)_2POCH(Et)$-$NHCH(^iBu)CO$—, IC_{50} = 1 μM). A related series of compounds containing aromatic residues at P'_2 in place of leucine has been reported by Hunter *et al.* (1989). This change has given only a slight improvement in activity.

Compounds with the phosphoramidate ligand $(HO)_2PONH$ were found to be very unstable and had little activity. Monoesters of phosphoramidate peptides are more stable, and a series of compounds exploring the effect of adding residues in the C-terminal direction up to P'_6 has been reported by Kortylewicz and Galardy (1990). The most active compound was *N*-(ethylphosphoryl)-L-isoleucyl-L-tryptophan methylamide (K_i = 1.5 μM). In a study of a series of phosphonamidate inhibitors $R(HO)PO.NH$— based on the Gly^P-Leu (P_1-P'_1) sequence, Mookhtiar *et al.* (1987) found that inhibition was enhanced by extending the peptide in either direction. In the C-terminal direction activity was greatest when both the P'_2 and P'_3 subsites were occupied (K_i = 14 μM), while in the N-terminal direction occupation of both P_3 and P_2 was required for the best result (K_i = 150 μM). None of the compounds studied were found to bind as tightly to collagenase as the natural substrate (K_m = 1.5 μM); however, no compounds were reported that take advantage of binding sites on both sides of the scissile bond. An analogue in which the NH group of the phosphon-amidate was replaced by oxygen was found to be 30 times less potent. The requirement for the presence of a basic nitrogen as a proton acceptor to mimic the binding of the NH group of the scissile bond was noted, in agreement with results reported previously (Thorsett *et al.* 1982). Clearly, however, other factors must be involved in view of the good potency observed for inhibitors where the scissile bond NH has been replaced by carbon.

A series of phosphinic acid derivatives which interact with binding sites on both sides of the scissile bond position has been reported (Broadhurst *et al.* 1988). Initial attempts to replace one of the hydroxyl groups of the phosphonic acid inhibitors, $R(OH)POCH_2CH(^iBu)CO—$ $(R = OH)$, with a variety of substituents $(R = H, MeNH, MeO, Me)$ met with little success. Some activity was restored when the methyl group of the phosphinic acid $(R = Me)$ was substituted with groups designed to utilize part of the P_1 and P_2 residue binding sites $(R = MeCONHCH_2, IC_{50} = 40 \ \mu M)$. The activity was further improved by replacement of the acetyl group by an aromatic residue $(R = PhCONHCH_2, IC_{50} = 12 \ \mu M)$. Extension to include the leucine (P_2) residue produced only a marginal improvement, but addition of N-protected proline derivatives (P_4P_3) with $(R = BzOCO.-Pro.Leu.NHCH_2)$ **(10)** resulted in a dramatic increase in activity $(IC_{50} = 45 \ nM)$. Of major importance was the discovery that the phthaloyl-protected aminomethyl derivative $(R = $ phthalimidomethyl, $IC_{50} \ 0.6 \ \mu M)$ was 20 times more potent than the corresponding *N*-benzoyl compound. Imides with larger aromatic groups, for example 1,8-naphthalimide, gave a further significant improvement in activity $(IC_{50} = 80 \ nM)$ which was enhanced by introduction of substituents into the aromatic ring $(R = $ 4-hydroxy-1,8-naphthalimidomethyl, $IC_{50} = 40 \ nM)$. In a later publication, a phthaloyl-protected phosphonamidate (phthaloyl-Gly^P-Ile.Trp.NHBzl) was reported to have similar activity (Kortylewicz and Galardy 1989).

15.3.4   Other ligands

Formyl hydroxylamine $HCO.N(OH)—$, a retro version of hydroxamic acid, is approximately six times less active than the corresponding hydroxamic acid (Johnson *et al.* 1987). Replacement of formyl by a larger acyl group (e.g. acetyl) destroys most of the activity. The carboxyalkylamino ligand $HOOC.CH(R).NH—$, which was very successful when used in the inhibition of ACE (Patchett *et al.* 1980), has only given moderate activity $(IC_{50} = 0.8 \ \mu M)$ against collagenase (McCullagh *et al.* 1984). Attempts to extend the R group in order to obtain additional binding from the S_1-S_4 subsites, has not improved the potency of these compounds (McCullagh *et al.* 1984; Johnson *et al.* 1987).

5.3.5   Peptide mimetics

There is now good agreement on the ligands, spacer groups, and subsite residues required for good inhibition of interstitial collagenase. However, these compounds are peptidic in nature, largely as a consequence of the substrate-based design strategy adopted (Schwartz and Van Wart 1991). Since peptides are easily hydrolysed in the gut, plasma, and other organs, protection against proteolytic destruction is essential for *in vivo* activity. Whilst there are many potential ways of modifying the peptidic nature of substrate analogues and therefore minimizing proteolytic destruction, one of the most successful strategies for collagenase inhibitors has been reported by Johnson *et al.* (1987). Using a computer graphics model of a C-terminal hydroxamate, derived from the structure of a collagen-like polymer (Gly.Pro.Hyp), together with structure–activity relationship data, they postulated that it would be possible to join the side-chain of P'_2 to the C-terminus of the P'_3 residue. This led to a series of lactams which, when the ring size was large enough (9) to accommodate a *trans* amide bond, had essentially the full activity of the linear inhibitor. Furthermore, incorporation of this lactam into a series of phosphinic acid transition state analogues led to a potent inhibitor Ro 31–7467 (11), which appeared to have complete metabolic stability.

Whilst such peptide mimetics may be metabolically stable there is no reason to assume that such molecules will have optimal pharmacokinetic properties *per se*. For example, oral bioavailability is likely to be a prerequisite for a collagenase inhibitor where long-term therapy is envisaged. The problems associated with meeting this requirement are significant, and they are compounded by a number of other factors. Plasma levels of a drug post-dose may be critical. The rate and route of excretion from plasma and the half-life of a drug need to be considered. Once in the plasma, the drug must be able to reach the site of action, which for arthritic disease processes is probably the cartilage within synovial joints. Thus distribution of the drug throughout the heterogeneous tissues of the joint, as well as cartilage penetration by the drug, may be pivotal to the clinical efficacy of a collagenase inhibitor.

It is possible for the medicinal chemist to modify the physicochemical properties (and thus, perhaps, the pharmacokinetic properties) of the inhibitors by judicious incorporation of different functional groups in a way that has little or no effect on the *in vitro* potency of the inhibitors. A series of hydroxamic acids which have different C-terminal end-groups, presumably to address some of these issues, has recently been described (Davidson *et al.* 1990). However, unless one can correlate improvements in a particular pharmacokinetic measurement with physicochemical parameters such as log P or pK_a, then finding a molecule with the 'ideal pharmacokinetic profile' is likely to remain an open ended, hit and miss affair.

15.4   Therapeutic uses of collagenase inhibitors

The exact role played by collagenase and other MMPs in normal physiological processes such as wound healing, ovulation, cell migration, and involution of the uterus after parturition and in disease processes such as arthritis, periodontal disease, tumour metastasis, and bone resorption is still poorly understood. However, the hypothesis that collagenase inhibitors will have a beneficial effect on excessive collagen turnover *in vivo* lies at the heart of whether a collagenase inhibitor will be therapeutically useful in diseases such as rheumatoid arthritis and osteoarthritis. Therefore evidence that collagenase inhibitors can inhibit collagen turnover *ex vivo*, or better still *in vivo*, is a crucial boundary between the many inhibitors with good *in vitro* potency and a therapeutically useful drug.

Nixon *et al.* (1991) have described the effect of two inhibitors, Ro 31–4724 (**7**, R = H) and Ro 31–7467 (**11**), on the degradation of collagen and proteoglycan from bovine nasal cartilage explants stimulated with interleukin-1α (IL-1α). The explants release glycosoaminoglycan (a measure of proteoglycan breakdown), followed by hydroxyproline (a measure of collagen turnover) in a dose-dependent manner upon stimulation with IL-1α. The phosphinic acid Ro 31–7467 inhibits the release of hydroxyproline, whilst the hydroxamic acid Ro 31–4724 inhibits the release of glycosoaminoglycan and hydroxyproline.

DiMartino *et al.* (1991) have reported the effects of a hydroxamic acid inhibitor BBL16 in the adjuvant model of arthritis. At intraperitoneal doses between 0.6 and 50 mg kg^{-1} there was a significant reduction of hindpaw swelling. However, the mechanism by which a collagenase inhibitor reduces paw swelling in adjuvant arthritis still remains unclear.

Although this review concentrates on the design of substrate derived inhibitors, there are an increasing number of reports of non-substrate-related compounds being active as collagenase inhibitors. Several tetracyclines have been shown to inhibit collagenase *in vitro* (Burns *et al.* 1989). They have been used in the treatment of rheumatoid arthritis (Greenwald *et al.* 1987), periodontal disease (Golub *et al.* 1985), and epidermolysis bullosa (White 1989). However, the clinical effects seen with these drugs have not been conclusively linked to their relatively weak collagenase inhibitory activity.

15.5   Conclusions

In this chapter it has been demonstrated that potent selective collagenase inhibitors have been designed from a knowledge of the substrate sequence and the catalytic mechanism.

A wealth of potent enzyme inhibitors are available and, provided that the pharmacokinetic hurdles can be overcome, the next few years should see significant progress in the clinical evaluation of such compounds in many disease states involving excessive turnover of collagen. These inhibitors should help to elucidate the role of collagenase in diseases such as arthritis and eventually lead to a new class of disease-modifying antirheumatic drugs (DMARDs).

References

Angel, P., Imagawa, M., Chiu, R., Stein, B., Imbra, R. J., Rahmsdorf, H. J., *et al.* (1987a). Phorbol ester-inducible genes contain a common *cis*-element recognised by a TPA-modulated trans-acting gene. *Cell*, **49**, 729–39.

Angel, P., Baumann, I., Stein, B., Delius, H., Rahmsdorf, H. J., and Herrlich, P. (1987b). 12-*O*-tetradecanoyl-phorbol-13 acetate (TPA) induction of the human collagenase gene is mediated by an inducible enhancer element located in the 5′-flanking region. *Molecular and Cellular Biology*, **7**, 2256–66.

Auble, D. T. and Brinckerhoff, C. E. (1991). The AP-1 sequence is necessary but not sufficient for phorbol induction of collagenase in fibroblasts. *Biochemistry*, **30**, 4629–35.

Brinckerhoff, C. E., Suzuki, K., Mitchell, T. I., Oram, F., Coon, C. I., Palmiter, R. D., and Nagase, H. (1990). Rabbit procollagenase synthesised and secreted by a high-yield mammalian vector requires stromelysin (matrix metalloproteinase-3) for maximal activation. *Journal of Biological Chemistry*, **265**, 22262–9.

Broadhurst, M. J., Handa, B. K., Johnson, W. H., Lawton, G., and Machin, P. J. (1988). Preparation and formulation of phosphinic acid derivatives as collagenase inhibitors. European Patent Application 276,436; *Chemical Abstracts*, **110**, 24085.

Burns, F. R., Stack, M. S., Gray, R. D., and Paterson, C. A. (1989). Inhibition of purified collagenase from alkali-burned rabbit corneas. *Investigative Ophthalmology and Visual Science*, **30**, 1569–75.

Cawston, T. E. and Barrett, A. J. (1979). A rapid and reproducible assay for collagenase using [1-^{14}C]acetylated collagen. *Analytical Biochemistry*, **99**, 340–5.

Cawston, T. E., Murphy, G., Mercer, E., Galloway, W. A., Hazleman, B. L., and Reynolds, J. J. (1983). The interaction of purified rabbit bone collagenase with purified rabbit bone metalloproteinase inhibitor. *Biochemical Journal*, **211**, 313–18.

Clark, I. M. and Cawston, T. E. (1989). Fragments of human fibroblast collagenase: purification and characterisation. *Biochemical Journal*, **263**, 201–6.

Darlak, K., Miller, R. B., Stack, M. S., Spatola, A. F., and Gray, R. D. (1990). Thiol-based inhibitors of mammalian collagenase. *Journal of Biological Chemistry*, **265**, 5199–205.

Davidson, A. H., Dickens, J. P., and Crimmin, M. J. (1990). Preparation and formulation of hydroxamic acid derivatives as collagenase inhibitors. International Patent Application 90,05716; *Chemical Abstracts*, **113**, 190468.

Dickens, J. P., Donald, D. K., Kneen, G., and McKay, W. R. (1986). Hydroxamic acid based collagenase inhibitors. US Patent 4,599,361; *Chemical Abstracts*, **105**, 153550.

DiMartino, M. J., Wolff, C. E., High, W., Crimmin, M. J., and Galloway, W. A. (1991). Anti-inflammatory and chondroprotective activities of a potent metalloproteinase inhibitor. *Journal of Cell Biochemistry*, **15E**, 179.

Docherty, A. J. P., Lyons, A., Smith, B. J., Wright, E. M., Stephens, P. E., Harris, T. J., *et al.* (1985). Sequence of human tissue inhibitor of metalloproteinases and its identity to erythoid-potentiating activity. *Nature, London*, **318**, 66–9.

Donald, D. K., Hann, M. M., Saunders, J., and Wadsworth, H. J. (1986).

N-(mercaptoalkanoyl) amino acid derivatives as collagenase inhibitors. US Patent 4,595,700; *Chemical Abstracts*, **105**, 209393.

Eastgate, J. A., Symons, J. A., Wood, N. C., Grinlinton, F. M., diGiovine, F. S., and Duff, G. W. (1988). Correlation of plasma interleukin 1 levels with disease activity in rheumatoid arthritis. *Lancet*, **ii**, 706–9.

Faucher, D. C., Lelievre, Y., and Cartwright, T. (1987). An inhibitor of mammalian collagenase active at micromolar concentrations from an actinomycete culture broth. *Journal of Antibiotics*, **40**, 1757–61.

Gadher, S. J., Eyre, D. R., Duance, V. C., Wotton, S. F., Heck, L. W., Schmid, T. M., and Woolley, D. E. (1988). Susceptibility of cartilage collagens Type II, IX, X and XI to human synovial collagenase and neutrophil elastase. *European Journal of Biochemistry*, **175**, 1–7.

Galloway, W. A., Murphy, G., Sandy, J. D., Gavrilovic, J., Cawston, T. E., and Reynolds, J. J. (1983). Purification and characterization of a rabbit bone metalloproteinase that degrades proteoglycan and other connective tissue components. *Biochemical Journal*, **209**, 741–52.

Gavrilovic, J. and Murphy, G. (1989). The role of plasminogen in cell-mediated collagen degradation. *Cell Biology International Reports*, **13**, 367–75.

Goldberg, G. I., Wilhelm, S. M., Kronberger, A-M., Bauer, E. A., Grant, G. A., and Eisen, A. Z. (1986). Human fibroblast collagenase. Complete primary structure and homology to an oncogene transformation-induced rat protein. *Journal of Biological Chemistry*, **261**, 6600–5.

Golub, L. M., Wolff, M., Lee, H. M., McNamara, T. F., Ramamurthy, N. S., Zambol, S., and Ciancio, S. (1985). Further evidence that tetracyclines inhibit collagenase activity in human crevicular fluid and from other mammalian sources. *Journal of Periodontal Research*, **20**, 12–23.

Gray, R. D., Saneii, H. H., and Spatola, A. F. (1981). Metal binding peptide inhibitors of vertebrate collagenase. *Biochemical and Biophysical Research Communications*, **101**, 1251–8.

Gray, R. D., Miller, R. B., and Spatola, A. F. (1986). Inhibition of mammalian collagenases by thiol-containing peptides. *Journal of Cellular Biochemistry*, **32**, 71–7.

Greenwald, R. A., Golub, L. M., Lavietes, B., Ramamurthy, N. S., Gruber, B., Laskin, R. S., and McNamara, T. F. (1987). Tetracyclines inhibit human synovial collagenase *in vivo* and *in vitro*. *Journal of Rheumatology*, **14**, 28–32.

Hasty, K. A., Pourmotabbed, T. F., Goldberg, G. I., Thompson, J. P., Spinella, D. G., Stevens, R. M., and Mainardi, C. L. (1990). Human neutrophil collagenase. A distinct gene product with homology to other matrix metalloproteinases. *Journal of Biological Chemistry*, **265**, 11421–4.

Hunter, D. J., Markwell, R. E., and Ward, R. W. (1989). N-(phosphonoalkyl)-dipeptide amides as collagenase inhibitors for treating arthritic diseases. European Patent Application 320,118; *Chemical Abstracts*, **112**, 56704.

Johnson, W. H., Roberts, N. A., and Borkakoti, N. (1987). Collagenase inhibitors: their design and potential therapeutic use. *Journal of Enzyme Inhibition*, **2**, 1–22.

Johnson-Wint, B. (1980). A quantitative collagen film collagenase assay for large numbers of samples. *Analytical Biochemistry*, **104**, 175–81.

Kortylewicz, Z. P. and Galardy, R. E. (1989). Phthaloyl-glycyl-isoleucyl-tryptophan benzylamide is a potent inhibitor of human skin fibroblast collagenase with a K_i of 25 nM. *Journal of Enzyme Inhibition*, **3**, 159–62.

Kortylewicz, Z. P. and Galardy, R. E. (1990). Phosphoramidate peptide inhibitors of human skin fibroblast collagenase. *Journal of Medicinal Chemistry*, **33**, 263–73.

Krane, S. M., Amento, E. P., Goldring, M. B., Goldring, S. R., and Stephenson, M. L. (1988). Modulation of matrix synthesis and degradation in joint inflammation. In *The control of tissue damage: research monographs in cell and tissue physiology* (ed. A. M. Glavert), Vol. 15, pp. 179–95. Elsevier, Amsterdam.

Lelievre, Y., Bouboutou, R., Boiziau, J., and Cartwright, T. (1989). Inhibition de la collagenase synoviale par 1′ actinonine etude de relations structure/activite. *Pathologie et Biologie*, **37**, 43–6.

Liotta, L. A., Steeg, P. S., and Stetler-Stevenson, W. G. (1991). Cancer metastasis and angiogenesis. An imbalance of positive and negative regulation. *Cell*, **64**, 327–36.

McCullagh, D., Wadsworth, H., and Hann, M. (1984). Carboxyalkyl peptide derivatives. European Patent Application 126,974; *Chemical Abstracts*, **102**, 221199.

Mainardi, C. L., Hasty, K. A., and Hibbs, M. S. (1988). Collagenolytic metalloproteinases of the human neutrophil. In *The control of tissue damage: research monographs in cell and tissue physiology* (ed. A. M. Glavert), Vol. 15, pp. 139–46. Elsevier, Amsterdam.

Markwell, R. E., Smith, S. A., and Hughes, I. (1988). *N*-(2-alkyl-3-mercapto-glutaryl) *a*-amino acid derivatives, process for their preparation and their use as collagenase inhibitors. European Patent Application 273,689; *Chemical Abstracts*, **110**, 232070.

Markwell, R. E., Smith, S. A., and Gaster, L. M. (1989). Preparation of *N*-(2-alkyl-3-mercapto-1,5-dioxoalkyl)glycinamides as collagenase inhibitors. European Patent Application 322,184; *Chemical Abstracts*, **112**, 36457.

Masui, Y., Takemoto, T., Sakakibara, S., Hori, H., and Nagai, Y. (1977). Synthetic substrates for vertebrate collagenase. *Biochemical Medicine*, **17**, 215–21.

Matthews, B. W. (1988). Structural basis of the action of thermolysin and related zinc peptidases. *Accounts of Chemical Research*, **21**, 333–40.

Mookhtiar, K. A., Marlowe, C. K., Bartlett, P. A., and Van Wart, H. E. (1987). Phosphonamidate inhibitors of human neutrophil collagenase. *Biochemistry*, **26**, 1962–5.

Moore, W. M. and Spilburg, C. A. (1986a). Purification of human collagenases with hydroxamic acid affinity column. *Biochemistry*, **25**, 5189–95.

Moore, W. M. and Spilburg, C. A. (1986b). Peptide hydroxamic acids inhibit skin collagenase. *Biochemical and Biophysical Research Communications*, **136**, 390–5.

Murphy, G. (1990). Purification of connective tissue metalloproteinases. In *Protein purification applications: a practical approach* (ed. E. L. V. Harris and S. Angal), pp. 142–6. IRL Press, Oxford.

Murphy, G. and Docherty, A. J. P. (1988). Molecular studies on the connective tissue metalloproteinases and their inhibitor TIMP. In *The control of tissue damage: research monographs in cell and tissue physiology* (ed. A. M. Glavert), Vol. 15, pp. 223–41. Elsevier, Amsterdam.

Murphy, G., Ward, R., Hembry, R. M., Reynolds, J. J., Kühn, K., and Tryggvason, K. (1989). Characterisation of gelatinase from pig polymorphonuclear leucocytes. *Biochemical Journal*, **258**, 463–72.

Nagai, Y., Masui, Y., and Sakakibara, S. (1976). Substrate specificity of verte-brate collagenase. *Biochimica et Biophysica Acta*, **45**, 521–4.

Netzel-Arnett, S., Fields, G., Birkedal-Hansen, H., and Van Wart, H. E. (1991a). Sequence specificities of human fibroblast and neutrophil collagenases. *Journal of Biological Chemistry*, **266**, 6747–55.

Netzel-Arnett, S., Mallya, S. K., Nagase, H., Birkedal-Hansen, H., and Van Wart, H. E. (1991b). Continuously recording fluorescent assays optimised for five human matrix metalloproteinases. *Analytical Biochemistry*, **195**, 86–92.

Nixon, J. S., Bottomley, K. M. K., Broadhurst, M. J., Brown, P. A., Johnson, W. H., Lawton, G., *et al.* (1991). Potent collagenase inhibitors prevent IL1-induced cartilage degradation *in vitro*. *International Journal of Tissue Reactions —Experimental and Clinical Aspects*, **13**, 237–41.

Odake, S., Okayama, T., Obata, M., Morikawa, T., Hattori, S., Hori, H., and Nagai, Y. (1990). Vertebrate collagenase inhibitor. I. Tripeptidyl hydroxamic acids. *Chemical and Pharmaceutical Bulletin*, **38**, 1007–11.

O'Hare, M. C., Clarke, N. J., Cawston, T. E., and Harper, G. P. (1991). Cloning of a cDNA for porcine type I collagenase and expression in *E. coli*. *Transactions of the Biochemical Society*, in press.

Ondetti, M. A., Rubin, B., and Cushman, D. W. (1977). Design of specific inhi-bitors of angiotensin-converting enzyme: a new class of orally active antihyper-tensive agents. *Science*, **196**, 441–4.

Ondetti, M. A., Condon, M. E., Reid, J., Sabo, E. F., Cheung, H. S., and Cushman, D. W. (1979). Design of potent and specific inhibitors of carboxy-peptidases A and B. *Biochemistry*, **18**, 1427–30.

Patchett, A. A., Harris, E., Tristram, E. W., Wyvratt, M. J., Wu, M. T., Taub, D., *et al.* (1980). A new class of angiotensin-converting enzyme inhibitors. *Nature, London*, **288**, 280–3.

Schechter, I. and Berger, A. (1967). On the size of the active site in pro-teases. I. Papain. *Biochemical and Biophysical Research Communications*, **27**, 157–62.

Schwartz, J.-C. (1989). Enkephalinase inhibitors as drugs. In *Design of enzyme inhibitors as drugs* (ed. M. Sandler and H. J. Smith), pp. 206–26. Oxford University Press.

Schwartz, M. A. and Van Wart, H. E. (1991). Synthetic inhibitors of bacterial and mammalian collagenases. In *Progress in medicinal chemistry* (ed. G. P. Ellis and G. B. West), Vol. 29, pp. 271–334. Elsevier, Amsterdam.

Schwartz, M. A., Venkataraman, S., Ghaffari, M. A., Libby, A., Mookhtiar, K. A., Mallya, S. K., and Van Wart, H. E. (1991). Inhibition of human colla-genases by sulfur-based substrate analogs. *Biochemical and Biophysical Research Communications*, **176**, 173–9.

Springman, E. B., Angleton, E. L., Birkedal-Hansen, H., and Van Wart, H. E. (1990). Multiple modes of activation of latent human fibroblast collagenase: Evi-dence for the role of Cys 73 active-site zinc complex in latency and 'Cysteine switch' mechanism for activation. *Proceedings of the National Academy of Sciences of the United States of America*, **87**, 364–8.

Stack, M. S. and Gray, R. D. (1989). Comparison of vertebrate collagenase and gelatinase using a new fluorogenic substrate peptide. *Journal of Biological Chemistry*, **264**, 4277–81.

Stricklin, G. P., Jeffrey, J. J., Roswit, W. T., and Eisen, A. Z. (1983). Human skin fibroblast procollagenase: mechanisms of activation by organomercurials and trypsin. *Biochemistry*, **22**, 63–8.

Sundeen, J. E. and Dejneka, T. (1981). Inhibitors of mammalian collagenase. US Patent Application 4,297,275; *Chemical Abstracts*, **96**, 104789.

Suzuki, K., Enghild, J. J., Morodomi, T., Salvesen, G., and Nagase, H. (1990). Mechanisms of activation of tissue procollagenase by matrix metalloproteinase 3 (stromelysin). *Biochemistry*, **29**, 10261–70.

Thorsett, E. D., Harris, E. E., Peterson, E. R., Greenlee, W. J., Patchett, A. A., Ulm, E. H., and Vassil, T. C. (1982). Phosphorus-containing inhibitors of angiotensin-converting enzyme. *Proceedings of the National Academy of Sciences of the United States of America*, **79**, 2176–80.

Weingarten, H., Martin, R., and Feder, J. (1985). Synthetic substrates of vertebrate collagenase. *Biochemistry*, **24**, 6730–4.

White, J. E. (1989). Minocycline for dystrophic epidermolysis bullosa. *Lancet*, **i**, 966.

Williamson, R. A., Marston, F. A. O., Angal, S., Koklitis, P., Panico, M., Morris, H. R., *et al.* (1990). Disulphide bond assignment in human tissue inhibitor of metalloproteinases (TIMP). *Biochemical Journal*, **268**, 267–74.

Windsor, L. J., Birkedal-Hansen, H., Birkedal-Hansen, B., and Engler, J. A. (1991). An internal cysteine plays a role in the maintenance of the latency of human fibroblast collagenase. *Biochemistry*, **30**, 641–7.

Inhibitors of aldose reductase

Dushan Dvornik

16.1   Introduction

Aldose reductase (AR) inhibitors are designed to interfere with the initiation and early development of secondary complications of chronic diabetes mellitus. The concept was deduced from the insight that, in diabetic tissues with insulin-independent glucose uptake, excess glucose is metabolized via the polyol (sorbitol) pathway.

16.2   Polyol pathway

The polyol pathway comprises two enzymatic reactions: in tandem, glucose is reduced to sorbitol by AR using NADPH, and sorbitol is oxidized to fructose by sorbitol dehydrogenase using NAD^+ (Fig. 16.1). According to Vander Jagt *et al.* (1990), AR functions as an NADPH-binding protein, thus facilitating oxidation of NADPH. In contrast with other aldehyde or ketone reductases, such as lactate dehydrogenase (LDH) or alcohol dehydrogenase (ADH), AR is almost exclusively a 'one-way catalyst, with a ratio of catalytic efficiency for the forward versus the reverse reaction that is 1000–100 000 times higher than that for either LDH or ADH (Grimshaw 1991).

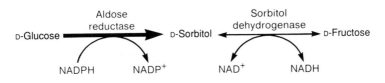

Fig. 16.1   Polyol (sorbitol) pathway.

The polyol pathway was first found by Hers (1956) in the seminal vesicles of sheep. However, current evidence does not support the earlier view that seminal fructose is related to sperm motility (Gonzales 1989). Interest in the polyol pathway was prompted by its detection in the lenses of rats with experimental diabetes or galactosaemia (van Heiningen 1959). While it is well known that sugar cataract formation is readily induced in rats by experimental galactosaemia or diabetes, our understanding of the pathogenesis of sugar cataract started to develop only after a primary role was assigned to AR. Kinoshita *et al.* (1962) postulated that the development of sugar cataract is initiated by the osmotic swelling of lens fibres caused by the intracellular accumulation of sugar alcohols (polyols) formed from the sugar by the action of AR. In order to validate the hypothesis, Kinoshita and colleagues attempted to prevent cataract formation by inhibiting aldose reductase. Indeed, tetramethyleneglutaric acid, the first experimentally useful AR inhibitor, prevented both polyol accumulation and the ensuing swelling and opacification of rabbit lenses incubated in sugar-rich medium in a concentration-dpendent fashion (Kinoshita *et al.* 1968).

Of greater importance was the recognition that, at hyperglycaemia-induced lenticular sugar concentrations above the binding capacity of the increased though rate-limiting hexokinase, the excess sugar is disposed of by AR (Sochor *et al.* 1990); this was also observed in other tissues not requiring insulin for glucose uptake, i.e. hyperglycaemic diabetic tissues susceptible to chronic complications (Gabbay 1975). Indeed, a considerable body of experimental and clinical results now supports the theory that, in such tissues, a cascade of metabolic abnormalities, progressing steadily to cellular dysfunction and structural lesions, is initiated by the disposal of excess tissue glucose by AR (Dvornik 1987a; Kinoshita and Nishimura 1988; Harrison *et al.* 1989; Stribling *et al.* 1989a,b, 1990).

16.3   Aldose reductase

AR belongs to a large family of aldehyde reductases (Carper *et al.* 1987; Bohren *et al.* 1989) which are cytosolic monomeric enzymes that stereo-selectively reduce aldehydes to their corresponding alcohols. Mammalian tissues contain two major aldehyde reductases: one predominates in the liver, brain, and kidney, and is referred to in this chapter as 'hexonate dehydrogenase', and the other, 'aldose reductase', is present in a variety of tissues, notably those susceptible to complications of long-term diabetes (Dvornik 1987c). Enzymes belonging to the 'super- family' of aldehyde reductases employ nicotinamide adenosine dinucleotides as cofactors; while AR has dual nucleotide specificity, hexonate dehydrogenase is NADPH specific.

AR is present in the paranodal cytoplasm of Schwann cells (Chakrabarti *et al*. 1987), in the terminal expansions of paranodal myelin lamellae and nodal microvilli (Powell *et al*. 1991), in Henle's loop, the collecting tubules, and the epithelial cells lining the pelvis of the inner medulla near the kidney papilla (Terubayashi *et al*. 1988), in the Muller cells of the retina (particularly near the inner limiting membrane), the pericytes, the retinal capillaries (but not the endothelial cells), some ganglion and cone cells, and the axon of the optic nerve (Akagi *et al*. 1984; Chakrabarti *et al*. 1987), and in many other locations (Dvornik 1987c). Increased AR activity was found in the lens, kidney, sciatic nerve, skeletal muscle, retina, and spinal cord of spontaneously diabetic BB rats (Ghahary *et al*. 1991) and in the kidney of experimentally diabetic rats (Ghahary *et al*. 1989. The increase was due to enhanced AR gene expression and was reversed by insulin treatment. While AR was immunohistochemically undetectable in retinal pigment epithelium of non-diabetic subjects, it was detected in 55 per cent of diabetic patients with background retinopathy; 87.5 per cent of patients with proliferative retinopathy showed bilateral staining of the pigment epithelium (Vinores *et al*. 1988).

All the tissues examined, except human skeletal muscle (Vander Jagt *et al*. 1990), also contained hexonate dehydrogenase (Sato and Kador 1991). Despite approximately 50 per cent homology in their amino acid sequences (Carper *et al*. 1987) and their partially overlapping substrate specificities, AR and hexonate dehydrogenase differ in molecular mass, isoelectric points, immunological cross-reactivities, and affinity for D-glucose, which is high for AR and very low for hexonate dehydrogenase (Kawasaki *et al*. 1989; Morjana and Flynn 1989; Ohta *et al*. 1990). Hexonate dehydrogenase derives its name from its high affinity for D-glucuronate. While all aldehyde reductases have a high proline content (7–8 per cent), AR has a higher cysteine content (Morjana and Flynn 1989). Topological differences at the active sites of the two enzymes became evident when they reacted with pyridoxal 5'-phosphate (PLP): while AR was activated in a concentration-dependent fashion, hexonate dehydrogenase was inactivated (Morjana *et al*. 1989). The reaction with PLP occurred at the lysine involved in the binding of the 2'-hydroxyl-phosphate of adenine ribose in NADPH. This finding was surprising in view of the virtually identical amino acid sequences around the reactive lysine in AR and hexonate dehydrogenase (Morjana *et al*. 1989).

Human AR (L-alditol, NADP$^+$ 1-oxidoreductase, EC 1.1.1.21) is a 316 amino acid protein with a molecular mass of 35 858 Da (Nishimura *et al.* 1988; Bohren *et al.* 1989; Grundman *et al.* 1990; Graham *et al.* 1991). Peptide sequencing of bovine AR (Schade *et al.* 1990) and complementary DNA sequencing of rat (Carper *et al.* 1987) and human AR (Bohren *et al.* 1989; Chung and LaMendola 1989; Graham *et al.* 1989; Grundmann *et al.* 1990) have been reported. Comparisons of the composite amino acid sequence for rat, rabbit, bovine, and human AR indicate that AR is structurally similar in different species and tissues (Carper 1990). The human enzyme has bee expressed in a *Baculovirus* system (Nishimura *et al.* 1991) and in *Escherichia coli* (Grundmann *et al.* 1990), and the structure of its gene determined (Graham *et al.* 1991). AR in crystalline form was obtained from porcine lens (Rondeau *et al.* 1987) and muscle (El-Kabbani *et al.* 1991).

The 'native' form of AR contains a tightly bound NADP$^+$; its binding depends on the reduced state of the seven cysteine residues of AR (Del Corso *et al.* 1990, Vander Jagt *et al.* 1990). In the absence of NADP$^+$, the 'native' enzyme is transformed by linking two cysteine residues at or near the coenzyme binding site (Liu *et al.* 1989); the transformation is prevented or reversed by dithiothreitol. The ensuing structural change results in a stereospecific decline in affinity for glyceraldehyde (Del Corso *et al.* 1989) and a decrease in susceptibility to AR inhibitors (Bhatnagar *et al.* 1989). The latter depends on the inhibitor's chemical structure, ranging from 8.8-fold for tolrestat to 6857-fold for ponalrestat (Vander Jagt *et al.* 1990) thus indicating that the AR inhibitors do not bind at the same site, at least on the 'modified' AR (Bhatnagar *et al.* 1989). These observations make it likely that the frequently reported differences in kinetic behaviour of AR preparations isolated from different species and tissues (Vander Jagt *et al.* 1990; Grimshaw 1990a,b) were due to mixtures of the two enzyme forms produced inadvertently during enzyme purification. It is not likely that the NADP$^+$-depleted form of AR occurs *in vivo* (Nishimura *et al.* 1991).

16.4 Aldose reductase inhibitors

Inspired by the results obtained in animal models of diabetic hyperglycaemia and in exploratory clinical studies with alrestatin, the first orally effective AR inhibitor (Dvornik *et al.* 1973), a pharmacological rationale was formulated for the development of AR inhibitors as drugs to control the development of diabetic complications in man (Dvornik 1978). Coupled with the availability of a simple, rapid, and readily reproducible procedure for the detection of AR inhibition *in vitro* (Hayman and Kinoshita 1965), the concept has attracted many investigators, and over the past 15 years scores of different substances have been found to inhibit AR

(Humber 1987; Larson *et al.* 1988) However, very few exhibited *in vivo* characteristics suitable for development into a clinically acceptable drug. Eventually it became clear that the lack of activity *in vivo* was due mainly to the inadequate tissue pharmacokinetics of the inhibitors (Dvornik *et al.* 1988). Virtually all experimental and clinical results have been generated with five orally active AR inhibitors: alrestatin (Dvornik *et al.* 1973), sorbinil (Peterson *et al.* 1979), epalrestat (Kikkawa *et al.* 1983), tolrestat (Sestanj *et al.* 1984), and ponalrestat (Stribling *et al.* 1985).

About 10 AR inhibitors have been tested in human subjects (Hotta and Sakamoto 1990) in investigations ranging from short pharmaco-kinetic studies (Gabbay *et al.* 1979; Foulds *et al.* 1981; Mizuno *et al.* 1990; Sawada *et al.* 1990; Brazzell *et al.* 1991) to chronic clinical trials (Dvornik 1987c; Hotta *et al.* 1990; Stribling 1990a) aimed at uncovering efficacy upon intervention with AR inhibitors in diabetic patients with clinically evident neuropathy (Krentz *et al.* 1989a; Greene *et al.* 1989b; Boulton *et al.* 1990; Dietrich *et al.* 1990; Gill *et al.* 1990; Green and Jaspan 1990; Greene *et al.* 1990; Masson and Boulton 1990; Florkowski *et al.* 1991; Gieron *et al.* 1991; Gonen *et al.* 1991; Greene and Sima 1991; Macleod and Sonksen 1991; Pinget *et al.* 1991; Sima and Greene 1991; Ziegler *et al.* 1991), keratopathy (Fukushi 1988), limited joint mobility (Eaton 1986), retinopathy (Hotta and Sakamoto 1990; Sorbinil Retinopathy Trial Research Group 1990), and incipient nephropathy (Sato *et al.* 1988; Blohme and Smith 1989; Jennings *et al.* 1990; Christiansen *et al.* 1991; Passariello *et al.* 1991; Pedersen *et al.* 1991).

16.4.1   Chemical structure and inhibitory activity

Chemically, the clinically tested AR inhibitors form two classes: aryl-substituted acetic acids, and acidic cyclic imides, mainly *spiro*-hydantoins or *spiro*-succinimides. Retrospective scrutiny of the pathways of chemical design of AR inhibitors suggests that, to some extent, they are all struc-turally related to alrestatin, sorbinil, or ponalrestat (Figs 16.2–16.4). The effect of chemical modifications of AR inhibitors on their intrinsic inhibitory activity is illustrated in Table 16.1. According to available data, all AR inhibitors in current use are either uncompetitive, i.e. sorbinil (Peterson *et al.* 1979), tolrestat (Simard-Duquesne *et al.* 1985), and epal-restat (Terashima 1988), or non-competitive, i.e. ponalrestat (Tuffin *et al.* 1989), FK-366 (Ao *et al.* 1991), zopolrestat (Mylari *et al.* 1991), SNK-860 (Mizuno *et al.* 1990), and AD-5467 (Ikeda 1990). This indicates that the inhibitors bind at allosteric sites (Grimshaw *et al.* 1989) that are dis-tinct from the catalytically active site. It is of practical importance that the extent of non-competitive inhibition is not influenced by substrate concentration, whereas the extent of uncompetitive inhibition would increase

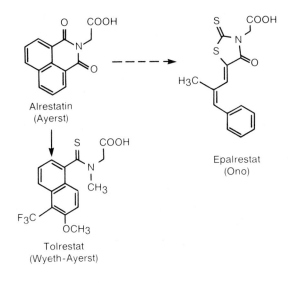

Fig. 16.2 Alrestatin-related AR inhibitors.

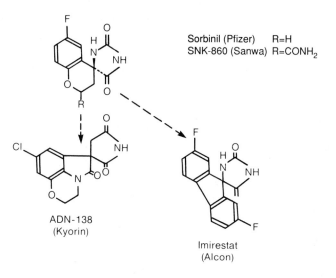

Fig. 16.3 Sorbinil-related AR inhibitors.

with substrate concentration. Therefore, in theory uncompetitive AR inhibitors would be preferred for therapeutic use (Terashima 1988).

Despite considerable differences in their chemical structure and ensuing physicochemical properties, effective AR inhibitors appear to possess some

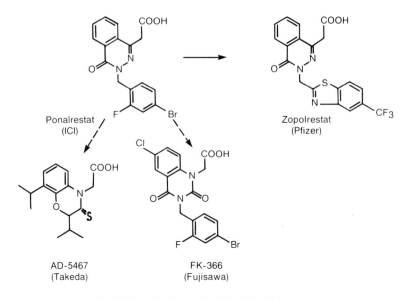

Fig. 16.4 Ponalrestat-related AR inhibitors.

Table 16.1 *In vitro* inhibitory activity of clinically tested AR inhibitors

AR inhibitor (originator)	Rat lens aldose reductase IC_{50} ($\times 10^{-9}$ M)	Reference
Alrestatin (Ayerst)	4000	Dvornik *et al.* 1987c
Tolrestat (Wyeth-Ayerst)	6	Dvornik *et al.* 1987c
Epalrestat (Ono)	14	Dvornik *et al.* 1987c
Sorbinil (Pfizer)	400	Dvornik *et al.* 1987c
SNK-860 (Sanwa)	20	Mizuno *et al.* 1990
Imirestat (Alcon)	16	Dvornik *et al.* 1987c
ADN-138 (Kyorin)	250	Hotta and Sakamoto 1990
Ponalrestat (ICI)	13	Dvornik *et al.* 1987c
FK-366 (Fujisawa)	4	Ao *et al.* 1991
Zopolrestat (Pfizer)	41	Mylari *et al.* 1991
AD-5467 (Takeda)	129	Ikeda 1990

common planar lipophilic regions and moieties that can undergo a reversible charge−transfer interaction (Kador *et al.* 1986). According to Kador (1990), AR inhibitors may induce conformational perturbation(s) of the

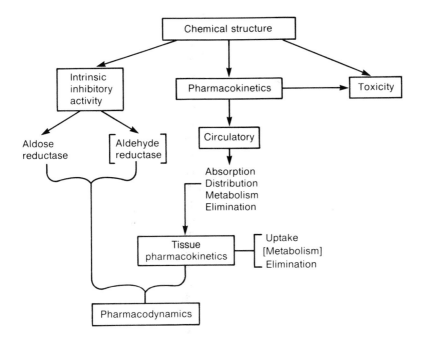

Fig. 16.5 Chemical structure determines the properties of AR inhibitors.

Table 16.2 Plasma half-lives of clinically tested AR inhibitors in human subjects

AR inhibitor	Plasma half-life (hours)	Estimated	
		No. of doses to attain steady state	Accumulation factor
Alrestatin	0.8 *	1	1.0
Tolrestat	9 − 13 †	2.5 − 4	1.2 − 1.4
Epalrestat	0.8 ‡	1	1.0
Sorbinil	68 ± 5 §	18	4.5
SNK-860	1.7 ¶	1	1.0
Imirestat	72 ± 21 ‖	20 ± 6	4.8 ± 1.8
Ponakrestat	15 − 51 **	4 − 14	1.5 − 3.6
Zopolrestat	27.5 ††	8	2.2

* Gabbay *et al.* 1979
† Hicks *et al.* 1984
‡ Sawada *et al.* 1990
§ Scott *et al.* 1987

¶ Mizuno *et al.* 1990
‖ Brazell *et al.* 1990
** Price *et al.* 1988
†† Mylari *et al.* 1991

enzyme either by creating a 'charge-transfer' bridge between the nucleophilic (carbonyl) moiety of the inhibitor and an 'acidic' residue or via an ionic interaction between inhibitor and enzyme.

Clearly, it is the chemical structure which, by determining the physico-chemical properties of a compound, enables it to inhibit AR and, by establishing the compound's pharmacokinetics, also establishes both its pharmacodynamics and its potential toxicity (Fig. 16.5). While the pharmacodynamics of an AR inhibitor corresponds to the degree of AR inhibition in a given tissue, its pharmacokinetics reflects how an organism, animal or human, acts upon the inhibitor. This is illustrated by the differences in plasma half-lives between the clinically tested AR inhibitors and the derived pharmacokinetic propensity to accumulation in plasma upon repetitive dosing (Welling 1986) (Table 16.2).

16.4.2   Chemical structure and tissue pharmacokinetics

Axiomatically, an effective AR inhibitor should interfere with AR activity in every hyperglycaemic diabetic tissue susceptible to developing chronic complication. In such tissues, the pharmacodynamics of an AR inhibitor corresponds to its concentration at the AR site(s). Such bioavailability is determined by the tissue pharmacokinetics of the inhibitor, i.e. by the processes determining the uptake and elimination, or perhaps metabolism, of the inhibitor in a relevant tissue (Dvornik 1987c). To assess the dependence of pharmacodynamic efficacy of an AR inhibitor on its circulatory and tissue pharmacokinetics, the dose and pharmacological effect are correlated with the drug concentrations in blood and in a selected tissue. Such a relationship was demonstrated in the sciatic nerves of severely galactosaemic rats and dogs treated with the AR inhibitor tolrestat (Dvornik et al. 1988). The localization of tolrestat at the AR site(s) in the sciatic nerves was established by the marked fall in nerve galactitol concentrations. Comparison of these results with those obtained in sural nerve biopsy specimens collected from patients with diabetic neuropathy and treated with tolrestat (Greene et al. 1990; unpublished results) indicates that, in all three species, similar decreases in nerve polyol levels were associated with comparable nerve drug levels (Table 16.3). This suggests that, in the three species, similar portions of the total drug levels (measured in the nerve samples) have reached the AR site(s). In diabetic patients, treatment with tolrestat resulted in improved nerve fibre pathology (Greene and Sima 1991). Lack of efficacy of ponalrestat (at 600 mg daily) (Price et al. 1989; Krentz et al. 1989a; Dietrich et al. 1990; Gill et al. 1990; Florkowski et al. 1991; Zegler et al. 1991) was attributed to insignificant nerve tissue penetration, and further clinical trials were discontinued (Kirchain and Rendell 1990).

Table 16.3 Comparative pharmacokineiics and pharmacodynamics of an AR inhibitor (tolrestat) in the peripheral nerve of galactosaemic rats and dogs, and in patients with advanced diabetic neuropathy

Species	Condition (duration)	n	Dose (mg kg^{-1} daily)	AR inhibitor concentration		
				Serum (free, ng ml^{-1} ± SE)	Nerve (μg g^{-1} ± SE)	Decrease in nerve polyol accumulation (%)
Rat[*]	Experimental galactosaemia (178 days)	5	7	7.5 ± 0.7	0.9 ± 0.1	58
Dog[*]	Experimental galactosaemia (4 days)	4	5	28 ± 8	0.5 ± 0.1	58
Man[†]	Diabetes mellitus[‡] (17.6 ± 2.9 years)	2	< 3	8,10[§]	1.0,0.6[§]	73,56[¶]
		9	< 6	23 ± 4[§]	1.1 ± 0.1[§]	60[¶]

[*] Dvornik et al. 1988
[†] Greene et al. 1990; unpublished results
[‡] Patients with neuropathy of 6.5 ± 0.6 years duration received tolrestat 200 or 400 mg daily) for an average of 5 years.
[§] Blood and sural nerve specimens obtained 25–32.5 hours after tolrestat dose.
[¶] Compared with diabetic patients given tolrestat for an average of 4 years, followed by tolrestat withdrawal for 1 year.

16.4.3 Chemical structure and side-effects

A Dilantin-like hypersensitivity reaction was produced in about 10 per cent of human subjects upon administration of AR inhibitors possessing a Dilantin-like *spiro*-hydantoin or *spiro*-succinimide structure, i.e. sorbinil (Pitts et al. 1986; Green and Jaspan 1990; Kirchain and Rendell 1990) and ADN-138 (Hotta and Sakamoto 1990). Therefore new clinical studies of sorbinil (Asbury 1988) and ADN-138 (Hotta and Sakamoto 1990) have been deferred. The hypersensitivity reaction was tentatively attributed to genetic abnormalities in the detoxification of reactive metabolites of Dilantin and sorbinil (Spielberg et al. 1991). Evidence that the hypersensitivity reactions to sorbinil and ADN-138 had no relation to AR inhibition was provided by the absence of such reactions in patients treated with non-hydantoin AR inhibitors such as tolrestat (Ryder et al. 1987; Boulton et al. 1990) and ponalrestat (Stribling 1988).

16.4.4 Clinical effectiveness

A number of clinical trials with AR inhibitors have been performed. According to Ward (1990), 'the role of AR inhibitors in the treatment of diabetic neuropathy remains the area of the greatest interest in neuropathy studies', particularly in view of encouraging evidence that treatment with systemically bioavailable AR inhibitors improved clinically relevant parameters of nerve fibre pathology in patients with advanced diabetic neuropathy (Sima *et al.* 1987, 1988b; Greene and Sima 1991). While clinical and functional improvement were not striking (Masson and Boulton 1990; Ward 1990), the results from randomized placebo-controlled multi-centre interventive trials of sorbinil (Greene *et al.* 1989b) and tolrestat (Boulton *et al.* 1989, 1990; Macleod and Sonksen 1991; Gonen *et al.* 1991) indicate benefits, notably in patients with milder neuropathy and poorer glycaemic control (Pinget *et al.* 1991). Supporting evidence was provided by relapse upon withdrawal of AR inhibitor treatment (Gonen *et al.* 1991). Interventive trials of intensified insulin therapy, the only alternative non-invasive method of metabolic control, have not shown greater improvement in nerve function; at best, an arrest of the small amount of decline was detectable over a period of 2 years (Watkins 1990). In fact, there is some disagreement (Zimmerman 1989) as to whether recent studies (Lauritzen *et al.* 1985; Mühlhauser *et al.* 1987; Brinchmann-Hansen *et al.* 1988; Kroc Collaborative Study Group 1988) have (Hanssen *et al.* 1986; Deckert 1988) or have not (DCCT Research Group 1988) demonstrated that intervention with intensive insulin therapy controls the development of diabetic complications. However, in insulin-dependent diabetics, effective glycaemic control initiated immediately after diagnosis prevented the early deterioration of nerve function (Ziegler *et al.* 1988), and 5 years of intensified conventional insulin treatment retarded the progression of microvascular complications (Reichard *et al.* 1991). The trials of both intensified insulin therapy and AR inhibitor treatment were hampered by similar problems, including methods of measurement with high coefficients of variation (Macleod and Sonksen 1991) which made it impossible to detect minor changes accurately, for example those during neuropathy itself (Watkins 1990), and difficult to define 'hard' end-points for all measures of nerve integrity (Masson and Boulton 1990). When combined, these findings suggest that the outcome of a trial was predestined by patient selection and duration of treatment. Given the inadequate understanding of the natural history of the disease (Stribling 1990b), it was extremely difficult to conduct properly designed clinical trials with treatments aimed at preventing the adverse progression of chronic diabetic complications (Feinstein 1989; Zimmerman 1989). This was particularly notable with respect to the extent of tissue damage at the time of intervention, the duration of therapy, for example in retinopathy (Sorbinil

Retinopathy Trial Research Group 1990), and the number of subjects needed to detect a treatment effect (Macleod and Sonksen 1991).

Thus, in retrospect, it is not surprising that the trials of AR inhibitors have failed to produce unequivocal evidence of clinical benefit to patients with clinically overt diabetic complications. A major hope for better natural history data lies with the Diabetes Control and Complication Trial (DCCT Research Group 1986) which was designed to assess both the parameters of subclinical nerve dysfunction and the appearance of clinically overt neuropathy in patients randomly assigned to conventional or intensive insulin therapy. It is hoped that the DCCT will establish the predictability of functional tests for the development of clinical neuropathy, as well as assessing the ability of strict metabolic control to prevent, delay, or ameliorate diabetic neuropathy. In the meantime, some of the best natural history data are emerging from controlled clinical trials with AR inhibitors (Krentz et al. 1989b; Boulton et al. 1990; Armstrong et al. 1991; Christiansen et al. 1991; Gonen et al. 1991; Greene and Sima 1991; Jennings et al. 1990; Passariello et al. 1991; Pedersen et al. 1991; Sorbinil Retinopathy Trial Research Group 1990).

Despite some encouraging results in exploratory trials of AR inhibitors (Cunha-Vaz et al. 1986; Hotta et al. 1988), no clinically important effect on the course of retinopathy was found with sorbinil in insulin-dependent diabetics with mild or no retinopathy (Sorbinil Retinopathy Trial Research Group 1990). However, the number of microaneurysms increased at a slightly lower rate in sorbinil-treated patients. In view of the negative trials of 2–5 years of intensified insulin therapy (Lauritzen et al. 1985; Kroc Collaborative Study Group 1988; Brinchmann-Hansen et al. 1988; Verillo et al. 1988), it is very likely that 2–3 years of AR inhibitor treatment was too short a time to detect any differences between the progression of retinopathy in treated and non-treated subjects (Frank 1990). Intensified insulin treatment for 5 years (Reichard et al. 1991) to 7 years (Dahl-Jorgensen et al. 1990) was needed to retard the progression of retinopathy in insulin-dependent diabetics.

Treatment of diabetic patients with AR inhibitors lowered the increased glomerular filtration rate (Blohme and Smith 1989; Christiansen et al. 1991; Pedersen et al. 1991) and decreased urinary protein excretion (Sato et al. 1988; Jennings et al. 1990; Passariello et al. 1991; Pedersen et al. 1991), thus suggesting a link between AR activity and some of the early changes in diabetic kidney function.

16.4.5 Aldose reductase inhibitors as pathobiochemical probes

As well as creating an incentive for drug-oriented research, the AR inhibition concept has instigated the use of AR inhibitors as probes to characterize the chronology of the metabolic, functional, and structural abnormalities triggered in diabetic tissues by the AR-catalysed disposal of excess glucose (Dvornik 1989). The role of AR in the initiation of the hyperglycaemia-induced cascade of diabetic tissue abnormalities was substantiated by the prevention of its occurrence in animal models of diabetic hyperglycaemia by treatment with effective AR inhibitors (Dvornik 1987b,c; Hotta and Sakamoto 1990). Selected representative findings are listed in Table 16.4. The fact that AR inhibitors prevented a number of abnormalities strongly suggests that the evolution of dysfunction in a hyperglycaemic diabetic tissue is not initiated by hyperglycaemia *per se*. Two points support this conclusion: first, essentially similar results were obtained with several structurally unrelated AR inhibitors; second, all effects occurred in the presence of highly elevated systemic sugar concentrations. The latter suggests that glycation is not involved in the initiation and early development of diabetic complications.

Of particular interest is the use of AR inhibitors as pathobiochemical probes to link the abnormalities occurring in hyperglycaemic diabetic tissues into plausible pathogenetic schemes (Finegold *et al.* 1983; Winegrad 1987; Tomlinson *et al.* 1988; Hotta and Sakamoto 1990). This is exemplified by the formulation and extension of the polyol pathway theory (Dvornik 1987a; Kinoshita 1988; Harrison *et al.* 1989) in the nerve by the 'myoinositol depletion' hypothesis (Greene *et al.* 1985, 1987a), and the 'myoinositol uptake/Na^+,K^+-ATPase dysfunction' hypothesis (Winegrad 1987). While it is readily demonstrable in peripheral nerves of acutely diabetic animals (Dvornik 1987a), myoinositol depletion was not found in fresh nerve tissue of diabetic subjects (Dyck *et al.* 1980, 1988; Hale *et al.* 1987; Willars *et al.* 1987; Greene *et al.* 1990). The myoinositol depletion hypothesis thus remains controversial (Lambourne *et al.* 1987, 1988; Llewelyn *et al.* 1987; Greene *et al.* 1989a; Miwa *et al.* 1989; Calcutt *et al.* 1990; Sredy *et al.* 1991) and unproven (Dyck *et al.* 1989; Tomlinson 1989; Hirata and Okada 1990). The pathogenetic scheme was expanded by connecting the impaired activation of the membrane Na^+,K^+-ATPase with sodium accumulation at the nodes of Ranvier, and the ensuing paranodal axonal swelling, axoglial dysjunction (Sima *et al.* 1988a), and paranodal demyelination (Greene *et al.* 1988). The link between nerve sorbitol accumulation and myelinated fibre atrophy, axoglial dysjunction, and nerve fibre degeneration was corroborated by their reversal in patients with diabetic neuropathy upon treatment with the systemically bioavailable AR inhibitors sorbinil (Sima *et al.* 1988b), and tolrestat (Greene *et al.* 1990; Greene and Sima 1991).

Results generated with AR inhibitors in animal models of diabetic hyperglycaemia and in diabetic subjects are also expanding our understanding of the natural history of diabetic complications. An appreciation of the stage of a tissue abnormality and its dependence upon metabolic control would be of particular importance for interventive therapy (by intensified

Table 16.4 Demonstration of the pivotal role of AR in hyperglycaemia-induced abnormalities in animal models of diabetic hyperglycaemia

Type of abnormality	Hyperglycaemia-induced abnormality prevented by AR Inhibitor treatment	Reference
Metabolic	Polyol accumulation	Dvornik 1987c
	Myoinositol depletion (nerve, glomeruli, retina)	Dvornik 1987c
	Na^+, K^+-ATPase impairment (nerve, glomeruli)	Dvornik 1987c
	Endoneurial Na accumulation	Dvornik 1987c
	Ascorbic acid depletion	McLennan et al. 1988; Yue et al. 1989
	Decreased nerve conduction velocity	Dvornik 1987c
	Glomerular hyperperfusion	Bank et al. 1989; Goldfarb et al. 1991; Oates et al. 1991
Functional	Decreased axonal transport	Dvornik 1987c
	Contractile dysfunction (skeletal, cardiac papillary, and atrial muscle)	Cameron et al. 1990; Colter et al. 1991
	Cardiac β-adrenoceptor supersensitivity	Austin and Chess-Williams 1991
	Decreased non-cholinergic motor transmission	Lukeshi and Zar 1990
	RBC swelling, decreased filterability	Kowluru et al. 1989
	Albuminuria	McCaleb et al. 1988, 1991; Tilton et al. 1989; Pugliese et al. 1990
	Delayed corneal re-epithelialization	Dvornik 1987c
Structural	Cataract	Dvornik 1987c
	Basement membrane thickening (retina)	Robinson et al. 1989a; McCaleb et al. 1991
	Pericyte loss, micro-aneurysm formation (retina)	Robinson et al. 1989b; 1990
	Endothelial abnormalities (cornea)	Datiles et al. 1990
	Paranodal axonal swelling	Greene et al. 1987b; Sima et al. 1990
	Axoglial dysjunction	Greene et al. 1987b; Sima et al. 1990

insulin treatment or with AR inhibitors). Clearly, metabolic control can prevent, arrest, or reverse an abnormality in a diabetic tissue only if the latter still depends on the underlying metabolic aberration that initiated it, thus suggesting the existence of a diabetic 'point of no return' (Viberti *et al.* 1983; Frank 1984; Verillo *et al.* 1988) or a 'point of little return' (Siegel 1990). Of particular interest was the finding that extended treatment with an effective AR inhibitor can 'improve clinically relevant parameters of nerve fibre pathology in diabetic patients with advanced neuropathy' (Greene and Sima 1991). The results suggest that, even in diabetics with neuropathy of long duration (6.5 ± 0.6 years), the morphometrically detectable nerve abnormalities were still dependent upon the metabolic aberrations caused by the AR-catalysed disposal of excess glucose in the nerve. The studies have also demonstrated a link between the degree of nerve fibre loss and the extent of sensory deficit (Sima and Greene 1991).

16.5   Role of aldose reductase in non-diabetic tissues

Despite wide tissue distribution, a vital role for AR non-diabetic tissue has not been found (Dvornik 1987c; Harrison *et al.* 1989; Masson and Boulton 1990). This is not surprising because, owing to its low affinity for glucose, at normal glucose concentrations AR cannot compete with hexokinase for glucose. This is reflected in barely detectable sorbitol levels in tissues of non-diabetic animals and human subjects (Dvornik 1987a,c) except in erythrocytes and the renal medulla. The coincident existence in the inner renal medulla of a gradient of both sorbitol content (Oates and Goddu 1987; Wirtensohn *et al.* 1987, 1989; Guder *et al.* 1988; Chauncey *et al.* 1988) AR activity (Chauncey *et al.* 1988; Sands *et al.* 1989) has led to the view that AR may play a unique osmoregulatory role in renal cells (Burg 1988; Bondy *et al.* 1990). The concept was based on the observation that renal papillary epithelial cells survived long-term exposure to hypertonic media by inducing AR to provide the osmolyte sorbitol in amounts adequate to counterbalance the high extracellular osmotic pressure (Bagnasco *et al.* 1987; Garcia-Perez *et al.* 1989). In fact, when cultured in hypertonic media, a variety of non-renal cells responded to osmotic stress by AR to produce sorbitol (Hohman *et al.* 1988; Kaneko *et al.* 1990). This suggests the existence of a vestigial adaptive mechanism no longer required in homeostasis. Of greater importance was the finding that the AR-catalysed supply of sorbitol was not essential for the survival of osmotically stressed cells because the cells had substituted other non-perturbing osmolytes (Yancey *et al.* 1982) for sorbitol to maintain proper cell volume (Moriyama *et al.* 1990, 1991). This conclusion was arrived at by using AR inhibitors to block sorbitol formation (Hohman and Carper 1990; Hohman *et al.* 1990; Moriyama *et al.* 1990, 1991). The finding was corroborated *in vivo* (Yancey *et al.* 1990) by showing that, in dehydrated rats treated with an

AR inhibitor, the decrease in renal medullary sorbitol was compensated by increased betaine levels (Moriyama *et al.* 1991). The view that osmoregulation in the kidney medulla is not a vital physiological role of AR is supported by the absence of unusual generic renal effects in long-term safety evaluation studies of AR inhibitors (Moriyama *et al.* 1990, 1991). In fact, no unusual generic toxicity of AR inhibitors has been observed to date across the animal species tested (Stribling 1988; Harrison *et al.* 1989). This supports the current view that AR does not appear to have a vital enzymatic function in non-diabetic tissues (Green and Jaspan 1990). It is tempting to suggest that AR normally functions as a structural protein, and starts acting as an enzyme only in the presence of high intracellular sugar concentrations and an adequate NADPH supply.

16.6 Conclusion

In animal models of diabetic hyperglycaemia, AR inhibitors have been shown to prevent the inception and early evolution of a cascade of metabolic, functional, and structural alterations which are characteristic of chronically hyperglycaemic diabetic tissues. Whereas animals used as models do not develop all human-type ultimate diabetic lesions, 'if any therapeutic manoeuvre inhibits the initial stage of the development, this is sufficient to warrant optimism about its long-term effect' (Osterby 1988). Indeed, in subjects with diabetic neuropathy, prolonged treatment with AR inhibitors (displaying adequate tissue pharmacokinetics) has produced evidence of benefit. The results have identified AR inhibitors as an important pharmacotherapeutic addition to glycaemic control in the early interventive treatment of diabetic neuropathy.

References

Akagi, Y., Yajima, Y., Kador, P. F., Kuwabara, T., and Kinoshita, J. H. (1984). Localization of aldose reductase in the human eye. *Diabetes*, **33**, 562–6.

Ao, S., Shingu, Y., Kikuchi, C., Takamo, Y., Nomura, K., Fujiwara, T., *et al.* (1991). Characterization of a novel aldose reductase inhibitor, FR 74366, and its effects on diabetic cataract and neuropathy in the rat. *Metabolism*, **40**, 77–87.

Armstrong, F. M., Bradburg, J. E., Ellis, S. H., Owens, D. R., Rosen, I., Sonksen, P., and Sundkvist, G. (1991). A study of peripheral diabetic neuropathy. The application of age-related reference values. *Diabetic Medicine*, *8 Symposium*, S 94–9.

Asbury, A. K. (1988). Understanding diabetic neuropathy. *New England Journal of Medicine*, **319**, 577–8.

Austin, C. E. and Chess-Williams, R. (1991). Diabetes-induced changes in cardiac β-adrenoceptor responsiveness: effects of aldose reductase inhibition with ponalrestat. *British Journal of Pharmacology*, **102**, 478–82.

Bagnasco, S. M., Uchida, S., Balaban, R. S., Kador, P. F., and Burg, M. B.

(1987). Induction of aldose reductase and sorbitol in renal inner medullary cells by elevated extracellular NaCl. *Proceedings of the National Academy of Sciences of the United States of America*, **84**, 1718–20.

Bank, N., Mower, P., Aynedjian, H. S., Wilkes, B. M., and Silverman, S. (1989). Sorbinil prevents glomerular hyperperfusion in diabetic rats. *American Journal of Physiology*, **256**, F1000–6.

Bhatnagar, A., Liu, S., Das, B., and Srivastava, S. K. (1989). Involvement of sulfhydryl residues in aldose reductase–inhibitor interaction. *Molecular Pharmacology*, **36**, 825–30.

Blohme, G. and Smith, V. (1989). Aldose reductase inhibition reduces urinary albumin excretion rate in incipient diabetic nephropathy. *Diabetologia*, **32**, 467A.

Bohren, K. M., Bullock, B., Wermuth, B., and Gabbay, K. H. (1989). The aldo-keto reductase superfamily. *Journal of Biological Chemistry*, **264**, 9547–51.

Bondy, C., Cowley, B. D., Lightman, S. L., and Kador, P. F. (1990). Feedback inhibition of aldose reductase gene expression in rat renal medulla. Galactitol accumulation reduces enzyme mRNA levels and depletes cellular inositol content. *Journal of Clinical Investigation*, **86**, 1103–8.

Boulton, A. J. M., Atiea, J., DeLeeuw, I. H., Lemkes, H., MacLeod, A. F., and MacRury, S. (1989). The efficacy and safety of the aldose-reductase inhibitor tolrestat in the treatment of chronic sensorimotor diabetic neuropathy, *Diabetologia*, **32**, 469A.

Boulton, A. J. M., Levin, S., and Comstock, J. (1990). A multicentre trial of the aldose-reductase inhibitor, tolrestat in patients with sympomatic diabetic neuropathy. *Diabetologia*, **33**, 431–7.

Brazzell, R. K., Park, Y. H., Woolbridge, C. B., McCue, B., Barker, R., and Couch, R. (1990). Interspecies comparison of the pharmacokinetics of aldose reductase inhibitors. *Drug Metabolism and Disposition*, **18**, 435–40.

Brazzell, R. K., Mayer, P. R., Dobbs, R., McNamarra, P. J., Teng, R., and Slattery, J. T. (1991). Dose-dependent pharmacokinetics of the aldose reductase inhibitor imirestat in man. *Pharmaceutical Research*, **8**, 112–18.

Brinchmann-Hansen, O., Dahl-Jorgensen, K., Hanssen, K. F., and Sandvik, L. (1988). The response of diabetic retinopathy to 41 months of multiple insulin injections, insulin pumps, and conventional insulin therapy. *Archives of Ophthalmology*, **106**, 1242–6.

Burg, M. B. (1988). Role of aldose reductase and sorbitol in maintaining the medullary intracellular milieu. *Kidney International*, **33**, 635–41.

Calcutt, N. A., Tomlinson, D. R., and Biswass S. (1990). Coexistence of nerve conduction deficit with increased Na^+-K^+-ATPase activity in galactose-fed mice. Implications for polyol pathway and diabetic neuropathy. *Diabetes*, **39**, 663–6.

Cameron, N. E., Cotter, M. A., and Robertson, S. (1990). Changes in skeletal muscle contractile properties in streptozotocin-induced diabetic rats and the role of polyol pathway and hypoinsulinemia. *Diabetes*, **39**, 460–5.

Carper, D. (1990). Comparison of deduced amino acid sequences of human aldose reductase from four different tissues. In *Current concepts of aldose reductase and its inhibitions* (ed. N. Sakamoto, J. H. Kinoshita, P. F. Kador, and N. Hotta), pp. 25–9. Elsevier, Amsterdam.

Carper, D., Nishimura, C., Shinohara, T., Dietzchold, B., Wistow, G., Craft, C., *et al.* (1987). Aldose reductase and ρ-crystallin belong to the same protein superfamily as aldehyde reductase. *Federation of European Biochemical Societies Letters*, **22**, 209–13.

Chakrabarti, S., Sima, A. A. F., Nakajima, T., Yagihashi, S., and Greene, D. A. (1987). Aldose reductase in the BB rat: isolation, immunological identification and localization in the retina and peripheral nerve. *Diabetologia*, **30**, 244–51.

Chauncey, B., Leite. M. V., and Goldstein, L. (1988). Renal sorbitol accumulation and associated enzyme activities in diabetes. *Enzyme*, **39**, 231–4.

Christiansen, J. S., Pedersen, M. M., and Mogensen, C. E. (1991). Reduction of GFR during short-term aldose reductase inhibition in Type-1 diabetes. *Diabetologia*, **34** (Suppl. 2), A28.

Chung, S. and LaMendola, J. (1989). Cloning and sequence determination of human placental aldose reductase gene. *Journal of Biological Chemistry*, **264**, 14775–7.

Cotter, M., Cameron, N., and Robertson, S. (1991). Polyol pathway mediated dysfunction in striated muscle of diabetic and galactosemic rats and the effects of ARI. *Aldose Reductase Workshop, Kona, HI*, Abstract S 4:4.

Cunha-Vaz., J. L., Mota, C., Leite, E. C., Abreu, J. R. F., and Ruas, M. A. (1986). Effect of sorbinil on blood-retinal barrier in early diabetic retinopathy. *Diabetes*, **35**, 574–8.

Dahl-Jorgensen, K., Brinchmann-Hansen, O., Sandvik, L., and Hanssen, K. F. (1990). Blood glucose control and progression of diabetic retinopathy: seven years results from the Oslo Study. *Diabetologia*, **33** (Suppl.), 4–68.

Datiles, M. B., Kador, P. F., Kashima, K., Kinoshita, J. H., and Sinha, A. (1990). The effects of sorbinil, an aldose reductase inhibitor, on the corneal endothelium in galactosemic dogs. *Investigative Ophthalmology and Visual Science*, **31**, 2201–4.

DCCT Research Group (1986). The diabetes control and complications trial (DCCT). Design and methodologic considerations for the feasibility phase. *Diabetes*, **35**, 530–45.

DCCT Research Group. (1988). Are continuing studies of metabolic control and microvascular complications in insulin-dependent diabetes mellitus justified? *New England Journal of Medicine*, **318**, 246–50.

Deckert, T. (1988). Glycemic control and complications. In *The diabetes annual*, Vol. 4 (ed. K. G. M. M. Alberti and L. P. Krall), pp. 496–518. Elsevier, Amsterdam.

Del Corso, A., Barsacchi, D., Giannessi, M., Tozzi, M. G., Camici, M., and Mura, U. (1989). Change in stereospecificity of bovine lens aldose reductase modified by oxidative stress. *Journal of Biological Chemistry*, **264**, 17653–5.

Del Corso, A., Barsacchi, D., Gianessi, M., Tozzi, M. G., Camici, M., Houben, J. H., *et al.* (1990). Bovine lens aldose reductase: tight binding of the pyridine coenzyme. *Archives of Biochemistry and Biophysics*, **283**, 512–18.

Dietrich, E., Stracke, H., and Federlin, K. (1990). The effects of the aldose reductase inhibitor 'Statil' on diabetic peripheral neuropathy. *Diabetologia*, **33** (Suppl.), A-167.

Dvornik, D. (1978). Chronic complications of diabetes. *Annual Reports of Medicinal Chemistry*, **13**, 159–66.

Dvornik, D. (1987a). Hyperglycemia in the pathogenesis of diabetic complications. In *Aldose reductase inhibition: an approach to the prevention of diabetic complications* (ed. D. Porte), pp. 69–151. BIC/McGraw-Hill, New York.

Dvornik, D. (1987b) Animal models of diabetic complications and their relation to aldose reductase inhibitions. In *Aldose reductase inhibition: an approach to the prevention of diabetic complications* (ed. D. Porte), pp. 152–219. BIC/McGraw-Hill, New York.

Dvornik, D. (1987c). Aldose reductase inhibitors. In *Aldose reductase inhibition, an approach to the prevention of diabetic complications* (ed. D. Porte), pp. 221–323. BIC/McGraw-Hill, New York.

Dvornik, D. (1989). Aldose reductase inhibition: an approach to prevention of diabetic complications. *Journal of the American College of Neuropsychiatrists*, **3**, 9–15.

Dvornik, D., Simard-Duquesne, N., Kraml, M., Sestanj, K., Gabbay, K. H., Kinoshita, J. H., *et al.* (1973). Polyol accumulation in galactosemic and diabetic rats: control by an aldose reductase inhibitor. *Science*, **182**, 1146–8.

Dvornik, D., Millen, J., Hicks, D., Cayen, M., and Sredy, J. (1988). The pharmacokinetics of aldose reductase inhibitors. In *Polyol pathway and its role in diabetic complications* (ed. N. Sakamoto, J. H. Kinoshita, P. F. Kador, and N. Hotta), pp. 61–71. Elsevier, Amsterdam.

Dyck, P. J., Sherman, W. R., Hallacher, L. M., Service, F. J., O'Brien, P. C., Grina, L. A., *et al.* (1980). Human diabetic endoneurial sorbitol, fructose, and myoinositol related to sural nerve morphometry. *Annals of Neurology*, **8**, 590–6.

Dyck, P. J., Zimmerman, B. R., Vilen, T. H., Minnerath, S. R., Karnes, J. L., Yao, J. K., and Poduslo, J. F. (1988). Nerve glucose, fructose, sorbitol, myoinositol, and fiber degeneration and regeneration in diabetic neuropathy. *New England Journal of Medicine*, **319**, 542–8.

Dyck, P. J., Zimmerman, B. R., Vilen, T. H., Minnerath, S., Karnes, J. L., Yao, J. K., and Poduslo, J. F. (1989). *Pathogenesis of diabetic neuropathy*. *New England Journal of Medicine*, **320**, 59.

Eaton, R. P. (1986). Aldose reductase inhibition and the diabetic syndrome of limited joint mobility: implication for altered collagen hydration. *Metabolism*, **35** (Suppl. 1), 119–21.

El-Kabbani, O., Narayana, S. V. L., Babu, Y. S., Moore, K. M., Flynn, T. G., Petrash, J. M., *et al.* (1991). Purification, crystallization and preliminary crystallographic analysis of porcine aldose reductase. *Journal of Molecular Biology*, **218**, 695–8.

Feinstein, A. R. (1989). Problems, pitfalls, and opportunities in long-term randomized trials. In *Drug research and drug development in the 21st century* (ed. H. P. Wolff, A. Fleckenstein, and E. Phillip), pp. 105–16. Springer, Berlin.

Finegold, D., Lattimer, S. A., Nolle, S., Bernstein, M., and Greene, D. A. (1983). Polyol pathway activity and myo-inositol metabolism: a suggested relationship in the pathogenesis of diabetic neuropathy. *Diabetes*, **32**, 988–92.

Florkowski, C. W., Rowe, B. R., Nightingale, S., Harvey, T. C., and Barnett, A. H. (1991). Clinical and neurophysiological studies of aldose reductase inhibitor ponalrestat in chronic symptomatic diabetic peripheral neuropathy. *Diabetes*, **40**, 129–33.

Foulds, G., O'Brien, M. M., Bianchine, J. R., and Gabbay, K. H. (1981). Kinetics of an orally absorbed aldose reductase inhibitor sorbinil. *Clinical Pharmacology and Therapeutics*, **30**, 693–700.

Frank, R. N. (1984). On the pathogenesis of retinopathy. *Ophthalmology*, **91**, 626–34.

Frank, R. N. (1990). Aldose reductase inhibition. The chemical key to the control of diabetic retinopathy? *Archives of Ophthalmology*, **108**, 1229–31.

Fukushi, S. (1988). Corneal epitheliopathy in diabetes. In *Polyol pathway and its role in diabetic complications* (ed. N. Sakamoto, J. H. Kinoshita, P. F. Kador, and N. Hotta), pp. 217–30. Elsevier, Amsterdam.

Gabbay, K. H. (1975). Hyperglycemia, polyol metabolism and complications of diabetes mellitus. *Annual Review of Medicine*, **26**, 521–35.

Gabbay, K. H., Spack, N., Loo, S., Hirsch, H., and Ackil, A. A. (1979). Aldose reductase inhibition: studies with alrestatin. *Metabolism*, **28** (suppl. 1), 471–6.

Garcia-Perez, A., Martin, B., Murphy, H. R., Uchida, S., Murer, H., Cowley. B. D., *et al.* (1989). Molecular cloning of cDNA coding for kidney aldose reductase: regulation of specific mRNA accumulation by NaCl-mediated osmotic stress. *Journal of Biological Chemistry*, **264**, 16815–21.

Ghahary, A., Luo, J., Gong, Y., Chakrabarti, S., Sima, A. A. F., and Murphy, L. (1989). Increased renal aldose reductase activity, immunoreactivity, and mRNA in streptozocin-induced diabetic rats. *Diabetes*, **38**, 1067–71.

Ghahary, A., Chakrabarti, S., Sima, A. A. F., and Murphy, L. J. (1991). Effects of insulin and Statil on aldose reductase-expression in diabetic rats. *Diabetes*, **40**, 1391–6.

Gieron, M. A., Malone, J. I., Lowitt, S., and Korthals, J. K. (1991). Improvement in peripheral nerve function after one year of sorbinil. *Neuro Report*, **2**, 348–50.

Gill, J. S., Williams, G., Ghatei, M. A., Hetreed, A. H., Mather, H. M., and Bloom, S. R. (1990). Effect of the aldose reductase inhibitor, ponalrestat, on diabetic neuropathy. *Diabète et Metabolisme*, **16**, 296–302.

Goldfarb, S., Ziyadeh, F. N., Kern, E. F. O., and Simmons, D. (1991). Effects of polyol-pathway inhibition and dietary myo-inositol on glomerular hemodynamic function in experimental diabetes mellitus in rats. *Diabetes*, **40**, 465–71.

Gonen, B., Bochenek, W., Beg, M., Graepel, J., and Tolrestat Study Group. (1991). The effect of withdrawal of tolrestat, an aldose reductase inhibitor, on signs, symptoms and nerve function in diabetic neuropathy. *Diabetologia*, **34** (Suppl. 2), A153.

Gonzales, G. F. (1989). Functional structure and ultrastructure of seminal vesicles. *Archives of Andrology*, **22**, 1–13.

Graham, A., Hedge, P. J., Powell, S. J., Riley, J., Brown, L., Gammack, A., *et al.* (1989). Nucleotide sequence of cDNA for human aldose reductase. *Nucleic Acids Research*, **17**, 8368.

Graham, A., Brown, L., Hedge, P. J., Gammack, A. J., and Markham, A. F. (1991). Structure of the human aldose reductase gene. *Journal of Biological Chemistry*, **266**, 6872–7.

Green, A. J. and Jaspan, J. B. (1990). Treatment of diabetic neuropathy with inhibitors of the aldose reductase enzyme. *Journal of Diabetic Complications*, **4**, 138–44.

Greene, D. A. and Sima, A. A. F. (1991). Aldose reductase inhibitor (ARI) treatment normalizes axo-glial dysjunction and improves nerve fiber pathology in advanced diabetic neuropathy. *Diabetes*, **40** (Suppl. 1), 9A.

Greene, D. A., Lattimer, S., Ulbrecht, J., and Carroll, P. (1985). Glucose-induced alterations in nerve metabolism: current perspective on the pathogenesis of diabetic neuropathy and future direction for research and therapy. *Diabetes Care*, **8**, 290–9.

Greene, D. A., Lattimer, S. A., and Sima, A. A. F. (1987a). Sorbitol, phospho-inositides, and sodium-potassium ATPase in the pathogenesis of diabetic complications. *New England Journal of Medicine*, **316**, 599–606.

Greene, D. A., Chakrabarti, S., Lattimer, S. A., and Sima, A. A. F. (1987b). Role of sorbitol accumulation and myo-inositol depletion in paranodal swelling of large myelinated nerve fibers in the insulin-deficient spontaneously diabetic Bio-Breeding rat. Reversal by insulin replacement, an aldose reductase inhibitor, and myo-inositol. *Journal of Clinical Investigation*, **79**, 1479–85.

Greene, D. A., Lattimer, S. A., and Sima, A. A. F. (1988). Are disturbances of sorbitol, phosphoinositide, and Na^+/K^+-ATPase regulation involved in the pathogenesis of diabetic neuropathy? *Diabetes*, **37**, 688–93.

Greene, D. A., Sima, A. A. F., Lattimer, S. A., Hachiya, H., Diaz, T. C., and Delmonte, M. (1989a). The elusive sorbitol-accumulation/myo-inositol-depletion hypothesis of diabetic complications is alive and well but in hiding. In *Diabetes 1988* (ed. R. Larkins, P. Zimmet, and D. Chisholm), pp. 45–53. Elsevier, Amsterdam.

Greene, D. A., Porte, D., Bril. V., Clements, R. S., Shamoon, H., and Ziedler, A. (1989b). Clinical response to sorbinil treatment in diabetic neuropathy. *Diabetologia*, **32**, 493A.

Greene, D. A., Bochenek, W., Harati, Y., Sima, A. A. F., Hohman, T., Hicks, D., *et al.* (1990). Biochemical and morphometric response to tolrestat in human diabetic nerve. *Diabetologia*, **33** (Suppl.), A-92.

Grimshaw, C. E. (1990a). A kinetic perspective on the peculiarity of aldose reductase. In *Enzymology and molecular biology of carbonyl metabolism*, Vol. 3 (ed. H. Weiner, B. Wermuth, and D. W. Crabb), pp. 217–28. Plenum Press, New York.

Grimshaw, C. E. (1990b). Chromatographic separation of activated and unactivated forms of aldose reductase. *Archives of Biochemistry and Biophysics*, **278**, 273–6.

Grimshaw, C. E. (1991). Mechanistic insights into the catalytic efficiency of aldose reductase. *Aldose Reductase Workshop, HI*, Abstract P20.

Grimshaw, C. E., Shahbaz, M., Jahangiri, G., Putney, C. G., McKercher, S. R., and Mathur, E. J. (1989). Kinetic and structural effects of activation of bovine kidney aldose reductase. *Biochemistry*, **28**, 5343–53.

Grundmann, U., Bohn, H., Obermeier, R., and Amann, E. (1990). Cloning and prokaryotic expression of a biologically active human placental aldose reductase. *DNA and Cell Biology*, **9**, 149–57.

Guder, W. G., Schmolke, M., and Wirthensohn, G. (1988). Zur physiologischen funktion des renalen Sorbitolstoffwechsels und seiner Veränderung beim experimentellen Diabetes mellitus. *Aktuelles in Endokrinologie und Stoffwechsel*, **9**, 88.

Hale, P. J., Nattrass, M., Silverman, S. H., Sennit, C., Perkins, C. M., Uden, A., and Sundquist, G. (1987). Peripheral nerve concentrations of glucose, fructose, sorbitol and myoinositol in diabetic and non-diabetic patients. *Diabetologia*, **30**, 464–7.

Hanssen, K. F., Dahl-Jorgensen, K., Lauritzen, T., Feldt-Rasmussen, B., Brinchmann-Hannsen, O., and Deckert, T. (1986). Diabetic control and microvascular complications: the near-normoglycaemic experience. *Diabetologia*, **29**, 677–84.

Harrison, H. E., Stribling, D., Armstrong, F. M., and Perkins, C. M. (1989). Aldose reductase in the etiology of diabetic complications. I. Introduction. *Journal of Diabetic Complications*, **3**, 6–11.

Hayman, S. and Kinoshita. J. H. (1965). Isolation and properties of lens aldose reductase. *Journal of Biological Chemistry*, **240**, 877–82.

Hers, H. G. (1956). Le mécanisme de la transformation de glucose en fructose par les vésicules seminales. *Biochimica et Biophysica Acta*, **22**, 202–3.

Hicks, D. R., Kraml, M., Cayen, M. N., Dubuc, J., Ryder, S., and Dvornik, D. (1984). Tolrestat kinetics. *Clinical Pharmacology and Therapeutics*, **36**, 493–9.

Hirata, Y. and Okada, K. (1990). Relation of Na^+,K^+-ATPase to delayed motor nerve conduction velocity: effect of aldose reductase inhibitor, ADN-138, on Na^+,K^+-ATPase activity. *Metabolism*, **39**, 563–7.

Hohman, T. C. and Carper, D. (1990). Hypertonic stress induces aldose reductase and myoinositol accumulation in lens epithelial, kidney endothelial and Chinese hamster ovary cells. In *Current concepts of aldose reductase and its inhibitions* (ed. N. Sakamoto, J. H. Kinoshita, P. F. Kador, and N. Hotta), pp. 31–41. Elsevier, Amsterdam.

Hohman, T. C., Millen, J., Bock, M. C., and Dvornik, D. (1988). Hypertonicity induces aldose reductase in cultured mesangial, endothelial and CHO cells. *Journal of Cell Biology*, **107**, 203A.

Hohman, T. C., Carper, D., Dasgupta, S., and Kaneko, M. (1990). Osmotic stress induces aldose reductase in glomerular endothelial cells. In *Enzymology and molecular biology of carbonyl metabolism* Vol. 3 (ed. H. Weiner, B. Wermuth, and D. W. Crabb), pp. 139–52. Plenum Press, New York.

Hotta, N. and Sakamoto, N. (1990). Aldose reductase inhibitors. In *The diabetes annual* Vol. 5 (ed. K. G. M. M. Alberti and L. P. Krall), pp. 330–61. Elsevier, Amsterdam.

Hotta, N., Kakuta, H., Ando, F., and Sakamoto, N. (1988). Clinical trial of aldose reductase inhibitor ONO-2235. In *Polyol pathway and its role in diabetic complications* (ed. N. Sakamoto, J. H. Kinoshita, P. F. Kador, and N. Hotta), pp. 253–66. Elsevier, Amsterdam.

Hotta, N., Kakuta, H., Ando, F., and Sakamoto, N. (1990). Current progress in clinical trials of aldose reductase inhibitors in Japan. *Experimental Eye Research*, **50**, 625–8.

Humber, L. (1987). The medicinal chemistry of aldose reductase inhibitors. In *Progress in medicinal chemistry* (ed. G. P. Ellis and G. B. West), pp. 299–343. Elsevier, Amsterdam.

Ikeda, H. (1990). Pharmacological profile of AD-5467, a new aldose reductase inhibitor. In *Current concepts of aldose reductase and its inhibitions* (ed. N. Sakamoto, J. H. Kinoshita, P. F. Kador, and N. Hotta), pp. 97–103. Elsevier, Amsterdam.

Jennings, P. E., Nightingale, S., LeGuen, C., Lawson, N., Williamson, J. R., Hoffman, P., and Barnett, A. H. (1990). Prolonged aldose reductase inhibition in chronic peripheral diabetic neuropathy: effects on microangiopathy. *Diabetic Medicine*, **7**, 63–8.

Kavor, P. F. (1990). Aldose reductase inhibitors. In *Current concepts of aldose reductase and its inhibitions* (ed. N. Sakamoto, J. H. Kinoshita, P. F. Kador, and H. Hotta), pp. 73–79. Elsevier, Amsterdam.

Kador, P. F., Kinoshita, J. H., and Sharpless, N. (1986). The aldose reductase inhibitor site. *Metabolism*, 35 (Suppl. 1), 109–13.

Kaneko, M., Carper, D., Nishimura, C., Millen, J., Bock, M., and Hohman, T. C. (1990). Induction of aldose reductase expression in rat kidney mesangial cells and Chinese hamster ovary cells under hypertonic conditions. *Experimental Cell Research*, 188, 135–40.

Kawasaki, N., Tanimoto, T., and Tanaka, A. (1989). Characterization of aldose reductase and aldehyde reductase from rat testis. *Biochimica et Biophysica Acta*, 996, 30–6.

Kikkawa, R., Hatanaka, I., Yasuda, H., Kobayashi, N., Shigeta, Y., Terashima, H., et al. (1983). Effect of a new aldose reductase inhibitor, (E)-3-carboxymethyl-5-[(2E)-methyl-3-phenylpropenylidene]rhodanine (ONO 2235) on peripheral nerve disorders in streptozotocin-diabetic rats. *Diabetologia*, 24, 290–2.

Kinoshita, J. H. (1988). History of aldose reductase. In *Polyol pathway and its role in diabetic complications* (ed. N. Sakamoto, J. H. Kinoshita, P. F. Kador, and N. Hotta), pp. 12–19. Elsevier, Amsterdam.

Kinoshita, J. H. and Nishimura, C. (1988). The involvement of aldose reductase in diabetic complications. *Diabetes/Metabolism Reviews*, 4, 323–37.

Kinoshita, J. H., Merola, L. O., Satoh, K., and Dikmak, E. (1962). Osmotic changes caused by the accumulation of dulcitol in the lenses of rats fed with galactose. *Nature, London*, 194, 1085–7.

Kinoshita, J. H., Dvornik, D., Kraml, M., and Gabbay, K. H. (1968). The effect of an aldose reductase inhibitor on the galactose-exposed rabbit lens. *Biochimica et Biophysica Acta*, 158, 472–5.

Kirchain, W. R. and Rendell, M. S. (1990). Aldose reductase inhibitors. *Pharmacotherapy*, 10, 326–36.

Kowluru, R., Bitensky, M. W., Kowluru, A., Dembo, M., Keaton, P. A., and Buican, T. (1989). Reversible sodium pump defect and swelling in the diabetic rat erythrocyte: effects on filterability and implications for microangiopathy. *Proceedings of the National Academy of Sciences of the United States of America*, 86, 3327–31.

Krentz, A. J., Honigsberger, L., Ellis, S. H., and Nattrass, M. (1989a). A 12 month randomised controlled study of ponalrestat in chronic symptomatic diabetic neuropathy. *Diabetic Medicine*, 6 (suppl. 2), 14A.

Krentz, A. J., Honigsberger, L., and Nattras, M. (1989b). Selection of patients with symptomatic diabetic neuropathy for clinical trials. *Diabète et Metabolisme*, 15, 416–19.

Kroc Collaborative Study Group. (1988). Diabetic retinopathy after two years of intensified insulin treatment. Follow-up of the Kroc Collaborative Study. *Journal of the American Medical Society*, 260, 37–41.

Lambourne, J. E., Tomlinson, D. R., Brown, A. M., and Willars, G. B. (1987). Opposite effects of diabetes and galactosemia on adenosine triphosphatase activity in rat nervous tissue. *Diabetologia*, 30, 360–2.

Lambourne, J. E., Brown, J. E., Calcutt, N., Tomlinson, D. R., and Willars, G. B. (1988). Adenosine triphosphatase in nerves and ganglia of rats with streptozotocin-induced diabetes or galactosemia; effects of aldose reductase inhibition. *Diabetologia*, 31, 379–84.

Larson, E. R., Lipinski, C. A., and Sarges, R. (1988). Medicinal chemistry of aldose reductase inhibitors. *Medicinal Research Reviews*, 8, 159–86.

Lauritzen, T., Frost-Larsen, K., Larsen, H. W., Deckert, T., and the Steno Study Group. (1985). Two-year experience with continous subcutaneous insulin infusion in relation to retinopathy and neuropathy. *Diabetes*, **34** (Suppl. 3), 74–9.

Liu, S., Bhatnangar, A., Das, B., and Srivastava, S. K. (1989). Functional cysteinyl residues in human placental aldose reductase. *Archives of Biochemistry and Biophysics*, **272**, 112–21.

Llewelyn, J. G., Patel, N. J., Thomas, P. K., and Stribling, D. (1987). Sodium, potassium adenosine triphosphatase activity in peripheral nerve tissue of galactosemic rats. Effect of aldose reductase inhibition. *Diabetologia*, **30**, 971–2.

Lukeshi, G. N. and Zar, M. A. (1990). Inhibitory effect of streptozotocin-induced diabetes on non-cholinergic motor transmission in rat detrusor and its prevention by sorbinil. *British Journal of Pharmacology*, **161**, 411–17.

McCaleb, M. L., Sredy, J., Millen, J., Ackerman, D. M., and Dvornik, D. (1988). Prevention of urinary albumin excretion in 6 month streptozotocin-diabetic rats with the aldose reductase inhibitor tolrestat. *Journal of Diabetic Complications*, **2**, 16–18.

McCaleb, M. L., McKean, M. L., Hohman, T. C., Laver, N., and Robison, W. G., Jr (1991). Intervention with the aldose reductase inhibitor, tolrestat, in renal and retinal lesions of streptozotocin-diabetic rats. *Diabetologia*, **34**, 695–701.

McLennan, S., Yue, D. K., Fisher, E., Capogreco, C., Heffernan, S., Ross, G., and Turtle, J. R. (1988). Deficiency of ascorbic acid in experimental diabetes. Relationship with collagen and polyol pathway abnormalities. *Diabetes*, **37**, 359–61.

Macleod, A. and Sonksen, P. (1991). The effect of the aldose reductase inhibitor tolrestat on diabetic polyneuropathy; a meta-analysis. *Diabetes*, **40** (Suppl. 1), 555A.

Masson, E. A. and Boulton, A. J. M. (1990). Aldose reductase inhibitors in the treatment of diabetic neuropathy. A review of the rationale and clinical evidence. *Drugs*, **39**, 190–202.

Miwa, I., Kaubara, M., and Okuda, J. (1989). Improvement of nerve conduction velocity in mutant diabetic mice by aldose reductase inhibitor treatment without affecting nerve myo-inositol content. *Chemical and Pharmaceutical Bulletin*, **37**, 1581–2.

Mizuno, K., Yamaguchi, T., Inoue, A., Tomiya, N., Unno, R., Miura, K., *et al.* (1990). Profile of a new aldose reductase inhibitor, (2S,4S-6-fluoro-2′,5′-dioxo-spiro-[chroman-4,4′-imidazoline]-2-carboxamide (SNK-860). In *Current concepts of aldose reductase and its inhibitions* (ed. N. Sakamoto, J. H. Kinoshita, P. F. Kador, and N. Hotta), pp. 89–96. Elsevier, Amsterdam.

Moriyama, T., Garcia-Perez, A., and Burg, M. B. (1990). Factors affecting the ratio of different organic osmolytes in renal medullary cells. *American Journal of Physiology*, **259**, F847–58.

Moriyama, T., Garcia-Perez, A., Olson, A. D., and Burg, M. B. (1991). Intracellular betaine substitutes for sorbitol in protecting renal medullary cells from hypertonicity. *American Journal of Physiology*, **260**, F494–7.

Morjana, N. A. and Flynn, T. G. (1989). Aldose reductase from human psoas muscle. Purification, substrate specificity, immunological characterization, and effect of drugs and inhibitors. *Journal of Biological Chemistry*, **264**, 2906–11.

Morjana, N. A., Lyons, C., and Flynn, T. G. (1989). Aldose reductase from human psoas muscle. Affinity labelling of an active site lysine by pyridoxal 5′-

phosphate and pyridoxal 5'-diphospho-5'-adenosine. *Journal of Biological Chemistry*, **264**, 2912–19.

Mühlhauser, I., Bruckner, J., and Howorka, I. (1987). Near-normoglycaemia and microvascular complications. *Diabetologia*, **30**, 47–8.

Mylari, B. L., Larson, E. R., Beyer, T. A., Zembrowski, W. J., Aldinger, C. E., Dee, M. F., *et al.* (1991). Novel, potent aldose reductase inhibitors: 3,4-dihydro-4-oxo-3[[5-(trifluoromethyl)-2-benzothiazolyl]methyl]-1-phthalazine-acetic acid (zopolrestat) and congeners. *Journal of Medicinal Chemistry*, **34**, 108–22.

Nishimura, C., Graham, C., Hohman, T., Nagata, M., Robison, W. G., Jr, and Carper, D. (1988). Characterization of mRNA and genes for aldose reductase in rat. *Biochemical and Biophysical Research Communications*, **153**, 1051–9.

Nishimura, C., Yamaoka, T., Mizutani, M., Yamashita, K., Akera, T., and Tanimoto, T. (1991). Purification and characterization of the recombinant human aldose reductase expressed in *Baculovirus* system. *Biochimica et Biophysica Acta*, **1078**, 171–8.

Oates, P. J. and Goddu, K. J. (1987). A soribitol gradient in rat renal medulla. *Kidney International*, **31**, 448.

Oates, P. J., Ellery, C. A., Inskeep, P. B., Reed, A. E., Beyer, T. A., and Hutson, N. J. (1991). Zopolrestat dose-dependently inhibits renal hyperperfusion in galactosemic rats. *Diabetes*, **40** (Suppl. 1), 131A.

Ohta, M., Tanimoto, T., and Tanaka, A. (1990). Characterization of aldose reductase and aldehyde reductase from the medulla of rat kidney. *Chemical Pharmaceutical Bulletin*, **38**, 1639–43.

Osterby, R. (1988). Glomerular structural abnormalities in early and late stages of experimental diabetes: models for diabetes nephropathy. In *Frontiers in diabetes research. Lessons from animal diabetes II* (ed. E. Shafrir and A. E. Renold), pp. 522–7. Libbey, London.

Passariello, N., Marazzo, G., Castellano, L., Peluso, A., Sepe, J., Sgambato, S., and D'Onofrio, F. (1991). Effect of tolrestat on urinary albumin excretion in patients with diabetic nephropathy. *Diabetologia*, **34** (Suppl. 2), A28.

Pedersen, M. M., Christiansen, J. S., and Mogensen, C. E. (1991). Reduction of glomerular hyperfiltration in normoalbuminuric IDDM patients by 6 mo of aldose reductase inhibition. *Diabetes*, **40**, 527–31.

Peterson, M. J., Sarges, R., Aldinger, C. E., and MacDonald, D. P. (1979). CP-45,634: A novel aldose reductase inhibitor that inhibits polyol pathway activity in diabetic and galactosemic rats. *Metabolism*, **28** (Suppl. 1), 456–61.

Pinget, M., Baudoin, C., and Waguet, J. C. (1991). Effects of a new aldose reductase inhibitor on nerve conduction in 409 patients with neuropathy. *Diabetologia*, **34** (Suppl. 2), A153.

Pitts, N. E., Vreeland, F., Shaw, G. L., Peterson, M. J., Mehta, D. J., Collie. J., and Gundersen, K. (1986). Clinical experience with sorbinil—an aldose reductase inhibitor. *Metabolism*, **35** (Suppl. 1), 96–100.

Powell, H. C., Garrett, R. S., Kador, P. F., and Mizisin, A. P. (1991). Fine structural localization of aldose reductase and ouabain-sensitive, K^+-dependent p-nitro-phenylphosphatase in rat peripheral nerve. *Acta Neuropathologica*, **81**, 529–39.

Price, D. E., Kemp, J. V., Perkins, C. M., Bastain, W., Airey, C. M., and Wales, J. K. (1988). The pharmacokinetics of ICI 128,436 during multiple oral dosing to diabetics. In *Polyol pathway and its role in diabetic complications* (ed. N. Sakamoto, J. H. Kinoshita, P. F. Kador, and N. Hotta), pp. 114–20. Elsevier, Amsterdam.

Price, D. E., Airey, C. M., Hampton, K. K., and Wales, J. K. (1989). Aldose reductase inhibition with ponalrestat improves nerve conduction velocity in diabetic patients with asymptomatic neuropathy. *Diabetic Medicine*, **6** (Suppl. 1), A-31.

Pugliese, G., Tilton, R. G., Speedy, A., Chang, K., Province, M. A., Kilo, C., and Williamson, J. R. (1990). Vascular filtration function in galactose-fed versus diabetic rats: the role of polyol pathway activity. *Metabolism*, **39**, 690–7.

Reichard, P., Berglund, B., Britz, A., Cars, I., Nilsson, B. Y., and Rosenqvist, U. (1991). Intensified conventional insulin treatment retards the microvascular complications of insulin-dependent diabetes mellitus (IDDM): the Stockholm Diabetes Intervention Study (SDIS) after 5 years. *Journal of Internal Medicine*, **230**, 101–8.

Robison, W. G., Jr, Nagata, M., Laver, N., Hohman, T. C., and Kinoshita, J. H. (1989a). Diabetic-like retinopathy in rats prevented with aldose reductase inhibitors. *Investigative Ophthalmology and Visual Science*, **30**, 2285–92.

Robison W. G., Jr., Nagata, M., Tillis, T. N., Laver, N., and Kinoshita, J. H. (1989b). Aldose reductase and pericyte-endothelial cell contacts in retina and optic nerve. *Investigative Ophthalmology and Visual Science*, **30**, 2293–9.

Robison, W. G., Jr., Tillis, T. N., Laver, N., and Kinoshita, J. H. (1990). Diabetes-related histopathologies of the rat retina prevented with an aldose reductase inhibitor. *Experimental Eye Research*, **50**, 355–66.

Rondeau, J. M., Samama, J. P., Samama, B., Barth, P., Moras, D., and Biellman. J. F. (1987). Crystallization and preliminary X-ray study of pig lens aldose reductase. *Journal of Molecular Biology*, **195**, 945–8.

Ryder, S., Sarokhan, B., Shand, D. G., and Mullane, J. F. (1987). Human safety profile of tolrestat: an aldose reductase inhibitor. *Drug Development Research*, **11**, 131–43.

Sands, J. M., Terada, Y., Bernard, L. M., and Knepper, M. A. (1989). Aldose reductase activities in microdissected rat renal tubule segments. *American Journal of Physiology*, **256**, F563–9.

Sato, S. and Kador, P. F. (1991). Is the inhibition of aldehyde reductase by aldose reductase inhibitors beneficial? *Aldose Reductase Workshop*, *Kona*, *HI*, Abstract S 7.5.

Sato, T., Fuji, S., Yamamoto, M., Morii, H., Shimojo, N., Kitahashi, E., *et al.* (1988). Effects of an aldose reductase inhibitor on urinary excretion of albumin, N-acetyl-β-D-glucosaminidase and alanine aminopeptidase in diabetic patients. In *Polyol pathway and its role in diabetic complications* (ed. N. Sakamoto, J. H. Kinoshita, P. F. Kador, and N. Hotta), pp. 348–53. Elsevier, Amsterdam.

Sawada, M., Terashima, H., Okegawa, T., and Kawasaki, A. (1990). Pharmacokinetic study of epalrestat (ONO-2235). In *Current concepts of aldose reductase and its inhibitions* (ed. N. Sakamoto, J. H. Kinoshita, P. F. kador, and N. Hotta), pp. 111–18. Elsevier, Amsterdam,

Schade, S. Z., Early, S. L., Williams, T. R., Kezdy, F. J., Heinrikson, R. L., Grimshaw, C. E., and Doughty, C. C. (1990). Sequence analysis of bovine lens aldose reductase. *Journal of Biological Chemistry*, **265**, 3628–35.

Scott, A. K., Webster, J., and Petrie, J. C. (1987). Sorbinil pharmacokinetics in male and female elderly volunteers. *British Journal of Clinical Pharmacology*, **23**, 495–7.

Sestanj, K., Bellini, F., Fung, S., Abraham, N., Treasurywala, A., Humber, L., et al. (1984). *N*-[[5-(trifluoromethyl)-6-methoxy-1-naphthalenyl]thioxomethyl]-*N*-methylglycine (tolrestat), a potent, orally active aldose reductase inhibitor. *Journal of Medicinal Chemistry*, **27**, 255–6.

Siegel, E. G. (1990). Normoglykämie als Therapieziel der Diabeiesbehandlung-Konzept und Realisierung. *Klinische Wochenschrift*, **68**, 306–12.

Sima, A. A. F. and Greene, D. A. (1991). Sural nerve density and normality predict clinical sensory deficits and electrophysiology in chronic diabetic neuropathy. *Diabetes*, **40** (Suppl. 1), 554A.

Sima, A. A. F., Nathaniel, V., Lattimer, S. A., and Greene, D. A. (1987). The effect of sorbinil treatment on diabetic neuropathy. In *Polyol pathway and its role in diabetic complications* (ed. N. Sakamoto, J. H. Kinoshita, P. F. Kador, and N. Hotta), pp. 416–21. Elsevier, Amsterdam.

Sima, A. A. F., Nathaniel, V., Bril, V., McEwen, T. A. J., and Greene, D. A. (1988a). Histopathological heterogeneity of neuropathy in insulin-dependent and non-insulin-dependent diabetes, and demonstration of axo-glial dysjunction in human diabetic neuropathy. *Journal of Clinical Investigation*, **81**, 349–64.

Sima, A. A. F., Bril, V., Nathaniel, V., McEwen, T. A. J., Brown, M. B., Lattimer, S. A., and Greene, D. A. (1988b). Regeneration and repair of myelinated fibers in sural-nerve biopsy specimens from patients with diabetic neuropathy treated with sorbinil. *New England Journal of Medicine*, **319**, 548–55.

Sima, A. A. F., Prashar, A., Zhang, W. X., Chakrabarti, S., and Greene, D. A. (1990). Preventive effect of long-term aldose reductase inhibition (ponalrestat) on nerve conduction and sural nerve structure in the spontaneously diabetic Bio-Breeding rat. *Journal of Clinical Investigation*, **85**, 1410–20.

Simard-Duquesne, N., Greselin, E., Dubuc, J., and Dvornik, D. (1985). The effects of a new aldose reductase inhibitor (tolrestat) in galactosemic and diabetic rats. *Metabolism*, **34**, 885–92.

Sochor, M., Baquer, T. Z., Hothersall, J. S., and McLean, P. (1990). Effect of experimental diabetes on the activity of hexokinase in tissues of the rat. *Biochemistry International*, **22**, 467–74.

Sorbinil Retinopathy Trial Research Group (1990). A randomized trial of sorbinil, an aldose reductase inhibitor, in diabetic retinopathy. *Archives of Ophthalmology*, **108**, 1234–44.

Spielberg, S. P., Shear, N. H., Cannon, M., Hutson, N., and Gunderson, K. (1991). *In-vitro* assessment of a hypersensitivity syndrome associated with sorbinil. *Archives of Internal Medicine*, **114**, 720–4.

Sredy, J., Flam, B. R., sand Sawicki, D. R. (1991). Adenosine triphosphatase activity in sciatic nerve tissue of streptozotocin-induced diabetic rats with and without high dietary sucrose: effect of aldose reductase inhibitors. *Proceedings of the Society for Experimental Biology and Medicine*, **197**, 135–43.

Stribling, D. (1988). The chemistry and properties of aldose reductase inhibitors. In *Polyol pathway and its role in diabetic complications* (ed. N. Sakamoto, J. H. Kinoshita, P. F. Kador, and N. Hotta), pp. 32–41. Elsevier, Amsterdam.

Stribling, D. (1990a). Clinical trials with aldose reductase inhibitors. *Experimental Eye Research*, **50**, 621–4.

Stribling, D. (1990b). Designing clinical trials with aldose reductase inhibitors.

In *Current concept of aldose reductase and its inhibitions* (ed. N. Sakamoto, J. H. Kinoshita, P. F. Kador, and N. Hotta), pp. 139–47. Elsevier, Amsterdam.

Stribling, D., Mirrlees, D. J., Harrison, H. E., and Earl, D. C. N. (1985). Properties of ICI 128,436, a novel aldose reductase inhibitor, and its effects on diabetic complications in the rat. *Metabolism*, **34**, 336–44.

Stribling, D., Armstrong, F. M., and Harrison, H. E. (1989a). Aldose reductase in the etiology of diabetic complications. 2. Nephropathy. *Journal of Diabetic Complications*, **3**, 70–6.

Stribling, D., Armstrong, F. M., Perkins, C. M., and Smith, J. C. (1989b). Aldose reductase in the etiology of diabetic complications. 3. Neuropathy. *Journal of Diabetic Complications*, **3**, 139–48.

Stribling, D., Armstrong, F. M., Hardman, M., and Perkins, C. M. (1990). Aldose reductase in the etiology of diabetic complications. 4. Retinopathy. *Journal of Diabetic Complications*, **4**, 102–7.

Terashima, H. (1988). Aldose reductase and pharmacokinetics. In *Polyol pathway and its role in diabetic complications* (ed. N. Sakamoto, J. H. Kinoshita, P. F. Kador, and N. Hotta), pp. 42–60. Elsevier, Amsterdam.

Terubayashi, H., Sato, S., Kador, P. F., and Kinoshita, J. H. (1988). Aldose and aldehyde reductase in the kidney. In *Polyol pathway and its role in diabetic complications* (ed. N. Sakamoto, J. H. Kinoshita, P. F. Kador, and N. Hotta), pp. 330–41. Elsevier, Amsterdam.

Tilton, R. G., Chang. K., Pugliese, G., Eades, D. M., Province, M. A., Sherman, W. R., and Williamson, J. R. (1989). Prevention of hemodynamic and vascular albumin filtration changes in diabetic rats by aldose reductase inhibitors. *Diabetes*, **37**, 1258–70.

Tomlinson, D. R. (1989). Polyols and myo-inositol in diabetic neuropathy—of mice and men. *Mayo Clinic Proceedings*, **64**, 1030–33.

Tomlinson, D. R., Willars, G. B., Robinson, J. P., Lambourne, J. E., Calcutt, N. A., and Compton, A. M. (1988). Experimental aspects of diabetic neuropathy: role of axonal transport disorders. In *Polyol pathway and its role in diabetic complications* (ed. N. Sakamoto, J. H. Kinoshita, P. F. Kador, and N. Hotta), pp. 385–96. Elsevier, Amsterdam.

Tuffin, D. P., Dingle, A., Sennitt, C. M., Mirrlees, D. J., and Ward, W. H. J. (1989). Ponalrestat: a potent and selective inhibitor of bovine lens aldose reductase. In *Enzymology and molecular biology of carbonyl metabolism* Vol. 2 (ed. H. Weiner and T. G. Flynn), pp. 221–35. Liss, New York.

Vander Jagt, D. L., Robinson, B., Taylor, K. K., and Hunsaker, L. A. (1990). Aldose reductase from human skeletal and heart muscle. *Journal of Biological Chemistry*, **265**, 20982–7.

van Heiningen, R. (1959). Formation of polyols by the lens of the rat with 'sugar' cataract. *Nature, London*, **184**, 194–5.

Verillo, A., DeTeresa, A., Martino, C., Verillo, L., and DiChiara, G. (1988). Long-term correction of hyperglycemia and progression of retinopathy in insulin-dependent diabetes. A five-year randomized prospective study. *Diabetes Research*, **8**, 71–6.

Viberti, G. C., Bilous, R. W., Mackintosh, D., Bending, J. J., and Keen, H. (1983). Long-term correction of hyperglycemia and progression of renal failure in insulin dependent diabetes. *British Medical Journal*, **286**, 598–602.

Vinores, S. A., Campochiaro, P. A., Williams, E. H., May, E. E., Green, R., and Sorenson, R. L. (1988). Aldose reductase expression in human diabetic retina and retinal pigment epithelium. *Diabetes*, **37**, 1658–64.

Ward, J. D. (1990). Diabetic neuropathy. In *The diabetes annual*, Vol. 5 (ed. K. G. M. M. Alberti and L. P. Krall), pp. 312–29. Elsevier, Amsterdam.

Watkins, P. J. (1990). Natural history of the diabetic neuropathies. *Quarterly Journal of Medicine, New Series* , **77**, 1209–18.

Welling, P. G. (1986). *Pharmacokinetics: processes and mathematics. ACS Monograph 185*, pp. 193–6. American Chemical Society, Washington, DC.

Willars, G. B., Newrick, P. G., Tomlinson, D. R., and Ward, J. D. (1987). Polyol metabolites and myo-inositol in sural nerve biopsies from diabetic patients. *Diabetic Medicine*, **4**, 382.

Winegrad, A. I. (1987). Does a common mechanism induce the diverse complications of diabetes? *Diabetes*, **36**, 396–406.

Wirtensohn, G., Lefrank, S., Guder, W. G., and Beck, F. (1987). Studies on the role of glycerophosphorylcholine and sorbitol in renal osmoregulation. In *Nephrology. Biochemical aspects of kidney function* (ed. Z. Kovacevic and W. G. Guder), pp. 321–7. DeGruyter, Berlin.

Wirtensohn, G., Lefrank, S., Schmolke, M., and Guder, W. G. (1989). Regulation of organic osmolyte concentrations in tubules from rat renal inner medulla. *American Journal of Physiology*, **256**, F128–35.

Yancey, P. H., Clark, M. E., Hand, S. C., Bowlus, R. D., and Samero, G. N. (1982). Living with water stress: evolution of osmolite systems. *Science*, **217**, 1214–22.

Yancey, P. H., Hauer, R. G., and Freudenberger, T. H. (1990). Effects of an aldose reductase inhibitor on organic osmotic effects in rat renal medulla. *American Journal of Physiology*, **259**, F733–8.

Yue, D. K., McLennan, S., Fisher, E., Heffernan, S., Capogreco, C., Ross, G. R., and Turtle, J. R. (1989). Ascorbic acid metabolism and polyol pathway in diabetes. *Diabetes*, **38**, 257–61.

Ziegler, D., Cicmir, I., Mayer, P., Wiefels, K., and Gries, F. A. (1988). The natural course of peripheral and autonomic neural function during the first two years after diagnosis of Type I diabetes. *Klinische Wochenschrift*, **66**, 1085–92.

Ziegler, D., Mayer, P., Rathmann, W., and Griess, F. A. (1991). One-year treatment with the aldose-reductase inhibitor, ponalrestat, in diabetic neuropathy. *Diabetes Research and Clinical Practice*, **14**, 63–74.

Zimmerman, B. R. (1989). Influence of the degree of control of diabetes on the prevention, postponement and amelioration of late complications. *Drugs*, **38**, 941–56.

17

Miscellaneous topics

Section 17A

'Atriopeptidase' (EC 3.4.24.11) inhibition and
protection of atrial natriuretic factor

J.C. Schwartz, C. Gros, P. Duhamel, L. Duhamel,
J.M. Lecomte, and J. Bralet

17A.1   Introduction

Two major hormonal peptide systems appear to play opposite roles in
the regulation of electrolyte balance and blood pressure, so that their
imbalance might be responsible for cardiovascular and salt-retention disorders affecting much of the population. The first is the renin–angiotensin–aldosterone system which several classes of established or potential
antihypertensive agents, namely the inhibitors of angiotensin-converting
enzyme (ACE; EC 3.4.15.1), tend to oppose. The second consists of atrial
natriuretic factor (ANF), also called atrial natriuretiic peptide (ANP), a
28 amino acid peptide (Fig. 17A.1) secreted by the heart into the circulation
to decrease blood pressure, raise the urinary excretion of water and sodium,
and lower plasma renin and aldosterone levels (Brenner *et al.* 1990). This
unusual combination of effects, as well as various clinical studies in which
the hormone was infused intravenously, suggest that ANF might prove
useful in the treatment of cardiovascular disorders such as hypertension

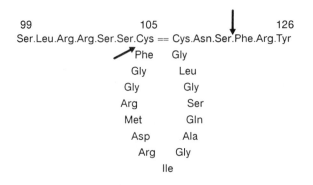

Fig. 17A.1 Amino acid sequence of human ANF and its main peptide bonds hydrolysed (arrows) by purified MEP.

and heart failure. However, its poor absorption *per os* and extremely rapid inactivation when injected, difficulties often encountered with the therapeutic application of peptides, have so far prevented its clinical use.

One approach to this problem involves delaying the inactivation of endogenous ANF which involves two distinct processes: (i) binding to so-called 'clearance receptors', which are devoid of guanylate cyclase activity like the so-called 'biological receptors' and presumably are responsible for ANF internalization; (ii) hydrolysis into inactive fragments. Indeed, blockade of the 'clearance receptors' by ANF analogues inactive at biological receptors seems to result in ANF-like responses in rodents (Koepke *et al.* 1989) but the blockers available so far are peptides, raising the same bioavailability problems as ANF itself.

In contrast, inhibition of endogenous ANF hydrolysis emerges to progressively as a practical therapeutic means of promoting ANF-like responses. It is based upon the utilization of enkephalinase inhibitors, a class of drugs designed a decade ago to delay enkephalin inactivation (Schwartz *et al.* 1981) and which, through this mechanism, have already found therapeutic application as antisecretory agents in gastroenterology (Erdös and Skidgel 1989; Schwartz 1989). Their possible use in the cardiovascular field derives from the recent demonstration that the zinc-containing peptidase enkephalinase, numbered 3.4.24.11 and named membrane metalloendopeptidase (MEP) by the Enzyme Commission (also known as atriopeptidase or neutral endopeptidase 24.11), is largely responsible for the inactivation not only of endogenous enkephalins but also of endogenous ANF. Whereas various other peptidases, for which ANF is also a substrate, were previously believed to play such a role, only MEP satisfies all the criteria (Schwartz 1989) which need to be met for this function (Schwartz *et al.* 1990; Carretero and Sicli 1991). Briefly stated, MEP efficiently cleaves the hormone into inactive fragments *in vitro*, and *in vivo* its inhibitors delay ANF metabolism, increase ANF level in plasma, and elicit renal and cardiovascular responses characteristically induced by exogenous ANF.

Several MEP inhibitors have currently submitted to clinical trials in both essential hypertension and congestive heart failure, and these drugs appear to constitute a promising new class of cardiovascular agent. In addition, a novel class of agent, mixed inhibitors of the two metallo-peptidases ACE and MEP, whose therapeutic potential remains to be assessed, has emerged even more recently.

17A.2 Inactivation of exogenous ANF by MEP *in vitro* and *in vivo*

The initial indication (Olins *et al*. 1986) that ANF can be efficiently cleaved by MEP was that a brush border membrane preparation from rabbit kidney, in which the peptidase is extremely abundant, rapidly hydrolyses the peptide at the level of the Cys^7-Phe^8 and the Ser^{25}-Phe^{26} amide bonds (Fig. 17A.1). MEP was identified as the responsible enzyme among the various peptidases present in the preparation: ANF hydrolysis is largely prevented by MEP inhibitors and, characteristically, the purified enzyme also cleaves ANF at the same bonds (Koehn *et al*. 1987; Olins *et al*. 1987; Stephenson and Kenny 1987; Sonnenberg *et al*. 1988; Sybertz *et al*. 1989). Hydrolysis of ^{125}I-hANF, a biologically active peptide, by the human recombinant peptidase also occurs at the same bonds (Gros *et al*. 1989) with a high 'specificity constant' (the ratio of k_{cat} to K_m) close to that of (Met^5)-enkephalin, one of its 'best' substrates (Schwartz 1989). Both hydrolysed bonds involve the amino group of an aromatic amino acid residue, which is consistent with the known substrate specificity of the enzyme except that shorter peptides and bonds located toward the C-terminal end are generally preferred. Therefore the efficient hydrolysis of the Cys^7-Phe^8 bond is somewhat unexpected, but presumably related to the ring structure of ANF. Cleavage of either of these two bonds, particularly the Cys^7-Phe^8 bond which destroys the tertiary structure of ANF by opening its intramolecular ring, leads to a loss of biological activity (Brenner *et al*. 1990). Brain natriuretic peptide (BNP) is a 26 amino acid polypeptide homologous to ANF, originally isolated from porcine brain but also present in heart and displaying ANF-like biological activity. Like ANF, BNP is hydrolysed at the level of the Cys-Phe amide bond by kidney enkephalinase (Vogt-Schaden *et al*. 1989). Nevertheless, these purely biochemical observations do not suffice to establish that MEP is responsible for the inactivation of the hormone circulating in the blood because the enzyme in brush borders may be responsible, at best, for ANF hydrolysis in the glomerular ultrafiltrate.

In fact, the crucial role of this peptidase in the inactivation of exogenous ANF *in vivo* was clearly demonstrated with the use of MEP inhibitors.

Injected ANF has a very short half-life in plasma and its metabolism is delayed in rodents treated with MEP inhibitors, as shown either directly by the enhanced hormone levels in plasma and tissues or indirectly by amplified hormonal responses.

For instance, in rats constantly infused with ANF various MEP inhibitors enhance the plasma level of the hormone by a factor of 2–3 (Olins *et al.* 1989; Trapani *et al.* 1989). In rats receiving a 200 ng bolus of ANF (Northridge *et al.* 1989) or mice receiving ^{125}I-ANF in tracer dosage (Gros *et al.* 1989, 1990a), MEP inhibitors enhance the half-life of the hormone in plasma, which otherwise is only about 1 minute, by a factor of 2. The rapid metabolism of ^{125}I-ANF is also demonstrated at the level of a target organ: 2 minutes after its intravenous injection in mice, most of the radioactivity in kidney is recovered in the form of free ^{125}I-tyrosine; pretreatment with MEP inhibitors enhances the kidney level of intact ^{125}I-ANF by about a factor of 6 (Gros *et al.* 1989, 1990b). The protective effect of MEP inhibitors is also demonstrated by measuring the *in vivo* binding of radioactivity to lung membranes of mice receiving ^{125}I-ANF intravenously in tracer dosage (Souque *et al.* 1992). This binding of the intact hormone which occurs at 'clearance receptors', i.e. a subtype of ANF recognition site devoid of guanylate cyclase activity and presumably responsible for ANF internalization (Brenner *et al.* 1990), is markedly and selectively enhanced by a variety of MEP inhibitors. In all these investigations the protection of exogenous ANF can clearly be attributed to inhibition of MEP, since several inhibitors of this peptidase, belonging to different chemical classes, share this action; protection also occurs with stereoselectivity, time course, and potency closely similar to those corresponding to occupancy of the membrane peptidase, as judged by an *in vivo* binding test (De La Baume *et al.* 1988). Furthermore, this protection of ANF seems largely restricted to MEP inhibitors since, among a large variety of peptidase inhibitors, only aminopeptidase inhibitors also displayed some, although marginal, protective effect (Gros *et al.* 1990b). However, plasma clearance of a 24 amino acid ANF peptide (shortened at its N-terminal end) was delayed not only by MEP inhibitors but also by aminopeptidase and ACE inhibitors (Krieter *et al.* 1989).

As a consequence of their protective effect, different MEP inhibitors (Fig. 17A.2) significantly amplify the magnitude and/or duration of typical responses induced by exogenous ANF in rodents such as diuresis, natriuresis, urinary excretion of cGMP, or decrease of arterial blood pressure in spontaneously hypertensive rats (Seymour *et al.* 1989a,b; Sybertz *et al.* 1989; Trapani *et al.* 1989; Webb *et al.* 1989).

Enkephalinase, i.e. MEP, is widely distributed among tissues (Llorens and Schwartz 1981; Ronco *et al.* 1988), and the above studies do not indicate which tissue is mainly responsible for the hydrolysis of circulating ANF. The following observations suggest that the kidney may not be

(1) Mercaptoalkyl inhibitors

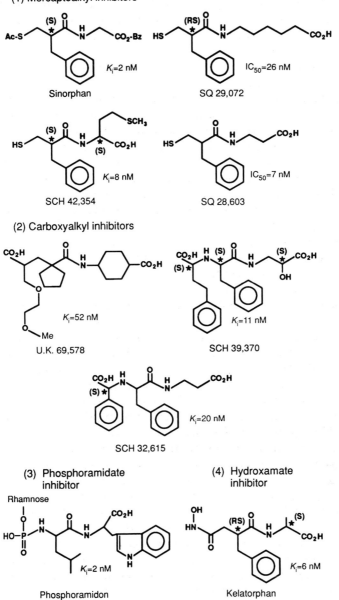

(2) Carboxyalkyl inhibitors

(3) Phosphoramidate inhibitor

(4) Hydroxamate inhibitor

Fig. 17A.2 Various MEP inhibitors used to assess ANF-protecting activity or ability to induce ANF-like responses in preclinical or clinical studies. All these compounds incorporate, in a dipeptide-like structure, a zinc-chelating group and a C-terminal carboxylate. K_i values as inhibitors of purified or recombinant MEP are reported. Sinorphan is a prodrug and the K_i value corresponds to that of (S)thiorphan, its de-esterified product.

primarily involved: (i) kidney MEP is mainly present in brush border membranes not in contact with the blood plasma (Schulz *et al.* 1988); (ii) after administration of ^{125}I-ANF, MEP inhibitors enhance not only the recovery of intact ^{125}I-ANF but also the total radioactivity in kidney, indicating that more intact hormone is reaching the organ (Gros *et al.* 1989, 1990b; Lafferty *et al.* 1989); (iii) nephrectomy reduces plasma ANF clearance only slightly and actually enhances the protective actions of MEP inhibitors (Sybertz *et al.* 1989; Barclay *et al.* 1991). Although blood plasma contains a soluble form of MEP (Schwartz 1989), the protective effect of MEP inhibitors is not attributable to its inhibition because the half-life of ^{125}I-ANF in blood *in vitro* is greater than *in vivo* and is not affected by MEP inhibitors (Gros *et al.* 1990a). Nevertheless, it seems likely that some renal actions of MEP inhibitors are related to inhibition of the peptidase, which is strongly expressed in brush borders of proximal tubules (see below).

17A.3 MEP inhibitors protect endogenous ANF and trigger ANF-like responses

In tissues such as brain, the metabolism of exogenous and endogenous messenger peptides may differ, mainly as a result of topographic factors (Schwartz *et al.* 1981). However, in the case of hormones, the metabolic fate of peptides either injected or secreted into the blood should be the same. Accordingly, after treatment with MEP inhibitors, ANF immuno-reactivity (ANF-ir) rises two- to threefold in the plasma of rats in which it is already elevated as a consequence of volume load (Bralet *et al.* 1991), cardiac insufficiency (Northridge *et al.* 1989; Wilkins *et al.* 1990), or reduced renal mass (Lafferty *et al.* 1989), and it is also enhanced in the urine of DOCA-Na or Dahl-S hypertensive rats (Sybertz *et al.* 1989). Unexpectedly, however, different MEP inhibitors do not enhance steady state plasma ANF-ir in normal rats (Olins *et al.* 1989; Sybertz *et al.* 1989; Bralet *et al.* 1991), although clearance of the exogenous hormone was shown to be delayed by these drugs. It is likely that, in rats, in-activation of the circulating hormone at normal plasma ANF levels predominantly involves its binding to clearance receptors: ANF-ir doubled after coadministration of a selective clearance receptor ligand and thiorphan, a prototypic MEP inhibitor, whereas each agent alone was inactive (Koepke *et al.* 1989).

In contrast, ANF inactivation in humans seems predominantly to involve its hydrolysis by MEP. In healthy human volunteers, either oral adminis-tration (Gros *et al.* 1989; Lecomte *et al.* 1990) or intravenous infusion of various MEP inhibitors (Northridge *et al.* 1990) enhances plasma ANF-ir by a factor of 2 to 3 for several hours. This limited rise is in the same range as those occurring under certain physiological conditions, such as head-out water immersion, which are sufficient to be accompanied by biological responses (Brenner *et al.* 1990). The duration of the rise of plasma ANF-ir is related to the oral dosage of MEP inhibitors and to the degree of inhibition of plasma MEP activity, so that an inhibition by about 50 per cent is accompanied by doubling of the hormone level (Gros *et al.* 1989; Lecomte *et al.* 1990).

Even more interestingly, sustained increases in plasma ANF-ir of similar magnitude, i.e. two- to threefold, still occur in patients with mild (Northridge *et al.* 1989) or even severe (Kahn *et al.* 1990) chronic heart failure, a condition in which baseline plasma ANF is already markedly elevated as a consequence of hypersecretion induced by the rise in atrial pressure. Enhanced plasma ANF levels are also found in patients with chronic renal failure (Dussaule *et al.* 1993) or cirrhosis with ascites (Dussaule *et al.* 1991) who are receiving sinorphan. These studies, performed with chemically distinct MEP inhibitors, suggest that their administration represents an effective means of enhancing plasma ANF in a sustained manner, whatever its baseline level.

When MEP inhibitors are administered alone to normal rats, only rather modest ANF-like effects occur. For instance, diuretic and natriuretic responses were either not significant (Lafferty *et al.* 1989; Seymour *et al.* 1989b) or rather limited (Ura *et al.* 1987; Bralet *et al.* 1990).

In contrast, MEP inhibitors elicit clear-cut responses in rats in which ANF secretion has been acutely or chronically enhanced by extracellular volume expansion. This is the case for rats in which the diuretic and natriuretic responses, which normally follow an intravenous saline load, are strongly enhanced by MEP inhibitors; this effect probably involves endogenous ANF since it is blocked in animals receiving antibodies raised against the hormone and used here as ANF antagonists (Bralet *et al.* 1990, 1991). In rats with experimentally reduced renal mass or cardiac insufficiency, in which ANF secretion is elevated, MEP inhibitors enhance the glomerular filtration rate by 25 per cent and the urine flow rate, $U_{Na}V$, FE_{Na}, or cGMP excretion by 200–300 per cent (Lafferty *et al.* 1989; Wilkins *et al.* 1990).

In healthy human volunteers receiving MEP inhibitors, such as sinorphan (Fig. 17A.2) orally (Lecomte *et al.* 1990) or candoxatrilat parenterally (Northridge *et al.* 1989), consistent ANF-like renal effects were recorded in three separate studies, whereas arterial blood pressure and cardiac variables were not significantly affected (Table 17A.1). Interestingly, these characteristic responses to MEP inhibitors appear to be both qualitatively and quantitatively very similar to those elicited by a constant infusion of ANF in moderate dosage, a treatment leading to a rise in plasma ANF-ir only slightly higher than that elicited by MEP inhibitors. Both approaches provide evidence that ANF acts as a natriuretic hormone at physiological plasma concentrations in man.

Table 17A.1 Summary of the cardiovascular and renal effects of MEP inhibitors

Variable	Change (%)
Plasma ANF-ir (human)	+ 100–200
Plasma ANF-ir (rodent)	0
Urinary ANF-ir (rodent)	+ 1000
Urinary cGMP (rodent, human)	+ 100
Urinary sodium (rodent, human)	+ 100
Plasma renin activity (human)	− 50
Mean blood pressure (rat, acute)	
normal	0
SHR	0
DOCA-Na, Dahl-S	− 20
Mean blood pressure (human, chronic)	
normal volunteers	0
mild hypertensive	− 20

Other characteristic ANF-like responses to MEP inhibitors are listed in Table 17A.1. Interestingly, in patients with congestive heart failure in which down-regulation of ANF receptors related to the high circulating level of the hormone has been hypothesized (Brenner *et al.* 1990), the natriuretic and diuretic responses to administration of MEP inhibitors seem unaltered.

17A.4   Mixed MEP–ACE inhibitors: a novel class of cardiovascular drug

The cell-surface zinc-containing peptidases ACE and MEP play a key role in the activation and inactivation respectively of the two major hormonal peptide systems which govern blood pressure and salt-water metabolism. Since the renin–angiotensin–aldosterone system and the natriuretic peptide system appear to play opposite roles at various physiological levels it seems reasonable to expect synergistic effects from the coinhibition of angiotensin II formation and ANF inactivation.

It seemed possible to obtain both effects in a single compound displaying mixed MEP–ACE inhibitory potency since some mercaptoalkyl derivatives display limited but significant cross-reactivity towards the two metallopeptidases (Gordon *et al.* 1983; Schwartz 1989). This partial overlap suggested that careful structure–activity analysis of compounds in this chemical series might lead to an agent with such properties. Glycoprilat and alatrioprilat (Table 17A.2), and their corresponding prodrugs glycopril

Table 17A.2 Glycoprilat and alatrioprilat, two mixed MEP–ACE inhibitors: structures, *in vitro* potencies and potential modes of interaction with the two metallopeptidases

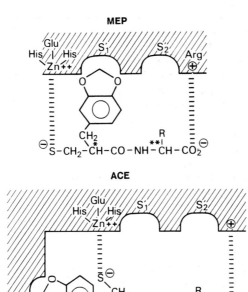

Compounds	Configuration ($*$, $**$)	R	K_i (nM)	
			Enkephalinase	ACE
I Glycoprilat	(S)	H	5.6 ± 1.0	6.5 ± 1.3
II	(R)	H	12.0 ± 2.0	420 ± 100
III Alatrioprilat	(S,S)	CH_3	5.1 ± 0.8	9.8 ± 1.3
IV	(R,S)	CH_3	13.7 ± 0.9	215 ± 30

and alatriopril, which display nanomolar inhibitory potency of both ACE or MEP, were designed in this way by a step-by-step modification of thiorphan, a prototypic enkephalinase inhibitor (Roques *et al*. 1980).

Although ACE (Soubrier *et al*. 1988) and MEP (Devault *et al*. 1987; Malfroy *et al*. 1987) display little overall amino acid sequence homology, they presumably share the same catalytic mechanism and their substrate specificities overlap to some extent since they hydrolyse some peptides, such as enkephalins, bradykinin, or substance P, at the same amide bonds

(Erdös and Skidgel 1989; Schwartz 1989). In addition, most inhibitors of the two peptidases incorporate essentially similar features, i.e. a zinc-chelating group borne by a modified dipeptide with a free C-terminal carboxylate interacting with a positively charged guanidinium residue (Malfroy and Schwartz 1982; Schwartz 1989) identified as belonging to Arg-95 in rabbit MEP (Bateman *et al.* 1989). However, the optimal dipeptide sequence binding to the S_1' and S_2' subsites differ in the two peptidases. For instance, a P_1' aromatic residue is strongly preferred in the case of MEP but only tolerated in the case of ACE, and an unsubstituted $CO-NH$ function is essential for binding to MEP but not to ACE, most inhibitors of which have a C-terminal proline. As a consequence of these main features, several compounds show cross-reactivity *in vitro*, and 'selective' mercapto inhibitors of one peptidase even display some inhibitory activity towards the other, with the selectivity ratio being, for instance, about 100 for the MEP inhibitor thiorphan (Roques *et al.* 1980) and about 1000 for the ACE inhibitor captopril (Swerts *et al.* 1979). However, similarly high *in vivo* potency towards the two enzymes is obviously required for thera-peutic application of mixed inhibitors, with their effective dosage being ultimately determined by their affinity for the less readily inhibited enzyme.

The observation that the S_1' hydrophobic pocket of MEP tolerates the phenyl ring of thiorphan in its two spatial orientations (Mendelsohn *et al.* 1985; Giros *et al.* 1987) suggests that this pocket is large enough to accomodate more bulky groups than a phenyl ring. In contrast, the high stereochemical preference of (*S*)thiorphan for ACE suggests that the phenyl ring can interact differently with a subsite of this enzyme and that this putative interaction can be optimized by substitution of the ring. In glyco-prilat, the methylenedioxy substitution provides a 10-fold increase in affinity towards ACE without significant loss in affinity toward MEP. Glycoprilat and alatrioprilat, its methylated analogue, inhibit both MEP and ACE at similar concentrations (in the nanomolar range) but with low and high stereospecificity ratios respectively (Table 17A.2). Analysis of molecular models suggests that, in a discrete configuration of these compounds, their methylenedioxy substituent binds to the S_1 subsite of ACE in the same way as the phenethyl group of enalapril. Indeed, in the enalapril series of ACE inhibitors, the high affinity of compounds is attributable to the presence of aromatic, aralkyl, or aliphatic groups in the (*S*)-configuration which are able to bind to this S_1' subsite (Wyvratt and Patchett 1985).

In vivo, glycopril and alatriopril, the corresponding diester prodrugs, showed occupation of ACE and MEP occurring at ED_{50} values of 0.2–0.5 mg kg^{-1} (Gros *et al.* 1991).

As expected, the mixed inhibitors display a combination of biological activities due to inhibition of either MEP or ACE alone (Table 17A.3). For instance, alatriopril enhances the recovery of intact ^{125}I-hANF in kidney or the binding of ^{125}I-rANF to lung membranes to the same extent as

Table 17A.3 Potencies of glycopril and alatriopril in various tests reflecting MEP or ACE inhibition *in vivo*

Test	ED_{50} or ID_{50} (mg kg^{-1})	
	Glycopril	Alatriopril
MEP occupation (mouse lung)	0.41 ± 0.15	0.42 ± 0.08
ACE occupation (mouse lung)	0.47 ± 0.09	0.19 ± 0.04
^{125}I-ANF protection (mouse kidney)	0.73 ± 0.09	0.23 ± 0.06
^{125}I-ANF protection (mouse lung)	3.7 ± 1.0	2.5 ± 1.2
Angiotensin I pressor response (rat)[*]	1.7 ± 0.2	0.9 ± 0.2

ED_{50} values corresponding to determinations performed 30 minutes after oral administration of glycopril or alatriopril.

[*]Glycoprilat and alatrioprilat administered intravenously 5 minutes before angiotensin II.

selective MEP inhibitors. Like the latter they also increase urinary excretion of water, Na$^+$ and cGMP in rats submitted to extracellular volume expansion. In addition, at doses in the low mg kg^{-1} range, atrioprilat and glycoprilat prevent the hypertensive action of angiotensin I in rats, a typical effect of selective ACE inhibitors (Gros *et al.* 1991).

Coinhibition of the two peptidases may result in several potentially useful therapeutic effects which mainly reflect the counterbalance, at various physiological levels, of the two functionally opposite hormonal systems that these enzymes control. First, vascular smooth muscle and aldosterone secretion are affected in opposite manner by angiotensin II and ANF, so that inhibition of their formation and degradation respectively may have synergistic consequences. Second, ANF reduces plasma renin activity, an effect which may facilitate the prevention of angiotensin II formation through ACE inhibition, particularly during chronic treatment regimens in which renin activity rises in compensation. Third, mixed inhibitors may facilitate the diuretic and natriuretic actions of intrarenal bradykinin, a peptide whose inactivation seems to depend on both ACE and MEP (Ura *et al.* 1987). Finally, in view of their diuretic–natriuretic activity (without kaliuresis) via protection of endogenous ANF, mixed inhibitors may be useful in the treatment of essential hypertension; in this condition, various diuretics potentiate the effects of ACE inhibitors.

17A.5   Conclusions: potential clinical applications

The diuretic, natriuretic, vasorelaxant, and renin- and aldosterone-suppressing effects of exogenous ANF can all be regarded as potentially beneficial in cardiovascular diseases, such as essential hypertension or congestive heart failure, as well as in various sodium-retaining states. The fact that MEP inhibitors significantly enhance plasma ANF levels in all these diseases suggests that these orally active drugs can be used in such conditions. Preliminary data obtained in humans seem to confirm such expectations.

In patients with essential hypertension, candoxatril has been shown to enhance plasma ANF and induce natriuresis (O'Connell *et al.* 1992). Neither this compound nor sinorphan decreased blood pressure after a single administration; in an open study, however, sinorphan significantly decreased blood pressure after about 2 weeks of treatment (Kahn *et al.* 1990).

In patients with mild and severe congestive heart failure receiving candoxatrilat intravenously (Northridge *et al.* 1989) or sinorphan orally respectively (Varin *et al.* 1989; Kahn *et al.* 1990), marked increases in plasma ANF levels, urinary cGMP, and natriuresis were accompanied by decreases in right atrial pressure and pulmonary capillary pressure.

In various sodium-retaining states such as nephrotic syndrome (Dussaule *et al.* 1993) and cirrhosis (Dussaule *et al.* 1991), the enhancement of plasma ANF levels elicited by sinorphan was accompanied by natriuresis.

In the case of the mixed MEP−ACE inhibitors, clinical data are not yet available. However, these drugs were recently found to prevent cardiac hypertrophy in rats with experimental myocardial infarction in a significantly more successful manner than captopril (Bralet *et al.*, in press, 1993).

It is clear that controlled clinical trials with these various representatives of new classes of drugs will be required to assess their therapeutic utility in the cardiovascular field.

References

Barclay, P. L., Bennett, J. A., Samuels, G. M., and Shepperson, N. B. (1991). The atriopeptidase inhibitor $(+/-)$candoxatrilat reduces the clearance of atrial natriuretic factor in both intact and nephrectomized rats: evidence for an extra-renal site of action. *Biochemical Pharmacology*, **41**, 841–4.

Bateman, R. C., Jackson, D., Slaugher, C. A., Unnithan, S., Chai, Y. G., Mooman, C., and Hersch, L. B. (1989). Identification of the active-site Arginine in rat neutral endopeptidase 24.11 (enkephalinase) as Arginine[102] and analysis of glutamine 102 mutant. *Journal of Biological Chemistry*, **264**, 6151–7.

Bralet, J., Mossiat, C., Lecomte, J. M., Charpentier, S., Gros, C., and Schwartz, J. C. (1990). Diuretic and natriuretic responses in rats treated with enkephalinase inhibitors. *European Journal of Pharmacology*, **179**, 57–64.

Bralet, J., Mossiat, C., Gros, C., and Schwartz, J. C. (1991). Thiorphan-induced natriuresis in volume expanded rats: roles of endogenous atrial natriuretic factor and kinins. *Journal of Pharmacology and Experimental Therapeutics*, **258**, 807–11.

Bralet, J., Marie, C., Mossiat, C., Lecomte, J. M., Gros, C., and Schwartz, J. C. (1993). Effects of alatriopril, a mixed inhibitor of atriopeptidase and angiotensin I-converting enzyme, on cardiac hypertrophy and hormonal responses in rats with myocardial infarction. Comparison with captopril. *Journal of Pharmacology and Experimental Therapeutics*, (In press.)

Brenner, B. M., Ballermann, B. J., Gunnning, M. E., and Zeidel, M. L. (1990). Diverse biological actions of atrial natriuretic peptide. *Physiological Reviews*, **70**, 665–99.

Carretero, O. A. and Sicli, A. G. (1991). Zinc metallopeptidase inhibitors. A novel antihypertensive treatment; editorial comment. *Hypertension*, **18**, 366–71.

De La Baume, Brion, F., Dam Trung Tuong, M., and Schwartz, J. C. (1988). Evaluation of enkephalinase inhibition in the living mouse, using [³H]acetorphan as a probe. *Journal of Pharmacology and Experimental Therapeutics*, **247**, 653–60.

Devault, A., Lazure, C., Nault, C., Lemoual, M., Seidam, N. G., Chretien, M., *et al.* (1987). Aminoacid sequence of rabbit kidney neutral endopeptidase 24.11 (enkephalinase) deduced from a complementary DNA. *EMBO Journal*, **6**, 1317–22.

Dussaule, J. C., Grange, J. D., Wolf, J. P., Lecomte, J. M., Gros, C., Schwartz, J. C., *et al.* (1991). Effect of sinorphan, an enkephalinase inhibitor, on plasma atrial natriuretic factor and sodium urinary excretion in cirrhotic patients with ascites. *Journal of Clinical Endocrinology and Metabolism*, **72**, 653–9.

Dussaule, C., Michel, C., Peraldi, M. N., Lecomte, J. M., Gros, C., Mignon, F., and Ardaillou, R. (1993). Inhibition of neutral endopeptidase stimulated renal sodium excretion in patients with chronic renal failure. *Clinical Science*, **84**, 31–9.

Erdös, E. G. and Skidgel, R. A. (1989). Neutral endopeptidase 24.11 (enkephalinase) and related regulators of peptides hormones. *FASEB Journal*, **3**, 145–51.

Giros, B., Gros, C., Schwartz, J. C., Danvy, D., Plaquevent, J. C., Duhamel, L., *et al.* (1987). Enantiomers of thiorphan and acetorphan: correlations between enkephalinase inhibitor protection of endogenous enkephalins and behavioural effects, *Journal of Pharmacology and Experimental Therapeutics*, **243**, 666–73.

Gordon, E. M., Cushman, D. W., Tung, R., Cheung, H. S., Wang, F. L., and Delaney, N. G. (1983). Rat brain enkephalinase: characterization of the active site using mercaptopropanol aminoacid inhibitors and comparison with angiotensin converting enzyme. *Life Sciences*, **33**, 113–16.

Gros, C., Souque, A., Schwartz, J. C., Duchier, J., Cournot, A., Baumer, P., and Lecomte, J. M. (1989). Protection of atrial natriuretic factor against degradation; diuretic and natriuretic responses after *in vivo* inhibition of enkephalinase (EC 3.4.24.11) by acetorphan. *Proceedings of the National Academy of Sciences of the United States of America*, **86**, 7580–4.

Gros, C., Souque, A., and Schwartz, J. C. (1990a). Degradation of atrial natriuretic factor in mouse refliood *in vitro* and *in vivo*: role of enkephalinase (EC 3.4.24.11). *Peptides*, **17**, 1–5.

Gros, C., Souque, A., and Schwartz, J. C. (1990b). Inactivation of atrial natriuretic factor in mice *in vivo*: crucial role of enkephalinase (EC 3.4.24.11). *European Journal of Pharmacology*, **179**, 45–56.

Gros, C., Noel, N., Souque, A., Schwartz, J. C., Danvy, D., Plaquevent, J. C., *et al.* (1991). Mixed inhibitors of angiotensin-converting enzyme (EC 3.4.15.1) and enkephalinase (EC 3.4.24.11): rational design, properties and potential cardiovascular applications of glycopril and alatriopril. *Proceedings of the National Academy of Sciences of the United States of America*, **88**, 4210–14.

Kahn, J. C., Patey, M., Dubois-rande, J. L., Merlet, P., Castaigne, A., Lim-Alexandre, C., *et al.* (1990). Sinorphan, an orally-active enkephalinase inhibitor, enhances plasma atrial natriuretic factor in severe congestive heart failure. *Lancet*, **335**, 112–19.

Koehn, J. A., Norman, J. A., Jones, B. N., Lesueur, L., Sakane, Y., and Ghai, R. D. (1987). Degradation of atrial natriuretic factor in kidney cortex membranes. *Journal of Biological Chemistry*, **262**, 11623–7.

Koepke, J. P., Tyler, L. D., Trapani, A. J., Bovy, P. R., Spear, K. L., Olins, G. M., and Blaine, E. M. (1989). Interaction of non guanylate cyclase-linked atriopeptin receptor ligand and endopeptidase inhibition in concious rats. *Journal of Pharmacology and Experimental Therapeutics*, **249**, 172–6.

Krieter, P. A., Olins, G. M., Verrett, S. P., and Durley, R. C. (1989). *In vivo* metabolism of atrial natriuretic peptide: identification of plasma metabolites and enzymes responsible for their generation. *Journal of Pharmacology and Experimental Therapeutics*, **249**, 411–17.

Lafferty, H. M., Gunning, M., Silva, P., Zimmermann, M. B., Brenner, B. M., and Anderson, S. (1989). Enkephalinase inhibition increases plasma atrial natriuretic peptide levels, glomerular filtration rates and urinary excretion in rats with reduced renal mass. *Circulation Research*, **65**, 640–6.

Lecomte, J. M., Baumer, P., Lim, C., Duchier, J., Cournot, A., Dussaule, J. C., *et al.* (1990). Stereoselective protection of exogenous and endogenous ANF by enkephalinase inhibitors in mice and humans. *European Journal of Pharmacology*, **179**, 65–73.

Llorens, C. and Schwartz, J. C. (1981). Enkephalinase activity in rat peripheral organs. *European Journal of Pharmacology*, **69**, 113–16.

Malfroy, B. and Schwartz, J. C. (1982). Properties of 'enkephalinase' from rat kidney: comparison of dipeptidyl carboxypeptidase and endopeptidase activities. *Biochemical and Biophysical Research Communications*, **106**, 276–85.

Malfroy, B., Schofield, P. R., Kuang, W., Seeburg, P., Mason, A. J., and Menzel, W. J. (1987). Molecular cloning and aminoacid sequence of rat enkephalinase. *Biochemical and Biophysical Research Communications*, **144**, 59–66.

Mendelsohn, L. G., Johnson, B. G., Scott, W. L., and Frederickson, R. C. A. (1985). Thiorphan and analogs: lack of correlation between potency to inhibit 'enkephalinase A' *in vitro* and analgesic potency *in vivo*. *Journal of Pharmacology and Experimental Therapeutics*, **234**, 386–90.

Northridge, D. B., Alabaster, J. M. C., Connell, S. G., Dilly, A. F., Lever, A. G., Jardine, P. L., *et al.* (1989). Effects of UK 69578: a novel atriopeptidase inhibitor. *Lancet*, **ii**, 591.

Northridge, D. B., Jardine, A. G., Findlay, I. N., Archibald, M., Dilly, S. G., and Dargie, H. J. (1990). Inhibition of the metabolism of atrial natriuretic factor causes diuresis and natriuresis in chronic heart failure. *American Journal of Hypertension*, **3**, 682–7.

O'Connell, J. E., Jardine, A. G., Davidson, G., and Connell, J. M. C. (1992). Candoxatril, an orally active neutral endopeptidase inhibitor raises plasma atrial natriuretic factor and its natriuretic in essential hypertension. *American Journal of Hypertension*, **10**, 271–7.

Olins, G. M., Spear, K. L., Siegel, N. R., Zurcher-Neely, H. A., and Smith, C. E. (1986). Proteolytic degradations of atriopeptin III by rabbit kidney brush border membranes. *Federation Proceedings, Federation of American Societies of Experimental Biology*, **45**, 427.

Olins, G. M., Spear, K. L., Seiger, N. R., and Zurcher-Neely, H. A. (1987). Inactivation of atrial natriuretic factor by the renal brush border. *Biochemical and Biophysical Research Communications*, **901**, 97–100.

Olins, G. M., Krieter, P. A., Trapani, A. J., Spear, K. L., and Bovy, P. R. (1989). Specific inhibitors of endopeptidase 24.11 inhibit the metabolism of atrial natriuretic peptides *in vivo* and *in vitro*. *Molecular and Cellular Endocrinology*, **61**, 201–8.

Ronco, P., Pollard, H., Galceran, M., Delauche, M., Schwartz, J. C., and Verroust, P. (1988). Distribution of enkephalinase (membrane metalloendopeptidase, EC 3.4.24.11). *Laboratory Investigation*, **58**, 210–17.

Roques, B. P., Fournie-Zaluski, M. C., Soroca, E., Lecomte, J. M., Malfroy, B., Llorens-Cortes, C., and Schwartz, J. C. (1980). The enkephalinase inhibitor thiorphan shows antinociceptive activity in mice. *Nature, London*, **288**, 286–8.

Schulz, W. W., Hagler, H. K., Buja, L. M., and Erdös, E. G. (1988). Ultra-structural localization of angiotensin I—converting enzyme (EC 3.4.15.1) and neutral metallopeptidase (EC 3.4.24.11) in the proximal tubercle of the human kidney. *Laboratory Investigation*, **59**, 789–97.

Schwartz, J. C. (1989). Enkephalinase inhibitors as drugs. In *Design of enzyme inhibitors as drugs* (ed. M. Sandler and H. J. Smith), pp. 206–20. Oxford University Press.

Schwartz, C., Malfroy, B., and De La Baume, S. (1981). Biological inactiva-tion of enkephalins and the role of enkephalin-dipeptidyl-carboxypeptidase ('enkephalinase') as neuropeptidase. *Life Science*, **29**, 1715–40.

Schwartz, J. C., Gros, C., Lecomte, J. M., and Bralet, J. (1990). Enkephalinase (EC 3.4.24.11) inhibitors: protection of endogenous ANF against inactivation and potential therapeutic applications. *Life Science*, **47**, 1279–97.

Seymour, A. A., Swerdel, J. N., Fennell, S. A., Druckman, S. P., Neubeck, R., and Delaney, N. G. (1989a). Potentiation of the depressor responses to atrial natriuretic peptides in conscious SHR rats by an inhibitor of neutral endo-peptidase. *Journal of Cardiovascular Pharmacology*, **14**, 194–204.

Seymour, A. A., Swerdel, J. N., and Swerdel, J. A. (1989b). Potentiation of renal effects of atrial natriuretic factor (99–126) by SQ 29,072. *Hypertension*, **14**, 87–97.

Sonnenberg, J. L., Sakane, Y., Jeng, A. Y., Koehn, J. A., Ansell, J. A., Wennogle, L. P., and Ghai, R. D. (1988). Identification of protease 3.4.24.11 as the major atrial natriuretic factor degrading enzyme in the rat kidney. *Peptides*, **9**, 173–80.

Soubrier, F., Alhenc-Gelas, F., Hubert, C., Allegrini, J., John, M., Tregear, G., and Corvol P. (1988). Two putative active centers in human angiotensin I converting enzyme revealed by molecular cloning. *Proceedings of the National Academy of Sciences of the United States of America*, **85**, 9386–90.

Souque, A., Gros, C., and Schwartz, J. C. (1992). Binding of [^{125}I]atrial natriu-retic factor to mouse lung membranes *in vivo*: characterization and effects of peptidase inhibitors. *Journal of Pharmacology and Experimental Therapeutics*, **260**, 1373–8.

Stephenson, S. L. and Kenny, A. J. (1987). The hydrolysis of *a*-human atrial natriuretic peptide by pig kidney microvillar membranes is initiated by endo-peptidase 24.11. *Biochemical Journal*, **243**, 183–7.

Swerts, J. P., Perdrisot, R., Patey, G., De La Baume, S., and Schwartz, J. C. (1979). Enkephalinase is distinct from brain angiotensin converting enzyme. *European Journal of Pharmacology*, **57**, 279–81.

Sybertz, E. J., Chiu, J. S., Vemulapalli, S., Pitts, B., Foster, C. J., Watkins, R. W., *et al.* (1989). SCH 39370 a neutral metalloendopeptidase inhibitor potentiates biological responses to atrial natriuretic factor and lowers blood pressure in desoxycorticosterone acetate-sodium hypertensive rats. *Journal of Pharmacology and Experimental Therapeutics*, **250**, 624–31.

Trapani, A. J., Smits, G. J., McGraw, D. E., Spear, K. L., Koepke, J. P., Olins, G. M., and Blaine, E. M. (1989). Thiorphan, an inhibitor of endopeptidase 24.11 potentiates the natriuretic activity of atrial natriuretic peptide. *Journal of Cardiovascular Pharmacology*, **14**, 419–24.

Ura, N., Carretero, O. A., and Erdös, E. G. (1987). Role of renal endopeptidase 24.11 in kinin metabolism *in vitro* and *in vivo*. *Kidney International*, **32**, 507–13.

Varin, J., Duboc, D., Lim, C., Weber, S., Mestre, G., Gros, C., *et al.* (1989). Enhancement of atrial natriuretic factor in congestive heart failure by sinorphan, an enkephalinase inhibitor. *Circulation*, **80**, 110.

Vogt-Schaden, M., Gagelmann, M., Hock, D., Herbst, F., and Forssmann, W. G. (1989). Degradation of porcine brain natriuretic peptide (pBNP-26) by endopeptidase 24–11 from kidney cortical membranes. *Biochemical and Biophysical Research Communications*, **161**, 1177–83.

Webb, R. L., Yasay, G. D., McMartin, C., McNeal, R. B., Jr, and Zimmerman, M. B. (1989). Degradation of atrial natriuretic peptide: pharmacologic effects of protease EC 24.11 inhibition. *Journal of Cardiovascular Pharmacology*, **14**, 285–93.

Wilkins, M. R., Settle, S. L., Stockmann, P. T., and Needleman, P. (1990). Maximizing the natriuretic effect of endogenous atriopeptin in a rat model of heart failure. *Proceedings of the National Academy of Sciences of the United States of America*, **87**, 6465–9.

Wyvratt, M. J. and Patchett, A. A. (1985). Recent developments in the design of angiotensin-converting enzyme inhibitors. *Medicinal Research Reviews*, **5**, 483–531.

Section 17B

Calpain inhibitors

James C. Powers

17B.1 Introduction

Calpain (EC 3.4.22.17) is a calcium-dependent cysteine protease which is widely distributed in mammalian cells, with platelets being a particularly rich source. There are two distinct classes of calpains: one requires micromolar concentrations of calcium for optimal enzymatic activity and is referred to as calpain I or μ-calpain; the other requires millimolar concentrations of calcium and is referred to as calpain II or m-calpain. With synthetic substrates such as Suc-Leu-Tyr-AMC, Boc-Leu-Thr-Arg-AMC, and Suc-Leu-Leu-Val-Tyr-AMC (AMC = 7-amino-4-methylcoumarin), half maximal activity requires 1.6–3.7 μM Ca^{2+} for μ-calpain and 200–560 μM Ca^{2+} for m-calpain (Barrett et al. 1991). A number of reviews of calpain have appeared in recent years (Melloni and Pontremoli 1989; Johnson 1990; Mellgren and Murachi 1990).

Calpain was orginally isolated from skeletal muscle and was thought to be responsible for muscle turnover. Calpains are now known to be exclusively intracellular enzymes which are widely distributed throughout the cytoplasm in a variety of cells (Goll et al. 1990). Calpains have many possible biological roles, including the development of long-term memory, the breakdown of neurofilaments at axon terminals, muscle protein turnover, breakdown of membrane proteins, cytoskeletal modification and cleavage of surface proteins during platelet activation, the metabolism of neuropeptides, and the regulation of meiosis. Calpain cleaves and activates a number of proteins, including protein kinase C, protein-activated kinase II, phosphorylase kinase, glycogen synthase, Ca^{2+}-dependent cyclic nucleotide phosphodiesterase, factor XIII, and the calmodulin-dependent protein phosphatase calcineurin, while inactivating others such as the myosin light-chain kinase and tryptophan hydroxylase. In addition to activating or altering the regulation of certain enzymes, calpains cleave a number of receptors, including the EGF receptor, the oestrogen receptor, the progesterone receptor, the glucocorticoid receptor, and the platelet-devoid growth factor receptor (Barrett et al. 1991).

Since calpain is involved in such a diversity of important physiological processes, calpain inhibitors should be useful for the treatment of a variety of disease states. Calpain's role in the degradation of myofibrillar proteins and other cytoskeletal proteins suggests that it initiates the turnover of contractile proteins. Thus inhibitors should be useful for the treatment of diseases such as muscular dystrophy. Calpain has also been implicated in the pathogenesis of stroke, where excitatory amino acids such as glutamate can trigger a dangerous cascade of events leading to the activation of calpain as calcium enters the cell (Bartus 1990; Melloni and Pontremoli 1989). Calpain can then degrade spectrin and other proteins, leading to destruction of the cytoskeleton of neurones and disintegration of neuronal membranes. This finding suggests that calpain inhibitors can be used to prevent the turnover of neural proteins and destruction of the nervous system which occurs during stroke. Calpain inhibitors may also prove useful in the prevention of other age-related neurodegeneratlve diseases, including Parkinson's disease, Alzheimer's disease (Nilsson *et al.* 1990), and multi-infarct dementia.

17B.2   Active-site structure and sequence

Unlike other cysteine proteases, μ-calpain and m-calpain are hetero-dimers composed of 80 kDa and 30 kDa subunits. The 80 kDa subunit is unique to each enzyme, while the 30 kDa regulatory subunit is common to both enzymes. The former is composed of a propeptide, a cysteine protease domain, another domain, and a calmodulin-like domain (Suzuki 1990). Both subunits undergo autolysis, with the loss of N-terminal fragments, to form other active forms of the enzyme (Edmunds *et al.* 1991; Zimmerman 1991). The cysteine protease domain is homologous to typical cysteine proteases, including papain and cathepsins B, H, and L, with homologies significantly higher around Cys-108 and His-265, the active site residues. Although the X-ray crystal structure of calpain has not yet been determined, the structures of papain and cathepsin B are available for molecular modelling.

Most mechanistic studies with cysteine proteases have been carried out with papain or other cysteine proteases such as cathepsin B. The active site contains a cysteine residue hydrogen bonded to a histidine residue. During substrate hydrolysis, the cysteine residue adds to the carbonyl group of the substrate to produce a tetrahedral adduct which then collapses to form an acyl enzyme, releasing the first product. The acyl enzyme is eventually hydrolysed to release the second product. Many interesting mechanistic questions involving calpain should be investigated. For example, it is possible that the calcium atom in calpain plays a mechanistic role, indirectly stabilizing the oxyanion, as has been observed with the phospholipase A_2 mechanism (Scott *et al.* 1990). Indeed, it appears likely that there are other mechanistic differences between calpains and cysteine proteases such as papain, but possible differences have not yet been investigated.

Calpain is found in most tissues together with a natural protein inhibitor known as calpastatin. There appear to be low and high molecular mass forms of calpastatin (70 kDa and 110 kDa) (Maki *et al.* 1990). The sequence of human calpastatin contains 673 amino acids and four repeating homologous sequences of 120–140 amino acids which have no homology with the cystatin family of cysteine protease inhibitors. The reactive site sequence has not yet been identified, although each domain contains a central conserved sequence which is essential for inhibition. The 27 residue peptide Ac-DPMSSTYIEELGKREVTIPPKYRELLA-NH$_2$ from one domain of calpastatin inhibits μ-calpain and m-calpain with IC$_{50}$ values of 20 nM and 80 nM respectively (Maki *et al.* 1989). Sasaki has recently shown that calpain is inhibited by Gln-Val-Val-Ala-Gly in domain 2 of high molecular mass kininogen (HMWK). Both calpains require calcium for complex formation with HMWK.

17B.3   Substrate specificity

The specificity of calpain has been studied with natural peptides, synthetic peptide substrates, and proteins (Sasaki *et al.* 1984; Takahashi 1990). With peptides, the site of cleavage indicates a preference for Leu or Val at P_2 and for Arg, Lys, Met, and Tyr at P_1. Phe, Trp, Leu, and Val predominate at P_3, while basic residues such as Arg and Lys seem to predominate at P_1'. Calpain will also cleave C-terminal amides when the appropriate P_1 residue is present in the substrate. Pro never appears in either P_1 or P_1'. Although inconclusive at this stage, the P_2 residue seems to be of more significance than P_1.

A few 7-amino-4-methylcoumarin substrates have been tested with calpains and some representative data are shown in Table 17B.1 (Sasaki *et al.* 1984). Suc-Leu-Met-AMC was 16 times better than Suc-Val-Met-AMC, indicating the importance of Leu at P_2. A similar trend was observed with Suc-Leu-Tyr-AMC and Suc-Val-Tyr-AMC. Tetrapeptide AMC derivatives were slightly better than the dipeptide derivatives, and Tyr is preferred over Met at P_1. The kinetic parameters for μ-calpain and m-calpain were quite similar with only small differences.

17B.4   Transition state inhibitors

Most classes of calpain inhibitor were initially described as inhibitors for other more widely studied cysteine proteases such as papain or cathepsin B.

Table 17B.1 Kinetic parameters for μ-calpain and *m*-calpain

Substrate	Enzyme	K_m (mM)	k_{cat} (s^{-1})	k_{cat}/K_m $(M^{-1}s^{-1})$
Suc-Leu-Met-AMC	μ-calpain	1.2	0.062	51
	m-calpain	4.8	0.19	41
Suc-Leu-Tyr-AMC	μ-calpain	4.7	0.37	78
	m-calpain	2.2	0.092	42
Suc-Leu-Leu-Val-Tyr-AMC	μ-calpain	0.20	0.029	140
	m-calpain	0.47	0.065	140
Boc-Val-Leu-Lys-AMC	μ-calpain	5.9	0.49	83
	m-calpain	7.1	0.81	110

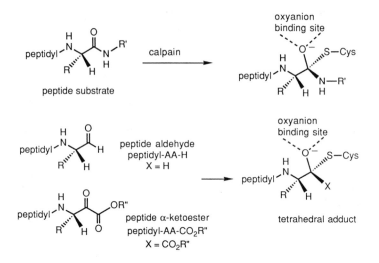

peptide substrate

peptide aldehyde
peptidyl-AA-H
X = H

peptide α-ketoester
peptidyl-AA-CO₂R"
X = CO₂R"

tetrahedral adduct

Fig. 17B.1 Tetradehral adduct formed in the hydrolysis of peptide substrates by calpain (top) and the tetrahedral adducts formed from transition state inhibitors with calpain (bottom).

Compounds with the appropriate sequence(s) were then synthesized as calpain inhibitors. Excellent reviews of cysteine protease inhibitors have appeared recently and should be consulted before embarking on a programme of calpain inhibitor design (Rich 1986; Shaw 1990; Crawford 1990; Demuth 1990; Wang 1990).

A number of carbonyl compounds have been found to be transition state inhibitors for cysteine proteases. These structures include peptide aldehydes, peptide α-ketoesters, and peptides containing other electronegative carbonyl groups. In each case, the enzyme is believed to form a hemithioacetal structure with the carbonyl group of the inhibitor similar to that formed in substrate hydrolysis (Fig. 17B.1).

17B.4.1 Peptide aldehydes

The peptide aldehydes leupeptin and antipain, from an *Actinomycete*, were initially found to inhibit calpain moderately (Sasaki *et al*. 1984). Subsequently, peptide aldehyde sequences based on the substrate specificity of calpain towards aminomethylcoumarin substrates were synthesized (Sasaki *et al*. 1990) and were found to be potent reversible inhibitors of μ-calpain and m-calpain with K_i values as low as 36 nM. Some representative data are given in Table 17B.2 (Sasaki *et al*. 1984, 1990; Higuchi *et al*. 1990).

The most potent inhibitors were dipeptide derivatives, and those with a P_1 Met were slightly more potent than the Nle and Phe derivatives. The

Table 17B.2 Inhibition of calpains by peptide aldehydes

	K_i (nM)	
	μ-calpain	m-calpain
Leupeptin	320	430
Antipain	1400	1500
Z-Leu-Nle-H(calpeptin)	67	62
PhCH$_2$CH$_2$CH$_2$CO-Leu-Nle-H	65	68
Ac-Leu-Leu-Nle-H	190	220
Z-Leu-Met-H	36	68
PhCH$_2$CH$_2$CH$_2$CO-Leu-Met-H	36	50
Ac-Leu-Leu-Met-H	120	230
Z-Leu-Phe-H	60	100
PhCH$_2$CH$_2$CH$_2$CO-Leu-Phe-H	38	78
	IC$_{50}$ (nM)	
Boc-Leu-Nle-H	30	120

inhibitors were quite specific and inhibited chymotrypsin, trypsin, cathepsin B, and cathepsin H poorly, while they were effective inhibitors of cathepsin L. Calpeptin (Z-Leu-Nle-H) is a membrane-permeant inhibitor and prevented Ca^{2+}-ionophore-induced degradation of proteins in intact platelets. It also inhibited thrombin-, ionomycin-, or collagen-stimulated phosphorylation in platelets (Tsujinaka et al. 1988). Z-Val-Phe-H, a potent inhibitor of calpain (K_i = 7 nM), also inhibits the proteolytic degradation of erythrocyte cytoskeletal proteins (Mehdi et al. 1988), and Ac-Leu-Leu-Nle-H prevents the rapid post-mortem degradation of benzodiazepine binding proteins (Reichelt et al. 1990).

17B.4.2 Peptide α-ketoesters and ketones

Peptide α-ketoester derivatives were initially described as potent inhibitors of serine proteases (Hori et al. 1985) and subsequently were also discovered to be cysteine protease inhibitors (Angelastro et al. 1990; Hu and Abeles 1990). In comparing a variety of electrophilic carbonyl-containing inhibitors of papain, Hu and Abeles (1990) found that α-ketoester and amide inhibitors were more potent than ketoacids, which in turn were better than ketones. Calpain has also been studied with a variety of electrophilic carbonyl derivatives and the data are shown in Table 17B.3 (Angelastro et al. 1990). Aldehydes are the best inhibitors for calpain, while they are the worst for chymotrypsin. The greatest discrimination between calpain

Table 17B.3 Inhibition of calpain and chymotrypsin by electrophilic carbonyl derivatives

	K_i (μM)	
	Calpain	Chymotrypsin
Z-Val-Phe-H	0.01	54
Z-Val-Phe-CO$_2$Me	0.4	0.06
Z-Val-Phe-CO$_2$Et	0.6	0.06
Z-Val-Phe-COMe	0.7	0.2
Z-Val-Phe-CF$_3$	>180	2.4

and chymotrypsin in this set of compounds was observed with the peptide aldehyde. Extending the chain from a single amino acid derivative to a dipeptide resulted in a 150–400-fold improvement in potency.

17B.5   Irreversible inhibitors

17B.5.1   Peptide chloromethyl ketones, peptide diazomethyl ketones, and peptide fluoromethyl ketones

The mechanisms of inhibition of cysteine proteases by peptide chloromethyl, fluoromethyl, and diazomethyl ketones have many similarities and some important differences (Shaw 1990). In each case, it is believed that the inhibitor forms a tetrahedral adduct with the inhibitor carbonyl group which then rearranges to the alkylated product (Fig. 17B.2). In the case of the diazomethyl ketone, protonation by the active site histidine is required for alkylation to occur.

Both calpains are effectively inhibited by H-Leu-Leu-Phe-CH$_2$Cl (Sasaki et al. 1986). Tripeptides with a P$_1$ Tyr or Lys were 3–15 times less effective and E-64 (see Table 17B.5 for formula) was much poorer. A wide variety of peptide chloromethyl ketones and diazomethyl ketones have been studied with m-calpain, and representative inhibitors are shown in Table 17B.4 (Crawford et al. 1988). The best inhibitors are Z-Leu-Leu-Phe-CH$_2$Cl and Z-Leu-Leu-Tyr-CHN$_2$. Using a set of dipeptide diazomethyl ketone inhibitors, the preference at P$_1$ was shown to be homoPhe > Met > Tyr > Tyr(I) > Trp > Leu. The preference at P$_4$ was Z > Ac > H.

Several diazomethyl and fluoromethyl ketones have been used to study calpain as a stimulus-response mediator in human platelets (Anagli et al. 1991). Z-Leu-Leu-Tyr-CHN$_2$ and Z-Leu-Leu-Tyr-CH$_2$F emerged as the most potent inhibitors of Ca^{2+}-dependent proteolysis in platelets, but did not inhibit changes in cell shape and aggregation, adhesion and spreading on glass, or 5-hydroxytryptamine release. A radiolabelled version (Z-Leu-

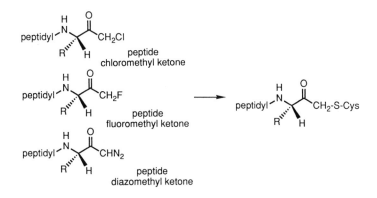

Fig. 17B.2 Inhibition of cysteine proteases by peptide chloromethyl ketones, peptide fluoromethyl ketones, and diazomethyl ketones.

Table 17B.4 Inhibition of m-calpain by peptide chloromethyl and diazomethyl ketone derivatives

	k_2/K_i $(\mathrm{M^{-1}s^{-1}})$
Z-Leu-Leu-Phe-CH$_2$Cl	>100 000
H-Leu-Leu-Phe-CH$_2$Cl	>100 000
Z-Leu-Leu-Tyr-CHN$_2$	230 000
Ac-Leu-Leu-Tyr-CHN$_2$	11 000
Boc-Lys(CF$_3$CO)-Leu-Tyr-CHN$_2$	13 000
Boc-Val-Lys(Z)-Leu-Tyr-CHN$_2$	21 000

Leu-Tyr(^{125}I)-CHN$_2$) was shown to label three major proteins of molecular mass 78, 40, and 23 kDa, and Z-Leu-Leu-Tyr(^{125}I)-CH$_2$F labelled an 80 kDa protein. Labelling of many of the proteins was calcium dependent.

17B.5.2   Epoxysuccinyl peptides

Epoxysuccinyl peptides (or E-64 derivatives) inhibit cysteine proteases by covalent bond formation with the active-site cysteine residue. The crystal structure of the papain E-64-c complex has been determined by X-ray crystallography (Yamamoto *et al.* 1991) and is shown schematically in Fig. 17B.3. Interestingly, the peptide chain of the inhibitor is interacting with the S$_2$ and S$_3$ subsites of papain, with the inhibitor peptide chain running in the opposite direction compared with normal substrates or inhibitors such as peptide chloromethyl ketones (Yamamoto *et al.* 1990).

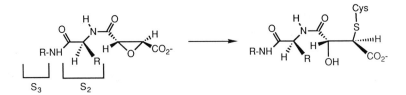

Fig. 17B.3 Mechanism of inhibition of cysteine proteases by epoxysuccinyl peptides.

Table 17B.5 Inhibition of m-calpain by epoxysuccinyl (Eps) peptides

		Rate constant $(M^{-1}s^{-1})$
HO-Eps-Leu-NH-(CH)$_4$-NH-Z	E-460	23 000
HO-Eps-Leu-NH-(CH$_2$)$_4$-NH-CH(=NH$_2$$^+$)NH$_2$	E-64	7 500
HO-Eps-Leu-NH-CH$_2$-CH$_2$-CHMe$_2$	E-475	7 500
HO-Eps-Leu-NH-(CH$_2$)$_7$-NH$_2$	E-479	5 000

Epoxysuccinyl peptides are potent inhibitors of m-calpain (Parkes *et al.* 1985), and some are shown in Table 17B.5. It is clear that the S_2 and S_3 subsites of calpain can tolerate both hydrophobic and cationic groups. A number of other derivatives which were tailored for cathepsin B were found to be poor inhibitors of m-calpain (Murata *et al.* 1991). E-64-d (E-64 with the D-isomer of HO-Eps) is a membrane-permeant calpain inhibitor and has been shown to inhibit calpain activity in intact platelets (McGowan *et al.* 1989).

17B.5.3   *S*-(3-nitro-2-pyridinsulphenyl) derivatives

A unique affinity labelling approach to calpain inhibition involves re-action with *S*-(3-nitro-2-pyridinesulphenyl) peptide derivatives (Matsueda *et al.* 1990). The best inhibitor discovered is Leu-Leu-Cys(Npys)-NH$_2$ which had a IC$_{50}$ of 0.18 μM with human platelet calpain. This inhibitor sequence was 1000-fold poorer at inhibiting cathepsin B and papain, and did not inhibit serine or aspartate proteases. Related sequences with P$_2$ and P$_3$ Ile, Val, or Phe residues had IC$_{50}$ values of 6–22 μM. The pro-bable mechanism of inhibition is shown in Fig. 17B.4, and in two cases the release of 3-nitrothiopyridone was detected by absorbance at 310 nm. The inhibitor Phe-Gln-Val-Val-Cys(Npys)-Gly-NH$_2$, which is related to the Gln-Val-Val-Ala-Gly sequence, believed to be the calpain inhibitory region of high molecular mass kininogen, had IC$_{50}$ = 4.1 μM and was a

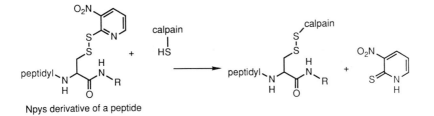

Fig. 17B.4 Mechanism of inhibition of calpain by Npys derivatives of peptides.

potent and specific inhibitor of thrombin- and plasmin-induced platelet aggregation.

17B.6 Therapeutic utility and perspectives

A wide variety of inhibitor structures have now been reported to inhibit calpain effectively. These include transition state inhibitors, a variety of irreversible inhibitors, calmodulin antagonists (Zhang and Johnson 1988a,b) and polyamines (Johnson and Hammer 1990). Calpain inhibitors which can penetrate cells are now available (Mehdi 1991). Several groups have shown that calpain inhibitors have the ability to prevent the activation and aggregation of platelets (Tsujinaka *et al.* 1988), and calpain may be involved in the activation of phospholipase C and thromboxane synthetase (Tsujinaka *et al.* 1990). A calpain inhibitor has been shown to initiate neurite formation in tissue culture, which suggests a role for calpain in the development of the nervous system (Saito and Kawashima 1989). Calpain has also been shown to degrade neurofilaments (Schlaepfer and Zimmerman 1990) and modify synaptic structure (Seubert and Lynch 1990), which indicates that calpain inhibitors might be useful for preventing or treating neurodegenerative diseases.

In summary, a number of fairly potent calpain inhibitors have been described and are being actively used to explore the role of calpain in numerous physiological processes, including muscular dystrophy, muscle denervation, hypertension, and platelet abnormalities. In the future, it is highly likely that calpain inhibitors will find utility in the treatment of human diseases, particularly in the area of neurodegenerative disease.

References

Anagli, J., Hagmann, J., and Shaw, E. (1991). Investigation of the role of calpain as a stimulus-response mediator in human platelets using new synthetic inhibitors. *Biochemical Journal*, **274**, 497–502.

Angelastro, M. R., Mehdi, S., Burkhart, J. P., Peet, N. P., and Bey, P. (1990). α-Diketone and α-keto ester derivatives of N-protected amino acids and peptides as novel inhibitors of cysteine and serine proteinases. *Journal of Medicinal Chemistry*, **33**, 11–13.

Barrett, M. J., Goll, D. E., and Thompson, V. F. (1991). Effect of substrate on Ca^{2+}-concentration required for activity of the Ca^{2+}-dependent proteases, μ- and m-calpain. *Life Sciences*, **48**, 1659–69.

Bartus, R. T. (1990). Drugs to treat age-related neurodegenerative problems. The final frontier of medical science? *Journal of the American Geriatrics Society*, **38**, 680–95.

Crawford, C. (1990). Protein and peptide inhibitors of calpains. In *Intracellular calcium-dependent proteolysis* (ed. R. L. Mellgren and T. Murachi), pp. 75–89. CRC Press, Boca Raton, FL.

Crawford, C., Mason, R. W., Wikstrom, P., and Shaw, E. (1988). The design of peptidyldiazomethane inhibitors to distinguish between the cysteine proteinases calpain II, cathepsin L and cathepsin B. *Biochemical Journal*, **253**, 751–8.

Demuth, H.-U. (1990). Recent developments in inhibiting cysteine and serine proteases. *Journal of Enzyme Inhibition*, **3**, 249–78.

Edmunds, T., Nagainis, P. A., Sathe, S. K., Thompson, V. F., and Goll, D. E. (1991). Comparison of the autolyzed and unautolyzed forms of μ- and m-calpain from bovine skeletal muscle. *Biochimica et Biophysica Acta*, **1077**, 197–208.

Goll, D. E., Kleese, W. C., Okitani, A., Kumamoto, T., Cong, J., and Kapprell, H.-P. (1990). Historical background and current status of the Ca^{2+}-dependent proteinase system. In *Intracellular calcium-dependent proteolysis* (ed. R. L. Mellgren and T. Murachi), pp. 3–24. CRC Press, Boca Raton, FL.

Higuchi, N., Saitoh, M., and Shibata, H. (1990). Proteinase inhibitors. European Patent Application 0 393 457.

Hori, H., Yasutake, A., Minematsu, Y., and Powers, J. C. (1985). Inhibition of human leukocyte elastase, pancreatic elastase and cathepsin G by peptide ketones. In *Peptides: structure and function. Proceedings of the Ninth American Peptide Symposium* (ed. C. M. Deber, V. J. Hruby, and K. D. Kopple), pp. 819–22. Pierce Chemical Co., Rockford, IL.

Hu, L.-Y. and Abeles, R. H. (1990). Inhibition of cathepsin B and papain by peptidyl α-keto esters, α-keto amides, α-diketones, and α-keto acids. *Archives of Biochemistry and Biophysics*, **281**, 271–4.

Johnson, P. (1990). Calpains (intracellular calcium-activated cysteine proteinases): structure–activity relationships and involvement in normal and abnormal cellular metabolism. *International Journal of Biochemistry*, **22**, 811–22.

Johnson, P. and Hammer, J. L. (1990). Inhibitory effects of spermine and spermidine on muscle calpain II. *Experientia*, **46**, 276–8.

McGowan, E. B., Becker, E., and Detwiler, T. C. (1989). Inhibition of calpain in intact platelets by the thiol protease inhibitor E-64d. *Biochemical and Biophysical Research Communications*, **158**, 432–5.

Maki, M., Bagci, H., Hamaguchi, K., Ueda, M., Murarchi, T., and Hatanaka, M. (1989). Inhibition of calpain by a synthetic oligopeptide corresponding to an exon of the human calpastatin gene. *Journal of Biological Chemistry*, **264**, 18866–69.

Maki, M., Hatanaka, M., Takano, E., and Murachi, T. (1990). Structure-function relationships of calpastatins. In *Intracellular calcium-dependent proteolysis* (ed.

R. L. Mellgren and T. Murachi), pp. 37–54. CRC Press, Boca Raton, FL.

Matsueda, R., Umeyama, H., Puri, R. N., Bradford, H. N., and Colman, R. W. (1990). Potent affinity labeling peptide inhibitors of calpain. *Chemistry Letters*, 191–4.

Mehdi, S. (1991). Cell-penetrating inhibitors of calpain. *Trends in Biochemical Sciences*, **16**, 150–3.

Mehdi, S., Angelastro, M. R., Wiseman, J. S., and Bey, P. (1988). Inhibition of the proteolysis of rat erythrocyte membrane proteins by a synthetic inhibitor of calpain. *Biochemical and Biophysical Research Communications*, **157**, 1117–23.

Mellgren, R. L. and Murachi, T. (1990). *Intracellular calcium-dependent proteolysis*. CRC Press, Boca Raton, FL.

Melloni, E. and Pontremoli, S. (1989). The calpains. *Trends in Neurosciences*, **12**, 438–44.

Murata, M., Miyashita, S., Yokoo, C., Tamai, M., Hanada, K., Hatayama, K., *et al.* (1991). Novel epoxysuccinyl peptides. Selective inhibitors of cathepsin B, *in vitro*. *Federation of European Biochemical Societies Letters*, **280**, 307–10.

Nilsson, E., Alafuzoff, I., Blennow, K., Blomgren, K., Hall, C. M., Janson, I., *et al.* (1990). Calpain and calpastin in normal and Alzheimer-degenerated human brain tissue. *Neurobiology of Aging*, **11**, 425–31.

Parkes, C., Kembhavi, A. A., and Barrett, A. J. (1985). Calpain inhibition by peptide epoxides. *Biochemical Journal*, **230**, 509–16.

Reichelt, R., Möhler, H., and Hebebrand, J. (1990). Calpain inhibitor I prevents rapid postmortem degradation of benzodiazepine binding proteins: fluorographic and immunological evidence. *Journal of Neurochemistry*, **55**, 1711–15.

Rich, D. H. (1986). Inhibitors of cysteine proteinases. In *Protinase inhibitors* (ed. A. J. Barrett and G. Salvensen), pp. 153–78. Elsevier, Amersterdam.

Saito, Y. and Kawashima, S. (1989). The neurite-initiating effect of a tripeptide aldehyde protease inhibitor on PC12h cells. *Journal of Biochemistry*, **106**, 1035–40.

Sasaki, T., Kikuchi, T., Yumoto, N., Yoshimura, N., and Murachi, T. (1984). Comparative specificity and kinetic studies of porcine calpain I and calpain II with naturally occuring peptides and synthetic fluorogenic substrates. *Journal of Biological Chemistry*, **259**, 12489–94.

Sasaki, T., Kikuchi, T., Fukui, I., and Murachi, T. (1986). Inactivation of calpain I and calpain II by specificity-oriented tripeptidyl chloromethyl ketones. *Journal of Biochemistry*, **99**, 173–9.

Sasaki, T., Kishi, M., Saito, M., Tanaka, T., Higuchi, N., Kominami, E., *et al.* (1990). Inhibitory effect of di- and tripeptidyl aldehydes on calpains and cathepsins. *Journal of Enzyme Inhibition*, **3**, 195–201.

Schlaepfer, W. W. and Zimmerman, U.-J. P. (1990). The degradation of neurofilaments by calpains. In *Intracellular calcium-dependent proteolysis*, (ed. R. L. Mellgren and T. Murachi), pp. 241–9. CRC Press, Boca Raton, FL.

Scott, D. L., White, S. P., Otwinowski, Z., Yuan, W., Gelb, M. H., and Sigler, P. B. (1990). Interfacial catalysis: The mechanism of phospholipase A_2. *Science*, **250**, 1541–6.

Seubert, P. and Lynch, G. (1990). Plasticity to pathology: brain calpains as modifiers of synaptic structure. In *Intracellular calcium-dependent proteolysis* (ed. R. L. Mellgren and T. Murachi), pp. 251–63. CRC Press, Boca Raton FL.

Shaw, E. (1990). Cysteinyl proteinases and their selective inactivation. *Methods in Enzymology*, **63**, 271–347.

Suzuki, K. (1990). The structure of calpains and the calpain gene. In *Intracellular calcium-dependent proteolysis* (ed. R. L. Mellgren and T. Murachi), pp. 25–35. CRC Press, Boca Raton, FL.

Takahashi, K. (1990). Calpain substrate specificity. In *Intracellular calcium-dependent proteolysis* (ed. R. L. Mellgren and T. Murachi), pp. 55–74. CRC Press, Boca Raton, FL.

Tsujinaka, T., Kajiwara, Y., Kambayashi, J., Sakon, M., Higuchi, N., Tanaka, T., and Mori, T. (1988). Synthesis of a new cell penetrating calpain inhibitor (calpeptin). *Biochemical and Biophysical Research Communications*, **153**, 1201–8.

Tsujinaka, T., Ariyoshi, H., Uemura, Y., Sakon, M., Kambayashi, J., and Mori, T. (1990). Potential participation of calpain in platelet activation studied by use of cell penetrating calpain inhibitor (calpeptin). *Life Sciences*, **46**, 1059–66.

Wang, K. K. W. (1990). Developing selective inhibitors of calpain. *Trends in Pharmacological Sciences*, **11**, 139–42.

Yamamoto, D., Ishida, T., and Inoue, M. (1990). A comparison between the binding modes of a substrate and inhibitor to papain as observed in complex crystal structures. *Biochemical and Biophysical Research Communications*, **171**, 711–16.

Yamamoto, D., Matsumoto, K., Ohishi, H., Ishida, T., Inoue, M., Katamura, K., and Mizuno, H. (1991). Refined X-ray structure of papain E-64-c complex at 2.1 Å. *Journal of Biological Chemistry*, **266**, 14771–7.

Zhang, H. and Johnson, P. (1988a). Effects of trifluoperazine and compounds W-7 and W-13 on chicken gizzard calpain II. *Biochemical Society Transactions*, **16**, 1043–4.

Zhang, H. and Johnson, P. (1988b). Inhibition of calpains by calmidazolium and calpastatin. *Journal of Enzyme Inhibition*, **2**, 163–6.

Zimmerman, U.-J. P. (1991). Two-stage autolysis of the catalytic subunit initiates activation of calpain I. *Biochimica et Biophysica Acta*, **1078**, 192–8.

Section 17C

Inhibitors of prolyl endopeptidase

Naoki Higuchi

17C.1 Clinical potential of the inhibitors
17C.2 Target enzyme
17C.3 Inhibitors
References

17C.1 Clinical potential of the inhibitors

Bohus *et al.* (1973) have reported that [Lys[8]]-vasopressin

$$\text{H-Cys}^1\text{-Tyr}^2\text{-Phe}^3\text{-Glu}^4\text{-Asn}^5\text{-Cys}^6\text{-Pro}^7\text{-Lys}^8\text{-Gly}^9\text{-NH}_2,$$

an antidiuretic cyclic nonapeptide hormone which constricts peripheral blood vessels, lending to the absorption of water in the kidney and the conservation of free water in the body, ameliorates impaired avoidance learning in a shuttle-box avoidance response task in hypophysectomized rats. The cyclic peptide both facilitates passive avoidance learning (Ader and de Wied 1972) and increases resistance to extinction of shuttle-box avoidance in a pole-jumping avoidance response in intact rats (de Wied 1971). It was also shown that removal of vasopressin from the cerebro-spinal fluid by vasopressin antiserum inhibits memory expression in Brattelboro strain rats with a hereditary blockade of vasopressin ([Arg^8]-vasopressin) synthesis which display a severe memory deficit in a single-trial passive avoidance situation (de Wied *et al.* 1975; van Wimersma Greidanus *et al.* 1975). Furthermore, Burbach *et al.* (1983) isolated a peptide that accumulated as a major product during the proteolysis of vasopressin by rat brain synaptic membranes, and showed that it was a hexapeptide, [Arg^8]-vasopressin$_{4-9}$:

$$\text{H-Cys}^1\text{-OH} \qquad \text{pGlu}^4\text{-Asn}^5\text{-Cys}^6\text{-Pro}^7\text{-Arg}^8\text{-Gly}^9\text{-NH}_2$$

When administered intracerebroventricularly in extremely low doses, this vasopressin fragment and its desglycineamide derivative [Arg^8]-vaso-pressin$_{4-8}$ facilitated memory consolidation in a passive avoidance situation at a concentration three to four orders lower than that of the native cyclic peptide. These vasopressin metabolites constitute highly potent neuropeptides with selective effects on memory and related processes. Because the behaviourally active metabolites are devoid of direct pressor activity on the peripheral vasculature, it was concluded that the memory effects of these metabolites are mediated by central rather than peripheral receptors (de Wied *et al.* 1984), and that these binding sites are present in the hilus of the hippocampal formation and other organs in the brain (Brinton *et al.* 1986)

Prolyl endopeptidase is highly active in the brain and readily degrades proline-containing low molecular mass neuropeptides such as vasopressin which is speculatively associated with memory, as described above. Some anti-amnesic drugs, such as aniracetam and pramiracetam, show weak inhibitory activity toward prolyl endopeptidase (Yoshimoto *et al.* 1987a).

These observations suggest the potential use of prolyl endopeptidase inhibitors as nootropic agents for preventing and/or alleviating amnesia.

17C.2 Target enzyme

Prolyl endopeptidase (EC.3.4.21.26, post-proline cleaving enzyme) is the only known endopeptidase specific for proline residues and it post-proline peptide bond (Yoshimoto *et al.* 1977, 1979, 1981; Walter and Yoshimoto 1978). The enzyme was discovered in the human uterus as an oxytocin-degrading enzyme (Walter *et al.* 1971), and was purified from lamb kidney and named post-proline cleaving enzyme (Koida and Walter 1976; Walter 1976). It is widely distributed in various mammalian tissues such as brain, testis, liver, skeletal muscle, and kidney (Yoshimoto *et al.* 1979), and is also found in microorganisms (Yoshimoto *et al.* 1980), plants, (Yoshimoto *et al.* 1987b) and fungi (Sattar *et al.* 1990). The enzyme was classified as a serine proteinase using active-site directed irreversible inhibitors Yoshimoto *et al.* 1977) and its substrate specificity was defined.

It catalyses the hydrolysis of peptides with the general structure X-Pro(Ala)-Y (where X is a peptide or N-protected amino acid, and Y is an amino acid moiety, peptide, amide or ester) on the carboxyl side of proline, and very weakly on the carboxyl side of alanine (Walter and Yoshimoto 1978; Yoshimoto *et al.* 1978). Some enzymatic properties of typical prolyl endopeptidases from a microorganism and from bovine brain are summarized in Table 17C.1 (Yoshimoto *et al.* 1980, 1988). The enzyme is highly active in the brain, as noted above, and degrades peptide hormones such as thyrotropin-releasing hormone (TRH) (Orlowski *et al.* 1979) luteinizing-hormone-releasing hormone (LH-RH) (Knisatschek and Bauer 1979), angiotensin II (Hersh and McKelvy 1979), brady-kinin (Rupnow *et al.* 1979), substance P (Taylor and Dixon 1980), and neurotensin (Kreider *et al.* 1981). Prolyl endopeptidase is considered to be the only endopeptidase which is able to degrade memory-related peptides [Arg[8]]-vasopressin$_{4-9}$ and [Arg[8]]-vasopressin$_{4-8}$ because they contain a C-terminal pyroglutamic residue and proline residue in their sequences.

Table 17C.1 Enzymatic and physicochemical properties of prolyl endopeptidase purified from bovine brain and *Flavobacterium meningosepticum*

	Bovine brain enzyme	*Flavobacterium* enzyme
Optimum pH	6.9	7.0
pH stability	5.5–5,9	5.0–9 0
Optimum temperature (°C)	40	40
Thermal stability *(°C)	47.5	42
Molecular weight (kDa)	76	74
Isoelectric point	4.8	9.6

*Residual activity was 50 per cent after 15 min of incubation at pH 7.0 and the temperature indicated.

Data from Yoshimoto *et al.* 1980, 1988.

17C.3   Inhibitors

Naturally occurring inhibitors of prolyl endopeptidase have been described. An endogeneous high molecular mass inhibitor of prolyl endopeptidase, which was very stable against temperature and pH, was isolated by Yoshimoto *et al.* (1982). The molecular mass was estimated to be 6.5 kDa by gel filtration. A low molecular mass inhibitor of the enzyme from *Streptomyces staurosporeus* was reported by Kimura *et al.* (1990) and named staurosporine. The chemical structure is shown in Fig. 17C.1. The IC_{50} and K_i values of staurosporine are 770 nM and 700 nM respectively.

Low molecular mass synthetic inhibitors of prolyl endopeptidase have been widely studied. Chloromethylketone derivatives of acyl-proline or acyl-peptidyl-proline inhibited the enzyme by alkylation of the active site with pseudo-first-order rate kinetics (Yoshimoto *et al.* 1977) and were considered to interact with a critical histidine residue of prolyl endopeptidase. The pseudo-first-order rate constants ($k_{obs}/[I]$ for a typical chloromethylketone derivative Z-Gly-L-Pro-CH$_2$Cl (**1**) are 56 $M^{-1}s^{-1}$ and 21 $M^{-1}s^{-1}$ for lamb kidney and *Flavobacterium* enzyme respectively (Yoshimoto *et al.* 1980).

Various acyl-peptidy prolinal derivatives were also synthesized (Yoshimoto *et al.* 1985) and tested as potential inhibitors of prolyl endopeptidase, and some were also tested as anti-amnesic agents *in vivo*. Nishikata *et al.* (1986) synthesized some prolinal derivatives (prolinal is a residue in which the carboxylic acid group of the C-terminal proline is reduced to a formyl group) and tested their inhibitory activity towards the ascidian and *Flavobacterium* enzymes (Table 17C.2). They showed that the best potential inhibitor in the series was Z-L-Val-L-Pro-H (**2**).

Yoshimoto *et al.* (1987a) found that an *in vitro* inhibitor could exert an *in vivo* anti-amnesic effect and reported the relationship between inhibitory activity and anti-amnesic effect for some inhibitors. They reported

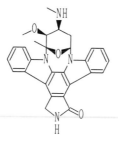

Fig. 17C.1 Chemical structure of staurosporine.

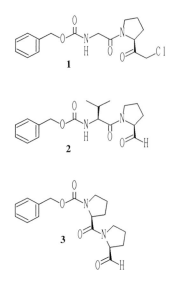

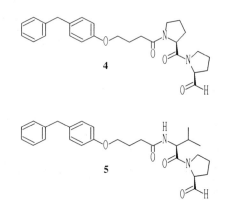

Table 17C.2 Inhibition of prolyl endopeptidase from an ascidian and from *Flavobacterium meningosepticum* by prolinal-containing peptides

Inhibitors	IC$_{50}$ (μM)	
	Ascidian enzyme	*Flavobacterium* enzyme
Z-L-Ala-L-Pro-H	2.0	1.0
Z-L-Val-L-Pro-H	0.01	0.03
Z-L-Ile-L-Pro-H	0.02	0.03
Z-L-Phe-L-Pro-H	0.2	0.6
Z-D-Phe-L-Pro-H	> 100	900
Z-L-Phe-D-Pro-H	> 50	800

From Nishikata *et al.* 1986.

that some of these compounds were more potent inhibitors of endo-peptidase than Z-Val-Pro-H (**2**), the most effective inhibitor *in vitro* ($K_i = 5$ nM). The most potent of these inhibitors was Z-Pro-Pro-H (**3**). A passive avoidance learning test using rats with amnesia experimentally induced with scopolamine showed that the prolinal derivatives prevented experimental amnesia at an intraperitoneal dose of 1 μM per animal (Table 17C.3.) The anti-amnesic effect of these compounds was approxi-mately parallel to their *in vitro* inhibitory activity on prolyl endopeptidase.

Table 17C.3 Inhibitory constants of prolinal derivatives towards bovine brain prolyl endopeptidase and their preventative action against scopolamine-induced amnesia

| Inhibitors | K_i (nM) | No. of rats | Dose (μM, i.p.) | Step-down latency (mean $\pm$ SEM) | | |
| | | | | Training trial | Test trial | |
					24 hours	48 hours
Control		23		3.7 ± 0.3	$262.3 \pm 83**$	$258.6 \pm 116**$
Scopolamine		25		2.7 ± 0.3	$183.7 \pm 88*$	$119.5 \pm 69*$
Z-Pro-Pro-H	9	10	1	5.3 ± 0.3	$296.7 \pm 3.5***$	$290.8 \pm 38***$
Z-Pro-Pro-H	15	8	1	5.3 ± 0.3	$296.7 \pm 3.5***$	$290.8 \pm 38***$
Z-Pyr-Pro-H	15	8	1	2.6 ± 0.1	$233.0 \pm 56**$	$247.2 \pm 76**$
Z-Val-Pro-H	5	10	1	4.6 ± 0.3	$296.7 \pm 10***$	$252.0 \pm 40***$
Boc-Pro-Pro-H	18	9	1	3.0 ± 0.2	$235.8 \pm 52**$	$243.2 \pm 73**$

$*\ p < 0.05$ vs control
$**\ p < 0.05$ vs scopolamine
$***\ p < 0.01$ vs scopolamine

From Yoshimoto et al. 1987a.

Saito *et al.* (1990) have also synthesized a number of prolinal derivatives and examined their inhibitory activity towards prolyl endopeptidase from *Flavobacterium* and bovine brain and their potential as nootropic agents. Almost all the compounds tested inhibited the activity of both enzymes with low IC_{50} values in the nanomolar range, but a specificity difference was observed with alkylacyl-prolinal derivatives which strongly inhibited the bacterial enzyme only (Table 17C.4). The most potent inhibitors towards bacterial and bovine brain enzymes were 4-(4-benzylphenoxy)-butyryl-Pro-Pro-H **(4)** $(IC_{50} = 0.20$ nM) and 4-(4-benzylphenoxy)butyryl-Val-Pro-H **(5)** $(IC_{50} = 2.0$ nM). Overall, prolyl-prolinal derivatives were the most effective inhibitors for both enzymes.

The same passive avoidance learning test using rats with amnesia induced by scopolamine was also performed (Table 17C.5). The prolinal derivatives with potent inhibitory activity towards brain prolyl endopeptidase also exhibited strong anti-amnesic activity at intraperitoneal doses of $0.01-1.0$ mg kg^{-1}. Interestingly, some of the compounds showed a bell-shaped dose dependence (Table 17C.5).

Interesting progress has recently been made with prolyl endopeptidase inhibitors employing pyrrolidine or thiazolidine moieties at the P_1 site (Saito *et al.* 1991; Yoshimoto *et al.* 1991). These compounds do not have a functional group such as formyl (aldehyde) or halomethylketone which reacts with the enzyme active site. Both groups of workers synthesized many derivatives of pyrrolidine or thiazolidine and examined their inhibitory activity towards prolyl endopeptidase.

Yoshimoto *et al.* (1991) generally used thioproline for the P_2 site and thiazolidine for the P_1 site in their inhibitors. They showed that replacement of L-proline by its D-isomer substantially reduced the inhibitory potency. Introduction of a sulphur atom in the proline (thioproline residue) and/or the penultimate pyrrolidine ring (thiazolidine ring) significantly increased the potency, but the introduction of oxygen (oxazolidine ring) diminished the activity to some extent. These workers also showed that a peptide linkage (acid–amide bond) between the proline and pyrrolidine ring was also required to retain inhibitory activity. A benzyloxycarbonyl group was most effective for blocking the N-terminal of the inhibitor. The most effective inhibitors are shown in Table 17C.6, and the most potent was benzyloxycarbonyl thioproly-thiazolidine **(6)**.

Saito *et al.* (1991) synthesized many inhibitors containing the pyrrolidine ring at the P_1 site and examined their inhibitory activity towards enzymes from both microorganisms and bovine brain. Almost all the compounds tested in the study inhibited both enzymes at very low IC_{50} values, similar to those for the prolinal derivatives, but a specificity difference was observed with alkylacyl-peptidyl-pyrrolidine derivatives which strongly inhibited only the bacterial enzyme (a similar observation was made for alkylacyl-prolinal derivatives and is included in Table 17C.4).

Table 17C.4 Inhibition of prolyl endopeptidase from bovine brain and *Flavobacterium meningosepticum* by acyl-peptidyl prolinal derivatives

Inhibitor	IC$_{50}$ (μM)	
	Flavobacterium enzyme	Bovine brain enzyme
4-Phenylbutyl-Ala-Pro-H	57.0	140
4-Phenylbutyl-Val-Pro-H	0.87	4.2
4-Phenylbutyl-Leu-Pro-H	1.2	12
4-Phenylbutyl-nLeu-Pro-H	1.7	250
4-Phenylbutyl-Met-Pro-H	2.7	79
4-Phenylbutyl-Phe-Pro-H	1.1	22
4-Phenylbutyl-Pro-Pro-H	0.87	8.7
Phenylacetyl-Pro-Pro-H	4.7	4.7
3-Phenylpropionyl-Pro-Pro-H	1.8	4.5
5-Phenylvaleryl-Pro-Pro-H	0.84	4.2
4-(2-Styrylphenoxy)butyryl-Val-Pro-H	0.25	19
4-(2-Styrylphenoxy)butyryl-Leu-Pro-H	6.2	32
4-(2-Styrylphenoxy)butyryl-Phe-Pro-H	0.27	20
4-(2-Styrylphenoxy)butyryl-Pro-Pro-H	0.23	6.5
4-(4-Benzylphenoxy)butyryl-Val-Pro-H	6.7	2.0
4-(4-Benzylphenoxy)butyryl-Leu-Pro-H	6.5	65
4-(4-Benzylphenoxy)butyryl-Phe-Pro-H	6.2	62
4-(4-Benzylphenoxy)butyryl-Pro-Pro-H	0.20	6.7
4-(5-Isoquinolinoxy)butyryl-Val-Pro-H	3.5	3.0
4-(5-Isoquinolinoxy)butyryl-Leu-Pro-H	3.5	6.0
4-(5-Isoquinolinoxy)butyryl-nLeu-Pro-H	3.5	69
4-(5-Isoquinolinoxy)butyryl-Phe-Pro-H	2.3	97
4-(5-Isoquinolinoxy)butyryl-Pro-Pro-H	1.1	7.2
Oleoyl-Ala-Pro-H	52	
Oleoyl-Val-Pro-H	2.2	320
Oleoyl-Leu-Pro-H	2.5	3200
Oleoyl-nLeu Pro-H	2.2	6200
Oleoyl-Phe-Pro-H	1.2	45000
Oleoyl-Lys(Z)-Pro-H	1.4	6000
Oleoyl-Glu(H)-Pro-H	0.94	190
Oleoyl-Phe-Pro-H	0.97	65
Linoleoyl-Leu-Pro-H	1.9	320
Stearoyl-Leu-Pro-H	3.0	170
Palmitoyl-Leu-Pro-H	2.3	6500

From Saito *et al*. 1990.

Table 17C.5 The preventive action of prolyl endopeptidase inhibitors toward scopolamine-induced retrograde amnesia in rats and their dose responses

Compound	No. of rats	Dose (mg kg^{-1} i.p.)	Training (Mean ± SE)		
			First step-down latency (seconds)	No. descending	Amnesia %
Saline	9		6.2 ± 1.7	2.3 ± 0.6	33
Scopolamine	10		2.7 ± 0.6	2.9 ± 0.3	80
4-Phenylbutyryl-Val-Pro-H	10	1000	3.8 ± 0.8	2.2 ± 0.2	60
	10	250	2.4 ± 0.6	2.4 ± 0.6	40
	10	100	3.2 ± 0.5	3.2 ± 0.5	0
	10	25	1.9 ± 0.6	2.2 ± 0.6	10
4-Phenylbutyryl-Leu-Pro-H	10	250	1.5 ± 0.6	3.0 ± 0.8	30
	10	100	2.5 ± 0.4	3.0 ± 0.5	0
	10	25	2.7 ± 0.9	2.4 ± 0.8	0
Oleoyl-Val-Pro-H	10	1000	3.5 ± 0.6	2.8 ± 0.9	50
	10	250	2.1 ± 0.3	2.8 ± 0.5	20
	10	100	1.8 ± 0.4	1.6 ± 0.2	10
Oleoyl-Leu-Pro-H	5	1000	9.4 ± 3.0	1.6 ± 0.9	60
	5	250	1.7 ± 0.8	2.4 ± 0.6	20
	5	100	3.1 ± 0.9	1.8 ± 0.7	0
	5	25	2.2 ± 0.8	2.0 ± 0.5	0
	5	10	4.7 ± 0.7	2.0 ± 0.9	40

From Saito *et al.* 1990.

Table 17C.6 Inhibition of prolyl endopeptidase from bovine brain by thiazolidine derivatives

	IC$_{50}$ (μM)
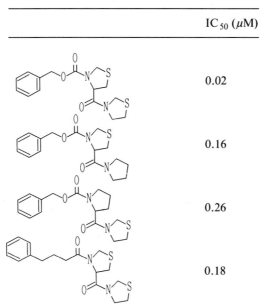	0.02
	0.16
	0.26
	0.18

From Yoshimoto *et al.* 1991

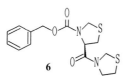

6

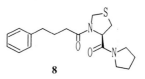

8

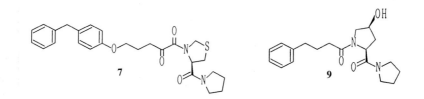

7

9

The most effective inhibitors have a proline residue at their P$_2$ subsite and a substituted or unsubstituted phenoxybutyryl moiety at their N-terminal (P$_3$ subsite). Thus phenoxybutyryl-prolyl-pyrrolidine is the most

Table 17C.7 Inhibitory activity of acyl-peptidyl-pyrrolidine derivatives on prolyl endopeptidase from *Flavobacterium* and bovine brain

Compound	Chemical structure	Prolyl endopeptidase	
		Flavobacterium IC$_{50}$ (μM)	Bovine brain IC$_{50}$ (μM)
4-(2-Styrylphenoxy)-butyryl-Pro-Py		0.0069	0.14
4-Phenoxybutyryl-Pro-Py		0.0045	0.45
4-(2-Benzylphenoxy)-butyryl-Pro-Py		0.0035	0.21
4-(2'-Chalconoxy)-butyryl-Pro-Py		0.0025	0.13
4-(2-Chalconoxy)-butyryl-Pro-Py		0.0032	0.13
4-(2-Phenethylphenoxy)-butyryl-Pro-Py		0.0067	0.20
4-(2-Benzoylphenoxy)-butyryl-Pro-Py		0.0035	0.17
4-(2-Allylphenoxy)-butyryl-Pro-Py		0.0079	0.27
4-(4-Benzylphenoxy)-butyryl-Pro-Py		0.0014	0.27

effective partial structure for the inhibitors. The best inhibitors were 4-(4-benzylphenoxy)butyryl-thioprolyl-pyrrolidine (**7**) for the bacterial enzyme (IC$_{50}$ = 1.4 nM) and 4-phenylbutyryl-thioprolyl-pyrrolidine (**8**) for

Table 17C.7 (*continued*)

Compound	Chemical structure	Prolyl endopeptidase	
		Flavobacterium IC$_{50}$ (μM)	Bovine brain IC$_{50}$ (μM)
4-Phenylbutyryl-Pro-Py		0.094	0.19
4-Phenylbutyryl-aHyP-Py		0.45	0.35
4-Phenylbutyryl-Thp-Py		0.89	0.067

bovine brain enzyme (IC$_{50}$ = 67 nM). Some potent inhibitors are listed in Table 17C.7. Among the other amino acid residues tested for the P$_2$ subsite, hydroxyproline (4-phenylbutyryl-allohydroxyprolyl-pyrrolidine (**9**) exhibits potent inhibition of bovine enzyme. This observation suggests the possibility of a potent inhibitor with a basic structure other than proline or thioproline. In the passive avoidance test using rats with amnesia experimentally induced by a drug, the pyrrolidine derivatives exhibiting potent inhibitory activity towards prolyl endopeptidase also showed anti-amnesic activity as good as that of prolinal derivatives. These results suggested that prolyl endopeptidase plays an important role in the regulation of learning and memory consolidation in the brain, and inhibitors of these enzymes are suggested as possible candidates for nootropic agents.

References

Ader, R. and de Wied, D. (1972). Retention of a passive avoidance response as a function of the intensity and duration of electric shock. *Psychonomic Sciences*, **26**, 125–8.

Bohus, B., Gispen, W. H., and de Wied, D. (1973). Effects of lysine vasopressin and ACTH$_{4-10}$ on conditioned avoidance behavior of hypophysectomized rats. *Neuroendocrinology*, **11**, 137–43.

Brinton, R. E., Cehlert, D. R., Wamsley, J. K., Wan, Y. P., and Yamamura, H. I. (1986). Vasopressin metabolite, AVP$_{4-9}$, binding sites in brain: distribution distinct from that of parent peptide. *Life Sciences*, **38**, 443–52.

Burbach, J. P. H., Kovacs, G. L., and de Wied, D. (1983). A major metabolite of arginine vasopressin in the brain is a highly potent neuropeptide. *Science*, **221**, 1310–12.

de Wied, D. (1971). Long-term effect of vasopressin on the maintenance of a conditioned avoidance response in rats. *Nature, London*, **232**, 58–60.

de Wied, D., Bohus, B., and van Wimersma Greidanus, T. B. (1975). Memory deficit in rats with hereditary diabetes insipidus. *Brain Research*, **85**, 1152–6.

de Wied, D., Gaffori, O., van Ree, J. M., and de Jong, W. (1984). Central target for the behavioural effects of vasopressin neuropeptides. *Nature, London*, **308**, 276–8.

Hersh, L. B. and McKelvy, J. F. (1979). Enzymes involved in the degradation of thyrotropin releasing hormone (TRH) and luteinizing hormone releasing hormone (LH-RH) in bovine brain. *Brain Research*, **168**, 553–64.

Kimura, K., Kawaguchi, N., Yoshihama, M., and Kawanishi, G. (1990). Staurosporine, a prolyl endopeptidase inhibitor. *Agricultural Biological Chemistry*, **54**, 3021–2.

Knisatschek, H. and Bauer, K. (1979). Characterization of 'thyroliberin-deamidating enzyme' as a post-proline-cleaving enzyme. *Journal of Biological Chemistry*, **254**, 10936–43.

Koida, M. and Walter, R. (1976). Post-proline cleaving enzyme. *Journal of Biological Chemistry*, **251**, 7593–9.

Kreider, M. S., Winokur, A., and Krieger, N. R. (1981). Pathways of TRH degradation in rat brain. *Neuropeptide*, **1**, 455–63.

Nishikata, M., Yokosawa, H., and Ishii, S. (1986). Synthesis and structure of prolinal-containing peptides, and their use as specific inhibitors of prolyl endopeptidase. *Chemical and Pharmaceutical Bulletin*, **34**, 2931–6.

Orlowski, M., Wilk, E., Pearce, S., and Wilk, S. (1979). Purification and properties of a prolyl endopeptidase from rabbit brain. *Journal of Neurochemistry*, **33**, 461–9.

Rupnow, J. H., Taylor, W. L., and Dixon, J. E. (1979). Purification and characterization of a thyrotropin-releasing hormone deamidase from rat brain. *Biochemistry*, **18**, 1206–12.

Saito, M., Hashimoto, M., Kawaguchi, N., Fukami, H., Tanaka, T., and Higuchi, N. (1990). Synthesis and inhibitory activity of acyl-peptidyl prolinal derivatives toward post-proline cleaving enzyme as nootropic agents. *Journal of Enzyme Inhibition*, **3**, 163–78.

Saito, M., Hashimoto, M., Kawaguchi, N., Shibata, H., Fukami, H., Tanaka, T., and Higuchi, N. (1991). Synthesis and inhibitory activity of acyl-peptidyl-pyrrolidine derivatives toward post-proline cleaving enzyme; a study of subsite specificity. *Journal of Enzyme Inhibition*, **5**, 51–75.

Sattar, A. K. M. A., Yamamoto, N., Yoshimoto, T., and Tsuru, D. (1990). Purification and characterization of an extracellular prolyl endopeptidase from *Agaricus bisporus*. *Journal of Biochemistry*, **107**, 256–61.

Taylor, W. L. and Dixon, J. E. (1980). Catabolism of neuropeptide by a brain prolyl endopeptidase. *Biochemical and Biophysical Research Communications*, **94**, 9–15.

van Wimersma Greidanus, T. B., Dogterom, J., and de Wied, D. (1975). Intraventricular administration of antivasopressin serum inhibits memory consolidation in rats. *Life Sciences*, **16**, 637–44.

Walter, R. (1976). Partial purification and characterization of post-proline cleaving enzyme: ezymatic inactivation of neurohypophyseal hormones by kidney preparations of various species. *Biochemical and Biophysical Research Communications*, **422**, 138–58.

Walter, R. and Yoshimoto, T. (1978). Postproline cleaving enzyme: kinetic studies of size and stereospecificity of its active site. *Biochemistry*, **17**, 4139–44.

Walter, R., Shlank, H., Class, J. D., Schwartz. I. L., and Keranyi, T. D. (1971). Leucylglycineamide released from oxytocin by human uterine enzyme. *Science*, **173**, 827–9.

Yoshimoto, T., Orlowski, R. C., and Walter, R. (1977). Postproline cleaving enzyme: identification as serine protease using active site specific inhibitors. *Biochemistry*, **16**, 2942–48.

Yoshimoto, T., Fischl, M., Orlowski, R. C., and Walter, R. (1978). Post-proline cleaving enzyme and post-proline dipeptidyl aminopeptidase. *Journal of Biological Chemistry*, **253**, 3708–16.

Yoshimoto, T., Ogita, K., Walter, R., Koida, M., and Tsuru, D. (1979). Post-proline cleaving enzyme. *Biochimica et Biophysica Acta*, **569**, 184–92.

Yoshimoto, T., Walter, R., and Tsuru, D. (1980). Proline-specific endopeptidase from *Flavobacterium*. *Journal of Biological Chemistry*, **255**, 4786–92.

Yoshimoto, T., Simmons, W. H., Kita, T., and Tsuru, D. (1981). Post-proline cleaving enzyme from lamb brain. *Journal of Biochemistry*, **90**, 325–34.

Yoshimoto, T., Tsukumo, K., Takatsuka, N., and Tsuru, D. (1982). An inhibitor for post-proline cleaving enzyme; distribution and partial purification from porcine pancreas. *Journal of Pharmacobio-Dynamics*, **5**, 734–40.

Yoshimoto, T., Kawahara, K., Matsubara, F., Kado, K., and Tsuru, D. (1985). Comparison of inhibitory effects of proline-containing peptide derivatives on prolyl endopeptidases from bovine brain and *Flavobacterium*. *Journal of Biochemistry*, **98**, 975–9.

Yoshimoto, T., Kado, K., Matsubara, F., Koriyama, N., Kaneto, H., and Tsuru, D. (1987a). Specific inhibitors for prolyl endopeptidase and their anti-amnesic effect. *Journal of Pharmacobio-Dynamics*, **10**, 730–5.

Yoshimoto, T., Sattar, A. K. M. A., Hirose, W., and Tsuru, D. (1987b). Studies on prolyl endopeptidase from carrot (*Daucus carota*): purification and enzymatic properties. *Biochimica et Biophysica Acta*, **916**, 29–37.

Yoshimoto, T., Oyama, H., Koriyama, N., and Tsuru, D. (1988). Prolyl endopeptidase from bovine testis: purification, characterization and comparison with the enzymes from other tissues. *Chemical and Pharmaceutical Bulletin*, **36**, 1456–62.

Yoshimoto. T., Tsuru, D., Yamamoto, M., Ikezawa, R., and Furukawa, S. (1991). Structure activity relationship of inhibitors specific for prolyl endopeptidase, *Agricultural Biological Chemistry*, **55**, 37–43.

Section 17D

Inhibitors of dihydropteridine reductase

Rong-Sen Shen

17D.1   Introduction
17D.2   Dihydropteridine reductase
17D.3   Inhibitors
References

17D.1   Introduction

Dihydropteridine reductase (NADH: 6,7-dihydropteridine oxidoreductase, EC 1.6.99.7) (DHPR) catalyses the reduction of quinonoid dihydrobiopterin (qBH_2, **1**) to L-*erythro*-5,6,7,8-tetrahydrobiopterin (BH_4, **2**) using NADH as the cofactor (Fig. 17D.1). BH_4 is the essential cofactor for Phe hydroxylase (EC 1.14.16.1) during the conversion of Phe to Tyr and for Tyr hydroxylase (EC 1.14.16.2) and Trp hydroxylase (EC 1.14.16.4) during the formation of biogenic amines (Kaufman and Fisher 1974). The essential role of DHPR in helping to maintain a catalytic pool of BH_4 for these three hydroxylases is demonstrated by the discovery that a defect in this enzyme causes hyperphenylalaninaemia (Kaufman *et al.* 1975; Smith *et al.* 1975). However, DHPR and BH_4 may have other physiological roles such as the transfer of electrons (Rembold and Buff 1972), the synthesis of nitric oxide (Kwon *et al.* 1989; Tayeh and Marletta 1989) which stimulates soluble guanylate cyclase, and the removal of oxygen radicals (Heales *et al.* 1988; Shen 1991; Shen and Zhang 1991). A potential clinical application of DHPR inhibitors is in the development of an animal model of hyperphenylalaninaemia.

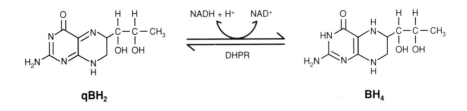

qBH₂   BH₄

Fig. 17D.1   Reaction catalysed by DHPR.

17D.2 Dihydropteridine reductase

DHPR is widely distributed in nature and has been found in almost all mammalian tissues, including human blood cells and skin fibroblasts (Shen and Abell 1981; Armarego *et al*. 1984). The enzyme uses quinonoid dihydropteridines, including qBH_2, as substrate. NADH is the preferred pyridine nucleotide cofactor, but an NADPH-specific DHPR has been found in bovine liver (Nakanishi *et al*. 1977). Mammalian DHPR is a dimeric protein consisting of two identical subunits with molecular masses ranging from 21.3 to 27.4 kDa (Armarego *et al*. 1984). Amino acid composition analyses of DHPR and cDNA clones encoding the enzyme indicate structural similarities among mammalian species (Dahl *et al*. 1987; Lockyer *et al*. 1987; Shahbaz *et al*. 1987). Human DHPR shows a small region of 50 per cent sequence identity with human dihydrofolate reductase (EC 1.5.1.3) (DHFR), which is also a pterin and pyridine nucleotide-requiring enzyme (Dahl *et al*. 1987). Morever, anti-idiotypic antibodies elicited by pterin recognize active-site epitopes in DHPR and DHFR, indicating a common topography at the pterin-binding sites (Ratnam *et al*. 1989; Jennings and Cotton 1990).

The active site of DHPR has not yet been defined. Amino acid modifications of the rat liver enzyme suggest that as many as four Cys residues per subunit may be involved in maintaining a catalytically functional tertiary structure (Webber and Whitely 1981). Mammalian DHPR binds up to two moles of NADH per mole of native enzyme. The reaction catalysed by DHPR may follow a sequential ordered mechanism with NADH binding first and NAD^+ dissociation last. The reaction probably involves a direct transfer of the pro-S hydrogen from the B face of NADH to N_3 or N_5 of the qBH_2 (Armarego *et al.* 1984).

17D.3 Inhibitors

Mammalian DHPR is inhibited by 'unconjugated' (**3–6**) and 'conjugated' (**7–12**) pteridines (Table 17D.1). Various types of inhibition with respect to pteridine substrate and NADH cofactor have been reported. The K_i values are in the range $10^{-4}-10^{-5}$ M which are approximately a factor of 10^4-10^5 higher than those for DHFR with these inhibitors (Craine *et al*. 1972). The substituents to the pteridine rings, particularly the C_6 atom, appear to have little effect on the inhibition potency of the compound. It is probably that these pteridines bind to the enzyme sufficiently tightly that they neither catalytically turn over nor allow binding of substrate.

The activity of mammalian DHPR has also been reported to be inhibited by catechol- and *p*-hydroxyphenyl-containing compounds such as catecholamines (Purdy and Blair 1980; Purdy *et at*. 1981; Shen 1983),

Table 17D.1 Pteridines as inhibitors of DHPR

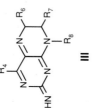 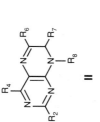 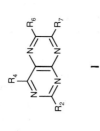

I   II   III

Structure	R_2	R_4	R_6	R_7	R_8	$K_i (I_{50})$, (μM)	Reference
3 **I**	H	H	CH_3	CH_3	–	300	Cheema et al. 1973
4 **I**	H	OH	CH_3	CH_3	–	50	Cheema et al. 1973
5 **I**	NH_2	NH_2	CH_3	CH_3	–	80	Cheema et al. 1973
6 **III**	–	OH	CH_3, CH_3	H,H	CH_3	(200)	Randles and Armarego 1985
7 **I**	NH_2	NH_2	CH_2-NH-C_6H_4-COOH	H	–	30	Lind 1972
8 **I**	NH_2	NH_2	CH_2-NH-C_6H_4-CO-Glu	H	–	10–24	Cheema et al. 1973; Lind 1972 Aksnes and Ljones 1980; Shen et al. 1982
9 **II**	NH_2	NH_2	CH_2-NH-C_6H_4-CO-Glu	H,H	H	23	Lind 1972
10 **III**	–	NH_2	CH_2-NH-C_6H_4-CO-Glu,H	H,H	H	22	Lind 1972
11 **I**	NH_2	OH	CH_2-NH-C_6H_4-CO-Glu	H	–	240	Cheema et al. 1973
12 **I**	NH_2	NH_2	CH_2-NCH_3-C_6H_4-CO-Glu	H	–	17–50	Craine et al. 1972; Webber et al. 1978; Chauvin et al. 1979

Table 17D.2 Catechol-containing compounds as inhibitors of DHPR

	R	R'	R"	$K_i(I_{50})$ (μM)	Reference
13	H	H,COOH	H,H	260	Shen 1984
14	H	H,H	H,H	14	Purdy et al. 1981, Shen 1983
15	CH$_3$	H,H	H,H	(27)	Shen 1983
16	H	H,H	H,OH	200–490	Shen 1983; Purdy and Blair 1980
17	CH$_3$	H,H	H,OH	130	Shen 1983

Table 17D.3 Dopamine-derived tetrahydroisoquinolines as inhibitors of DHPR

	R	R'	R"	$K_i(I_{50})$ (μM)	Reference
18	H	CH$_3$	H	90	Shen et al. 1982
19	H	H	CH$_3$	(52)	Shen (unpublished)
20	H	C$_6$H$_3$(OH)$_2$	H	8	Shen and Abell 1987
21	COOH	CH$_2$-C$_6$H$_5$	H	14	Shen et al. 1982
22	COOH	CH$_2$-C$_6$H$_4$OH	H	4.5	Shen et al. 1982
23	H	CH$_2$-C$_6$H$_4$OH	H	1.5	Shen et al. 1982
24	H	CH$_2$-C$_6$H$_3$(OH)$_2$	H	0.5	Shen and Abell 1987
25	H	CH$_2$-C$_6$H$_3$(OH)$_2$	CH$_3$	(4.5)	Shen (unpublished)

dopamine-derived tetrahydroisoquinolines (Shen *et al.* 1982), and apor-phines (Shen *et al.* 1984) (Table 17D.2 and 17D.3). The K_i values are in the range 10^{-4}–10^{-6} M. The type of inhibition is non-competitive with respect to pterin and NADH in all cases. The inhibitory potency increases with increasing number of hydroxyl groups in the catechols and decreases progressively as the hydroxyl groups are methylated. The most potent inhibitor is tetrahydropapaveroline (24) with a K_i of 0.5 μM.

The active species of these inhibitors (13–25) are probably o-quinones (Armarego and Waring 1983; Shen and Abell 1983; Milstien and Kaufman 1987) because DHPR activity was assayed in a reaction mixture containing either horseradish peroxidase and H_2O_2 or 2,6-dichlorophenol indophenol, conditions which favour oxidation of the catecholic inhibitors. This interpretation is consistent with the observation that aminochromes, the oxidation products of catecholamines, inhibit DHPR (Armarego and Waring 1983; Waring 1986).

A quantitative structure–activity relationship study of some hydroxylated 4-phenyl-1,2,3,6-tetrahydropyridines, 4-phenylpyridines, and 4-phenylpiperidines as inhibitors of DHPR has been reported by Babbar et al. (1989). The inactivation mechanism may involve the attack of nucleophilic residues, such as the sulphydryl of Cys, in the enzyme molecules by the quinone (Shen and Abell 1983). However, disulphide cross-linking of DHPR molecules at or near the active site to form inactive polymers has been proposed as the mechanism of DHPR inactivation by aminochromes (Waring 1986).

One of the potential clinical applications of DHPR inhibitors is to develop an animal model of hyperphenylalaninaemia. However, the inhibition of DHPR alone is probably not sufficient to deplete intracellular BH_4, because BH_4 is synthesized de novo by GTP cyclohydrolase I (EC 3.5.4.16, GTP-CH) and three other enzymes, and by DHFR through a salvage pathway (Nichol et al. 1985). Since pteridines also inhibit DHFR (Craine et al. 1972) and GTP-CH (Bellahsene et al. 1984; Shen et al. 1988, 1989), the use of one pteridine to inhibit all these enzymes selectively remains a challenge to the design of drugs with high efficacy.

References

Aksnes, A. and Ljones, T. (1980). Steady state kinetics of dihydropteridine reductase: Initial velocity and inhibition studies. *Archives of Biochemistry and Biophysics*, **202**, 342–7.

Armarego, W. L. F. and Waring, P. (1983). Inhibition of human dihydropteridine reductase by the oxidation products of catecholamines, the aminochromes. *Biochemical and Biophysical Research Communications*, **113**, 895–9.

Armarego, W. L. F., Randles, D., and Waring, P. (1984). Dihydropteridine reductase (DHPR), its cofactors, and its mode of action. *Medical Research Reviews*, **4**, 267–321.

Babbar, R., Gupta, J. K., and Gupta, S. P. (1989). Quantitative structure–activity relationship study on some dihydropteridine reductase inhibitors. *Journal of Enzyme Inhibition*, **2**, 231–7.

Bellahsene, Z., Dhondt, J.-L., and Farriaux, J.-P. (1984). Guanosine triphosphate cyclohydrolase activity in rat tissues. *Biochemical Journal*, **217**, 59–65.

Chauvin, M. M., Korri, K. K., Tirpak, A., Simpson, R. C., and Scrimgeour, K. G. (1979). Purification of dihydropteridine reductase using immobilized Cibacron Blue. *Canadian Journal of Biochemistry*, **57**, 178–87.

Cheema, S., Soldin, S. J., Knapp, A., Hofmann, T., and Scrimgeour, K. G. (1973). Properties of purified quinonoid dihydropterin reductase. *Canadian Journal of Biochemistry*, **51**, 1229–39.

Craine, J. E., Hall, E. S., and Kaufman, S. (1972). The isolation and characterization of dihydropteridine reductase from sheep liver. *Journal of Biological Chemistry*, **247**, 6082–91.

Dahl, H.-H. M., Hutchison, W., McAdam, W., Wake, S., Morgan, F. J., and Cotton, R. G. H. (1987). Human dihydropteridine reductase: characterization of a cDNA clone and its use in analysis of patients with dihydropteridine reductase deficiency. *Nucleic Acid Research*, **15**, 1921–32.

Heales, S. J. R., Blair, J. A., Meinschad, C., and Ziegler, I. (1988). Inhibition of monocyte luminol-dependent chemiluminescence by tetrahydrobiopterin, and the free radical oxidation of tetrahydrobiopterin, dihydrobiopterin and dihydroneopterin. *Cell Biochemistry and Function*, **6**, 191–5.

Jennings, I. and Cotton, R. (1990). Structural similarities among enzyme pterin binding sites as demonstrated by a monoclonal anti-idiotypic antibody. *Journal of Biological Chemistry*, **265**, 1885–9.

Kaufman, S. and Fisher, D. B. (1974). Pterin-requiring aromatic amino acid hydroxylases. In *Molecular mechanisms of oxygen activation* (ed. O. Hayaishi), pp. 285–369. Academic Press, New York.

Kaufman, S., Holtzman, N. A., Milstien, S., Butler, I. J., and Krumholz, A. (1975). Phenylketonuria due to a deficiency of dihydropteridine reductase. *New England Journal of Medicine*, **293**, 785–90.

Kwon, N. S., Nathan, C. F., and Stuehr, D. J. (1989). Reduced biopterin as a cofactor in the generation of nitrogen oxides by murine macrophages. *Journal of Biological Chemistry*, **264**, 20496–501.

Lind, K. E. (1972). Dihydropteridine reductase. Investigation of the specificity for quinonoid dihydropteridine and the inhibition by 2,4-diaminopteridines. *European Journal of Biochemistry*, **25**, 560–2.

Lockyer, J., Cook, R. G., Milstien, S., Kaufman, S., Woo, S. L. C., and Ledley, F. D. (1987). Structure and expression of human dihydropteridine reductase. *Proceedings of the National Academy of Sciences of the United States of America*, **84**, 3329–33.

Milstien, S. and Kaufman, S. (1987). The oxidation of apomorphine and other catechol compounds by horseradish peroxidase: relevance to the measurement of dihydropteridine reductase activity. *Biochimica et Biophysica Acta*, **923**, 333–8.

Nakanishi, N., Hasegawa, H., and Watabe, S. (1977). A new enzyme, NADPH-dihydropteridine reductase in bovine liver. *Journal of Biochemistry*, **81**, 681–5.

Nichol, C. A., Smith, G. K., and Duch, D. S. (1985). Biosynthesis and metabolism of tetrahydrobiopterin and molybdopterin. *Annual Review of Biochemistry*, **54**, 729–64.

Purdy, S. E. and Blair, J. A. (1980). Rat liver dihydropteridine reductase inhibition. *Biochemical Society Transactions*, **8**, 565–6.

Purdy, S. E., Blair, J. A., and Barford, P. A. (1981). Inhibition of dihydropteridine reductase by dopamine. *Biochemical Journal*, **195**, 769–71.

Randles, D. and Armarego, W. L. F. (1985). Reduced 6,6,8-trimethylpterins.

Preparation, properties and enzymatic reactivities with dihydropteridine reductase, phenylalanine hydroxylase and tyrosine hydroxylase. *European Journal of Biochemistry*, **146**, 467–74.

Ratnam, S., Ratnam, M., Cotton, R. G. H., Jennings, I. G., and Freisheim, J. H. (1989). Anti-idiotypic antibodies elicited by pterin recognize active site epitopes in dihydrofolate reductase and dihydropteridine reductase. *Archives of Biochemistry and Biophysics*, **275**, 344–53.

Rembold, H. and Buff, K. (1972). Tetrahydrobiopterin, a cofactor in mitochondrial electron transfer. *European Journal of Biochemistry*, **28**, 586–91.

Shahbaz, M., Hoch, J. A., Trach, K. A., Hural, J. A., Webber, S., and Whiteley, J. M. (1987). Structural studies and isolation of cDNA clones providing the complete sequence of rat liver dihydropteridine reductase. *Journal of Biological Chemistry*, **262**, 16412–16.

Shen, R.-S. (1983). Inhibition of dihydropteridine reductase by catecholamines and related compounds. *Biochimica et Biophysica Acta*, **743**, 129–35.

Shen, R.-S. (1984). Potent inhibitory effects of tyrosine metabolites on dihydropteridine reductase from human and sheep liver. *Biochimica et Biophysica Acta*, **785**, 181–5.

Shen, R.-S. (1991). Inhibition of dopamine autoxidation by tetrahydrobiopterin and NADH in the presence of dihydropteridine reductase. *Neurotoxicology*, **12**, 201–8.

Shen, R.-S. and Abell, C. W. (1981). Purification of dihydropteridine reductase from human platelets. *Journal of Neuroscience Research*, **6**, 193–201.

Shen, R.-S. and Abell, C. W. (1983). Inhibition of dihydropteridine reductase by catechol estrogens. *Journal of Neuroscience Research*, **10**, 251–9.

Shen, R.-S. and Abell, C. W. (1987). Rat striatal synaptosomes as a model system for studying the inhibition of dihydropteridine reductase. *Journal of Enzyme Inhibition*, **1**, 223–9.

Shen, R.-S. and Zhang, Y. (1991). Antioxidation activity of tetrahydrobiopterin in pheochromocytoma PC 12 cells. *Chemico-Biological Interactions*, **78**, 307–19.

Shen, R.-S., Smith, R. V., Davis, P. J., Brubaker, A., and Abell, C. W. (1982). Dopamine-derived tetrahydroisoquinolines. Novel inhibitors of dihydropteridine reductase. *Journal of Biological Chemistry*, **257**, 7294–7.

Shen, R.-S., Smith, R. V., Davis, P. J., and Abell, C. W. (1984). Inhibition of dihydropteridine reductase from human liver and rat striatal synaptosomes by apomorphine and its analogs. *Journal of Biological Chemistry*, **259**, 8994–9000.

Shen, R.-S., Alam, A., and Zhang, Y. (1988). Inhibition of GTP cyclohydrolase I by pterins. *Biochimica et Biophysica Acta*, **965**, 9–15.

Shen, R.-S., Zhang, Y., and Perez-Polo, J. R. (1989). Regulation of GTP cyclohydrolase I and dihydropteridine reductase in rat pheochromocytoma PC 12 cells. *Journal of Enzyme Inhibition*, **3**, 119–26.

Smith, I., Clayton, B. E., and Wolff, O. H. (1975). New variant of phenylketonuria with progressive neurological illness unresponsive to phenylalanine restriction. *Lancet*, **i**, 1108–11.

Tayeh, M. A. and Marletta, M. A. (1989). Macrophage oxidation of L-arginine to nitric oxide, nitrite, and nitrate. *Journal of Biological Chemistry*, **264**, 19654–8.

Waring, P. (1986). The time-dependent inactivation of human brain dihydropteridine reductase by the oxidation products of L-dopa. *European Journal of Biochemistry*, **155**, 305–10.

Webber, S. and Whiteley, J. (1981). The effect of specific animo acid modifications on the catalytic properties of rat liver dihydropteridine reductase. *Archives
of Biochemistry and Biophysics*, **206**, 145–52.
Webber, S., Deits, T. L., Snyder, W. R., and Whiteley, J. M. (1978). The purification of rat and sheep liver dihydropteridine reductases by affinity chromatography on Methotrexate-Sepharose. *Analytical Biochemistry*, **84**, 491–503.

Section 17E

Inhibitors of aldehyde dehydrogenase: anticancer drug resistance

Ronald Lindahl

17E.1   Introduction

The role of aldehyde dehydrogenases in the metabolism of certain families
of anticancer drugs is now well established. The effects of aldehyde dehydrogenase inhibitors in modulating the therapeutic effectiveness of
these agents is an area of current active interest. In this chapter we briefly
review the mammalian aldehyde dehydrogenases, discuss the roles of aldehyde dehydrogenase in antitumour drug metabolism, and examine the
ability of several aldehyde dehydrogenase inhibitors to affect cell-killing by
chemotherapeutic agents. References to the primary literature are limited
to recent key studies. The reader is referred to these and the several excellent
reviews cited for additional relevant work and background.

17E.2   Aldehyde dehydrogenase

Mammalian aldehyde dehydrogenases (ALDHs, E.C. 1.2.1.3) are a family
of NAD^+-dependent enzymes which catalyse the irreversible oxidation
of aldehydes to their corresponding carboxylic acids (Ehrig *et al.* 1990;
Yoshida *et al.* 1991; Lindahl 1992). Substrates for the ALDHs are produced endogenously from amino acid, biogenic amine, and lipid metabolism
(Schauenstein *et al.* 1977; Esterbauer *et al.* 1990). The metabolism of
xenobiotics, including ethanol, pharmaceuticals, and procarcinogens, is a

major exogenous source of aldehydes (Sladek *et al*. 1989; Lindahl 1992). Consistent with the ubiquitous distribution of their substrates, ALDHs exist in virtually every tissue. Within a cell, one or more ALDHs are located in mitochondrial, microsomal, and/or cytosolic compartments.

The primary sequences of 13 mammalian ALDHs are known (Lindahl and Hempel 1991; Lindahl 1992). Based on this information, three major classes of ALDHs have been defined (Anonymous 1989). (Table 17E.1). Class 1 ALDHs are found in the cytosol, class 2 ALDHs are found in the mitochondria, and class 3 ALDHs are microsomal or cytosolic. Class 2 forms are constitutive, being found in mitochondria of all cells. Both constitutive and inducible class 1 ALDHs are known. One class 1 ALDH is a constitutive cytosolic enzyme found in virtually all tissues. A second, closely related, class 1 ALDH appears in liver and other tissues after induction by phenobarbital. Class 3 ALDHs also consist of constitutive and inducible forms. The constitutive microsomal ALDH is a class 3 enzyme. The second class 3 ALDH is the form inducible in several tissues by polycyclic aromatic hydrocarbons and dioxins.

The constitutive class 1, 2, and 3 ALDHs are tetramers of identical subunits of approximately 480 (class 3 microsomal) or 500 (classes 1 and 2) amino acids per subunit (subunit molecular mass, 55 kDa). The inducible class 1 ALDH is a dimer of identical 55 kda subunits, each containing 501 amino acids. The Class 3 inducible ALDH is also a dimer of identical subunits (453 residues, 50 kDa).

The mechanism of catalysis by ALDH is similar to that of glyceraldehyde-3-phosphate dehydrogenase. The reaction is ordered: coenzyme

Table 17E.1 Nomenclature of Mammalian aldehyde dehydrogenases

---

Class aldehyde dehydrogenase (ALDH 1)
Members of the Class 1 ALDHs are the constitutive and inducible CYTO-PLASMIC ALDHs of *human*, *horse*, beef, *rat*, mouse, sheep, and dog liver and the ALDH inducible by phenobarbital

Class 2 adehyde dehydrogenase (ALDH 2)
Members of the class 2 ALDHs are the mitochondrial ALDHs isolated from *human*, *horse*, *beef*, *rat*, mouse, sheep, and dog liver

Class 3 aldehyde dehydrogenase (ALDH 3)
Members of the Class 3 ALDHs are the rat liver *dioxin-inducible* cytoplasmic ALDHs. Also included in this class are the major constitutive or inducible ALDHs from liver microsomes, mammalian cornea, stomach, lung, and urinary bladder.

Sources identified in italics are considered the prototype enzyme of the class based on primary structure determination. Other representatives are based on kinetic, physical and immunological properties. See Lindahl and Hempel (1991) for details.

binding precedes aldehyde binding and acid release precedes reduced co-enzyme release. The aldehyde forms a hemiacetal with an active site nucleophile; this complex is then oxidized by coenzyme to an acyl form, which is hydrolysed to produce the acid product. A fully conserved cysteine (Cy-302 in the human enzyme numbering system) has been implicated as the critical enzyme nucleophile. However, evidence also exists for a critical role for a conserved glutamate (Glu-268) in the active site. For the class 1 enzyme, the rate-limiting step is the release of reduced coenzyme. For the class 2 enzyme, it is acyl intermediate hydrolysis.

Until recently, interest in ALDH has been related to its role in the oxidation of acetaldehyde derived from ethanol. Because alcohol metabolism occurs primarily in the liver, most studies have been performed with hepatic ALDHs. In man, liver ALDH is distributed approximately equally between class 1 and class 2 constitutive forms. For other large mammals, such as the horse, sheep, and cow, a similar hepatic ALDH distribution is seen. For rats and mice, the majority of the liver ALDH activity is class 2 and the constitutive class 3 microsomal ALDH. In rodents, constitutive class 1 activity is much lower than in human liver. Induction of class 1 and class 3 ALDHs is most frequently observed in the liver.

Tissues other than liver also possess significant ALDH activity. Haematopoietic stem cells and their progeny, brain, and kidney all possess significant ALDH activity. The subcellular distribution in these tissues is similar to that of liver, with constitutive class 1 and class 2 forms predominant.

For other tissues, most notably the eye, stomach, and urinary bladder, the ALDH subcellular distribution and activity profiles are different from liver. In these cases, cytosol possesses a large amount of ALDH activity and total specific activity may be many times greater than in liver. For example, more than 90 per cent of the ALDH in cornea is cytosolic. In stomach and urinary bladder, the contribution of the cytosol approaches 50 per cent. This difference is particularly striking in a species such as the rat or mouse, where the liver has relatively little constitutive cytosolic ALDH activity. Of particular interest is the fact that the major constitutive ALDH in tissues such as the cornea, stomach, and bladder are the class 1 and/or class 3 ALDHs inducible in liver.

For most aldehydes, at least one ALDH catalyses its oxidation with a K_m in the low (1–10) micromolar range. Small aliphatic aldehydes, such as acetaldehyde and propionaldehyde, are excellent substrates for both Class 1 and Class 2 constitutive ALDHs. Malondialdehyde, derived from lipid peroxidation, is oxidized primarily by class 1 ALDH. Biogenic aldehydes derived from neurotransmitter metabolism and 4-hydroxyalkenals from lipid peroxidation are also substrates for various class 1 or class 2 forms, but class 2 ALDHs seem to play major roles in the oxidation of these aldehydes. Class 3 ALDHs are responsible for the oxidation of medium chain length (C6−C9) aliphatic aldehydes derived from lipid peroxidation. Large aldehyde-containing molecules, such as corticosteroid aldehydes, are oxidized effectively by both class 1 and class 2 ALDHs. Benzaldehyde-like aromatic aldehydes are oxidized primarily by class 3 ALDHs. However, phenylacetaldehyde-like substrates are metabolized exclusively by class 1 forms.

17E.3   Role of aldehyde dehydrogenase in the metabolism of anticancer drugs

One established physiological role for ALDH is in the metabolism of certain chemotherapeutic agents. ALDH activity is critical in determining the levels of putative active metabolites of oxazaphosphorines, such as cyclophosphamide (CP) (Sladek 1988), and substituted hydrazines such as procarbazine (PCZ) (Erikson *et al.* 1992). Cyclophosphamide is a widely used antineoplastic agent, effective against certain leukaemias and lymphomas, neuroblastoma, retinoblastoma, and carcinomas of the lung, ovary, breast, and cervix. Cyclophosphamide is also an effective immunosuppressant. Procarbazine is effective against Hodgkin's lymphoma and certain brain tumours. Often CP and PCZ are part of a combination chemotherapy regimen, as in COPP (cyclophosphamide, vincristine, prednisone, procarbazine).

Cyclophosphamide and procarbazine are prodrugs, requiring hepatic mixed-function oxidase-mediated metabolic activation to generate transport metabolites which are further metabolized by target cells to alkylating cytotoxic species (Figs. 17E.1 and 17E.2). The transport form for CP is 4-hydroxycyclophosphamide, which exists in equilibrium with its open, ring tautomer aldophosphamide (Sladek 1988). In target cells, aldophosphamide undergoes β elimination to produce the cytotoxic metabolite phosphoramide mustard (Fig. 17E.1). The role of ALDH in CP metabolism is the oxidation of aldophosphamide to carboxyphosphamide, which is not cytotoxic (Fig. 17E.1). This reaction is catalysed by a constitutive class 1 ALDH (Russo and Hilton 1988; Manthey *et al.* 1990; Dockham *et al.* 1992). Since oxidation to carboxyphosphamide is a detoxification reaction, the chemotherapeutic effectiveness of CP should be inversely correlated with target cell class 1 aldehyde dehydrogenase activity. This is indeed the case (Sladek and Landkamer 1985; Kohn *et al.* 1987).

Azoprocarbazine, the transport form of PCZ undergoes further cytochrome P450 mediated oxidation to azoxy PCZ isomers (Fig. 17E.2) (Weinkam and Shiba 1978; Tweedie *et al.* 1991; Erikson *et al.* 1992). The azoxy PCZ isomers, particularly azoxy 2 PCZ, exhibit greater anticancer effects than their precursors. ALDH is involved in the further metabolism of azoxy 2 PCZ through an aldehyde intermediate, *N*-isopropyl-*p*-formyl-benzamide, to a carboxylic acid derivative which is a major

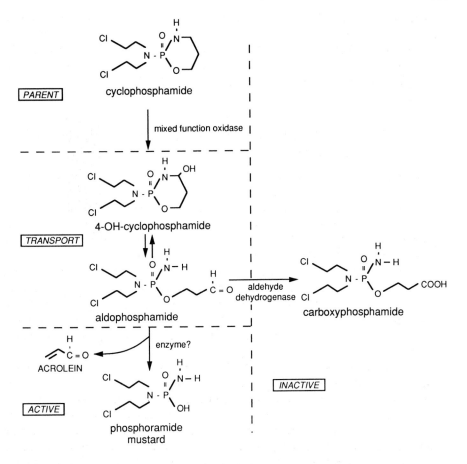

Fig. 17E.1 Metabolism of cyclophosphamide. From Sladek (1988).

urinary metabolite of PCZ (Fig. 17E.2). The relevant ALDH is the phenobarbital-inducible class 1 enzyme (Tweedie *et al.* 1991).

However, the metabolism of azoxy 2 PCZ is complex. Azoxy 2 PCZ is unstable and may decompose to the aldehyde and an ultimately cytotoxic metabolite. The class 1 ALDH mediated procarbazine reaction involves two steps catalysed by a single enzyme and is unique among the ALDHs (Tweedie *et al.* 1991). The first reaction, the conversion of azoxy 2 PCZ to the aldehyde, is NAD$^+$ independent and involves the inherent esterase activity of class 1 ALDH (Fig. 17E.2). The oxidation of the aldehyde to the carboxylic acid is NAD$^+$ dependent. Both the spontaneous and enzyme-catalysed processes produce the ultimate cytotoxic alkylating species of procarbazine. Azoxy 2 PCZ and the aldehyde intermediate are potent

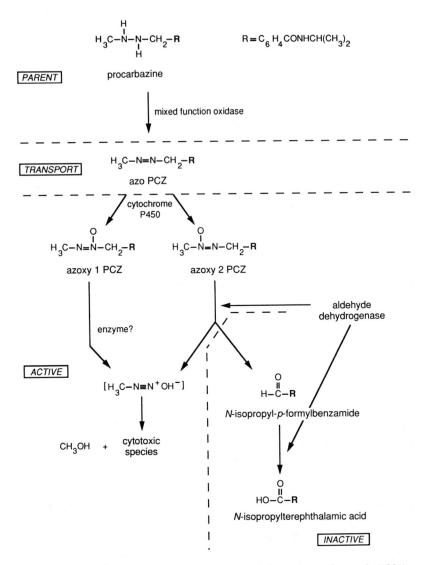

Fig. 17E.2 Metabolism of procarbazine. Modified from Tweedie *et al.* (1991) and Erikson *et al.* (1992).

inhibitors of both the dehydrogenase and esterase activities of class 1 ALDH. This may explain the potentiation of mafosfamide (a CP analogue) cytotoxicity for cultured leukaemia cells treated with both mafosfamide and procarbazine (Maki and Sladek 1991). These results also indicate that the role of ALDH in procarbazine metabolism is not yet clear. Since

ALDH catalyses the activation of azoxy 2 PCZ to more cytotoxic metabolites, cell killing should directly correlate with target cell ALDH activity.
However, in model systems, cells without measurable ALDH activity are
sensitive to PCZ (Tweedie *et al*. 1991). Alternatively, the inhibition of
ALDH by azoxy 2 PCZ or the aldehyde may reduce the production of
cytotoxic metabolites, reducing the therapeutic effectiveness of PCZ.

17E.4 Inhibitors

Inhibition of ALDH activity is the basis of many alcohol aversion therapies. The two most widely used alcohol-deterrent drugs are disulfiram
(tetraethylthiuram disulphide) and cyanamide (calcium carbimide) (Peachey
and Naranjo 1983; Brien and Loomis 1985). Both act by inhibiting the
ALDH involved in acetaldehyde metabolism, the class 2 ALDH. The
elevation of blood acetaldehyde produced by ALDH inhibition causes a
set of symptoms, collectively called the 'disulfiram-like reaction', which
may include severe headache, nausea, vomiting, flushing of the skin, hypotension, tachycardia, tachypnoea, and palpitations.

Other drugs produce a disulfiram-like reaction in some patients who
consume ethanol while taking the drug. Among those known to inhibit
ALDHs are the monoamine oxidase inhibitor pargyline (Lebsack *et al*.
1977), the sedative chloral hydrate (Crow *et al*. 1974), the oral hypo-
glycaemics chlorpropamide and tolbutamide (Nagasawa *et al*. 1988), and
some of the cephalosporin antibiotics (Kitson 1987). While any of these
drugs could alter the effectiveness of antitumour drugs when coadministered, certain cephalosporins are of particular interest in the present context.

For anticancer drugs such as cyclophosphamide and procarbazine, inhibition of ALDH activity may have two major effects. For CP, tumour
cells with little or no relevant ALDH activity should be most sensitive to
these agents. Tumours may develop resistance to CP as the proportion
of tumour cells possessing the relevant ALDH activity increases. Thus
inhibition of the relevant ALDH activity in tumour cells should potentiate
the cell-killing ability of CP. On the basis of model systems, this situation
appears to be of clinical importance. For procarbazine, target cells should
possess the relevant ALDH and inhibition of this activity may reduce the
effectiveness of the drug.

Conversely, inhibition of the relevant ALDH activity in proliferating
normal cells would place them at risk of being killed by active forms of
CP. For PCZ, inhibition of ALDH in critical normal cells would protect
them from the cytotoxic effects of the drug. Therefore the need is for
inhibitors that are specific for, or at least preferentially inhibitory of, the
ALDH activity in the relevant cells. In the remainder of this chapter we
shall discuss some ALDH inhibitors that may be useful in modulating the
effects of various antitumour drugs.

Disulfiram (Fig. 17E.3) is the 'classical' ALDH inhibitor, even though it is not specific for ALDH and has significant side-effects. Most interest has focused on the effect of disulfiram on class 2 ALDH because of its role in acetaldehyde oxidation. However, all three classes of aldehyde dehydrogenases are inhibited. In fact, class 1 ALDHs appear to be most sensitive to disulfiram *in vivo*, followed by class 3 and then class 2.

Disulfiram has little effect on ALDHs *in vitro*, and disulfiram metabolites are the active inhibitors *in vivo* (Kitson 1983; Johansson *et al.* 1989; Hart *et al.* 1990). Although some uncertainty remains, the diethyldithiocarbamate methyl ester

$$[(C_2H_5)_2N-\overset{\overset{\displaystyle O}{\displaystyle \|}}{C}-S-CH_3]$$

may be the physiologically important inhibitory species (Johansson *et al.* 1989; Hart *et al.* 1990). Disulfiram is an irreversible inhibitor with a slow onset (12 hours) and long duration (7 days). The target residue is a

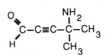

Disulfiram

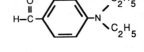

Cyanamide

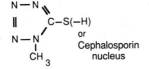

Methyltetrazolethiol
(MTT)

4-(Diethylamino)benzaldehyde
(DEAB)

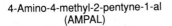

4-Amino-4-methyl-2-pentyne-1-al
(AMPAL)

Fig. 17E.3 Structure of relevant aldehyde dehydrogenase inhibitors.

critical enzyme sulphydryl, probably the conserved active-site cysteine-302 (Vallari and Pietruszko 1982; Kitson 1983). The exact mechanism by which disulfiram metabolites interact with Cys-302 is yet to be elucidated. One possibility is that disulfiram or its metabolites catalyse the formation of an intramolecular disulphide bond between Cys-302 and another enzyme — SH group (Vallari and Pietruszko 1982; Kitson 1983). It has also been suggested that the methyl ester acts as a suicide inhibitor (Johansson *et al.* 1989). A third possibility is that diethyldithiocarbamate methyl ester is metabolized further to an ultimate inhibitory species (Hart *et al.* 1990).

As a sulphydryl-directed reagent, disulfiram inhibits a number of other enzymes (Brien and Loomis 1985) including dopamine hydroxylase, hexokinase, 5-lipoxygenase, cholesterol hydroxylase, and the cytochrome P450 dependent mixed-function oxidase system. Inhibition of some of these enzymes, the mixed-function oxidases for example, could result in significant drug–drug interactions. Both CP and PCZ require cytochrome P450 activity for activation. The use of disulfiram to inhibit ALDH as a means of potentiating antitumour drug cytotoxicity could be counterproductive owing to decreased metabolic activation of the anticancer prodrug because of disulfiram effects on the mixed-function oxidases.

Disulfiram side-effects include hepatotoxicity, neurotoxicity, elevation of blood pressure, drowsiness and depression, and elevation of serum cholesterol (Brien and Loomis 1985). Considerable individual variation in the effectiveness of disulfiram as an alcohol aversive drug, coupled with the severity of its side effects and slow onset of inhibition, have limited its clinical usefulness.

Cyanamide (Fig. 17E.3) also causes a disulfiram-like reaction (Brien and Loomis 1985; Nagasawa *et al.* 1990). It is used in alcohol aversion therapy in Europe, Canada and Japan, but not in the United States. Cyanamide acts by inhibiting class 2 ALDHs preferentially, although class 1 forms are also inhibited. The effect of cyanamide on class 3 ALDH is not known.

The precise mechanism of ALDH inhibition by cyanamide is unknown. Cyanamide requires bioactivation and an essential role is played by catalase (Nagasawa *et al.* 1990; Prunonosa *et al.* 1991). Cyanamide is oxidized by catalase to an unstable intermediate which decomposes to produce nitroxyl and cyanide, of which nitroxyl is believed to be the inhibitory species (Nagasawa *et al.* 1990). *In vivo*, cyanamide inhibition can be reversed by subsequent ethanol exposure, suggesting that inhibition is competitive with aldehyde substrate (Brien and Loomis 1985). An ionizable group, presumably a histidine, has also been implicated (Prunonosa *et al.* 1991). Inhibition is rapid (1 hour) and lasts about a day.

Cyanamide is a more specific inhibitor of ALDHs than disulfiram. It has no effect on the enzymes inhibited by disulfiram or several others. Therefore there are few reports of drug–drug interactions caused by cyanamide. There are also few reports of significant side-effects associated with cyanamide.

Certain cephalosporin antibiotics, including moxalactam, cefamandole, and cefoperazone, elicit a disulfiram-like reaction (Kitson 1983; Lipsky 1989). These compounds possess a methyltetrazolethiol (MTT) group attached to the β-lactam-dihydrothiazine ring complex (Fig. 17E.3). Class 1 and class 2 ALDHs are both inhibited by MTT and MTT-containing antibiotics, although class 2 forms may be more sensitive. Because the metabolisms of MTT and disulfiram are similar, one would also expect class 3 ALDH to be inhibited by MTT-containing drugs (see below).

Inhibition of ALDH by methyltetrazolethiol-containing drugs requires metabolic activation. The first step is the release of the MTT group, which is further metabolized to the ultimate inhibitory species (Kitson 1983; Lipsky 1989). Subsequent steps in the activation and the mechanism of inhibition remain largely undefined but are believed to be very similar to disulfiram. *In vivo*, methyltetrazolethiol may form a disulphide-linked dimer, dithiobis(1-methyltetrazole) (DTMT), which is structurally similar to disulfiram. Evidence also exists for a methyl mixed disulphide metabolite, methyl-(1-methyltetrazole) disulphide, which is structurally similar to the active disulfiram metabolite diethyldithiocarbamate methyl ester. Therefore the same mechanisms proposed for disulfiram inhibition of ALDH, i.e. involvement of a critical enzyme sulphydryl such as Cys-302, probably apply to MTT-catalysed enzyme inhibition. Like disulfiram, MTT inhibition of ALDH is irreversible. However, its onset is relatively rapid (2–3 hours) and its action is of long duration (2–5 days).

Significant drug–drug interactions are possible when patients receive both antitumour drugs such as CP or PCZ and an MTT-containing cephalosporin antibiotic to prevent infection. Potentiation of CP and inhibition of PCZ effectiveness may occur if MTT inhibits the activity of the relevant tumour cell ALDH activity. Conversely, CP-induced cytotoxicity to essential normal cells may be increased significantly, and PCZ cytotoxicity to the same cell reduced, by MTT inhibition of ALDH.

Recently, attempts have been made to identify ALDH inhibitors that are specific to the particular forms involved in antitumour drug metabolism. One candidate compound has been identified: 4-(diethylamino)-benzaldehyde (DEAB) (Fig. 17E.3) (Russo *et al.* 1988, 1989). The class 1 ALDH involved in cyclophosphamide metabolism is preferentially inhibited by low concentration of DEAB *in vitro*. Moreover, treatment of CP-resistant leukaemia cells with DEAB makes them sensitive to CP. Finally, DEAB potentiates the cytotoxicity of CP in mouse normal intestinal crypt cells *in vivo* (Russo *et al.* 1989).

Structure–activity studies indicate that both the aldehyde and dialkyl-amino groups are necessary for DEAB function (Russo *et al.* 1988). Inhibition appears to be partially competitive and reversible, with activity returning to uninhibited levels within 30 minutes. These properties, combined with the fact that DEAB does not require metabolic activation, indicate that it may be possible to develop dialkylamino aldehydes that are clinically useful ALDH inhibitors.

A second, little studied, ALDH inhibitor, which may useful as an antitumour drug proper, is 4-amino-4-methyl-2-pentyne-1-al (AMPAL) (Ogier *et al*. 1989; Quemener *et al*. 1990). However, rather than acting as an inhibitor of ALDH-mediated anticancer drug activation, AMPAL itself acts as an antitumour agent by inhibiting the activity of the ALDHs involved in malondialdehyde oxidation (class 1 ALDH). Malondialdehyde is cytotoxic, and inhibition of the relevant ALDH activity has potentiated the cell-killing ability of AMPAL and elevated malondialdehyde levels in a human glioma tumour cell model (Quemener *et al*. 1990). However, nothing is currently known about the mechanism or specificity of AMPAL inhibition. While the situation is promising, much more information is needed before the clinical usefulness of this inhibitor can be assessed.

This brief discussion has focused on only five of the more than 30 pharmaceuticals causing a disulfiram-like reaction. It is not known how many of these agents brings about disulfiram-like effects by inhibiting aldehyde dehydrogenases and therefore may also modulate the effectiveness of chemotherapeutic agents metabolized by ALDHs. However, the variety of roles played by ALDHs in the metabolism of various chemotherapeutic agents (activation or inhibition) must also be considered when ALDH inhibitors are to be employed to improve the effectiveness of these agents. Further, the identification of DEAB and AMPAL as specific aldehyde dehydrogenase inhibitors indicates that development of additional inhibitors based on knowledge of the structural and functional properties of the enzymes may be a useful future approach.

References

Anonymous (1989). Nomenclature of mammalian aldehyde dehydrogenase. In *Enzymology and molecular biology of carbonyl metabolism*, Vol. 2 (ed. H. Weiner and T. G. Flynn), pp. xix-xxi. Liss, New York.

Brien, J. F. and Loomis, C. W. (1985). Aldehyde dehydrogenase inhibitors as alcohol-sensitizing drugs: A pharmacological perspective. *Trends in Pharmacological Science*, **6**, 477–80.

Crow, K. E., Kitson, T. M., MacGibbon, A. K. H., and Batt, R. D. (1974). Intracellular localization and properties of aldehyde dehydrogenase from sheep liver. *Biochimica et Biophysica Acta*, **350**, 121–8.

Dockham, P. A., Lee, M.-O., and Sladek, N. E. (1992). Identification of human liver aldehyde dehydrogenases that catalze the oxidation of aldophosphamide and retinaldehyde. *Biochemical Pharmacology*, **43**, 2453–69.

Ehrig, T., Bosron, W. F., and Li, T.-K. (1990). Alcohol and aldehyde dehydrogenases. *Alcohol and Alcoholism*, **25**, 105–16.

Erikson, J. M., Tweedie, D. J., and Prough, R. A. (1993). Metabolism of the hydrazine anti-cancer agent, procarbazine. *Pharmacology and Therapeutics*, in press.

Esterbauer, H., Zollner, H., and Schaur, R. J. (1990). Aldehydes formed by lipid peroxidation: Mechanisms of formation, occurrence and determination, In *Membrane lipid oxidation*, Vol. 1 (ed. C. Vigo-Pelfrey), pp. 239–68. CRC Press, Boca Raton, FL.

Hart, B. W., Yourick, J. J., and Faiman, M. D. (1990). S-methyl-N,N-diethyl-thiolcarbamate: a disulfiram metabolite and potent rat liver mitochondrial low K_m aldehyde dehydrogenase inhibitor. *Alcohol*, 7, 165–9.

Johansson, B., Petersen, E. N., and Arnold, E. (1989). Diethylthiocarbamic acid methyl ester. A potent inhibitor of aldehyde dehydrogenase found in rats treated with disulfiram or diethylthiocarbamic acid methyl ester. *Biochemical Pharmacology*, 38, 1053–9.

Kitson, T. M. (1983). Mechanism of inactivation of sheep liver cytoplasmic aldehyde dehydrogenase by disulfiram. *Biochemical Journal*, 213, 551–4.

Kitson, T. M. (1987). The effect of cephalosporin antibiotics on alcohol metabolism: a review. *Alcohol*, 4, 143–8.

Kohn, F. R., Landkamer, G. J., Manthey, C. L., Ramsey, N. K. C., and Sladek, N. E. (1987). Effect of aldehyde dehydrogenase inhibitors on the *ex vivo* sensitivity of human multipotent and committed hematopoietic progenitor cells and malignant blood cells to oxazaphosphorines. *Cancer Research*, 47, 3180–5.

Lebsack, M. E., Peterson, D. R., Collins, A. C. and Anderson, A. D. (1977). Preferential inhibition of low K_m aldehyde dehydrogenase activity by pargyline. *Biochemical Pharmacology*, 26, 1151–4.

Lindahl, R. (1992). Aldehyde dehydrogenases and their role in carcinogenesis. *CRC Critical Reviews in Biochemistry and Molecular Biology*, 27, 283–335.

Lindahl, R. and Hempel, J. (1991). Aldehyde dehydrogenases: What can be learned from a baker's dozen sequences? In *Enzymology and molecular biology of carbonyl metabolism*, Vol. 3 (ed. H. Weiner, B. Wermuth, and D. W. Crabb), pp. 1–8. Plenum Press, New York.

Lipsky, J. J. (1989). Ability of 1-methyltetrazole-5-thiol with microsomal activation to inhibit aldehyde dehydrogenase. *Biochemical Pharmacology*, 38, 773–9.

Maki, P. A. and Sladek, N. E. (1991). Potentiation of the cytotoxic action of mafosfamide by N-isopropyl-p-formylbenzamide, a metabolite of procarbazine. *Cancer Research*, 51, 4170–5.

Manthey, C. L., Landkamer, G. J., and Sladek, N. E. (1990). Identification of mouse liver aldehyde dehydrogenases important in aldophosphamide detoxification. *Cancer Research*, 50, 4991–5002.

Nagasawa, H. T., Elberling, J. A., Shirota, F. N., and DeMaster, E. G. (1988). A nonhypoglycemic chlorpropamide analog that inhibits aldehyde dehydrogenase. *Alcoholism: Clinical and Experimental Research*, 12, 563–9.

Nagasawa, H. T., DeMaster, G. G., Redfern, B., Shirota, F. N., and Goon, D. J. (1990). Evidence for nitroxyl in the catalase-mediated bioactivation of the alcohol deterrent agent cyanamide. *Journal of Medicinal Chemistry*, 33, 3120–2.

Ogier, G., Chantepie, J., Quash, G., Doutheau, A., Gore, J., and Marion, C. (1989). The effect of a novel inhibitor of aldehyde dehydrogenase on viral replication. *Biochemical Pharmacology*, 38, 1335–43.

Peachey, J. E. and Naranjo, C. A. (1983). The use of disulfiram and other alcohol-sensitizing drugs in the treatment of alcoholism. In *Research advances in alcohol and drug problems*, Vol. 7 (ed. R. G. Smart, F. B. Glaser, Y. Israel, H. Kalant, R. E. Popham, and W. Schmidt), pp. 397–431. Plenum Press, New York.

Prunonosa, J., Sagrista, M. L., and Bozal, J. (1991). Inactivation mechanism of low K_m rat liver mitochondrial aldehyde dehydrogenase by cyanamide *in vitro*. *Drug Metabolism and Disposition*, **19**, 787–92.

Quemener, V., Moulinoux, J.-P., Martin, C., Darcel, F., Guegan, Y., Faivre, J., and Quash, G. A. (1990). Aldehyde dehydrogenase activity in xenografted human brain tumor in nude mice. Preliminary results in human glioma biopsies. *Journal of Neuro-oncology*, **9**, 115–23.

Russo, J. E. and Hilton, J. (1988). Characterization of cytosolic aldehyde dehydrogenase from cyclophosphamide resistant L1210 cells. *Cancer Research*, **48**, 2963–8.

Russo, J. E., Hauquitz, D., and Hilton, J. (1988). Inhibition of mouse cytosolic aldehyde dehydrogenase by 4-(diethylamino)benzaldehyde. *Biochemical Pharmacology*, **37**, 1639–42.

Russo, J. E., Hilton, J., and Colvin, O. M. (1989). The role of aldehyde dehydrogenase isozymes in cellular resistance to the alkylating agent cyclophosphamide. In *Enzymology and molecular biology of carbonyl metabolism*, Vol. 2 (ed. H. Weiner and T. G. Flynn), pp. 65–79. Liss, New York.

Schauenstein, E., Esterbauer, H., and Zollner, H. (1977). *Aldehydes in biological systems: their natural occurrence and activities*. Pion, London.

Sladek, N. E. (1988). Metabolism of oxazaphosphorines. *Pharmacology and Therapeutics*, **37**, 301–55.

Sladek, N. E. and Landkamer, G. J. (1985). Restoration of sensitivity to oxazaphosphorines by inhibitors of aldehyde dehydrogenase activity in cultured oxazaphosphorine-resistant L1210 and cross-linking agent resistant P388 cell lines. *Cancer Research*, **45**, 1549–55.

Sladek, N. E., Manthey, C. L., Maki, P. A., Zhang, Z., and Landkamer, G. J. (1989). Xenobiotic metabolism catalzed by aldehyde dehydrogenases. *Drug Metabolism Reviews*, **20**, 697–720.

Tweedie, D. J., Fernandez, D., Spearman, M. E., Feldhoff, R. C., and Prough, R. A. (1991). Metabolism of azoxy derivatives of procarbazine by aldehyde dehydrogenase and xanthine oxidase. *Drug Metabolism and Disposition*, **19**, 793–803.

Vallari, R. C. and Pietruszko, R. (1982). Human aldehyde dehydrogenase: mechanisms of inhibition by disulfiram. *Science*, **216**, 637–9.

Weinkam, R. J. and Shiba, D. A. (1978). Metabolic activation of procarbazine. *Life Sciences*, **22**, 937–46.

Yoshida, A., Hsu, L. C., and Yasunami, M. (1991). Genetics of human alcohol-metabolizing enzymes. In *Progress in nucleic acid research and molecular biology*, Vol. 40 (ed. W. E. Cohn and K. Moldave), pp. 255–87. Academic Press, New York.

Section 17F

Enzyme inhibition mediated toxic effects of drugs

M. Pirmohamed and B. K Park

7F.1   Introduction

The purpose of this chapter is to review adverse drug reactions which are caused by inhibition of an enzyme by a drug, but are not related to the principal pharmacological activity of the drug. Thus the toxicities associated with chemotherapeutic agents and antiviral drugs, in which the toxic effects and the therapeutic effects are the consequence of the same initial biochemical effect, will be excluded. Broadly speaking, there are two main groups of enzymes, together with their normal substrate(s) and inhibitors, that must be considered (Fig. 17F.1): (a) enzymes which are responsible for the metabolism, anabolism, and catabolism of endogenous compounds, where enzyme inhibition may lead to a deficiency of an essential metabolite, production of abnormal and biologically inactive metabolites, or accumulation of intermediary products which become toxic when present in excess; (b) those enzymes responsible for the metabolism, and thus the clearance of foreign compounds, where enzyme inhibition may lead to a reduced rate of clearance of a pharmacologically active substance and hence toxicity mediated by supratherapeutic plasma concentrations. Alternatively, enzyme inhibition may alter the route rather than the rate of metabolism of a drug or chemical and thus lead to a greater body burden of a toxic metabolite.

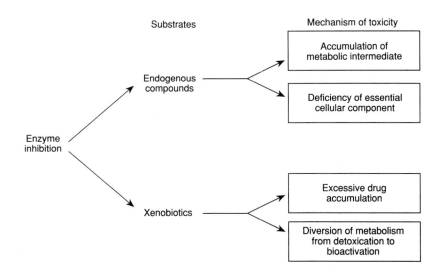

Fig. 17F.1 Schematic representation of the possible consequences of enzyme inhibition on the metabolism of endogenous and exogenous compounds.

17F.2   Fundamental considerations

The toxicological impact of enzyme inhibition will be dependent upon two sets of independent factors. The first set which depend mainly on the characteristics of the inhibitor, are those which determine the degree and duration of enzyme inhibition. They include the following:

(1) potency K_i of the inhibitor compared with K_m of the substrate;

(2) whether inhibition is competitive or non-competitive;

(3) whether inhibition is reversible or irreversible;

(4) the pharmacokinetics of the enzyme inhibitor.

In the case of reversible competitive inhibition, the concentration and rate of formation of the substrate must be taken into account. If there is irreversible enzyme inhibition, the extent and duration of toxicity will be partly dependent upon the rate of enzyme synthesis.

The second group of factors will reflect the biological importance of the enzyme in the target tissue, and the ability of the tissue to overcome the inhibition by either synthesis of more enzyme (e.g. enzyme induction) or utilization of alternative biochemical pathways.

Generally speaking, most biological enzyme systems operate with enzyme reserve and therefore the toxic effects of drugs are usually only noted at or around complete enzyme inhibition, in contrast with pharmacological effects which are often achieved by modulation of enzyme activity. Therefore, in the majority of cases of clinically important drug–drug interactions, which are the direct result of enzyme inhibition, competition for the same substrate binding site seems the most likely mechanism, given the broad substrate specificity of the enzymes responsible for xenobiotic metabolism.

As mentioned above, the potency K_i of the inhibitor relative to the Michaelis constant K_m of the drug whose metabolism is being inhibited is an important determinant of the efficacy of a drug as an inhibitor of drug metabolism. In addition, the relative maximal velocity V_{max} of the metabolism of the inhibitor and the drug is also important; the inhibitory capacity will increase towards maximum as V_{max} for metabolism of the inhibitor approaches zero. An important aspect of drug metabolism as a cause of toxicity is that many drugs can undergo several routes of metabolism. The effect of enzyme inhibition on the ratio R of the new half-life of a drug in the presence of the inhibitor to the normal half-life is given by the expression (Rowland 1975)

$$R = \frac{t_{1/2}\ (\text{inhibited})}{t_{1/2}\ (\text{normal})}$$

$$= \frac{1}{f_m/(1 + I/K_i) + (1 - f_m)} \tag{17F.1}$$

The impact of enzyme inhibition on drug half-life is very sensitive to the fraction f_m of the dose normally metabolized via the inhibited pathway. According to this model, the ratio R changes dramatically with increasing inhibitor concentration when $f_m = 1$. Thus drugs such as tolbutamide, which are dependent upon a single metabolic pathway for their clearance, are particularly sensitive to this type of interaction. For example, coadministration of the sulphonamide sulphaphenazole may cause a fivefold increase in tolbutamide half-life, occasionally precipitating hypoglycaemia (Hansen and Christensen 1977; Pond *et al.* 1977). In contrast, when $f_m < 0.5$ the maximum increase in the ratio is twofold and therefore inconsequential from a clinical standpoint, unless the therapeutic index of the drug is small. The most important and interesting clinical examples of this type are those with drugs which have a steep dose–response relationship and/or narrow therapeutic margin, such as warfarin and phenytoin, where relatively modest changes in plasma levels mediated by enzyme inhibition may result in a shift from a therapeutic response to a toxic effect (Fig. 17F.2).

A number of these concepts can be illustrated by consideration of the pharmacological effects of the anticoagulant warfarin which inhibits the enzyme vitamin K_1 2,3-epoxide reductase, thus reducing levels of

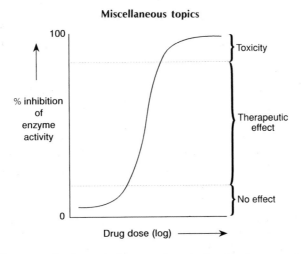

Fig. 17F.2 Conceptualized graph showing the relationship between drug dose and enyme inhibilion as exemplified by the relationship between the dose of warfarin and inhibition of the enzyme vitamin K_1 2,3-epoxide reductase (Choonara *et al.* 1988). Of particular importance is the steepness of the dose–response curve, where small alterations in drug dose can lead to large changes in the inhibition of enzyme activity, which in the case of warfarin could result in either under-anticoagulation (leading to thrombosis) or over-anticoagulation (leading to haemorrhage).

hepatic vitamin K, an essential cofactor for the post-ribosomal synthesis of clotting factors (Choonara *et al.* 1988). Low doses (0.2 mg) of warfarin have no measurable effect on clotting factor synthesis, despite inhibition of the enzyme epoxide reductase (as measured by plasma levels of vitamin K_1 2,3-epoxide). In contrast, therapeutic levels not only inhibit the enzyme but also cause a partial reduction in clotting factor synthesis, while supratherapeutic levels caused by inappropriate dose or drug interaction can completely abolish clotting factor synthesis, predisposing to a bleeding tendency (Fig. 17F.2).

17F.3   Endogenous compounds

Various drugs designed as enzyme inhibitors to achieve their therapeutic actions may also result in the interruption of the metabolism of other closely related endogenous compounds or the same endogenous compound but at a different site in the body, resulting in drug toxicity. The enzymes inhibited and the endogenous compounds thus affected are discussed below.

17F.3.1   Angiotensin-converting enzyme

Angiotensin-converting enzyme (ACE) inhibitors such as captopril and enalapril, which inhibit the conversion of angiotensin I to the potent vasoconstrictor, angiotensin II, are widely used in the treatment of hypertension and heart failure. In addition, the C-terminal cleavage of bradykinin by kininase II (which is identical with (ACE) can also be inhibited by ACE inhibitors, resulting in elevated bradykinin concentration, particularly in the tissues (William 1988).

Cough is a common adverse effect of all ACE inhibitors, occurring in 15 per cent of all patients (Yeo *et al.* 1991). Although the pathogenesis of the side-effect is unknown, it is thought to be secondary to ACE inhibition resulting in interruption of the metabolism of endogenous compounds. Three such compounds acting either individually or collectively, may be responsible for the increased frequency of cough. Firstly, bradykinin, whose local pulmonary concentration is increased, may cause coughing directly by stimulating unmyelinated afferent sensory c nerve fibres (Kaufman *et al.* 1980). Secondly, bradykinin indirectly increases the rate of formation of vasodilatory prostaglandins (PGE_2 and PGI_2) (McGiff *et al.* 1972), and thus an increase in their local concentration may cause cough by a direct stimulant action on afferent c fibres (Coleridge *et al.* 1976; Berkin and Ball 1988). Thirdly, ACE is also known to inhibit the hydrolysis of substance P (Casceiri *et al.* 1983), and increased local concentration of such tachykinins could also produce coughing (Morice *et al.* 1987).

Angioedema has also been reported with ACE inhibitors (Dixon *et al.* 1987), although this is less common than coughing. This severe adverse effect which is occasionally fatal, occurs soon after the start of therapy and is thought to be due to inhibition of bradykinin metabolism (Dixon *et al.* 1987). It is more common with the longer-acting ACE inhibitors (enalapril and lisinopril) than with captopril (Williams 1988).

17F.3.2   Cholinesterase

The action of acetylcholine at cholinergic nerve endings is terminated by the enzyme cholinesterase. Since the discovery of the first anticholinesterase, physostigmine, chemical modification has resulted in the production of a large number of such compounds with varying properties, ranging from the short-acting drug edrophonium to irreversible inhibitors such as the organophosphorus compounds which are used as insecticides and in chemical warfare. The toxicity of these compounds is a function of their dose and mechanism of enzyme inhibition. Thus the clinically used compounds such as neostigmine can cause abdominal cramps, excessive salivation, and diarrhoea (Taylor 1985), while accidental poisoning with the organophosphorus compounds can result in respiratory failure (Taylor 1985) due to acetylcholine build-up.

17F.3.3 Cyclo-oxygenase

Non-steroidal anti-inflammatory drugs (NSAIDs) are widely used for the treatment of rheumatological disorders. They act by inhibiting the enzyme cyclo-oxygenase, thereby interfering with prostaglandin synthesis. As the enzyme inhibition is not organ specific, interference with prostaglandin production in extra-articular tissues, particularly the kidney, has been implicated in various adverse effects (Table 17F.1) (Clive and Stoff 1984).

In acute renal insufficiency secondary to NSAIDs, several factors influence the likelihood of occurrence of such toxicity. First, the vasodilatory prostaglandins are important for the maintenance of renal haemodynamics under disease conditions rather than under normal circumstances (Clive and Stoff 1984). Thus renal failure with NSAIDs is more likely to develop when there is renal hypoperfusion, for example in heart failure or liver cirrhosis (Stillman et al. 1984), or in the presence of pre-existing primary renal disease such as lupus nephritis (Stillman et al. 1984; Clive and Stoff 1984). In these conditions, prostaglandins are required to counteract the renal vasoconstriction from increased circulating angiotensin II and catecholamine levels (Stillman and Schlesinger 1990). Secondly, glomerular filtration rate (GFR) declines with age (Davies and Shock 1950), and thus nephrotoxicity is more common in the elderly. Thirdly, drugs such as diuretics (Favre et al. 1982) and ACE inhibitors (Seelig et al. 1990), used concurrently with NSAIDs, will increase the incidence of renal impairment. Finally, inhibition of prostaglandin synthesis is dose dependent,

Table 17F.1 Renal syndromes which can be produced by NSAIDs as a result of the inhibition of prostaglandin synthesis

Renal syndrome	Mechanism
Acute renal insufficiency	Diminished renal prostaglandin synthesis reducing GFR and renal blood flow
Nephrotic syndrome	Increased production of inflammation inducing leucotrienes with secondary recruitment and activation of T-cells
Water retention	Increased medullary interstitial osmotic gradient resulting in maximal urinary concentration
Sodium retention	Inhibition of the natriuretic effects of prostaglandins
Hyperkalaemia	Hyporeninaemic hypoaldosteronism

Adapted from Clive and Stoff 1984.

and thus the higher the dose of the NSAID, the higher the incidence of nephrotoxicity (Stillman and Schlesinger 1990).

Sulindac, a prodrug which is converted to its active sulphide metabolite in the liver, is said to have a 'renal sparing' effect (Patrono and Dunn 1987). The mechanism of this is unclear, although it has been hypothesized that a selective sparing of prostacyclin production in the renal cortex is responsible (Patrono and Pierucci 1986). However, impairment of renal function has been reported with sulindac, particularly when high doses are used (Blackshear et al. 1983).

17F.3.4   Cytochrome P450 enzymes

Ketoconazole, a systemic antimycotic agent, inhibits adrenal (Pont et al. 1982a), testicular (Pont et al. 1982b) and ovarian (Weber et al. 1991) steroidogenesis by non-specifically inhibiting the cytochrome P450 enzymes (Loose et al. 1983). The effect of ketoconazole on adrenal steroid synthesis is dose dependent, although even single doses (400 mg) can suppress the cortisol response to exogenous corticotrophin for up to 8 hours (Pont et al. 1982a). High doses of ketoconazole, used for the treatment of systemic fungal infections and prostatic carcinoma, can lead to more pronounced adrenal suppression, occasionally resulting in adrenal hypofunction (Trachtenberg and Pont, 1984) which may be manifested particularly at times of stress (White and Kendall-Taylor 1985), necessitating corticosteroid replacement therapy. The adrenal hypofunction may even occur in patients being treated for Cushing's syndrome, a condition characterized by hypercortisolaemia (McCance et al. 1987). Ketoconazole can affect testicular function, producing adverse effects such as gynaecomastia, oligospermia, azoospermia, impotence, and reduced libido (Pont et al. 1984).

17F.3.5   Dihydrofolate reductase

Dihydrofolate reductase (DHFR) is a ubiquitous enzyme, essential for the conversion of folates present in food to their active form, tetrahydrofolic acid, which alternately acts as an acceptor and a donor of one-carbon units essential for the synthesis of purines, pyrimidines, and certain amino acids. Known inhibitors of DHFR include trimethoprim, pyrimethamine, and methotrexate. With trimethoprim and pyrimethamine, the selectivity of inhibition varies according to the species; thus pyrimethamine, an antimalarial, is a selective inhibitor of the DHFR in *Plasmodium* sp. (Burchall and Hitchings 1965; Ferone et al. 1969), while the concentration of trimethoprim necessary to inhibit *E. coli* DHFR by 50 per cent is 50 000 times less than that required for the same degree of inhibition of the mammalian enzyme (Brumfitt et al. 1973). Nevertheless, folate deficiency in man, manifested as a megaloblastic marrow or in some cases frank megaloblastic anaemia, has been reported with both drugs (Chanarin 1964; Jewkes *et al*. 1970; Magee *et al*. 1981), particularly in patients who may be nutritionally deficient (for example, the elderly, patients with malabsorption, and chronic alcoholics) and when the drugs are used for prolonged periods at high dosages. In the latter context, patients with AIDS are treated with high doses of trimethoprim in combination with sulphamethoxazole for *Pneumocystis carinii* pneumonia, and thus may be susceptible to the adverse effects of DHFR inhibition.

Methotrexate, in contrast with trimethoprim and pyrimethamine, inhibits all forms of DHFR, but its selectivity in malignant disease is achieved by virtue of the high proliferative capacity of the neoplastic cells. However, more recently, methotrexate has been used at low dosages for prolonged periods in non-neoplastic conditions such as psoriasis and rheumatoid arthritis, and not surprisingly such patients have been reported to develop folate deficiency (Fulton 1986; Morgan *et al*. 1987; Weinblatt and Fraser 1989).

17F.3.6   HMG CoA reductase

HMG CoA reductase catalyses the conversion of HMG CoA to mevalonic acid, the rate-limiting step in cholesterol synthesis (Tobert 1987; Grundy 1988). Inhibitors of this enzyme (simvastatin, lovastatin, pravastatin) are used for the treatment of hypercholesterolaemia. Cholesterol is the precursor of steroid hormones, bile acids, dolichol (a glycoprolein precursor), and ubiquinone (which mediates electron transport). Theoretically, inhibition of the formation of cholesterol may interfere with the production of these compounds, with resultant drug toxicity. However, studies so far have not shown changes in the level of steroids (Illingworth and Corbin 1985), bile acids (Grundy 1988), or other endogenous compounds, although clinical experience with these drugs is limited. Myopathy, which is seen with all drugs in this class, may also be the result of inhibition of the enzyme (Smith *et al*. 1991), although the exact mechanism is unknown.

17F.3.7   Monoamine oxidase

Monoamine oxidases (types A and B) are mitochondrial enzymes responsible for (1) regulation of free intraneuronal concentrations of catecholamines and serotonin, and (2) the inactivation of trace amines such as tyramine formed in the body or absorbed from the gut. Nowhere is the importance of selectivity of inhibition in the avoidance of drug toxicity better illustrated than in the case of monoamine oxidase (MAO) inhibitors. The non-specific MAO inhibitors such as iproniazid and phenelzine are used more rarely now because of the potential to cause dangerous hypertensive reactions with tyramine containing foods such as cheeses and yeast extracts ('cheese reaction'). In contrast, the specific MAO-B inhibitor selegiline, which is being increasingly used in the treatment of Parkinson's disease, does not cause the 'cheese reaction' (Pickar *et al.* 1981) since it does not affect tyramine metabolism by MAO-A in the gut.

17F.4   Exogenous compounds

The rate of elimination of a lipophilic drug is governed largely by its rate of metabolism. Therefore the ability of an individual to metabolize a particular drug will be an important determinant of drug efficacy and drug toxicity. Metabolism, which in most cases involves a combination of phase I oxidation reactions and phase II conjugation reactions, is usually associated with an increase in the water solubility of the compound and enhanced clearance, and, thus can be regarded as a detoxication process (Park 1986). However, in certain circumstances normal metabolic processes, and in particular oxidation, may produce a chemically reactive metabolite which, if inadequately detoxified by enzymes such as epoxide hydrolase and gluta-thione transferase, may cause tissue injury (Park 1986). Therefore enzyme inhibition may lead to drug toxicity through a change in either the rate or route of drug metabolism.

17F.4.1   Drug oxidation

Phase I oxidation reactions occur predominantly in the liver and are cata-lysed by the cytochrome P450 enzymes located in the endoplasmic reti-culum. Several P450 enzymes have been isolated; each is believed to be encoded by a separate gene. A nomenclature for the P450 gene super-family, based on the homology of the amino acid sequences of the different enzymes, has been proposed by Nebert *et al.* (1989) and has recently been updated (Nebert *et al.* 1991). Despite the fact that this nomenclature does not depend on the P450 catalytic activity or function, it provides us with a framework whereby we can classify functional activity with respect to substrates of pharmacological and toxicological interest. In this context, although eight P450 families are known to exist in man, only three are thought to be of particular importance.

It is well established that each P450 enzyme has a wide substrate speci-ficity (Brosen 1990), i.e. it can metabolize several drugs, and thus wide overlap in the substrate specificities of different enzymes is not uncommon, even among P450 enzymes from separate subfamilies. However, despite this wide substrate specificity, many P450 enzyme inhibitors have been described which may be of toxicological interest. Such inhibitors can be either selective, inhibiting only one enzyme, or non-selective, inhibiting several P450 enzymes. The selective inhibitors may give rise to important and otherwise unexpected drug toxicities (Table 17F.2), which are often not identified until the drug is clinically established. The non-selective inhibitors may non-specifically bind to the haem moieties of the P450 enzymes, resulting in inhibition of several enzymes. They can cause problems with a wide range of drugs (Table 17F.3); however, this type of inhibitor can now be easily identified in clinical pharmacological screens and therefore should not represent a problem in practice.

Toxicity may also ensue from inhibition of other oxidative biotransformations. The drug disulfiram, used to treat alcoholism, acts by inhibiting the enzyme aldehyde dehydrogenase which is responsible for the conversion of ethanol into acetic acid. Alcohol intake while an alcoholic is on disulfiram therapy results in acetaldehyde accumulation (Hald and Jacobsen 1948) which causes nausea and flushing. A second example is allopurinol, an inhibitor of the enzyme xanthine oxidase, which is used for the treatment of gout. Apart from catalysing the conversion of hypoxanthine to xanthine and of xanthine to uric acid, this enzyme is also involved in the metabolism of synthetic xanthine analogues used in chemotherapy such as 6-mercaptopurine; allopurinol has been shown to increase both the toxicity and therapeutic actions of 6-mercaptopurine (Rundles *et al.* 1969).

17F.4.2 Drug conjugation

Multiple forms of UDP-glucuronyl transferases (UDPGT), encoded by a multigene family, have been observed in most species, including man, on the basis of biochemical characterization (Tephly and Burchell 1990). Most xenobiotics react with more than one isoform of UDPGT, and thus it is not possible to use a single substrate, even in *in vitro* studies, to evaluate the activity of a single transferase enzyme. The low substrate selectivity of the transferase enzymes, taken together with the high capacity of the glucuronidation system, suggests that serious drug toxicity by competitive inhibition for glucuronyl transferase is unlikely. Nevertheless, recent studies have shown that probenecid, which is metabolized by glucuronidation (Cunningham *et al.* 1981), significantly reduces the *in vivo* glucuronidation of paracetamol (Abernethy *et al.* 1985), lorazepam (Abernethy *et al.* 1985), and zidovudine (AZT) (Miranda *et al.* 1989), presumably by acting as an alternative substrate. The increase in half-life for each drug was approximately twofold. Probenecid not only inhibits the glucuronidation of AZT but also impairs the renal excretion of the glucuronide. *In vitro* studies with human liver microsomes have also shown that the glucuronidation of AZT can be inhibited by NSAIDs and chloramphenicol (Sim *et al.* 1991), although whether this would be of significance *in vivo* requires further study. Lamotrigine, a triazine anticonvulsant which undergoes extensive glucuronidation, has a half-life of 25 hours when given as sole therapy. However, coadministration of valproic acid more than doubles

Table 17F.2 Specific inhibitors and substrates of the cytochrome P450 isozymes

Isozyme	Substrates	Inhibitors	Toxicological consequences
CYP1A2	Phenacetin (O-de-ethylation) Caffeine (demethylation) Theophylline	Furafylline Quinolone antibiotics Mexiletine	Dose-dependent theophylline toxicity, e.g. arrhythmias, tremor, nausea, and convulsions
CYP2C8/9	Tolbutamide Phenytoin	Sulphaphenazole	Tolbutamide: hypoglycaemia Dose-dependent phenytoin toxicity: ataxia, drowsiness, and nystagmus
CYP2D6	Debrisoquine Sparteine Tricyclic antidepressants Metoprolol Phenacetin Thioridazine Flecainide and propafenone Perhexiline	Quinidine Fluoxetine	Altered (exaggerated) pharmacological response
CYP2E1	Paracetamol Nitrosamines	Disulfiram	

Table 17F.2 (*continued*)

Isozyme	Substrates	Inhibitors	Toxicological consequences
CYP3A3/4	Warfarin Oestrogens Corticosteroids Erythromycin Cyclosporin Nifedipine Progestogens Tamoxifen Lignocaine	Gestodene Troleandomycin	Altered (exaggerated) pharmacological response

Derived from Jacqz *et al.* (1986), Nebert *et al.* (1989, 1991), Brosen (1990), Eichelbaum and Gross (1990), and Gonzalez *et al.* (1991). Nomenclature according to Nebert *et al.* (1991).

Table 17F.3 Non-specific inhibitors of cytochrome P450 enzymes

Non-specific cytochrome P450 inhibitors	
Cimetidine	Chloramphenicol
Erythromycin	Isoniazid
Ketoconazole	Verapamil

Drugs whose metabolism can be inhibited	Toxicological consequence
Warfarin	Haemorrhage
Phenytoin	Ataxia, drowsiness
Carbamazepine	Ataxia, drowsiness
Theophylline	Arrhythmias, convulsions
Prednisolone	Exaggerated pharmacological response

the half-life to 55 hours (Jawad *et al.* 1987). A recent study in volunteers has shown that this may partly be due to inhibition of the glucuronidation of lamotrigine by valproate (Yuen *et al.* 1991).

Like glucuronidation, sulphation is catalysed by a family of trans-ferases (Falany 1991), but differs in that it is a capacity-limited process, suggesting a higher possibility of drug interactions based on competition for either the transferase or cofactors. However, it is common for drugs to undergo simultaneous conjugation with sulphate and glucuronic acid, with sulphation usually predominating at low concentrations of substrate and glucuronidation becoming a major metabolic pathway at higher sub-strate concentrations.

Both fenoldopam and paracetamol undergo conjugation with sulphate and glucuronic acid in man (Ziemniak *et al.* 1987). Fenoldopam undergoes extensive presystemic conjugation as well as systemic metabolism. Con-comitant dosing with paracetamol resulted in significant but modest (*c.* 50 per cent) increases in fenoldopam plasma concentrations and a decrease in fenoldopam's sulphated metabolites, suggesting that the basis for the interaction was through competition for inorganic sulphates. A further consequence of this interaction was a shift in metabolism of fenoldopam from sulphation to glucuronidation. These elevated plasma fenoldopam levels may lead to a more pronounced pharmacodynamic action of the drug but are unlikely to produce serious toxicity.

Indeed, no clinically important drug toxicities have been observed as a result of inhibition of either sulphation or glucuronidation. This is because of the relatively modest elevation of plasma concentrations com-pared with the normal inter-individual variation in plasma levels of the drug concerned. Thus toxicity is only likely to occur in certain individuals taking drugs with a narrow therapeutic index, such as AZT.

17F.4.3 Drug (metabolite) detoxication

Although the enzymes involved in drug oxidation and drug conjugation reactions can be considered to be detoxication enzymes, those considered in this section are involved in the detoxication of electrophilic reactive metabolites, namely the glutathione-S-transferases and epoxide hydrolases.

Glutathione-S-transferases are a family of multifunctional proteins whose main function is the detoxication of reactive metabolites (Boyer 1989). At least three forms, which have wide and overlapping substrate specificities, are known to exist in man (Mannervik and Danielson 1988). Drugs which have been reported to inhibit these enzymes include indomethacin (Wu and Matthews 1983), sulphasalazine (Bach et al. 1985), and diuretics (frusemide, bumetanide, tienilic acid) (Ahokas et al. 1985); however, whether such inhibition is of any toxicological significance is unknown, although it is unlikely in view of the overlapping substrate specificities of the different isozymes.

At least four different epoxide hydrolases exist, three of which are of relatively minor toxicological significance (Guenthner 1990). The enzyme which is located in the endoplasmic reticulum (termed microsomal epoxide hydrolase (mEH) in this section) is of toxicological importance since it catalyses the hydrolysis of numerous epoxides, including arene oxides (Seidegard and DePierre 1983). Many inhibitors of mEH have been identified: these are either epoxides (Oesch et al. 1971; Oesch 1983) or unsubstituted amides (Kerr and 1990). Such inhibitors may be present in the environment as pollutants and thus, the potential for inhibition of mEH exists, although methods to assess such inhibition in vivo are not available and, furthermore, the long-term in vivo toxicological consequences of enzyme inhibition are largely unknown.

More recently, three drugs used in the treatment of epilepsy, valpromide (Meijer et al. 1984; Pacifici et al. 1985), valproic acid (Kerr and Levy 1989; Kerr et al. 1989), and progabide (Kutt et al. 1984), have been found to be inhibitors of mEH at therapeutic concentrations. Concurrent administration of any of these mEH inhibitors with carbamazepine can result in elevation of plasma levels of carbamazepine and its 10,11-epoxide, resulting in dose-dependent toxic manifestations such as ataxia and drowsiness (Meijer et al. 1984; Robbins et al. 1990). Of greater importance is the increased risk of teratogenicity in female patients on combination anti-epileptic therapy which includes either valpromide or valproic acid. Lindhout et al. (1984) reported a 58 per cent rate of fetal malformations associated with combination therapy (which included valproic acid); inhibition of fetal mEH by valproic acid, thus increasing fetal exposure to reactive epoxides has been suggested to be the mechanism (Kerr and Levy 1989).

References

Abernethy, D. R., Greenblatt, D. J., Ameer, B., and Shader, R. I. (1985). Probenecid impairment of acetaminophen and lorazepam clearance: direct inhibition of ether glucuronide formation. *Journal of Pharmacology and Experimental Therapeutics*, **23**, 345–9.

Ahokas, J. T., Nicholls, F. A., Ravenscroft, P. J., and Emmerson, B. T. (1985). Inhibition of purified rat liver glutathione-*S*-transferase isozymes by diuretic drugs. *Biochemical Pharmacology*, **34**, 2157–61.

Bach, M. K., Brashler, J. R., and Johnson, M. A. (1985). Inhibition by sulfasalazine of LTC synthetase and of rat liver glutathione-*S*-transferases. *Biochemical Pharmacology*, **34**, 2695–704.

Berkin, K. E. and Ball, S. G. (1988). Cough and angiotensin converting enzyme inhibition. *British Medical Journal*, **296**, 1279–80.

Blackshear, J. L., Davidman, M., and Stillman, M. T. (1983). Identification of risk factors for renal insufficiency from NSAID. *Archives of Internal Medicine*, **143**, 1130–4.

Boyer, T. D. (1989). The glutathione-*S*-transferases: an update. *Hepatology*, **9**, 486–96.

Brosen, K. (1990). Recent developments in hepatic drug oxidation. Implications for clinical pharmacokinetics. *Clinical Pharmacokinetics*, **18**, 220–39.

Brumfitt, W., Hamilton-Miller, J. M. T., and Kosmidis, J. (19733. Trimethoprim-sulfamethoxazole: the present position. *Journal of Infectious Diseases*, **128**, 778–91.

Burchall, J. J. and Hitchings, G. H. (1965). Inhibitor binding analysis of dihydrofolate reductase from various species. *Molecular Pharmacology*, **1**, 126–36.

Casceiri, M. A., Bull, H. G., Mumford, R. A., Patchett, A. A., Thornberry, N. A., and Liang, T. (1983). Carboxyl-terminal tripeptidyl hydrolysis of substance P by purified rabbit lung angiotensin converting enzyme and the potentiation of substance P activity *in vivo* by captopril and MK 422. *Molecular Pharmacology*, **25**, 287–93.

Chanarin, I. (1964). Studies in drug-induced megaloblastic anaemia. *Scandinavian Journal of Haematology*, **1**, 280–8.

Choonara, I. A., Malia, R. G., Haynes, B. P., Hay, C. R., Cholerton, S., Breckenridge, A. M., et al. The relationship between inhibition of Vitamin K1 2,3-epoxide reductase and reduction of clotting factor activity with warfarin. *British Journal of Clinical Pharmacology*, **25**, 1–7.

Clive, D. M. and Stoff, J. S. (1984). Renal syndromes associated with non-steroidal anti-inflammatory drugs. *New England Journal of Medicine*, **310**, 563–72.

Coleridge, H. M., Coleridge, J. C. G., Ginzel, K. H., Baker, D. G., Banzett, R. B., and Morrison, M. A. (1976). Stimulation of 'irritant' receptors and afferent c fibres in the lungs by prostaglandins. *Nature, London*, **264**, 451–3.

Cunningham, R. F., Israili, Z. H., and Dayton, P. G. (1981). Clinical pharmacokinetics of probenecid. *Clinical Pharmacokinetics*, **6**, 135–51.

Davies, D. F. and Shock, N. W. (1950). Age changes in glomerular filtration rate, effective renal plasma flow and tubular excretory capacity in adult males. *Journal of Clinical Investigation*, **29**, 496–507.

Dixon, C. M., Fuller, R. W., and Barnes, P. J. (1987). The effect of angiotensin converting enzyme inhibitor, ramipril, on bronchial responses to inhaled histamine and bradykinin in asthmatic subjects. *British Journal of Clinical Pharmacology*, **23**, 91–3.

Eichelbaum, M. and Gross, A. S. (1990). The genetic polymorphism of debrisoquine/sparteine metabolism—clinical aspects. *Pharmacology and Therapeutics*, **46**, 377–94.

Falany, C. N. (1991). Molecular enzymology of human liver cytosolic transferases. *Trends in Pharmacological Sciences*, **12**, 255–9.

Favre, L., Glasson, P., and Valhotton, M. B. (1982). Reversible acute renal failure from combined triamterene and indomethacin: a study in healthy subjects. *Annals of Internal Medicine*, **96**, 317–20.

Ferone, R., Burchall, J. J., and Hitching, G. H. (1969). *Plasmodium berghei* dihydrofolate reductase; isolation, properties and inhibition by antifolates. *Molecular Pharmacology*, **5**, 49–59.

Fullon, R. A. (1986). Megaloblastic anaemia and methotrexate treatment. *British Journal of Dermatology*, **114**, 267–8.

Gonzalez, F. J., Crespi, C. L., and Gelboin, H. V. (1991). cDNA-expressed human cytochrome P450s: a new age of molecular toxicology and human risk assessment. *Mutation Research*, **247**, 113–27.

Grundy, S. M. (1988). HMG-CoA reductase inhibitors for treatment of hypercholesterolaemia. *New England Journal of Medicine*, **319**, 24–33.

Guenthner, T. M. (1990). Epoxide hydrolases. In *Conjucation reactions in drug metabolism: an integrated approach* (ed. G. J. Mulder), pp. 365–404. Taylor & Francis, London.

Hald, J. and Jacobsen, E. (1948). The formation of acetaldehyde in the organism after ingestion of antabuse (tetraethylthiuram-disulphide) and alcohol. *Acta Pharmacologica et Toxicologica*, **4**, 305–10.

Hansen, J. M. and Christensen, L. K. (1977). Drug interactions with oral sulphonylurea hypoglycaemic drugs. *Drugs*, **13**, 24–34.

Illingworth, D. R. and Corbin, D. (1985). The influence of mevinolin on the adrenal cortisol response to corticotrophin in heterozygous familial hypercholesterolemia. *Proceedings of the National Academy of Sciences of the United States of America*, **82**, 6291–4.

Jacqz, E., Hall, S. D., and Branch, R. A. (1986). Genetically determined polymorphisms in drug oxidation. *Hepatology*, **6**, 1020–32.

Jawad, S., Yuen, W. C., Peck, A. W., Hamilton, M. J., Oxley, J., and Richens, A. (1987). Lamotrigine: single dose pharmacokinetics and initial one week experience in refractory epilepsy. *Epilepsy Research*, **1**, 194–201.

Jewkes, R. F., Edwards, M. S., and Grant, D. J. B. (1970). Haematological changes in a patient on long-term treatment with a trimethoprim-sulphonamide combination. *Postgraduate Medical Journal*, **46**, 723–6.

Kaufmann, M. P., Coleridge, H. M., Coleridge, J. C. G., and Baker, D. G. (1980). Bradykinin stimulates afferent vagal c fibres in intrapulmonary airways of dogs. *Journal of Applied Physiology*, **48**, 511–17.

Kerr, B. M. and Levy, R. H. (1989). Inhibition of epoxide hydrolase by anticonvulsants and the risk of teratogenicity. *Lancet*, **i**, 610–11.

Kerr, B. M. and Levy, R. H. (1990). Unsubstituted amides: a new class of potent inhibitors of human microsomal epoxide hydrolase. *Drug Metabolism and Disposition*, **18**, 540–2.

Kerr, B. M., Rettie, A. E., Eddy, C., Loiseau, P., Guyot, M., Wilensky, A. J., and Levy, R. H. (1989). Inhibition of human liver microsomal epoxide hydrolase by valproate and valpromide: *in vitro/in vivo* correlation. *Clinical Pharmacology and Therapeutics*, **46**, 82–93.

Kutt, H., Solomon, G. E., Dhar, A. K., Resor, S. R., Jr, Krall, R. L., and Morselli, P. L. (1984). Effects of progabide on carbamazepine epoxide and carbamazepine concentrations in plasma. *Epilepsia*, **25**, 674.

Lindhout, D., Hoppener, R. J. E. A., and Meinardi, H. (1984). Teratogenicity of anti-epileptic drug combinations with special emphasis on epoxidation (of carbamazepine). *Epilepsia*, **25**, 77–83.

Loose, D. S., Kun, P. B., Hirst, M. A., Marcus, R. A., and Feldman, D. (1983). Ketoconazole blocks adrenal steroidogenesis by inhibiting cytochrome P450 dependent enzymes. *Journal of Clinical Investigation*, **71**, 1495–9.

McCance, D. R., Ritchie, C. M., Sheridan, B., and Atkinson, A. B. (1987). Acute hypoadrenalism and hepatotoxicity after treatment with ketoconazole. *Lancet*, **i**, 573.

McGiff, J. C., Terragno. N. A., Malik, K. O., and Lonigno, A. J. (1972). Release of a prostaglandin E-like substance from canine kidney by bradykinin. *Circulation Research*, **31**, 36–43.

Magee, F., O'Sullivan, H., and McCann, S. R. (1981). Megaloblastosis and low-dose trimethoprim-sulfamethoxazole. *Annals of Internal Medicine*, **95**, 657.

Mannervik, B. and Danielson, U. H. (1988). Glutathione transferases—structure and catalytic activity. *CRC Critical Reviews in Biochemistry*, **23**, 283–337.

Meijer, J. W. A., Binnie, C. D., Debets, R. M. C., Van Parrys, J. A. P., and De Beer-Pawlikowski, N. K. B. (1984). Possible hazard of valpromide-carbamazepine combination therapy in epilepsy. *Lancet*, **i**, 802.

Miranda, P., Good, S. S., Yarchoan, R., Thomas, R. V., Blum, R., Myers, C. E., and Broders, S. (1989). Alteration of zidovudine pharmacokinetics in patients with AIDS or AIDS-related complex. *Clinical Pharmacology and Therapeutics*, **46**, 494–500.

Morgan, J. L., Baggott, J. E., and Altz-Smith, M. (1987). Folate status of rheumatoid arthritis patients receiving long-term, low-dose methotrexate therapy. *Arthritis and Rheumatism*, **30**, 1348–56.

Morice, A. H., Lowry, R., Brown, M. J., and Higenbottam, T. (1987). Angiotensin converting enzyme and the cough reflex. *Lancet*, **ii**, 1116–18.

Nebert, D. W., Nelson, D. R., Adesnik, M., Coon, M. J., Estabrook, R. W., Gonzalez, F. J., *et al.* (1989). The P450 gene superfamily. Update on the naming of new genes and nomenclature of chromosomal loci. *DNA*, **8**, 1–13.

Nebert, D. W., Nelson, D. R., Coon, M. J., Estabrook, R. W., Feyereisen, R., Fujii-Kuriyama, Y., *et al.* (1991). The P450 superfamily: update on new sequences, gene mapping, and recommended nomenclature. *DNA and Cell Biology*, **10**, 1–14.

Oesch, F. (1983). Drug detoxification: epoxide hydrolase. *Progress in Clinical and Biological Research*, **135**, 81–105.

Oesch, F., Kaubisch, N., Jerina, D. M., and Daly, J. W. (1971). Hepatic epoxide hydrase. Structure–activity relationships for substrates and inhibitors. *Biochemistry*, **10**, 4858–66.

Pacifici, G. M., Tomson, T., Bertilsson, L., and Rane, A. (1985). Valpromide/carbamazepine and risk of teratogenicity. *Lancet*, **i**, 397–8.

Park, B. K. (1986). Metabolic basis of adverse drug reactions. *Journal of the Royal College of Physicians*, **20**, 195–200.

Patrono, C., and Dunn, M. J. (1987). The clinical significance of inhibition of renal prostaglandin synthesis. *Kidney International*, **32**, 1–12.

Patrono, C. and Pierucci, A. (1986). Renal effects of nonsteroidal anti-inflammatory drugs in chronic glomerular disease. *American Journal of Medicine*, **81** (Suppl. 2B), 71–83.

Pickar, D., Cohen, R. M., Jimerson, D. C., and Murphy, D. L. (1981). Tyramine infusions and selective monoamine oxidase inhibitor treatment. I. Changes in pressor sensitivity. *Psychopharmacology*, **74**, 4–7.

Pond, S. M., Birkett, D. J., and Wade, D. N. (1977). Mechanisms of inhibition of tolbutamide metabolsm: phenylbutazone, oxyphenbutazone, sulfaphenazole. *Clinical Pharmacology and Therapeutics*, **22**, 573–9.

Pont, A., Williams, P. L., Loose, D. S., Feldman, D., Reitz, R. E., Bochra, C., and Stevens, D. A. (1982a). Ketoconazole blocks adrenal steroid synthesis. *Annals of Internal Medicine*, **97**, 370–2.

Pont, A., Williams, P. L., Azhar, S., Reitz, R. E., Bochra, C., Smith, E. R., and Stevens, D. A. (1982b). Ketoconazole blocks testosterone synthesis. *Archives of Internal Medicine*, **142**, 2137–40.

Pont, A., Graybill, J. R., Craven, P. C., Galgiani, J. N., Dismukes, W. E., Reitz, R. E., and Stevens, D. A. (1984). High dose ketoconazole therapy and adrenal and testicular function in humans. *Archives of Internal Medicine*, **144**, 2150–3.

Robbins, D. K., Wedlund, P. J., Kuhn, R., Baumann, R. J., Levy, R. H., and Chang, S.-L. (1990). Inhibition of epoxide hydrolase by valproic acid in epileptic patients receiving carbamazepine. *British Journal of Clinical Pharmacology*, **29**, 759–62.

Rowland, M. (1975). Kinetics of drug–drug interactions. In *Pharmacology and pharmacokinetics* (ed. T. Teorell, R. L. Dedrick, and P. G. Condliffe), pp. 321–8. Plenum Press, London.

Rundles, R. W., Wyngaarden, J. B., Hitchings, G. H., and Elton, G. B. (1969). Drugs and uric acid. *Annual Reviews in Pharmacology*, **9**, 345–62.

Seelig, C. B., Maloley, P. A., and Campbell, J. R. (1990). Nephrotoxicity associated with concomitant ACE inhibitor and NSAID therapy. *Southern Medical Journal*, **83**, 1144–8.

Seidegard, J. and DePierre, J. W. (1983). Microsomal epoxide hydrolase: properties, regulation and function. *Biochimica et Biophysica Acta*, **695**, 251–70.

Sim, S. M., Back, D. J., and Breckenridge, A. M. (1991). The effect of various drugs on the glucuronidation of zidovudine (azidothymidine; AZT) by human liver microsomes. *British Journal of Clinical Pharmacology*, **32**, 17–21.

Smith, P. F., Eydelloth, R., Grossman, S. J., Stubbs, R. J., Schwartz, M. S., Germerhausen, J. I., *et al.* (1991). HMG-CoA reductase inhibitor-induced myopathy in the rat: cyclosporin A interaction and mechanism studies. *Journal of Pharmacology and Experimental Therapeutics*, **257**, 1225–35.

Stillman, M. T. and Schlesinger, P. A. (1990). Nonsteroidal anti-inflammatory drug nephrotoxicity. Should we be concerned? *Archives of Internal Medicine*, **150**, 268–70.

Stillman, M. T., Napier, J., and Blackshear, J. L. (1984). Adverse effects of non-steroidal anti-inflammatory drugs on the kidney. *Medical Clinics of North America*, **68**, 371–85.

Taylor, P. (1985). Anticholinesterase agents. In *The pharmacological basis of therapeutics* (ed. A. G. Gilman, L. S. Goodman, T. W. Rall, and F. Murad), pp. 110–29. MacMillan, New York.

Tephly, T. R. and Burchell, B. (1990). UDP-glucuronyl transferases: a family of detoxifying enzymes. *Trends in Pharmacological Sciences*, **11**, 276–9.

Tobert, J. A. (1987). New developments in lipid-lowering therapy the role of inhibitors of hydroxymethyl glutaryl-coenyme A reductase. *Circulation*, **76**, 534–8.

Trachtenberg, J. and Pont, A. (1984). Ketoconazole therapy for advanced prostate cancer. *Lancet*, **ii**, 433–5.

Weber, M. M., Will, A., Adelmann, B., and Engelhardt, D. (1991). Effect of keto-conazole on human ovarian C17, 20-desmolase and aromatase. *Journal of Steroid Biochemistry and Molecular Biology*, **38**, 213–18.

Weinblatt, M. E. and Fraser, P. (1989). Elevated mean corpuscular volume as a predictor of haematologic toxicity due to methotrexate therapy. *Arthritis and Rheumatism*, **32**, 1592–6.

White, M. C. and Kendall-Taylor, P. (1985). Adrenal hypofunction in patients taking ketoconazole. *Lancet*, **i**, 44–5.

Williams, G. H. (1988). Converting enzyme inhibitors in the treatment of hypertension. *New England Journal of Medicine*, **319**, 1517–25.

Wu, C. and Matthews, K. P. (1983). Indomethacin inhibition of glutathione S-transferases. *Biochemical and Biophysical Research Communications*, **112**, 980–5.

Yeo, W. W., Ramsay, L. E., and Morice, A. H. (1991). ACE inhibitor cough: a genetic link? *Lancet*, **i**, 187.

Yuen, A. W. C., Land, G., Weatherley, B. C., and Peck, A. W. (1991). Sodium valproate inhibits lamotrigine metabolism. *Fundamental Clinical Pharmacology*, **5**, 468.

Ziemniak, J. A., Allison, N., Boppana, U. K., Dubb, J., and Stote, R. (1987). The effect of acetaminophen on the disposition of fenoldopam: competition for sulfation. *Clinical Pharmacology and Therapeutics*, **41**, 275–81.

Index